PEDIATRIC
Physical Therapy

FOURTH EDITION

PEDIATRIC
Physical Therapy

FOURTH EDITION

Jan S. Tecklin

Professor
Department of Physical Therapy
Arcadia University
Glenside, Pennsylvania

Lippincott Williams & Wilkins
a Wolters Kluwer business
Philadelphia • Baltimore • New York • London
Buenos Aires • Hong Kong • Sydney • Tokyo

Acquisitions Editor: Peter Sabatini
Managing Editor: Andrea M. Klingler
Marketing Manager: Allison M. Noplock
Production Editor: Sally Anne Glover
Designer: Stephen Druding
Compositor: Circle Graphics, Inc.

Fourth Edition

Library of Congress Cataloging-in-Publication Data

Pediatric physical therapy / [edited by] Jan Tecklin.—4th ed.
   p. ; cm.
   Includes bibliographical references and index.
   ISBN-13: 978-0-7817-5399-9
   ISBN-10: 0-7817-5399-6
   1. Physical therapy for children. I. Tecklin, Jan Stephen.
   [DNLM: 1. Physical Therapy Modalities. 2. Child. 3. Infant. WB 460 P371 2008]
   RJ53.P5P43 2008
   615.8'20832—dc22

                                    2007019782

DISCLAIMER

Care has been taken to confirm the accuracy of the information present and to describe generally accepted practices. However, the authors, editors, and publisher are not responsible for errors or omissions or for any consequences from application of the information in this book and make no warranty, expressed or implied, with respect to the currency, completeness, or accuracy of the contents of the publication. Application of this information in a particular situation remains the professional responsibility of the practitioner; the clinical treatments described and recommended may not be considered absolute and universal recommendations.

The authors, editors, and publisher have exerted every effort to ensure that drug selection and dosage set forth in this text are in accordance with the current recommendations and practice at the time of publication. However, in view of ongoing research, changes in government regulations, and the constant flow of information relating to drug therapy and drug reactions, the reader is urged to check the package insert for each drug for any change in indications and dosage and for added warnings and precautions. This is particularly important when the recommended agent is a new or infrequently employed drug.

Some drugs and medical devices presented in this publication have Food and Drug Administration (FDA) clearance for limited use in restricted research settings. It is the responsibility of the health care provider to ascertain the FDA status of each drug or device planned for use in their clinical practice.

To purchase additional copies of this book, call our customer service department at **(800) 638-3030** or fax orders to **(301) 223-2320**. International customers should call **(301) 223-2300**.

Visit Lippincott Williams & Wilkins on the Internet: http://www.lww.com. Lippincott Williams & Wilkins customer service representatives are available from 8:30 am to 6:00 pm, EST.

In loving memory of my parents

Coleman J. Tecklin
5/20/24–1/26/72

Natalie Rosen Tecklin
8/20/25–2/28/92

Olev HaShalom

In loving thanks to the Sprouls
To Gayle, Ed, Sophie, Molly, and Harry

Heather Atkinson, PT, DPT, NCS
Team Leader—In-Patient Rehabilitation
Children's Hospital of Philadelphia
Philadelphia, PA

Emilie Aubert, PT, DPT, MA
Associate Professor
Department of Physical Therapy
Marquette University
Milwaukee, WI

Dolores Bertoti, PT, MS, PCS
Dean of Center for Academic Advancement
Associate Professor
Alvernia College
Reading, PA

Amy Both, PT, MHS, ACCE
Assistant Professor and ACCE
Department of Physical Therapy
Health Science Campus
University of Toledo
Toledo, OH

Heather Brossman, PT, MS, DPT, CCS
Brossman Physical Therapy
Richboro, PA

Jean M. Flickinger, MPT, PCS
Physical Therapist
Children's Hospital of Philadelphia
Philadelphia, PA

Rita Geddes, PT, MEd, DPT
Bucks County Schools Intermediate Unit #22
Doylestown, PA

Allan Glanzman, PT, DPT, PCS, ATP
Clinical Specialist
Physical Therapy Department
The Children's Hospital of Philadelphia
Philadelphia, PA

Maria Hanna, MS, RD, LDN
Clinical Nutritionist
Cystic Fibrosis Center
Children's Hospital of Philadelphia
Philadelphia, PA

Susan E. Klepper, PhD, PT
Assistant Professor of Physical Therapy
Physical Therapy Program
Columbia University
New York, NY

Karen Yundt Lunnen, PT, EdD
Associate Professor and Head
Department of Physical Therapy
Western Carolina University
Cullowhee, NC

Victoria Gocha Marchese, PT, PhD
Assistant Professor
Physical Therapy Department
Lebanon Valley College
Annville, PA

Donna L. Merckel, PT, MS, SCS, CSCS
Lead Physical Therapist
The Chester County Hospital
West Chester, PA

Sue Migliore, PT, DPT, MS, PCS
Clinical Practice Coordinator
Physical Therapy Department
The Children's Hospital of Philadelphia
Philadelphia, PA

Joseph Molony, Jr., PT, MS, SCS, CSCS
Program Manager
Sports Medicine and Performance Center
The Children's Hospital of Philadelphia
Philadelphia, PA

Dale E. Smith, EdD
Assistant Professor of Education
Alvernia College
Reading, PA

Elena McKeogh Spearing, MA, DPT, PCS
Physical Therapist and former Physical Therapy Manager
Children's Hospital of Philadelphia
Philadelphia, PA

Meg Stanger, PT, PCS
Director
Department of Physical Therapy
Children's Hospital of Pittsburgh
Pittsburgh, PA

Jane L. Styer-Acevedo, PT
Senior Adjunct Faculty
Arcadia University
Pediatric Coordinator-Instructor of the
Neuro-Developmental Treatment Association
KenCrest Infant & Toddler Services
Upper Darby, PA

Elena Tappit-Emas, PT, MHS
Staff Therapist, School District of Philadelphia
Former Senior Therapist
Myelomeningocele Clinic
Children's Memorial Hospital, Chicago, IL
Private practice, Philadelphia, PA

Jan Stephen Tecklin, PT, MS
Professor
Department of Physical Therapy
Arcadia University
Glenside, PA

Diane Versaw-Barnes, PT, MS, PCS
Clinical Specialist-NICU
The Children's Hospital of Philadelphia
Philadelphia, PA

Audrey Wood, PT, MS
OT/PT Clinical Specialist
Ken-Crest Services
Philadelphia, PA

This is the fourth edition of *Pediatric Physical Therapy*—how the years have flown by since the first edition was conceived in 1987. That this text has become so well received and regularly adopted by many entry-level physical therapy programs in the United States and abroad is a testament primarily to the contributors, some of whom have been with the text through each of its four editions. The provision of a current description of the major areas of pediatric physical therapy for the new practitioner is the continuing goal that has guided the editor and many contributors through each of the editions. The "functional goal" is to prepare entry-level students and new practitioners who decide to enter pediatric care with a content that is supported by the literature, provides knowledge and insight within the diagnostic areas, and offers the tools by which to initiate and continue sound practice for the children with whom we work.

Organization

The book is organized into several sections based on the more common groups of disorders seen in infants and children. Chapter 1 is new to the text and presents the important issues of cultural sensitivity and family-centered care, both of which are critical areas of understanding when working with a child because the family is virtually always involved and we depend so often on a family's support and adherence with interventions. Chapters 2 through 7 discuss development and include chronologic motor development with a strong emphasis on biomechanical aspects of that development. An update on tests and measures of development follows.

Neurologic and neuromuscular diseases and injuries serve as the focus for the next section of the text. The eight chapters in this section include one with a new title, Chapter 8 (Traumatic and Atraumatic Spinal Cord Injury in Pediatrics), and new authors for Chapter 4 (The Infant at High Risk for Developmental Delay) and Chapter 9 (Neuromuscular Disorders in Childhood: Physical Therapy Intervention). Chapters 10 through 12 discuss common musculoskeletal disorders and include one entirely new chapter. Chapter 13 (Traumatic Disorders and Sports Injuries) is a major addition in which a multitude of common injuries are explored.

The final five chapters encompass several diverse groups of disorders. Chapter 15 (Pediatric Oncology) and Chapter 16 (Rehabilitation of the Child with Burns) have new authors. Also, Chapter 17 (Cardiac Disorders) is new to this edition. The other chapters include updates to the previous edition.

Features

We have included extensive **Chapter Outlines** in order to help the student and the instructor focus on specific areas of information in the chapter. **Displays** have been included in an effort to provide greater depth of information, allowing information to be more inclusive without necessarily lengthening the text of the chapters. **Chapter Summaries** encapsulate and recapitulate the major points of information presented in each chapter. **Nutrition Boxes** are a unique feature to this new edition. Over the past decade, the importance of nutrition and the work of our colleagues in the nutritional field have improved and enhanced the lives of children with significant illness and injury. Although not suggesting that physical therapists have the wherewithal to offer nutritional counseling, it seems that an overview of the nutritional needs of children with various diseases and disabilities can only improve our understanding of the importance and work of nutritionists and the needs of the children.

Ancillaries

An interactive website is also included with this edition of *Pediatric Physical Therapy*. Instructors will have access to an Image Bank and PowerPoint lecture outlines. All of these resources are available at thePoint.lww.com/ Tecklin4e.

The fourth edition of *Pediatric Physical Therapy* is much more than a timely update. It includes four entirely new chapters and major updates for virtually all other chapters. In addition to the updates, the new authors in this edition have extensive experience in clinical care and regularly teach at the full-time faculty level or as an associated faculty member, and most have participated in clinical research. The authors represent the best in pediatric practice.

I would like to acknowledge the skill, creativity, knowledge, and determination of each of the authors who have contributed chapters to this edition. Elena Spearing added to the four new chapters by writing Chapter 1, Providing Family-Centered Care in Pediatric Physical Therapy, and coauthoring Chapter 8, Traumatic and Atraumatic Spinal Cord Injury in Pediatrics, along with Heather Atkinson. Emilie Aubert has provided a wonderful new Motor Development chapter that includes a strong biomechanical approach as well as an extensive array of supportive photographs. Emilie also authored Chapter 11, Adaptive Equipment and Environmental Aids for Children with Disabilities. These two chapters represent an incredible professional and personal investment by Dr. Aubert and I am very grateful for her keen interest and participation. Diane Versaw-Barnes and Audrey Wood completely rewrote Chapter 4, The Infant at High Risk for Developmental Delay. As I have told them both during the writing process, this extraordinarily complete and comprehensive chapter could serve as the basis for a textbook on its own. My good friend Jane Styer-Acevedo continues to update and enhance her chapter on The Infant and Child with Cerebral Palsy (Chapter 5), and has been with the text for three editions. Chapter 6, Spina Bifida, represents the fourth version of this comprehensive chapter by Elena Tappit-Emas, who, along with Dolores Bertoti (coauthor of Chapter 10 with Dale E. Smith), has been with the text since the first edition in 1989. Amy Both again tackles the group of children with Traumatic Injury to the Central Nervous System: Brain Injury in Chapter 7, just as she did so successfully in the third edition. Allan Glanzman, and Jean Flickinger, have coauthored an entirely new Chapter 9, Neuromuscular Disorders in Childhood: Physical Therapy Intervention. Meg Stanger has updated Chapter 12 on Orthopedic Management, which has been complemented by Chapter 13, Traumatic Disorders and Sports Injuries, by the husband/wife team of Joe Molony and Donna Merckel. Susan Klepper has again presented the Juvenile Idiopathic Arthritis chapter (Chapter 14), which updates the third edition. Victoria (Tori) Gocha Marchese provides a very contemporary perspective in the Pediatric Oncology chapter (Chapter 15), which was written during her time at St. Jude's Hospital in Memphis. Chapter 16, Rehabilitation of the Child with Burns, by Suzanne Migliore offers a thorough discussion of the acute and long-term rehabilitation following these serious injuries. A new chapter on Cardiac Disorders (Chapter 17) by Heather Brossman adds a new perspective to the book and places much emphasis on the child who has had heart transplantation. I have updated the Pulmonary Disorders chapter (Chapter 18). Karen Lunnen, a friend since the early days of the Section on Pediatric Physical Therapy in the 1970s, and Rita Geddes have made the chapter on Physical Therapy in the Educational Environment (Chapter 19) and the IDEA laws more friendly and clinically relevant.

In addition to each chapter, I thank my friend and colleague Maria Hanna from the Cystic Fibrosis Center at Children's Hospital for both writing and helping secure the several Nutrition boxes throughout the text.

I am deeply indebted to each author for the untold number of hours, moments of aggravation, and requests for the chapters to have been submitted "yesterday." I have incredible respect for each of these learned individuals who are also outstanding clinicians, mentors, and caregivers to children. I am pleased to have had at least eight authors as colleagues during my recent years of part-time work at the Children's Hospital of Philadelphia; the physical therapy program here has become so very well known throughout the world. On a personal note, one of the most enjoyable parts of editing this edition was to have the gratification of working with two former students, Diane Versaw-Barnes and Heather Baj Atkinson, both of whom have become extremely accomplished professionals after their entry-level education at Beaver College/Arcadia University.

I would be remiss to not acknowledge the support of the staff at Lippincott Williams & Wilkins. Notable among these folks has been Ms. Andrea Klingler, our Managing Editor, who has nudged, pushed, cajoled, encouraged, and been largely responsible for the ultimate production of this book. To each and all of the folks above I offer my heartfelt appreciation and thanks.

Jan Tecklin

CONTENTS

Providing Family-Centered Care in Pediatric Physical Therapy

Elena M. Spearing

Family-Centered Care
  Barriers to Family-Centered Care
Family Response to Illness and Disability
  Coping Strategies
  Illness/Disability
Culture
  Diversity Versus Sensitivity
  Influences on Cultural Identity
  Culture and Parental Expectations
  Illness
  Disability
  Death and Dying

Providing Family-Centered Intervention
  Cultural Desire
  Cultural Awareness
  Cultural Knowledge
  Cultural Skill
Benefits to Providing Family-Centered Care
Summary

Family-Centered Care

The notion of family-centered care was first presented in the 1980s. It began in children's hospitals and pediatrics units. This philosophy of care then spread to cancer units, maternity wards, mental health units, and various adult health care practices, where it is referred to as patient-centered care. Family-centered care is a philosophy recognizing that the family plays a vital role in ensuring the health and well-being of its members. Family-centered care also empowers the family to participate fully in the planning, delivery, and evaluation of health care services. It supports families in this role by building on family members' individual strengths.[1]

Family-centered care is the foundation of pediatric physical therapy. Since a child is dependent on a caretaker, we must address both the child and the caretaker when we interact with a child receiving physical therapy.

The definition of family, in today's society, respects the notion that each family has unique characteristics and variables. Today, the family unit consists of "those significant others who profoundly influence the personal life and health of the individual over an extended period of time."[2] Families today come in all configurations and sizes and are not all traditional, married, two–biologic parent families. The 2000 U.S. Census reports the number of traditional families in the United States to be 38.9% of all families.[3] There are single-parent families, dual-income families, adoptive

families, same-sex-parent families, and intergenerational families, just to name a few.

Additionally, there is a "melting pot" of various cultural identities represented in the United States. The U.S. Census Bureau reported that the minority population grew from 20% in 1980 to 31% in 2000.[4] Of this minority population, 31.8 million spoke a language other than English in their homes. From 1980 through 2000, the three fastest growing racial categories were Asian and Pacific Islander (up 204%), Hispanic (up 141.7%), and "other" (up 127.3%).[4] This cultural factor presents additional challenges to health care providers who care for people with varying cultural and ethnic backgrounds.[5]

Historically, there has been a change in the developmental theory behind how pediatric physical therapy is provided (Display 1.1). The change has resulted in a shift from a reflex hierarchy model where a child develops based on a set of primitive reflexes to one where a child develops as a result of the interaction of different systems that affect one another in the development of the child. The child's family is one of those systems. Similarly, pediatric care has shifted from being child focused, as in the 1980s, to being currently family focused.[1,6] Also, many centered-based physical therapy service delivery models have been replaced by physical therapy service in the natural environment of the home and school. These initiatives help to promote family-centered care practice by the physical therapist.

Physical therapists who practice in the early intervention setting are mandated by law to provide care that respects a

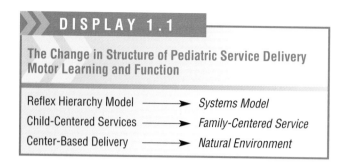

DISPLAY 1.1

The Change in Structure of Pediatric Service Delivery Motor Learning and Function

Reflex Hierarchy Model	→	*Systems Model*
Child-Centered Services	→	*Family-Centered Service*
Center-Based Delivery	→	*Natural Environment*

family's individualism. Those therapists have been charged with providing family-centered care since the initiation of Public Law 99-142 in 1975, Public Law 99-457 in 1986, and, most recently, Public Law 102-119 in 1991.[1] These laws placed focus on revising and enhancing parents' involvement in the habilitation and education of the child.[1,7] Early studies showed that it was difficult to achieve this role based upon white middle-class families, and little attention was paid to social or ethnic differences. Additionally, enhancing parents' involvement is based on the assumption that the parents can participate in formal processes and, when necessary, draw on the availability of due process of the law. Family-centered care processes are also central to the development of the individualized family service plan (IFSP), the required documentation for early intervention.

Physical therapists who practice in other pediatric settings, including the medically based inpatient and outpatient arenas, may be bound by health care accreditation standards, which recognize the importance of family-centered care. The Joint Commission on the Accreditation of Health Care Organizations has standards of care initiatives in place to address the needs of the family.[8]

Collectively, the vision for family-centered care has included increasing support for the emotional and developmental needs of the child. Strategies for this include pre-hospitalization visits, presurgical education and preparation, 24-hour parental visitation and sibling visitation guidelines, and home care services. These initiatives have shifted from not only placing the family central to the child, but also placing the family central to the child's plan of care.[9] Ultimately, this type of care results in a respect and a value for the parents as the ultimate experts in caring for their child.

Family-centered care involves the following themes[10,11]:

1. Respecting each child and his or her family
2. Honoring racial, ethnic, cultural, and socioeconomic diversity and its effect on the family's experience and perception of care
3. Recognizing and facilitating choice for the child and family even in difficult and challenging situations
4. Facilitating and supporting the choices of the child and family about approaches to their care
5. Ensuring flexibility in organizational policies, procedures, and provider practices so services can be tailored

to the needs, beliefs, and cultural values of each child and family
6. Sharing honest and unbiased information with families on an ongoing basis and in ways they find useful and affirming
7. Providing and ensuring formal and informal support for the child and parent and/or guardian during pregnancy, childbirth, infancy, childhood, adolescence, and young adulthood
8. Collaborating with families in the care of their individual child at all levels of health care including professional education, policy making, and program development
9. Empowering each child and family to discover their own strengths, build confidence, and make choices and decisions about their health care

The purpose of this chapter is to describe the examination, assessment, and intervention techniques that will enable pediatric physical therapists to incorporate principles of family-centered care into their service delivery, regardless of the pediatric practice setting. Themes of family-centered care cross not only practice settings, but also age and diagnosis. As these themes are threads across the pediatric spectrum of care, they are also threaded throughout the chapters of this textbook.

BARRIERS TO FAMILY-CENTERED CARE

Role conflict between families and health care professionals can impede the implementation of family-centered care. Often, this is very evident in the acute care setting. In the past, parents were expected to hand over the care of their children to the professionals and remain separate from them. Today, parents are expected to stay with their child and participate in the care. This example is also seen in the home care environment where parents are not afforded the respite care that they once were.

Role conflict contributes to role stress. Role stress is defined as "a subjective experience that is associated with lack of role clarity, role overload, role conflict, or temporary role pressures."[9] This stress can affect the communication process between health care provider and parent by causing one or the other to focus on the source of the stress as opposed to the underlying issues. Parents can be subjected to role stress due to their child being ill with exacerbation of that stress being associated with the child being hospitalized (Display 1.2).[9] The hospitalization of a child can be extremely stressful for even the most well-organized family. Studies show that a professional can ease this stress by helping the parents understand the illness, help provide familiarity and comfort with the hospital setting, and encourage negotiating care of the child with health professionals.[9]

DISPLAY 1.2

Stress-Limiting Strategies

Newton defines strategies that health care providers can do to limit stress for a family by using the acronym LEARN[9]:

Listen sympathetically and with understanding of the family's perception of the situation.

Explain your perception of the situation.

Acknowledge and discuss the similarities and differences between the two perceptions.

Recommend interventions.

Negotiate an agreement on the interventions.

Family Responses to Illness and Disability

When parents are faced with the fact that their child has an illness or disability, their lives must change immediately. Some changes include readjusting the family's expectations and dealing with financial difficulties and health care systems and professionals. The most common initial responses include shock, disbelief, guilt, a sense of loss, and denial. After the period of denial, some parents may experience anger due to the stress of the medical issues as well as spousal disagreement or individual feelings of fault and guilt.[12]

As a result of these things, there are many stresses for families with a child with a disability. Families respond and adapt differently to raising a child with a disability. Factors that affect how a family responds include past life experiences, familial reactions to the child and the disability, and knowledge about health care and support systems. Supports can also vary. Sometimes there is a lack of understanding of the medical implications from those outside the family. There can also be feelings of embarrassment for the family. Professionals can use a cognitive approach to problem solving to help families examine their feelings and develop solutions for their own needs.

The effects of having a child with a disease or disability can not only affect the parents' relationship, but it can also have varied effects on siblings who also have individualized needs based on gender, birth order, and temperament. Siblings can also have mixed feeling toward their disabled sibling.[13]

A child may experience different effects as a result of the disability. By school age, most children are aware of their disability and may need help dealing with their feelings as they transition to school. The transition to school can be eased with education to the classmates prior to the disabled child entering school. Parents and professionals can assist with this planning. During adolescence, there may be particular new issues that emerge for a child with a disability. Feelings of comparing themselves and being part of a peer group are important for all adolescents and can present new challenges for those with chronic or new disabilities. Adolescents should also be acknowledged as having sexual interests. They should be educated on these feelings as well as trained in social skills. They also should be exposed to age-appropriate recreational skills, such as dancing, listening to music, and sports activities. Programs of inclusion help children to develop socialization skills and a good self-image.

The transition to adulthood is both important and difficult for patients and parents. Those individuals who remain dependent through adolescence tend to remain dependent through adulthood.[14] Adolescents who have the potential for independence but are having difficulties with separation may need assistance. Likewise, the family members may need assistance in supporting their child during this difficult time. Professionals should be partners with the family members and empower them to make decisions.

Disability as defined by the Americans with Disabilities Act is "physical or mental impairment that substantially limits one of more of the life activities of an individual, a record of such an impairment, or being regarded as having such an impairment."[15] Advances in medical technology, diagnosis, and treatment have resulted in decreased mortality rates for children with life-threatening conditions to survive well into adulthood.[14] The diagnosis of chronic illness or disability clearly impacts a family. How families respond to the diagnosis is a function of their adaptive capabilities.[12] What makes some families reorganize and become stronger while others decline in function, become symptomatic, and sometimes disintegrate depends on family resilience according to Ferguson.[12] He describes eight aspects of resilient family processes as:

1. Balancing the illness with other family needs
2. Developing communication competence
3. Attributing positive meaning to the situations
4. Maintaining clear family boundaries
5. Maintaining family flexibility
6. Engaging in active coping efforts
7. Maintaining social integration
8. Developing collaborative relationships with professionals

A family's ability to be resilient or the extent of its resiliency is largely defined by society, time, place, and culture.[12]

COPING STRATEGIES

In cross-cultural studies dealing with disability, when looking at reaction to disability, there are three issues considered to be universal. They are[16]:

1. The culturally perceived cause of a chronic illness or disability will play a significant role in determining family and community attitudes toward the individual.

2. The expectations for physical survival for the infant or the child with a chronic disability will affect both the immediate care the child receives and the amount of effort expended in planning for future care and education.
3. The social role(s) deemed appropriate for disabled or chronically ill children and adults will help determine the amount of resources a family and community invests in an individual. This includes issues of education and training, participation in family and social life, and the long-range planning done by, or undertaken for, the individual over the course of a lifetime.

Cultural sensitivity refers to understanding that cultural differences exist. These differences are not necessarily better or worse, right or wrong, or more or less intelligent, but rather simply differences.[17] It is necessary to examine, in detail, attitude, behavior, and communication, which directly affect health care. It is important to realize that each person within a culture is an individual and should not be characterized or stereotyped on the basis of his or her cultural association. It is only through generalizations that one can gain a frame of reference and become more culturally aware.

ILLNESS/DISABILITY

In the history of literature on family reactions to having a child with a disability there has been a shift in thinking. In the 19th century, with the flourish of specialization, the moral blame for disabilities often was placed on the parents. This set of beliefs most often placed the blame on poor mothers who made bad judgments. Reform schools, asylums, and residential schools all became apparent in the 19th century. This movement also led to special education schools after the turn of the century. The only way to deal with children that weren't "normal" was to turn the parenting over to professionals within the walls of these facilities.[12]

There was a major shift in thinking throughout the 20th century that included a reversal of the above assumptions. Professionals shifted to focusing on the damage that children with disabilities caused their families. The medical model began to analyze the family unit with terms such as *guilt, denial,* and *grief* and *role disruption, marital cohesiveness,* and *social withdrawal.*

Over the past two decades, a new approach has developed regarding the impact of a child's disability on the family. The recent approach includes models of stress and coping (adaptation) and models of family life course development. The adaptive family describes X—the potential family crisis—as an interaction of three factors: A, an initial stressful event, combined with B, a family's resource for dealing with the crisis, and C, the family's definition of the stressor.[12] This approach has allowed researchers to focus on the resiliency of the family and its ability to cope with a potentially stressful situation. There is a level of con-

sensus today that identifies the varying ways that families with children with disabilities deal with stressful situations. There is great similarity to the way that families with children without disabilities deal with similar issues. There are also varying responses to how some deal with stressors. Sometimes, others can view stressors as benefits. Also, the response to stressors is cyclic and cumulative. Each stressor response affects others' responses.[12]

The evolving family concept also accepts that families evolve over time and tries to identify where they are in their developmental process. This line of thinking also allows families to be considered across the continuum of care. This is especially true as their younger children age and approach adulthood. This line of thinking has allowed researchers to look at how and why some families are more resilient than others and also how extended coping with chronic disabilities affects families over time.

The supported family members look at internal and external resources that are available to them. How family members respond to difficulties depends on their supports. This also has root in societal and cultural assumptions. Recent research on family adaptation shows the following key themes[12]:

- There is a dominant body of literature that shows patterns of adjustment and well-being to be similar across groups of families of children with and without disabilities. This does show, however, that there are some developmental differences over the family life course.
- Additionally, there is an increasing recognition and growing research that a significant number of parents actually report numerous benefits and positive outcomes for their family associated with raising a child with a disability. These include coping skills (adaptability), family harmony (cohesiveness), spiritual growth or shared values, shared parenting roles, and communication.
- There are, obviously, stressors associated with having a child with a disability. The research continues to refine our understanding of why some families are more resilient than others in adapting to stress. Some research has suggested that the level of disability or family structure may not be as crucial as other factors (income, self-injurious behaviors, etc.). There are also differing patterns of adaptations along ethnic and cultural lines.[12]

◆ Culture

Culture affects how others view disability, how people with disabilities view themselves, and how people with disabilities are treated. The cultural context within which a disability is perceived is important to understanding the meaning of disability for a person or his or her family. It is also important to know the kinds of services to be provided to families and people with disabilities.

Culture can be defined in many ways. O'Connor defines culture as "the acquired knowledge people use to interpret experience and generate social behavior."[18] Other definitions include "the ever changing values, traditions, social and political relationships and a world view shared by a group of people bound together by a number of factors that can include a common history, geographic location, language, social class and/or religion."[19] An analysis of the various studies of culture yields the emergence of various similar themes[18]:

1. Culture is not innate or biologically inherited but, in fact, learned patterns of behavior.
2. Culture is transmitted from the older people to the young, from generation to generation.
3. Culture serves as a group identity and is shared by other members of the group.
4. Culture provides the individual or the members of a group with an effective mechanism for interacting with each other and their environment.

DIVERSITY VERSUS SENSITIVITY

There are many terms that are used today to refer to the impact of culture on health care. It is necessary to describe the two most common terms and their fundamental differences. *Cultural diversity* refers to having a range of cultures represented in an organization. This leads to a workforce that is more representative of the general population. In health care, diversity in the workplace leads to the increased potential of having similar cultures represented. By comparison, *cultural sensitivity* and effectiveness is a process of becoming "culturally competent" and striving toward the ability and availability to work effectively within the cultural context of a client, individual, family, or community regardless of the cultural background.[19]

INFLUENCES ON CULTURAL IDENTITY

There are various things that influence who we are and how we view illness and disability. These include our nationality, our race, and our ethnicity. Similarly, our socioeconomic status and education also play a role. Our society's view of illness and disability also influences our perception of the same. Other things like age, religion, and past experience shape our beliefs.

In addition to these, health care providers who were brought up in the U.S. culture are finding that their medical views are in conflict with the views of their patients from differing cultural backgrounds. Care provided in the past was monocultural and suited for the Euro-American culture. Traditionally, in medicine we have functioned under a "medical culture," one that values a "cure" and the expertise of those in the medical profession.[7]

This traditional model, however, is not as appropriate or relevant for those who are not of that "medical" cultural identity.[7] When this cultural disconnect occurs, the consequence is often disparities in the quality of care received by racial and ethnic minority populations. One example of this is the Tuskegee Syphilis Research Experiment, which occurred during the years between 1932 and 1972. Three hundred and ninety-nine poor African-American sharecroppers who were identified as having syphilis were told that they were being treated for the disease when they were unaware that they were control subjects.[20] This legacy has continued to affect the credibility and reputation of the medical industry for many African Americans who believe there are continuing racial and ethnic disparities in the health care system and mistrust the medical community.[20]

CULTURAL AND PARENTAL EXPECTATIONS

Many studies reveal that culture and acculturation are strong predictors of parental expectations of cognitive and social development. Most studies point to ethnic origin as the differentiating factor. More contemporary literature has determined that Western education and socioeconomic status was more predictive of differential beliefs than ethnic origin. This demonstrates that acculturation has a powerful effect on parenting styles and on parental beliefs about child development. What is even more profound is the difference between the description of mildly retarded, behaviorally disordered, and learning disabled between the parents and the professionals. Ethnographic studies have shown that there are sometimes differences related to culture, which emphasized that for some parents, a child's cognitive and social functioning has to be more limited for the concept of handicap or disabled to be applied. These statements are then interpreted by the professional as families being in "denial."[17] The following themes occur in a review of the literature on culturally appropriate services in the special education literature[7]:

1. There are cultural differences in definitions and interpretations of disability.
2. There are cultural differences in family coping styles and responses to disability-related stress.
3. There are cultural differences in parental interaction styles, as well as expectations of participation and advocacy.
4. There are differences in cultural groups' access to information and services.
5. There are negative professional attitudes to, and perceptions of, families' roles in the special education processes.
6. There is dissonance in the cultural fit of educational programs.

There are traditional cultural patterns associated with particular cultural groups. One example is that Asian groups attribute disability to spiritual retribution or reward. Similarly, there is an emphasis on the wholeness of the spirit within a disabled body. This is powerfully described in the novel *When the Spirit Catches You, and You Fall Down* by Anne Fatiman. It is demonstrated throughout the novel that this Hmong family attributed epilepsy to spiritual phenomena within the individual.[21]

ILLNESS

How one views and responds to health, illness, and death is largely defined by his or her cultural values. Before detailing this, a distinction between disease and illness must be made.

Physicians diagnose and treat diseases, which can be defined as abnormalities in the structure and function of body organs and systems. Illnesses, on the other hand, are experiences of disvalued changes in states of being and cultural reactions to disease or discomfort.[22]

How a person understands and responds to illness is determined by what Kleinman calls "explanatory models." These are defined as "notions about an episode of sickness and its treatment that are employed by all those engaged in the clinical process."[22] Explanatory models address five major issues:

1. Etiology of the problem
2. Time and mode of onset
3. Pathophysiology of illness
4. Course of illness and degree and severity
5. Type of treatment that should be sought[23]

"Illness is culturally shaped in how we perceive, experience, and cope with disease based on our explanations of sickness, explanations specific to the social positions we occupy and systems of meanings we employ."[22] The role of traditional medicine and folk healing is based on cultural values. An estimated 70% to 90% of self-recognized episodes of sickness are managed outside of the formal health care system.[22] As Kleinman states, "folk healers deal with the human experience of illness." They seek to provide meaningful explanations for illness and respond to personal, family, and community issues surrounding illness.[22] Illness referred to as "folk illness" (i.e., illnesses that are recognized within a cultural group), may sometimes conflict with the biomedical paradigm.[24]

It is important to understand folk illness because people who experience "folk illness" may present to a medical practitioner and a "folk healer." Additionally, some "folk treatments" may be potentially hazardous. Finally, folk illness may be cultural interpretations of states of pathophysiology that may require medical attention. For many chronic problems, patients have reported greater improvement with marginal folk healers than with medical physicians. Kleinman attributes this improvement to folk healers' increased emphasis on "explanation" and a greater concordance of explanatory systems between healer and patient.[22]

For more serious illness, values and beliefs become even more crucial to understanding. Although the biologic manifestations of diseases are the same among cultural groups, individuals differ in the way they experience, interpret, and respond to illness. Explanatory models as well as coping styles have been shown to influence perceptions of illness.[23] It has been suggested that meanings are assigned using characteristic themes that are the result of individual coping styles, knowledge, beliefs, and cultural background.[23] Viewing illness as a challenge regards the illness as something to be approached internally and mastered. The proper authorities are consulted, advice is followed, and life goes on. Illness as God's will emphasizes resignation. Illness is perceived as beyond human control and when illness is perceived as God's will, it may result in passive acceptance of what cannot be changed. This may result in less interest in aggressive procedures or may produce depression. Illness as a "strategy" describes using illness to secure attention or nurturing from parents, family, or health care professionals. Illness as a "value" may be the "highest form" of coping where illness is viewed as an opportunity that can result in important insight into the meaning of life. Although meanings may be influenced by culture, they are not culture specific.[23]

Our expectations and perceptions of symptoms, as well as the labels we attach to sickness behaviors, are influenced by environment, family, and explanatory models. In addition, the way in which problems are communicated, how symptoms are presented, when and who is visited for care, how long one remains in care, and how care is evaluated are all affected by cultural beliefs.[25] Likewise, culture dramatically influences the reaction and expression of pain. This is learned throughout childhood.[25]

DISABILITY

Research gives strong support to the argument that definitions of disability are socially constructed.[7,17] When disability is severe, the studies show that although all groups recognize gross developmental, behavioral, or sensory impairments, their attributions differ widely as does the extent of stigma or value associated with that condition.[7,26] Responses to impairments vary through time, place, and culture. Over the course of history, societies have defined what did and did not constitute a disability or handicap. The past decade has seen changes in the conceptualization of the meaning of disability and the interplay between the possibility that an impairment becomes a physical handicap. Even more than physical limitations placed on the individual with a disability, attitudinal concepts and images affect treatment of an individual with a disability. The sources of the concepts and images they produce are found in literature and art, television and movies, and religious texts and school books. Since these sources are all artifacts of culture, it is impossible to separate culture from attitudes toward disability.

For children with disabilities, the culturally perceived cause of a chronic illness or disability affects aspects of a family and community's attitudes toward that child.[16] In some cultures disability is viewed as a form of punishment. Depending on the belief system, the individual with a disability, the family, or an ancestor has been targeted by God or a god for having sinned or violating a taboo. Witchcraft may also be strongly linked to disability as well as associated with that person who has been bewitched.[16]

Similarly, inherited disorders are frequently attributed to "running in the blood" or caused by a curse.[16,22] Closely related to this is the traditional belief that a disabled child may be the product of an incestuous relationship. In societies where there is a belief in reincarnation, disability may be seen as the result of a transgression in a previous life by parents of a child with a disability or the child him- or herself. Some belief systems may emphasize the imbalance of humeral elements in the body as cause for disability.[16]

All of these perceived causes identify the individual with the disability as responsible for that disability and suggests likely consequences on the person's place in the family. Additionally, where disability is seen as a punishment, the presence of a child with a disability may be a source of embarrassment to the family. Various types of neglect may be apparent, including isolation. In many cultures, the idea of early intervention is not in the mindset for medical and educational professionals.[16] There also may be incredible social pressures placed on the family in these instances. Families may be reluctant to participate in therapeutic programs, fearing that these will call attention to their family member's physical and intellectual limitations.[16]

An understanding of traditional expectations for survival is also important. For some cultures, the belief that severely disabled children will simply not survive makes the allocation of medical and parental attention to healthy children more practical. Either neglecting a disabled child or overprotecting him or her because he or she is alive for only a short period of time can have serious implications for both health care services and psychological development. Moreover, how one is believed to be restored to health can have implications on long-term planning or arranging for special care, with members of some cultures feeling that "maybe God will make your baby all better on its own."[16]

Societies that limit occupational roles and social roles for individuals with disabilities can affect the time, energy, and expense invested in educating a child with a disability. Additionally, a gender bias, common in some cultures, may affect the degree to which a family is willing to spend money in order to obtain medical care. In these cultures it may be perceived less justifiable to expend vast amounts of family resources on female disabled children than male disabled children.[16]

Failure to fully understand cultural beliefs and values toward disability may influence a family's care toward its disabled child. Consider the family members whose cultural beliefs lead them to feel that it is their responsibility to provide complete and total care for their disabled child. They may prefer to keep their child at home, unseen by even neighbors. They may hesitate to come forward for aid or advice, for various reasons, which may include poverty, fear, language barriers, or faith in traditional medical practices. When not viewed in a cultural context, this may be construed as neglect—the failure of parents to nurture and provide adequate ongoing education and emotional support.[17]

DEATH AND DYING

Death and the customs surrounding it need to be addressed as they are highly influenced by cultural values. Expressions of grief and coping mechanisms vary from person to person but are related to cultural background.[27] The meaning of death, family patterns including family roles during periods of grief, and the family's expectations for professional health care need to be understood.

 Providing Family-Centered Intervention

The nursing literature has explored the process of cultural competence in the delivery of health care service including a model for providing culturally competent interventions. This model for cultural competence includes cultural desire, cultural awareness, cultural knowledge, and cultural skill.[28]

CULTURAL DESIRE

The first requirement for cultural competence is "cultural desire." This is the motivation to "want to" engage in the process of becoming culturally aware, becoming culturally knowledgeable, becoming culturally skillful, and seeking cultural encounters.[28] Rather than doing it because it is required, cultural desire involves doing it because it is personally desired. It includes a genuine passion to be open and flexible with others, to accept differences and build on similarities, and to be willing to learn from others as cultural informants.

CULTURAL AWARENESS

The next step is cultural awareness. Cultural awareness is the self-examination and in-depth exploration of one's own cultural background.[28] This involves the recognition of one's biases, prejudices, and assumptions about individuals who are different. Without this self-awareness, there is a risk of imposing one's own beliefs, values, and patterns of behavior on one from another culture.

CULTURAL KNOWLEDGE

Cultural knowledge is the process of seeking and obtaining a sound educational foundation about diverse cultural and ethnic groups.[28] Obtaining this information does not refer to learning generalizations but to learning individual differences. Learning generalizations about specific cultural subgroups leads to the development of stereotypes. Understanding that there is as much intracultural difference and intercultural difference due to life experiences, acculturation to other cultures, and diversity within cultures will prevent us from imposing stereotypic patterns on our patients and families.

CULTURAL SKILL

Cultural skill is the ability to collect cultural data regarding the patient's problem as well as performing a culturally based physical assessment.[28] There are many tools available to help collect this information via questions. One must also remember that it is a developmental skill to ask questions in a way that does not offend the patient or family. Listening and remaining nonjudgmental are effective and sensitive ways to obtain information. Additionally, having multiple cultural encounters is the way to refine or modify one's own belief about a cultural group and prevent stereotyping. Linguistic assessment is necessary to facilitate accurate communication. The use of specifically medically trained interpreters is important to the assessment process. Untrained interpreters, family members, and specifically children and siblings may pose a problem due to lack of medical knowledge. We must provide not only care that is culturally competent, but also care that provides for low literacy skills. It is documented that people who have limited English proficiency experience obstacles when accessing health care.[29] They may experience delays in making appointments, and are also more likely to have misunderstandings regarding time, place, date, and location of appointment. People with low literacy skills may have difficulty communicating with the health care professional and employees in the health care institution. These issues are more likely to exacerbate medical problems that require timely treatment or follow-up.[29]

In 1999, the U.S. Department of Health and Human Services (HHS) office of Minority Health developed standards of care within these areas. In addition, the Office of Civil Rights (2003) and HHS enforce federal laws that prohibit discrimination by health care providers who receive funding from the HHS. Antidiscrimination laws are established by Section 504 of the Rehabilitation Act of 1973, title VI of the Civil Rights Act of 1964, title II of the Americans with Disabilities Act of 1990, Community Service Assurance provisions of the Hill-Burton Act, and the Age Discrimination Act of 1975. The laws mandate that providers who accept federal money must "ensure meaningful access to and benefits from health services for individuals who have limited English proficiency."[30] Using interpreters and translating materials into languages and levels that can be read by those who have literacy deficiencies are important mandated tools.

Adults who have literacy deficiencies face many problems in understanding written and verbal materials that are provided to them. It is important to remember that while some readily admit their limitations regarding understanding verbal and written information, others may feel shameful and use strategies to hide their limitations. In these situations, one can use oral explanation and demonstration. Pictures, photographs, and visual cues also help to reinforce the information. Some people will also use family members to assist them with reading and these family members may be important in the education process.

One can identify people with low literacy skills by looking for clues. An example is someone who gives excuses for not being able to read something or who cannot read back information that is provided. Some other strategies to providing information to those with low literacy skills include[31]:

- Remaining nonjudgmental
- Involving the patient/family
- Asking the patient simple questions
- Simplifying instructions
- Repeating the information many times
- Finding various ways to give the same message
- Organizing information so that the most important information is provided first
- Using audio-visual information
- Involving family and friends in the learning and reinforcing of information
- Asking the patient to recall the message in his or her own words or demonstrate the skill that is being taught
- Empowering individuals and families and fostering independence in their programs

Health care professionals and physical therapists should promote the sharing of information and collaboration among patients, families, and health care staff. Offering places such as a family resource center will give families opportunities to educate themselves around their child's needs. Also, developing programs that provide support to families in the community is an important related activity.

Some institutions have instituted family faculty.[32] These families have often been in similar situations and can act to encourage and facilitate parent-to-parent support. They also provide a network for families. Additionally, one must support family caregiving and decision making and help give them the tools to do so, even if one does not agree with the decision that is made. Institutions must involve patients and families in the planning, delivery, and evaluation of health care services. They should take feedback from families and incorporate that into program planning. They should also consider the family needs as well as the child's needs.

In summary, one provides culturally competent intervention by the following acronym: Have I "ASKED" the right questions?[19]

*A*wareness: Am I aware of my personal biases and prejudices toward cultural groups different from mine?

*S*kill: Do I have the skill to conduct a cultural assessment and perform a culturally based physical assessment in a sensitive manner?

*K*nowledge: Do I have knowledge of the patient's world view and the field of biocultural ecology?

*E*ncounters: How many face-to-face encounters have I had with patients from diverse cultural backgrounds?

*D*esire: What is my genuine desire to "want to be" culturally competent?

Benefits to Providing Family-Centered Care

Health care practitioners who practice family-centered care are aware that it can enhance parents' confidence in their roles and, over time, increase the competence of children and young adults to take responsibility for their own health care, particularly in the anticipation of the transition to adult services.[32] Family-centered care can improve patient and family outcomes, increase patient and family satisfaction, build on the child and family strengths, increase professional satisfaction, decrease health care costs, and lead to more effective use of health care resources, as shown in the following examples from the literature[32]:

- Family presence during health care procedures decreases anxiety for the child and the parents. Research indicates that when parents are prepared, they do not prolong the procedure or make the provider more anxious.
- Children whose mothers were involved in their post-tonsillectomy care recovered faster and were discharged earlier than were children whose mothers did not participate in their care.
- A series of quality improvement studies found that children who had undergone surgery cried less, were less restless, and required less medication when their parents were present and assisted in pain assessment and management.
- Children and parents who received care from child life specialists did significantly better than did control children and parents on measures of emotional distress, coping during the procedure and adjustment during the hospitalization, the posthospital period, and recovery, including recovery from surgery.

- A multisite evaluation of the efficacy of parent-to-parent support found that one-on-one support increased parents' confidence and problem-solving abilities.
- Family-to-family support can have beneficial effects on the mental health status of mothers of children with chronic illness.
- Family-centered care has been a strategic priority at children's hospitals all over the country. Families participated in design planning for the new hospital, and they have been involved in program planning, staff education, and other key hospital committees and task forces.

Staff satisfaction also improves with family-centered care initiatives. The following points have been found:

- Staff report valuable learning experiences.
- A Vermont program has shown that a family faculty program, combined with home visits, produces positive changes in medial student perceptions of children and adolescents with cognitive disabilities.
- When family-centered care is the cornerstone of culture in a pediatric emergency department, staff members have more positive feelings about their work than do staff members in an emergency department that does not emphasize family-centered care.
- Coordination for prenatal care in a manner consistent with family-centered principles for pregnant women at risk of poor birth outcomes at a medical center in Wisconsin resulted in more prenatal visits, decreased rate of tobacco and alcohol use during pregnancy, higher infant birth rates and gestational ages, and fewer neonatal intensive care unit days. All these factors decrease health care costs and the need for additional services.
- After redesigning their transitional care center in a way that is supportive of families, creating 24-hour open visiting for families, and making a commitment to information sharing, a children's hospital in Ohio experienced a 30% to 50% decrease in their infants' length of stay.
- In Connecticut, a family support service for children with HIV hired family support workers whose backgrounds and life experiences were similar to those of the families served by the program. This approach resulted in decreases in HIV-related hospital stays, missed clinic appointments, and foster care placement.
- King County, Washington, has a children's managed care program based on a family participation service model. Families decide for themselves how dollars are spent for their children with special mental health needs as long as the services are developed by a collaborative team created by the family. In the 5 years since the program's inception, the proportion of children living in communication homes instead of institutions has increased from 24% to 91%. The number of children attending community schools has grown from 48% to

95%, and the average cost of care per child or family per month has decreased from approximately $6,000 to $4,100.

Benefits to the health care professional include[32]:

- A stronger alliance with the family in promoting each child's health and development
- Improved clinical decision making on the basis of better information and collaborative processes
- Improved follow-through when the plan of care is developed by a collaborative process
- Greater understanding of the family's strengths and caregiving capacities
- More efficient and effective use of professional time and health care resources
- Improved communication among members of the health care team
- A more competitive position in the health care marketplace
- An enhanced learning environment for future pediatricians and other professionals in training
- A practice environment that enhances professional satisfaction
- Greater child and family satisfaction with their health care

SUMMARY

It is important for us to examine our own belief systems to provide family-centered culturally competent care. First, we need to recognize the vital role families play in ensuring the health and well-being of its family members. It has been proposed that family members are equal members of the team.

Next, we need to acknowledge that emotional, social, and developmental supports are integral components of health care. Third, we need to respect the patient's and the family's choices and their values, beliefs, and cultural backgrounds. This can be accomplished by asking questions.

Finally, we can assume that families, even those living in difficult circumstances, bring important and unique strengths to their health care experiences.

"Family-centered care is a service delivery model that includes the manner in which the services match the needs identified by the family."[1] Though many people practice family-centered care, it is not widespread. Heath care professionals must adopt new practices and policies and families and patients must learn new skills.

In an attempt to educate professionals around principles of family-centered care, in 1998, then Vice President Al Gore held a conference in Nashville in 1998 regarding Families and Health. This conference set the stage for initiatives nationwide for recognizing the value of family-centered care in our health system. Recommendations include that training programs should be in place to include educating professionals both pre- and postprofessionally about their role in fostering family-centered care. The Family Bill of Rights was developed by President Clinton at this conference. Posting this Bill of Rights in public areas in health care practices in multiple languages and making them available to families are necessary.[10] At the family reunion conference, Vice President Gore outlined a five-step action plan for bringing the powers of families into our health care system. This action plan can be used as a summary for this chapter. The plan is SMART. Its principles are as follows[10]:

Support families with information, education, understanding, and resources. Some examples of this are family resource centers, family advocacy groups, and family faculty.

Measure the effectiveness of programs. This can be done with outcome measures, qualitatively and quantitatively.

Ask the right questions. Determine the individual needs of the patient and family. This will decrease the tendency to make generalizations based on culture.

Respect that individual differences do occur and that they may be different from our own.

Train early on in the health care profession. Recognize that training is lifelong and ongoing.

Training programs should be in place to educate health care workers both pre- and postprofessionally about their role in fostering family-centered care. There is an urgent need for preservice training in multicultural practices.[10] Coursework for special educators and health professionals should be part of the preprofessional curriculum. There has been much published about specific cultural groups. This type of approach is promising for professionals who are being trained to work with specific groups of people. There is danger, however, in this method of training. It risks the development of stereotypes and assumptions that are not true. No individual training program can possibly address all the differences that are possible within groups. More effective methods of teaching cultural effectiveness include processes for a much broader conceptual approach. Many programs have developed their own methods. All have common themes: self-assessment, culturally effective knowledge of language, and the ability to apply the knowledge at both interpersonal and systems levels. Harry recommends an approach that is a habit of reflective practice that will lead to effective parent–professional collaboration without having a great deal of culturally specific information.[10] The approach includes developing culturally appropriate observation and interviewing skills, including asking questions that are open-ended. The Federal government will continue to look at funding systems for programs and enact legislation to ensure that principles are being respected.

CASE STUDIES

CASE STUDY 1

Roselyn

Roselyn is an 8-year-old girl with cerebral palsy. She lives with her mother, father, two brothers, one sister, grandmother, aunt, and four cousins in a small home in an urban environment. Roselyn's parents moved to the United States when they were teenagers. They have learned to speak English, but it is not their primary language that is spoken in the home. Roselyn is unable to walk and does not attend school. Her family takes care of her every need. She rarely leaves the house except to go to church where she is carried and doesn't have many friends her own age. She has a close family and enjoys many visits from friends and neighbors. Her family takes her regularly to the major medical center for all her medical care.

The professionals have recommended a special educational setting for Roselyn where she would receive all her educational needs and therapies. The family has declined such a placement and prefers to home-school her. She is not receiving any therapy at this time.

Many of the professionals that have seen Roselyn have tried to get the family to agree to outside help for Roselyn. They have stressed the importance of teaching her how to function independently. The family members insist that she does not need to do anything, because they will take care of her. They do not even want to get any type of special equipment to help them to take care of her. Roselyn has not had any acute medical issues; however, the team feels that Roselyn could do more for herself.

After many years of team recommendations not being followed by Roselyn's family, a new physical therapist offered to make a visit to the family's home to assess the situation. When she arrived, she found a very crowded living arrangement within a very small home. As she stayed to "visit" she observed a typical day in the life of Roselyn. She was amazed to see the whole family involved. One family member bathed and dressed her. Another family member fed her along with the rest of the family. When the other children went off to school, Roselyn's mother spent a few hours teaching her math and reading and doing "exercises" to make her strong. After lunch, Roselyn was carried outside and taken for a walk around the neighborhood and accompanied her father to the store for some groceries in a homemade wagon. After the children returned from school, Roselyn sat outside on the porch and watched the children as they played. They all included her in their games.

The physical therapist realized that Roselyn's family and neighbors had embraced her care as a team. They had developed strategies to care for her and included her in the family's activities. When speaking to Roselyn's mother, she sensed an enormous amount of sense of responsibility for Roselyn's disability, even referred to "punishment for sins that had been committed by her parents." It was obvious that Roselyn's family took great pride in her care taking.

When the physical therapist returned from her visit, she shared the information that she received with the team. She took photos and video of the house and the equipment that the family used. All agreed that Roselyn was being cared for, but that perhaps they were going about helping her in the wrong way. They decided to have a social worker, who was of the same ethnic group, to work with the family on changing its understanding of the disability. Instead of focusing on changing what the family was doing, the team worked to support the family members in what they were doing. Very soon, the family accepted some help from the team. The team was able to give the family members suggestions to make it easier for them to care for Roselyn and gave them suggestions for how she could play a more active role in the family and the community.

Clinic visits were not frustrating anymore as the team took a new approach to making recommendations to the family.

Points to Ponder

Was the team being family centered when they first worked with Roselyn and her family?

How did the therapist's visit change the perception of the team?

Why was the family so resistant to the recommendations that they made as a team?

How should the team proceed with their recommendations as Roselyn gets older?

CASE STUDY 2

Daniel

Daniel is a 4-year-old boy who was admitted to the hospital for "a bad cough." His parents were not born in this country and spoke little English. There was no other family member with Daniel who spoke English, so the nurses and doctors attempted to get information to complete their assessment using gestures, pictures, and simple English. It appeared from the examination that Daniel had been ill for quite some time, without medical care. He was malnourished and had a severe productive cough with bloody sputum. He also had marks on his chest that appeared to be caused by a small object being rubbed on it. The professionals who examined Daniel felt that he had been neglected and discussed whether the authorities should be notified. The attending physicians decided to admit Daniel to the hospital for a workup. He called Social Services because of his concerns about the family and refused to allow the parents to accompany Daniel to his room. The family was left in the emergency room while Daniel was wheeled away and security was called to restrain them there until Social Services arrived.

The social worker arrived to the situation and first went to speak to the doctor. The doctor said that he felt the parents neglected Daniel's needs and he was very concerned for Daniel's welfare. He added that Daniel had signs of abuse on his chest and was malnourished. It was his duty to call child protective services. In the meantime, Daniel was undergoing tests to determine what was wrong with him. The physician left to attend to Daniel as the social worker returned to the emergency room to speak with the parents.

The social worker met the parents and found out by simple cards with different languages what language they spoke. She then was able to get an interpreter through a language service. She collected basic facts about the boy and his current medical situation. She was also able to get a phone number to a neighbor of the family who was bilingual. She was able to convey to the parents that their son was going to have some medical tests to determine why he is sick and how to make him better.

The family's neighbor was able to come to the hospital to help to communicate with the family. It turned out that the boy had been sick for a few weeks and the family members were using traditional means to care for their son. "Coining," where a coin is rubbed on the ailing part of the body, was performed by the mother to "drive out the cough." The family also believed that a special diet of herbs and natural foods would cleanse his body and bring him back to health. It was very apparent to the social worker that they loved their son very much and were doing everything in their means to make him well.

She determined that they were not neglectful, but did not understand Western medicine and the importance that we as Americans place on our medical system. She spoke with the doctor and relayed, through the family interpreter, that the boy needed special treatment with medication. The family was scared as they did not trust the medical system. With the help of the interpreter, the nurses spent some time teaching the family some techniques, using pictures. The parents were allowed to be with their son. The nurses allowed the family to set up the child's room to allow "spiritual healing" to occur. They also took the time to explain everything that they were doing to the family.

A member of the family's church came to visit the boy and spoke with the nurses and doctor about some of the family's traditions, and they all decided on a few that the family would be able to carry out in the hospital room. For example, instead of prayer with the use of candles, the nurses obtained a battery-operated candle that used a light bulb for the flames. The family also was shown manual airway clearance techniques to perform in place of coining to assist Daniel with coughing.

The team held family meetings with Daniel's family frequently during his admission, with the use of medical interpreters. A mutual trust developed between the team and the family. Daniel began to get well and was discharged home with his family. He was followed as an outpatient and continued to enjoy a healthy and happy life.

Points to Ponder

How could the emergency room situation have been handled differently?

How did the social worker's behavior change the situation?

Do you think that the family of Daniel was negligent? Why or why not?

Did the doctor provide family-centered care? Why or why not?

What would you do if you were responsible for the care of this child?

REFERENCES

1. O'Neil ME. Palisano R. Attitudes toward family centered care and clinical decision making in early intervention among physical therapists. Pediatr Phys Ther 2000;12:173–182.
2. Sparling JW, Sekarek DK. Embedding the family perspective in an entry level physical therapy curriculum. Pediatr Phys Ther 1992;4:116–122.
3. Census 2000 Profile. Washington, DC: U.S. Department of Commerce, Economics, and Statistics Administration, U.S. Census Bureau, July 2002.
4. Hobbs F, Stoops N. US Census Bureau, Census 2000 Special Reports, Series CENSR-4. Demographic Trends in the 20th Century. Washington, DC: US Government Printing Office, 2000.
5. Reynolds D. Improving care and interactions with racial and ethnically diverse populations in healthcare organizations. J Healthcare Manage 2004;49:4.
6. Iverson M, Shimmel J, Ciacera S, et al. Creating a family-centered approach to early intervention services—perceptions of parents and professionals. Pediatr Phys Ther 2003;15:23–31.
7. Harry B. Trends and issues in serving culturally diverse families of children with disabilities. J Special Educ 2002;36:131–138.
8. The Joint Commission on the Accreditation of Healthcare Organizations. Comprehensive Accreditation Manual for Hospitals. Oak Brook, IL: Joint Commission Resources, Inc., 2006.
9. Newton M. Family-centered care: current realities in parent participation. Pediatr Nurs 2000;26:164–169.
10. Harvey J. Proceedings from the Family Re-Union 7 conference. Nashville, TN: Vanderbilt University, 1998. Available at: http://www.familycenteredcare. Accessed October 7, 2006.
11. The Institute for Family Centered Care. Patient and Family-Centered Care. Bethesda, MD. Available at: http://www.familycenteredcare. Accessed October 7, 2006.
12. Ferguson P. A place in the family: an historical interpretation of research on parental reactions to having a child with a disability. J Special Educ 2002;36:124–130.
13. Suris JC, Michaud PA, Viner R. The adolescent with a chronic condition. Part I: developmental issues. Arch Disabled Child 2004;89:938–942.
14. Blum R. A consensus statement on health care transitions for young adults with special health care needs. Pediatrics 2002;110:1304–1307.
15. PL 101-336 Americans with Disabilities Act of 1990.
16. Groce E, Irving Z. Multiculturalism, chronic illness and disability. Pediatrics 1993;91(5):1048–1055.
17. Anderson PP, Fenichel ES. Serving Culturally Diverse Families of Infants and Toddlers with Disabilities. Arlington: National Center for Clinical Infant Programs, 1989.
18. McMillan A. Relevance of culture on pediatric physical therapy: a Saudi Arabian experience. Pediatr Phys Ther 1995;7(3):138–139.
19. Camphina-Bacote J. Many faces: addressing diversity in health care. Online J Issues Nurs 2003;8:1.
20. Thomas SB, Quinn SC. The Tuskegee Syphilis Study, 1932–1972: implications for HIV education and AIDS risk programs in the Black community. Am J Public Health 1991;81:1503.

21. Taylor J. The story catches you and you fall down: tragedy, ethnography, and cultural competence. Med Anthropol Qtly 2003;2:159–181.

22. Kleinman A. Patients and Healers in the Context of Culture: An Exploration of the Borderline Between Anthropology, Medicine, and Psychiatry. Berkeley, CA: University of California Press, 1980.

23. Parry K. Patient-therapist relations: culture and personal meanings. Phys Ther 1994;2(10):88–345.

24. Pachtner LM. Culture and clinical care: folk illness beliefs and their implications for health care delivery. JAMA 1994;271:690–694.

25. Munet-Vilaro F, Vessey JA. Children's explanation of leukemia: a Hispanic perspective. Adv Nurs Sci 1990;15(2):76–79.

26. Spearing E, Devine J. A qualitative analysis of attitudes towards disability between Hispanic And Anglo-American families of children with chronic disabilities. Pediatr Phys Ther 2004;16:65.

27. Lawson LV. Culturally sensitive support for grieving parents. MCN Am J Matern Child Nurs 1990;15(2):76–79.

28. Gartner A, Lipisky D, Turnball A. Supporting Families with a Child with a Disability. Baltimore: Paul H. Brooks Publishing Co., 1991.

29. Camphina-Bacote J. A model and instrument for addressing cultural competence in health care. J Nurs Educ 1999;38:203–207.

30. Byrd W, Clayton LA. An American Health Dilemma. A Medical History of African Americans and the Problem of Race. New York: Routledge, 2000.

31. National Standards for Culturally Linguistically Appropriate Services in Health Care. Washington, DC: U.S. Department of Health and Human Services, March 2001.

32. Bronheim S, Goode T, Jones W. Policy Brief: Cultural and Linguistic Competence in Family Supports. Washington, DC: National Center for Cultural Competence, 2006. Available at: http://gucchd.georgetown.edu. Accessed October 7, 2006.

Development

Motor Development in the Normal Child

Emilie J. Aubert
Photo credit to Ryan C. Aubert

N ormal or typical development of abilities and skills in humans begins at the moment of conception. In normal conception and pregnancy, the **embryo** (conception through 8 weeks' gestation) and the **fetus** (9 weeks' gestation until birth) develop according to a sequence and timing common to all humans.[1] Birth typically occurs at 40 weeks' gestation or 10 lunar months after conception, plus or minus 2 weeks.[2,3] Infants considered to be **term** or **full term** are then born after 38 to 42 weeks of gestation.[2,3] Postpartum development of human behaviors is the continuation of that which began at conception. A person's development occurs over his or her lifespan as the body undergoes change. It has been said that human development is an ongoing process from the womb to the tomb.

After a child is born, change occurs at a relatively rapid rate compared to many changes in adulthood. Particularly notable during the first 24 months of life are the acquisition of and changes in gross and fine motor skills.

New gross and fine motor skills are definitely learned and refined after age 2, but many of these new and refined motor behaviors occur as the child or adult learns new skills needed for play, sports, and/or work. Also, new motor skills are acquired and refined as needed when the individual has particular age-appropriate functional requirements. Dr. Milani-Comparetti has referred to these as *appointments with function*.[4] Some of these appointments with function occur at relatively typical times in life, such as learning to independently don and doff one's jacket in time to begin kindergarten, learning to drive at age 16, or

learning to tie one's own necktie when moving away from home to attend college. The chronologic ages of achievement of motor behaviors and skills are influenced by these appointments with function and numerous intrinsic and extrinsic factors, both prenatally and postnatally.[5]

Gestational and postgestational motor development usually occur according to a typical sequence, pattern, and timing. However, after birth, extrinsic factors such as opportunity to learn and practice a skill, exposure to environmental pollutants, inadequate nurture and bonding, and parental and cultural childrearing practices may modify age of skill acquisition and possibly the sequence and pattern of the motor behaviors. As the child ages, more latitude must be allowed for the expression of differences in development as a result of the many and varied extrinsic factors (see Table 2.1).

Behaviors that develop in the human include gross motor, fine motor, cognitive, language, and personal–social behaviors. Although the emphasis of this chapter is on chronologic motor development, a thorough appreciation for and understanding of a child's development stems from knowledge regarding all developmental domains, as well as growth parameters such as strength and range of motion. Additionally, one must consider the development of and changes in the various systems of the body. All of these areas interact together as the child matures, grows, and develops.

The focus of this chapter is on normal or typical gross and fine motor development in the infant and toddler. The motor developmental sequence offers physical therapists a

TABLE 2.1	
Examples of Extrinsic Factors That Affect Motor Development	
Factor	**Example**
Opportunity	Stair climbing develops earlier in a child who must contend with stairs in the home, compared to children who are not permitted on stairs.
Environmental pollutants	Children raised in an environment of smoke from cigarette smoking may be delayed in developing motor skills and may have stunted growth.
Inadequate nurture and bonding	Infants who are not held to be fed may experience motor delay as well as failure to thrive.
Parental and cultural childrearing practices	Children placed supine to sleep may be slower to develop head control in prone and upright, prone-on-elbows posture, and rolling prone to supine.

foundation for studying and understanding not only typical development, but also aberrant or atypical development of the child. This developmental sequence may be used as a basis for evaluating, assessing, and treating motor delays and deficiencies in both children and adults. The sequence, in particular, can play an important role in evaluating and treating people of all ages because identifiable components of motor behavior begin to evolve in specific aspects of the sequence. For example, in the prone-on-elbows or -forearms position typical of a 4-month-old infant, once able to assume the posture, the child begins to shift weight while maintaining the posture. This shifting of weight contributes the beginnings of movement components such as elongation of the trunk on the side bearing more weight (i.e., to the side the weight is shifted), unilateral weight bearing in the upper extremities to allow for visually directed reaching, and early accidental rolling from prone to supine. If the prone-on-elbows posture is not achieved or is delayed, the evolution of some of the mentioned movement components may be delayed, or the components may not develop.

Each stage of the motor developmental sequence has purpose and contributes to the overall development of the child. Therefore, various aspects of the sequence can be used in therapy, for adults and children, to facilitate the evolution of different movement components. In the evaluation and assessment of children, the typical timing of the acquisition of specific motor skills is linked to the determination of a **motor age.** Ideally, as an infant or toddler develops, the assessed motor age will be congruent with the child's chronologic age. A gap between the child's chronologic age and motor age, assessed according to established standards for age of skill or **milestone** development, is undesirable.[6–8] The greater the gap between chronologic age and motor age, the more likely that the child is exhibiting a possible developmental problem.

In the **habilitation** of a developing child, established norms for the sequence, timing, and patterns of motor behaviors can be used not only to evaluate and assess the child, but also to set treatment goals and develop a treatment plan. This is not to say that the sequence must be followed in some strict manner when habilitating or rehabilitating a child or adult. Rather, the sequence can be used as a guide, and it informs our understanding of the need for particular movement components in order to develop and refine particular functional motor skills.

Care must be taken when using the terms *normal* and *typical* when speaking about the motor development of a child, especially regarding age of milestone acquisition. Normal is defined as conformity with the established standards for humans.[9] Typical is defined as having the qualities of a particular group, in this case, human infants and children, so completely as to be representative of that group.[9] The reader should keep in mind that what is normal or typical motor behavior of humans at various ages is generally described in ranges. Such ranges exist because both motor development and individual motor skills are affected by numerous factors, in addition to the intrinsic biologic nature of the human. Even the intrinsic anatomy and physiology of a human is, in many ways, uniquely his or her own. For the purposes of this chapter, the terms normal and typical will be used synonymously.

Normative values for age of skill acquisition, based on a defined subject pool, are set forth in numerous norm-referenced developmental instruments.[6–8] Because the norms are based on a limited, albeit large, group of subjects and therefore established with certain cultural bias, extrinsic factors such as cultural customs, parental practices, and opportunity to learn skills may detract from or improve a child's score. Therefore, this text emphasizes a rather broad range of achievement ages, based on several norm-referenced evaluation and assessment tools. Also, it is important to note that typical ages of achievement are usually based on full-term gestation in humans, which is 40 weeks.[2,3] Table 2.2 shows approximate expected ages of acquiring specific motor milestones for full-term infants.

The Variability of Human Growth and Development

Although human birth, growth, and development have long histories, our understanding of these processes has

TABLE 2.2

Ages of Motor Milestone Acquisition in Typical Full-Term Infants

Milestone	Typical Age	Age Range
Physiologic flexion	Birth	N/A
Turns head to side in prone	Birth	N/A
Attempts to lift head in midline	1 mo	1–2 mo
Automatic stepping	Birth	N/A
Fencer's posture	2 mo	N/A
Astasia	2 mo	N/A
Abasia	2 mo	N/A
Rolling supine to side-lying nonsegmentally	3 mo	2–4 mo
Beginning midline head control	3 mo	2–3 mo
Prone on elbows, head to 90 degrees, chin tuck	4 mo	3–5 mo
Hands to midline	4 mo	3–5 mo
Unilateral reaching prone on elbows	5 mo	4–6 mo
Prone on extended arms	5 mo	4–6 mo
Pivot prone posture	5 mo	4–6 mo
Beginning intra-axial rotation	5 mo	4–5 mo
Rolling prone to supine, segmentally	5 mo	4–6 mo
Head lifting in supine	5 mo	4–6 mo
Supine, hands to knees and feet	5 mo	4–6 mo
Supine, hands to feet	5 mo	4–6 mo
Supine, feet to mouth	5 mo	4–6 mo
Propped sitting	5 mo	5–6 mo
Supine bridging	5 mo	5–7 mo
Rolling supine to prone, segmentally	6 mo	5–7 mo
Ring sitting, unsupported with full trunk extension and high guard	6 mo	5–7 mo
Transferring objects hand to hand	6 mo	5–7 mo
Independent sitting with secondary curves	8 mo	7–9 mo
Beginning quadruped	8 mo	7–9 mo
Beginning pull to standing	8 mo	7–9 mo
Creeping	10 mo	9–11 mo
Plantigrade posture	10 mo	10–12 mo
Plantigrade creeping	10 mo	10–12 mo
Pulling to standing and lowering self	10 mo	10–12 mo
Cruising	10 mo	9–11 mo
Pulling to standing through half-kneeling	12 mo	11–13 mo
Walking independently	12 mo	10–15 mo
Creeping up stairs*	15 mo	14–18 mo
Walking up stairs with help or handrail*	18 mo	16–20 mo

*Age of achievement of ascending and descending stairs depends greatly on motivation, opportunity, and experience.

increased and been refined over time. As we continue to study all aspects of human development, one characteristic of human development clearly stands the test of time. Human development is characterized by variability. In fact, lack of variability, either within one individual or when comparing an individual to textbook standards, is often a red flag.

Motor development and motor behaviors vary because of the influence of numerous intrinsic (endogenous) and extrinsic (exogenous) factors, many of which we cannot influence or control. However, many intrinsic and extrinsic factors can be controlled and manipulated to optimize fetal and infant development. For example, it is now known that fetal exposure to alcohol of unknown quantities can result in a child who has fetal alcohol effects or

fetal alcohol syndrome.[10,11] Children 3 years of age who were exposed to alcohol or illicit drugs in utero have been found to exhibit delayed mental, motor, and behavioral development when compared to standardized norms for children at age 3.[12,13] Furthermore, prenatal alcohol effects on fetal, infant, and child development are not totally known, and the effects can be compounded by other pre-, peri-, and postnatal risk factors.[13,14] Fetal alcohol exposure is something that can be controlled (i.e., eliminated) during pregnancy, thereby effectively eliminating the potential adverse effects of alcohol on growth and development. To the contrary, if a woman unexpectedly develops a disease process during pregnancy, the disease may impact the fetus and child negatively. However, this insult to the developing embryo or fetus may not have been preventable.

The variability of human motor development has been the subject of much study. Scientists and therapists have attempted to explain the differences in motor development between one person and another, and have tried to discover ways to optimize those factors that produce healthy motor behaviors and minimize those that have a negative impact.

A number of theories about how humans develop motor and other behaviors have been proposed. Brief descriptions of some of these theories follow. The reader should keep in mind that just as no two humans develop exactly alike, it is most likely that no single theory can explain developmental fact.

 ## Developmental Theories

Developmental theories have been applied to all aspects of infant and child development including physical, psychosocial, and cognitive. To effectively work with children, physical therapists need to have a broad understanding of all areas of infant and child development. However, physical therapists most definitely need a broad and deep understanding of the physical aspects of growth and development. Therefore, those developmental theories that adequately address a child's physical development are easiest to apply in physical therapy. Those theories will be emphasized in this brief discussion.

MATURATIONAL THEORIES

Maturational theories, also referred to as hierarchical theories, have been developed and advanced by people with familiar names such as Piaget, Gesell, Bayley, and McGraw, beginning in the early 1900s. The works of these developmental theorists continue to contribute heavily to our understanding of child development today.[6,11,15–19] Their legacies are seen in the clinic worldwide. For example, Nancy Bayley's early work from the 1930s produced standardized scales for mental and motor development.[20–22] Her work continues to be a powerful clinical tool for assessing a child's mental and/or motor development, with a third edition of the *Bayley Scales of Infant Development* having been published recently.[23]

Maturational theories of development emphasize a *normal developmental sequence* that is common to all fetal, infant, and child mental and motor development. According to *maturationists*, the normal sequence of development evolves as the central nervous system (CNS) matures, and the CNS is the major driving force of development.[19,24,25] Hierarchical theory has been interpreted by some to suggest a strict, invariant sequence of development in all *normal* children.[19,20] However, others have interpreted hierarchical development in a less stringent manner, including many physical therapists that have practiced since the 1970s who understand the hierarchy of motor skills to be merely, but consistently, a roadmap. Nonetheless, many of these same therapists believe in the primacy of the CNS in dictating developmental sequence and timing.

BEHAVIORAL THEORIES

A behavioral theory of development is rooted in the works of Pavlov, Skinner, and Bandura, with emphasis on conditioning behavior through the use of a stimulus-response approach.[20,25] Behavior theory advocates modifying behavior through manipulating stimuli in the environment to create a response that positively or negatively reinforces a particular behavior.[20] This type of theory is used by physical therapists when they control the environment to elicit a predictable behavior. For example, a therapist may move a very distractible child from the physical therapy gym to a quiet room, in order to control or improve the child's ability to stay on task. Therapists also use a stimulus-response approach when they manipulate parameters such as intensity, rate, and frequency of application of a given treatment modality.[26] Regarding motor development, some of a child's motor behaviors (responses) are conditioned by positive or negative feedback to particular behaviors. For example, one typically developing child evaluated by this author spent very little time creeping on hands and knees, showing a preference for plantigrade creeping on hands and feet. Engaging in the plantigrade creeping as a major form of locomotion seemed to be the result of conditioning. During this prewalking stage of development, which happened to occur during the summer, the child spent considerable time playing outdoors on the family's concrete patio and sidewalk. It did not take him long to *learn* that the trio of rough surfaces, shorts, and creeping on hands and knees could cause great discomfort and even injury. The stimulus of the rough surface, with *givens* of hot weather and summertime apparel, conditioned a movement response that kept his bare knees off the rough surface, yet still allowed him to locomote and explore his environment.

DYNAMIC SYSTEMS THEORIES

The third and final developmental theory to be addressed here is the dynamic systems theory. This theory is based on the original work of Bernstein in 1967 and has been modified by numerous others more recently, including Thelen et al., Horak, Heriza, and Shumway-Cook and Wollacott.[5,19,20,24,25] Unlike the longitudinal and hierarchical maturation theories, which consider the CNS to be the predominate factor and manager, organizer, and regulator of development, dynamic systems theories see infant and child development as nonlinear and the result of many factors, both intrinsic and extrinsic, that impact the developing fetus and child. According to the dynamic systems theory, no one system (such as the CNS in the maturational theories) is the pre-eminent director of development. Instead, each fetus and child develops certain characteristics and skills based on the confluence of many factors.[5,19,20,24,25] While motor behaviors do seem to develop in the fetus, infant, and toddler according to a basic scheme, the sequence, timing, and quality of developmental milestones may be modified by numerous factors in any one fetus or child.

Factors that influence motor development in the human include genetic inheritance, errors and mutations in genetic transmission, poor maternal/fetal and child nutrition, fetal and infant exposure to toxins and other chemical substances, race, ethnicity, presence or absence of quality prenatal care, childrearing practices, socioeconomic level (which may have immense bearing on several of the other factors mentioned here), disease processes, and trauma. In addition, opportunity, cognitive abilities, level of stimulation, and motivation affect the learning of new motor skills in children and adults, as do the motor task at hand, the functional outcome desired, and the context for using a particular motor skill.[5,10–12,14,15,18–20]

In a dynamic systems view of growth and development, the CNS is merely one, albeit very important, influential system. Unlike a purely hierarchical or maturational viewpoint, a dynamic systems approach to development considers the profound influences of other body systems on the anatomic, physiologic, and behavioral qualities of the fetus and child (the organism). These other systems include the peripheral nervous, musculoskeletal, cardiopulmonary, and integumentary systems.

CENTRAL PATTERN GENERATORS

"Today the existence of networks of nerve cells producing specific, rhythmic movements, without conscious effort and without the aid of peripheral afferent feedback, is indisputable for a large number of vertebrates. These specialized neural circuits are referred to as 'neural oscillators' or 'central pattern generators' (CPGs)."[27] It is known that the brainstem has central pattern generators for rhythmic functions such as chewing, breathing, and swallowing.[19,27–29] The spinal cord has CPGs for functional locomotion.[27,30]

In the absence of afferent input, the CPGs can still produce stereotypic, rhythmic movements such as locomotion. This is not to say that sensory feedback is not an important factor in normal locomotion.[27] However, the idea that motor output can occur without first having sensory input is contrary to early thinking in this field of study.[26]

WHICH DEVELOPMENTAL THEORY IS CORRECT?

Motor development in humans and motor behaviors have been shown to be under the influence of supraspinal structures, spinal structures, peripheral sensory input, central pattern generators, dynamic environmental features, and neuromodulatory influences. Supraspinal centers that con-

trol human locomotion include the sensorimotor cortex, cerebellum, and basal ganglia.[27] Sensory afferents, from the periphery, are important regulators of movement, helping modify the patterns generated centrally so that movements can be constantly adapted to the environment, task, and task context.[27] Neuromodulators such as serotonin and dopamine are also thought to influence centrally generated locomotion in some vertebrates, but their role is not yet completely understood.[27]

Among the many theories of development, including those affecting motor development, probably no one theory can ever be considered the one and only correct theory. Rather, many different theories can be called upon to explain and predict fetal and child motor development. Principles from different theories can be combined to analyze, interpret, and even predict motor development. Many aspects of the dynamic systems approach probably come the closest to being the dominant theory of motor development used by physical therapists in the 21st century, because this approach, in itself, considers the impact of many variables on the creation, growth, and development of a human biologic system. Having said that, it is this author's opinion that many contemporary physical therapists, in an effort to de-emphasize the hierarchical aspect of development, risk underconsideration of the basic motor development sequence that has characterized fetal and child development for thousands of years. Given the multitude of environments in which children have grown and developed over time, the similarities in the *normal developmental sequence* and motor milestone acquisition among infants and toddlers are simply too great to be ignored.

 ## Preterm Infants

Preterm or **premature** infants, defined as those with a gestational age of less than 38 weeks, may not exhibit motor skills consistent with the child's chronologic age because of the prematurity.[3] The child born too early may demonstrate motor delays equivalent to the number of weeks premature. In order to distinguish between delays that are the natural result of not having enough in utero time and delays caused by abnormal pathophysiology, the premature infant is evaluated and assessed according to an **adjusted age.** Adjusted age is determined by subtracting the **gestational age** of the child, the number of weeks and days in utero, from 40 weeks. This remainder is then subtracted from the child's actual **chronologic age,** which is calculated from the date of the child's birth.[31] A sample adjusted age calculation is shown in Display 2.1.

 ## Developmental Direction

Studying the typical sequence of motor development reveals a developmental direction that applies to most of development, although there are exceptions. Pertinent exceptions will be noted in the following discussion. Ten sequences of developmental direction are listed in Table 2.3, with examples of how these sequences are revealed in normal development. A few of these principles deserve additional attention to develop an understanding of the typical emergence of motor skills in humans.

Motor behavior in humans is at first a reflex in nature. As the organism matures, motor behaviors become more complex and eventually come under **cortical** or **volitional** control. This is an example of **reflex to cortical** developmental direction. Additionally, primitive reflex responses tend to be more generalized rather than localized responses. This **generalized or total movement before the development of localized movement** in a given area of the body is another example of developmental direction. A good example of a generalized response is the response seen in the **flexor withdrawal reflex.** This reflex is a **primitive reflex** that is present at birth and produces a total flexion response in the limb, either upper or lower, when the hand or foot, respectively, is exposed to a **noxious** or **nociceptive** stimulus (Fig. 2.1). The response to the stimulus in this reflex, because it is primitive and generalized, does not permit selective or isolated movements at the various joints of the limb when elicited.

>> **TABLE 2.3**

Examples Reflecting Principles of Developmental Direction

Principle	Earliest Control/Response	Control/Response with Maturation
Reflex control before cortical control	Asymmetric tonic neck reflex causes limbs to move in response to the head position.	Child volitionally moves limbs independent of head position.
Total response before localized response	Neonate moves upper extremities in wide sweeps and at random.	Child gains control of individual joints to stabilize the shoulder for precise, visually directed reach and grasp.
Proximal control before distal control	Child develops shoulder and hip stability.	Elbow, then wrist, and knee, then ankle, stability develop.
Cephalic control before caudal control	Shoulders develop control and stability.	Hips develop control and stability.
Medial control before lateral control	Three ulnar fingers dominate first grasp.	Thumb and index finger dominate pincer grasp. Forefinger dominance develops.
Cervical control before rostral control	Child has motor control of mouth at birth.	Child develops ability to fix eyes and focus.
Gross motor control before fine motor control	Child stabilizes the shoulders and holds a baby bottle with both hands.	Child picks up tiny pellets and puts them in a small bottle.
Flexor muscle tone before extensor muscle tone	Neonate is dominated by physiologic flexion.	Flexor tone loses dominance, and extensor tone is more manifest to balance tone.
Extensor antigravity control before flexor antigravity control	Child lifts head in prone at 4 months of age.	Child lifts head in supine at 5 months of age.
Weight bearing on flexed extremities before on extended extremities	Child bears weight on upper extremities flexed at elbows in prone on elbows.	Child bears weight on extended elbows in prone on extended arms and quadruped.

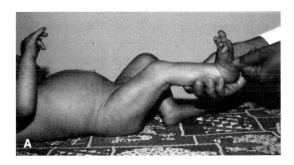

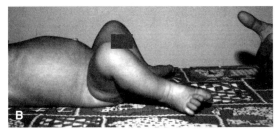

Figure 2.1 ▪ Flexor withdrawal reflex. **(A)** Nociceptive stimulus to the sole of the foot. **(B)** Flexor withdrawal response, total lower extremity flexion.

The flexor withdrawal reflex is present at birth and becomes partially integrated by 2 months of age. However, vestiges of this reflex remain throughout life as a protective mechanism for the hands and feet. The flexor withdrawal reflex is controlled at the level of the spinal cord in the central nervous system.[15] Most early or primitive reflexes are spinal cord reflexes, whereas the mature postural and balance responses are mediated in the midbrain and the cortex of the brain. The stimulus for a spinal cord reflex is an **exteroceptive** stimulus.[5] The receptors for exteroceptive stimuli are "peripheral end organs of the afferent nerves in the skin or mucous membrane, which respond to stimulation by external agents."[1,5,32,33] Another example of a **total response** developing before **localized response** is neonatal kicking. When the infant is first born, he or she moves in very random total patterns. In fact, full-term neonates, when compared to preterm neonates, exhibit a variety of neonatal kicking patterns, with differences in frequency, reciprocal movements, and intralimb *coupling*.[34–36] Coupling is defined by Heathcoch et al. as similar timing of movement between joints within the same limb.[34] Heathcoch et al. also found that full-term neonates were able to exhibit task-specific and purposeful lower extremity control compared to their preterm cohorts.[34] When some **neonates** kick, both lower limbs often move together, the infant being unable to consistently **dissociate** one lower extremity from the other. Also, when kicking, the pelvis frequently moves with the lower extremities, another example of lacking dissociation. In this case, the lack of dissociation is between the hips and pelvis. As the infant matures, he or she consistently is able to move the lower extremities while keeping the pelvis stable, and

right and left limbs can move independently of each other as well as reciprocally, all examples of dissociation. The ability to move the limbs independent of each other allows for **reciprocal kicking,** alternating kicks of the lower extremities. At this point, the infant is also able to move one lower extremity without moving the other and to move a joint within an extremity independent of the other joints in that extremity.

A third principle of developmental direction is **cephalocaudal** development. Generally, this principle is true in the development of motor control in that the head, upper trunk, and upper extremities develop motor control before the lower trunk and lower extremities. An example of cephalocaudal development of motor control is the development of stability of the scapulae and shoulders to maintain the prone-on-elbows posture, before the development of stability of the pelvis and hips as needed for the quadruped position (Fig. 2.2). An exception to cephalocaudal development is the development of muscle tone in the fetus. Studies of premature infants have shown that muscle tone develops in the lower extremities and lower body before tone in the upper extremities and upper body develops.[37]

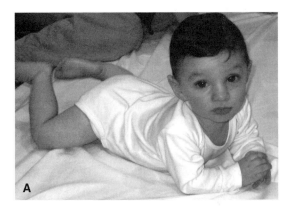

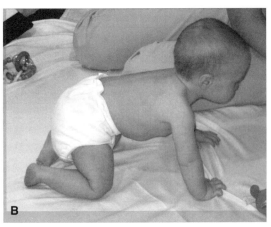

Figure 2.2 ▪ Cephalocaudal development in prone. **(A)** Prone-on-elbows posture with prestance positioning of lower extremities; the more cephalic shoulder girdle exhibits stability. **(B)** Quadruped posture; the more caudal hip exhibits stability.

Motor control also develops from **medial to lateral;** that is, control develops close to the median or midline of the body before developing more laterally. Midline stability of the neck and trunk develop before the more lateral shoulder and hip stability. During the first few weeks of life the infant is relatively symmetric, with the exception of the head, which is turned to one side or the other in prone and supine. The second through fourth months of life are characterized in the term infant by asymmetry, as a result of the influence of reflex activity, most notably the **asymmetric tonic neck reflex (ATNR)** (Fig. 2.3). The ATNR influence diminishes over those first months, thereby reducing reflex dominance and allowing the development of volitional control as noted previously. Volitional control and developing stability begin medially in what is termed **midline activity.** As the ATNR wanes, the child is able to bring his head into midline and maintain it there, instead of being in the asymmetric cervical extension pattern of the ATNR, by 4 months of age. In addition, the child begins bringing his hands to midline, relying on the newly developed shoulder stability to use his hands together in midline (Fig. 2.4). Thus, by 6 months of age, the child demonstrates great symmetry.

Another example of this medial-to-lateral development is the development of grasp. To understand this, one must visualize the body in anatomic position. The ability to grasp and manipulate objects with the hands begins with predominant use of the ulnar fingers, which are more medial, before using the more lateral index finger (radial finger) and thumb.[38]

Control of the two major muscle groups, the flexors and extensors, also develops in a particular developmental direction and occurs in a general sequence. However, development of flexors and extensors differs depending on

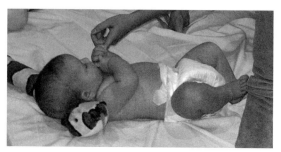

Figure 2.4 ■ Notable symmetry of infant; head and hands are stable in midline.

whether the infant is developing muscle tone, antigravity control, or weight-bearing function. Dominant **muscle tone** throughout the body develops in flexor muscles before extensor muscles, as readily seen in the full-term neonate who is born with **physiologic flexion.**[16,17,39] This physiologic flexion is a dominant flexor tone in all postures when at rest and with passive or active movement. Even in the absence of physiologic flexion, as seen in infants born preterm, extensor tone is relatively low.

In each posture, the development of antigravity movements and control occurs first in extensor muscles at a particular joint, prior to the development of the antagonist flexor muscles at that joint. For example, the infant learns to use his cervical extensors in the controlled anti-gravity movement of lifting his head in prone before he is able to lift his head against gravity in supine, which requires antigravity flexor control. However, to develop full and balanced control at a joint, both antigravity extensors and antigravity flexors are needed. Cephalocaudally developing trunk extensors for antigravity work develop before the flexors of the trunk. Therefore, the child is able to get into a prone-on-elbows posture by 4 months of age, using midline antigravity extensors, before he is able to bring his feet to his mouth in supine at 5 months of age. The foot-to-mouth activity requires anti-gravity flexor control of the trunk.

The weight-bearing function of the extremities occurs on flexed extremities before weight bearing occurs on extended limbs. In prone on elbows, the infant bears weight on flexed upper extremities, with relatively passive lower extremities. This developmental posture occurs before quadruped, wherein weight bearing is on extended upper extremities (the elbows) and on flexed lower extremities (knees and hips) (refer again to Fig. 2.2). The plantigrade creeping posture calls for weight bearing on the open hands and soles of the feet (Fig. 2.5). This posture is an example of weight bearing on extended upper extremities (elbows) and extended lower extremities (knees). In addition to exemplifying the rule of weight bearing, this progression from prone-on-elbows to the plantigrade creeping posture is also an example of cephalocaudal development.

Gross motor skills develop before fine motor skills, the infant being able to stabilize the shoulder with the large

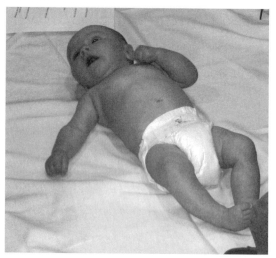

Figure 2.3 ■ Asymmetric tonic neck reflex (fencer's posture) with head turned to right; note the extension of the face-side limbs and flexion of the skull or occiput-side limbs. Fencer's posture seen here in an infant 2 months of age.

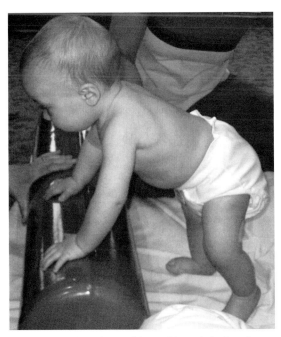

Figure 2.5 ■ Plantigrade position with weight bearing on palms of hands and soles of feet; this is a transition posture between being on the floor and erect standing and may also be used as a locomotive form called plantigrade creeping.

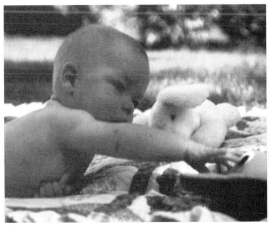

Figure 2.6 ■ Unilateral weight bearing in prone-on-elbows posture with weight shift to the skull side and one upper extremity freed for reaching.

muscles of the shoulder before gaining control of the small muscles of the fingers and hand for fine motor skills. This exemplifies not only the **gross-to-fine** principle of developmental direction, but also the **proximal-to-distal** principle. Proximal refers to the part of an extremity, upper or lower, that is closest to the midline of the body. Distal means the part of the extremity farthest from the midline.

The neck and trunk muscles and all major joints of the extremities (i.e., shoulders, elbows, wrists, hips, knees, and ankles) develop according to certain stages of motor control. They develop mobility, stability, controlled mobility, and skill, as described by Sullivan et al.[33] This sequence was first described, using slightly different terminology, in the early 1960s by Margaret Rood.[26] In the upper extremity, the sequence unfolds in the following manner. The shoulder first develops mobility, the ability to move the upper extremity in space with the distal end, the hand, free. This is referred to as an **open-chain** movement.[40] The early movement of the infant is random and poorly controlled initially but evolves over the first few weeks of life. Success with this ability to move the upper extremity at the shoulder in an open-chain activity paves the way for the shoulder to stabilize in the **closed-chain** activity of prone on elbows and forearms.[40] Now, the distal segments of the extremity (i.e., the forearm, hand, and fingers) are not free in space. Rather, the extremity is performing a weight-bearing function, described by Rood as the stability aspect of motor behavior. Next, the infant demonstrates the ability to move the proximal joint, the shoulder in this exam-

ple, over the distal extremity while the extremity is in a closed chain. This movement is seen as the development of weight shifting in the various weight-bearing postures of the upper extremities. Rood and others have described this phase as mobility superimposed on stability.[26,33] Eventually the child is able to shift his weight entirely onto one or the other upper extremities for unilateral weight-bearing. Then he begins to stabilize the non–weight-bearing shoulder with the hand free (open-chain activity), as the fingers move to grasp and manipulate an object, as seen in Figure 2.6. This represents the skill level denoted by Rood.[26,33]

The lower extremities follow the same sequence for developing mobility, stability, controlled mobility, and functional distal control. This sequence plays out again and again, for both the upper and lower extremities, in each of the developmental postures of prone on elbows, prone on extended arms, sitting, quadruped, and erect standing. In sitting without support and erect standing, the upper extremities play a vital role in providing stability of the upper body, even though they are not performing a weight-bearing function. This will be described later in this chapter when the sitting and erect standing sequences are explained.

 The Neonate

The neonatal period in the infant is the first 28 days of post-partum life.[3] Full-term infants are born with **physiologic flexion** as described earlier, a prime example of muscle tone developing in flexor muscles before extensor muscles. This results in generalized moderate flexion in all positions of the neonate, prone, supine, held in sitting, vertical or horizontal suspension, and held in standing.[16,17,38,39] This flexor tone gradually diminishes over the first month of life in these full-term babies.

Babies who are preterm exhibit less physiologic flexion or the flexion is absent, depending on the child's gestational age.[41,42] The more weeks the child is preterm, the less likely he is to have the physiologic flexion. Instead, preterm infants are born with limbs and trunk relatively extended. This extension is not a dominance of extensor tone, but rather a lack of or diminished flexor tone. The reasons for this lack of flexor tone in the preterm infant are unknown. Several theories have been suggested, including intrauterine positioning and maternal hormonal influences.

In addition to lack of physiologic flexion in preterm neonates, other differences between full and preterm infants are noted at birth. These differences have been well described by Dubowicz, and a few of the major differences are shown in Table 2.4.[2]

 ## Motor Development Goals

One goal of normal motor development is control of the body against gravity.[4] These antigravity movements generally develop first in the head, followed by development in the trunk (cervical to thoracic to lumbosacral), then in the lower extremities. Antigravity control in the lower extremities includes control at the three major joints of the hip, knee, and ankle. While the overall development of antigravity control is cephalocaudal, as revealed by the development of head control, then midline trunk control, and then lower extremity control, control at the various joints of the lower extremities may be occurring simultaneously, very close together in timing, or with the ankle being the lead joint.

Antigravity movements must develop in both extension movements and flexion movements. However, in mature, erect standing, the major body extensor groups are the antigravity muscles, as compared to their flexor antagonists. That is, the midline neck and trunk extensors, hip extensors, and knee extensors are the primary muscle groups that keep humans from surrendering to the force of gravity when upright.

A second goal of development is the ability to maintain the body's center of mass within the base of support.[4] The center of mass when standing is gradually and progressively rising as humans grow in height. Learning to maintain the body's center of mass within the base of support is accomplished as the infant and toddler develop righting, equilibrium, and tilting reactions. While these reactions develop and continue to be activated automatically, the typically developing individual eventually can control these automatic responses volitionally, as long as there are no intrinsic or extrinsic barriers to such control.

A third goal of motor development is the performance of intrasegmental and intersegmental isolated movements.[4] For example, even though various joints of the upper extremity move in a coordinated manner to pro-

TABLE 2.4		
Differences Between Full-Term and Preterm Neonates		
Tone and Movement Patterns	**Preterm Neonate (<32 wk)**	**Full-Term Neonate (>36 wk)**
Posture	Full extension	Physiologic flexion (full flexion)
Scarf sign: arm passively moved across chest of child in supine with head midline	No resistance to passive movement	Resistance to passive movement before reaching midline
Popliteal angle: passively moves knee to chest; extend knee	Angle of extension between lower leg and thigh 135 to 180 degrees	Angle of extension between lower leg and thigh 60 to 90 degrees
Ankle dorsiflexion: infant supine, passively flexes foot against shin	Angle between lower leg and foot 60 to 90 degrees	Angle between lower leg and foot <30 degrees
Slip through: infant in vertical suspension, holding under axillae	Completely slips through hands, does not set shoulders	Sets shoulders and does not slip through
Pull to sit: child supine, pull to sitting by pulling gently on both upper extremities	Complete head lag	Head held in alignment with body
Rooting reflex: child supine in midline, stroke corner of mouth	Absent	Head turns toward stimulus and mouth opens
Sucking reflex: put nipple or clean finger in child's mouth	Weak or absent sucking response	Strong rhythmic sucking
Grasp reflex: place finger horizontally in child's palm	Absent	Sustained flexion and traction
Asymmetric tonic neck reflex: child supine with head in midline, passively turn head to one side	Absent	Upper and lower extremities on face side extend, extremities on skull side flex

duce an upper extremity functional skill, the individual joints, such as the elbow joint, must learn to move independently while the other upper extremity joints do not move. This is intrasegmental dissociation. Intersegmental dissociation, such as moving the head without moving the extremities or moving one lower extremity into flexion while moving the contralateral lower extremity into extension, must develop as well.

◆ The Developmental Progressions

Rather than discussing motor development as a timeline of chronologically occurring events, this text will present the sequence of occurrences that leads to the development of various components of movement. This sequence includes various motor milestones and postures and movement within these postures. Because these events in the normal infant and toddler develop in an orderly sequence in each posture, these sequences will be referred to as **progressions.** One of the earliest developmentalists, Myrtle McGraw, defined these progressions.[16] Prone, supine, rolling, sitting, and erect standing progressions will be presented, as well as various forms of locomotion in each progression.

Stabilizing in various postures is termed static posture and is in contrast to dynamic posture, the translation of those static postures into movement for locomotion, transitions between postures, and prehension.[17] These static and dynamic postures are often referred to as motor milestones. Particularly significant ages of performing certain milestones will be discussed. More detail of the age ranges for the achievement of these motor milestones can be found in Table 2.2. An important point to note is that the ages of acquisition of certain skills fall within ranges rather than at exact points in the developing child. Each developing child is unique, both in the intrinsic factors, biologic structure and function, and in the extrinsic factors that affect his or her development. This uniqueness must be remembered and considered, even though basic commonalities of anatomy, physiology, sequential development, and pathology exist.

PRONE PROGRESSION

PRONE LYING

At birth, the healthy, full-term neonate has physiologic flexion, which dominates the prone position. In prone the head is turned to one side. This turning of the head to one side is the result of two primary influences. The first influence is a survival instinct, which allows the infant to turn his head to the side to clear his mouth and nose so he can breathe in prone, and the second is the influence of the

ATNR.[15,43] Although the normal infant can be moved out of this pattern easily, the ATNR continues to influence head position in all postures, including prone, until the influence has completely subsided by approximately 4 months of age. Encountering considerable resistance to moving the child out of the fencer's posture may be an indication of atypical sensorimotor development.

The hip flexion aspect of physiologic flexion is particularly strong in prone lying and is accompanied by a relative anterior tilt of the pelvis. The infant's knees are drawn underneath him with buttocks up in the air, and the exaggerated hip flexion and anterior tilt are preventing the pelvis from lying flat on the surface (Fig. 2.7). His weight is shifted forward onto his upper chest and face. When his head is turned to one side, the weight shifted onto the head is borne by the child's cheek on that side. The upper extremities are adducted into the side of the body with the elbows caudal to the shoulders. Hands are generally fisted, due to the strong influence of the hand grasp reflex. However, the hands frequently and spontaneously will open and can be opened passively in the normally developing infant. Persistently fisted hands that never open may indicate abnormal sensorimotor development. Persistently fisted hands with the thumb flexed into the palm and held by the fingers is often a sign of pathology.

As physiologic flexion diminishes over the first month, the infant begins falling more and more into gravity in both prone and supine. In prone, hip flexion decreases, allowing the buttocks to come down and the pelvis to lie flat against the surface (Fig. 2.8). Weight shifts away from the face, back toward the trunk and lower extremities. However, a relative anterior pelvic tilt is still present, albeit decreased (Fig. 2.9). The diminished nature of the anterior pelvic tilt is not due to an active posterior tilt at this point but results simply from the loss of the physiologic flexion that kept the hips and knees flexed underneath the child's body.

As physiologic flexion disappears completely, the child lies flat on the surface in prone (Fig. 2.10). The hips are now passively extended and prepared for the beginning of active posterior pelvic tilt, which is an indication of the activation and development of the abdominal muscles (the trunk flexors) and the hip extensors. Without the buttocks

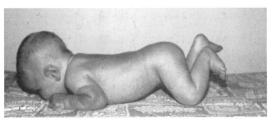

Figure 2.7 ■ Neonate in prone; note anterior pelvic tilt and hip flexion, with buttocks up in the air; position prevents infant from lifting his head from the surface.

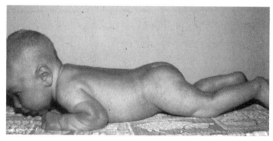

Figure 2.8 ■ Diminishing physiologic flexion; as pelvis comes down to the mat with decreasing hip flexion and anterior pelvic tilt, infant's weight shifts posteriorly making it easier for the child to lift his head in prone (compare to Figure 2.7).

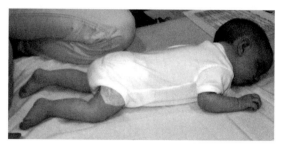

Figure 2.10 ■ Physiologic flexion is gone; infant is flat in prone with elongated hip flexors and a relatively neutral pelvis.

in the air, the child's weight is no longer shifted forward onto the chest and cheek but instead is borne over all the body segments that are in contact with the surface. The infant at this point has no active antigravity control.

In the ensuing prone posture the lower extremities are positioned in hip abduction, partial extension, and external rotation (Fig. 2.11). Knees are semi-flexed and feet are dorsiflexed. This position of the lower extremities is the precursor to the position of the lower extremities in initial standing. Beginning at approximately 5 months of age, the child will stand, with hands held or holding onto something such as the crib rails, with this same wide base of support, hips, knees, and feet mimicking the early lower extremity position seen in prone.

PRONE ON ELBOWS

To achieve the **prone-on-elbows** or prone-on-forearms posture, the next step in the prone progression, three things must happen: (1) stabilization of the pelvis; (2) head lifting with cephalocaudally progressing antigravity extensor control; and (3) movement of the upper extremities out of the neonatal position.

Head control in prone is the earliest antigravity control to develop. In order for the infant to begin experiment-

ing with head control, he must move the head away from the support of the surface. To lift his head he must actively contract his cervical extensors. At birth he was able to lift his head only briefly in prone to turn his head for breathing. The first truly active attempts at lifting his head in prone are tenuous, at best (see Fig. 2.8). Body proportions of infants are different than older children and adults. In the infant, the head makes up approximately one-quarter of the body in length, causing the head to be proportionately large and heavy.[44] This compares to the body proportions of an adult, in whom the head is only one-eighth of height.[44] Maturation and practice of the skill of head lifting strengthens the cervical extensor muscles so that the infant can eventually lift his heavy head (Fig. 2.12). This ability depends on the cervical flexors, the anterior muscles, to lengthen through reciprocal inhibition.

Even with cervical extensors increasing in strength, the child is not able to lift his head without stabilizing in another part of his body. When the buttocks were up and the head was down, weight was shifted toward the head.

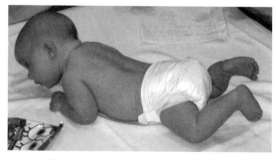

Figure 2.9 ■ Attempt to lift head and attain prone on elbows, but pelvis is still in a relative anterior tilt, and upper extremities are held close to the sides with the elbows too caudal.

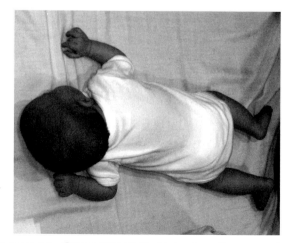

Figure 2.11 ■ Once physiologic flexion has disappeared, lower extremities exhibit a prestance position in prone, which includes hip external rotation with slight flexion and abduction, slight flexion of the knee, and dorsiflexion of the ankle.

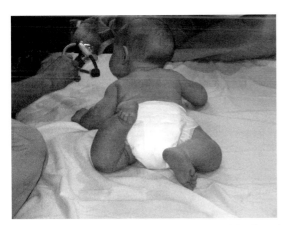

Figure 2.12 ■ Infant has a relative posterior pelvic tilt, which promotes the use of the antigravity cervical extensors for head lifting in prone; note the more abducted and forward position of the upper extremities and the prestance position of the lower extremities.

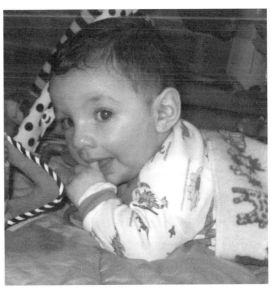

Figure 2.13 ■ At 3 months of age child attains prone on elbows with the head lifted so that the face is at a 45-degree angle; note forward position of elbows.

If the head is to be up, the buttocks must be down, the weight must be shifted caudally, and the pelvis must stabilize for head and midline upper trunk lifting. If one thinks of the child's head and upper trunk as being a lever arm, the fulcrum around which the lever arm turns for this movement is the pelvis, so the pelvis must be stabilized. This stabilization of the pelvis is achieved by recruiting abdominal muscles to tilt the pelvis posteriorly and hold it stable in a posterior tilt. With the help of the abdominal muscles to stabilize the pelvis in a relative posterior tilt, the infant begins actively lifting the head at approximately 2 months of age. By 3 months, cervical extension is adequate to lift the head such that the baby's face is at a 45-degree angle with the surface, and head control is mostly due to antigravity extensor muscles (Fig. 2.13). As development of the spinal extensors progresses cephalocaudally, the upper thoracic extensors begin to strengthen and gain antigravity control. By 4 months, the baby is able to lift the head to 90 degrees. However, the chin of the infant who is able to lift his head to 90 degrees tends to jut forward slightly, with the neck hyperextended, during early successes in the prone-on-elbows and prone-on-extended arms postures (Fig. 2.14). Although the infant has control of his cervical and upper thoracic antigravity extensors to lift the head to this face vertical position, one element of head control is still missing. Control at any joint in the body depends on a balance of muscles surrounding that joint. Therefore, head control is not complete until the antigravity cervical flexors have been activated and strengthened.

The child's ability to use his midline cervical extensors to lift his head is a sign of the diminishing ATNR and the development of active cervical flexors. Although the strength of the ATNR diminishes during the first 4 months, the waning influence continues to provide slight cervical asymmetric extension. Once the child begins to develop active cervical flexors to balance those extensors, the head is more easily brought to midline for lifting in prone. Continued strengthening of the cervical flexors, along with the activation of the serratus anterior muscles in the prone-on-elbows posture, contributes to what Bly refers to as a **chin tuck** when the head is lifted to 90 degrees, so that the face is vertical (Fig. 2.2A).

The infant who is 4 months of age and has stable control of the head at 90 degrees, with the chin tucked, displays balanced cervical extensors and flexors. By comparison, head control of the 3-month-old child during head lifting is dominated by extensors that are not balanced by antigravity flexors, helping produce a chin that is not tucked.

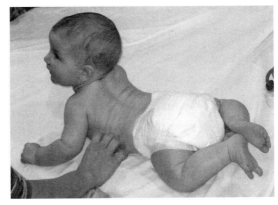

Figure 2.14 ■ Infant prone on extended arms with face vertical (at 90 degrees) but with mild cervical hyperextension and without chin tuck.

Chin tuck appears, therefore, as a result of three developmental occurrences: activation and strengthening of the cervical flexors; reduction of the ATNR; and activation and strengthening of the serratus anterior muscles. The infant uses the serratus anterior muscles to protract the shoulder girdle and work the elbows into the surface. Without the protraction provided by these muscles, the child may exhibit what Bly and others have termed *TV shoulders*.[45] In TV shoulders, the child's upper extremities are not worked into the surface. Rather, the shoulders elevate and the neck hyperextends, with the infant's occiput resting on his posterior cervical soft tissue, chin jutting forward. The face, in this position, is not at 90 degrees or vertical, and the child does not have active head control. With the shoulders elevated at the sides of the head, close to the ears, the head is passively supported. Consequently, persistence of the TV shoulders interferes with the development of active, antigravity head control and lateral head righting. TV shoulders also make it difficult to swallow, talk, and breathe, because of the cervical hyperextension.

If at 4 months of age the child exhibits cervical hyperextension with the occiput of the skull resting on the upper back, the cervical flexors and/or serratus anterior muscles are not activated or have insufficient strength. This is an example of how the developmental sequence and the movement components might be used to determine a plan of treatment. If a child exhibits TV shoulders while prone on elbows, strength of the serratus anterior muscles as well as the strength of the cervical flexor and extensor muscles should be tested. If any of these muscles are weak, this may account for the cervical hyperextension, at least in part. If the cervical extensors are weak, it is likely that they are too weak to maintain the head upright, and once the head is lifted, the child compensates for the inability to actively stabilize the neck. His head falls backward into hyperextension as a response to gravity. This is a pattern frequently seen in children who have delayed or abnormal sensorimotor development, such as children with cerebral palsy or other brain disorders. In such a case, one part of the physical therapy treatment plan would include strengthening the muscles that are weak and practicing control over those muscles.

The third element necessary for the child to achieve the prone-on-elbows milestone is a forward position of the elbows. The upper extremities, in the full-term neonate, are adducted closely into the body, or even slightly under the body, and extended at the shoulders, causing them to have a mechanical disadvantage in trying to lift the upper trunk and head. During the second month, at the time when the infant is first attempting to lift his head, upper extremity control at the shoulder begins to develop. The infant gradually abducts and flexes the shoulders, bringing the elbows from underneath his body forward, more to a position underneath or just anterior to the shoulders. This enables the baby to bear weight on his elbows and forearms when he lifts his head. Figures 2.7 through 2.9, 2.12, and 2.13 show this progression. One important component of movement that begins to develop in this process is **scapulohumeral** elongation. Scapulohumeral elongation refers to the ability of elongation of the axillary region as the humerus is flexed and/or abducted away from the body and therefore away from the scapulae. Without the ability to elongate this region, the child will not be able to get the elbows into position underneath the shoulders for the prone-on-elbows posture. Failure to elongate the axillary region will also interfere with reaching out in space, such as when a child reaches out to grasp an object while sitting at his desk.

While the upper extremities are typically envisioned as limbs with important mobility functions, such as reach and grasp, and the lower extremities are visualized in terms of their weight-bearing functions, such as standing, all four extremities have both weight-bearing and mobility functions to perform. Prior to assuming the prone-on-elbows posture, the upper extremities have exhibited only mobility functions. The prone-on-elbows posture is the first call for the upper extremities to be weight bearing. This ability to weight-bear through the forearms, elbows, and shoulders foreshadows the weight bearing that will follow in the quadruped position.

Once the infant has achieved a stable prone-on-elbows position, in order to be functional he must be able to translate the position into movement while maintaining stability at the proximal joint, the shoulder. He begins to shift his weight from side to side, increasing the amount of weight bearing on each upper extremity as the weight is shifted to that side. Shifting weight side to side soon becomes shifting of weight in all directions, including forward, back, and diagonally. This weight shifting is a feature of all the milestone postures once the stability of each posture has been established. It is critical for the development of equilibrium and tilting responses for maintaining balance, as well as for functional use of the upper extremity. In the prone-on-elbows posture, if the baby does not learn to shift his weight, his upper extremities will not be able to develop controlled mobility functions. Essentially, he will be stuck. Without the appropriate development of weight-shifting, the controlled mobility functions of reaching (open chain) and the closed-chain propulsion function of the upper extremities, needed for crawling and creeping, will not develop.

Weight shift is necessary for reasons other than just to free a limb for controlled mobility. Weight shift encourages elongation of muscles on one side of a joint or joints while the antagonist muscles shorten. In typical sensorimotor development, this elongation during weight shift occurs in the lateral trunk muscles on the side that is weight bearing or bearing most of the weight. For example, when the child shifts his weight while in quadruped such that he unilaterally weight-bears on an upper extrem-

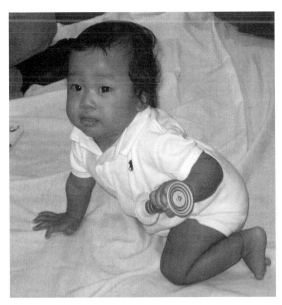

Figure 2.15 ■ *Unilateral weight bearing in the upper extremities from quadruped with elongation of the child's trunk on the side bearing the most weight, in this case his right side.*

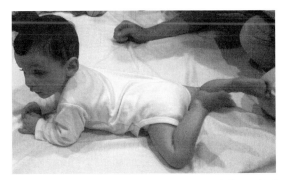

Figure 2.17 ■ *Prone on elbows with weight shift to skull side and elongation on the weight-bearing side.*

ity, the lateral trunk on the side bearing the weight is elongated (relaxed and stretched) while the lateral trunk on the side of the free upper extremity shortens (contracts), with lateral bending or flexion to that side (Fig. 2.15). Figures 2.16 through 2.21 show this elongation on the weight-bearing side in different postures and at different ages.

Weight shift also introduces the infant to vestibular stimulation, which is under his control, as opposed to the vestibular stimulation of being moved by another person or an object (rocking chair) or watching another person or object move (the crib mobile). Finally, when in full unilateral weight bearing, weight shift increases the weight borne, and therefore, joint compression, on a particular side or limb up to twice the normal customary weight and compression. This increased weight on one limb or one side of the trunk facilitates the recruitment of motor units in the working muscles.[26,46]

Weight shifting in prone on elbows has another subtle, yet significant, effect on the baby's development. Babies are born with their forearms in relative pronation and are unable to supinate the forearms actively, even though the forearms can be moved passively into supination. As the baby shifts from side to side in prone on elbows, the weight shifting causes the forearm on the side to which he shifts his weight to supinate, and the forearm on the side away from which he shifts pronates. The proprioceptive feedback from this reciprocal pronation and supination lays the foundation for emerging, active supination. Without the ability to supinate the forearms, the infant would not develop the ability to reach for, grasp, and visually engage an object. With the forearm in

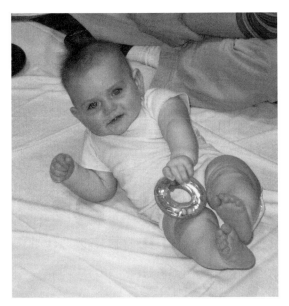

Figure 2.16 ■ *Weight shift to side-lying with elongation on the weight-bearing side.*

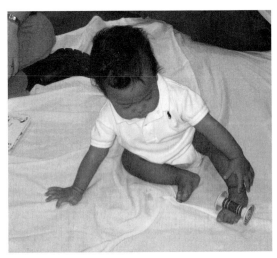

Figure 2.18 ■ *Half–ring sitting with weight shifted to child's right side and elongation of the weight-bearing side.*

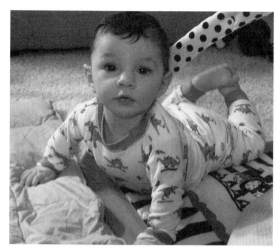

Figure 2.19 ▪ Prone on extended arms with muscles on the weight-bearing side elongated, in this case the muscles of the anterior trunk and lower extremities.

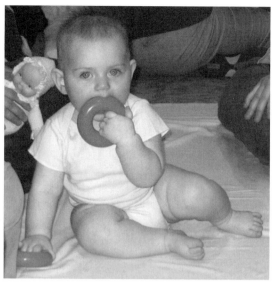

Figure 2.21 ▪ Side sitting with elongation on weight-bearing side.

pronation the first two steps can be accomplished, but the dorsum of the hand blocks the child's view of the object grasped (Fig. 2.22). Lack of supination of the forearm is also responsible for spillage when children first attempt to feed themselves with a spoon. The child holds the spoon and captures the food with the forearm in pronation. As she brings the spoon toward her mouth,

she needs to supinate in order to keep the bowl of the spoon level. Until she develops full active supination, spillage will continue to occur (Fig. 2.23). Many other functional activities across the lifespan depend on the ability to supinate the forearms, such as donning a shirt, buttoning and unbuttoning a shirt, turning a door knob, turning a steering wheel, and tying a bow.

As the child practices weight shift in prone on elbows, he begins to take an interest in reaching for toys from this

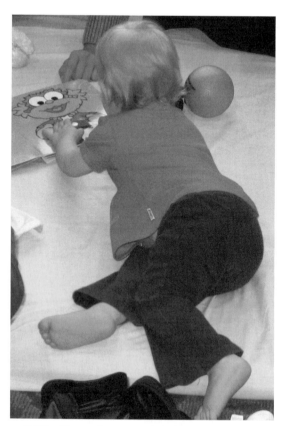

Figure 2.20 ▪ Elongation on weight-bearing side, child's right side here; note the high degree of intra-axial rotation.

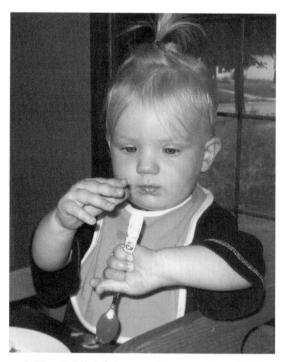

Figure 2.22 ▪ Child's left forearm is pronated as she holds the spoon, blocking her view of the object.

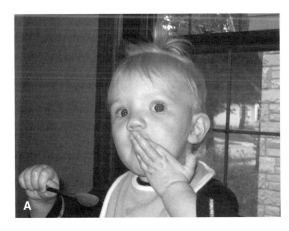

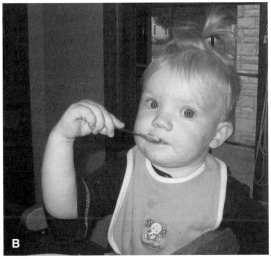

Figure 2.23 ■ **(A)** Lack of forearm supination when bringing the spoon to her mouth causes spillage. **(B)** With the development of forearm supination a child is able to use a spoon with very little spillage.

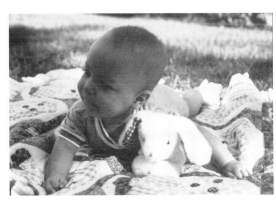

Figure 2.24 ■ First attempts at visually directed reaching in prone on elbow or extended arms are often unsuccessful because the child shifts his weight in the direction that he is looking, and the arm nearest the object is not freed.

position. First attempts at reaching while prone on elbows often fail because the child shifts his weight onto the side to which he is looking (Fig. 2.24). Eventually, the child learns from the error of his ways that his weight is shifted onto the very limb he needs to unweight in order to reach for the toy he sees. With practice of weight-shifting in this posture and through trial and error, the child eventually is able to shift his weight to one elbow and forearm while looking in the opposite direction, thereby establishing visually directed reaching (Fig. 2.25).

PRONE ON EXTENDED ARMS

Having secured the prone-on-elbows posture and having learned to shift his weight in different directions, the baby begins to lift himself farther from the surface. He pushes himself up into prone on extended arms, working his open hands into the surface, using his triceps to extend his elbows, and actively using the serratus anterior muscles to protract and stabilize the shoulder girdle (Fig. 2.26A).

The trunk extensors, continuing to activate and strengthen in a cephalocaudal direction, assist in this antigravity movement. The anterior thoracic muscles must elongate. The elbows, in the prone-on-extended arms posture, illustrate the principle of weight bearing on extended limbs after first weight bearing on flexed limbs. In addition to the extended elbows, this posture is noted for increased antigravity extension using midline thoracic extensors, increased scapulo-humeral elongation, a pelvis still in a relative posterior tilt in order to stabilize the lifted head and upper trunk, and comparatively passive lower extremities.

Although the lower extremities are decidedly passive in prone on elbows and prone on extended arms, the position assumed by the lower extremities in these postures is predictive of later development and active use of the lower extremities. It is the same lower extremity position seen in the infant after the loss of physiologic flexion (Figs. 2.2A and 2.26A).

Once the child has begun to push into prone on arms with extended elbows, he begins to weight-shift in that

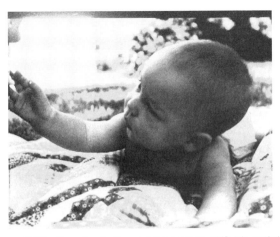

Figure 2.25 ■ Eventually the child learns to shift his weight to the skull-side limb, freeing the appropriate arm for reaching the object as he looks at it.

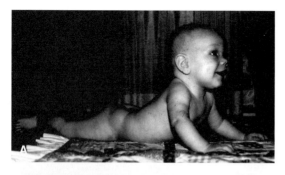

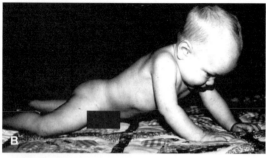

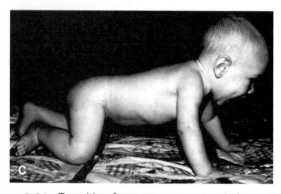

Figure 2.26 ■ Transition from prone on extended arms to quadruped. **(A)** Prone on extended arms. **(B)** Push-up transition position. **(C)** Quadruped.

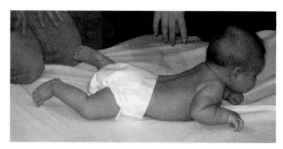

Figure 2.27 ■ Pivot prone posture with elongation of anterior trunk and lower extremity musculature and retraction of shoulder girdle; only mid- and lower trunk are in contact with the supporting surface.

PIVOT PRONE

At approximately 5 months of age the child develops an interesting skill that contributes to his pelvic and scapular mobility. The pivot prone posture or pattern, as seen in Figure 2.27, uses cephalocaudally progressing extension to extend the child's neck, midline trunk, and lower extremities. The pelvis is in an anterior tilt with hips hyperextended. The upper extremities assume the **high guard** position with the scapulae adducted by the rhomboid muscles. The upper limbs are horizontally abducted at the shoulders and flexed at the elbows. This **retraction** of the shoulder girdle with the posturing of the upper extremities enhances the trunk extension. To assume the pivot prone pattern, the anterior musculature must elongate.

Once the child develops stability in the pivot prone position, he playfully moves alternately between pivot prone and prone on elbows. In this manner, he practices scapular and pelvic mobility. The shoulder girdle alternates between **protraction** in prone on elbows and retraction in pivot prone. The pelvic girdle moves between the posterior tilt of prone on elbows and the anterior tilt of pivot prone. Often, in his exuberance, the child actually pivots his body in a circle as he kicks his legs or quickly alternates between these two postures.

QUADRUPED

As in other postures, early attempts at the hands-and-knees posture are generally not refined, often because the lower extremities are not positioned optimally to accept weight (Fig. 2.28). But with practice the child soon masters another new skill. Refer again to Figure 2.2B. His open hands are aligned under flexed shoulders, and his knees are aligned under flexed hips. The active participation of the lower extremities in **quadruped,** also called **four-point,** requires stability around the hip joints caused by cocontraction of the hip musculature. The principles of developmental direction are well illustrated in quadruped. Weight bearing on flexed elbows has given way to weight bearing on extended elbows. True to cephalocaudal development,

posture, just as he did in prone on elbows. Weight shifting produces increased stability at the shoulder joints as more weight is accepted onto one or the other shoulder during weight shifting. Weight shifting to the side eventually produces unilateral weight bearing with the ability to reach and grasp, with the accompanying elongation of the trunk on the weight-bearing side. Posterior weight shift may actually cause him to move himself backward in this position, increasing scapulohumeral elongation. While pushing backward the child may lift his buttocks from the surface, continuing to push his weight backward over the knees and into the quadruped posture, with weight on open hands. If he pushes with enough force, he may shift his weight backward onto his toes, rather than his flexed knees, in a "push-up" position (Fig. 2.26B). Eventually the child succeeds in getting his weight shifted posteriorly onto his knees for hands and knees weight-bearing (quadruped or four-point). He is definitely pleased with his accomplishment (Fig. 2.26C).

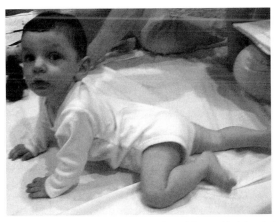

Figure 2.28 ■ Immature quadruped position with hip abduction and external rotation, lower extremities in poor weight-bearing alignment; reciprocal and contralateral movement of extremities; note the lumbar lordosis, an indication in quadruped that the abdominals are weak or not being activated.

the lower extremities now participate actively, unlike when in prone on elbows. Stability in quadruped increases, as it does in prone on elbows and prone on extended arms, as the child moves into the weight-shifting phase of the quadruped posture. When weight is shifted posteriorly, with the upper extremities fixed in a closed chain, scapulohumeral elongation is facilitated. The base of support in quadruped may be wide in initial attempts, particularly because of excessive abduction of the lower extremities. This wider base of support helps the child to be more stable. However, it interferes with adequate lateral weight shift, which is needed to achieve unilateral weight bearing. Unilateral weight bearing is necessary in both the upper and lower body to free one upper and one lower limb for the forward movement of creeping.

A stable quadruped position requires not only stable hips and shoulders, but also a stable trunk. Trunk flexors and extensors must balance each other to produce a flat back in the four-point position. When the child first achieves the quadruped posture, he generally displays the lumbar lordosis of the young infant whose abdominal musculature is not yet developed and strong. This is due to under-developed abdominal muscles as well as strong contraction of his hip flexors in order to stabilize. Overly active hip flexion is progravity fixing to increase muscle tone around the hip joints, and therefore stability. Increased hip flexion posturing leads to increased lumbar lordosis or anterior pelvic tilt. Development of the abdominals begins when the child first acquires the posterior tilt, which was essential for lifting of the head in prone. Concurrent with the achievement of a stable prone-on-elbows posture, with its posterior pelvic tilt resulting from activation of abdominal muscles, changes are taking place in the supine position to further recruit and strengthen abdominal muscles. Abdominal musculature continues to develop to balance the extensors of the trunk. With the balance of lumbar flexors and exten-

sors, the quadruped position with a flat back is achieved (refer once again to Fig. 2.2B).

LOCOMOTION IN PRONE

Locomotion is defined as movement from one place to another.[1] Six modes of locomotion develop in the prone position typically. In the order of development, they are scooting, crawling, pivoting in prone, rolling, creeping, and plantigrade creeping. Some locomotive forms may develop and be used nearly simultaneously, such as crawling and pivoting in prone, at approximately 5 months of age. Also, it is not unusual for one or more modes of locomotion not to develop in a given child. No long-term negative effects result from such failure. However, it is important for the child to develop, in other ways, any components of movement that typically develop or improve in the different forms of prone locomotion.

As early as a few days of age, the infant is able to move in the crib by wiggling and scooting. This is his first form of locomotion. Inevitably, an infant placed in the middle of a crib for a nap will find his way to a corner of the crib. It is thought that the closeness and security offered by a corner is comforting to the child, especially after 40 weeks in the close spaces of the womb. Because infants are able to wiggle and scoot, not even the youngest of babies should be left unattended on a raised surface such as a sofa, adult bed, changing table, or mat table, unless sufficient barriers of pillows and rolls have the infant contained.

During the first 2 months, when the infant is in prone or supine, he will wiggle and scoot as his chief form of locomotion. Once he attains and is stable in the prone-on-elbows position, he may locomote by crawling, moving his body forward by digging his elbows and forearms into the surface and extending his shoulders. **Crawling** is a locomotive form that infants may use from 3 months to 8 or 9 months of age. Crawling is defined as moving "slowly by dragging the body along the ground."[9,16,17] First attempts at crawling often produce a backward motion as the infant flexes his shoulders, instead of extending them. Once he achieves a forward progression, he may crawl by moving both forearms forward at the same time, or he may crawl by using reciprocal motions of the upper extremities (Fig. 2.29). This reciprocal motion is a precursor to reciprocal creeping, plantigrade creeping, and walking with reciprocal arm swing.

The defining component of crawling is that the child's belly is in contact with the floor. This compares to **creeping,** which means to move across the floor on hands and knees without the trunk being in direct contact with the surface.[9,15–18,47] While this distinguishing component may seem inconsequential, especially when the lay public often uses the terms synonymously, differentiating between crawling and creeping is important in the health care professions so that terminology is used consistently, leaving no room for misunderstanding.

In crawling, the lower extremities are basically passive while the upper extremities move either together or

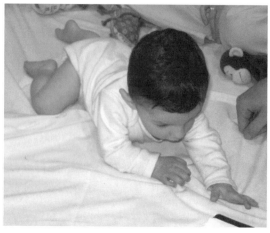

Figure 2.29 ■ Crawling with reciprocal use of upper extremities.

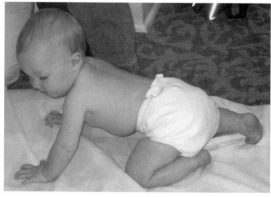

Figure 2.30 ■ Creeping with reciprocal use of upper and lower extremities; note loss of lumbar lordosis, an indication that lumbar flexors and extensors are cocontracting (compare to Fig. 2.28).

reciprocally. Crawling with nonreciprocal use of the upper extremities requires no trunk rotation, while reciprocal crawling does require rotation within the body axis. In **rotation** of the trunk, either the upper or the lower trunk moves while the rest of the trunk remains stable. Rotation of the upper trunk means the upper trunk moves on a stable, nonmoving lower trunk. The converse is true as well. Reciprocal, contralateral creeping requires counterrotation, a progressively more complex movement. This contralateral movement requires counterrotation within the trunk. **Counterrotation** is defined as rotating the upper trunk to one side while rotating the lower trunk in the opposite direction. Counter-rotation of the trunk is a different movement from simple rotation of the trunk.

Pivoting in prone, as described previously, is a form of locomotion that some infants use in conjunction with crawling or rolling to move intentionally in a particular direction. For example, if the child wants to reach a toy that is out of his immediate space, he will often use a combination of these movements to direct himself appropriately to reach his goal.

Rolling from prone to supine and supine to prone, another means of locomotion, develops in the infant by 5 to 6 months of age. Still lacking an efficient locomotive form, once he achieves rolling from prone to supine and supine to prone, he may use a combination of rolling and crawling to move in a specific direction across the floor. The evolution of rolling will be discussed in a later section of this chapter.

At 6 to 7 months of age, while prone on extended arms, he begins pushing his body backward, raising his buttocks into the air in attempts to get into quadruped (hands-and-knees posture). This position, also called four-point, is the position from which his next locomotive form, **creeping,** will develop. Both the upper and lower extremities participate equally in creeping (Fig. 2.30).

Once he is stable on hands and knees, the usual process of weight shifting in various directions occurs.

With controlled weight shift he is able to lift one limb at a time, eventually lifting one upper extremity and the opposite lower extremity at once. This movement leads to creeping on hands and knees at approximately 8 to 10 months of age. Typical, refined creeping is reciprocal and contralateral. In other words, the child advances one arm and the opposite leg at the same time (contralateral), reciprocating with the other arm and leg, which also move together. This contralateral movement requires not only rotation of the trunk, but also counterrotation. The reciprocal activity of creeping helps to refine intra-axial rotation and reciprocal use of the limbs, strengthening counterrotation for use in the higher levels of locomotion.

Plantigrade creeping, sometimes referred to as bear walking, is more of a transitional posture than a form of locomotion. However, some children do use the plantigrade position, open hands and plantar surfaces of the feet in closed-chain contact with the ground, to locomote. In many cases, this type of creeping may be the result of an environmental factor. For example, the child may choose plantigrade creeping over creeping in quadruped if he has bare knees and is on a concrete or other rough surface (see Fig. 2.31). This illustrates the dynamic nature of develop-

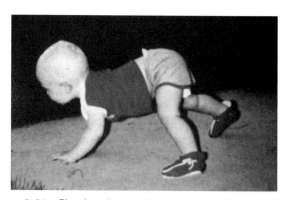

Figure 2.31 ■ Plantigrade creeping, also called bear walking.

ment. Many factors, in addition to maturation, influence the development of motor skills.

As a transitional posture, the plantigrade position is used by the child as one means of getting to standing from the prone position. In early attempts the child may rely on being near furniture or a wall for assistance as he rises to standing, going through the plantigrade position to the upright standing posture.

SUPINE PROGRESSION

SUPINE LYING AND PULL TO SITTING

Like the prone progression, development in the supine position proceeds in a known sequence. The full-term neonate in supine has physiologic flexion, expressed in slight cervical flexion, with the head held toward midline, elbow flexion, posterior pelvic tilt, hip adduction, and hip and knee flexion. The feet are typically in the air and not touching the table surface (Fig. 2.32). When the infant is **pulled to sitting,** the examiner gently pulling the infant's upper extremities at the wrists, the head is held in plane with the body and exhibits no **head lag,** mimicking active head control. Over the first month, as the physiologic flexion gradually disappears, the head falls away from midline to the side, elbows relax, and the hip and knee flexion dissipate, bringing the infant's feet down to the surface (Fig. 2.33). As the feet come down to the surface, the pelvis is pulled into a relative anterior tilt by gravity, now unopposed by physiologic flexion. Increasing hip abduction and external rotation begin to evolve. When pulled to sitting, head lag is present. This means that the infant's head, no longer being supported by the physiologic flexion, lags behind the rest of the body as the child is pulled toward the sitting posture. Antigravity flexors have yet to develop. Without active head control, the child's head falls backward into gravity when he is pulled toward the sitting posture. Over time, as the antigravity cervical flexors become stronger and active head control develops, the infant

exhibits less and less head lag when pulled to sitting. After the initial period of head lag, which follows the loss of physiologic flexion, he will begin to hold his head in alignment with the body, in the same plane as the body. Then he learns to lead with his head as soon as the stimulus of being pulled to sitting occurs. Next in the sequence, the lower extremities begin to flex actively at the hips during the pull-to-sitting maneuver. Finally, the pull-to-sit stimulus recruits cervical flexors, trunk flexors, and hip flexors. Figure 2.34 shows the pull-to-sitting sequence.

In supine, after the first month, the infant usually has his head turned to one side or the other, influenced by the ATNR. The ATNR is manifested in infants during wakefulness and sleep and diminishes over time, as seen in Figure 2.3. This reflex begins prenatally and is manifested by asymmetric extension of the neck, with accompanying predictable limb movements. Under the influence of the ATNR, when the head is turned to one side in slight hyperextension, cervical proprioceptors are stimulated. This causes the **face limbs,** the ipsilateral upper and lower extremities on the side to which the head is turned, to extend. The contralateral limbs, the **skull limbs** or **occiput limbs,** flex. The upper extremity manifestations of the ATNR are usually stronger than the lower extremity manifestations. The ATNR is seen in normal infants during the first 4 months of life, more as an attitude or assumed posture than a strong obligatory position. This posture is frequently termed the fencer's posture (refer again to Fig. 2.3). Although this fencer's posture is evident in nearly all infants during this time period and is seen repeatedly in supine and supported sitting, the ATNR is not so strong in typical infants that it limits voluntary or passive movement of the extremities or head. If the ATNR presents stereotypically, is obligatory during those first months, or produces strong flexor or extensor tone in the extremities, this may be an indication of atypical neuromotor development. In the typical infant, the strength of the ATNR reflex is noted to diminish over time such that by 4 months it is evident inconsistently and finally disappears.[48]

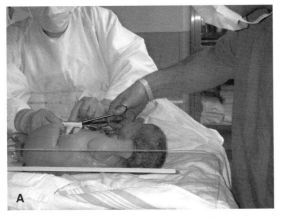
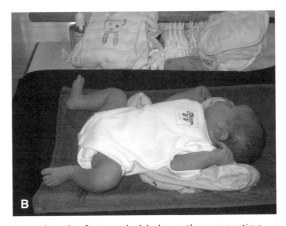

Figure 2.32 ■ Physiologic flexion in the full-term neonate; note that the feet are held above the supporting surface. **(A)** Physiologic flexion seen in infant only minutes old. **(B)** Same infant at 12 days of age.

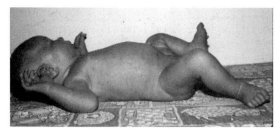

Figure 2.33 ❚ As physiologic flexion diminishes, the hip and knee flexion decrease, allowing the feet to rest on the supporting surface.

The ATNR is evidence of the infant's lack of dissociation. **Dissociation** is the ability of the human to move limbs independently from the head, move limbs independently from each other, move joints within the same limb independently, and move the body independently from the head. Head and limbs lack dissociation in a child manifesting an ATNR. The proprioceptors of the neck influence the position of the limbs, resulting in the posture as described. As the child matures and the ATNR loses its influence, the limbs no longer assume specific postures based on the position of the head, thereby demonstrating dissociation.

Another reflex that affects the supine and prone postures, although not well understood in normal development, is the tonic labyrinthine reflex. The tonic labyrinthine reflex provides underlying tone tendencies of flexion in prone and extension in supine.[48] The receptors for this reflex are in the labyrinths of the ears and are responsive to the continuous forces of gravity. The basic functional skills of lifting the head in prone and supine, performing total body antigravity extension in prone (the pivot prone pattern) and antigravity flexion in supine (the feet-to-mouth pattern), are accommodated in the typical infant because resting tone and tone with initiation of movement are not excessive. If the child is influenced negatively by the tonic labyrinthine reflex in motor development, extensor or flexor **hypertonus** may prevent the development of antigravity contraction of the antagonist muscles in either or both postures. If tone is excessive in extensors in supine, for example, the flexor antagonists are not able to contract because the extensor muscles are not able to relax. This loss of **reciprocal inhibition,** the ability of antagonist muscles to relax or lengthen while agonist muscles contract or shorten, may be strong enough to cause sensorimotor impairment.

As the ATNR diminishes, the infant begins to appear more symmetric in supine (Fig. 2.35). The ability to bring

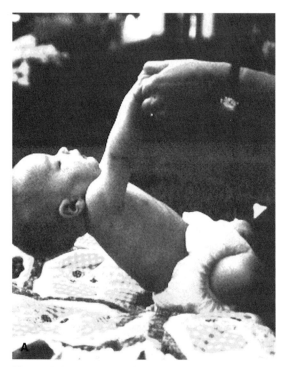

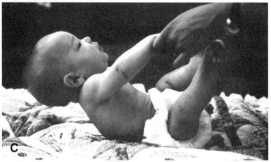

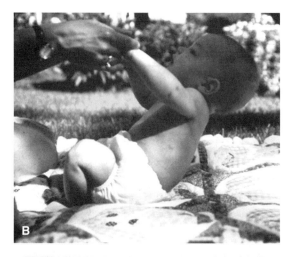

Figure 2.34 ❚ Pull-to-sitting sequence. **(A)** Head lag when pulled to sitting, denoting lack of antigravity control of cervical flexor muscles. **(B)** No head lag when pulled to sitting; as child matures and control of antigravity cervical flexors develops child holds head in the same plane as his body. **(C)** Cervical, trunk, and hip flexors exhibit active antigravity control when child is pulled to sitting.

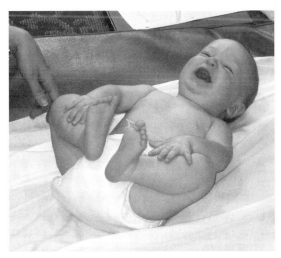

Figure 2.35 ■ Postural symmetry exhibited by 6 or 7 months of age.

his head to midline and hold it there is a significant milestone. Two processes interact to allow head-to-midline movement. Because the ATNR is an asymmetric influence on the posture of the head, as the ATNR diminishes the cervical extensors no longer contract as a reflex response. Rather, they relax, no longer keeping the head to one side. At the same time this passive factor occurs in supine, the cervical flexors begin to work as antigravity muscles, helping to actively bring the head to midline. Eventually, the cervical flexors are strong enough to bring the head to midline and to lift the infant's head from the surface in supine (Fig. 2.36). These developmental achievements in supine are occurring during the second to fourth months, at the same time that the cervical extensors are emerging as antigravity muscles in prone. Lifting of the head in prone develops shortly before lifting of the head in supine. When the cervical flexors contract to lift the head into flexion while in supine, the cervical extensors must elongate. This is another example of reciprocal inhibition. Children with neuromotor pathologies may lack the ability to lengthen or relax the cervical extensors.

As cephalocaudal development continues in supine, controlled movement of the upper extremities begins with volitional movement and subsequent stabilization of the

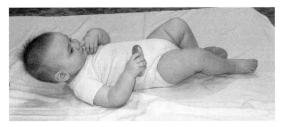

Figure 2.36 ■ Lifting head in supine, an indication of well-developed antigravity cervical flexion.

shoulder joints. Whereas the achievement of prone on elbows develops the stability of the shoulder girdle in a weight-bearing function (closed chain), the supine position permits the development of shoulder stability for non–weight-bearing function (open chain).

During the first 3 months of life, the infant has little control over the placement and holding of the upper extremities in space. Attempts at grasping an object are made with the hands close to the body, because the child lacks the shoulder girdle stability and the strength to use his hands in space (see Fig. 2.4). With shoulder adduction, the upper extremities are held against the sides of the infant's body, providing stability in the only way the infant knows at this point. This process is referred to as **fixing.** Fixing is a normal process of development that occurs with first attempts to stabilize the body, relative to gravity, in all postures. These first attempts, this fixing, are not true antigravity stability. Instead, they are a temporary means of stabilizing by fixing into gravity (**progravity**), until the appropriate muscles in a particular posture learn to stabilize or fix against gravity (**antigravity**).

Without the eventual emergence of muscle groups strong enough to work as antigravity muscles, development will be delayed. Fundamentally, antigravity muscle work is what keeps a person upright against gravity, whether in sitting, kneeling (tall kneeling or knee standing), quadruped, or standing erect. In normal mature movement, extensor muscles are the main antigravity muscles. Consider the erector spinae, gluteus maximus, proximal hamstrings, and quadriceps muscles. In the supine position, however, the flexors act as antigravity muscles. Consider the cervical flexors, abdominal muscles, and hip flexors.

Once the infant develops shoulder stability using cocontraction of all of the muscles around the shoulder joint, he is able to reach out to grasp a toy (Fig. 2.37A), and thus begin the skills of grasp and manipulation. This process of fine motor development will take approximately 18 months to refine and will not be complete until approximately 30 months of age. Development of grasp and prehension will be discussed elsewhere in this chapter.

HANDS TO KNEES AND FEET, FEET TO MOUTH

Another developmental landmark occurs when the child reaches upward against gravity while in supine. As the pectoral muscles are being activated, so are the abdominals. The pectoral muscles are partially responsible for reaching the upper extremity toward the ceiling in supine (Fig. 2.37B). In order for this movement to occur, the serratus anterior muscles act in synergy, and the rhomboid muscles must elongate. These muscles, acting in concert, cause the shoulder girdle to protract. It is now that one sees the child's ability to reach for his mother or father's face while being diapered or dressed. Active use of the pectorals with reciprocal inhibition of the rhomboids, along with the recent

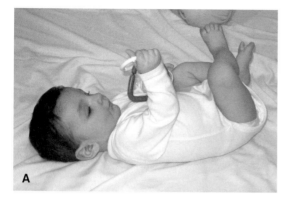

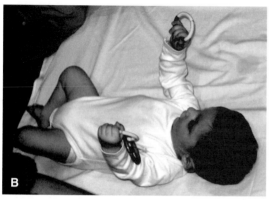

Figure 2.37 ■ Reaching with upper extremities. **(A)** Once stability is achieved in the shoulder girdle, the child can reach into space to grasp a toy; note the midline head and hands. **(B)** Reaching well into space using antigravity control of the serratus anterior muscles; note supine symmetry and concurrent but separate use of hands.

inhibition of the ATNR, allows the child to reach upward and also to bring his hands to midline.

In supine at 5 months of age, as the child continues to gain ever-increasing control of his antigravity flexors, with reciprocal lengthening of antagonist extensor muscles, he begins to actively lift his lower extremities from the surface. Some foot-to-foot contact usually occurs (Fig. 2.38). Next he begins to reach for his knees and then his feet. At

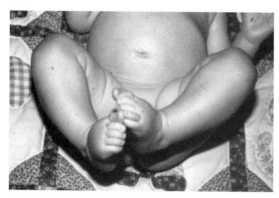

Figure 2.38 ■ Supine at 5 months, foot-to-foot contact.

first he reaches his hand to the ipsilateral knee and foot, as seen in Figure 2.35. Eventually he is able to cross midline with his upper extremities, placing a hand on the contralateral knee and/or foot (Fig. 2.39). This contact of the infant with his own body is important to the process of developing **body image** or **body scheme**.[43]

As the child flexes his hips to bring his feet toward his hands and head, his abdominals and hip flexors are gaining strength. Active contraction of the abdominal muscles causes the pelvis to tip posteriorly and the gluteus maximus and proximal hamstrings to elongate. The hips are in moderate flexion, abduction, and external rotation. His knees are flexed, and his feet are dorsiflexed and supinated (Fig. 2.40A).

The natural progression of hands to knees and hands to feet leads to the infant bringing his feet to his mouth. At 5 months of age a child is very interested in oral stimulation. No longer under the influence of the rooting and sucking reflexes, he begins to use his mouth for more than eating. As he brings a foot toward his mouth, he exhibits feed-forward anticipation of putting his toes in his mouth (Fig. 2.40B). Putting his feet in his mouth, seen here in Figure 2.40C, further develops body image. This activity also facilitates cognitive development. Infants learn about objects through touch, including the touch that accom-

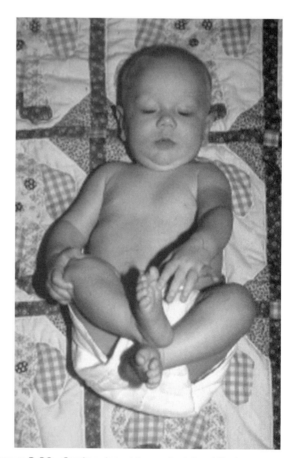

Figure 2.39 ■ Supine, hand to contralateral foot.

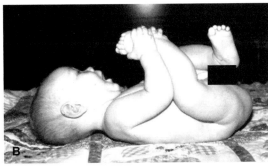

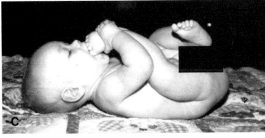

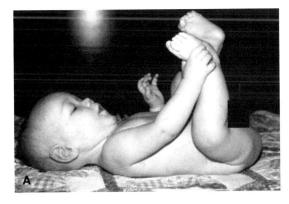

Figure 2.40 ■ Foot-to-mouth sequence at 5 months of age. **(A)** Note elongation of posterior musculature and visually directed reaching to foot. **(B)** Movement of foot toward mouth, child opening his mouth with feed-forward anticipation. **(C)** Child puts foot into his mouth, one way of learning about his body.

panies placing objects in the mouth, a process referred to as **mouthing** (Fig. 2.40).

Pelvic stability, in a posterior pelvic tilt, is needed in prone for the infant to begin lifting his head in prone. In supine, at 5 months of age, the child puts his feet in his mouth, further enhancing the posterior pelvic tilt. Once the posterior pelvic tilt is achieved and strengthened, the child begins to develop pelvic mobility. That is, he moves back and forth in supine between a posterior pelvic tilt and an anterior pelvic tilt. This is often observed during spontaneous play in supine, as the child brings his feet to his mouth with a posterior pelvic tilt. Then he lowers his feet to the surface, with a relative anterior tilt. Sometimes when he lowers his feet to the surface, he continues with active lumbar extension into the **bridging** posture, which requires more of the relative anterior tilt. In doing this, he works his

feet into the surface. Developing pelvic mobility in supine allows the child to move back and forth between these two postures, in tandem with activities occurring in prone (Fig. 2.41A and B). At about the same time in development, approximately 5 months of age, the child practices pelvic mobility in prone. This requires alternating between the posterior tilt of prone on forearms and the anterior tilt of the pivot prone posture, as discussed previously.

ROLLING PROGRESSION

NONSEGMENTAL ROLLING

Rolling develops in a two-stage progression. From birth to 6 months of age the child performs **nonsegmental rolling.**

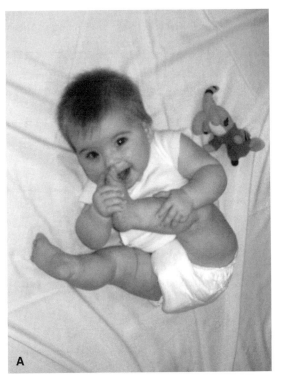

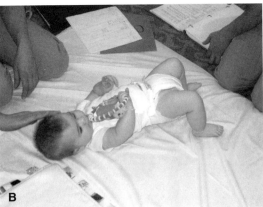

Figure 2.41 ■ Development of pelvic mobility in supine. **(A)** Feet to mouth with posterior pelvic tilt. **(B)** Bridging with anterior pelvic tilt.

Segmental rolling develops at approximately 6 months of age. Nonsegmental rolling, also referred to as **log rolling,** allows the child to roll from supine to side-lying. This movement is based on one of the infant reflexes, the **neck-righting reaction.** In the neck-righting reaction, the stimulation of proprioceptors in the neck as the child's head is turned actively or passively to one side causes the body to follow in one complete unit, without rotation within the vertebral column.[15,48] The neck-righting reaction gradually diminishes over time as another reaction, the **body-righting reaction acting on the body,** evolves.[15,48]

SEGMENTAL ROLLING

The body-righting reaction acting on the body is a predominant factor in movement by 6 months of age. When the head is rotated to one side, the body reacts to the proprioceptive stimulus to the neck by following in the direction of the head turning, thus rolling toward that side. Now the movement within the vertebral column is segmental. That is, the different segments, the trunk, shoulder girdle, and pelvic girdle, as well as the upper and lower extremity on one side, are seen to respond sequentially, rather than moving as one unit (Fig. 2.42). The sequence of movement of the various body segments is not identical in all people, nor is it always the same sequence in an individual. The baby may lead with the head, a lower extremity, an upper extremity, the pelvic girdle, or the shoulder girdle, and the other segments follow the lead segment. Segmental rolling requires rotation within the body axis, the vertebral column. This rotation is referred to as **intra-axial rotation** and is facilitated by the body-righting reaction acting on the body, permitting the infant to roll from prone to supine and supine to prone.

ROLLING PRONE TO SUPINE

Before the infant attempts to roll volitionally, rolling from prone to supine and supine to prone often occurs acciden-

tally. Early on, the infant may roll accidentally from prone to supine because he pulls his knees underneath him and his buttocks are elevated. If the center of mass gets high enough, as a result of the elevated buttocks, the child may roll accidentally (Fig. 2.43). Accidental rolling, from prone to supine, may also occur as spinal extension progresses caudally, and the child achieves prone on elbows and prone on extended arms. In this case, his center of mass becomes higher through the lifting of the head and upper trunk. Experimenting with the prone-on-elbows and prone-on-extended arms postures, he becomes rather top heavy and therefore may roll to supine accidentally. When this happens, the child may attempt to replicate the movement. Once able to replicate the movement, the child will practice this movement. Through trial and error and the increasingly strong body-righting reaction acting on the body, the child learns to roll segmentally from prone to supine, usually by 5 months of age (Fig. 2.44).

Rolling supine to prone also may occur as an involuntary movement initially. When the child is in supine around the age of 4 or 5 months, he may lift his pelvis from the surface on which he rests by plantar flexing his feet, working his feet into the surface. This bridging type of maneuver raises the center of mass, through the lower trunk, and may cause the infant to roll to one side or the other as he pushes a little harder into the surface with one foot, the foot contralateral to the direction to which he accidentally rolls. Trial-and-error practice, along with the strong body-righting reaction acting on the body, combines with

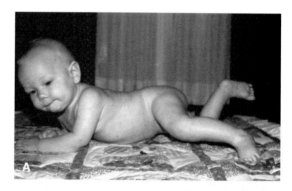

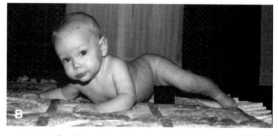

Figure 2.43 ▪ Accidental rolling prone to supine. **(A)** In prone, child lifts buttocks from the surface. **(B)** As he lifts buttocks higher off the surface and pushes into the supporting surface with his foot, child may accidentally roll prone to supine.

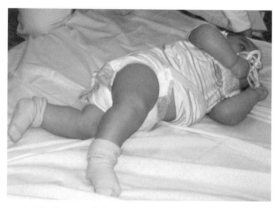

Figure 2.42 ▪ Intra-axial rotation develops, in part, as the result of the body righting acting on the body response.

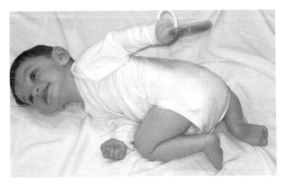

Figure 2.44 ■ Segmental rolling prone to supine, leading with upper extremity.

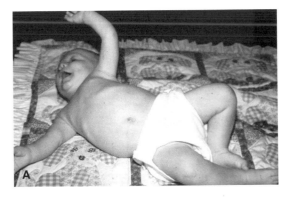

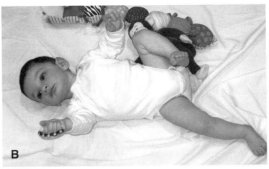

Figure 2.45 ■ Segmental rolling supine to prone using intra-axial rotation. **(A)** Rolling leading with upper extremity; note the scapulohumeral elongation. **(B)** Segmental rolling leading with lower extremity; note the crossing of midline.

other factors such as motivation, allowing the child to volitionally roll supine to prone by 6 months of age, using intra-axial rotation. Although the age of acquisition of rolling skills may vary slightly, volitional rolling usually occurs from prone to supine before supine to prone, at 5 and 6 months, respectively.

Once a child is able to roll volitionally, it is important that he learn to roll toward both left and right sides when in prone or supine. This will occur naturally in most cases, unless the infant encounters an obstacle to rolling to both left and right. Furniture, the side of the crib, or other environmental barriers may cause the child to always roll toward the same side. However, if such is the case, attentive parents and other caregivers can make sure the child is placed away from environmental obstacles and encouraged to roll toward both left and right sides. A child unable to roll toward one or the other side in the absence of environmental barriers or lack of opportunity may be exhibiting signs of neuromotor or musculoskeletal pathology. In such cases, the inability to roll in both directions should be viewed as a red flag, but is not in itself diagnostic.

The functional activity of rolling helps develop and secure several components of movement, as well as being a functional motor milestone in its own right. As the child learns to roll segmentally from prone to supine, the asymmetric cervical extension that he uses to initiate rolling during early attempts gives way to extension of the neck with lateral flexion and rotation. As the child gets to supine, he completes the roll using slight cervical flexion.

If the infant leads with the upper extremity when rolling supine to prone, he typically will bring one upper extremity across his chest, reaching toward the side to which he is rolling. This movement requires and encourages scapulohumeral elongation at the shoulder of the extremity with which he leads (Fig. 2.45). Rolling supine to prone using intra-axial rotation also requires the lead upper or lower extremity, along with the other ipsilateral extremity, to cross midline (Fig. 2.45). The ability to roll demonstrates dissociation of the right and left extremities as well as dissociation of the extremities and the head. If

the upper or lower extremities are dependent on movements of the head in order to function, segmental rolling cannot occur. In such a case, the asymmetric tonic neck reflex may be influencing the limb movements. Turning of the head to one side in order to roll supine to prone causes the face-side extremities, upper more than lower, to extend in a pathologic pattern that blocks the ability to roll toward that side. Persistence of a primitive or obligatory ATNR may contribute to a child's inability to roll supine to prone. However, such reflex activity may actually be used by the child to roll prone to supine, using the abnormal asymmetric extensor tone of the ATNR and an elevated center of mass. This is also an atypical and pathologic pattern and is another red flag, particularly if the child does not have dissociation of the head and extremities and/or intra-axial rotation.

SITTING PROGRESSION

SUPPORTED SITTING

Preparation for sitting begins in the prone and supine positions as the child develops early components such as cephalocaudally progressing antigravity extension of the spine, pelvic mobility, intra-axial rotation, scapular mobility, and weight bearing on the upper extremities. During the neonatal period when the child is held in sitting, his posture is remarkable for extreme flexion of the spine, caused by the lack of antigravity extensor muscle control. In this posture, seen in Figure 2.46, the infant's trunk exhibits what is termed a complete C-curve. The head is forward, with chin resting on the chest. Even though the child is at the mercy of gravity at this time and must be supported in sitting, the pelvis of the typical child is perpendicular to the surface on which he sits. That is, he should be bearing weight on his ischial tuberosities. If the pelvis is perpendicular to the surface, the very top portion of the gluteal cleft is visible. If the child is bearing his weight, instead, on the sacrum, the pelvis is not perpendicular and the gluteal cleft is hidden from view. This weight bearing on the sacrum, referred to as **sacral sitting,** is a red flag and may be indicative of pathology. Regardless of a child's age and stage of development, it is atypical to be in the extreme posterior pelvic tilt exhibited in sacral sitting, even when the spine is in the immature C-curve characteristic of the neonate. Note the position of the pelvis in all of the figures of children sitting in this chapter.

As the neonate develops, antigravity extension of the neck and trunk in sitting begins to appear. First, the cervical spine develops antigravity control, counteracting the infant's forward head position and lifting the head so that the face is vertical and the mouth is horizontal. As head control develops in supported sitting over the first 3 to 4 months, the child also is gaining increased anti-gravity extension in the prone position. At the same time, in the supine position, he is developing antigravity flexion control. Thus, head control, as provided by a balance of cervical flexors and extensors, evolves to keep the head upright against gravity when sitting. Additionally, the development of the chin tuck in the prone and supine positions secures the stable head in sitting by 4 months of age, even though the child still depends on external support to remain in a sitting position (Fig. 2.47).

PROPPED SITTING

At approximately 5 months of age, the child begins to exhibit his first abilities for sitting without the external support of either being held or sitting with a backrest. When put in the sitting position, the child attempts to prop with his upper extremities. With his weight shifted forward the child's hands are able to make contact with the surface. The **hand grasp reflex** has diminished and generally disappeared by 4 months of age, allowing the child's open hands to be placed on the floor in front of him. Thus, he begins the adventure of sitting, with his lower extremities out in front of him and his upper extremities once again performing in a major weight-bearing role. The two hands and the buttocks create a tripod base, which gives the infant a larger and more stable base of support than if he were to attempt to sit without the propping support of his upper extremities. This **propped sitting** posture is typical of an infant who is 5 months of age. As the infant feels increasingly secure in this posture, he will begin to rotate his neck to look around at his surroundings (Fig. 2.48). During propped sitting the child fixes pro-gravity, strongly contracting his hip flexors to increase his stability. He has not learned yet that his antigravity extensors will serve him better for remaining upright by assuming an antigravity role.

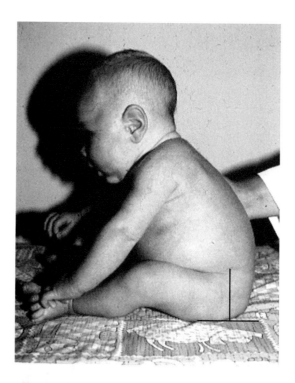

Figure 2.46 ■ *Supported sitting posture of neonate; note the lack of antigravity spinal extension and that the pelvis is perpendicular to the supporting surface.*

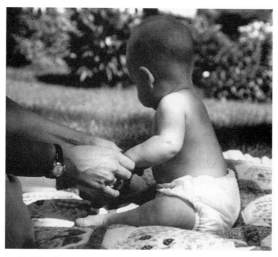

Figure 2.47 ■ *Supported sitting with full spinal extension; note position of pelvis.*

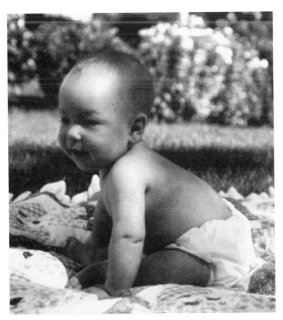

Figure 2.48 ■ *Propped sitting using the upper extremities to create a large base of support; note that pelvis is perpendicular to the supporting surface.*

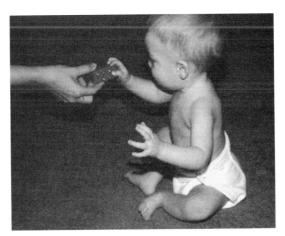

Figure 2.49 ■ *Independent ring sitting; note the high guard position of the upper extremities, used by the child to enhance trunk stability.*

Mature stability against the forces of gravity in upright postures such as sitting and erect standing is attained through activation and strength of extensor muscles primarily. This antigravity extension of the trunk, hips, and knees develops over time in various postures. However, initial attempts at stability in upright postures are through the use of progravity contractions of trunk, hip, and knee flexors. Using progravity stabilizing motor behaviors is referred to as **fixing into gravity** rather than **fixing against gravity.**

RING SITTING

One major disadvantage of propping with the upper extremities while sitting is that the child cannot use his upper extremities for reaching and grasping objects. As his trunk extension becomes stronger, the child eventually is able to rely less on the upper extremity support and the wide base, until he finally lifts his hands from the surface on which he sits. This new sitting posture is termed **ring sitting** because of the position of the lower extremities (Fig. 2.49).

Now the child is sitting more erect, pelvis still perpendicular to the surface, utilizing his ever-increasing trunk extension to remain upright against gravity. Although by this time, approximately 6 months of age, the child has adequate spinal extension to resist the pull of gravity while in sitting, he probably feels less stable in that posture than he is in actuality. In order to further secure his trunk extension when sitting without propping or other external support, the child holds his upper extremities in the high guard position (see Fig. 2.49). The retraction of the shoulders in this position is analogous to the positioning

of the upper extremities in the pivot prone posture and serves as an adjunct to the spinal extension. Contraction of the rhomboids increases the overall muscular activity in the child's posterior trunk, better securing him against gravity. This high guard position, using the rhomboid muscles to increase midline trunk stability against the pull of gravity, is seen again in the initial performance of tall kneeling and erect standing, as the child's center of mass moves higher in space relative to the supporting surface. However, the upper extremities, in the high guard position, are rendered virtually useless in terms of reaching for, grasping, and manipulating objects.

The lower extremities in ring sitting are flexed and externally rotated at the hips and flexed at the knees. The plantar surfaces of the feet are near to or touching each other. Ring sitting provides a relatively wide base of support as the externally rotated hips allow the lower extremities to rest on the floor. With the wider base of support and the high guard position, the child is able to sit independent of external support at this point, but he lacks the ability to independently achieve the sitting posture from the prone or supine positions. Rather, when placed in sitting, he is able to remain stable without falling as long as he does not attempt much movement while in this posture, lest he disturb his balance.

OTHER INDEPENDENT SITTING POSTURES

As the child experiences increasing stability in independent sitting, he begins to move his lower extremities out of the ring position, into either a **half-ring** position or **long sitting** (Figs. 2.50 and 2.51). His ability to have one lower extremity in front of him with relatively neutral hip rotation and an extended knee, while the other hip is still in flexion and external rotation with a flexed knee, is a sign of developing dissociation between the two lower limbs. The child moves in and out of this position, varying

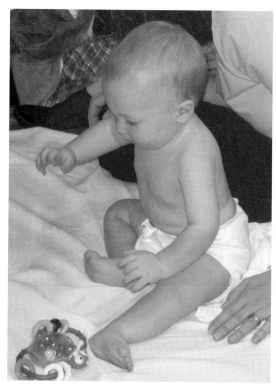

Figure 2.50 ■ *Half–ring sitting.*

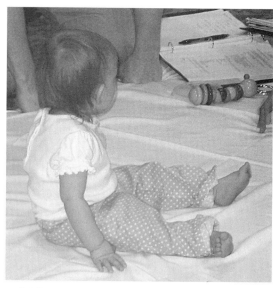

Figure 2.52 ■ Mature long sitting with narrowed mediolateral base of support.

which leg is extended, and is often seen to be in simple long sitting. In mature long sitting, the base of support is narrowed mediolaterally, allowing lateral weight shifting with ease (Fig. 2.52).

The child develops a series of increasingly advanced sitting postures that do not require external support, including ring sitting, half–ring sitting, long sitting, and side sitting. He also develops short sitting (sitting with knees and hips flexed to approximately 90 degrees) on a child-size chair, getting into and sitting on an adult-size chair, and climbing onto higher surfaces such as a child's highchair to sit (Fig. 2.53). Depending on the environment and the individual child's motivation and opportunity, once the child achieves propped sitting followed by ring sitting, these various, more mature sitting postures may develop at different times for each child, sometimes

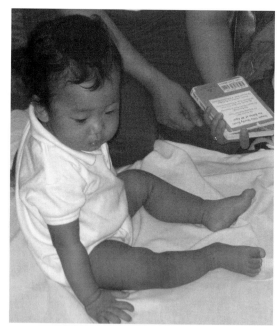

Figure 2.51 ■ Long sitting.

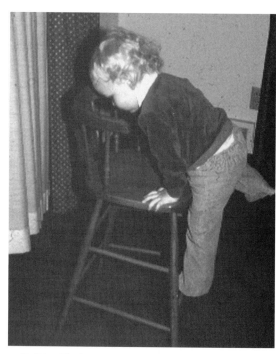

Figure 2.53 ■ Climbing onto a high chair.

nearly concurrently. In each new sitting posture, the child repeats a series of motor behaviors that take him from a stable posture when placed, through being able to move in and out of the posture (the **transition**), to using his hands for prehension and object manipulation in each posture. These motor behaviors include antigravity performance, antigravity stabilization, weight shifting, intra-axial rotation, and transition between postures. Weight shifting in each posture is accompanied by elongation on the weight-bearing side.

As the child becomes more secure in ring sitting, he gradually relaxes the rhomboid muscles and lowers his upper extremities. No longer dependent on the upper extremities for stability in sitting, he is able to volitionally protract and retract the shoulder girdle in order to reach for and grasp objects (Fig. 2.54). At about the same time, he feels confident enough in his sitting that he is able to rotate his head and neck to look around and begin performing visually directed reaching. The stability that results from the wide base of support in ring sitting, however, is gained at the expense of lateral weight shifting. The wider the base of support in any posture, the more difficult it is to shift weight. Consequently, the child must move beyond ring-sitting to sitting postures with narrower bases of support.

At 6 months of age the child's forearms are pronated such that, as he looks toward and reaches for an object, he grasps the object with his forearm pronated. Being

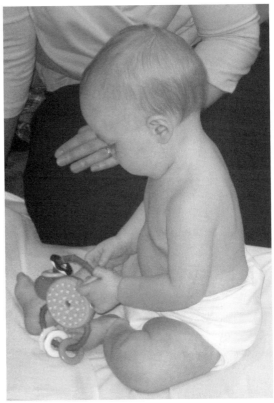

Figure 2.54 ■ Ring sitting with no guard; note bilateral use of hands in midline.

unable to supinate volitionally, he is unable to inspect the object once it is in his hand (Fig. 2.49). By 8 months of age, he develops volitional supination and reciprocal pronation and supination of the forearms and is able to look at the object he has secured. The ability to reach, grasp, and supinate with either upper extremity makes it possible for him to take an object presented to him, inspect it, and manipulate it by transferring the object from one hand to the other. This bilateral hand activity also requires working in midline and crossing the midline of his body with his upper extremities, head, and eyes. By the time the typical child has achieved the ring-sitting posture, he is no longer influenced by the ATNR, so keeping his head in midline, using two hands in midline, and crossing midline with the head, eyes, and hands are easily achieved.

In propped sitting and ring sitting, the feet and ankles are notable for their passive positioning in supination (see Figs. 2.48 and 2.49). Therefore, at 5 and 6 months of age, these sitting positions reflect the supinated feet, hip flexion and external rotation, and knee flexion seen in the supine position when the child is bringing his feet to his mouth at 5 months of age. Also notable in the propped and ring-sitting postures is the child's tendency for pro-gravity stabilization, using the hip flexors and abdominal muscles.

Once the child is stable in ring sitting and is able to move the head and limbs, he begins to use intra-axial rotation in sitting. This intra-axial rotation develops and strengthens by 5 to 7 months of age in prone and supine, allowing for segmental rolling. The intra-axial rotation also allows him to make transitions between postures, thus broadening his repertoire of sitting positions and increasing his independence as he learns to move from supine and prone to sitting and vice versa, using intra-axial rotation. See Figure 2.55 for one example of this transition from sitting to prone. Intra-axial rotation also serves to increase the accessibility of the space around the child, making more of his environment available for interaction (Fig. 2.56).

By 8 months of age the child is able to sit independently. He has developed not only full antigravity extension of the back, but by the eighth month, sitting posture is characterized by the completion of the secondary curves of the spine (Fig. 2.57). These anterior-posterior curves, developing cephalocaudally, are the **cervical lordosis** and the **lumbar lordosis.** Now the child is able to move from prone or supine to sitting and return to prone or supine. He also is able to move in and out of the various sitting postures using the intra-axial rotation and can pull himself to standing.

Side sitting is a mature sitting posture that requires a number of motor components and abilities, including intra-axial rotation, dissociation, weight shifting, and elongation of the trunk on the weight-bearing side (Fig. 2.58). In side sitting dissociation of the lower extremities is evidenced by the hip external rotation and abduction on one side with internal rotation and adduction of the other

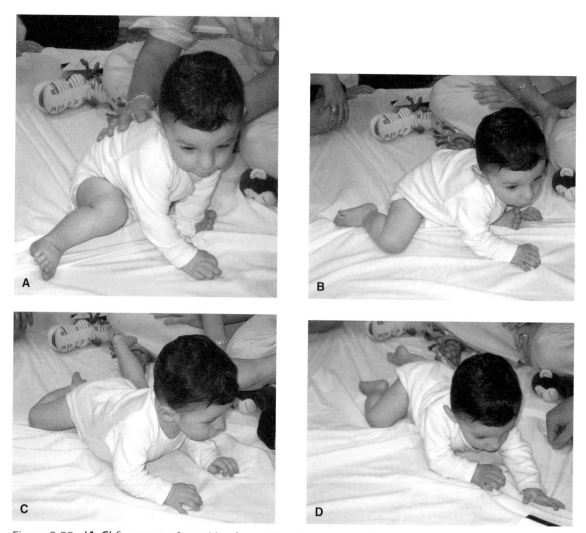

Figure 2.55 ▪ **(A–C)** Sequence of transition from sitting to prone on elbows using intra-axial rotation. **(D)** Reciprocal and contralateral crawling.

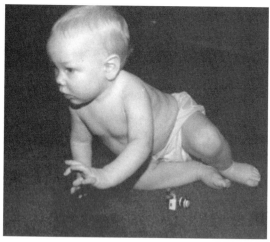

Figure 2.56 ▪ Intra-axial rotation is also used to increase the accessibility of the child's environment and for the transition between sitting and quadruped.

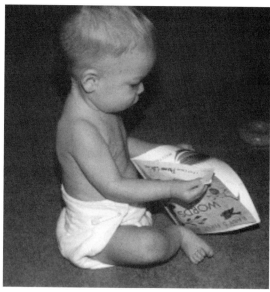

Figure 2.57 ▪ Sitting independently with secondary curves, the cervical and lumbar lordoses.

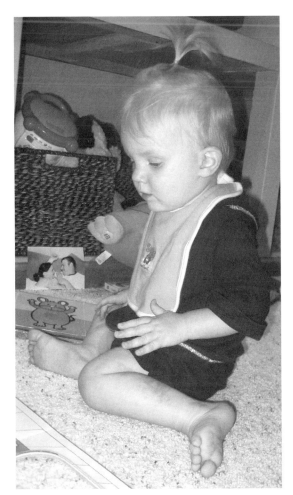

Figure 2.58 ■ Side sitting; note the dissociation of the lower extremities.

hip. Sitting on a child-size chair requires the child to use another component of movement, eccentric contractions. Eccentric or lengthening contractions of the quadriceps, proximal hamstrings, and gluteus maximus muscles allow the child to lower himself slowly to the chair. As he lowers himself to sit, he shifts his weight posteriorly from the forefoot to the heel of the foot. Rising to standing from a small chair requires an anterior weight shift and concentric contractions of these same muscles.

Sitting on an adult-size chair, such as a sofa, is accomplished through a combination of several movements. This activity is often the first function that reveals a child's developing climbing skills. When a child begins to climb onto an adult-size chair, he usually uses considerable lateral trunk flexion to one side while he abducts and flexes the opposite hip. After months of practice, he begins to use more weight shifting to one side with accompanying elongation of the lateral trunk on that weight-bearing side, intra-axial counterrotation, and hip flexion of the opposite lower extremity. Figure 2.59 shows a series of movements used by a child to get into an adult-sized chair.

LOCOMOTION IN SITTING

Once children exhibit dissociation of the two lower extremities and are stable in half–ring sitting, some children actually develop a locomotive form in this posture called **hitching.** Hitching is when a child, while sitting on the floor, uses either foot to dig into the surface in order to scoot forward on his buttocks. Many children use hitching as a means of moving around in their environments before they learn to creep efficiently and can become quite adept at this form of locomotion.

ERECT STANDING PROGRESSION

SUPPORTED STANDING

When held in standing during the neonatal period, the child bears partial weight on his lower extremities. His legs may be stiff with cocontraction, and the base of support is very narrow, with the feet supinated. Head control is absent, and his neck is flexed with the chin resting on the chest (Fig. 2.60). While in supported standing, tilting the child forward slightly will produce reflex stepping (automatic stepping) (Fig. 2.61).

By the end of 2 months of age, most infants lose the reflex stepping ability. Early developmentalists believed that the cessation of automatic stepping was simply a function of maturation of the child's central nervous system. However, the groundbreaking studies of Esther Thelen in the early 1980s found that reflex stepping in infants whose lower extremities were weighted artificially was diminished. Babies who were held standing in water increased their stepping, and the stepping persisted beyond the usual time of dissolution. On the other hand, babies who were held standing in water increased their stepping, presumably due to the effect of buoyancy on the lower extremities, and the stepping persisted beyond the usual age of dissolution. The conclusion drawn from these studies was that reflex stepping ceased at approximately 2 months of age, not because of programming and maturation of the central nervous system, but because the mass of the infant's lower extremities became such that it was too difficult for the infant to lift the heavy lower extremities.[49]

Regardless of the theory that one accepts for the cessation of automatic stepping, by the end of 2 months the typical child no longer produces this reflex stepping and often will cease to take weight on the lower extremities when held in standing. This absence of automatic stepping is referred to as **abasia,** derived from the Greek words that mean *without step.*[1] The next stepping abilities will be volitional. The lack of weight bearing through the lower extremities, which occurs typically during the third and fourth months, is the stage of **astasia,** literally meaning *without standing.*[1] This stage is temporary during normal development and may not be seen in all children.

During the first 4 months, head control has been developing in all postures, as control and balance of the

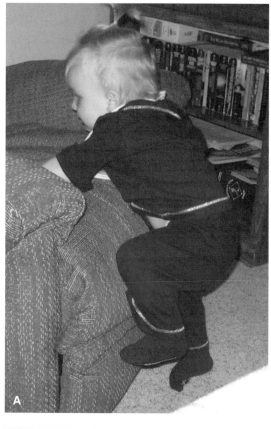

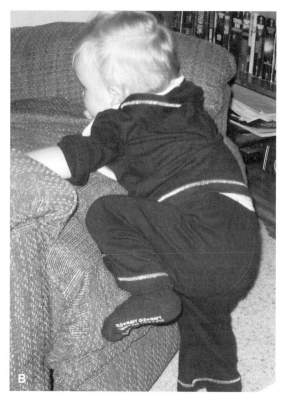

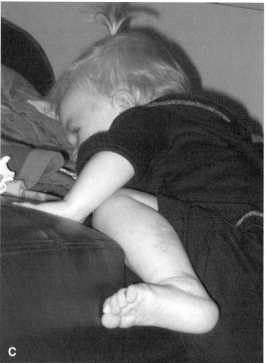

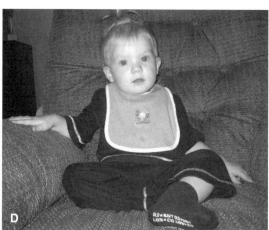

Figure 2.59 ■ Climbing onto adult-sized chair, early sequence; note the lateral flexion of the trunk to the right (instead of shifting of weight to the right, which would cause lateral trunk flexion to the left) and the extreme abduction of the left hip.

antigravity cervical extensors and flexors progressed. By 5 months of age, his head secure in space, the infant volitionally begins to accept partial weight on the lower extremities during supported standing (Fig. 2.62). This milestone is characterized by moderate abduction, flex-

ion, and external rotation of the hips, with knee flexion and pronation of the feet. This 5-month posture becomes even more exaggerated by 7 months of age, at which time the child is bearing full weight on his lower extremities (Fig. 2.63).

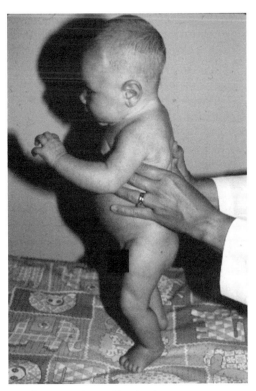

Figure 2.60 ■ Supported standing in the neonate.

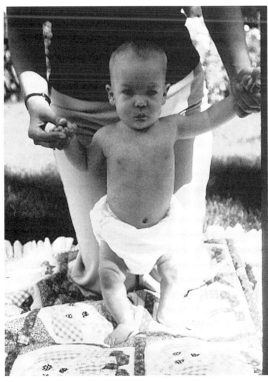

Figure 2.62 ■ Supported standing at 5 months of age; note the flexed hips and knees.

At 7 months, the child's poor anterior-posterior weight-bearing alignment and underdeveloped balance responses prevent him from standing alone without external support. He can stand and walk with his hands held (Fig. 2.63). His gait is characterized by hip external rotation and moderate

abduction, giving him a wide base of support, and extremely pronated feet. The greater the abduction and external rotation of the hips, the more pronated the feet are. Typically, a fat pad masks the longitudinal arch of each foot, in babies and toddlers, increasing the pronated appearance of the

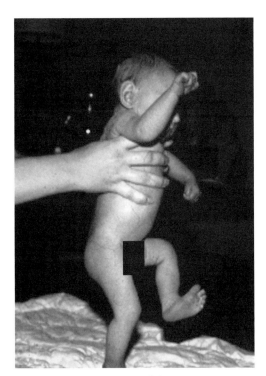

Figure 2.61 ■ Automatic stepping of the neonate.

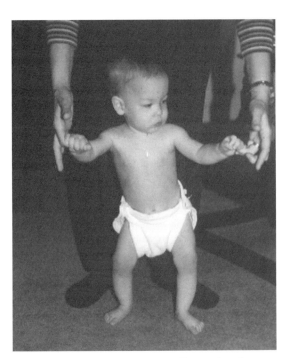

Figure 2.63 ■ Supported standing at 7 months of age; note wide base of support, hip and knee flexion, and pronation of feet.

feet. Hips and knees are flexed, creating continued poor anterior-posterior alignment for standing without support. In proper, mature weight-bearing alignment, an imaginary straight line can be drawn in a parasagittal plane through the ear, shoulder, hip, knee, and lateral malleolus. In the immature standing posture, the imaginary line falls through the ear and shoulder but anterior to the hip joint and often slightly posterior to the knee joint (Fig. 2.64).

The child begins pulling himself to standing in his crib at about this time (7 to 8 months). At first, this is accomplished by using the newly developed strength of the upper extremities, while the lower extremities remain essentially passive. Once standing, the child frequently will hold onto the crib rails for support while he bounces and experiments with this newly discovered standing ability. During his earliest attempts at supported standing in the crib, he finds that he is unable to get down. Lowering himself slowly to the mattress requires strong eccentric control of his hips and knees, something that he has not developed. Frustrated

and tired of standing, he may simply let go of the crib rails and drop to sitting, thanks to gravity, or he may begin to cry, signaling to his parent his need for help. A parent will come and either take the child from the crib or put him down in prone or supine. Once this has happened, the child seems to realize that his actions were attention getting, so he will pull to standing once again, and the sequence of events repeats. This is great fun for the child to repeat these behaviors, as he discovers that his actions cause effects, oftentimes predictable effects.

INDEPENDENT STANDING

By 10 months of age the child pulls himself to standing at furniture such as a sofa or low table. As seen in Figure 2.65, now he gets to standing by going through the knee-standing (tall kneeling) and half-kneeling postures and is adept at getting down with control. In the tall kneeling posture, the base of support is kept relatively wide as the child's cen-

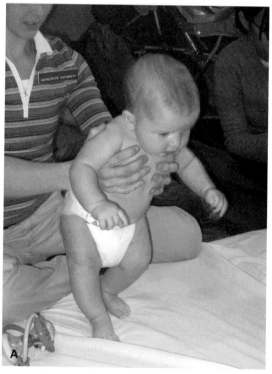

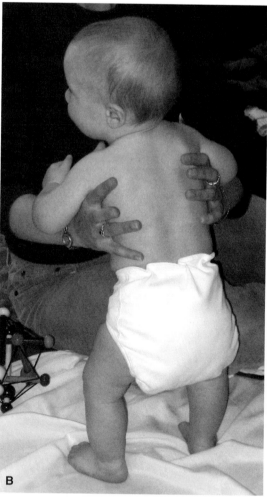

Figure 2.64 ■ Ear-to-heel postural alignment for standing. **(A)** Inadequate and immature weight-bearing alignment for independent standing; note that the ear-to-heel weight line falls anterior to the hips and posterior to the knees; note the narrow base of support with supination of the feet. **(B)** Improved postural alignment, but alignment is still inadequate for standing independently.

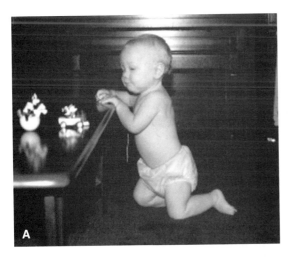

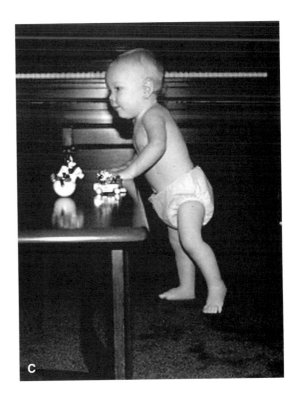

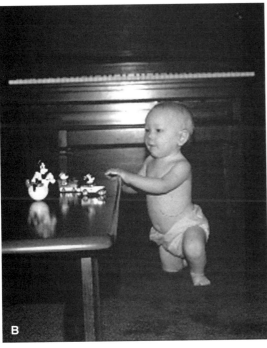

Figure 2.65 ■ Pull-to-standing at furniture sequence. **(A)** Tall kneeling. **(B)** Half-kneeling; note the intra-axial rotation and the dissociation of the lower extremities. **(C)** Erect standing at low table with cruising.

ter of mass moves farther away from the floor. In order to achieve the half-kneeling posture, he must shift his weight to one side, elongating the trunk on that side, so that he is able to bring the unweighted limb forward and put his foot flat on the floor. This action, the transition between the tall kneeling and standing postures, requires intra-axial rotation, just as all transitional postures do. Once in half-kneeling, he uses his lower extremity muscles, particularly the hip extensors and knee extensors, to raise himself against gravity. He relies very little on the strength of the upper extremities as in past pulling-to-standing attempts. Instead, the lower extremities do most of the work and the upper extremities help with balance. The same half-kneeling and tall kneeling positions are used to get down to the floor from standing. With practice, these movements become very controlled and fast. Occasionally, he simply may let go of his support and drop quickly to the floor.

CRUISING

Once standing at furniture, the child will play for long periods of time, going back and forth between the floor and the furniture, squatting and rising to stand repeatedly. He moves in and out of the various postures. Soon he begins stepping sideways while holding onto the furniture. This supported walking at 10 months of age is called **cruising** (Fig. 2.65C). He is able to work his way back and forth along the sofa or table and eventually begins to reach to other pieces of furniture to make his way around the room. Meanwhile, his anterior-posterior alignment is improving, with decreasing hip and knee flexion.[43] While standing at furniture, he can be seen to lift one or the other hand from the support, sometimes rotating his trunk to one side or the other while still maintaining his balance. Often, as he cruises around the furniture and reaches for the next piece of furniture, he briefly stands and maybe even takes one or two steps without support from either upper extremity. At times he stands briefly without touching the supporting surfaces. However, when walking without furniture for support, he still needs someone to hold his hand, but he is fast approaching the day when he will walk forward without holding the furniture or someone's hand. During the cruising phase of development, in addition to practicing his walking, the child's cruising movements contribute to the development and strengthening of hip abduction/adduction and eversion/inversion of the feet as he side-steps. Even though the child walks, supported by holding onto furniture or someone's hand, the **plantar grasp reflex** may still be positive at 10 months of age, although considerably diminished and present inconsistently. The plantar grasp reflex is manifested by curling of the toes when the examiner places a finger horizontally at the base of the toes (Fig. 2.66). A positive plantar grasp causes the toes to flex or curl.[15,48] This reflex can also be observed spontaneously as curling of the toes when the child is in supported standing. Usually the complete dissolution of this reflex must occur before independent walking without support will develop. Gradually, over the next several weeks, he lets go of the adult's hand or the furniture, often standing independently for brief periods. When this happens his upper extremities usually assume the high guard position for increased trunk stability.

During the development of standing, cruising, and walking, the child develops the ability to squat to play as well as squatting to pick up an object (Fig. 2.67). Often while standing at furniture, such as a sofa, the child can be seen to squat to pick up a toy, stand and place the toy on the sofa, and repeat this process many times. Also, she is able to spend great lengths of time in the squat position while playing. Squatting, therefore, is both a movement used to transition between postures and a posture in itself. Some have theorized that the active squat-to-stance-to-squat sequence facilitates cocontraction, and therefore stability, of the muscles surrounding the ankle joint. The theory is that the prolonged and maximal stretch to the muscle spindles of the ankle musculature fires both primary and secondary afferent endings.[26]

INDEPENDENT BIPEDAL LOCOMOTION

First independent forward walking generally occurs between 10 and 15 months of age, with the typical child walking at 12 months of age, plus or minus a month. At first, the child holds his upper extremities in the high guard position, the same position in which he held his arms during first independent sitting, in an attempt to increase stability against gravity by adducting the scapulae (Fig. 2.68). Posture is characterized by improving but continuing poor, vertical alignment, with hips and knees flexed. Abduction and external rotation of the hips continue to provide a wide base of support. The child does not have heel strike initially, and the feet are still in considerable pronation.

As forward independent gait progresses over the next months, the shoulders lose much of the flexion of the high guard position, assuming a low guard position with elbows still flexed and hands just above the waist; fingers may be pointed upward or shoulders are adducted and the hands are stabilized against the body as in Figure 2.69. Then the upper extremities relax into full shoulder extension and hang at the child's sides. Over the next few weeks, reciprocal arm swing during gait is attained (Fig. 2.70).

With practice, the anterior-posterior postural alignment continues to improve with increasing hip and knee extension, decreasing hip abduction with narrowing of the base of support, and lessening of external rotation of the hips. Eventually the child walks with good postural alignment, a narrow base of support, neutral pronation/supination of the feet, heel strike, push off, and reciprocal arm swing. The plantar fat pad does not completely disappear until approximately 2 years of age, at which time the longitudinal arches become visible.

Bipedal locomotion will continue to improve and progress over the next 2 to 4 years. Gait parameters for the 3-year-old child differ from early gait parameters at age 1 year.[50] These parameters include alignment of the lower extremities as well as various aspects of the gait cycle. As the child's gait matures, mediolateral alignment at the hip progresses from hip abduction to adduction, until the feet are approximately shoulders' width apart. At the knees, mediolateral alignment moves from genu varus at birth to approximately 12 degrees of genu valgus at 3 years of age. Then between 4 and 7 years of age, the valgus resolves to only 7 to 10 degrees. This change in alignment of the knees affects the mediolateral align-

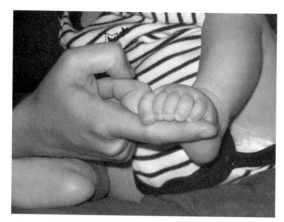

Figure 2.66 ■ Plantar grasp, positive response.

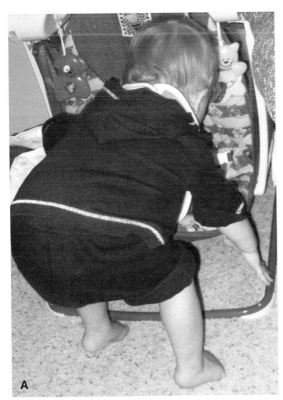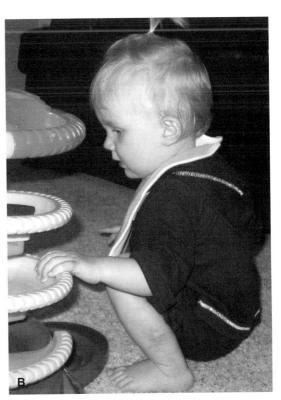

Figure 2.67 ■ Squatting. **(A)** Active squatting. **(B)** Squat position, a frequent play position.

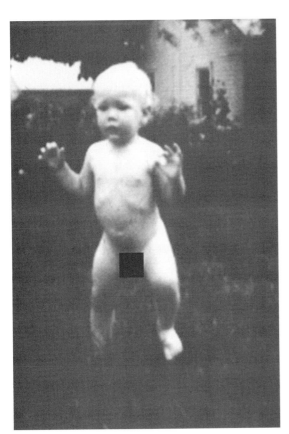

Figure 2.68 ■ First independent walking with high guard positioning of upper extremities.

ment of the hips, ankles, and feet as well.[50] Other gait parameters that change with growth and maturation are cadence, step and stride length, and velocity.[50] **Cadence,** the number of steps per minute, starts out very high in first independent walking. The 1-year-old child spends a decreased amount of time in single limb stance, compared to the 3-year-old and the adult. This is because the 1-year-old child has less strength and stability in his hips. Consequently, he takes more steps per minute and spends less time in single limb support.[50]

Gait **velocity,** the distance one covers in a specified amount of time, starts low and increases as the child ages.[50] Velocity is related to the length of one's step or stride. A **step** is measured from heel strike of one lower extremity to heel strike of the opposite lower extremity. **Stride length,** measured from heel strike of one foot to heel strike of the same foot, is usually twice the step length.[50] In a case where step length of the two extremities differs, because of pathology affecting only one limb, both step and stride length must be measured, instead of calculating stride length by multiplying the step length by two.

From 1 to 3 years of age, a child's step length and stride length increase, as do velocity and single limb stance time.[50] Single limb stance increases with increasing strength and balance abilities. Length of step and/or stride, and therefore gait velocity, increases as the child's lower extremities continue to grow in length, even well

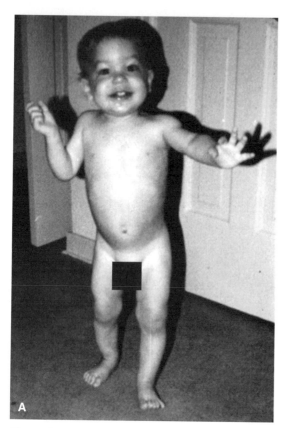 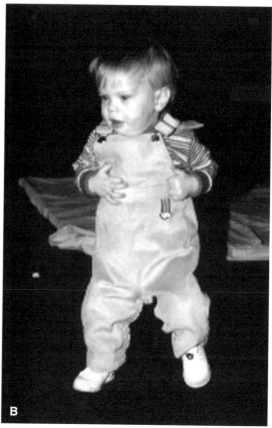

Figure 2.69 ■ Independent walking. **(A)** Note that the high guard position is decreasing, with the right upper extremity still in high guard, the left upper extremity being lowered with shoulder girdle protraction. **(B)** Walking independently with low guard to enhance upright trunk stability.

after age 3. Otherwise, gait at age 3 is considered to have parameters similar to those of an adult.[50] Various gait parameters at ages 1 year and 3 years are shown in Table 2.5.

Even though a toddler is able to walk fast, and his parents will often insist he is running, true running does not develop until 3 to 4 years of age. A **true run** is characterized by having both feet off the ground at the same time, unlike walking, where one foot does not leave the ground until the other foot makes initial contact.

STAIR CLIMBING

Stairs present a considerable challenge to toddlers, as one might imagine. The typical **rise** of a step in a flight of stairs is 7 to 8 inches. For a 15-month-old child to negotiate stairs in erect standing would be the equivalent of an adult attempting to climb stairs with a knee-high rise (Fig. 2.71).

The ability to ascend and descend stairs is affected by a number of factors, most particularly, opportunity. Therefore, the age of achieving this milestone has considerable variability, although the sequence of achievement is much the same from one child to the next. A

child who lives in a home without stairs, or at least without stairs that the child is permitted to climb, usually develops stair-climbing skills at a later age than the child who has frequent daily encounters with stairs to get to and from his bedroom and/or toys.

The first ability to ascend and descend stairs is usually in the quadruped position (Fig. 2.72). The child learns to go up the stairs on his hands and knees, followed soon by coming down the stairs backward on his hands and knees. Sometimes children, in their first attempts at descending stairs, will try to do so in quadruped, but head first, with disastrous results if a caregiver is not nearby. With a bit of coaching, the child quickly learns through trial and error to descend the stairs backward on his hands and knees.

Ascending stairs generally develops to a more skillful level before descending stairs develops to the same level of skill. This sequence generally repeats itself in bipedal locomotion after the child has developed the ability to go up and down stairs using quadrupedal locomotion. Another feature of stair climbing that develops in a rather typical pattern is apparent once the child is climbing stairs while standing. Initially, bipedal stair climbing is performed by

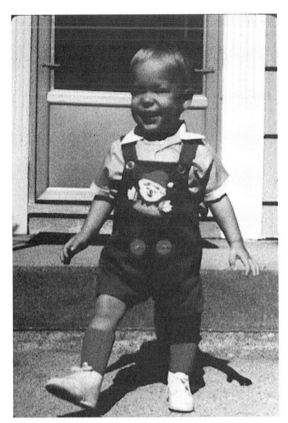

Figure 2.70 ■ Mature independent walking with heel strike and reciprocal arm swing.

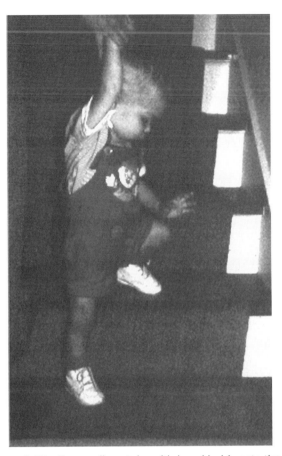

Figure 2.71 ■ Descending stairs with hand held; note the height of the step in relationship to the length of the child's lower extremity.

placing both feet on each step, in a manner that is called **marking time.**[17] Generally, the child will not begin doing steps one over one (i.e., only one foot to each step) until he is close to 3 years of age, depending of course on how much trial and error and practice on stairs he has been afforded. This pattern of the feet is also dependent on the type of upper extremity support that is available. Stair climbing progresses as the upper extremity support decreases from using one handrail and/or an adult hand for support, to needing a handrail but no adult, and finally to needing

no upper extremity support (Fig. 2.73). Of course, the speed with which the child develops increasingly more skillful stair-climbing abilities varies greatly, and like other skills, the ability to locomote on stairs may temporarily digress as unique and/or challenging circumstances, such as unusually steep stairs or the absence of a handrail, present themselves.

TABLE 2.5

Gait Parameters in 1- and 3-Year-Old Children[a]

Gait Parameter	1 Year of Age	3 Years of Age	Direction of Change
Base of support (pelvic span to ankle spread)	<1	≥1	↓
Step length	20 cm	33 cm	↑
Stride length (double the step length)	40 cm	66 cm	↑
Single limb stance	32% of gait cycle	35% of gait cycle	↑
Cadence (step frequency)	180 steps per minute	154 steps per minute	↓
Velocity (speed)	60 cm/sec	105 cm/sec	↑

From Long TM, Toscano K. *Handbook of Pediatric Physical Therapy.* Philadelphia: Lippincott Williams & Wilkins, 2001.

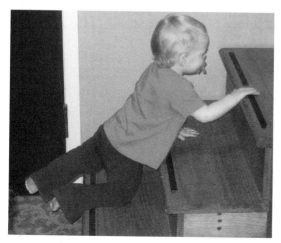

Figure 2.72 ■ *Ascending stairs in quadruped.*

 ## Balance

Maintaining one's balance, that is, keeping one's center of mass within the base of support and effectively compensating when balance is disturbed, is a challenge to the devel-

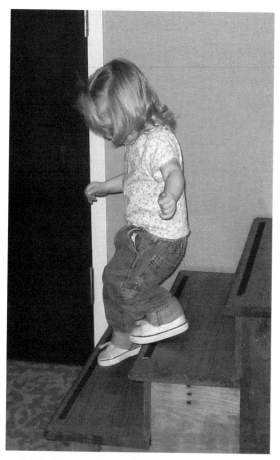

Figure 2.73 ■ *Descending stairs without upper extremity support.*

oping child as he attempts and learns new motor skills. Following the achievement of a particular milestone or posture, a child must develop the ability to maintain his balance in that posture. Usually, as the child is bravely moving toward the next posture in the hierarchy, he continues to practice the newest learned posture, thereby developing new balancing skills in each successive posture. Balance skills make up the normal postural reflex mechanism. These balance skills are divided into four subgroups: righting reactions, tilting reactions, equilibrium reactions, and protective reactions. Each subgroup has a defined aspect of balance for which it is responsible. These subgroups operate on a continuum such that when one's balance is challenged, the reactions occur in a predictable order (see Display 2.2).

Righting reactions are responsible for securing the head in space and develop in all planes.[15,48] When there is a disturbance in one's center of mass in any posture, **head-righting reactions,** also termed **labyrinthine righting reactions,** come into play first. If the disturbance is only slight and does not come close to moving the child's center of mass outside the base of support, the head-righting reactions suffice in bringing the body back into balance. When an individual's body is tilted in any direction, the head automatically rights itself; that is, no matter what the position of the body, the head moves to an upright position wherein the mouth is horizontal and the face is vertical, referenced to the floor or ground[15,48] (Fig. 2.74). If the disturbance is large enough to move the center of mass very near the edge of the child's base of support, then head righting occurs automatically, but it is not enough to maintain balance. Help is needed from the tilting or equilibrium reactions.

Tilting and equilibrium reactions, responsible for securing the position of the body in space when balance is challenged, are identical responses but are elicited by slightly different stimuli. A **tilting reaction** is the correct term to use when the surface on which the child is seated or otherwise positioned is moved, thus causing the child's center of mass to shift. When this happens, head righting occurs immediately. If the body senses that head righting is insufficient in itself, the tilting reactions are elicited. The response looks like this. When on a balance board, ball, or other moveable surface, if the child is tilted to his left far enough to elicit the tilting reactions, lateral bending toward the right side occurs. If viewing the spine from a posterior vantage point, the vertebral column curves to the right, away from the direction toward which the child was tilted (Fig. 2.75). The concavity of the curved spine is on the right side (the direction opposite the direction the child was pushed), with the convex side on the left. This returns the body's mass toward the center of the base of support. If the stimulus and the response are strong enough, the limbs enter into the response. In this case, the right shoulder and hip abduct, in an effort to help bring the

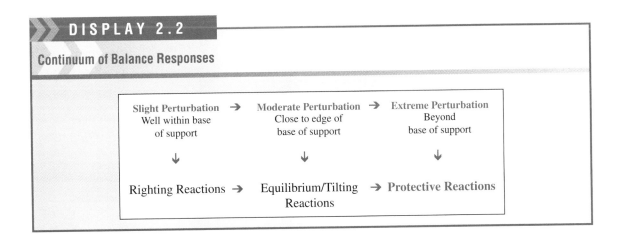

Continuum of Balance Responses

Slight Perturbation → Moderate Perturbation → Extreme Perturbation
Well within base   Close to edge of   Beyond
of support   base of support   base of support
↓   ↓   ↓
Righting Reactions → Equilibrium/Tilting → **Protective Reactions**
                     Reactions

body mass into the center of the base of support once again. An **equilibrium reaction** is identical to the tilting reaction, but the stimulus differs in that the individual is on a stationary surface instead of a mobile surface, and the force of the perturbation is directed at the child's body rather than the surface.[15,48] Tilting and equilibrium reactions develop in each successive posture shortly after the child develops stability in that posture and while he is beginning to experiment with and work on the next higher posture.

The final type of balance response is the protective response. In normal development, the protective response is responsible for regaining balance when the center of mass has been pushed beyond the borders of the base of support. When this happens, head-righting and tilting/equilibrium responses are elicited but are insufficient to regain control. Automatically, the child protects himself from the inevitable fall by sticking out his hand or foot (Fig. 2.76). This motion effectively moves the borders of the base of support out-ward, enlarging the base. In this manner, the body's mass is once again within the base of support, not because the body returned to being inside the base of support, as in the tilting/equilibrium reactions, but because the base of support has enlarged to once again capture the center of mass within its borders. The following example shows how protective responses are used in one of two ways to maintain balance and sometimes prevent injury. When one is standing in the aisle on a moving bus, and the driver suddenly slams on the brakes, if head-righting and tilting responses, both of which are elicited first, do not suffice in regaining balance, a person probably will do one of two things. Either he will take a step with one foot in order to increase the size of the base of support enough to regain balance within the base of support, or he will fall forward. If he falls, as he nears the floor of the bus, one or both arms will reach out to help break the fall, creating a new and larger base of support and hopefully protecting the head and face from the potential impact. This second response is the reason people often fracture the distal end of the radius, the well-known Colles fracture, in a fall.[1]

 Fine Motor Development

GRASP

A discussion about motor development cannot be complete without attention to the development of grasp. Earlier in this chapter, the importance of proximal stability to the development of grasp and prehension was discussed. Like gross motor development, fine motor development occurs, in most typical cases, in a predictable order.

At birth, the full-term neonate has a hand grasp reflex. This reflex, which began in utero, is a reflex closing of the hand when stimulated by touch to the palmer surface with stretch of the intrinsic muscles of the hand. The response to this two-part stimulus is reflex grasping of the stimulating object. As long as the stimulus is in contact with the infant's hand, the fist remains closed. The grasp reflex is

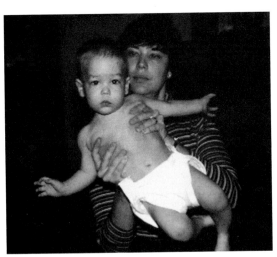

Figure 2.74 ■ Positive labyrinthine righting reflex (head righting); face is maintained vertical with mouth horizontal in response to a lateral tilt to the child's right.

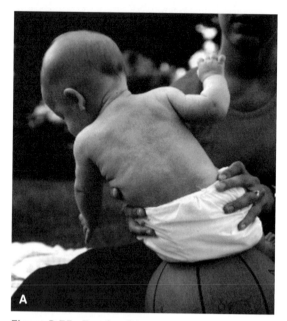
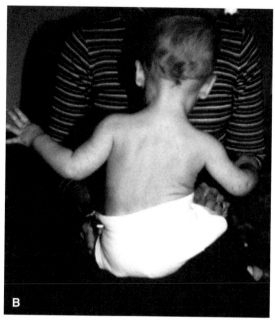

Figure 2.75 ■ *Test for tilting reaction in sitting.* **(A)** *Response to a tilt to the left is negative because child does not right his trunk.* **(B)** *Response to same tilt is positive in older child because he laterally flexes his trunk away from the direction of the tilt.*

usually tested by the examiner placing his index finger into the infant's palm[15,48] (Fig. 2.77).

During the early months of life, the grasp reflex is intact, although it gradually weakens until disappearing at approximately 4 months of age. This means that until the reflex becomes naturally inhibited with time, anything that stimulates the palm of the infant's hand will elicit a reflex behavior. Such reflex grasp pre-empts voluntary grasping of objects. Therefore, attempts by the infant at voluntary

grasp will not be successful until the hand grasp reflex has diminished and then disappeared. Even though this may mean that the child's early attempts at voluntary grasp are essentially thwarted, little is lost during those 4 months of active reflex behavior. This is because until approximately 3 to 4 months of age, the child still lacks the stability in the shoulder joint needed for skillful reaching for and grasping of objects at will.

During the first 4 months, while the infant's grasp reflex diminishes, the child is gradually developing the ability to stabilize his shoulders in order to reach for objects with some degree of accuracy and hold the upper extremity

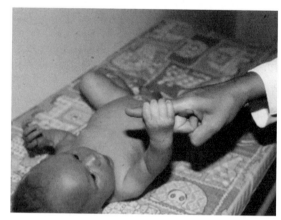

Figure 2.76 ■ Protective extension of the upper extremity to the side.

Figure 2.77 ■ Hand grasp reflex is positive in response to tactile and proprioceptive stimuli from examiner's finger being placed in the infant's palm.

stable while grasping an object. The development of this shoulder stability is followed by the development of the child's ability to control the extremity enough to bring the object toward him for a closer look, to put it in his mouth, or to examine it with two hands (Fig. 2.78). Shoulder stability and the ability to perform a controlled reach arise from the infant's increasingly skillful weight bearing and weight shifting in the prone-on-elbows posture. It is complemented by such activities in supine as bringing the hands to midline (inhibition of the ATNR), reaching hands to knees and eventually hands to feet, and reaching up to touch the caregiver's face during dressing and feeding activities. Accomplishing these motor behaviors in prone and supine requires activation of the pectoralis major and serratus anterior muscles, with concurrent lengthening of the rhomboid muscles, allowing protraction of the shoulders. Prior to the development of these particular components of motor behavior, the infant is unable to reach into space and stabilize the shoulder for grasp and prehension. Consequently, at 3 months of age, the child will take a toy such as a rattle only if it is presented close to his body, within 2 or 3 inches. This is because he cannot stabilize the shoulders when reaching into space, but he can stabilize them by adducting and fixing his upper arms into his body.

At 4 to 5 months of age, the child actively and successfully reaches for objects in space and can grasp them, at will, using the whole hand in a palmar grasp. The thumb is inactive initially. Once he grasps the object, he can bring it close to his face but is not able to put it into his mouth or inspect it. This is because he has not developed the ability to actively supinate his forearm (Fig. 2.79). Conse-

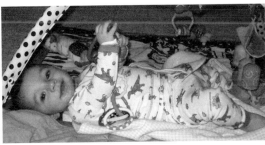

Figure 2.79 ■ Supine, reaching into space with pronation of the forearm.

quently, the dorsum of his hand is between his mouth and/or eyes and the object, and the object is essentially hidden from view. At 4 months of age, with a stable prone-on-elbows position, the child is beginning to shift weight. As mentioned earlier in this chapter, weight shifting in prone on elbows is the beginning of supination, as well as the ability to pronate and supinate the forearm reciprocally. As active, controlled supination develops and improves, the child begins to engage an object with his eyes, reach for the object, and grasp it. He then supinates his forearm as he brings the object close to his face. Now he can put it into his mouth, visually inspect it, touch it with both hands at once, and/or transfer the object from one hand to the other. Victory!

Although voluntary grasp at first is crude and palmar, the development of refined grasp progresses rather quickly in the large scheme of things. Sitting in a high chair with an object on the chair tray, a child at first will pick up the object by crudely raking it into his palm, using just his fingers, with the ulnar two fingers predominating.[17,51] This ulnar activity occurs long before the active participation of the thumb (radial activity), and it is a good example of the medial-to-lateral principle of developmental direction. In anatomic position, the ulnar fingers are medial and the thumb is lateral.

As grasp develops and becomes more refined, the child continues to use the fingers to palm the object, ulnar fingers still predominating, but radial fingers participating. The thumb is still inactive. This type of grasp progresses to increasing dominance by the first two fingers. By 10 months of age, the child begins using a very active forefinger (index finger or first finger), and loves to poke and prod with that index finger.[17,51] This is the time when babies poke their fingers in noses, eyes, and ears. They begin pointing at and poking nearly everything in sight. This poking with the forefinger continues to dominate fine motor activities for many months, as seen in this 15-month-old child in Figure 2.80. This obsession with the forefinger occurs at about the same time the thumb is becoming very active. At 10 months of age the child has a well-developed pincer grasp, using the thumb and finger pad to pad.[17,51] Finger foods are very important to the child at this time as he develops the ability to pick up Cheerios and put them in his mouth with

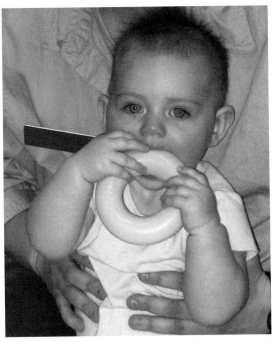

Figure 2.78 ■ Bilateral use of hands in midline with mouthing; note supination of forearms.

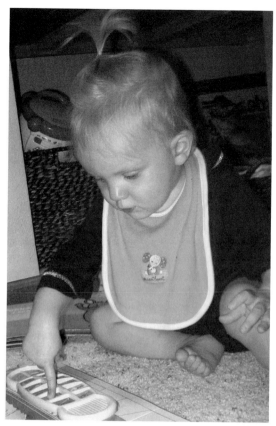

Figure 2.80 ■ Forefinger (index finger) dominance, poking and prodding.

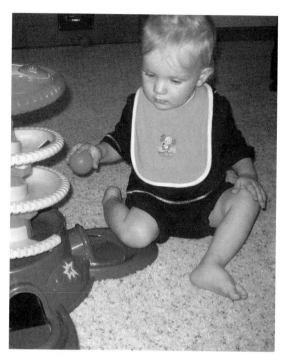

Figure 2.81 ■ Three jaw chuck grasp, using thumb, index finger, and second finger in a triangular pattern.

considerable accuracy. Also around 10 months of age, the child begins to use a *three-jaw chuck* type of grasp, using the thumb, index, and second finger[17,51] (Fig. 2.81).

RELEASE

The development of release lags somewhat behind the development of grasp. Volitional release begins at approximately 11 months of age. Until that time, a child lets go of an object simply by relaxing the finger flexion. Not until 11 months of age does the child begin to intentionally release by actively extending his fingers.[17] The inability to actively and accurately release an object during those first 10 to 12 months of life is the root cause of the tendency to knock down the tower when trying to stack blocks. Until the child begins to gain some control over the release, he is able to place one block on top of another but causes the tower to fall when he tries to withdraw his hand.[17]

By 18 months of age a child can grasp a pencil in the center using the pads of his fingers, put tiny pellets in a small bottle, stack a tower of three blocks, and mark with a crayon while holding the paper with the other hand.[6,17,51] See Table 2.6 for approximate times of development of various fine motor skills.

 The 2- to 7-Year-Old Child

During the first 2 years of life, the typical child develops the motor skills required for ordinary mobility and prehension. Further gross and fine motor development occur after the first 2 years, but these later attained skills are more specific to an individual's play and work. These more advanced motor skills are developed and perfected more intentionally by each individual. Table 2.7 lists some of these more advanced skills and the approximate ages of acquisition.

SUMMARY

Normal motor development in humans usually occurs according to a particular sequence and timing. The sequence and timing are important to the clinician and can be used as guides in the physical therapy evaluation and treatment of children and adults. A thorough understanding of normal motor development is particularly germane to the study of abnormal neuromotor development in children. Although all humans share a common anatomy, physiology, and developmental sequence, one must keep in mind that many intrinsic and extrinsic factors, including pathology and culture, affect the sequence and timing of motor development in an individual.

TABLE 2.6

Development of Fine Motor Skills

Skill	Age of Achievement
Hand grasp reflex	Birth–4 to 5 mo
Visual regard	Birth–2 mo
Swipes with whole hand	2–3 mo
Visually directed reaching	3–5 mo
Midline clasping of hands	2–5 mo
Reaches out to grasp object	4–5 mo
Plays with feet; bangs objects together	5 mo
Crude palming, ulnar fingers predominating	5–7 mo
Transfers object one hand to the other	6 mo
Lateral scissors grasp	8–9 mo
Pincer grasp, forefinger and thumb in opposition	10–11 mo
Forefinger dominance: poking and prodding with index finger	10–11 mo
Holds crayon	11 mo
Beginning voluntary release	11 mo
Uses graded pressure; varies pressure depending on object; uses fingertip with thumb opposition in fine pincer grasp	12 mo
Precision grasp with fine pincer and controlled release	15 mo
Scribbles on paper	15–18 mo
Holds paper with other hand when scribbling	18 mo
Puts object in container and dumps contents	18 mo
Builds tower of three cubes	18 mo
Turns pages of book, perhaps two or three at a time	21 mo
Turns page of a book one at a time	24 mo
Unscrews jar lid	24 mo
Builds tower with eight cubes	30 mo

TABLE 2.7

Advanced Motor Skills and Approximate Ages of Acquisition

Motor Skill	Age of Acquisition
Stands on low balance beam	2 yr
Walks straight line	3 yr
Walks circular line	4 yr
Balances on one foot for 3–5 sec	5 yr
Walks backward	18 mo
Jumps from bottom step	2 yr
Jumps off floor with both feet	28 mo
Hops three times	3 yr
Hops eight to 10 times on same foot	5 yr
Hops distance of 50 feet	5 yr
Gallops	4 yr
Skips	6 yr
Catches ball using body and hands	3 yr
Catches ball using hands only	5 yr
Attempts to kick ball	18 mo
Kicks ball	2–3 yr
Hurls ball 3 feet	18 mo
Throws ball	2–3 yr
Fast walk	18 mo
True run with nonsupport phase	2–3 yr

REFERENCES

1. Dirckx JH. Stedman's Concise Medical Dictionary for the Health Professions: Illustrated 4th Ed. Baltimore: Lippincott Williams & Wilkins, 2001.
2. Cowlin AF. Women's Fitness Program Development. Champaign, IL: Human Kinetics, 2002.
3. Bale JR, Stoll BJ, Lucas AO, eds. Improving Birth Outcomes: Meeting the Challenge in the Developing World. Washington, DC: The National Academies Press, 2003. Available at: http://www.iom.edu/CMS/3783/3915/16191.aspx. Accessed January 2, 2006.
4. VanSant AF. Should the normal motor developmental sequence be used as a theoretical model to progress adult patients? In: Contemporary Management of Motor Control Problems: Proceedings of the II STEP Conference. Fredricksburg, VA: Bookcrafters, Inc, 1991:95–97.
5. Shumway-Cook A, Woollacott M. Motor Control: Theory and Practical Applications. Baltimore, MD: Williams & Wilkins, 1995.
6. Bayley Scales of Infant Development. 2nd Ed. The Bayley II. The Psychological Corporation. San Antonio, TX: Harcourt Brace & Co, 1993.
7. Stuberg WA, Dehne P, Miedaner J, White P et al. The Milani-Comparetti Motor Development Screening Test. 3rd Ed. Rev. Omaha, NE: University of Nebraska Medical Center, 1992.
8. Piper MC, Darrah J. Alberta Infant Motor Scale. Philadelphia: WB Saunders, 1995.
9. Friend JH, Guralnik DB, eds. Webster's New World Dictionary of the American Language. College Ed. Cleveland, OH: The World Publishing Company, 1960.

10. Streissguth AP. Fetal Alcohol Syndrome: A Guide for Families and Communities. Baltimore, MD: Paul H. Brookes, 1997.

11. Edelman C, Mandle CL. Health Promotion Throughout the Lifespan. 5th Ed. St. Louis: Mosby, Inc, 2002.

12. Kartin D, Grant TM, Streissguth AP, et al. Three-year developmental outcomes in children with prenatal alcohol and drug exposure. Pediatr Phys Ther 2002; 14:145–153.

13. U.S. Department of Health and Human Services. Healthy People 2010. Washington, DC: U.S. Department of Health and Human Services/Office of Public Health and Science, 1998.

14. LaGasse LL, Seifer R, Lester BM. Interpreting research on prenatal substance exposure in the context of multiple confounding factors. Clin Perinatal 1999; 26:39–54.

15. Illingworth RS. The Development of the Infant and Young Child: Normal and Abnormal. New York: Churchill Livingstone, 1980.

16. McGraw MB. The Neuromuscular Maturation of the Human Infant. New York: Hafner Publishing, 1945.

17. Gesell A, Ilg FL. Infant and Child in the Culture of Today. New York: Harper and Brothers Publishers, 1943.

18. Cech DJ, Martin ST. Functional Movement Development across the Life Span. 2nd Ed. Philadelphia: W. B. Saunders Company, 2002.

19. Keshner EA. How theoretical framework biases evaluation and treatment. In: Lister MJ, ed. Contemporary Management of Motor Control Problems: Proceedings of the II STEP Conference. Fredricksburg, VA: Bookcrafters, Inc, 1991:37–47.

20. Effgen SK. Meeting the Physical Therapy Needs of Children. Philadelphia: F. A. Davis Company, 2005.

21. Bayley N. The California Infant Scale of Motor Development. Berkeley, CA: University of California, 1936.

22. Tecklin JS, ed. Pediatric Physical Therapy. 3rd Ed. Philadelphia: Lippincott Williams & Wilkins, 1998.

23. Bayley N. Bayley Scales of Infant and Toddler Development. 3rd Ed. San Antonio, TX: Harcourt Assessment, Inc, 2006.

24. Heriza C. Motor development: traditional and contemporary theories. In: Lister MJ, ed. Contemporary Management of Motor Control Problems: Proceedings of the II STEP Conference. Fredricksburg, VA: Bookcrafters, Inc, 1991:99–126.

25. Horak FB. Assumptions underlying motor control for neurologic rehabilitation. In: Lister MJ, ed. Contemporary Management of Motor Control Problems: Proceedings of the II STEP Conference. Fredricksburg, VA: Bookcrafters, Inc, 1991:11–27.

26. Stockmeyer SA. An interpretation of the approach of Rood to the treatment of neuromuscular dysfunction. Am J Phys Med 1967;46:900–956.

27. MacKay-Lyons M. Central pattern generation of locomotion: a review of the evidence. Phys Ther 2002;82:69–83.

28. Marder E, Calabrese RL. Principles of rhythmic motor patter generation. Physiol Rev 1996;76:687–717.

29. Jordan M, Brownstone RM, Noga BR. Control of functional systems in the brainstem and spinal cord. Curr Opin Neurobiol 1992;2:794–801.

30. Grillner S. Locomotion in vertebrates: central mechanisms and reflex integration. Physiol Rev 1975;55: 247–304.

31. Folio MR, Fewell RR. Examiner's Manual: Peabody Developmental Motor Scales. 2nd Ed. Austin, TX: PRO-ED, 1999.

32. Edwards S, ed. Neurological Physiotherapy. 2nd Ed. New York: Churchill Livingstone, 2002.

33. Sullivan PE, Markos PD, Minor MAD. An Integrated Approach to Therapeutic Exercise: Theory & Clinical Application. Reston, VA: Reston Publishing Company, 1982.

34. Heathcoch JC, Bhat AN, Lobo MA, et al. The relative kicking frequency of infants born full-term and preterm during learning and short-term and long-term memory periods of the mobile paradigm. Phys Ther. 2005 Jan; 85(1):8–18.

35. Piek JP, Carman R. Developmental profiles of spontaneous movements in infants. Early Hum Dev 1994; 39:109–126.

36. Thelen E. Ridley-Johnson R, Fisher D. Shifting patterns of bilateral coordination and lateral dominance in the leg movements of young infants. Dev Psychobiol 1983;16:29–46.

37. Morgan A. Neuro-Developmental Approach to the High-Risk Neonate. (Notes from a seminar presented in Williamsburg, VA; November 3–4, 1984.) Cited in Tecklin JS. Pediatric Physical Therapy. Philadelphia: Lippincott Williams & Wilkins, 1999.

38. Saint-Anne Dargassies. Neurological Development in the Full Term and Premature Neonate. Amsterdam: Elsevier, 1977. Cited in Bly L. Motor Skills Acquisition in the First Year: An Illustrated Guide to Normal Development. Tucson, AZ: Therapy Skill Builders, 1994.

39. Guzzetta A, Haataja L, Cowan F, et al. Neurological examination in healthy term infants aged 3–10 weeks. Biol Neonate 2005;87:187–196.

40. Oatis CA. Kinesiology: The Mechanics and Pathomechanics of Human Movement. Philadelphia: Lippincott Williams & Wilkins, 2004:106.

41. Piek JP. Infant Motor Development. Champaign, IL: Human Kinetics, 2006.

42. Dubowitz LMS, Dubowitz V, Mercuri E. The Neurological Assessment of the Preterm and Full-term Newborn Infant. 2nd Ed. London: MacKeith Press, 1999.

43. Bly L. Motor Skills Acquisition in the First Year: An Illustrated Guide to Normal Development. Tucson, AZ: Therapy Skill Builders, 1994.

44. Haywood KM, Getchell N. Life Span Motor Development. 3rd Ed. Champaign, IL: Human Kinetics, 2001.

45. Bly L. Normal and Abnormal Components of Movement. Course notes presented in September 1984, Milwaukee, WI.

46. Umphred DA. Neurological Rehabilitation. 4th Ed. St. Louis: Mosby, Inc., 2001.

47. Norton ES. Developmental Muscular Torticollis and Brachial Plexus Injury. In Campbell SK, Vander Linden DW, and Palisano RJ, eds. Physical Therapy for Children, 2nd Ed. Saunders, Philadelphia; 2000 p. 291.

48. Fiorentino M. Reflex Testing Methods for Evaluating CNS Development. Springfield, IL: Charles C. Thomas, 1972.

49. Thelen E, Fisher DM. Newborn stepping: an explanation for a "disappearing" reflex. Dev Psychol 1982; 18:760–775.

50. Long TM, Toscano K. Handbook of Pediatric Physical Therapy. Philadelphia: Lippincott Williams & Wilkins, 2001.

51. Erhardt RP. Erhardt Developmental Prehension Assessment. Laurel, MD: Ramsco Publishing, 1984. Cited in Bly L. Motor Skills Acquisition in the First Year: An Illustrated Guide to Normal Development. Tucson, AZ: Therapy Skill Builders, 1994.

SUGGESTED READING

Allen MC, Capute AJ. Tone and reflex development before term. Pediatrics 1990;85:393–399.

Campbell SK, Levy P, Zawacki L, et al. Population-based age standards for interpreting results on the test of motor infant performance. Pediatr Phys Ther. 2006; 18:119–125.

Cintas HM. The accomplishment of walking: aspects of the ascent. Pediatr Phys Ther. 1993;5(2):61–68.

Clopton NA, Duvall T, Ellis B, et al. Investigation of trunk and extremity movement associated with passive head turning in newborns. Phys Ther. 2000;80: 152–159.

DiFranza JR, Aligne CA, Weitzman M. Prenatal and postnatal environmental tobacco smoke exposure and children's health. Pediatrics. 2004;113;1007–1015.

Dusing S, Mercer V, Yu B, et al. Trunk position in supine of infants born preterm and at term: an assessment using a computerized pressure mat. Pediatr Phys Ther. 2005;17:2–10.

Groome LJ, Swiber MJ, Holland SB, et al. Spontaneous motor activity in the perinatal infant before and after birth: stability in individual differences. Dev Psychobiol. 1999;35:15–24.

Hill S, Engle S, Jorgensen J, et al. Effects of facilitated tucking during routine care of infants born preterm. Pediatr Phys Ther. 2005;17:158–163.

Jaffe M, Tal Y, Dabbah H, et al. Infants with a thumb-in-fist posture. Pediatrics 2000;105:41–43.

Jeng SF, Chen LC, Tsou KI, et al. Relationship between spontaneous kicking and age of walking attainment in preterm infants with very low birth weight and full-term infants. Phys Ther. 2004;84(2):159–172.

Keller H, Yovsi RD, Voelker S. The role of motor stimulation in parental ethnotheories: the case of Cameroonian Nso and German women. J Cross Cult Psychol 2002;3:398–414.

Kolobe THA. Childrearing practices and developmental expectations for Mexican-American mothers and the developmental status of their infants. Phys Ther 2004;84:439–453.

Lee LLS, Harris SR. Psychometric properties and standardization samples of four screening tests for infants and young children: a review. Pediatr Phys Ther 2005;17:140–147.

Little RE, Northstone K, Golding J, ALSPAC Study Team. Alcohol, breastfeeding, and development at 18 months. Pediatrics 2002; 109:72–77.

Marsala G, VanSant AF. Age-related differences in movement patterns used by toddlers to rise from a supine position to erect stance. Phys Ther 1998;78(2): 149–159.

McEwen IR. "STEPS" in practice. Phys Ther 2004;84(7):606–607.

Monson RM, Deitz J, Kartin D. The relationship between awake positioning and motor performance among infants who slept supine. Pediatr Phys Ther 2003;15: 196–203.

Mulligan L, Specker BL, Buckley DD, et al. Physical and environmental factors affecting motor development, activity level, and body composition of infants in child care centers. Pediatr Phys Ther 1998;10:156–161.

Rose-Jacobs R, Cabral H, Beeghly M, et al. The movement assessment of infants (MAI) as a predictor of two-year neurodevelopmental outcome for infants born at term who are at social risk. Pediatr Phys Ther 2004;16:212–221.

Sanhueza AD. Psychomotor development, environmental stimulation, and socioeconomic level of preschoolers in Temuco, Chile. Pediatr Phys Ther 2006;18: 141–147.

Smith MR, Danoff JV, Parks RA. Motor skill development of children with HIV infection measured with the Peabody Developmental Motor Scales. Pediatr Phys Ther 2002;14:74–84.

Stanton WR, McGee R, Silva PA. Indices of perinatal complications, family background, child rearing, and health as predictors of early cognitive and motor development. Pediatrics 1991;88(5): 954–959.

Wiepert SL, Mercer VS. Effects of an increased number of practice trials on Peabody Developmental Gross Motor Scale scores in children of preschool age with typical development. Pediatr Phys Ther 2002;14: 22–28.

3

Assessment and Testing of Infant and Child Development

Susan K. Brenneman and Jan Stephen Tecklin

P hysical therapists are important members of the professional team working with disabled children. They must have the skill and knowledge to contribute to the assessment of children, as the assessment process is a professional responsibility that serves the purpose of keeping the therapist's work current. *Assessment* is a continuing process of collecting and organizing relevant information in order to plan and implement effective treatment. It is important for therapists to base their treatment recommendations on appropriate tools of assessment.

A broad view of the child's difficulty and its functional significance is the most important aspect of the assessment. Children may present with a wide variety of behavioral difficulties, and the physical therapist must determine how best to help them function to their fullest potential. Although some aspects of the disability may be better dealt with by other disciplines whereas other aspects are best handled by physical therapists, rigid division of labor among professionals is unwise. Depending on training and competence, the traditional roles of physical therapist, occupational therapist, and speech therapist may overlap. Most physical therapists, however, will be concerned mainly with the child's basic gross motor adaptation to the environment.[1]

The challenge for the physical therapist is to assess accurately and comprehend the significance of any delay that falls outside the limits of normal variability. Knowledge of the normal, orderly sequence of developmental achievement and patterns of integration is the basis upon which

significant deviation in maturation is gauged.[2] The physical therapist, therefore, must be knowledgeable about normal development, as presented in Chapter 2. Understanding this broad developmental scope forms the basis for therapeutic intervention. Developmental milestones present the major clinical parameter of progressive growth and integration in the central nervous system (CNS). It is important to focus on those aspects of motor behavior that are of greatest concern. Because of the focus of their education, most physical therapists' emphasis is on muscles and joints, rather than on total patterns of motor behavior. However, it is not acceptable to deal with isolated parts, such as a foot, gait, or the spine.[1]

A battery of tests is required to assess a child adequately. Developmental assessment tests are only one type of test used. Another category of assessment that is addressed in this chapter is that of functional capabilities. Subsequent chapters will address assessments that are unique to a particular disability, completing the total assessment for the child with that disability.

Purposes of Developmental Testing

Use of developmental tests as screening tools promotes early intervention for deviations from normal growth and development in young children. Early identification of deviations facilitates the provision of anticipatory advice to parents, clinicians, and caregivers for future planning. Early recognition and a focused plan for intervention may prevent severe disability.

Developmental tests can assist in determining a diagnosis. Comprehensive scales, such as the Gesell scale,[3] specify problem areas and indicate whether a developmental problem is likely to include all areas of development or one focal area, such as gross motor development.

Developmental tests also facilitate the planning of a treatment program. Developmental scales provide valuable information about the level of operation of the child or the milestones reached. Developmental tests indicate where treatment should begin, and they provide information by which the progression of a therapeutic regimen can be guided. An explanation of developmental tests and their results may help parents understand the child's limitations—what can and cannot be expected—making it possible to establish common goals and to plan for the future. The results of developmental testing may reveal specific areas of deficit that require additional evaluation to discover the underlying cause of the delay.

Subsequent assessments will reveal the rate and trend of development of a child. After determining goals for the child, tests can be used to monitor progress and determine whether and when the child has achieved the goals. Therapists involved in research rely on developmental assessments to evaluate strategies for treatment and means of intervention. Research continues to evaluate the assessments themselves to ensure their reliability and validity. Developmental assessments, as well as being used as a clinical research tool, can also be used for evaluation of a program.

The ways in which test data are to be used should be determined before testing so that one can avoid the collection of superfluous data and so that all necessary information is obtained. It is a waste of time and effort to perform extensive tests just to be thorough, unless all the information gained will be used. As a therapist becomes skilled in the administration of developmental assessments, the ability to test what is appropriate will improve.

 ### Basic Methods of Assessment

Decisions regarding intervention are usually based on information from various resources. Several basic methods are used to collect information about a child. A questioning mind is important in this process. Therapists must know what questions to ask both of themselves and of others. Guiding questions during clinical observation provides the foundation for all further screening or formal evaluation.

Among the most valuable skills a therapist can possess are the abilities to observe, to be flexible and spontaneous, and to be creative with play and other activities that foster intrinsic motivation in children.[4] Different methods and adaptations must be used for assessment because children are different from adults.

Orientation of the child and the parents to the environment is crucial. Both parent and child must feel comfortable with the therapist and the setting. This orientation is often best achieved by proceeding with the evaluation at a slow pace, and by adapting one's approach according to the reaction of the child.

During the assessment, the therapist needs to take a broad view of the child, whatever the disability. The child should not merely be labeled a "crutch walker," a "hemi," or "clumsy." Rather, the child is a person with a suspected disability, and the therapist's initial task is to be thorough and sensitive in discovering whether a disability or sensorimotor delay exists and what can be done to reduce the effects of the disability.[4]

INTERVIEW

An interview with the child and the parents provides important information about the development of the child. In many cases because of the young age of the child, the interview will be conducted exclusively with the parents. An interview should be friendly and informal rather than impersonal and inquisitive. The purpose of the interview should be clear, and the interviewer should know specifically what information is desired. A skillful and well-directed interview will help fill in the gaps of an assessment. The therapist should be able to determine the area of greatest concern to the parents, and should note the age and circumstances in which the problem was first discovered.

HISTORY

A review of the child's developmental and medical history provides valuable information. A developmental history can be obtained through a questionnaire or an interview. The possible lack of reliability and bias of the parent should be considered in assessing the information gained in the history.

The medical records of a child may provide information regarding precautions, patient health status, previous medical history, suspected diagnosis, prognosis, medications, and other factors impacting the child's health. The therapist should obtain information about the family and its genetic history; the pregnancy, labor, and delivery of the child; and the perinatal and neonatal events. This information will be useful in performing a comprehensive assessment.

CLINICAL OBSERVATION

Assessment begins by observation of the child at rest in various positions and during unstructured movement, as presented in Chapter 4. The therapist should also observe the child interacting with the environment, the child's social responses and communication, and the child's cognition. This observation can be done in a nonthreatening manner while the therapist is talking with the parents and establishing rapport with the child.

TOOLS FOR ASSESSMENT

After interviewing and observing the child, the administration of standardized and criterion- and norm-referenced assessments will yield an overall picture of the child's level of functioning. Tests of developmental assessment will help identify which specific tests of functioning (e.g., goniometry, manual testing of muscles, or assessment of activities of daily living [ADLs]) are needed. Those specific tests and methods used to evaluate disabilities in childhood are reviewed in subsequent chapters.

 Definitions

TERMS FOR UNDERSTANDING STANDARDIZED ASSESSMENTS[5]

An *age-equivalent score* is the mean chronologic age represented by a certain test score. For example, a raw score of 52 on the Bayley Mental Scales represents an age equivalent of 4.5 months. Age-equivalent scores may be especially useful with developmentally delayed children for whom it may be impossible to derive a meaningful developmental index. Age-equivalent scores are easy for parents to understand, but they must be interpreted carefully because they can be misleading. Usually these children have qualitative differences in their behaviors, as well as a wide mixture of successes and failures on developmental tests.

The *criterion-referenced test* is one in which scores are interpreted on the basis of absolute criteria (e.g., the number of items answered correctly) rather than on relative criteria, such as how the rest of the normal group performed. Such tests are usually developed by the teacher or researcher and can be used for research involving a comparison of groups, just as norm-referenced tests are used. Criterion-referenced tests are used to measure a person's mastery of a set of behavioral objectives. The tests represent an attempt to maximize the validity or appropriateness of the content based on that set of objectives. The *developmental quotient* is the ratio between the child's actual score (developmental age) on a test and the child's chronologic age. An example is motor age/chronologic age equal to the motor quotient (MQ).

Norm-referenced or *standardized tests* use normative values as standards for interpreting individual test scores. The purpose of standardized tests is to make a comparison between a particular child and the "norm" or "average" of a group of children. Norms describe a person's test score relative to a large body of scores that have already been collected on a defined population. Examples of norm-referenced tests include the Bayley Scales of Infant

Development,[6] the Denver II Screening Test,[7] and the Gesell Developmental Scales.[3]

The *percentile score* indicates the number of children of the same age or grade level (or whatever is used for a source of comparison) who would be expected to score lower than the child tested. For example, a child who scores in the 75th percentile on a norm-referenced test has done better than 75% of the children in the norm group.

A *raw score* is the total of individual items that are passed or correct on a particular test. On many tests, this will require establishing a basal and ceiling level of performance. The number of items required to achieve a basal or ceiling level varies from one test to another.

Reliability refers to consistency or repeatability between measurements in a series. Types of reliability include interobserver and test–retest. Interobserver reliability describes the relationship between items passed and failed, or the percentage of agreement, between two independent observers. Simply stated, interobserver reliability is an index of whether two different testers obtain the same score on a test. Test–retest reliability is the relationship of a person's score on the first administration of the test to the score on the second administration. Simply stated, this type of reliability determines whether the same or similar scores are achieved when the test is repeated under identical conditions.

Standard error of measurement (SEM) is a measure of reliability that indicates the precision of an individual test score. The SEM gives an estimate of the margin of error associated with a particular test score. For example, a Mental Development Index (MDI), from the Bayley Developmental Scales, at 12 months has an associated SEM of 6.7 points. This SEM means that one is 67% certain that the child's true MDI falls within 6.7 points of the obtained score.

Standard scores are expressed as deviations or variations from the mean score for a group. Standard scores are expressed in units of standard deviation. When using standard scores, information is needed concerning the mean and standard deviation of the standard score.

Validity is an indication of the extent to which a test measures what it purports to measure. *Construct validity* is an examination of the theory or hypothetical constructs underlying the test. *Content validity* assesses the appropriateness of the test or how well the content of the test samples the subject matter or behaviors about which conclusions must be drawn. The sample situations measured in the test must be representative of the set from which the sample is drawn. There are two types of *criterion-related validity*. *Concurrent validity* relates the performance on the test to performance on another well-known and accepted test that measures the same knowledge or behavior. *Predictive validity* means that the child's performance on the test predicts some actual behavior.

Sensitivity can be defined as the ability of a test to identify correctly those who actually have a disorder. High sensitivity results in few false-negative scores.

Specificity refers to the ability of the test to identify correctly those who do not have the disorder. High specificity results in few false-positive scores.

The *positive predictive value* of a test is defined as the proportion of true positives among all those who have positive results. The *negative predictive value* is the proportion of true negatives among all those who have negative screening results.

Guidelines for Selection of Tests

There is no lack of tests that purport to measure motor abilities of children. The problem is not quantity but quality.[8] Careful and knowledgeable selection of tests is, therefore, important. If evaluators are unaware of the strengths, weaknesses, limitations, and restrictions of the tests being used, there is a high probability that an inappropriate test could be used, thus resulting in inaccurate or misinterpreted information.[9] Most published tests have some limitations or restrictions to their use, particularly regarding the ages and populations for whom they were developed and on whom they were standardized. The result of disregarding these restrictions could be the misuse of the test or misinterpretation of the outcomes.

In order to choose an appropriate test, some guidelines by which to evaluate a test are needed. Stangler and associates[10] have proposed six criteria for evaluating a screening test that can be applied to any assessment test: (1) acceptability; (2) simplicity; (3) cost; (4) appropriateness; (5) reliability; and (6) validity. Every test may not fulfill each criterion; however, the test may be used knowledgeably if a therapist is aware of the limitations.

Acceptability is defined as acceptance to all who will be affected by the test, including the children and families screened, the professionals who receive resulting referrals, and the community. *Simplicity* is the ease by which a test can be taught, learned, and administered. *Appropriateness* of screening tests is based on the prevalence of the problem to be screened and on the applicability of the test to the particular population. *Cost* includes the actual cost of equipment, preparation and payment of personnel, the cost of inaccurate results, personal costs to the person being screened, and the total cost of the test in relation to the benefits of early detection.[10] In addition, tests must show both *reliability* and *validity,* as discussed previously.

USING QUESTIONS AS GUIDELINES

A therapist can further ensure appropriate selection of the test by posing several questions regarding the test:

1. *For what purpose will the test be used?*
   * For diagnosis
   * For program planning
   * For research

2. *Who is the child?*
   * Age
   * Suspected diagnosis
   * Presenting disability
3. *What content areas need to be assessed?*
   * Gross motor
   * Fine motor
   * Speech
   * Muscle strength
   * Comprehensive assessment of functional capabilities
4. *What are the constraints for the examiner?*
   * Time
   * Training
   * Space and equipment
   * Money

TEST ANALYSIS FORMAT

The Test Analysis Format developed by Clark and associates is another method for evaluating a test[4] (Display 3.1). An adapted version of this format is used to review the assessment tools in this chapter. After careful consideration of the aforementioned questions and criteria, the therapist

---

DISPLAY 3.1

Test Analysis Format*

Title and authors:

What the test proposes to measure:

Population for whom the test was developed:

Test format
A. Type of instrument
B. Content of test
C. Administration
D. Scoring
E. Interpretation

Include information about the basic type of instrument that is being used—for example, interview or criterion-referenced or standardized test. Briefly discuss the basic guidelines for administration that pertain to the entire test. For example, is information obtained by a report from parents or by presenting tasks to children? How is the test set up? In general, are there time limits for items? Include basic information about procedures for scoring and interpretation.

Advantages of the test:

Disadvantages of the test:

Purchasing information:

References:

*Adapted by permission from Pratt PN, Allen AS. Occupational Therapy for Children. 2nd Ed. St. Louis: CV Mosby, 1989.

should consult sources, including catalogs, books, and other therapists, to locate possible choices. The therapist should be sure to review several manuals thoroughly, to learn the tests and use them, and to evaluate the results.

 ## Overview of Tests

Assessment may be considered in several broad categories. Screening tests are used to identify deficits in a child's performance that indicate the need for further services. Assessments of component functions address specific areas of functioning (e.g., gross motor ability or reflex status). Comprehensive developmental scales evaluate all areas of development. Functional assessments evaluate the essential skills that are required in the child's natural environments of home and school.

The rest of the chapter reviews selected tests that are available. Some of the more widely known standardized evaluative procedures are presented, as are some tests that are not standardized but that have proven useful in clinical practice. The categories just mentioned are used for organization.

SCREENING TESTS

Screening tests are intended to differentiate between those persons who are normal and healthy in a particular respect from those who are not.[9] These tests typically raise more questions than answers, but the questions raised can be used to guide the selection of formal measures for evaluation.

MILANI-COMPARETTI MOTOR DEVELOPMENT SCREENING TEST

The Milani-Comparetti Screening Test was developed by Italian neurologists Milani-Comparetti and Gidoni.[11] The original score form was modified by the staff at Meyer Children's Rehabilitation Institute, University of Nebraska Medical Center.[12] The current test manual, which is in its third edition,[13] was written to provide additional clarification of the testing and scoring procedures, to document reliability data, and to revise the developmental milestones of the original score form to reflect a normative sample.

TEST MEASURES AND TARGET POPULATION   Motor development is evaluated on the basis of a correlation between the functional motor achievement of the child and the underlying reflex structures.[11] The appropriate population for testing comprises children from birth to approximately 2 years of age.

TEST CONSTRUCTION   The items included on the chart were not randomly selected or based on the statistical difference between normal and abnormal. Rather, Milani-Comparetti selected a parameter for study that involved items that were interrelated. This interrelatedness is described by a correlation between functional motor achievement and underlying reflex structures. The parameter chosen is called "standing," and is better translated from Italian to English to mean antigravity control of the body axis. This control includes head control and control while sitting, as well as control while standing. "Standing" was found to be a suitable parameter because it includes as essential and significant components a limited number of specific reactions, such as righting, parachute, and tilting reactions.[11] The original chart used in administering the test was developed after 5 years of experience in a child welfare clinic.

TEST FORMAT

Type   The test is criterion referenced, and the third edition of the test manual provides normative data.[13] The examiner physically manipulates the child for a particular motor response. Parents can provide information if the child is uncooperative.

Content   The illustrated manual developed by Meyer Rehabilitation Center provides instructions for test administration and scoring. The score chart can be reused at successive examinations (Fig. 3.1).

Administration   The original scoring chart developed by Milani-Comparetti has been revised to permit smoother, more rapid administration of the test. All of the original test procedures and scoring mechanisms are retained in the revision; they are simply placed in a different order for more efficient testing.[13] The chart integrates spontaneous behavior and evoked responses in a manner that is easy to follow and is based on the examination sequence. The child should be positioned for only the test items relevant to a particular age, expressed in months. Experienced observers can give the test in 4 to 8 minutes.

Scoring   The chart is a shaded graph indicating the time span during which a reflex or reaction is expected to be present. The child's age in months is used to score each item tested and is placed on the age line at which the child performs. Responses are judged as being either absent or present. Completion results in a graphic profile of the child's motor development (see Fig. 3.1). A narrative summary of additional observations may be included.

Interpretation   Age levels for stages of development are inherent in the test. Normal results are shown by a vertical alignment of notations that are consistent with the child's chronologic age. Motor retardation usually appears as a homogeneous shift of notations toward the left side of the graph, but the vertical alignment is maintained. A wider scattering of findings usually indicates a more

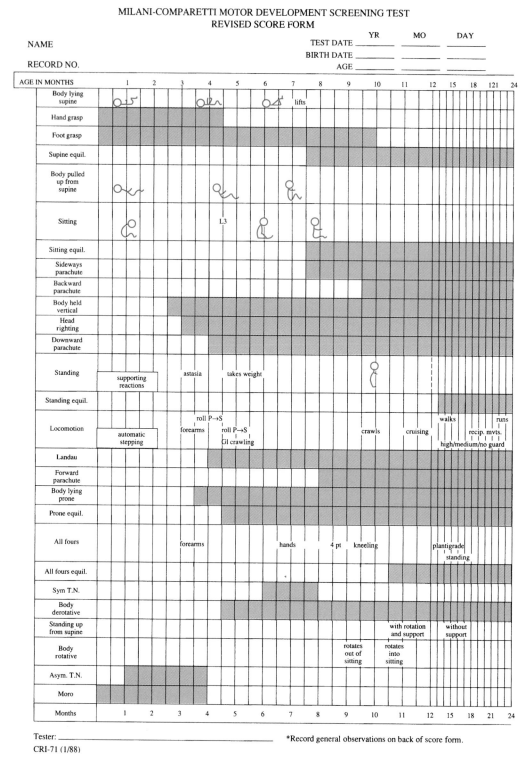

Figure 3.1 ■ Revised scoring chart used for the Milani-Comparetti Motor Development Screening Test. (Stuberg W. The Milani-Comparetti Motor Development Screening Test. 3rd Ed. Appendix B. Omaha: University of Nebraska Medical Center, 1992.)

severe, or possibly more specific, motor dysfunction, such as cerebral palsy.

RELIABILITY AND VALIDITY Interobserver reliability results of one study[14] showed a high percentage of agreement,

ranging from 79% to 98%. The most consistently high level of agreement was noted for active movement and postural control items. Overall, equilibrium reactions demonstrated lower levels of agreement, with standing equilibrium being the lowest scored item at 79%. Test–

retest reliability results[14] showed percentages of agreement ranging from 82% to 100%.

ADVANTAGES This screening test is practical and useful. It can be given quickly and does not require any special equipment or setting. The test can be learned quickly and is easily scored. By providing a developmental profile, it can provide early evidence of neuromotor delay or deficits, possibly indicating a need for further evaluation. The test relies on objective observations, rather than reports by the parents. Normative data have been provided with the third edition. Although the Milani-Comparetti Motor Development Screening Test continues in use, there has been virtually no additional research published in recent years.

DENVER II

The Denver Developmental Screening Test (DDST),[15] developed by Frankenburg and Dodds in 1967, has been widely used by health care providers to screen for developmental delays. It has been adapted for use and restandardized in many countries. Both despite and because of its widespread usage, there have been many criticisms of this tool, prompting a major revision and restandardization of the test. The result is the Denver II test.[7,16]

The reasons for updating the DDST included (1) the need for additional language items; (2) questionable appropriateness of 1967 norms for 1990; (3) changes in items that were difficult to administer or score; (4) appropriateness of the test for various subgroups and for predicting later performance in children; and (5) new methods for ensuring accurate administration and scoring of the test.[17]

The major additions to and differences between the Denver II and the DDST are (1) an 86% increase in language items; (2) two articulation items; (3) a new age scale; (4) a new category of item interpretation to identify milder delays; (5) a behavior rating scale; and (6) new training materials.[17]

TEST MEASURES AND TARGET POPULATION The Denver II screens general development in four areas:

1. Personal–Social: Getting along with people and caring for personal needs
2. Fine Motor–Adaptive: Eye–hand coordination, manipulation of small objects, and problem solving
3. Language: Hearing, understanding, and use of language
4. Gross Motor: Sitting, walking, jumping, and overall large muscle movement

Also included are five items documenting "test behavior" to be completed after administration of the test.

The Denver II is not an IQ test, nor is it designed to generate diagnostic labels or predict future adaptive and intellectual abilities. The test is best used to compare a given child's performance on a variety of tasks to the performance of other children of the same age.

The appropriate population for the test is children between birth and 6 years of age who are apparently well.

TEST CONSTRUCTION AND STANDARDIZATION The Denver II was developed by administering 326 potential items (including several modifications of the original 105 DDST items) to more than 2000 children who were considered to be representative of demographic variables within the Colorado population. Each item was administered an average of 540 times. Composite norms for the total sample and norms for subgroups (based on gender, ethnicity, maternal education, and place of residence) were used to determine new age norms. The *Denver II Technical Manual*[17] contains details of the standardization process.

TEST FORMAT

Type The test is norm referenced, with data presented as age norms, similar to physical growth curve.[16] Subnorms for various subgroups that differ in a clinically significant manner from norms depicted on the reference chart are presented in the technical manual.[17]

Content The Denver II has 125 items arranged on the test form in four sections: Personal–Social, Fine Motor–Adaptive, Language, and Gross Motor (Fig. 3.2). Age scales across the top and bottom of the test form depict ages, expressed in months and years, from birth to 6 years. Each test item is represented on the form by a bar that spans the ages at which 25%, 50%, 75%, and 90% of the standardization sample passed that item.[7] A standardized test kit, forms, and manuals are purchased to administer the Denver II.

Administration This test generally depends on the examiner's observation of the child. Although certain items may be scored based on the verbal report of a parent (as indicated on the test form by an "R"), observation of the particular task is a more reliable method of scoring. Correct calculation of the child's age is important because correct interpretation of test results depends on accuracy of the age. Although the order of presenting the test items is flexible, the items must be given in the manner specified in the manual. The number of items given varies with the age and abilities of the child. The examiner should begin by administering every item intersected by the age line and at least three items nearest to and totally to the left of the age line. Continued testing depends on whether the goal is to identify developmental delays or the relative strengths of the child.[7] "Test Behavior" ratings are scored after the completion of the test.

Scoring Each item given should be scored on the bar at the 50% hatch mark. Items are scored as a pass (P), failure (F), no opportunity (N.O.), or refusal (R).

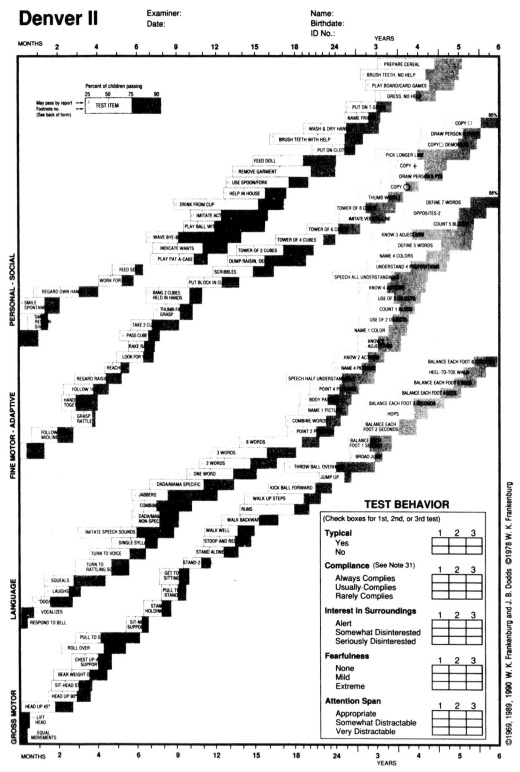

Figure 3.2 ■ Test form for the Denver II Screening test. (Frankenburg WK, Dodds J, Archer P, et al. Denver II Training Manual. Denver, CO: Denver Developmental Materials, Inc., 1992.)

Interpretation   The Denver II identifies the child whose development appears to be delayed in comparison to that of other children and identifies changes in development within one child over time. Individual items should be interpreted first, with the entire test being interpreted last.

Individual items are interpreted as "advanced," "normal," "caution," "delayed," or "no opportunity." The entire Denver II test is interpreted as "normal," "suspect," or "untestable." A child whose scores are interpreted as suspect or untestable on the first test should be screened again before referral for further diagnostic evaluation.

The *Denver II Technical Manual* contains data regarding the results that might be expected so that, in cases when marked deviation is noted, the evaluator may compare with other experiences.

RELIABILITY AND VALIDITY   Thirty-eight children from 10 age groups were tested twice on each of two occasions separated by an interval of 7 to 10 days. The mean examiner-observer reliability was found to be 0.99, with a range of 0.95 to 1.00 and a standard deviation of 0.016. The mean 7- to 10-day test–retest reliability for the same items was 0.90, with a range of 0.50 to 1.00 and a standard deviation of 0.12.[17]

The validity of the Denver II rests on its standardization, not on its correlation with other tests, as all tests are constructed slightly differently.[17]

ADVANTAGES   Administration and scoring is done quickly, and the test is acceptable to both children and parents. The *Denver II Training Manual*[7] gives detailed instructions for proper administration and interpretation of the tests. The *Denver II Technical Manual*[17] contains information on training personnel in the administration of the test and on the establishment of a community screening program. A videotaped instructional program and proficiency test have also been developed for the Denver II. This test is excellent for identifying children who are at risk for developmental problems and for monitoring a child longitudinally.

The authors of the Denver II stress that care should be taken not to use the test to generate diagnostic labels. Rather, it is more appropriately used as a "first step in tackling the problems of early detection, diagnosis, and treatment of developmental deviations in children."[17]

Recent clinical evidence regarding use of the Denver II has suggested that the test may be oversensitive when compared to the Child Development Review when used for children living in rural settings.[18] Hallioglu et al. used the Denver II to predict the likelihood of developing a major neurologic deficit following hypoxic-ischemic encephalopathy. Their results showed that when administered at 6 months of age, the Denver II yielded a very high predictive accuracy (sensitivity, 100%; specificity, 95%) for such major neurologic deficits.[19] Finally, on a less positive note, for the past decade some authors have called into question the cost effectiveness of the Denver II and other testing instruments that require direct examination of the child.[20–22]

TESTS OF MOTOR FUNCTION

The physical therapist is concerned primarily with motor behavior. A large number of assessment tools are available that examine gross and fine motor function. The Movement Assessment of Infants, the Alberta Infant Motor Scale, the Test of Infant Motor Performance, Gross Motor Function Measure and Gross Motor Performance Measure, Peabody Developmental Motor Scales, and Bruininks-Oseretsky Test of Motor Proficiency are described.

MOVEMENT ASSESSMENT OF INFANTS

The Movement Assessment of Infants (MAI) test was developed by Chandler and associates in response to the need for a systematic approach to the evaluation of motor function in infants who had been treated in a neonatal intensive care unit.[23]

TEST MEASURES AND TARGET POPULATION   The test evaluates muscle tone, primitive reflexes, automatic reactions, and volitional movement in the first year of life. The MAI test, when given to infants at 4 months of age, provides an assessment of risk for motor dysfunction. According to the authors, the purposes of the test are to (1) identify motor dysfunction in infants up to 12 months of age; (2) establish the basis for an early intervention program; (3) monitor the effects of physical therapy on infants and children whose motor behavior is at, or below, 1 year of age; (4) aid in research on motor development by using a standard system of assessment of movement; and (5) teach skillful observation of movement and motor development through an evaluation of normal and handicapped children.[23] The test should not be used to identify the cause of any delay or to make a diagnosis.

The appropriate population for testing using the MAI is children ages birth through 12 months.

TEST CONSTRUCTION AND STANDARDIZATION   The MAI test was created because of a need for a uniform approach to the evaluation of the high-risk infant. Over a period of 5 years of development and use, the MAI test was constantly modified and refined in order to improve its accuracy. When initially available, the test was still being developed and was distributed with a request by the authors for more research and revisions. Subsequent research studies[24–28] continue to refine and suggest revisions for the MAI.

TEST FORMAT

Type   The test is criterion referenced. Results are obtained by direct handling and observation.

Content   The test includes 65 items divided into four subtests: muscle tone, primitive reflexes, automatic reactions, and volitional movement. Muscle tone refers to the readiness of muscles to respond to gravity. Primitive reflexes are evaluated from fully integrated to reflex domination of movement. Automatic reactions include righting reactions, equilibrium reactions, and protective extension reactions. Volitional movement includes response to visual and auditory stimuli, production of sound, and typical motor milestones, such as hands to midline, fine grasp, rolling, and walking.

Administration The MAI test is designed for use by physical and occupational therapists, physicians, nurses, psychologists, and others who have experience in the development of infants. Formal training is recommended for examiners using the MAI test in research projects. A pleasant room with open space is needed, but little special equipment is required. The test manual describes the specific equipment needed. The MAI test requires 90 minutes for testing and scoring.

There is no particular order for giving items in the test. Items should be grouped by position in the test, by the amount of concentration required, and by the amount of distress. Observation of spontaneous activity and handling to assess postural tone and evoked behaviors are techniques used in testing.

Scoring Numeric rating scales, which indicate the expected sequence of development, have been designed for each subtest. Each item has its own set of scoring criteria. Scoring should be done only by applying the criteria for the specific item. Scoring of all items must be based on the performance actually observed by the examiner.

Interpretation At this point in the development of the MAI test, no method is available for calculating a developmental score. A profile of a typical 4-month-old child is presented by the authors. This profile can be used for a comparison with the scores received by another child. An overall score indicating "degree of risk" of deviance from the norm is computed. At the 4-month examination, the potential scores range from 0 to 48, with higher sores indicating greater deviance. The MAI authors suggest that children with total-risk scores of greater than 7 be identified as "at risk" in terms of motor development. Recent data on full-term 4-month-old infants indicate a normal range of 0 to 13, with a mean of 6.0 and one standard deviation of 3.[26] An 8-month profile[28] and a 6-month profile[29] have been developed by additional researchers.

RELIABILITY AND VALIDITY The test authors found an interobserver reliability of more than 90%.[23] Another study by Harris and associates showed an interobserver reliability of 0.72 and a test–retest reliability of 0.76.[30] Swanson and colleagues established interobserver reliability at a level of 0.90 agreement.[28] Subsequent reliability study of the standard and revised version of the 4-month MAI resulted in excellent interrater and test–retest reliabilities on both the standard (0.91 and 0.79, respectively) and revised (0.93 and 0.83, respectively) MAI.[31]

Harris and associates studied the predictive validity of the MAI test by comparing test scores in infants at 4 months with specific diagnoses at 12 months of age.[32] They found an 11% rate of overreferrals and no under-

referrals based on the MAI test scores at 4 months. Swanson and coworkers found strong correlations between MAI scores at 4 and 8 months and performance on the Bayley Scales at 18 months.[28] Sensitivity of the MAI was 83% at 4 months and 96% at 8 months. The specificity of the MAI at 4 months was 78%; this decreased to 65% at 8 months.

When working with at-risk infants, the most relevant information is afforded by the positive and negative predictive values of the test, which indicate the likelihood of normal or abnormal outcomes. The negative predictive value of the MAI is 85% and 91% at 4 and 8 months, respectively. The positive predictive value is 59% and 52% at 4 and 8 months, respectively, but is increased to 70% with sequential examinations.[28]

ADVANTAGES The MAI test is a comprehensive and qualitative test of motor development. It is one of few assessment tools that consider the quality of movement. Recent studies show a high predictive validity for the MAI.

DISADVANTAGES The MAI test is lengthy to administer and requires extensive handling of the infant. Normative data are required to strengthen the ability to interpret and score the results. Studies have reported that numerous items have questionable reliability[24,26,30]; therefore, continued reliability and validity studies are needed to improve the usefulness of the MAI as a clinical tool.

Recent publications on the MAI have increased the knowledge of the predictive validity of the test. Salokorpi and colleagues examined the predictive validity of the MAI in identifying the development of neurologic disorders in infants born at extremely low birth weight. They found that for predicting cerebral palsy, the sensitivity of the MAI was 64%; specificity 91%; and the positive and negative predictive values 78% and 84%, respectively. Results for minor neurologic disorders were not as strong.[33] More recently, Rose-Jacobs et al. used the MAI to examine its predictive value on 2-year cognitive and motor developmental status as measured by the Bayley Scales of Infant Development on 134 infants born at term but determined to be at risk for developmental delay. Based upon the total risk scores, the MAI appears to be valid in predicting cognitive functioning falling within normal limits for term infants born at risk of developmental delay.[34]

TEST OF INFANT MOTOR PERFORMANCE

The Test of Infant Motor Performance (TIMP) developed by Campbell and colleagues[35] was developed for use by physical and occupational therapists for the purpose of capturing the components of postural and selective control of movement that are important for function in early infancy.

TEST MEASURES AND TARGET POPULATION The test was constructed to assess specifically the postural control and alignment needed for age-appropriate functional activities involving movement in early infancy. These functions include changing positions and moving against the force of gravity, adjusting to handling, self-comforting, and orienting the head and body for looking, listening, and interacting with caregivers. The items in the test were designed to reflect the full range of motor maturity from 32 weeks' gestational age to 3.5 months after full-term delivery.

TEST CONSTRUCTION AND STANDARDIZATION The TIMP was initially developed by Girolami for use in a controlled clinical trial assessing the efficacy of neuro-developmental treatment in promoting motor development in prematurely born high-risk infants from 34 to 35 weeks' postconceptual age.[36] A revised research version of the TIMP was reviewed by 21 experts in early infant motor development, who suggested additional revision of item descriptors and rated each item for ability to assess developmental change and effects of therapeutic intervention. After administration to a population of 76 infants, including both prematurely born and full-term infants, the data were analyzed for conformity to a Rasch model, resulting in minor changes to the examination. Subsequent research continues to refine and suggest revisions for the TIMP.

TEST FORMAT

Type   The test is criterion referenced. Results are obtained by direct handling and observation.

Content   The current version of the TIMP has 27 observed items and 25 elicited items, six of which are repeated on both sides of the body. The items in the test emphasize the development of head and trunk control, use of handling techniques for precocious elicitation of postural control, and observation of spontaneously emitted behaviors, such as isolated movements of the hands and feet, antigravity movements, and the ballistic and oscillatory movements indicative of developing coordination of activity in muscle synergists and antagonists. According to the test authors, the processes tested by the items include:

1. The ability to orient and stabilize the head in space and in response to auditory and visual stimulation in supine, prone, side-lying, and upright positions, and during transitions from one position to another
2. Body alignment when the head is manipulated
3. Distal selective control of the fingers, wrists, hands, and ankles
4. Antigravity control of arm and leg movements

Administration/Scoring   The test takes from 25 to 40 minutes to administer, depending on the child's abilities, behavioral state, physiologic stability, and level of cooperation. Observed items are rated present or absent on the basis of continuous observation of spontaneously emitted behaviors throughout the course of the examination, including brief periods when the child is observed without handling. These items were designed to represent skills that should be present in a majority of normal full-term infants. Elicited items are administered according to standardized instructions and involve direct handling of the infant. Responses to these items are scored on 5- or 6-point scales that describe specific behaviors to be noted, ranging from less mature or minimal response to mature or full response, as defined individually for each test item.

Interpretation   Preliminary analysis, using a Rasch model, of the items on the TIMP demonstrates that a hierarchy of difficulty exists and adequately separates infants by ability. The scale reflects both maturational level of subjects and degree of medical risk for mortality and morbidity across the range of age from 32 weeks' postconceptional age to 3.5 months postterm.

RELIABILITY AND VALIDITY According to the test author, items are internally consistent (0.97). Intra- and inter-rater reliabilities are high, as demonstrated by Rasch model assessment of 5% or fewer misfitting ratings by each of five experienced examiners on 14 videotaped tests.[37] Construct validity was assessed by determining the test's sensitivity for assessing age-related changes in motor skills and correlation with risk for developmental abnormality. The correlation between postconceptual age and TIMP performance measures was 0.83. Risk and age together explained 72% of the variance in TIMP performance ($r = 0.85$; $p < 0.00001$).[38]

ADVANTAGES/DISADVANTAGES Development of the TIMP has followed recommended procedures for assessing reliability and validity properties. Interested users of the test are encouraged to obtain the published reports of these issues and make informed decisions as to the appropriateness of the test for their population.

RECENT RESEARCH Campbell and Hedeker attempted to find if the TIMP could discriminate among infants with varying degrees of risk for motor developmental morbidity on the basis of perinatal medical complications. They tested 98 infants each week following birth until 4 months of age. They found that the TIMP can discriminate among infants with differing risks for motor developmental delay with particular effectiveness for those with brain injury.[39] Campbell et al. attempted to correlate scores on the TIMP given at 7, 30, 60, and 90 days with percentile ranks (PRs) on the Alberta Infant Motor Scale (AIMS). The authors concluded that TIMP scores significantly predict AIMS PRs 6 to 12 months later. The greatest degree of validity for predicting motor performance on the AIMS at 12 months was shown by the TIMP at 3 months of age and that TIMP score can be used clinically to identify infants likely to benefit from intervention.

Flegel and Kolobe attempted to determine the predictive validity of the TIMP and Problem-Oriented Perinatal Risk Assessment System (POPRAS) to identify motor impairment in older children. The TIMP was performed on a stratified random sample of 35 infants with a mean postterm age of 10 days. These children were tested again using the Bruininks-Oseretsky Test of Motor Proficiency at 5.75 years of age. The TIMP's sensitivity, specificity, and positive and negative predictive values were 0.50, 1.00, 1.00, and 0.87, respectively. The authors concluded that the TIMP and POPRAS may be viable instruments that can be used together to identify infants who are at risk for poor long-term motor performance.[41] Kolobe et al. performed a study similar to the Campbell study previously noted that compared the TIMP to the AIMS, only Kolobe et al. compared the TIMP to the Peabody Developmental Motor Scales, second edition. The findings showed that the TIMP results were similar to results on the Peabody given to children 6 months of age and above. The authors spoke of the need for age-appropriate testing.[12]

ALBERTA INFANT MOTOR SCALE

The AIMS,[43] an observational assessment scale, was constructed by Piper and Darrah to measure gross motor maturation in infants from birth through independent walking. The overall objectives of the AIMS are to (1) identify infants whose motor performance is delayed or aberrant relative to a normative group; (2) provide information to the clinician and parent(s) about the motor activities the infant has mastered, those currently developing, and those not in the infant's repertoire; (3) measure motor performance over time or before and after intervention; (4) measure changes in motor performance that are quite small and thus not likely to be detected using more traditional motor measures; and (5) act as an appropriate research tool to assess the efficacy of rehabilitation programs for infants with motor disorders.

TEST MEASURES AND TARGET POPULATION The test is an assessment of gross motor performance designed for the identification and evaluation of motor development of infants from term (40 weeks after conception) through the age of independent walking (0 to 18 months of age). The focus of the assessment is on the evaluation of the sequential development of postural control relative to four postural positions: supine, prone, sitting, and standing.

TEST CONSTRUCTION AND STANDARDIZATION Test items were obtained through an exhaustive review of existing instruments and descriptive narratives of early motor development. Content validation of the instrument was accomplished through meetings with and a mail survey of Canadian pediatric physical therapists and consultation with an international panel of experts. A total of 58 items were included in the provisional test for reliability and validity testing. Five hundred and six infants, age stratified from birth through 18 months, participated in the reliability and validity testing of the AIMS. Scale properties were examined using the following techniques: multidimensional scaling, item response theory, and Guttman scaling. In addition, 20 infants who were experiencing abnormal motor development and 50 infants at risk for motor disorders were assessed and compared with the results of the full-term sample. The establishment of norms for the AIMS involved data collection on 2200 Albertan infants stratified by age and sex.[44]

TEST FORMAT

Type The test is criterion referenced with normed percentile ranks to allow for the determination of where an individual stands on the ability or trait being measured compared with those in the reference group.

Content The test includes 58 items organized into four positions: prone, supine, sitting, and standing. The distribution of these items is as follows: 21 prone, 9 supine, 12 sitting, and 16 standing. For each item, certain key descriptors are identified that must be observed for the infant to pass the items. Each item describes three aspects of motor performance—weight bearing, posture, and antigravity movements.

Administration/Scoring The administration of the test involves observational assessment with minimal handling required. The surface of the body bearing weight, posture, and movement are assessed for each item. The scoring is pass/fail. Scores in each area (prone, supine, sitting, standing) are summed to one total score of items passed.

Interpretation Age levels for stages of development are inherent in the test. Percentiles derived from the norming sample provide a comparison for monitoring a child's motor maturation over time.

RELIABILITY AND VALIDITY The original sample consisted of 506 (285 male, 221 female) normal infants, age stratified from birth through 18 months. One hundred twenty infants were scored on the AIMS, Peabody, and Bayley Scales for an assessment of concurrent validity, and 253 infants were each scored two or three times on the AIMS to assess the interrater and test–retest reliability of the AIMS.[44] The authors found an interrater reliability of 0.99 and a test–retest reliability of 0.99. Correlation coefficients reflecting concurrent validity with the Bayley and Peabody scales were determined to be $r = 0.98$ and $r = 0.97$, respectively.[44]

ADVANTAGES AND DISADVANTAGES The AIMS provides the ability to detect, as early as possible, any deviations from the norm, thereby permitting early intervention to remediate or minimize the effects of dysfunction. Use of percentile ranking should be done with caution because a small change in raw score can result in a large change in percentile ranking.[45]

RECENT RESEARCH Darrah et al. attempted to ascertain the predictive validity of the AIMS by identifying cutoff points for the 10th percentile at 4 months and the fifth percentile at 8 months and comparing these to the Peabody Developmental Motor Scales and the MAI. The best specificity was shown at 4 months for the MAI and at 8 months for the AIMS.[46] Bartlett and Fanning used the AIMS in an effort to characterize infants born preterm as neurologically "normal," "suspect," or "abnormal" at 8 months corrected age. Physicians evaluated the same group of infants for inclusion in the various categories noted. The AIMS was able to differentiate among these three conditions by virtue of differences in the infant's motor behaviors at the 8 month follow-up.[47] A study by Blanchard et al. examined interrater reliability on individuals using the AIMS and the effect of training on that reliability. Interrater reliability was very good (intraclass correlation coefficients (ICC) of 0.98 to 0.99) before and after training. Training had a small effect on a discreet subscale of the test as well as identifying the children as normal or abnormal based upon motor rankings.[48] Liao and Campbell examined the items on the AIMS by testing 97 infants. They found that gaps existed in several areas at 9 months of age, and also showed a ceiling effect in items for each of the four scoring positions. They concluded that the AIMS was best for infants from 3 to 9 months of age and cautioned about drawing clinical impressions when the precision of the testing is low.[49]

GROSS MOTOR FUNCTION MEASURE

The Gross Motor Function Measure (GMFM),[50,51] developed by the Gross Motor Measures Group, was designed for use by pediatric therapists as an evaluative measure for assessing change over time in gross motor function of children with cerebral palsy.

TEST MEASURES AND TARGET POPULATION The test is designed to assess motor function, or how much of an activity a child can accomplish. It is an evaluative index of gross motor function and changes in function over time, or after therapy, specifically for children with cerebral palsy (CP) or head injuries.

TEST CONSTRUCTION AND STANDARDIZATION The GMFM was developed and tested according to contemporary principles of measurement design through a process of item selection, reliability testing, and validation procedures. The selection of items was based on a literature review and the judgment of pediatric clinicians. Items were judged to have the potential of showing change in

the function of children. All items usually could be accomplished by a 5-year-old with normal motor abilities.[50,51]

TEST FORMAT

Type The GMFM is a criterion-based observational measure.

Content The test includes 88 items that assess motor function in five dimensions: (1) lying and rolling; (2) sitting; (3) crawling and kneeling; (4) standing; and (5) walking, running, and jumping. Because the aim of treatment is to maximize the child's potential for independent function, it was considered important to determine whether a child could complete the task independently (with or without the use of aids), without any active assistance from another person.

Administration/Scoring For ease of administration, the items are grouped on the rating form by test position and arranged in a developmental sequence. For scoring purposes, items are aggregated to represent five separate areas of motor function. Each GMFM item is scored on a 4-point Likert scale. Values of 0, 1, 2, and 3 are assigned to each of the four categories; 0 = cannot do; 1 = initiates (<10% of the task); 2 = partially completes (10 to <100% of the task); and 3 = task completion. A one-page score sheet is used to record results. Specific descriptions for how to score each item are found in the administration and scoring guidelines contained within the test manual.[51]

Interpretation Each of the five dimensions contributes equal weight to the total score; therefore, a percent score is calculated for each dimension (child's score/maximum score × 100%). A total score is obtained by adding the percent scores for each dimension and dividing by five. A "goal score" can also be calculated in order to increase the responsiveness of the GMFM: For this score only those dimensions identified as goal areas by the therapist at time of evaluation are included. (For example, if standing as well as walk, run, and jump activities were treatment goals, the goal total score is calculated by adding the percent score obtained for both these dimensions and dividing by two.[50])

RELIABILITY AND VALIDITY The test authors found intraobserver reliability for each dimension and the total score to range from 0.92 to 0.99 and interobserver reliability to range from 0.87 to 0.99 (ICC).[50] A subsequent study using videotapes resulted in ICCs of 0.75 to 0.97.[51]

Construct validity was assessed by establishing the GMFM responsiveness to change over time.[50] Four hypotheses were tested: (1) that if the measure were responsive, it should be capable of detecting change in children judged by their parents and therapists; (2) that children with "mild" CP should show more change per unit of time than age-matched children with "severe" CP; (3) that younger children with CP should change more than older children in the same time period; and (4) that children recovering from acute head injury should show more change than children with CP. The scale was applied to 140 children of various ages with a wide range of neuromotor disabilities and to 30 healthy preschool-aged children on two occasions separated by a 3- to 6-month interval.

To address the concern of reliable use of the GMFM, the effects of training pediatric developmental therapists to administer and score the GMFM were examined.[51] The authors found that clinicians who attended a 1-day GMFM training workshop improved their scoring reliability significantly when tested using videotaped assessments. To make training more accessible to therapists who are unable to attend a workshop, the Gross Motor Measures Group has developed a videodisc training package that contains videotape examples of children similar to those used for a workshop, along with a written commentary.

ADVANTAGES/DISADVANTAGES   The GMFM is based on comprehensive development and testing and continues to be refined as it is used and studied. Clear administration and scoring guidelines are available, as well as training workshops and videotapes. It is designed to assess function in a quantitative manner, without regard to the quality of performance; therefore, it is likely that the changes detected by the GMFM reflect only part of the "real" change in motor behavior over time. For that reason, the Gross Motor Measures Group developed the Gross Motor Performance Measure.

RECENT RESEARCH   The most significant work on the GMFM in recent years relates to the development of a new version of the GMFM that includes 66 rather than the original 88 test items. The validity, reliability, and responsiveness to change of the new version were reported by Russell et al. The authors reported that the GMFM-66 provided hierarchical structure and interval scoring that provides a better understanding of motor development in children with CP than the older GMFM-88.[52] In more recently published work, Avery et al. presented their conclusions following a Rasch analysis of the original GMFM-88. They agreed with the notion that the GMFM-66 provided a test with interval-level measures that should improve scoring, interpretation, and utility of the previous GMFM-88.[53]

GROSS MOTOR PERFORMANCE MEASURE

TEST MEASURES AND TARGET POPULATION   The Gross Motor Performance Measure (GMPM)[54-56] was developed to evaluate the quality of movement of children with CP. This measure was developed to be used in conjunction with the GMFM. The distinction between the two measures is that the GMFM measures how much a child can do, whereas the GMPM measures quality of performance, or how well a child performs a subset of the same gross motor tasks.

TEST CONSTRUCTION   Principles of contemporary test construction were used in the development of the GMPM: (1) a collaborative multicenter and multidisciplinary approach; (2) use of standard methodologic steps in instrument development; and (3) use of consensual methods with therapists and experts.[54] After reviewing the literature relative to attributes of gross motor performance, definitions were written for 33 attributes. Through nominal group process meetings, the number of attributes was reduced to five and attribute scales were developed. An international panel of experts provided the basis for content validity of the GMPM. Assessment of construct validity and reliability were performed.[55,56] The authors state that further work is required to add to the evidence of the validity and reliability of the GMPM.

TEST FORMAT

Type   The GMPM is a criterion-referenced observational instrument.

Content   The measure consists of 20 items derived from the GMFM, each of which is matched with three designated attributes of performance. Possible attributes to be assessed include (1) alignment; (2) stability; (3) coordination; (4) weight shift; and (5) dissociation. Definitions are provided for each of the attributes.

Administration/Scoring   The instrument can be administered with a minimum of equipment in less than 1 hour, depending on assessor skill, developmental stage, and cooperation of the child. Children are assessed only on items in which they can achieve at least a partial GMFM score, meaning that they can initiate an activity, thereby allowing an assessment of motor quality. Some children have motor performance assessed on all 20 items, whereas others are assessed on as few as two or three items.

A 5-point scale (1 = severely abnormal, 2 = moderately abnormal, 3 = mildly abnormal, 4 = inconsistently normal, and 5 = consistently normal) is used to score each attribute.[37-39] In total, a maximum of 60 GMPM items (three attributes for each of 20 GMFM items) can be scored. The mean score obtained for each attribute is calculated and converted to a percentage. This is referred to as the attribute percent score. The mean of the five attribute percent scores is then computed to give a total percent score.

Interpretation   Scores are used to track change over time and as a result of therapeutic intervention. At this stage of development, the GMPM scores have been correlated with therapists' global ratings of change and with varying severity of disability.

RELIABILITY AND VALIDITY   During development testing the ICCs for the total percent scores varied from

0.92 to 0.96 for intrarater, interrater, and test–retest reliability. The ICCs for the five attribute percent scores varied from 0.90 to 0.97 for intrarater reliability, from 0.84 to 0.94 for interrater reliability, and from 0.89 to 0.96 for test–retest reliability.[55]

Concurrent and construct validity and responsiveness of the GMPM were investigated.[56] Five hypotheses were tested: (1) that children will show different change according to diagnosis; (2) that children with CP will show different change according to severity classification; (3) that younger children with CP will show more change than older children; (4) that GMPM scores will correlate with GMFM scores; and (5) that change scores on the GMPM will correlate with therapist ratings of change. A measure of responsiveness was obtained by relating the variability in test scores of stable children to the scores of children who were identified as changing.

Results show that the GMPM is sensitive to diagnostic differences and severity of CP differences. Correlation between GMFM and GMPM was inconsistent across age groups and diagnoses. Differential change according to age was not supported, nor was the relationship between GMPM scores and therapist ratings of change. Responsiveness to change was supported with changes in GMPM total scores accurately reflecting therapist judgments of overall change in performance in children with CP.

ADVANTAGES/DISADVANTAGES The GMPM represents an important attempt to construct and validate an observational measure of quality of movement for use with children with CP. According to the authors, there are advantages in utilizing an existing measure of gross motor function as a source of observable activities. There are also difficulties, however, for observers to distinguish between motor function and performance in scoring activities.[56] The authors state that "future work may involve refinement of the GMPM measure as a clinical tool and evaluation of observer training techniques to ensure that potential users are capable of learning and applying the instrument to the complex patterns of motor behavior in children with CP."[56] Therefore, the reader who is interested in this instrument should obtain the original reports and contact the authors directly for the most current edition. There has been limited research on the GMPM in recent years. Thomas and colleagues examined the interrater reliability of the GMPM. They determined this reliability to be in the "fair to good" category initially, but it improved over time.[57]

PEABODY DEVELOPMENTAL MOTOR SCALES

The Peabody Developmental Motor Scales (PDMS) and Activity Cards[58] represent a comprehensive program combining in-depth assessment with instructional programming. The test was developed by Folio and Fewell between 1969 and 1982. A new edition, the Peabody Developmental Motor Scales, second edition (PDMS2), was published in 2000.

TEST MEASURES AND TARGET POPULATION The PDMS provides a comprehensive sequence of gross and fine motor skills from which the therapist can determine the relative developmental skill level of a child, identify skills that are not completely developed or not in the child's repertoire, and plan an instructional program to develop those skills.[58]

Children from birth through 83 months of age are candidates for the test. The PDMS can be used with both able-bodied and disabled children.

TEST CONSTRUCTION AND STANDARDIZATION The PDMS was developed to improve on the existing instruments used for motor evaluation. Test items were obtained from validated motor scales, and new items were created based on studies of children's growth and development. The test was standardized on a sample of 617 children considered to be representative of the American population by geographic region, race, and sex. The second edition included new normative data gathered in late 1997 and early 1998. Characteristics of the normative sample are therefore representative of the current U.S. population and have been stratified by age. Studies showing the absence of gender and racial bias have been added. Reliability coefficients were computed for subgroups of the normative sample (e.g., individuals with motor disabilities, African Americans, Hispanic Americans, females, and males) as well as for the entire normative sample. New validity studies have been conducted; special attention has been devoted to showing that the test is valid for a wide variety of subgroups as well as for the general population.[59]

TEST FORMAT

Type The PDMS is an individually administered test. Instructions are provided that enable examiners to give the test to groups of children in a station-testing format. Although the PDMS is norm referenced, it can be used as a criterion-referenced measure of motor patterns and skills.

Content The PDMS is divided into two components: the Gross Motor Scale and the Fine Motor Scale. The Gross Motor Scale contains 170 items divided into 17 age levels. The items are divided into five categories of skills: reflexes, balance, nonlocomotor, locomotor, and receipt and propulsion of objects.

The Fine Motor Scale contains 112 items divided into 16 age levels. The items are classified into four skill categories: grasping, use of hands, eye–hand coordination, and manual dexterity. Norms are provided for each skill category at each age level, as well as for total scores.

The second edition includes six subtests:

1. Reflexes (eight items)
2. Stationary (30 items)
3. Locomotion (89 items)
4. Object Manipulation (24 items)
5. Grasping (26 items)
6. Visual-Motor Integration (72 items)

These subtests are considered in three composite scores:

1. Gross Motor Quotient
2. Fine Motor Quotient
3. Total Motor Quotient

Administration   Both scales can be given to a child in approximately 45 to 60 minutes. Basal (item preceding earliest failure) and ceiling (item representing the most difficult success) rules are provided to eliminate unnecessary administration of items, thereby reducing the time taken for testing.

No specialized training is required to administer the scales and implement the activities, although the examiner should be thoroughly familiar with and have had practice in giving the test. In order to use the PDMS norms for valid interpretation of a child's performance, the scales must be given exactly as specified, including the presentation of materials, verbal instructions to the child, and adherence to basal and ceiling rules.[58] When instructional programming is the main purpose for testing, the directions can be adapted to fit the child's handicapped condition while retaining the intent of the item.

Scoring   The norms of the PDMS are based on scoring each item as 0, 1, or 2. Specific criteria are given for each item, as are the general criteria for the numeric scores. Scores are assigned as follows:

0—The child cannot or will not attempt the item.
1—The child's performance shows a clear resemblance to the item criterion but does not fully meet the criterion. (This value allows for emerging skills.)
2—The child accomplishes the item according to the specified item criterion.

Interpretation   Raw scores are determined and can be converted, by using the norms tables, to normative scores, which included percentile rank scores, standard scores, age-equivalent scores, and scaled scores. After the standard scores have been determined, they may be plotted on the Motor Development Profile. This profile provides a means of visually comparing performance on the Gross Motor Scale and Fine Motor Scale and on the skill categories in each scale. The second edition provides a computer-based PDMS2 Software Scoring and Report System. The software converts item scores or subtest raw scores into standard scores, percentile ranks, and age equivalents, and

generates composite quotients and several other activities including provision of a printed report.

RELIABILITY AND VALIDITY   Test–retest reliability for the total score is 0.99 for both scales. The test–retest reliability is 0.95 for items given on the Gross Motor Scale and 0.8 for the Fine Motor Scale.[58] Interobserver reliability for total scores is 0.99 for both scales. When calculated on an item-by-item basis, the reliability coefficients are 0.97 for the Gross Motor and 0.94 for the Fine Motor Scale.[58] Subsequent research has shown similar results for interobserver reliability.[60] The strong reliability data indicate that the PDMS is a highly stable assessment instrument.

According to the authors, the content validity of PDMS is based on established research on normal children's motor development and on other validated tests assessing motor development.[58] All of the data related to construct validity indicate that the PDMS is a valid instrument for assessing motor development and it can discriminate motor problems from normal developmental variability.[58] Reliability and new validity studies have been performed as part of the new edition. In addition, Provost et al. explored the concurrent validity of the age-equivalent and standard scores of the Bayley Scales of Infant Development II Motor Scales and the PDMS2. With limited exceptions, the results showed poor agreement among standard scores and low concurrent validity between the two instruments.[61]

ADVANTAGES   The PDMS is a standardized, reliable, and valid assessment tool that is both norm referenced and criterion referenced and that allows the scales to meet the needs of various users. The 3-point scoring system enables examiners to identify emerging skills and to measure progress in children who are slow in acquiring new skills. The scales are translated into a specific instructional program—the activity cards. Administration can be adapted for disabled children.

DISADVANTAGES   Several drawbacks of the PDMS have been identified by its researchers and users.[60,62] The Peabody kit does not provide all of the items necessary for administration of the Fine Motor and Gross Motor scales, thus threatening standardization. The test manual does not provide clear criteria for each item for assigning a score of 1, thereby leaving the raters to decide whether there is a resemblance to the criteria needed for a successful performance.

BRUININKS-OSERETSKY TEST OF MOTOR PROFICIENCY

The Bruininks-Oseretsky Test (BOT) of Motor Proficiency was developed by Dr. Robert H. Bruininks and is based partly on the American adaptation of the Oseretsky Tests of Motor Proficiency.[63] Although some similarity exists between the items in the two tests, the revised test reflects important advances in content, structure, and technical qualities.[63]

TEST MEASURES AND TARGET POPULATION The BOT is designed to assess gross and fine motor functioning in children so that a decision can be made about appropriate educational and therapeutic placement. The Complete Battery—eight subtests comprising 46 separate items—provides a comprehensive index of motor proficiency, as well as separate measures of both gross and fine motor skills.

This test is appropriate for children from 4 to 14 years of age. This test is designed for use with normal and developmentally disabled populations.

TEST CONSTRUCTION AND STANDARDIZATION Development and evaluation of the BOT has been extensive. The test has been standardized on a sample of 765 children who were carefully selected on the basis of age, sex, size of their community, and geographic location based on the 1970 Census in the United States.

TEST FORMAT
Type The BOT is norm referenced, and it involves individually administered tasks with direct observation and assessment of a child in a structured environment.

Content Each of the eight subtests is designed to assess an important aspect of motor development. The fine motor tests include coordination of the upper limbs, speed of response, visuomotor control, and speed and dexterity of the upper limbs. The subtests for gross motor skills assess speed and agility while turning, balance, bilateral coordi-

nation, and strength. The relationship of the eight subtests to the composites is shown in Figure 3.3.

Administration The entire battery can be given in 45 to 60 minutes. Two short testing sessions are recommended for young children. A large area, relatively free from distraction, is required. Examiners do not need special training, but they must be familiar with the directions for giving the test. Procedures for administration and scoring of the test are well written and are shown in the manual. All of the materials needed to administer the BOT are provided in the standardized test kit. In addition to the Complete Battery of the BOT, a Short Form is also available. The Short Form is designed for use when a brief survey of general motor proficiency is required, or when a large number of children must be tested in a limited amount of time. Each of the eight subtests is represented in the 14-item Short Form.

Scoring The person's raw scores are recorded during the administration of the test and are converted first to point scores, then to standard scores and approximate age equivalents (see Fig. 3.4 for a sample record form).

Interpretation Tables of norms are provided, and by comparing derived scores with the scores of subjects tested in the standardization program, users can interpret a person's performance in relation to a national reference group.

RELIABILITY AND VALIDITY Test–retest reliability scores average 0.87 for the complete battery. Interobserver reliability is excellent, with the results of two studies showing a reliability of 0.98 and 0.90.[63] The validity of the BOT, according to Bruininks, "is based on its ability to assess the construct of motor development or proficiency."[63] In terms of motor proficiency, as measured

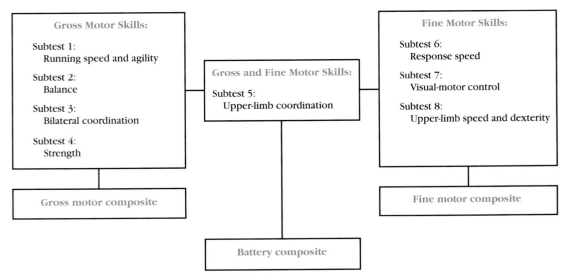

Figure 3.3 ■ Relationship of the eight subtests of the Bruininks-Oseretsky Test of Motor Proficiency to the composite test. (Adapted from Bruininks RH. Examiner's Manual for Bruininks-Oseretsky Test of Motor Proficiency. Circle Pines, MN: American Guidance Service, 1978:12.)

SUBTEST 1: Running Speed and Agility

1. Running Speed and AgilitySF*

TRIAL 1: ___8.7___ seconds　　TRIAL 2: ___7.5___ seconds

Raw Score	Above 11.0	10.9 11.0	10.5 10.8	9.9 10.4	9.5 9.8	8.9 9.4	8.5 8.8	7.9 8.4	7.5 7.8	6.9 7.4	6.7 6.8	6.3 6.6	6.1 6.2	5.7 6.0	5.5 5.6	Below 5.5
Point Score	⓪	①	②	③	④	⑤	⑥	⑦	⑧	⑨	⑩	⑪	⑫	⑬	⑭	⑮

RECORD POINT SCORES FOR COMPLETE BATTERY ▼ ⑧ POINT SCORE SUBTEST 1 (Max: 15)

RECORD POINT SCORES FOR SHORT FORM ▼ □

SUBTEST 2: Balance

1. Standing on Preferred Leg on Floor (10 seconds maximum per trial)

TRIAL 1: ___10___ seconds　　TRIAL 2: _____ seconds

Raw Score	0	13	45	68	9 10
Point Score	⓪	①	②	③	④

④

2. Standing on Preferred Leg on Balance BeamSF (10 seconds maximum per trial)

TRIAL 1: ___2___ seconds　　TRIAL 2: ___4___ seconds

Raw Score	0	12	34	56	78	9	10
Point Score	⓪	①	②	③	④	⑤	⑥

② □

3. Standing on Preferred Leg on Balance Beam—Eyes Closed (10 seconds maximum per trial)

TRIAL 1: ___2___ seconds　　TRIAL 2: ___5___ seconds

Raw Score	0	13	45	6	7	8	9	10
Point Score	⓪	①	②	③	④	⑤	⑥	⑦

②

4. Walking Forward on Walking Line (6 steps maximum per trial)

TRIAL 1: ___6___ steps　　TRIAL 2: _____ steps

Raw Score	0	13	45	6
Point Score	⓪	①	②	③

③

5. Walking Forward on Balance Beam (6 steps maximum per trial)

TRIAL 1: ___2___ steps　　TRIAL 2: ___4___ steps

Raw Score	0	13	4	5	6
Point Score	⓪	①	②	③	④

②

6. Walking Forward Heel-to-Toe on Walking Line (6 steps maximum per trial)

TRIAL 1: [|//bb//b] = ___2___ steps　　TRIAL 2: [|//bb/b] = ___3___ steps

Raw Score	0	13	45	6
Point Score	⓪	①	②	③

①

7. Walking Forward Heel-to-Toe on Balance BeamSF (6 steps maximum per trial)

TRIAL 1: [|//bbb] = ___1___ steps　　TRIAL 2: [|//bb/b] = ___3___ steps

Raw Score	0	13	4	5	6
Point Score	⓪	①	②	③	④

① □

8. Stepping Over Response Speed Stick on Balance Beam

TRIAL 1: Fail (Pass)　　TRIAL 2: Fail Pass

Raw Score	Fail	Pass
Point Score	⓪	①

①

⑯ POINT SCORE SUBTEST 2 (Max: 32)

*SF and the box in left-hand margin indicate short form.

Figure 3.4 ■ Recording form for the eight subtests of the Bruininks-Oseretsky Test of Motor Proficiency. (Adapted from Bruininks RH. Examiner's Manual for Bruininks-Oseretsky Test of Motor Proficiency. Circle Pines, MN: American Guidance Service, 1978:37.)

by the performance of a particular child on a particular day, the BOT is a valid test.[8] The tests discriminate well between nonhandicapped populations and children who are learning disabled or mentally retarded.

ADVANTAGES AND DISADVANTAGES The testing procedure is standardized and scores are normed. This is an excellent instrument for evaluating school-aged children who show motor problems but who do not have an obvious physical handicap. The test is valuable as a research tool because of the ability to differentiate between populations. One of the potential disadvantages of this test is that the space required to administer the BOT may limit its usefulness.

RECENT RESEARCH Duger et al.[64] examined the relationship between motor abilities and various demographic characteristics in 120 school-aged children. The BOT was the instrument used to assess gross and fine motor skills. The study showed that both gross and fine motor skills varied among age, gender, and academic learning and noted that the BOT was a useful device to investigate unexplored aspects of motor development.[64] Maccobb and colleagues[65] tested 76 Irish children at about 9 years of age with the BOT in an effort analyze the division of gross and fine motor subtests. The authors had neonatal and infancy measures for these children and focused upon appropriateness of gross and fine motor tests from the BOT. A prestudy statistical analysis demonstrated poor support for the current division of the BOT gross and fine motor subtests, although the longitudinal study demonstrated continuity in measured motor proficiency from birth through prepubertal years.[65]

COMPREHENSIVE DEVELOPMENTAL SCALES

A basic component of any physical therapy assessment is a developmental evaluation. Developmental testing looks at the whole child, across all areas of development. These developmental areas include language, personal–social, fine motor, gross motor, self-help, and cognitive development. By using a comprehensive assessment, the therapist can develop strategies for treatment that address the whole child.

GESELL DEVELOPMENTAL SCHEDULES

The Gesell Developmental Schedules were developed by Arnold Gesell and his associates beginning in the 1920s. The original test items and procedures have been modified and updated through the years.[3] The Gesell schedules are the basis for future developmental scales.

TEST MEASURES AND TARGET POPULATION The test assesses behavior in the areas of adaptive, gross motor, fine motor, language, and personal–social development. It can be used to identify even minor deviations in children, and to determine the maturity and integrity of an individual's CNS.

The test is appropriate for children ages 4 weeks to 36 months. Additional schedules are available to test children up to 60 months of age.

TEST CONSTRUCTION AND STANDARDIZATION During years of studying a large number of normal children, Gesell mapped the development of fetal, infant, and early behavior in children. The schedules have been standardized by Gesell and associates.

TEST FORMAT

Type The Gesell test is norm referenced and involves direct assessment and observation by the examiner of the quality of and integration of behaviors.

Content Standardized materials can be obtained, or substitutes can be made according to the directions provided.[3] Developmental schedules show the behavioral characteristics of a key age and its two adjacent ages in three vertical columns. The key age occupies the central position (see Fig. 3.5 for an example of the key age of 16 weeks). Horizontally, the characteristics of behavior are grouped according to the five major behavioral fields.

Administration As far as is possible, the standard sequences should be followed in the administration of the examination. The standard sequence differs depending on the maturity and age of the child. Examination procedures used in administering the individual items are well described and should be given in the prescribed, standardized manner[3] (Display 3.2).

Scoring Two columns are provided on the developmental schedules for scoring: H for history and O for observation. Some information is available only by report, particularly when it concerns language and personal–social behavior. A minus sign (−) indicates that the behavior does not occur, a plus sign (+) signifies the behavior occurs, and a plus/minus (±) notation is made if the behavior is just emerging but has not yet been fully integrated. A double plus sign (++) is recorded if a more mature pattern is observed.

Interpretation The final estimate of developmental maturity is based on the distribution of pluses and minuses. This estimate is not achieved merely by adding the pluses and minuses, but by determining how well a child's behavior fits one age level rather than another. In any field of behavior, the child's maturity level is that point at which the aggregate of plus signs changes to an aggregate of minus signs.[3] The examiner assigns a representative age to each of the four areas, as well as an overall age. The ages can then be used to work out a developmental quotient (DQ), which is the age of maturity divided by the chronologic age.[66]

RELIABILITY AND VALIDITY Knobloch and Pasamanick reported that, on more than 100 clinical observations, a correlation of 0.98 was found between the DQs assigned by 18 pediatricians and those assigned by their instructor.[3] Test–retest reliability is reported to be 0.82 for 65 infants examined within 2 to 3 days of the initial date of testing.[3] Correlations between infant and later examinations range from 0.5 to 0.85.[32]

ADVANTAGES AND DISADVANTAGES The test's reliability and validity are generally excellent, and it is a good diagnostic tool. Testing procedures are standardized. This test is especially useful in research.

One disadvantage of the test is that the directions for testing are quite involved and require extensive practice and use in order to ensure valid results.

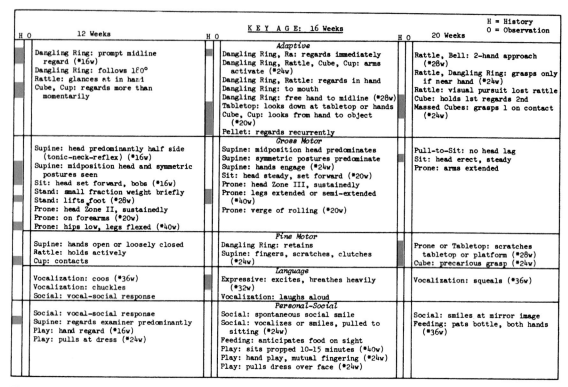

H O	12 Weeks	H O	K E Y A G E: 16 Weeks	H O	20 Weeks	H = History O = Observation
			Adaptive			
	Dangling Ring: prompt midline regard (*16w) Dangling Ring: follows 180° Rattle: glances at in hand Cube, Cup: regards more than momentarily		Dangling Ring, Ra: regards immediately Dangling Ring, Rattle, Cube, Cup: arms activate (*24w) Dangling Ring, Rattle: regards in hand Dangling Ring: to mouth Dangling Ring: free hand to midline (*28w) Tabletop: looks down at tabletop or hands Cube, Cup: looks from hand to object (*20w) Pellet: regards recurrently		Rattle, Bell: 2-hand approach (*28w) Rattle, Dangling Ring: grasps only if near hand (*24w) Rattle: visual pursuit lost rattle Cube: holds 1st regards 2nd Massed Cubes: grasps 1 on contact (*24w)	
			Gross Motor			
	Supine: head predominantly half side (tonic-neck-reflex) (*16w) Supine: midposition head and symmetric postures seen Sit: head set forward, bobs (*16w) Stand: small fraction weight briefly Stand: lifts foot (*28w) Prone: head Zone II, sustainedly Prone: on forearms (*20w) Prone: hips low, legs flexed (*40w)		Supine: midposition head predominates Supine: symmetric postures predominate Supine: hands engage (*24w) Sit: head steady, set forward (*20w) Prone: head Zone III, sustainedly Prone: legs extended or semi-extended (*40w) Prone: verge of rolling (*20w)		Pull-to-Sit: no head lag Sit: head erect, steady Prone: arms extended	
			Fine Motor			
	Supine: hands open or loosely closed Rattle: holds actively Cup: contacts		Dangling Ring: retains Supine: fingers, scratches, clutches (*24w)		Prone or Tabletop: scratches tabletop or platform (*28w) Cube: precarious grasp (*24w)	
			Language			
	Vocalization: coos (*36w) Vocalization: chuckles Social: vocal-social response		Expressive: excites, breathes heavily (*32w) Vocalization: laughs aloud		Vocalization: squeals (*36w)	
			Personal-Social			
	Social: vocal-social response Supine: regards examiner predominantly Play: hand regard (*16w) Play: pulls at dress (*24w)		Social: spontaneous social smile Social: vocalizes or smiles, pulled to sitting (*24w) Feeding: anticipates food on sight Play: sits propped 10-15 minutes (*40w) Play: hand play, mutual fingering (*24w) Play: pulls dress over face (*24w)		Social: smiles at mirror image Feeding: pats bottle, both hands (*36w)	

Figure 3.5 ■ Key age chart from the Gesell Developmental Schedules for a 16-week-old child. (Knobloch H, Pasamanick B. Gesell and Armatruda's Developmental Diagnosis. 3rd Ed. Philadelphia: JB Lippincott, 1974:42.)

DISPLAY 3.2

Prescribed and Standardized Examination Sequence for the Administration of Test Items for the Gesell Developmental Schedules*

Age: 12–16–20 Weeks	Situation No. (Appendix A-4)
Supine	1
Dangling ring	2
Rattle	3
Social stimulation	4
Bell ringing	5
Pull to sitting	6
Sitting supported	50
Chair—tabletop	
Cube 1, (2)	7,8
Massed cubes	11
(Cup)	16
Pellet	18
(Bell)	22
Mirror	24
Standing supported	51
Prone	52

Note: Italicized items appear for the first time in this sequence. Items in parentheses refer to situations sometimes omitted for special reasons.

Normative behavior characteristic of the *key age: 16 weeks* and adjacent age levels is codified by the Developmental Schedule.

*Adapted from Knobloch H, Pasamanick B. Gesell and Armatruda's Developmental Diagnosis. 3rd Ed. Philadelphia: JB Lippincott, 1974:43.

BAYLEY SCALES OF INFANT DEVELOPMENT

The Bayley Scales of Infant Development (BSID) were devised by Nancy Bayley and associates and are essentially a revision of Bayley's earlier work.[6]

TEST MEASURES AND TARGET POPULATION The Bayley Scales are a comprehensive means of evaluating a child's current developmental status at a particular age. The scales are composed of three parts, each of which is designed to assess a separate component of the child's total development. The Mental Scale is designed to assess sensory-perceptual acuities, discrimination, and the ability to respond to these; the early acquisition of object constancy and memory, learning, and problem-solving ability; vocalization and the beginnings of verbal communication; and early evidence of the ability to form generalizations and classifications, which is the basis for abstract thinking. The Motor Scale is designed to provide a measure of the degree of control of the body and coordination of the large muscles and finer manipulative skills of the hands and fingers. The Infant Behavior Record assesses the nature of the child's social and objective orientations toward the environment as expressed in attitudes, interests, emotions, energy, activity, and tendencies to approach or withdraw from stimulation. The appropriate population for the BSID includes infants and toddlers between the ages of 1 and 30 months.

TEST CONSTRUCTION AND STANDARDIZATION The current scales represent the culmination of more than

40 years of research and clinical practice with small children.[6] The test has been standardized on a sample of 1262 children, distributed in approximately equal numbers among 14 age groups ranging from 2 to 30 months. The sample was selected to be representative of the population in the United States, as described in the 1960 United States Census of Population.

TEST FORMAT

Type   The test is norm referenced. Information is obtained by direct observation and interaction with the child.

Content   All materials needed for the test are included in the test kit except for stairs and a balance board. Materials have been selected carefully, and casual substitutions are discouraged. A manual describes the procedures and progression of the test.

Administration   The time required for administration of the BSID varies with the number and complexity of items that must be presented. An average testing time for the Mental and Motor Scales is approximately 45 minutes, with some children occasionally requiring 75 minutes or more. After the child leaves, the researcher completes the Infant Behavior Record.

Changes may be made in the order of presentation, but no changes should be made in the specified manner of presenting test stimuli, as any such change would invalidate scoring. The Mental Scale is usually administered before the Motor Scale because the change in pace from sitting to moving about is the preferred sequence.

Scoring and Interpretation   Individual record forms are used to record a response on the test. For each item, the child is graded as follows: pass (P), fail (F), omit (O), refuse (R), or reported by mother (RPT). Only those items noted as passed are credited in scoring the test, but other results are useful in reviewing the adequacy of the test as an accurate measure of the child's performance. A basal level (item preceding earliest failure) and a ceiling level (item representing the most difficult success) are determined. The raw scores are changed to the Mental Development Index (MDI) and the Psychomotor Development Index (PDI) by consulting the norms for the child's particular age as derived by Bayley. An intelligence quotient should not be computed, because there is no evidence to support the interpretation of a figure of this kind derived from the BSID.[6]

RELIABILITY AND VALIDITY   The reliability of the 1958 to 1960 version of the Mental and Motor Scales, the immediate predecessor of the current version of the BSID, was assessed by Werner and Bayley. Interobserver reliability rates for the Mental Scale and the Motor Scale were 89.4% and 93.4%, respectively. Test–retest reliability was 76.4% for the Mental Scale and 75.3% for the Motor Scale.

The correlation between results derived from the BSID and the Stanford-Binet Scale has ranged from minimal to moderate. Because the scales have limited value as predictors of future abilities, they are most useful in ascertaining the developmental status of a particular child at a particular age.

ADVANTAGES   Collectively, the BSID probably represent the best standardized techniques for behavioral assessment available for infants. These scales have been used extensively as an instrument for research, and are helpful in determining the developmental status of infants at a particular age.

DISADVANTAGES   To administer the Bayley Scales, one must undergo training sessions and be validated as an examiner. The Bayley Motor Scale contains a small number of items for each level of development and omits stages that are generally accepted in the motor developmental sequence. For example, the Bayley Scales contain no items for running or kicking, and a single item incorporates all methods of the progression to walking. The Bayley Motor Scales, therefore, do not provide in-depth motor assessment, nor do they delineate gross and fine motor development.[67]

BAYLEY II

After 24 years of use, the BSID were revised. The changing nature of child care and the accumulation of information regarding children's abilities led to the revision. The *Bayley II*[68] reflects current norms and allows diagnostic assessment at an earlier age.

The fundamentals of the test remain unchanged. It is a norm-referenced, standardized, three-part evaluation of the developmental status of children. The three parts are the Mental Scale, the Motor Scale, and the Behavior Rating Scale (formerly the Infant Behavior Record).

The revisions include (1) revised norms; (2) age range extended downward to 1 month and upward to 42 months; (3) new items measuring a broader skill range; (4) updated stimulus materials that are more attractive and durable; (5) improved psychometric properties and improved clinical utility; and (6) new scoring procedures.

STANDARDIZATION   The *Bayley II* has been renormed on a stratified random sample of 1700 children (850 boys and 850 girls) ages 1 month to 42 months, grouped at 1-month intervals. The children came from all four geographic regions of the United States and closely parallel the 1988 U.S. Census statistics on the variables of age, gender, region, ethnicity, and parental education. These normative data enable the clinician to compare the infant's performance with same-age peers and, if needed, help initiate intervention.

CLINICAL VALIDITY   The Bayley Scales were originally designed to assess normal development in infants and young children. Because the primary use of developmental scales today is with children who are at risk or suspected of being at risk, an effort was made to gather more information about the use of the test with clinical samples. The *Bayley II Manual* contains data for the following groups of children: children who were born prematurely, have the HIV antibody, were prenatally drug exposed, were asphyxiated at birth, are developmentally delayed, have frequent otitis media, are autistic, and/or have Down syndrome.

ADMINISTRATION AND SCORING Although the fundamentals of the test remain unchanged, there have been some changes that facilitate the administration of the test. A second level of scoring was developed that is facet based to match the content areas of cognition, language, personal–social, and motor development. A developmental age for each facet can be obtained. This complements the traditional Mental/Motor Scale scoring.

RECENT RESEARCH Schuler et al.[69] compared scores from the Bayley and Bayley II in a group of high-risk, drug-exposed children. The Bayley was given at 12 and 18 months and the Bayley II at 24 and 30 months. The children scored higher on the Bayley II for both the Mental and Psychomotor parts of the tests.[69] Karmel et al.[70] examined 780 infants including a group of normal children and groups with various at-risk features. The Bayley and Bayley II were given to each child and there were notable differences in the scores with the Bayley II resulting in lower values for all groups including the normals.[70] The reader is also referred to the Provost et al. study described previously under the Peabody Developmental Motor Scales because of the findings related to the Bayley II.[61]

NEONATAL BEHAVIORAL ASSESSMENT SCALE

The Neonatal Behavioral Assessment Scale (NBAS), third edition,[71] was first developed by T. Berry Brazelton and published in 1973[72] with the help of many people who collaborated directly and indirectly. The second edition contains some additions and a few revisions designed to allay some of the criticisms of the first edition, as well as to restate some of the original purposes of the scale.

TEST MEASURES AND TARGET POPULATION The NBAS closely approximates a developmental evaluation of the neonate. It is intended to be a means of scoring interactive behavior rather than a formal neurologic evaluation, although the neurologic implications of such a scale make inclusion of some basic neurologic items necessary. The evaluation is primarily behavioral and is an attempt to score the infant's available responses to the environment and, indirectly, the infant's effect on the environment.[71]

The NBAS is appropriate for the testing of children ages newborn to 1 month of age. It has been used to study both normal and premature infants, as well as infants from different national and ethnic groups.

TEST CONSTRUCTION AND STANDARDIZATION No formal standardization sample has been used in the development of the NBAS. As yet, the normative base for the NBAS is relatively limited.[71] Researchers using the scale have provided their own normative data with the population for which they were using the NBAS.

TEST FORMAT

Content The score sheet includes 28 behavioral items and nine supplementary items (Display 3.3) that assess the neonate's capacity to organize states of consciousness, habituate reactions to disturbing events, attend to and process simple and complex events in the environment, control motor activity and postural tone while attending to these environmental events, and perform integrated motor acts.[71,73] The supplementary items have been developed for use with preterm, sick, fragile, and stressed infants, as well as to capture some of the more general characteristics of the infant's behavior in addition to the response of the examiner to the infant.[71] The test also includes 20 elicited (neurologic) responses (Display 3.4) that are based on Prechtl and Beintema's neurologic assessment of the infant.[74]

Administration An important consideration throughout the tests is the state of consciousness or "state" of the infant,[71] classified according to six stages: (1) deep sleep; (2) light sleep; (3) drowsy or semidozing; (4) alert; (5) active; and (6) crying. The examiner attempts to bring the baby through an entire spectrum of states in each examination.

The examination usually takes 20 to 30 minutes and involves about 30 different tests and maneuvers. The examiner tries to elicit the best performance rather than an average performance from the infant; therefore, the examiner attempts to verify that the infant is incapable of a better response. The examiner must be flexible in the sequence of item administration to allow most of the items to be given at a time when the best performance will be achieved. Use of the NBAS requires direct training by experienced examiners. There are seven established reliability training centers.[71]

Scoring Most of the items are scored at the end of the examination. The elicited neurologic items are scored on a 3-point scale designating low, medium, or high intensity of response. Asymmetry of response can also be noted. The behavioral items are each rated on a 9-point scale, with most of the items rated as optimal at the midpoint of the scale. A 9-point scale allows for a range of behavior that can bring out subtle differences among different groups of babies.

Interpretation The NBAS does not yield an overall score for an infant. Rather, the results of the test are the

>> **DISPLAY 3.3**

Neonatal Behavioral Assessment Scale (NBAS)*

1. Response decrement to light (1,2)
2. Response decrement to rattle (1,2)
3. Response decrement to bell (1,2)
4. Response decrement to tactile stimulation of foot (1,2)
5. Orientation—inanimate visual (4,5)
6. Orientation—inanimate auditory (4,5)
7. Orientation—inanimate visual and auditory (4,5)
8. Orientation—inanimate visual (4,5)
9. Orientation—animate auditory (4,5)
10. Orientation—animate visual and auditory (4,5)
11. Alertness (4 only)
12. General tonus (4,5)
13. Motor maturity (4,5)
14. Pull to sit (4,5)
15. Cuddliness (4,5)
16. Defensive movements (3,4,5)
17. Consolability (6 to 5,4,3,2)
18. Peak of excitement (all states)
19. Rapidity of build-up (from 1,2 to 6)

20. Irritability (all awake states)
21. Activity (3,4,5)
22. Tremulousness (all states)
23. Startle (3,4,5,6)
24. Lability of skin color (from 1 to 6)
25. Lability of states (all states)
26. Self-quieting activity (6,5 to 4,3,2,1)
27. Hand-to-mouth facility (all states)
28. Smiles (all states)

Supplementary Items
29. Alert responsiveness (4 only)
30. Cost of attention (3,4,5)
31. Examiner persistence (all states)
32. General irritability (5,6)
33. Robustness and endurance (all states)
34. Regulatory capacity (all states)
35. State regulation (all states)
36. Balance of motor tone (all states)
37. Reinforcement value of infant's behavior (all states)

*The behavior scale of the NBAS identifies the items examined and, in parentheses, the numbers of the appropriate states in which the assessment of each item on the scale can be made.

---

scores for each of the items. The mean is related to the expected behavior of an "average" full-term, normal, white infant weighing 7 lb or more whose mother has not received more than 100 mg of barbiturates and 50 mg of other sedative drugs before delivery; whose Apgar scores

were no less than 7 at 1 minute, 8 at 5 minutes, and 8 at 15 minutes after delivery; who needed no special care after delivery; and who had an apparently normal intrauterine experience.[72]

RELIABILITY AND VALIDITY The reliability of independent testers trained at the same time is reported to range from 0.85 to 1.[25] Testers can be trained to a 0.9 criterion of reliability, and the level of reliability is still determined to be 0.9 or higher for a prolonged time.[71]

According to the author, test–retest reliability must be viewed in terms of the kinds of questions being posed when the NBAS is employed. It is clear that the standard psychometric criterion of a Pearson product moment correlation coefficient will yield low to moderate day-to-day stabilities. Conversely, an individually derived measure of day-to-day stability reveals quite a different and much more variable picture. Patterns of score changes over repeated examinations may well reveal important characteristics about individual infants and about groups of infants.[71]

In terms of validity, studies have shown that individual differences, as measured by the NBAS, are related to later individual differences.[71,72]

ADVANTAGES The NBAS is an effective predictor of neurologic problems, as well as an effective teaching tool for parents. It is a valuable technique for differentiating the behavioral characteristics of normal neonates for research and clinical purposes.

>> **DISPLAY 3.4**

Elicited Responses of the Neonatal Behavioral Assessment Scale*

1. Plantar grasp
2. Hand grasp
3. Ankle clonus
4. Babinski's response
5. Standing
6. Automatic walking
7. Placing
8. Incurvatum
9. Crawling
10. Glabella
11. Tonic deviation of head and eyes
12. Nystagmus
13. Tonic neck reflex
14. Moro reflex
15. Rooting (intensity)
16. Sucking (intensity)
17–20. Passive movements: right arm; left arm; right leg; left leg

*Items the examiner attempts to elicit during the examination.

DISADVANTAGES Among the disadvantages of the NBAS is that it is a difficult test to learn, and the tester must guard against overinterpretation when discussing test results with physicians and parents.[25] When the time required for scoring, interpretation of the test, and writing of the report is considered, the test becomes a lengthy process. The relationship between results on the NBAS and those derived from later functional testing has yet to be demonstrated.

RECENT RESEARCH Ohgi et al.[75] used the NBAS to assess the likelihood of developmental disability occurring in 209 low-birth-weight or premature infants at 5 years of age. These infants were examined using the NBAS at 36 to 38 (NBAS36), 40 to 42 (NBAS40), and 44 to 46 weeks (NBAS44) of postmenstrual age, and their developmental outcome was measured using standardized assessments at 5 years. Motor, orientation, and reflex scores from the NBAS were useful in predicting the outcomes for infants grouped in the normal, mild disability, and severe disability categories at 5 years of age.[75] An interesting, and some might say surprising, finding was determined by Myers and colleagues when they studied 137 infants assessed using the NBAS. The infants were born to three groups of low-income mothers—cocaine and poly–drug-using mothers in a drug user treatment group ($n = 76$) and in a treatment rejecter group ($n = 18$), and a nonuser group ($n = 43$)—were examined at 2 days and 2 to 4 weeks. No group differences could be identified by the NBAS between drug-exposed and nonexposed infants at either testing session.[75]

EARLY INTERVENTION DEVELOPMENTAL PROFILE

The Early Intervention Developmental Profile (EIDP) was developed by an interdisciplinary team at the University of Michigan under the direction of Schafer and Moersch.[77]

TEST MEASURES AND TARGET POPULATION The EIDP is an infant assessment-based programming instrument made up of six scales that provide developmental norms and milestones in the following areas: perceptual or fine motor, cognition, language, social or emotional, self-care, and gross motor development. The profile should not be used to diagnose handicapping conditions, nor does it supply data that can predict future capabilities or handicaps. However, by examining a child's skills in six different areas, the profile helps describe the child's comprehensive function, identifying relative strengths and weaknesses.[77]

Designed for children from birth to 36 months, the EIDP yields information that can be used to plan comprehensive developmental programs for children with all types of handicaps who function below the 36-month level.

TEST CONSTRUCTION AND STANDARDIZATION Test items were selected from well-known, standardized instruments for the evaluation of infants, including general developmental scales, motor scales, and language scales. Some original profile items were based on current developmental theories. The profile has not been standardized. Assignment of items to specific age ranges was based on standardizations or research from other instruments. The age-norm suggestions derived from the original source (i.e., Piaget) were used for original items.

TEST FORMAT

Content Each section of the profile is divided into age groupings, each of which covers 3 months within the first year of life and 4 months within the second and third years. No consistent attempt was made to arrange items within age ranges in a developmental sequence.

The gross motor scale reflects a body of knowledge that constitutes the basis for the current treatment of cerebral palsy in infants and young children (e.g., Bobath and Fiorentino). There is an emphasis on neurodevelopmental theories of reflex development and integration of primitive reflexes into higher order righting reactions, protective responses, and equilibrium responses.[77]

The cognitive scale reflects the theories of Piaget, whereas, the social–emotional scale reflects current theory on the emotional attachment between the mother and child and the child's gradual acquisition of ego functions during the first 36 months of life.[77]

Administration The profile was designed to be given by a multidisciplinary team that includes a psychologist or special educator, a physical or occupational therapist, and a speech and language therapist. Each member of the team can learn to give the entire profile, rather than being limited to only certain scales by one's chosen discipline. Administration of test items is thoroughly explained in the evaluation manual. References for each item are well documented. Test items are given until the child fails either six consecutive items or all items in two consecutive age ranges. The total time required for administration of the test may vary from 30 minutes to several hours. The materials needed for administration are described in the manual and should be available.

Scoring Items are scored as a "pass" (P) when the criteria are met; however, when the child's behavior on an item does not meet scoring criteria, it is scored as a "fail" (F). A score of "pass-fail" (PF) indicates the emergence of a skill. An item is scored as "omitted" (O) when the evaluator must exclude an item.

Interpretation Ceiling levels (the age range containing the child's highest passed item) and basal levels (the age range preceding the child's earliest failure) are determined for each section. The ceiling and basal levels define a range of items on which the child's performance is inconsistent, which will provide the focus for programming efforts. Age levels for each area of performance are recorded on a composite table to yield a profile. Each testing booklet can be used for several subsequent evaluations, with the composite profile recorded with a different color or line notation for each item to document the child's progress.

RELIABILITY AND VALIDITY Interobserver and test–retest reliability values were assessed using small sample sizes; however, the results were generally excellent. Interobserver reliability ranged from a low of 80% to a high of 97%. Test–retest reliability ranged from 93% to 98%.[51]

Significant correlations were found between children's scores on the EIDP, the BSID, the Vineland Society Maturity Scale, and clinical motor evaluations. Thus, strong validity of content was found for the EIDP.

ADVANTAGES AND DISADVANTAGES The combined results of the six scales provide a comprehensive record of the child's skills. Moreover, the completed profile lends itself well to the formulation of individualized objectives. The third volume of *Developmental Programming for Infants and Children: Stimulation Activities* is a comprehensive collection of sequenced activities designed to complement the Developmental Profile.[78] The EIDP reflects current developmental theory in the motor, cognitive, and social areas and is best used as a clinical instrument for interdisciplinary team planning.

The sample sizes for reliability and validity testing were small. Thus, the EIDP cannot be used for diagnosis or for predicting future capabilities or handicaps.

ASSESSMENT OF FUNCTIONAL CAPABILITIES

Functional capabilities are viewed as skills that are essential within the child's natural environments of home and school. According to Haley,[79] the concept of disability and functional assessment incorporates the following key concepts:

1. A child may have serious motor impairments that are not always reflected by the level of functional limitation or disability.
2. Functional deficits may or may not lead to a restriction in social activities and important childhood roles.
3. Environmental factors, family expectations, and contextual elements of functional task requirements play an important role in the eventual level of disability and handicap of the child.

Comprehensive functional assessment instruments contain mobility, transfer, self-care, and social function items; they include measurement dimensions of assistance and adaptive equipment; and they incorporate developmental stages of functional skill attainment.[80] Pediatric physical therapists have long expressed the need for a functional approach to the assessment of children with movement disorders.

PEDIATRIC EVALUATION OF DISABILITY INVENTORY

The Pediatric Evaluation of Disability Inventory (PEDI)[81] was developed to meet the need for a reliable, valid, and norm-referenced instrument for assessing functional status in infants and young children by physical therapists and other rehabilitation personnel. The PEDI was designed to be a comprehensive yet clinically feasible instrument that can be used for clinical assessment, program monitoring, documentation of functional progress, and clinical decision making.[82]

TEST MEASURES AND TARGET POPULATION The PEDI measures both the capability and performance of functional activities in three content domains: (1) self-care; (2) mobility; and (3) social function. Capability is measured by the identification of functional skills for which the child has demonstrated mastery and competence (Display 3.5). Functional performance is measured by the level of caregiver assistance and environmental modifications needed to accomplish major functional activities (Display 3.6).

Children ranging in age from 6 months to 7.5 years may be tested. The PEDI is primarily designed for the evaluation of young children, but it can be used to evaluate older children whose functional abilities fall below those expected of 7.5-year-old children with no disabilities.

TEST CONSTRUCTION AND STANDARDIZATION The content and measurement scales of the PEDI underwent numerous revisions prior to the publication of the final version. Initially, content was identified based on the available literature, previous functional and adaptive tests, and the clinical experience of the authors and consultant involved. A Development Edition was field-tested on more than 60 handicapped children and their families. The scales' comprehensiveness and representativeness was evaluated by external content experts. Revisions based on the field testing and the content validity study were then incorporated into the final PEDI items to establish the Standardization Version.

Normative data for the PEDI were gathered from 412 children and families distributed throughout Massachusetts, Connecticut, and New York. The sample closely approximated most of the demographic characteristics of the U.S. population as defined by the 1980 U.S. Census data. Additionally, three groups of children (totaling 102) with disabilities made up clinical samples for validation purposes.

TEST FORMAT

Type The test is norm referenced, and it can also be used as a criterion-referenced measure of functional status.

Content The PEDI includes three sets of measurement scales: Functional Skills, Caregiver Assistance, and

>> **DISPLAY 3.5**

Functional Skills Content of the Pediatric Evaluation of Disability Inventory*

Self-Care Domain	Mobility Domain	Social Function Domain
Types of food textures	Toilet transfers	Comprehension of word meaning
Use of utensils	Chair/wheelchair transfers	Comprehension of sentence complexity
Use of drinking containers	Car transfers	Functional use of expressive communication
Toothbrushing	Bed mobility/transfers	Complexity of expressive communication
Hairbrushing	Tub transfers	Problem resolution
Nose care	Method of indoor locomotion	Social interactive play
Handwashing	Distance/speed indoors	Peer interactions
Washing body and face	Pulls/carries objects	Self-information
Pullover/front-opening garments	Method of outdoor locomotion	Time orientation
Fasteners	Distance/speed outdoors	Household chores
Pants	Outdoor surfaces	Self-protection
Shoes/socks	Upstairs	Community function
Toileting tasks	Downstairs	
Management of bladder		
Management of bowel		

*Used with permission from Haley SM, Coster WJ, Ludlow LH, et al. Pediatric Evaluation of Disability Inventory (PEDI): Development, Standardization and Administration Manual. Boston: New England Medical Center Hospital and PEDI Research Group, 1992:13.

Modifications. These scales are used to assess the three content areas of self-care, mobility, and social function. The Functional Skills Scales were designed to reflect meaningful functional units within a given activity. The Caregiver Assistance Scales measure disability of children with respect to the amount of help they need to carry out functional activities. The Modifications section is not a true measurement scale, but rather a frequency count of the type and extent of environmental modifications the child depends on to support functional performance.

Administration The PEDI can be administered by clinicians and educators who are familiar with the child, or by structured interview of the parent. The PEDI's focus on typical performance requires the respondent to have had the opportunity to observe the child on several different occasions in order to gain an accurate picture of the child's typical performance.[81] Administration guidelines, criteria for scoring each item, and examples are provided in the accompanying manual. Specific training is required to ensure that examiners are knowledgeable about the item criteria used in the instrument and the methods employed in determining the child's level of assistance.

Scoring Scores are recorded in a booklet that also contains a summary score sheet that is used to construct a profile of the child's performance across the different domains

>> **DISPLAY 3.6**

Complex Activities Assessed with Caregiver Assistance and Modification Scales*

Self-Care Domain	Mobility Domain	Social Function Domain
Eating	Chair/toilet transfers	Functional comprehension
Grooming	Car transfers	Functional expression
Bathing	Bed mobility/transfers	Joint problem solving
Dressing upper body	Tub transfers	Peer play
Dressing lower body	Indoor locomotion	Safety
Toileting	Outdoor locomotion	
Bladder management	Stairs	
Bowel management		

*Used with permission from Haley SM, Coster WJ, Ludlow LH, et al. Pediatric Evaluation of Disability Inventory (PEDI): Development, Standardization and Administration Manual. Boston: New England Medical Center Hospital and PEDI Research Group, 1992:13.

and scales. A summary of rating criteria for the three sets of measurement scales is provided in Display 3.7.

Interpretation The PEDI provides two types of transformed summary scores: normative standard scores and scaled scores. Separate summary scores are calculated for Functional Skills and for Caregiver Assistance in each of the three domains, thus yielding six normative standard scores and six scaled scores. Normative standard scores are transformed scores that take into account the child's chronologic age, thereby providing an indication of the child's relative standing in relation to age expectations for functional skills and performance. Scaled scores, distributed along a scale from 0 to 100, provide an indication of the performance of the child along the continuum of relatively difficult items in a particular domain on the PEDI. Scaled scores are not adjusted for age and, therefore, can be used to describe the functional status of children of all ages. In addition, frequency totals of the four levels of modifications can be calculated. These totals provide descriptive information on the frequency and the degree of modifications a child uses.

RELIABILITY AND VALIDITY The internal consistency reliability coefficients obtained from the normative sample range between 0.95 and 0.99. Inter-interviewer reliability in the normative sample was very high (ICCs = 0.96 to 0.99) for the Caregiver Assistance Scales. Agreement on Modifications was also quite high, except for Social Function, where it was still adequate (ICC = 0.79).[81] Further studies are planned to assess test–retest reliability and interobserver reliability between rehabilitation team members.

Content validity was examined using a panel of 31 experts[82] to validate and confirm the functional content of the PEDI. Data related to construct validity and concurrent validity[54] indicate that the PEDI is a valid measure of pediatric function. Preliminary data also support the discriminant and evaluative validity of the PEDI.[81]

ADVANTAGES AND DISADVANTAGES The PEDI represents a standardized clinical instrument for pediatric functional assessment. Rigorous methodology during its development has resulted in an instrument that is both valid and reliable. The authors welcome input and feedback from users of the PEDI that will be useful to the authors as updated and revised versions are made available in the future.

RECENT RESEARCH The PEDI has gained great acceptance in recent years both in the United States and in other countries.[83–85] In addition, the PEDI has been shown to be a discriminating tool in children with acquired brain injury[86] and spina bifida,[87] and to evaluate functional aspects of using a Lycra garment in children with CP and Duchenne dystrophy.[88]

FUNCTIONAL INDEPENDENCE MEASURE FOR CHILDREN

The Functional Independence Measure for Children (WeeFIM) builds on the conceptual framework and is an adaptation of the Functional Independence Measure (FIM) for adults of the Uniform Data System for Medical Rehabilitation (UDS).[89] The WeeFIM was developed to assess and track development of functional independence in children with disabilities. Key characteristics of the WeeFIM are the minimal data set, emphasis on consistent actual patient performance, and use by any trained health or educational professional.

TEST MEASURES AND TARGET POPULATION The WeeFIM consists of 18 items within six domains—self-care, sphincter control, mobility, locomotion, communication, and social cognition—and is designed for use

---

>> **DISPLAY 3.7**

Rating Criteria for the Three Types of Measurement Scales*

Part I: Functional Skills	Part II: Caregiver Assistance	Part III: Modification
(197 discrete items of functional skills) Self-care, Mobility, Social function 0 = unable, or limited in capability to perform item in most situations 1 = capable of performing item in most situations, or item has been previously mastered and functional skills have progressed beyond this level	(20 complex functional activities) Self-care, Mobility, Social function 5 = Independent 4 = Supervise/Prompt/Monitor 3 = Minimal Assistance 2 = Moderate Assistance 1 = Maximal Assistance 0 = Total Assistance	(20 complex functional activities) Self-care, Mobility, Social function N = No Modifications C = Child oriented (non-specialized) R = Rehabilitation Equipment E = Extensive Modifications

*Used with permission from Haley SM, Coster WJ, Ludlow LH, et al. Pediatric Evaluation of Disability Inventory (PEDI): Development, Standardization and Administration Manual. Boston: New England Medical Center Hospital and PEDI Research Group, 1992:16.

with children between the ages of 6 months and 7 years and individuals of all ages with developmental and mental disabilities of ages less than 7 years.

TEST CONSTRUCTION AND STANDARDIZATION To develop the appropriate levels of performance of daily living tasks for children for the WeeFIM, an interdisciplinary team, knowledgeable in the use of traditional developmental scales, reviewed developmental pediatric, developmental psychological, pediatric physical, occupation, speech-language, and preschool educational scales. Pilot testing was performed with two groups of well children in Buffalo and Chicago ($n = 111$ and $n = 170$, respectively).[90] Content validity was assessed and reported by McCabe and Granger.[91] Additionally, two groups of children (totaling 58) with motor impairments and a group of 66 survivors of extreme prematurity (less than 29 weeks' gestation) composed clinical samples for validation purposes.

TEST FORMAT

Type The test is criterion based and is a descriptive measure of the caregiver and special resources that are required because of functional limitations.

Content The test consists of six domains as shown in Display 3.8.

Administration/Scoring Assessment is based on direct observation of the child by an individual clinician or a team or by interviewing an informant who is knowledgeable about the usual and consistent performance of the child. Learning to use the WeeFIM correctly is important and is facilitated by a guide to its use,[89] an introductory videotape,[92] and training workshops. Performance of the child on each of the items is assigned to one of seven levels of an ordinal scale that represents the range of function from complete and modified independence (levels 7 and 6) without a helping person to modified and complete dependence (levels 5 to 1) with a helping person (Display 3.9).

Interpretation The WeeFIM measures disability, not impairment. The focus of the assessment is on the impact that a disorder has on the degree of independent performance of daily living tasks. The WeeFIM is a minimum data set and is not intended to supplant detailed clinical assessment of component parts of motor, sensory, cognitive, or communicative abilities. It is designed to track functional status and outcomes over time both in preschool years and in the early elementary school years.

RELIABILITY AND VALIDITY The test–retest reliability coefficients (Pearson's correlation) for the six domains range from $r = 0.83$ for sphincter control to $r = 0.99$ for mobility, communication, and social cognition. Interrater

reliability coefficients (Pearson's correlation) range from 0.74 for mobility to 0.96 for communication and social cognition. Test–retest and interrater reliability for the total WeeFIM are 0.99 and 0.95, respectively. Data related to construct and discriminative validity[57] indicate that the WeeFIM is a valid measure of disability related to func-

---

>> **DISPLAY 3.8**

WeeFIM Domains

Self-Care
1. Eating
2. Grooming
3. Bathing
4. Dressing—upper body
5. Dressing—lower body
6. Toileting

Sphincter Control
7. Bladder management
8. Bowel management

Mobility
9. Transfer chair, wheelchair
10. Transfer toilet
11. Transfer tub

Locomotion
12. Crawl/walk/wheelchair
13. Stairs

Communication
14. Comprehension
15. Expression

Social Cognition
16. Social interaction
17. Problem solving
18. Memory

>> **DISPLAY 3.9**

Levels of Function for the WeeFIM

No Helper
  7 = Complete independence (timely, safely)
  6 = Modified independence (device needed)

Helper
Modified dependence
  5 = Supervision
  4 = Minimal assist (child = 75%–99%)
  3 = Moderate assist (child = 50%–74%)
Complete dependence
  2 = Maximal assistance (child = 25%–49%)
  1 = Total assistance (child = 0%–24%)

tional independence. Additional work with the WeeFIM including a normative sample ($n = 413$) and samples of children with a variety of developmental disabilities contribute to the validation of the measure.[93–98]

ADVANTAGES AND DISADVANTAGES The WeeFIM can be used by health and educational providers, resulting in a common language to describe the child's ability to cope with daily living tasks and to set habilitation goals across health, educational, and community settings.

GROSS MOTOR FUNCTION CLASSIFICATION SYSTEM FOR CEREBRAL PALSY

The Gross Motor Function Classification System for Cerebral Palsy (GMFCS), developed by Palisano and colleagues in 1997, attempts to classify motor function in children with CP into one of five clinically meaningful levels.[99]

TEST MEASURES AND TARGET POPULATION The test was developed to describe distinct and meaningful levels of motor function based on functional limitations with particular emphasis on truncal control and walking. The authors' intent was to provide a classification system that facilitated prognostic counseling for parents of children with CP and as a means of planning for clinical management.

TEST FORMAT The GMFCS is a classification system developed to include five different levels of severity for children with CP at varied ages. One of the major goals was to standardize the manner in which the severity level was designated. The authors drafted the system using content developed from other classifications systems, from videotapes of children with CP whose severity of involvement was characterized by their physical therapists, and from extensive discussions among the authors. Upon development of the five levels, content validity of the system was examined using the modified nominal group consensus method. A two-round Delphi survey was employed using a panel of experts with an average of 20 years of professional experience. The GMFCS was the outcome of these several processes.

RELIABILITY AND VALIDITY Reliability of the GMFCS was established by Wood and Rosenbaum, who examined interrater and test–retest reliability and predictive validity of the instrument. Interrater reliability and test–retest reliability were judged to be high at $G = 0.93$ and $G = 0.79$, respectively. The positive predictive value of the GMFCS at 1 to 2 years of age to predict walking by age 12 years was 0.74. The negative predictive value was 0.90.[100] Palisano et al. validated the GMFCS classification levels for 586 children with CP by comparing them to their gross motor function measured by the GMFM.

The authors concluded that gross motor classification with the GMFCS is predictive of gross motor function.[101]

ADVANTAGES AND DISADVANTAGES The GMFCS is easily administered and is based on self-initiated movement. There is strong emphasis on sitting and walking with the differences in the five levels of classification at each age being clinically meaningful and emphasizing function rather than disability. Disadvantages include the fact that this is a broad classification system and the differences between levels 1 and 2 are not as pronounced as differences between the other levels.

 Integration of Information

Throughout the process of evaluation, physical therapists compile extensive information concerning their young clients. The final component of a thorough assessment is to organize, synthesize, and use the data to guide intervention. There are four possible uses for the information gained from evaluation[67]:

1. To plan a treatment program
2. To identify areas of progress or lack of progress
3. To identify or rule out the existence of a specific problem
4. To provide diagnostic information

Physical therapists are primarily involved with the first two areas. The way in which test data are to be used should help determine the data needed, thus ensuring the collection of necessary data while avoiding superfluous information. As a result of the procedure for assessment, the physical therapist identifies specific areas of dysfunction in a particular child. Program goals and objectives can then be developed to address these areas of dysfunction. *Program goals* describe long-term expectations of treatment and relate to general areas of development. *Objectives* are short-term accomplishments, written in behavioral terms, which enable the child to progress toward achievement of the long-term goals. A program for therapy is designed to meet the objectives identified by focusing on the activities required for the child to achieve the objectives. The assessment process can be seen as an ongoing cycle. The information gathered from the formal assessment is used in the development of goals and objectives that guide the treatment program. Reassessments are periodically performed to review the appropriateness of the treatment program and to monitor the progress of the child. Reports of physical therapy assessments are usually presented in narrative form. The purposes of a report are to clarify what has been heard and observed, to give the data on which recommendations for treatment are based, and to transmit this information in a clear and understandable way to others. Certain information is included for all patients, but each child's report should provide a specific description of the distinctive

>>> **DISPLAY 3.10**

Suggested Outline for a Narrative Report on the Results of Development Testing

1. Identification information: child's name, date of birth, current age, date of evaluation
2. Reason for evaluation and source of referral
3. History
   A. Perinatal history
   B. Significant medical history
   C. Developmental history as presented by parents or other historian
4. Clinical observations
   A. Neurologic development: reflex development, muscle tone, equilibrium, and protective responses
   B. Musculoskeletal status: range of motion, manual muscle test, anthropometric measurements
   C. Sensory status: results of sensory testing, visual ability, and auditory ability
   D. Functional abilities: daily activities (e.g., feeding, toileting, dressing), assistive devices
5. Results of developmental assessments: include developmental age
6. Summary of findings
7. Recommendations

abilities and disabilities of that child.[3] An outline of a narrative report is given in Display 3.10.

SUMMARY

Several clinically useful and commonly used tools for assessment have been described, among them screening tests, tests of motor function, and comprehensive developmental assessments. The information gained from these assessments, when combined with the information obtained from an interview, medical and developmental history, and clinical observation, completes the comprehensive evaluation of a child. The guidelines presented for the selection of specific tests will aid the therapist in choosing the test most appropriate for the population to be assessed. The therapist should remember that a questioning attitude, based on and supported by knowledge of human growth and development, is necessary for a comprehensive evaluation.

REFERENCES

1. Semans S. Specific tests and evaluation tools for the child with central nervous system deficit. Phys Ther 1965;45:456–462.
2. Scherzer AL, Tscharnuter I. Early Diagnosis and Therapy in Cerebral Palsy. New York: Marcel Dekker, 1982.
3. Knobloch H, Pasamanick B, eds. Gesell and Armatruda's Developmental Diagnosis: The Evaluation and Management of Normal and Abnormal Neuropsychologic Development in Infancy and Early Childhood. Hagerstown, MD: Harper & Row, 1974.
4. Clark PN, Coley LI, Allen AS, et al. Basic methods of assessment and screening. In: Clark PN, Allen AS, eds. Occupational Therapy for Children. St. Louis: CV Mosby, 1985.
5. Connolly B, Harris S. Survey of assessment tools. Totline 1983;9:8–9.
6. Bayley N. Bayley Scales of Infant Development. New York: The Psychological Corporation, 1969.
7. Frankenburg WK, Dodds J, Archer P, et al. Denver II Training Manual. Denver, CO: Denver Developmental Materials, Inc, 1992.
8. Gallahue D. Assessing child's motor behavior. In: Understanding Motor Development in Children. New York: John Wiley, 1982.
9. Lewko JH. Current practices in evaluating motor behavior of disabled children. Am J Occup Ther 1976;30:413–419.
10. Stangler SR, Huber CJ, Routh DK. Screening Growth and Development of Preschool Children: A Guide for Test Selection. New York: McGraw-Hill, 1980.
11. Milani-Comparetti A, Gidoni EA. Routine developmental examination in normal and retarded children. Dev Med Child Neurol 1967;9:631–638.
12. Trembath J, Kliewer D, Bruce W. The Milani-Comparetti Motor Development Screening Test. Omaha, NE: University of Nebraska Medical Center, 1977.
13. Stuberg WA, Dehne P, Miedaner J, et al. The Milani-Comparetti Motor Development Screening Test. 3rd Ed Rev. Omaha, NE: University of Nebraska Medical Center, 1992.
14. Stuberg WA, White PJ, Miedaner JA, et al. Item reliability of the Milani-Comparetti Motor Development Screening Test. Phys Ther 1989;69:328–335.
15. Frankenburg WK, Dodds JB, Fandel AW. Denver Developmental Screening Test Manual. Denver, CO: LADOCA Project & Publishing Foundation, 1973.
16. Frankenburg WK, Dodds J, Archer P, et al. The Denver II: a major revision and restandardization of the Denver Developmental Screening Test. Pediatrics 1992;89:1.
17. Frankenburg WK, Dodds J, Archer P. Denver II Technical Manual. Denver, CO: Denver Developmental Materials, Inc, 1990.
18. Brachlow A, Jordan AE, Tervo R. Developmental screenings in rural settings: a comparison of the child development review and the Denver II Developmental Screening Test. J Rural Health 2001;17(3): 156–159.
19. Hallioglu O, Topaloglu AK, Zenciroglu A, et al. Denver developmental screening test II for early identification of the infants who will develop major neurological deficit as a sequalea of hypoxic-ischemic encephalopathy. Pediatr Int 2001;43(4): 400–404.
20. Glascoe FP, Foster EM, Wolraich ML. An economic analysis of developmental detection methods. Pediatrics 1997;99(6): 830–837.
21. Dobrez D, Sasso AL, Holl J, et al. Estimating the cost of developmental and behavioral screening of preschool children in general pediatric practice. Pediatrics 2001;108(4):913–922.
22. Developmental surveillance and screening of infants and young children. Pediatrics 2001;108(1):192–196.
23. Chandler LS, Andrews MS, Swanson MW. Movement Assessment of Infants—A Manual. Rolling Bay, WA: Chandler, Andrews, and Swanson, 1980.
24. Haley SM, Harris SR, Tada WL, et al. Item reliability of the movement assessment of infants. Phys Occup Ther Pediatr 1986;6(1):21–38.
25. Harris SR. Early neuromotor predictors of cerebral palsy in low birthweight infants. Dev Med Child Neurol 1987;29:508–519.
26. Schneider JW, Lee W, Chasnoff IJ. Field testing of the Movement Assessment of Infants. Phys Ther 1988;68:321–327.

27. Piper MC, Pinnell LE, Darrah J, et al. Early developmental screening: sensitivity and specificity of chronological and adjusted scores. Dev Behav Pediatr 1992;13:95–101.

28. Swanson MW, Bennett FC, Shy KK, et al. Identification of neurodevelopmental abnormality at four and eight months by the Movement Assessment of Infants. Dev Med Child Neurol 1992;34: 321–337.

29. Washington K, Deitz JC. Performance of full-term 6-month-old infants on the movement assessment of infants. Pediatr Phys Ther 1995;7(2):65–74.

30. Harris SR, Haley SM, Tada WL, et al. Reliability of observational measures of the Movement Assessment of Infants. Phys Ther. 1984;64:471–475.

31. Brander R, Kramer J, Dancsak, et al. Inter-rater and test-retest reliabilities of the movement assessment of infants. Pediatr Phys Ther 1993;5(1):9–15.

32. Harris SR, Swanson MW, Andrews MS, et al. Predictive validity of the movement assessment of infants. J Dev Behav Pediatr 1984;5:336–343.

33. Salokorpi T, Rajantie I, Kivikko I, et al. Predicting neurological disorders in infants with extremely low birth weight using the movement assessment of infants. Pediatr Phys Ther 2001; 13(3):106–109.

34. Rose-Jacobs R, Cabral H, Beeghly M, et al. The Movement Assessment of Infants (MAI) as a predictor of two-year neurodevelopmental outcome for infants born at term who are at social risk. Pediatr Phys Ther 2004;16(4):212–221.

35. Campbell SK, Osten ET, Kolobe THA, et al. Development of the Test of Infant Motor Performance. Phys Med Rehab Clin North Am 1993;4(3): 541–550.

36. Girolami GL, Campbell SK. Efficacy of a neuro-developmental treatment program to improve motor control in infants born prematurely. Pediatr Phys Ther 1994;6(4):175–184.

37. Campbell SK. The child's development of functional movement. In: Campbell SK, ed. Physical Therapy for Children. Philadelphia: WB Saunders, 1994.

38. Campbell SK, Kolobe TH, Osten ET, et al. Construct validity of infant motor performance. Phys Ther 1995;75(7):585–596.

39. Campbell SK, Hedeker D. Validity of the Test of Infant Motor Performance for discriminating among infants with varying risk for poor motor outcome. J Pediatr 2001;139(4):546–551.

40. Campbell SK, Kolobe TH, Wright BD, et al. Validity of the Test of Infant Motor Performance for prediction of 6-, 9- and 12-month scores on the Alberta Infant Motor Scale. Dev Med Child Neurol 2002;44(4):263–272.

41. Flegel J, Kolobe TH. Predictive validity of the test of infant motor performance as measured by the Bruininks-Oseretsky test of motor proficiency at school age. Phys Ther 2002; 82(8):762–771.

42. Kolobe TH, Bulanda M, Susman L. Predicting motor outcome at preschool age for infants tested at 7, 30, 60, and 90 days after term age using the Test of Infant Motor Performance. Phys Ther 2004; 84(12):1144–1156.

43. Piper MC, Darrah J. Alberta Infant Motor Scale. Philadelphia: WB Saunders, 1995.

44. Piper MC, Pinnell LE, Darrah J, et al. Construction and validation of the Alberta Infant Motor Scale (AIMS). Can J Public Health. 1992;83(Suppl 2): S46–50.

45. Fetters L, Tronick EZ. Neuromotor development of cocaine-exposed and control infants from birth through 15 months: poor and poorer performance. Pediatrics. 1996;98(5):938–943.

46. Darrah J, Piper M, Watt MJ. Assessment of gross motor skills of at-risk infants: predictive validity of the Alberta Infant Motor Scale. Dev Med Child Neurol 1998;40(7):485–491.

47. Bartlett DJ, Fanning JE. Use of the Alberta Infant Motor Scale to characterize the motor development of infants born preterm at eight months corrected age. Phys Occup Ther Pediatr 2003;23(4): 31–45.

48. Blanchard Y, Neilan E, Busanich J, et al. Interrater reliability of early intervention providers scoring the Alberta Infant Motor Scale. Pediatr Phys Ther 2004;16(1):13–18.

49. Liao PM, Campbell SK. Examination of the item structure of the Alberta Infant Motor Scale. Pediatr Phys Ther 2004; 16(1):31–38.

50. Russell DJ, Rosenbaum PL, Cadman DT, et al. The Gross Motor Function Measure: a means to evaluate the effects of physical therapy. Dev Med Child Neurol 1989;31:341–352.

51. Russell DJ, Rosenbaum PL, Lane M, et al. Training users in the Gross Motor Function Measure: methodological and practical issues. Phys Ther 1994;74(7): 630–636.

52. Russell DJ, Avery LM, Rosenbaum PL, et al. Improved scaling of the gross motor function measure for children with cerebral palsy: evidence of reliability and validity. Phys Ther 2000;80(9):873–885.

53. Avery LM, Russell DJ, Raina PS, et al. Rasch analysis of the Gross Motor Function Measure: validating the assumptions of the Rasch model to create an interval-level measure. Arch Phys Med Rehabil 2003;84(5): 697–705.

54. Boyce WF, Gowland C, Hardy S, et al. Development of a quality-of-movement measure for children with cerebral palsy. Phys Ther 1991;71(11): 820–828.

55. Gowland C, Boyce WF, Wright V, et al. Reliability of the Gross Motor Performance Measure. Phys Ther 1995;75(7):597–602.

56. Boyce WF, Gowland C, Rosenbaum PL, et al. The Gross Motor Performance measure: validity and responsiveness of a measure of quality of movement. Phys Ther. 1995;71(7):603–613.

57. Thomas SS, Buckon CE, Phillips DS, et al. Interobserver reliability of the gross motor performance measure: preliminary results. Dev Med Child Neurol 2001;43(2):97–102.

58. Folio MR, Fewell PR. Peabody Developmental Motor Scales and Activity Cards Manual. Allen, TX: DLM Teaching Resources, 1983.

59. Folio MR, Fewell RR. Peabody Developmental Motor Scales. 2nd Ed. Austin, TX: Pro-Ed, 2000.

60. Stokes NA, Deitz JL, Crowe TK. The Peabody Developmental Fine Motor Scale: an interrater reliability study. Am J Occup Ther. 1990;44:334–340.

61. Provost B, Heimerl S, McClain C, et al. Concurrent validity of the Bayley Scales of Infant Development II Motor Scale and the Peabody Developmental Motor Scales-2 in children with developmental delays. Pediatr Phys Ther 2004;16(3):149–156.

62. Harris SR, Heriza CB. Measuring infant movement: clinical and technological assessment techniques. Phys Ther 1987;67: 1877–1880.

63. Bruininks RH. Bruininks-Oseretsky Test of Motor Proficiency: Examiners' Manual. Circle Pines, MI: American Guidance Services, 1978.

64. Duger T, Bumin G, Uyanik M, et al. The assessment of Bruininks-Oseretsky test of motor proficiency in children. Pediatr Rehabil 1999;3(3):125–131.

65. Maccobb S, Greene S, Nugent K, et al. Measurement and prediction of motor proficiency in children using Bayley Infant Scales and the Bruininks-Oseretsky test. Phys Occup Ther Pediatr 2005;25(1–2):59–79.

66. Self PA, Horowitz FD. The behavioral assessment of the neonate: an overview. In: Osofsky JD, ed. Handbook of Infant Development. New York: Wiley, 1979.

67. Palisano RJ. Concurrent and predictive validities of the Bayley Motor Scale and the Peabody Developmental Motor Scales. Phys Ther 1986;66:1714–1719.

68. Bayley Scales of Infant Development, 2nd Ed. The Bayley II. The Psychological Corporation. San Antonio, TX: Harcourt Brace & Co, 1993.

69. Schuler ME, Nair P, Harrington D. Developmental outcome of drug-exposed children through 30 months: a comparison of Bayley and Bayley-II. Psychol Assess 2003;15(3):435–438.

70. Karmel BZ, Gardner JM, Freedland RL. Neonatal neurobehavioral assessment Bayley I and II scores of CNS-injured and cocaine-exposed infants. Ann N Y Acad Sci 1998;846:391–395.

71. Brazelton TB. Neonatal Behavioral Assessment Scale. Clin Dev Med 1984:88.

72. Brazelton TB. Neonatal Behavioral Assessment Scale. Clin Dev Med 1973:50.

73. Stengel TJ. The Neonatal Behavioral Assessment Scale: description, clinical uses, and research implications. Phys Occup Ther Pediatr 1980;1:39–57.

74. Prechtl HFB, Beintema B. The neurological examination of the full-term infant. Clin Dev Med 1964:12.

75. Ohgi S, Arisawa K, Takahashi T, et al. Neonatal behavioral assessment scale as a predictor of later developmental disabilities of low birth-weight and/or premature infants. Brain Dev 2003;25(5):313–321.

76. Myers BJ, Dawson KS, Britt GC, et al. Prenatal cocaine exposure and infant performance on the Brazelton Neonatal Behavioral Assessment Scale. Subst Use Misuse 2003;38(14):2065–2096.

77. Rogers SJ, D'Eugenio DB. Assessment and application. In: Schafer DS, Moersch MS, eds. Developmental Programming for Infants and Young Children. Vol I. Ann Arbor, MI: The University of Michigan Press, 1977.

78. Brown SL, Donovan CM. Stimulation activities. In: Schafer DS, Moersch MS, eds. Developmental Programming for Infants and Young Children. Vol 3. Ann Arbor, MI: The University of Michigan Press, 1977.

79. Haley SM. Motor assessment tools for infants and young children: a focus on disability assessment. In: Forssberg H, Hirschfeld H, eds. Movement Disorders in Children. Basel: S. Karger, AG, 1992: 278–283.

80. Feldman AB, Haley SM, Coryell J. Concurrent and construct validity of the Pediatric Evaluation of Disability Inventory. Phys Ther 1990;70:602–610.

81. Haley SM, Costern J, Ludlons LH, et al. Pediatric Evaluation of Disability Inventory (PEDI): Development, Standardization and Administration Manual. Boston: New England Medical Center Hospitals and PEDI Research Group, 1992.

82. Haley SM, Coster WJ, Faas RM. A content validity study of the Pediatric Evaluation of Disability Inventory. Pediatr Phys Ther 1991;3:177–184.

83. Nordmark E, Orban K, Hagglund G, et al. The American Paediatric Evaluation of Disability Inventory (PEDI). Applicability of PEDI in Sweden for children aged 2.0–6.9 years. Scand J Rehabil Med 1999;31(2):95–100.

84. Wassenberg-Severijnen JE, Custers JW, Hox JJ, et al. Reliability of the Dutch Pediatric Evaluation of Disability Inventory (PEDI). Clin Rehabil 2003; 17(4):457–462.

85. Berg M, Jahnsen R, Froslie KF, et al. Reliability of the Pediatric Evaluation of Disability Inventory (PEDI). Phys Occup Ther Pediatr 2004;24(3): 61–77.

86. Kothari DH, Haley SM, Gill-Body KM, et al. Measuring functional change in children with acquired brain injury (ABI): comparison of generic and ABI-specific scales using the Pediatric Evaluation of Disability Inventory (PEDI). Phys Ther 2003;83(9):776–785.

87. Tsai PY, Yang TF, Chan RC, et al. Functional investigation in children with spina bifida—measured by the Pediatric Evaluation of Disability Inventory (PEDI). Childs Nerv Syst 2002;18(1–2):48–53.

88. Rennie DJ, Attfield SF, Morton RE, et al. An evaluation of Lycra garments in the lower limb using 3-D gait analysis and functional assessment (PEDI). Gait Posture 2000;12(1):1–6.

89. Data Management Service of the Uniform Data System for Medical Rehabilitation and the Center for Functional Assessment Research: Guide for Use of the Uniform Data System for Medical Rehabilitation, Including the Functional Independence Measure for Children (WeeFIM). State University of New York at Buffalo, 82 Farber Hall, SUNY South Campus, Buffalo, version 1.5, July 1991.

90. Msall ME, DiGaudio KM, Duffy LC. Use of assessment in children with developmental disabilities. Phys Med Rehab Clinics North Am 1993;4(3): 517–527.

91. McCabe MA, Granger CV. Content validity of a pediatric functional independence measure. Appl Nurs Res 1990;3:120–122.

92. Msall ME, Braun S, Granger CV. Use of the functional independence measure for children (WeeFIM: an interdisciplinary training tape [abstract].) Dev Med Child Neurol 1990;62:46.

93. Msall ME, Braun SL, Duffy L, et al. Normative sample of the Pediatric Functional Independence Measure: a uniform data set for tracking disability [abstract]. Dev Med Child Neurol 1992;66:19.

94. Msall ME, Heffner H, DiGaudio K, et al. Functional independence in school age children with lower extremity neurological impairment: use of WeeFIM in spastic diplegia and paraplegia [abstract]. Dev Med Child Neurol Suppl 1992;66:21.

95. Msall ME, Monti DA, Duffy LC, et al. Measuring functional independence in children with spina bifida [abstract 60]. Pediatr Res. 1992;31:12A.

96. Msall ME, Roehmholdt SJ, DiGaudio KM, et al. Functional independence of school age children with Down syndrome [abstract 61]. Pediatr Res. 1992;31:13A.

97. Msall ME, Rogers BT, Buck GM, et al. Functional status of extremely preterm infants at kindergarten entry. Dev Med Child Neurol 1993;35:312–320.

98. Msall ME, Rosenberg S, DiGaudio KM, et al. Pilot testing of the WeeFIM in children with motor impairments [abstract]. Dev Med Child Neurol Suppl 1990;32:41.

99. Palisano R, Rosenbaum P, Walter S et al. Gross motor function classification system for cerebral palsy. Dev Med Child Neurol 1997;39:214–223.

100. Wood E, Rosenbaum P. The gross motor function classification system for cerebral palsy: a study of reliability and stability over time. Dev Med Child Neurol 2000;42(5):292–296.

101. Palisano RJ, Hanna SE, Rosenbaum PL, et al. Validation of a model of gross motor function for children with cerebral palsy. Phys Ther 2000; 80(10): 974–985.

102. Stockmeyer S. A pattern for evaluation in the assessment of motor performance. Phys Ther 1965; 45: 453–455.

Neurological Disorders

4

The Infant at High Risk for Developmental Delay

Diane Versaw-Barnes and Audrey Wood

History and Evolution of the Philosophy of Care in the Neonatal Intensive Care Unit

he technologic advances of the 20th century have affected the lifestyles of all, including babies. In 1880, the first preterm babies were cared for in France in incubators modeled after incubators for egg hatching. Within 20 years, the first hospital nursery designed to care for preterm infants opened and the first textbook delineating the state-of-the-art care for "weaklings," as these preterm babies were called, was published.[1] As the term *weakling* implies, the competence of newborn babies was not appreciated at that time. Newborn babies were considered to be helpless, "mewling," and "puking," regarding the world as "blooming buzzing confusion" and waiting to have the adults around them write on the blank tablets of their minds.[2] In the first 50 to 60 years of the 20th century the medical care for babies focused on temperature regulation, infection control, feeding, and minimal handling. Mortality rates were nevertheless very high for these fragile infants.[1,3]

The medical and technologic advances in the mid- to late 1900s, such as radiant warmers, ventilators, total parental nutrition, and central line access, led to the regionalization of increasingly specialized and costly neonatal care. The American Academy of Pediatrics added neonatology to the subspecialties with board certification in 1970, and in 1975 the Committee on Perinatal Health published guidelines for regional perinatal centers. Very-low-birthweight (i.e., less than or equal to 1500 g or 3 lb, 5 oz) infants were surviving, however, with increased incidences of cerebral palsy, respiratory disorders, blindness, cognitive delays, and hearing impairments. Early intervention programs emerged in the mid-1970s to address the developmental needs of these survivors of neonatal intensive care with the goals of stimulating and normalizing their development. The womb was thought to provide a rich sensory environment of which the preterm infant was deprived. The pendulum had swung from the initial philosophy of "minimal handling" to one of simulating the varied tactile, vestibular, proprioceptive, and auditory conditions of the womb. Brazelton's[4] *Neonatal Behavioral Assessment Scale,* first published in 1973, led to a fuller understanding of the competence of the newborn infant and the plasticity of the neonatal brain. Transport teams to shuttle newborns to the hospital where the most appropriate level of care could be provided further supported the regionalization of intensive care.[1] The medical advances of the 1980s and 1990s brought sophisticated respiratory monitors and therapies, such as nitric oxide, extracorporeal membrane oxygenation (ECMO), pulse oximetry, and surfactant replacement therapy. These interventions led to further regionalization of newborn intensive care. In the 1980s, as neonatal intensive care unit (NICU) graduates demonstrated developmental outcomes that were frequently atypical, infant follow-up programs were formalized and infant stimulation programs proliferated. The Education for All Handicapped Children Amendments, passed in 1986, required states to provide early intervention services for infants with developmental delays or infants at risk for delays and their families.

Also in the 1980s, the amount of sensory stimulation appropriate for a preterm and/or critically ill infant was questioned and reconceptualized. The conditions in the NICUs were seen as aversive and excessive, producing stress and overload in the infants. Environmental modification of the constant lighting, excessive noise, and intrusive procedures ("environmental neonatology") became important in the philosophy for high-risk infants. With the need to balance the cost with the benefits of providing care for these frail babies and with the advent of health maintenance organizations (HMOs), the regionalization of highly specialized newborn intensive care has been reinforced.[1,3]

Levels of Newborn Intensive Care and the Role of the Physical Therapist

Today there are four levels of newborn intensive care. A level I nursery is a well-baby nursery where healthy newborns or newborns who require minimal observation or care such as warming in an isolette, phototherapy, circumcision, or limited diagnostic testing are taken. Small community hospitals where babies are routinely delivered have this level of newborn nursery. A level II nursery is considered to be an intermediate or step-down from a level III nursery and provides continuing care, intravenous medications or alimentation, tube feedings, and oxygen support. Neonatologists and neonatal nurses staff these intermediate-level nurseries, which are usually contained in regional or community hospitals. A level III nursery is a neonatal intensive care unit that provides highly specialized services for the sickest and most fragile infants. Level III units are usually part of teaching hospitals and affiliated with a medical school.

Neonatologists, neonatology fellows, clinical nurse specialists, neonatal nurse practitioners, and specially trained nurses staff level III nurseries and provide complex medical interventions, advanced diagnostic testing, surgery, and respiratory support for technologically dependent and medically fragile infants. A level IV nursery refers to a level III nursery that also is equipped to provide ECMO.[3]

Therapists are rarely consulted to see babies in level I nurseries, but may be consulted for a specific musculoskeletal issue. In level II nurseries, physical therapy intervention may involve handling for specific developmental needs. When working with fragile infants and their families in level III or IV nurseries, the therapist needs to use skilled ongoing observation to discern the needs of the baby and provide recommendations regarding positioning, energy conservation, pain management, environmental design, caregiving, and medical management. These observational skills are essential so that the baby is not further stressed by unnecessary handling.

In order to implement care in this way, therapists working in the NICU must have a good knowledge base and strong understanding of the theoretical and developmental frameworks that guide therapy, and the medical framework that drives care (Display 4.1). These areas will be addressed in this chapter; however, developmental intervention in a NICU is a complex subject, and the reader is referred to the list of additional reading materials in the references section at the end of this chapter.

Roles and Competencies of the Therapist in the Neonatal Intensive Care Unit

The role of the therapist working in the neonatal intensive care unit is very different from most other areas of physical therapy practice. The neonatal therapist provides consul-

DISPLAY 4.1

Areas of Knowledge for Neonatal Therapist

- Typical and atypical infant development
- Fetal and newborn development
- Development and interaction of sensory systems in preterm and full-term neonates
- Medical conditions of preterm and full-term neonates and interventions
- Neonatal preterm and full-term behaviors and social development
- Family dynamics, grief/loss process, parenting in the neonatal intensive care unit (NICU)
- Ecology and culture of the NICU
- Theoretical frameworks supporting care in the NICU
- Risk factors associated with developmental outcome

tation, diagnosis, intervention, and family support to extremely fragile infants and families within a very stressful and fast-paced intensive care environment. In addition to understanding a wide range of neonatal conditions, medical interventions, and their potential to impact future development, the neonatal therapist must be a careful observer, good collaborator, and effective communicator.[3,5–8] The ability to make decisions quickly in terms of an infant's stability and need for external supports is necessary, as an infant's status can change rapidly. In this environment, interventions that might otherwise be considered benign may have serious immediate and far-reaching consequences.[3,5,7]

Therapy in the NICU is considered to be an advanced level of pediatric practice[3,6–8] that needs to be achieved through education and mentored clinical practice. The American Association of Physical Therapy has established guidelines for therapists practicing in the NICU,[6] which include specific roles, competencies, knowledge areas, and precepted clinical training.

Theoretical Frameworks to Guide Therapy

DYNAMIC SYSTEMS THEORY

Dynamic systems theory describes a model of human development in which behaviors emerge due to the interaction of many subsystems.[10–14] There is no hierarchy; all subsystems are on an equal level, each complex, composed of many elements and unique to the individual. Both internal and external elements affect development; the environment is as equally important as the individual. In this model, the infant is not a passive recipient of information or change, but rather an active participant in which a developmental behavior assembles from the interaction of the many subsystems within the context of the environment and specific to the task. The progression of development is nonlinear; instead, there are series of states of stability, instability, and reorganization.[10–12,14–16] The individual is always trying to move toward homeostasis and reorganizes around the shift from stability to instability. These periods of instability or transition are important as the system has sufficient flexibility to explore and select new solutions or develop new behaviors. Therapeutic interventions are considered to be most effective at this time as the system can more easily be influenced or shifted.[10,12,14]

The dynamic systems framework can be used to evaluate and establish care for the high-risk infant in the NICU (Fig. 4.1).[6] The interaction of the multiple subsystems within the infant as well as the interaction of the infant and the environment influence the health and development of the individual infant. The infant subsystems include body structure, physiology, and behavior. The environment includes the physical environment of the nursery, multiple

caregivers and support personnel, and family. Changes to the intrinsic systems or the environment can have either positive or negative effects. These changes can produce stability to support function or interfere to cause disorganization and potentially maladaptive behaviors. A small change in one system component can have a large effect on another system and ultimately affect function.[6,10,15,16]

The therapist must understand the history, current status of the infant's system, and the environment, taking into consideration the effect caregiving/therapy will have on that particular infant.[6,12] The therapist must support the interactions that allow functional behaviors to develop, decrease infant stress, and understand the implications of the environment. At the same time, the therapist must assist the family and other caregivers in recognizing how they too can be supportive to the infant's health and development. The therapist needs to be aware of transition periods when developmental interventions can be safely implemented and guide families to utilize these same strategies.

MODELS OF ENABLEMENT

Models of enablement fit well with systems theory as they relate to human development and function. These models present interrelated frameworks for describing the many factors that influence not only an individual's health, but also how the environment influences health and function or participation. The *Guide to Physical Therapy Practice*,[17] based on the National Center for Medical Rehabilitation and Research (NCMRRI)[18] model of disability, views the enabling–disabling process as that in which disease, injury, or congenital anomaly affects function. Another model developed by the World Health Organization (WHO) is the *International Classification of Functioning, Disability, and Health* (ICF), which emphasizes health and functioning rather than disability.[19] Both models look at development and function as a multilevel, multifactorial process and emphasize the need to consider the effects of the environment on the process.[20,21]

As with other theoretical models discussed in this chapter, the *Guide to Physical Therapy* and the ICF view development as a nonlinear, dynamic process that is influenced by intrinsic and extrinsic factors. The *Guide to Physical Therapy* includes the following elements: pathophysiology, impairments, functional limitations, and disability. Using this framework, impairments are the loss or abnormality of body structures or physiologic function; functional limitations include the inability to perform a physical action or task, and disability is the inability to participate in age-appropriate activities. The components of the ICF are presented in a slightly different perspective and include body function and structures, activities and tasks, and participation. Instead of starting with the pathophysiology, the ICF looks at what the individual wants or needs to do and then considers the individual factors that support or interfere

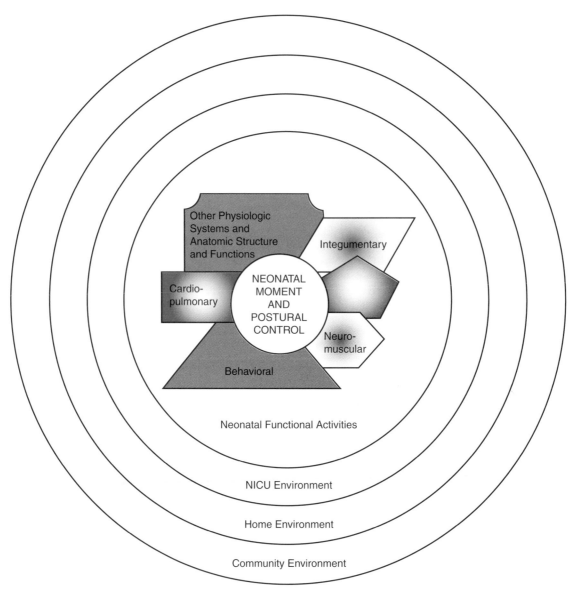

Figure 4.1 ■ Dynamic systems theory in the neonatal intensive care unit (NICU). (Reprinted with permission from Sweeney JK, Heriza CB, Reilly MA, et al. Practice guidelines for the physical therapist in the NICU. Pediatr Phys Ther 1999;11[3]:120.)

with participation. In both frameworks, the contextual factors of the individual and the environment are taken into consideration. They both acknowledge that the environment may need to be adapted in order to better support function/participation.

Although the setting of the NICU is a unique setting for physical therapy practice, the models of enablement can be applied to guide assessment and intervention.[6] The physical therapist working with high-risk infants in the NICU uses these frameworks to guide him or her in addressing functional and structural integrity of body parts and systems, promoting the development of postural and motor activities, and promoting appropriate interaction between the infant, the physical environment, and the family, NICU staff, and consultants. For exam-

ple, the functional goal for an infant may be to socially interact with his or her family while being held. After a thorough assessment, the therapist needs to consider what components are required for this activity to be successful for the infant and family as well as those components that may interfere. The therapist may assist the family in positioning the infant in optimal alignment to support physiologic functions such as respiration and in swaddling to maintain the posture, and may assist the infant in bringing his or her hands to his or her face for calming and behavioral organization; the therapist may also dim the lights, reduce the sound in the area to decrease stress and promote arousal, and support the family in recognizing the infant's cues for interaction. In addition, the therapist, family, and NICU staff can work together to find the most optimal times for the infant to be successful in these interactions.

SYNACTIVE THEORY

The synactive theory of infant development, proposed by psychologist Heidelise Als, is a model to understand and interpret the behavior of preterm infants and is similar to the dynamic systems approach in that multiple influences contribute and mutually influence the baby's functioning. The fetus from conception onward is thought to be organizing five distinct but interrelated subsystems: autonomic (governing basic physiologic functioning, e.g., heart rate, respiratory rate, visceral functions); motor (governing postures and movements); state (governing ranges of consciousness from sleep to wakefulness); attention/interaction (governing the ability to attend to and interact with caregivers); and self-regulatory (governing the ability to maintain balanced, relaxed, and integrated functioning of all four subsystems). These subsystems continually react

and influence each other, thus the term *synactive*.[22–26] Babies born at term have completed the maturation of these subsystems to the degree that, in general, they are able to demonstrate brief periods of social interaction with a caregiver while maintaining stability in the physiologic, motoric, and state subsystems (Fig. 4.2). They also can utilize strategies to regulate the various subsystems when the environment poses a threat to their stability; for example, when eye contact with a parent becomes too intense, a term infant may yawn, look away briefly, stretch, tuck his or her head to his or her trunk, and bring his or her hands together (strategies represented by the attention/interaction and motor subsystems) before returning to gaze again at a parent's face.

In babies born before term the maturation of the five subsystems is interrupted. In addition, babies born before term have lost the uterine supports for these subsystems (autonomic supports like temperature regulation, placental nutrition delivery, waste removal, oxygen delivery, and carbon dioxide removal; motoric supports like the

MODEL OF THE SYNACTIVE ORGANIZATION OF BEHAVIORAL DEVELOPMENT

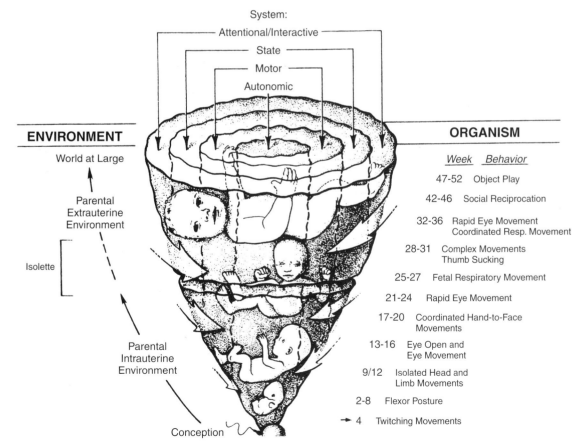

Figure 4.2 ■ Model of the synactive organization of behavioral development. (Reprinted with permission from Als H. Toward a synactive theory of development: promise for the assessment and support of infant individuality. Infant Ment Health J 1982;3[4]:234.)

containment of the uterine wall and the buoyancy of the amniotic fluid; state supports like the diurnal cycles of the mother's sleep–wake cycle; and attention/interaction supports like diminished visual and auditory input). Babies born before term are required to complete the maturation of each subsystem while also negotiating more independent functioning, such as breathing, feeding, eliminating wastes, maintaining postures, and moving against gravity, and while also enduring bright lighting, harsh noises, frequent handling, and multimodal stimulation. The preterm baby is adapted for functioning in the womb but is required to function outside the womb at a crucial time in his or her development and, therefore, faces a very challenging existence.[22,23,25,26]

DEVELOPMENTAL CARE

Applying this synactive theory of infant development through systematic serial observations of the baby is a very helpful way to identify the baby's areas of success at coping and areas of vulnerability. It is important to communicate these strengths and vulnerabilities to the parents and caregivers and to identify strategies to support the baby as he or she receives this necessary intensive care.[22,23,25–28] The process of systematic serial observations has led to a broad array of interventions to minimize the stress of the NICU for the infant and to individualize the caregiving to the infant's tolerance. These interventions include strategies to decrease noise and light levels, minimize handling of the infant, protect infant sleep states, promote understanding of infant behavioral cues, and promote relationship-based caregiving.[29] This approach to newborn intensive care is called the Newborn Individualized Developmental Care and Assessment Program (NIDCAP).[27] Ideally NIDCAP observations are scheduled every 7 to 10 days and include viewing the baby at a baseline for 10 to 20 minutes before nursing care or procedure, throughout the care session or procedure, and after the session or procedure until the baby returns to baseline functioning[27,30] (Fig. 4.3). During this time the observer is watching for signs of stability and stress from each subsystem (Table 4.1) while recording environmental events and care-taking tasks. The infant's strategies for self-regulation, whether successful or unsuccessful, are then noted, and recommendations to support the infant in his or her attempts at organizing and self-soothing are made as well as recommendations for environmental modification, caregiving, and parental involvement.[22,24,25–28] Formal training through the NIDCAP regional training centers is required for reliability and certification in NIDCAP. However, using the principles and applying the synactive model to understand a baby's behavior is a helpful way to guide caregivers in developmentally supportive interventions through observations of nursing care.

The synactive model of preterm behavior identifies the autonomic subsystem and the motoric subsystem as the two core subsystems on which the rest of the infant's functioning is based (Fig. 4.4). Together these two subsystems are the basis for the baby to achieve higher functioning like awaking (state subsystem) and gazing at a parent's face (attention/interaction subsystem). A therapist can recommend and intervene to support the motor system through positioning and containment and in so doing can support the autonomic subsystem as well as the state and interactional subsystems as each system continually interacts and influences the others.[22,23,25,26] The systematic individualization of caring for an infant is the root of developmentally supportive care.[29,31] The knowledge and understanding of how one baby differs from another can only be gleaned by intense observation of the infant in interaction with his or her environment. Using this individualized knowledge of the baby's strengths and vulnerabilities to guide the provision of care has been shown to result in short-term benefits to the baby such as shorter hospitalization resulting in less costly care, decreased use of ventilator, earlier attainment of oral feeds, and improved growth. Long-term benefits include improved neurobehavioral functioning and enhanced brain structure in later infancy, advantages in expressive language and neurologic organization and function at 3 years, and improved attention and visual/spatial perception at 8 years.[24,26,28–30,32–37] Critics of the research on developmental care point out that studies have shown conflicting results, have utilized small sample sizes, and have demonstrated outcomes that may not be clinically significant. Some studies also have serious methodologic flaws in the designs, such as neglecting to blind the outcome assessors and allowing the control and experimental groups to receive the same interventions. The critics of developmental care have not found harmful effects to result from the application of the developmental care philosophy in the NICU, but question whether the benefits are real.[38,39] It is not prudent to implement a philosophy because it does no harm if there are no substantial benefits, as this may detract from other approaches that may prove truly beneficial. Given the abstract nature of the developmental care philosophy and relationship-based caregiving, it is no surprise that it is difficult to study, let alone to teach and implement. During NIDCAP observations the authors have observed infants becoming progressively exhausted, limp, and passive during routine care, as their attempts to organize are continually thwarted by the noncontingent responses of the caregivers. In contrast, infants have been observed to maintain behavioral and physiologic stability when their caregivers are attentive and responsive to their cues. In addition, research on some specific techniques of supporting a baby during care (e.g., facilitated tucking and nonnutritive sucking) have shown significant positive results.[40–48] It is not surprising that preterm infants would also need extra and special supports in order to cope with intensive care, given the emotional dependency that characterizes the infant and toddler periods.

OBSERVATION SHEET Name: ______________ Date: ______________ Sheet Number ______________

	Time:	0-2	3-4	5-6	7-8	9-10
Resp:	Regular					
	Irregular					
	Slow					
	Fast					
	Pause					
Color:	Jaundice					
	Pink					
	Pale					
	Webb					
	Red					
	Dusky					
	Blue					
	Tremor					
	Startle					
	Twitch Face					
	Twitch Body					
	Twitch Extremities					
Visceral/ Resp:	Spit up					
	Gag					
	Burp					
	Hiccough					
	BM Grunt					
	Sounds					
	Sigh					
	Gasp					
Motor:	Flaccid Arm(s)					
	Flaccid leg(s)					
	Flexed/ Tucked Arms Act.					
	Flexed/ Tucked Arms Post.					
	Flexed/ Tucked Legs Act.					
	Flexed/ Tucked Legs Post.					
	Extend Arms Act.					
	Extend Arms Post.					
	Extend Legs Act.					
	Extend Legs Post.					
	Smooth Mvmt. Arms					
	Smooth Mvmt. Legs					
	Smooth Mvmt. Trunk					
	Stretch/Drown					
	Diffuse Squirm					
	Arch					
	Tuck Trunk					
	Leg Brace					
Face:	Tongue Extension					
	Hand on Face					
	Gape Face					
	Grimace					
	Smile					

	Time:	0-2	3-4	5-6	7-8	9-10
State:	1A					
	1B					
	2A					
	2B					
	3A					
	3B					
	4A					
	4B					
	5A					
	5B					
	6A					
	6B					
	AA					
Face (cont.):	Mouthing					
	Suck Search					
	Sucking					
Extrem.:	Finger Splay					
	Airplane					
	Salute					
	Sitting On Air					
	Hand Clasp					
	Foot Clasp					
	Hand to Mouth					
	Grasping					
	Holding On					
	Fisting					
Attention:	Fuss					
	Yawn					
	Sneeze					
	Face Open					
	Eye Floating					
	Avert					
	Frown					
	Ooh Face					
	Locking					
	Cooing					
	Speech Mvmt.					
Posture:	(Prone, Supine, Side)					
Head:	(Right, Left, Middle)					
Location:	(Crib, Isolette, Held)					
Manipulation:						
	Heart Rate					
	Respiration Rate					
	$TcPO_2$					

Figure 4.3 ■ Newborn Individualized Developmental Care and Assessment Program (NIDCAP) observation sheet. (Reprinted with permission from Als H. Reading the premature infant. In: Goldson E, ed. Nurturing the Premature Infant. Developmental Intervention in the Neonatal Intensive Care nursery. New York: Oxford University Press, 1999:37.)

FAMILY-CENTERED CARE

Family-centered care is a philosophy of patient care delivery for the maternal–child health division based on respect, collaboration, and support between health care professionals and patients' families. It is a philosophy that recognizes the family (defined as parents, children, and significant others) as the constant in the child's life and strives to include the family as partners in choosing and implementing the plan of care for the patient. Family-centered care also acknowledges that hospitalization is stressful for families and can potentially alter the integration of the child into the family and the development of the parental role.[49,50] In order to provide family-centered care in a

TABLE 4.1

Signs of Stability and Stress in the Preterm Infant

System	Signs of Stability	Signs of Stress
Autonomic	Smooth, regular respirations Pink, stable coloring	Respiratory pauses, tachypnea, gasping Paling, perioral duskiness, mottled, cyanotic, gray, flushed, ruddy
	Stable digestion	Hiccups, gagging, grunting, emesis, tremors, startles, twitches, cough, sneeze, yawn, sigh, gasp
Motor	Smooth, controlled posture and muscle tone	Fluctuating muscle tone
	Smooth movements of extremities and head	Flaccidity of trunk, extremities, and face
	Hand/foot clasp, leg brace, finger fold, hand to mouth, grasp, suck, tuck, hand hold	Hypertonicity of trunk and extremities
		Frantic diffuse activity
State	Clear, well-defined sleep states	Diffuse sleep with twitches, jerky movement, irregular breathing, whimpering sounds, grimacing, and fussing
	Focused alertness with animated facial expression	Diffuse wakeful periods with eye floating, glassy-eyed, strained appearance, staring, gaze aversion, panicked, dull look, weak cry

Adapted from Als H. Toward a synactive theory of development: promise for the assessment and support of infant individuality. *Infant Ment Health J* 1982;3(4):237–238.

NICU, a clinician must be knowledgeable about and sensitive to both the psychological tasks of pregnancy and the grief process.

PSYCHOLOGICAL TASKS OF PREGNANCY

In American culture pregnancy is typically and naively regarded as a happy time of anticipation, and although that may be partially true, pregnancy also is a time of psychological turmoil. The 40 weeks of pregnancy provide a

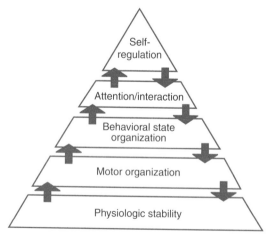

Figure 4.4 ■ Pyramid of the synactive theory of infant behavioral organization with physiologic stability at the foundation. (Used with permission from Sweeney JK, Swanson MW. Low birth weight infants: neonatal care and follow-up. In: Umphred DA, ed. Neurological Rehabilitation. 4th Ed. St. Louis: Mosby, 2001:205.)

physical as well as a psychological preparatory period for the expectant parents. When this period is shortened, the baby and the parents may suffer from the incompletion of the pregnancy.[51–54] Bibring[55,56] has identified three psychological tasks of pregnancy, correlating with the three trimesters.[52,54] In the first trimester, parents accept the overwhelming news that their lives have begun a new phase of responsibility for a child (first task). Euphoria, inventorying one's childhood to evaluate his or her own parents' job at childrearing, maternal ambivalence, paternal ambivalence and exclusion, feelings of helplessness and inadequacy, and fantasizing about the perfect baby and the perfect parent characterize this period.[52,57–59]

During the second trimester, the mother-to-be is confronted with the separateness of the baby as she begins to feel his or her movements (second task). Although she feels a personal closeness to the baby, the mother's bodily changes and the baby's burgeoning movements make the individuality of the baby more real and apparent. She may enjoy the attention she receives from her changing shape. During this time, the mother continues to question herself about her adequacy as a parent. Concerns regarding the health and the potential to inflict harm on the fetus are prominent. Ambivalence toward the baby is still very much present for both parents, with fathers struggling with feelings of resentment and rivalry. Attachment to a baby requires time to develop.[52,54,57–59]

In the third trimester, the baby begins to be personified as names are chosen and rooms painted. In addition, the expectant mother recognizes patterns in fetal movement and is able to assign the baby a temperament and/or a gender based on these patterns, further personifying the baby. The baby's individuality, revealed in his or her differing responses to the mother's music, food, or other environmental conditions, confirms his or her competence and capabilities, as well as demonstrates to the parents his or her ability to handle the rigors of labor and delivery.[52] Simultaneously, the mother-to-be is physically becoming increasingly uncomfortable and has difficulty sleeping, breathing, eating, and moving. She cannot get a break from being pregnant and this physical state leads to the third psychological task: being ready to give up the fetus.[54–56]

A full-term birth prepares the mother to cope with the shock of the separation of the baby from her body, and both parents to interact and bond with a particular baby. Parents who give birth prematurely are ill-prepared for these psychological tasks,[52] just as their babies are ill-prepared for independent living.[53] In addition, when a pregnancy or birth deviates from the expected, parents often feel guilty about failing to complete the pregnancy or about any complications the baby may experience.[53,60] The precariousness and unpredictability of a NICU have been shown to detract from completing the psychological tasks necessary for taking on the role of a parent. Instead, the psychological focus becomes the uncertainty and unpredictability of the situation, which distracts from the psychological task of preparing for a new family member and assuming the parental role.[59]

When babies are hospitalized at the critical time when parents should be establishing their relationships with their newborns and learning their parental roles, it is especially stressful.[61] The effects of this stress can continue for months after the NICU experience has ended and can pose severe threats to the parents individually and as a couple.[62] Indeed, the experience of having a baby who requires intensive care is a stressor significant enough to cause symptoms of post-traumatic stress disorder.[63–67] The development of post-traumatic stress disorder after life-threatening illnesses and medical procedures has been reported in the literature.[62] Research has shown that the families who endure the hospitalization and develop a positive outlook about the experience have children who develop better in the years after birth. Likewise, poor coping can have lasting detrimental effects on the child's development.[68,69] Therefore, it is important that clinicians working in the NICU recognize the stress families experience and establish supportive relationships with the families in an effort to support their individual coping styles. In order to do this, a clinician must understand the coping and grieving processes.

COPING AND GRIEVING

Both coping and grieving have been described as a linear progression through distinct stages (e.g., shock, denial, anger, guilt, adjustment, and acceptance). However, this linear progression has not been validated empirically.[68,70] Instead, it is more helpful to understand grief and coping as ongoing processes involving circular progressions where previous issues and losses are resurrected and revisited.[68,70] The beneficial effects of plain old social support cannot be underestimated in the NICU setting. Approaching families with stereotyped expectations of a rigid time frame regarding their coping and grieving will result in the family feeling judged and will prevent the development of supportive relationships between families and staff, to the ultimate detriment of the baby.[68]

PROVIDING FAMILY-CENTERED CARE IN THE NEONATAL INTENSIVE CARE UNIT

The shock of a pregnancy, labor, and/or delivery gone awry, whether resulting in a fragile preterm baby or a full-term baby who requires intensive medical/surgical care, can linger with parents indeterminately. Parents of babies in a NICU are in crisis and should be cared for sensitively. It is important to understand the families' backgrounds (previous losses due to deaths, infertility, miscarriages, assistive reproductive technology, financial situation, current work and/or school responsibilities, current relational situations, and other life stressors). This can be accomplished by reading the social work consults and speaking directly with the social workers, nurses, psychologists, and families. The NICU therapist should not ignore this social history because it "does not change what I do with the baby." Rather, this background knowledge should guide how the therapist interacts with the family.

Every family in the NICU is grieving something, maybe the loss of the expected labor/delivery plan or perhaps the loss of the perfect child. This grief will resurrect past losses and can limit the parents' availability to establish an emotional bond with their infant. In addition, the interactional deprivation imposed by the intensive care the baby requires can prevent the families from knowing and connecting with their infant. The high-tech, crisis-prone NICU environment shocks and intimidates families. The families must ask permission to enter the unit as well as to touch or hold their infant, which creates a sense of lost ownership of their infant. Families may not want to risk emotional involvement with their fragile newborn who may later die.

Developmental care of an infant grows out of establishing a supportive and nurturing relationship with the infant. Likewise, family-centered care grows out of establishing a supportive and empowering relationship with the family. One of the goals of family-centered care is to facilitate the bonding process between the infant and the child and to assist the family in establishing emotional ties with their infant.[54,71] In order to be effective in this goal, therapists must be mindful of their own attitudes and nonverbal behaviors and must congruently communicate nonjudgmental acceptance of the family's emotions, coping methods, and pace. Therapists are responsible for crafting the relationship with the family and supporting and empathizing with their emotions while reflecting the strengths they observe in the family and the infant. Some suggestions to accomplish this include using the baby's name when talking about him or her; commenting on the baby's accomplishments; stating the baby's strengths; stating that the baby is attractive; commenting on the positive interactions between the baby and the family; emphasizing the parents' importance to the infant; pointing out the baby's preference for the parents; and emphasizing the parents' competence with tasks related to the infant's care.[54,71]

A family's human tendency to maintain hope for the future, that the professionals may be wrong, and that miracles can occur should be preserved. Hope is a motivating emotion, providing the energy to cope, work, strive, and stay involved with the infant. It sustains the impetus to maintain the emotional bond to the baby through visiting and interacting. Hope should not be destroyed, but neither should it be falsely fed with unrealistic expectations. Families in crisis with babies in a NICU deserve to hear congruent information from the medical team and the therapy team. This requires sensitivity, diplomacy, and good communication skills.[54]

Developmental Foundations to Guide Therapy

EMBRYOGENESIS AND NEONATAL DEVELOPMENT

In this section, embryogenesis and the current understanding of muscle tone and sensory responses in the second half of gestation are discussed. The evolution of primitive reflexes is left out as it would not be prudent for a therapist today to try to elicit these reactions in a preterm infant for any reason, as it may cause unnecessary stress for the preterm infant. In addition, there is no benefit to a preterm infant to assess his or her muscle tone or sensory reactions solely to determine whether development is occurring appropriately. Rather, this information is included here to provide the neonatal therapist with an understanding of the preterm infant's development and struggle with the intrusiveness of the extrauterine environment at a critical time in his or her development.

Embryogenesis is a remarkable series of events. In 266 days, a 0.1-mm single large cell at fertilization increases in length by a factor of 5000, in surface area by a factor of 61 million, and in weight by a factor of 6 billion. During the pre-embryonic period, the first 2 weeks after fertilization of the oocyte by the sperm, cell division in the zygote forms three primary germ layers whose segmentation and axis formation are essential to the development of the human baby.[72] The ectoderm evolves into the skin, spinal cord, and teeth, the mesoderm into the blood vessels, muscles, and bone, and the endoderm into the digestive

system, lungs, and urinary tract.[73] During the embryonic period (weeks 3 through 8), the mass of cells divides and differentiates into the more than 200 different cell types comprising the various organs of the body.[72] This is a result of amazing and complex processes that are precisely timed and interwoven. In the embryonic period, the cells initially are homogenous, but increasing differentiation determines an exact biologic function for each cell. By the end of this period, the embryo has a heterogenous structure. Any misstep in this process can result in demise or a major morphologic malformation in the embryo.[73] The nervous system, the first organ to initiate development and the last to complete development continuing well after birth, is very susceptible to insult. Other systems have shorter critical periods where an interruption or insult can cause a congenital anomaly[72] (see Fig. 4.5 for timing of major/minor anomalies).

In the first week after fertilization, the fertilized egg travels from the fallopian tube and reaches the uterus. In the second week, the fertilized egg, having undergone several mitotic cell divisions to reach the blastocyst stage, implants into the rich vascular wall of the uterus and by the end of the second week forms a primitive placenta. By the end of the third week, the embryo's blood is circulating in a U-shaped tube that later fuses to a single tube and undergoes partitioning into four chambers during weeks 4 to 7. In the fourth week, the embryo is now less than a half a centimeter long. In 35 days a single cell has grown and been transformed into more than 10,000 different cells. The changes are swift and the process so precise and predictable that the timing of a congenital defect can be pinpointed.[73] In addition, an ultrasound during the embryonic period can be used to date the pregnancy within 7 days.[75]

During the fetal period, weeks 9 through 36, the established organs and body parts of the embryo become refined and enlarged. The placenta serves as a barrier, removes wastes, and provides nutrition for the growing fetus, fulfilling the function of the fetal lungs, kidneys, intestines, and liver. In the third month, unbeknownst to the mother, the fetus is quite active, kicking and turning in its 8 oz of amniotic fluid.[73,75] All movement patterns present in a term newborn have been initiated by 15 weeks' gestation, including sucking, swallowing, breathing, and grasping the umbilical cord. Fetal responses to extrauterine stimuli (e.g., turning to auditory or visual stimulation, heart rate changes to environmental stimulation, and habituation to repeated stimuli) have been documented for decades.[76–78] Fetal activity also demonstrates cyclic fluctuations and circadian rhythms.[78]

THE COMPETENCE OF THE TERM NEWBORN

Before the 1900s, there were no formal structured examinations for the newborn; the newborn was perceived as disorganized, unstructured, and lacking in sensory and motor capacities. In the early 1900s, under the prevailing

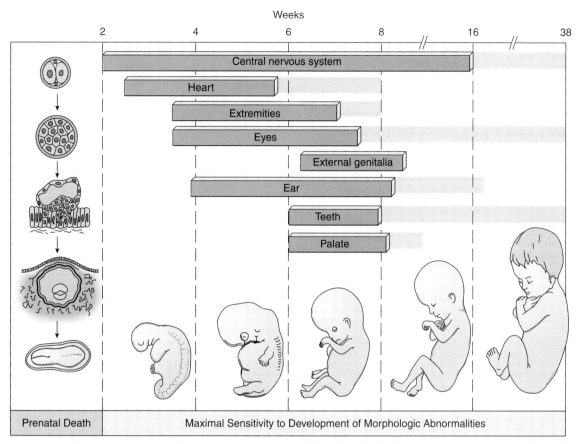

Figure 4.5 ■ Embryogenesis and fetal development. (Modified from Rubin E, Gorstein F, Schwarting R, et al. Pathology. 4th Ed. Baltimore: Lippincott Williams & Wilkins, 2005.)

Sherrington reflex model, newborn reflexes were investigated and a standard neurologic test for newborns was published. In the mid-1900s, the reflex model was expanded to include generalized motor functioning. Researchers looked at infants' active and passive muscle tone and considered infants as able to modulate their behavior. Prechtl and Beintema[79] introduced the concept of infant state as distinct organizations of the brain and associated physiology, affecting how an infant responded to a stimulus. The infant was seen as actively generating responses and modulating performances. In the latter half of the 20th century, more complex infant functioning was appreciated. Infants demonstrated preferential gaze, sound discrimination, affective behaviors, coordination of movements and speech, and differing cries, and were considered "social beings."[80] With this newfound appreciation, the infant was perceived as "competent," no longer a passive recipient or blank slate on which the environment and the baby's caregivers could write.[2,80] Comparetti[76] wrote of fetal competencies for induction and participation in labor/delivery (automatic walking and positive support to locate and engage the baby's head in the birth canal and collaborate in the expulsion process from the womb) and for survival (rooting and sucking for feeding). Brazelton saw the baby

as an active participant in the social tasks of eliciting caregiving and initiating the bonding process, organizing his or her own autonomic and state responses in order to modify the stimulation from the environment while maintaining his or her own stability.[4]

Likewise, Heidelise Als[22–27] has written numerous articles portraying the preterm infant as striving to initiate and maintain his or her own stability while completing the maturation of his or her organ systems in the high-stress environment of intensive care. Dr. Als has passionately worked to teach caregivers to recognize the attempts of the preterm infant to self-regulate, to support these efforts so that the baby not only succeeds at self-regulation but learns to trust his or her caregivers and him- or herself.

The neonatal competencies of a term baby allowing survival can be grouped into four categories: physiologic, sensorimotor, affective/communication, and complex. Physiologic competencies include the functional maturity and capability of all organ systems to allow breathing, feeding, and growing. Sensorimotor competencies include rooting, sucking, grasping, clearing the airway in prone, and horizontal and vertical tracking.[81] Affective/communication competencies include crying, self-consoling, eye contact, facial animation, and eye aversion. Complex competencies include the newborn's auditory preferences (mother's voice), taste preferences (mother's breast milk), visual preferences (faces), and imitative capacities (sticking tongue out).[82] Brazelton[52,83] has characterized the newborn as being on a mission to get his or her parents to care for him or her. The healthy term newborn is a full partner in the work of establishing a bond with the caregiver. Contrast this with the preterm infant, who is a weak partner in this task. A preterm infant is perceived as small and unattractive and is less responsive and more difficult to calm, and his cry elicits negative emotions in the caregiver. Mothers of preterm infants experience less synchronous interactions, play fewer games, work harder to engage, and derive less gratification from their infants.[84] Thus, the bonding process is at risk between a preterm infant and his or her family.

A COMPETENT FEEDER

Feeding has been described as the infant's "primary work"[3] and the coordination of sucking, swallowing, and breathing requires considerable skill as well as energy.[85] Nevertheless, every day, term newborn infants feed successfully. It is a typical and basic competency of a newborn term baby, who plays a very active role in the whole process, from waking and crying to communicate hunger, rooting to find the feeding source, pacing and coordinating sucking with swallowing and breathing, and digesting and eliminating a volume of food, to gaining weight and growing. In a preterm or sick full-term baby, failure with feeding can occur in any one or more of these areas. Sick or preterm babies may have learned an oral aversion as a result of their NICU care. A sick or preterm infant may lack the balance of flexion/extension to attain the appropriate alignment of neck extension and chin tuck to assist sucking and swallowing and breathing, or his or her residual lung disease may cause him or her to breathe too fast to allow time for sucking and swallowing. A preterm baby may not self-regulate his or her physiologic capacities so that he or she is calm and awake and can soothe him- or herself when the environment produces a stressor. A preterm infant may experience periodic breathing apnea, or bradycardia and be unable to manage the coordination of sucking, swallowing, and breathing without becoming physiologically unstable. Other potential obstacles to feeding involve immaturity or problems of the gastrointestinal tract including reflux and malabsorption.[85] Feeding is one of the primary functional tasks of a newborn infant and generally a requirement for discharge to home. Feeding problems not only delay hospital discharge, but can also be a major source of frustration and feelings of failure for parents and caregivers. Feeding interventions for babies in the NICU are beyond the scope of this chapter. Readers are referred to the recommendations for additional reading at the end of this chapter.

EVOLUTION OF TONE, REFLEXES, AND MUSCULOSKELETAL DEVELOPMENT

Due to the increasing sophistication of technology, younger preterm infants, just beyond the halfway mark of gestation, are surviving.[86] The preterm age of viability is now 23 to 24 weeks' gestation. A therapist working in a NICU must be intimately acquainted with fetal development in the last half of gestation in order to understand the behavior of the preterm infant and to intervene with and assess him or her. Suzanne Saint-Anne Dargassies[87] in 1955 studied 40 nonviable and previable fetuses from 20 to 27 weeks' gestation to determine the neurologic characteristics of fetal maturation. (At that time viability threshold was 27 weeks' gestation, and Dargassies studied these premature infants before they died.) She found that periods of 1 week were long enough to distinguish one stage from another, until 26 weeks, and then the rate of change slowed down. Dargassies observed spontaneous facial activity (excluding tongue and lips) very early; distal responses were manifest before proximal; gallant reflex (trunk incurvation) was completely present at 20 weeks; and active movements, elicited movements, and primary reflexes improved slowly in quality, duration, and completeness. She saw a complete lack of passive muscle tone in extremities and trunk, although this was hard to investigate because of "edema, sclerema, and death agony,"[87] and she observed babies from 21 weeks responding differently to tactile and painful stimuli.[87]

Dargassies[87] also studied 100 viable preterm infants from 28 weeks' to 41 weeks' gestation and observed maturational stages in 2-week segments during this time period. She created "maturative" criteria for infants at 28, 30, 32, 35, and 37 weeks and analyzed differences between term newborns and former preterms at 40 weeks' gestation. According to Dipietro,[77] the period between 28 and 32 weeks' gestation is a transitional one for a fetus. Heart rate, activity, state organization, responses to vibroacoustic stimulation, and the coupling between fetal activity and heart rate are variable with peaks and plateaus in presentation. By gestational weeks 31 to 32, the variability has stabilized and the rate of development has slowed, so that a baby at 32 weeks' gestation will demonstrate less startle responses, increasing periods of quiescence, increasing state organization, mature levels of vibroacoustic responsiveness, and increasing abilities to habituate to stimuli. These patterns continue to mature through term age; however, a 32-week fetus behaves more like a term infant than a younger fetus. This transitional period parallels the period of rapid increases in neural development and myelination, including cortical vagal responses and sulcation.[77]

Allen and Capute[86] studied 42 preterm infants, none who developed cerebral palsy, from 24 to 32 weeks' gestation with weekly neurodevelopmental examinations, and found that flexor tone, recoil, and hyperreflexia appeared

2 to 3 weeks earlier in the lower extremities (33 to 35 weeks) than the upper extremities (35 to 37 weeks). Trunk tone (measured on ventral suspension) was manifest at 36 to 40 weeks. Neck tone was poor with greater than one-half the babies at term corrected age continuing with a head lag in pull to sit. Primitive reflexes and deep tendon reflexes (DTRs) appeared in lower extremities before upper extremities. (Presence of asymmetric tonic neck reflex [ATNR] was detected in lower extremities first at 31 weeks and in upper extremities at 34 weeks.) They found that the evolution of tone, DTRs, and primitive and pathologic reflexes proceeded in an orderly sequential pattern (i.e., lower extremities to upper extremities and distal to proximal).[86]

Preterm infants, in addition to the previously described hypotonia, also have a decreased ratio of type I (slow twitch) muscle fibers to type II (fast twitch) compared to infants at term. This results in muscular fatigue (particularly respiratory muscles) in preterm infants. Preterm infants also demonstrate incomplete ossification of bones, ligamentous laxity, and connective tissue elasticity compared to term infants. The combination of these unique characteristics of preterm infants places them at the mercy of gravity and the surfaces on which they lie. Just as fetal movements or lack thereof are thought to contribute to the shaping of joints, skulls, and spinal curves of babies in utero, preterm infants can fall victim to positionally induced deformities in the NICU. These include skull shaping abnormalities like dolichocephaly (increased anterior–posterior diameter of the head) and plagiocephaly (flattening of posterior–lateral skull due to preferred head and neck rotation to one side), as well as extremity misalignment.[88]

Research comparing former preterm infants at term age (37 to 42 gestational weeks) and term newborns has demonstrated differences in tone and reactivity in the two groups. Unlike infants born at term, preterm infants miss the experience of a crowded uterus to limit their range of active movement and to support the development of flexor tone. In contrast to term infants who are tucked and contained in utero, preterm infants experience gravity, as well as intravenous lines, support boards, and other restraints, during this period of maturational-related hypotonia. For these reasons, at term age a former preterm infant and a term newborn will demonstrate differences in muscle tone. Former preterm infants at term age demonstrate less flexor tone of extremities and poorer flexor/extensor balance of head and neck, and in addition have greater range of motion in French angles, as well as greater active range of motion, than their term newborn counterparts.[89,90] Former preterm infants at term age are more reactive, demonstrating more startles, tremors, brisk reflexes, and a shorter attention span than their term counterparts.[87,90] Former preterms may also demonstrate toe walking during automatic walking, while their full-term counterparts demonstrate heel–toe walking.[87]

In addition, brain development of former preterm infants at term corrected age differs from brain development of babies born at term. Newborn term infants show better behavioral functioning of autonomic, motoric, state, and attention/interactional subsystems, as well as higher amplitudes in electroencephalography (EEG) and photic-evoked responses and increased gray/white matter differentiation and myelination, than healthy former preterm infants at term age. Some of these differences may be explained by the cumulative complications of preterm birth; however, the developmentally inappropriate sensory stimulation of a NICU may also affect preterm brain development.[91–93]

EVOLUTION OF SENSORY RESPONSES

Research demonstrates neurosensory development in animals to follow a sequential pattern, first touch, then movement, smell and taste, hearing, and lastly sight. Stimulation of a particular system during development can be essential for the development of that system. However, if the stimulus is too intense or is atypically timed, it can interfere with the development of that and other sensory systems.[94] Preterm infants are forced to complete the development and maturation of their sensory systems while in an intensive care environment. The effects of this environment on the developing brain are not fully understood and are only beginning to be studied.

TACTILE SYSTEM

Four different sensory abilities comprise the tactile system: touch, temperature, pain, and proprioception. The first three sensory receptors are housed in the skin and the last is composed of receptors from not only the skin, but also joints and muscles. The skin is the largest organ, and therefore touch is the largest sensory system as well as the first to develop.[95,96]

THE PROBLEM OF PAIN Pain comprises a component of the tactile sensory system and has recently become a focus of attention in the hospitalized infant. At one time it was standard practice for infants to have no anesthesia or analgesia for painful procedures like circumcision, central line placement, or patent ductus arteriosus ligation[44] as babies were believed to be incapable of feeling or remembering pain. However, research demonstrates both short-term and long-term consequences to pain in infancy. Infants exposed to painful and noxious stimuli show different behavioral and physiologic responses to pain, are less reactive to painful stimuli, and demonstrate more somatization as toddlers than infants not exposed to painful stimuli. At 8 to 10 years, children who were exposed to painful and noxious stimuli as infants rated medical pain significantly higher than psychosocial pain.[97]

Pain receptors appear initially around the mouth at 7 weeks' gestation and spread to the entire body, and pain pathways are myelinated by 22 weeks' gestation.[95] The neuroanatomic, neurophysiologic, and neuroendocrine systems are developed enough to allow the perception of pain in preterm and term infants, and their physiologic and hormonal pain responses are similar or exaggerated compared with adults or older children.[95,97-99]

Routine medical touch by staff members, as opposed to contacts with family, is typically experienced by hospitalized infants. Medical touch consists of repositioning, temperature taking, palpation to reinforce taping or to check the status of intravenous lines and organ systems, etc. Infants in a NICU experience an average of 40 to 70 contacts, with some infants experiencing 100 contacts per 24 hour period.[100-104] These infants are also subjected to repeated painful procedures and noxious stimuli, such as heel sticks, intravenous line placement, and suctioning of endotracheal tubes, which are completed on a routine basis in addition to frequent handling.[43,44,105] One researcher reported an average of 134 painful procedures for newborn babies in a NICU in the first 2 weeks of life,[106] whereas an infant born at 23 weeks' gestation had a documented 488 procedures.[107] Although the frequency of painful procedures is recognized, there is little understanding about the pain experienced from medical conditions associated with prematurity or a NICU stay (like necrotizing enterocolitis or intraventricular hemorrhage).[107] Unfortunately, pain and medical contacts are integral experiences of babies in a NICU.

THE PROBLEM OF PAIN ASSESSMENT Since babies are unable to report pain, comprehensive, valid, and reliable pain assessment in a NICU is complex and requires the identification of multiple responses, both physiologic and behavioral.[97,107-109] Term and preterm babies respond differently to pain, a fact that adds to the difficulty with pain assessment in babies in a NICU. Preterm babies are less robust than full-term infants in expressing pain through crying or moving; therefore, gestational age is an important consideration when assessing pain in an infant.[108-110] Critically ill infants may mimic preterm infants in their incapacity to display vigorous pain responses; therefore, a lack of behavioral pain responses should not be interpreted as a lack of pain.[97,99,109] The Joint Commission on Accreditation of Healthcare Organizations (JCAHO) standard of care now requires routine assessment of neonatal pain utilizing a standardized assessment scale of neonatal pain[111] and appropriate interventions to reduce and alleviate pain (see Table 4.2 for commonly used methods of pain assessment in newborns). Despite this recommendation and the understanding of the infant's capability to feel pain, strategies to manage pain are underemployed in NICUs.[97,107,112] Obstacles to implementation of nonpharmacologic and pharmacologic pain supports include health practitioners' concerns regarding side effects, toxicity, and physiologic dependence for pharmacologic agents and lack of understanding of effectiveness of nonpharmacologic supports in pain reduction.[97,107,112] Nonpharmacologic interventions are strategies to relieve pain while promoting the infant's self-regulatory capacities.[113] Physical therapists working in a NICU need to be familiar with the assessment of pain in young infants, as well as with a variety of environmental and behavioral strategies to reduce pain. They also need to be vigilant in anticipating the potential for pain for babies in the NICU and to advocate for early and aggressive intervention to minimize pain for these patients.[107]

ENVIRONMENTAL AND BEHAVIORAL STRATEGIES FOR PAIN REDUCTION Nonpharmacologic interventions are the bases for pain management and ideally should be implemented consistently for any painful procedure or noxious touch in the NICU.[97] However, they should not substitute for pharmacologic therapy, which should be utilized in addition to nonpharmacologic pain supports for prolonged or moderate to severe pain in the infant.

Environmental strategies reduce pain indirectly by reducing the level of noxious stimuli present to the infant.

TABLE 4.2

Common Neonatal Pain Assessment Scales

	CRIES	Premature Infant Pain Profile (PIPP)	Neonatal Facial Coding Scale (NFCS)	Neonatal Infant Pain Scale (NIPS)
Characteristics assessed	Crying Requires additional O$_2$ Increased vital signs Expression Sleeplessness	Gestational age Behavioral state Heart rate O$_2$ saturation Brow bulge Eye squeeze Nasolabial furrow	Brow bulge Eye squeeze Nasolabial furrow Open lips Stretched mouth Lip purse Taut tongue Chin quiver Tongue protrusion	Facial expression Cry Breathing patterns Arms Legs State of arousal

From Anand KJS, International Evidence-Based Group for Neonatal Pain. Consensus statement for the prevention and management of pain in the newborn. Arch Pediatr Adolesc Med 2001;155:173–180.

Environmental strategies include dimming the lights or shading the eyes of the infant and reducing the noise around the infant's bed space by keeping pagers on vibrate mode, silencing alarms, shutting drawers and porthole doors softly, and talking in soft voices away from the bedside. Other environmental strategies include reducing frequency of handling and painful procedures.[40]

Nonpharmacologic interventions include positioning via swaddling or facilitated tucking, nonnutritive sucking (NNS), skin-to-skin holding (kangaroo care), and sucrose.[97,105,114] Facilitated tucking is a manual technique where a support person holds the baby's flexed limbs close to the baby's body during a noxious or painful procedure. Facilitated tucking has been demonstrated to minimize physiologic indices of pain, shorten cry, maintain sleep state, and reduce scores on the premature infant pain profile (PIPP) during heel stick, endotracheal suctioning, and routine caregiving.[41–45] Swaddling an infant can also provide the bodily containment important for pain relief in infants undergoing painful procedures.[43]

Nonnutritive sucking has been demonstrated to reduce hospital stay and decrease fussing/crying and physiologic arousal during heel stick.[46–48,107,108] Kangaroo care, or skin-to-skin holding, demonstrates marked reductions in crying, grimacing, and heart rate during heel sticks in newborn infants.[115] The practice of giving sucrose with or without NNS has been shown to decrease physiologic and behavioral pain indices as well as pain scores for babies undergoing heel stick or venipuncture and is considered safe and effective in reducing procedural pain.[116] Physical therapists along with the nursing and medical teams in the NICU should be vigilant for the expression of stress and pain in the infant, as well as for opportunities to implement environmental and behavioral strategies to reduce neonatal pain and stress from noxious stimuli.

VESTIBULAR SYSTEM

The sensory end organs of the vestibular system, the three semicircular canals, and the otolith are housed inside the skull cavity (vestibule), which also contains the hearing sense organ, the cochlea. Both the hearing and the vestibular systems convert stimuli into electrical signals via the cilia. In the vestibular system, these signals are carried by the vestibular nerve to the brainstem and relayed to a variety of areas so that information regarding the baby's position in space can be interpreted, integrated, and used to guide movement and function.[96]

The vestibular system is one of the first to develop in utero and the vestibular nerve is the first fiber tract to begin myelination at the end of the first trimester. By 20 weeks' gestation, this nerve has reached its full-size shape and the other vestibular tracts have begun to myelinate.[96] The vestibular system is thought to be responsible for the fetus orienting to the head-down position prior to birth. The vestibular system is mature in the full-term newborn,[100] but modifications and growth in the synapses and dendrites of the vestibular pathways continue until puberty as the child learns to move and adapts to his or her changing body size and shape.[96]

The womb provides almost constant vestibular stimulation to the developing fetus, some contingent (fetal movement) and some noncontingent (maternal movements).[96,117] The preterm baby in a NICU experiences primarily immobilization and therefore reduced vestibular stimulation. The consequences of the constant vestibular stimulation a term baby experiences in utero and the lack of such with a preterm baby are unclear and there is little information to guide interventions with the vestibular system. Research on vestibular stimulation on the preterm infant is often carried out with other modes of stimulation, making it difficult to understand the effects of pure vestibular stimulation. Vestibular stimulation is known to enhance behavioral states; for example, slow rhythmic rocking is soothing and promotes quiet sleep, and fast arrhythmic vestibular stimulation increases activity and agitation.[3] Vestibular stimulation has not been demonstrated to affect feeding, weight gain, length of stay, or neurodevelopmental outcomes in hospitalized infants.[38] More research is needed in this area; however, gentle vestibular stimulation within the infant's tolerance levels and for a developmentally appropriate reason may be implemented in the NICU.[117]

OLFACTORY AND GUSTATORY DEVELOPMENT

Taste and smell are both chemical senses, initiated in response to specific molecules in the immediate environment and transmitted into electrical signals by neurons. Olfactory development begins at 5 weeks' gestation with the appearance of the nasal pit. At 8 weeks, the neurons in the olfactory bulb begin to develop and are mature by 20 weeks. By 11 weeks, the nostrils are replete with olfactory epithelia. The ability to smell begins at 28 weeks when the biochemical development of olfactory epithelia and neurons is completed.

Taste buds begin to mature at approximately 13 weeks when the fetus begins to suck and swallow. At term age approximately 7000 taste buds are present over the perimeter of the tongue, soft palate, and upper throat.[96] Sucking and swallowing amniotic fluid stimulates the taste buds and influences their synaptic connections. The amniotic fluid is constantly changing, reflecting the mix of the maternal diet with the fetus' urination. The fetus experiences a variety of tastes and smells while in utero. Likewise, breast milk is flavored by maternal diet and the newborn is able to recognize his or her mother's breast milk, as its smell and taste are familiar to him or her. From 24 weeks until term, a fetus swallows approximately 1 L of amniotic fluid per day. Contrast this with the experiences of the preterm baby, who frequently has an orogastric tube and/or endotracheal tube in his or her mouth, tape on his or her face, and the taste of a rubber glove, medications, or vitamins in his or her mouth. In addition, the preterm infant does not get this constant swallowing practice, making the necessary coordination of sucking, swallowing, and breathing a challenge.[96]

AUDITORY SYSTEM

By 24 weeks' gestation, the development of the cochlea and peripheral sensory end organs is complete and the first blink/startle responses to vibroacoustic stimulation can be elicited. By 28 weeks, these responses are consistent; the hearing threshold is approximately 40 dB and decreases to 13.5 dB (approximating the adult levels) by 42 weeks' postconceptual age, demonstrating the continuing maturation of the auditory pathways. A preterm infant in the NICU is subjected to the noise of a NICU during the normal development and maturation of hearing. Exposure to this NICU noise may cause cochlear damage as well as cause sleep disturbances and disrupt the growth and development of the baby.[94,118] The bubbling of water inside a ventilator tubing or tapping on the outside of the incubator can result in noise that is 70 to 80 dB inside an incubator, whereas closing the porthole doors or the drawers under the incubator or dropping the head of the mattress can result in 90 to 120 dB noise.[118] Incubator covers reduce only the noise of objects striking the incubator. However, most noise in an incubator comes from the motor, drawer and door closures, and the infant's own crying.[119] Other common NICU sounds include alarms, overhead pages, beepers, telephones, traffic, and conversations. In one study, peak noise was in the 65- to 75-dB range, and most noise was due to human activity.[120] Normal conversation is typically at the 60-dB range and whispering is between 20 to 30 dB.[118]

Contrast this with the sounds of pregnancy inside the womb (i.e., muffled maternal speech, maternal heart rate, and gastrointestinal sounds), which are structured or patterned but not continuous or fixed. These sounds may also be contingent on maternal or fetal behavior and typically affect more than one sensory organ.[81] Background noise in the human uterus allows low frequencies of maternal speech to be discriminated. In utero the maternal tissues attenuate sound frequencies greater than 250 Hz and thus shield the developing fetus. The sound environment of a NICU has levels of low- and high-frequency sound and this may diminish the babies' exposure to maternal speech. The NICU provides a very different auditory sensory experience for the developing baby than the womb.

The American Academy of Pediatrics (AAP)[118] recommends that noise levels in a NICU should not exceed 45 dB; in order to accomplish this, staff must be cooperative and NICU design and construction must support this. In addition to strategies to reduce noise from human or mechanical sources, new alternatives to the crowded and noisy state of current NICU designs have been suggested by Evans and Philbin,[121,123] White,[122] and Philbin and Evans.[124]

VISUAL SYSTEM

Vision is the most complex human sense and the least mature at term birth. By 23 to 24 weeks' gestation the major eye structures and the visual pathways are in place; however, the eyelids are fused, the optic media is cloudy, and there are remnants of embryonic tissue in the eye globe. A few immature photoreceptor cells occupy the retina, and retinal blood vessels in the posterior retina have begun to develop. From 24 weeks to term, the retina and visual cortex undergo extensive maturation and differentiation. At 24 to 28 weeks the eyelids separate. However, the pupillary reflex is absent; the lid will tighten to bright light, but this fatigues easily. By 34 weeks, the pupillary reflex is present and bright light causes lid closure without fatigue. Brief eye opening and fixation on a high-contrast form under low illumination may occur. Morante et al.[125] found that most 32-week gestation premature infants could perceive ½-inch stripes at 12 inches, and by 35 to 36 weeks most could perceive ¼-inch stripes. At term most infants could distinguish ⅛-inch stripes. Also, pattern preference matured from 34 weeks on as well. Unlike Saint-Anne Dargassies,[87] Morante et al.[125] found that former premature infants at 40 weeks did less well with visual acuity and pattern preference than term newborns. By 36 weeks, the infant will orient toward a soft light and demonstrate saccadic visual following horizontally and vertically. At term, infants see with acuity estimates of 20/400. They are far-sighted with poor focusing for objects up close.[81]

Typically, visual maturation occurs in a dark womb and does not require light exposure. However, the infants born prematurely are subjected to the harsh bright lighting of the NICU, which produces phototoxic effects in animals and can potentially impact brain development. Bilirubin lights to treat hyperbilirubinemia can produce light equivalent to greater than 10,000 footcandles. Because of their visual immaturity, preterm infants should be shielded from ambient and supplementary light sources. Five footcandles is desirable to encourage spontaneous eye opening. Although preterm infants will attend to black and white patterns, this can be stressful for them. Prolonged attention to black and white patterns has been associated with lower IQ in childhood. Visual stimulation may also interfere with typical auditory dominance, resulting in decreased attending to speech, and may disrupt the emergence of hand regard and visually directed reaching.[3,81,96]

EVOLUTION OF STATE DIFFERENTIATION

True behavioral states in terms of a set of characteristic variables linked together may not be present in infants less than 36 to 37 weeks' gestational age,[86,126] and preterm infants younger than 36 weeks do not possess a full capacity for control over states of arousal.[3] Brazelton and Nugent[127] define six states in their newborn assessment and pay close attention to the range, variety, and duration of the states a baby exhibits during an assessment (Table 4.3).

TABLE 4.3

State-Related Behaviors*

Sleep State	Behaviors
State 1A	Infant in deep sleep with obligatory regular breathing or breathing in synchrony with only the respirator; eyes closed; no eye movements under closed lids; quiet facial expression; no spontaneous activity; typically pale color.
State 1B	Infant in deep sleep with predominately modulated regular breathing; eyes closed; no eye movement under closed lids; relaxed facial expression; no spontaneous activity except isolated startles.
State 2A	Light sleep with eyes closed; rapid eye movements can be seen under closed lids; low-amplitude activity level with diffuse and disorganized movements; respirations are irregular and there are many sucking and mouthing movements, whimpers; facial, body, and extremity twitchings, much grimacing; the impression of a "noisy" state is given. Color is typically poor.
State 2B	Light sleep with eyes closed; rapid eye movements can be seen under closed lids; low activity level with movements and dampen startles; movements are likely to be of lower amplitude and more monitored than in state 1; infant responds to various internal stimuli with dampened startle. Respirations are more regular; mild sucking and mouthing movements can occur off and on; one or two whimpers may be observed, as well as infrequent sighs or smiles.

Transitional (Drowsy) States

State 3A	Drowsy or semi-dozing; eyes may be open or closed; eyelids fluttering or exaggerated blinking; if eyes are open, glassy veiled look; activity level variable with or without interspersed startles from time to time; diffuse movement; fussing and/or much discharge of vocalization, whimpers; facial grimace.
State 3B	Drowsy, same as above but with less discharge of vocalization, whimpers, facial grimace, etc.

Awake States†

State 4AL	Awake and quiet, minimal noisy activity, eyes half open or open but with glazed or dull look, giving the impression of little involvement and distance, or focused yet seeming to look through rather than at object or examiner, or the infant is clearly awake and reactive but has eyes closed intermittently.
State 4AH	Awake and quiet; minimal motor activity; eyes wide open, "hyperalert" or giving the impression of panic or fear; may appear to be hooked by the stimulus; seems to have difficulty in modulating or breaking the intensity of the fixation to the object or move away from it.
State 4B	Alert with bright shiny animated facial expression; seems to focus attention on source of stimulation and appears to process information actively and with modulation; motor activity is at a minimum.

Active States

State 5A	Eyes may or may not be open but infant is clearly aroused as is dictated by motor arousal, tonus, and distressed facial expression, grimacing, or other signs of discomfort. Fussing, if present, is diffuse or strained.
State 5B	Eyes may or may not be open but infant is clearly awake and aroused, with considerable, yet well-defined, motor activity. Infant may also be clearly fussing but not crying robustly.

Crying States

State 6A	Intense crying, as indicated by intense grimace and cry face, yet cry sound may be very strained or weak or absent; intensity of upset is greater than fussing.
State 6B	Rhythmic, intense, lusty crying that is robust, vigorous, and strong in sound.

*These are subgrouped into the states themselves and specific, typically attention-related behaviors. Various configurations of behaviors encompassing eye movements, eye opening and facial expressions, gross body movements, respirations, and tonus aspects are used in specific temporal relationships to one another to determine at what level of consciousness an infant is at a particular time. It is possible to make meaningful, systematic distinctions between dynamic transformations of various behavioral configurations that appear to correspond to varying states of availability and conscious responsiveness. The following spectrum of observable states is suggested: States labeled as A states are "noisy," unclean, and diffuse; states labeled as B states are clean, well-defined states.

†For 4A two types of diffuse alertness are distinguished, 4 AL and 4 AH. L or H is marked instead of a check mark.

AA: Should the infant move into prolonged respiratory pause (e.g., beyond 8 seconds). AA should be marked. The infant has removed him- or herself from the state continuum.

More than one box per 2-minute time block can be marked, depending on the fluctuation and behavior the infant shows.

Operationally, typically a 2- to 3-second duration of a behavioral configuration is necessary to be registered as a distinct state; however, even briefer excursions, especially into states 4 and 6, can be recorded reliably.

Reprinted with permission from Als H. Reading the premature infant. In: Goldson E, ed. Nurturing the Premature Infant. Developmental Intervention in the Neonatal Intensive Care nursery. New York: Oxford University Press, 1999:82–84.

Als[128] modifies these states for preterm infants, describing them as less well organized and less clearly defined than states a healthy term baby demonstrates. In preterm infants, sleep states predominate and wakeful periods emerge for brief periods around 28 weeks and become more numerous at 30 weeks.[87] Preterm infant sleep states are disorganized with more motoric responses during sleep. Wakeful periods in preterm infants are brief and sporadic. The proportions of sleep and wake periods change as babies' mature. Quiet alert times appear in preterm infants who are close to term age and have a degree of physiologic and motoric stability. Because the state system is foundational for attending and interacting, it is important to be familiar with and to assess the range and robustness of states available to an infant, as well as the ease of transition between states.[128]

Medical Foundations to Guide Therapy

LANGUAGE OF THE NEONATAL INTENSIVE CARE UNIT

The language of the NICU also reflects the crisis-driven nature of the intensive care required by these critically ill infants. Many complex procedures and diagnoses are referred to by acronyms, and the language can be intimidating for those who do not know what the terms mean. There is a list of commonly used abbreviations in Addendum A at the end of this chapter. In addition, a few key terms will be defined below.

Gestational age refers to the length of time the baby was in the womb and is counted in weeks from the mother's last menstrual period to the baby's birth.[129] Term gestation is 37 to 41½ weeks, and a baby born before 37 weeks is considered preterm. A baby born at 42 weeks or more is considered postterm.[130]

Correcting a baby's age is an important skill to understand and to teach to parents. The 40 weeks of gestation are so critical to development that it is unfair to ignore the time lost in utero when a preterm birth occurs. It is important that both the therapist and the family develop expectations for a baby that are based on corrected age and not chronologic age. Chronologic age (CA) is defined as the age the baby is based on his or her birthday. Corrected or adjusted age (AA) is defined as the age the baby is from his or her due date; a baby born at 28 weeks whose chronologic age is 8 weeks would have an adjusted age of 36 weeks' postconceptual age (PCA = GA + CA or 28 weeks + 8 weeks). That same baby 4 weeks later would be considered 40 weeks PCA, or term. Once the baby has reached his term age, the number of weeks the baby missed in utero is subtracted from his chronologic age, so that, at 5 months chronologic age, the baby's adjusted age is 3 months (6 months–3 months [12 weeks is 3 months early]). This age adjustment is important for assessing a former preterm infant's growth and development until 2 to 3 years as most catching up is completed by then.[131]

AGA, SGA, and LGA are acronyms for appropriate for gestational age, small for gestational age, and large for gestational age, respectively. These terms refer to the weight of the baby at birth. AGA refers to an infant whose weight at birth falls within the 10th and 90th percentiles for his or her age. A baby born 12 weeks early can be AGA, or a baby born at term can be AGA if his or her weight is within two standard deviations of the mean (10th to 90th percentiles) for babies born at that gestational age. A baby who is SGA has a weight that is below the 10th percentile (or below two standard deviations from the mean) for his or her age, and a baby who is LGA weighs above the 90th percentile (or above two standard deviations from the mean) for his or her age at birth (Fig. 4.6). SGA infants can also be called IUGR, or intrauterine growth restricted. The etiology for this may be a chromosomal abnormality in the baby, congenital malformation, or congenital infection.[75] LGA may be due to large parents, maternal diabetes, or postmaturity (greater than 42 weeks' gestation), or the baby may have other genetic syndromes. Babies born LGA are at risk for birth trauma, especially brachial plexus injury or perinatal depression. They may also be more likely to have hyperinsulinism or polycythemia.[130]

Research correlating birth weight with outcome is common, and has led to additional acronyms referring to weight such as NBW, LBW, MLBW, VLBW, and ELBW. Normal birth weight (NBW) is 2500 to 3999 g (5 lb 8 oz to 8 lb 13 oz). Low birth weight (LBW) is defined as less than 2500 g (5 lb 8 oz). Moderately low birth weight (MLBW) is defined as 1500 to 2500 g (3 lb 5 oz to 5 lb 8 oz). Very low birth weight (VLBW) is defined as less than 1500 g (3 lb 5 oz). Extremely low birth weight (ELBW) is less than 1000 g (2 lb 3 oz). Infants less than 750 g (1 lb 10 oz) are micropreemies, and infants weighing more than 4000 g (8 lb 13 oz) have macrosomia.[3,130]

The medical chart may describe the mother as a 32-year-old G5 P1223. G stands for gravida and P for para. These terms describe the number of maternal pregnancies and pregnancy outcomes, respectively. The mnemonic "Florida Power And Light" can be used to remember what the numbers following P mean. The first number stands for number of *f*ull-term births, the second for number of *p*reterm births, the third for number of *a*bortions (whether spontaneous or therapeutic), and the fourth for number of *l*iving children. In the case of G5 P1223, the mother had five pregnancies; one full-term infant, two preterm babies, two abortions, and a total of three living children. When only a single number follows the P, it represents the number of living children.

A scoring system to evaluate the physical condition of newborn infants after delivery was developed by Virginia Apgar[132] in 1953, and the name APGAR has evolved into an acronym for this scale. A is for appearance, P is for pulse,

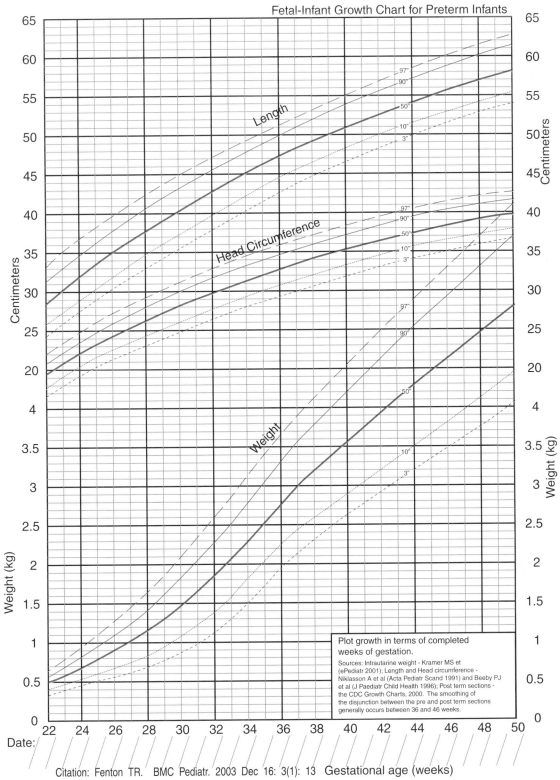

Date:

Citation: Fenton TR. BMC Pediatr. 2003 Dec 16: 3(1): 13   Gestational age (weeks)

Figure 4.6 ■ Premature infant growth chart. (Adapted with permission from Babson SG, Benda GI. Growth graphs for the clinical assessment of varying gestational age. J Pediatr 1976;89:814–820. Used with permission from Ross Products.)

TABLE 4.4						
Apgar Score						

	Score		
Sign	**0**	**1**	**2**
Heart rate	Absent	<100 bpm	100–140 bpm
Respiratory effort	Absent	Slow, shallow	Good, crying irregular
Reflex irritability	No response	Grimace	Cough or sneeze
Muscle tone	Flaccid	Some flexion	Active motion of extremities
Color	Blue	Pink body, blue extremities	All pink

From Apgar V. A proposal for a new method of evaluation of the newborn infant. Anesth Analg 1953;32(4):260–267.

G is for grimace, A is for activity, and R is for respiration (Table 4.4). These scores are generally assigned for the first and fifth minute of life if the baby does not require extensive resuscitation. Should the score reflect apnea or bradycardia with an Apgar score of less than 6, resuscitation is begun. A score in the range of 3 to 4 indicates the need for bag and mask ventilation; a score of 5 to 7 requires blow-by oxygen; and a score of 8 to 10 is considered typical for term newborns and the infant does not require resuscitation. An example of an Apgar score as recorded in the medical history is 8^195. The Apgar score after 1 minute indicates the infant's changing condition and whether resuscitative efforts are adequate or need to be increased. For infants who require extensive resuscitation, Apgar scores may be taken every 5 minutes until the score is greater than 6 (i.e., $0^10^52^{10}5^{15}6^{20}$).

ENVIRONMENTAL ASPECTS OF INTENSIVE CARE: EQUIPMENT AND TECHNOLOGIC SUPPORTS

The NICU is built around the highly technical supports that can sustain an infant's life. This technology has exploded in the latter half of the 20th century, allowing more babies to survive. This technology also influences the climate, culture, and workspace of the NICU, and can give the NICU a much cluttered, very cold, and metallic appearance. Equipment commonly found in the NICU to support a baby is listed in Table 4.5 (Figs. 4.7 and 4.8).

The primary objective of assisted ventilatory support in high-risk infants is to optimize the infant's cardiopulmonary status while minimizing trauma to the airways and lungs. This is done by working to improve gas exchange at the lowest amount of inspired oxygen (FiO_2) and the lowest pressures and tidal volume. The individual infant's condition will dictate how ventilatory support is provided.[135]

Continuous positive airway pressure (CPAP) provides a continuous flow of warmed, humidified gas at a set pressure to maintain an elevated end-expiratory lung volume while the infant breathes spontaneously.[135–138] CPAP can be delivered by mask, nasal prongs, or less frequently through an endotracheal tube.

The gas mixture delivered via CPAP can be either continuous flow or variable flow. In continuous flow the system provides a noninterrupted supply of gas to the infant. Bubble or water seal CPAP is a type of continuous flow. The blended gas is delivered to the infant after being heated and humidified. The distal end of the tubing is immersed in sterile water or acetic acid to a specific level to provide the desired amount of CPAP.[137] Bubble CPAP can generate vibrations in the infant's chest at frequencies similar to those used in high-frequency ventilation.[139] Variable flow nasal CPAP (NCPAP) uses injector jets to deliver gas at a constant pressure through nasal prongs into each nares. The flow is able to change so that the infant doesn't have to exhale against the CPAP.[137]

CPAP is used to prevent alveolar and airway collapse and to reduce the barotrauma caused by mechanical ventilation. Indications for CPAP include the early treatment of respiratory distress syndrome (RDS), moderately frequent apneic spells, recent extubation, weaning chronically ventilator-dependent infants, and early treatment to prevent atelectasis in premature infants with minimal respiratory distress and minimal need for supplemental oxygen. Negative aspects of NCPAP include gastric distension with high flows and excoriation or breakdown of the nasal septum.[136–138]

The most common approach in the United States for treating respiratory failure in the NICU is with positive pressure ventilation.[140,141] The two types of positive pressure mechanical ventilators are volume controlled or pressure limited. Volume-controlled ventilators deliver the same tidal volume of gas with each breath regardless of how much pressure is needed. While rarely used with newborn infants, volume ventilators designed specifically for neonates can be used in the presence of rapidly changing lung compliance.[135] Pressure-limited ventilators deliver gas until a preset limiting pressure is reached. The peak pressure delivered to the airway is constant but the tidal volume with each breath is variable. Synchronized intermittent mandatory ventilation (SIMV), assist/control, and pressure support are adaptations of conventional pressure-limited ventilators and are also used in the NICU.

High-frequency ventilation (HFV) utilizes extremely rapid ventilatory rates to deliver tidal volumes equal to or

TABLE 4.5	

Common Medical Equipment in the Neonatal Intensive Care Unit (NICU)

Radiant warmer	Open bed with low, adjustable, Plexiglas side rails on a height and angle adjustable table with overhead heat source, temperature monitor, and procedure lights
Isolette	Enclosed incubator. Clear plastic unit or box enclosing the mattress with heat and humidity control. Access to infant is through side port holes or side opening
Open crib	Small bassinet-style bed or small metal crib without a heat source
Bag and mask	Ventilating system consisting of self-inflating bag with reservoir, flow meter, pressure manometer connected to a mask that fits over the infant's nose and mouth
Oxy hood	Plexiglas hood that fits over the infant's head and provides controlled oxygen and humidification
Nasal cannula	Humidified gas delivered via flexible tubing with small prongs that fit into the nares
HFNC	Humidified gas (may be highly humidified) delivered at high flow rates via a nasal cannula
CPAP	Continuous or variable flow of warmed humidified gas at a set pressure generated by a CPAP unit or mechanical ventilator and delivered by mask, nasal prongs, or less frequently through an endotracheal tube (for infants with spontaneous breathing)
Vapotherm	Highly humidified, high flow system of delivering gas via nasal prongs
Mechanical ventilation	
CMV	Conventional mechanical ventilation. Positive-pressure ventilators are more commonly used in the NICU and are constant-flow, time-cycled, pressure-limited devices
HFJV	High-frequency jet ventilation delivers short pulses of heated, pressurized gas directly into the upper airway through a jet injector
HFOV	High-frequency oscillating ventilator has a piston pump or vibrating diaphragm that produces a sinusoidal pressure wave that is transmitted through the airways to the alveoli
iNO	Nitric oxide is an inspired gas delivered in combination with mechanical ventilation that acts as a vasodilator and vascular smooth muscle relaxant
ECMO	Extracorporeal membrane oxygenation is a heart and lung bypass procedure that involves draining venous blood, supplementing it with O_2, and removing CO_2 by means of a membrane oxygenator and returning the blood to either venous or arterial circulations
Vital signs monitor	Unit that displays monitoring of HR, RR, BP, and Sao_2
Pulse oximeter	Measures oxygen concentration in the peripheral circulation with a bandage-type light sensor attached to the infant's arm or leg, which provides a pulse-by-pulse readout of percent oxygen saturation on the screen of the monitor
Transcutaneous oxygen and carbon dioxide monitor	Noninvasive method for monitoring concentrations of O_2 and CO_2 through the skin
Infusion pumps	Electric infusion pump that controls the flow and rate of fluids, intralipids, and transpyloric feedings
Phototherapy	Fiberoptic or overhead bank or spot lights or fiberoptic blanket used to reduce hyperbilirubinemia
Gavage tube	Oral or nasogastric tube used for feeding directly into the stomach. Transpyloric tubes are used for infants who can't tolerate oral or nasal tubes, have severe GER, or are at risk for aspiration
PIV	Peripheral intravenous line, which may be used for fluids, nutrition, or antibiotics
CVL	Central venous line used for prolonged parental feeding or antibiotics, or to draw blood
PICC	Percutaneous inserted central catheter. Long, flexible catheter inserted through a peripheral antecubital vein and threaded centrally to the superior vena cava. PICC lines are used for prolonged parental feeding or antibiotics or to draw blood
UA	Umbilical arterial line inserted through the umbilical artery into the abdominal aorta and is used for first 5–7 days of life for monitoring arterial blood gases, infusion of fluids, and continuous blood pressure monitoring
UV	Umbilical venous line inserted into umbilical vein and is used for first 7–14 days of life and as the initial venous access, to infuse vasopressors, and for exchange transfusions, monitoring of central venous pressure, and infusion of fluids

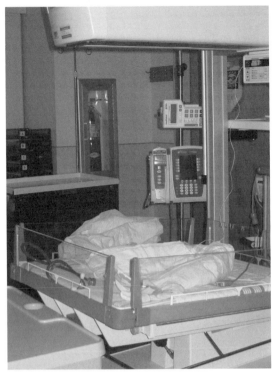

Figure 4.7 ▪ Radiant warmer bed set up for an admission to the neonatal intensive care unit.

smaller than anatomic dead space. Continuous pressures are applied to maintain an elevated lung volume with superimposed tidal volumes provided at a rapid rate. The advantages of HFV over conventional ventilation are to provide adequate gas exchange at lower proximal airway pressures in lungs already damaged by barotrauma and volutrauma, and to preserve normal lung structure in the relatively uninjured lung.[142–145]

The three types of HFV used in the NICU are high-frequency positive pressure ventilation (HFPPV), high-frequency jet ventilation (HFJV), and high-frequency oscillating ventilation (HFOV).[142,145] HFPPV is produced by conventional ventilators or modified conventional ventilators set at a high rate.[144] HFJV delivers short pulses of heated, pressurized gas directly into the upper airway through a narrow cannula or jet injector.[144–146] The HFJV can maintain oxygenation and ventilation to wide ranges of lung compliance and patient size. HFOV has a piston pump or vibrating diaphragm that produces a sinusoidal pressure wave that is transmitted through the airways to the alveoli.[144,145] Small tidal volumes are superimposed over a constant airway pressure at a high respiratory rate.[147]

HFV is used primarily for infants who are failing conventional ventilation.[135,142] While outcome studies have been unable to demonstrate clear benefits of HFV over conventional mechanical ventilation (CMV), clinically HFV has been helpful in airleak syndromes, pulmonary interstitial emphysema (PIE), pre-/postcongenital diaphragmatic hernia (CDH) repair, meconium aspiration syndrome (MAS), and some forms of pulmonary hypoplasia.[144,145,147] HFV can also be used as a bridge to ECMO for infants with severe respiratory failure and may eliminate the need for ECMO in some infants.[144] Neonatal RDS is the most common lung disease treated with HFV in the NICU. HFJV has been shown to be most successful in the treatment of airleak syndromes, while HFOV has shown better outcomes for infants with CDH, RDS, and persistent pulmonary hypertension of the newborn (PPHN).[144] The most serious side effect of HFV is an increase in long-term neurologic injury due to early periventricular leukomalacia (PVL) or severe intraventricular hemorrhage (IVH).[145] Some studies have found increased severe IVH in very premature infants treated with HFV versus CMV.[145,148] Other studies found no difference when other confounding variables were taken into consideration such as gestational age, type of delivery, early large patent ductus arteriosus (PDA), and decreased superior vena cava blood flow (Fig. 4.9).[135,149]

Another form of ventilatory support that is beginning to be used with greater frequency in the NICU is high-flow nasal cannula. Studies have shown the high nasal cannula to be as effective as NCPAP in providing positive end-

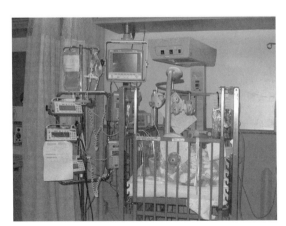

Figure 4.8 ▪ Crib with radiant warmer, infusion pumps, and monitor.

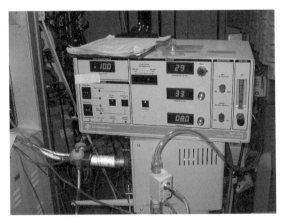

Figure 4.9 ▪ High-flow oscillating ventilator.

distending pressure to the lungs of some infants with mild respiratory disease. The advantage of nasal cannula over NCPAP is less irritation to the nasal septum.[150–152] The nasal cannula allows for greater comfort on the part of the infant and greater ease for the family or nurses to hold and care for the infant than mask or nasal prongs. Highly humidified high-flow nasal cannula is also used to provide higher flows of gas without the usual negative side effects of nasal cannula (i.e., drying, bleeding, or nasal septal breakdown due to the addition of high humidity).[153–157] Limited research is currently available regarding use of Vapotherm/highly humidified high-flow nasal cannula.

In December 1999, the U.S. Food and Drug Administration approved the use of inhaled nitric oxide (iNO) for the treatment of near-term and term infants with hypoxic respiratory failure. PPHN, RDS, aspiration syndromes, pneumonia, sepsis, and congenital diaphragmatic hernia are conditions that can cause hypoxic respiratory failure. The primary actions of nitric oxide are vasodilation and the relaxation of vascular smooth muscle, which increases blood flow to alveoli, improving oxygen and carbon dioxide exchange. Nitric oxide is a short-lived molecule, so that it affects the pulmonary vascular smooth muscle without affecting systemic vasculature. Airway smooth muscle is also affected by nitric oxide, and the combined action of airway and vascular smooth muscle relaxation has been effective in the treatment of infants with ventilation–perfusion abnormalities (Fig. 4.10).[158,159]

Infants in the first week of life, who are 34 weeks' or greater gestational age with progressive hypoxic respiratory failure, meet the criteria for use of iNO as an adjunct to therapeutic interventions. The degree of illness and/or the modalities tried prior to the initiation of nitric oxide have not been clearly delineated. Nitric oxide is contraindicated for infants with congenital heart disease whose cardiopulmonary function depends on a right-to-left shunt or who have severe left heart failure.[160] While inhaled nitric oxide has not been effective in treating infants with congenital diaphragmatic hernia, multicenter clinical trials have shown that iNO improves oxygenation and the outcome of near-term and term infants with hypoxic respiratory failure due to other conditions such as PPHN. Studies have also shown that iNO reduces the need for ECMO without increasing neurodevelopmental, behavioral, or medical abnormalities[161–164]

The use of iNO in preterm infants is controversial and there is no consensus on the timing for initiation, dosage, and length of time for iNO therapy with infants less than 34 weeks. In two studies of infants less than 32 weeks' GA and body weight less than 1250 grams requiring mechanical ventilation, those who received iNO demonstrated decreased incidence of bronchopulmonary dysplasia (BPD), less severe lung disease, decreased length of time requiring supplemental oxygen, decreased incidence of death, and no increased risk of brain injury. The benefits of iNO may be due to decreased airway resistance, which results in decreased need for supplemental oxygen, mechanical ventilation, and oxidative stress.[165,166]

ECMO is similar to a heart-lung bypass machine and provides rest and support for the baby's heart and lungs. ECMO is utilized with patients with cardiac and pulmonary dysfunction whose hypoxia is refractory to conventional therapies like conventional mechanical ventilation and high-frequency ventilation. In the last decade the use of surfactant, inhaled nitric oxide, and high-frequency ventilation has replaced ECMO with patients with RDS, MAS, or pulmonary hypertension. ECMO continues to be implemented with patients with CDH, PPHN, and sepsis (Fig. 4.11).[167–170,172]

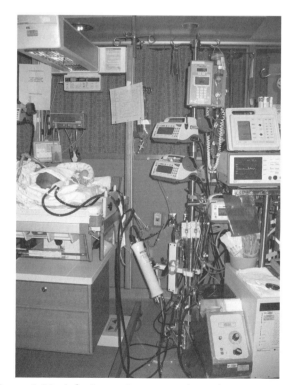

Figure 4.11 ■ Infant on extracorporeal membrane oxygenation.

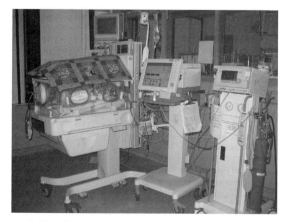

Figure 4.10 ■ Conventional ventilator with nitric oxide tank.

To initiate ECMO, catheters are inserted into the right side of the baby's neck and threaded to the heart in a process called "cannulation." The baby's unoxygenated blood drains via gravity (therefore, the baby's bed is elevated) through the catheters to the ECMO pump. The ECMO pump pushes the baby's blood through the ECMO circuit, where a membrane oxygenator acts as an artificial lung, removing carbon dioxide and providing oxygen to the blood. The oxygenated blood is then returned through the catheter into the baby. Babies receiving ECMO are sedated, paralyzed, and given pain medication. They are generally positioned in supine with their heads rotated to the left to allow access to the right neck vessels. These infants also are on large amounts of heparin in order to prevent the blood from clotting when it contacts the catheters and the ECMO circuit.[173] The heparin, used to prevent clot formation, may cause the baby to bleed, the most significant complication of ECMO. Babies receive daily head ultrasounds to assess if an intracranial hemorrhage (ICH) has occurred. If present, the ICH may be the reason to discontinue ECMO.[174] Babies who have received ECMO are at risk to develop atypical postures, tone, and movement patterns and require close developmental follow-up.[167–170,172] Babies post-ECMO frequently demonstrate difficulties with oral feeding. Other neurodevelopmental morbidity includes seizures, hearing loss, hyperactivity, behavioral problems, cerebral palsy, school failure, and developmental delay.[174] Although patients present with a variety of primary diagnoses requiring ECMO, after ECMO these patients demonstrate similar functional and neurodevelopmental outcomes, with the exception of babies with CDH. Patients with CDH have lower survival rates and higher morbidity, particularly in respiratory and digestive function, than other patients after ECMO.[169,171]

MEDICAL ISSUES OF PREMATURITY

Infants born prematurely are some of the most fragile in the NICU. They are at risk for multiple medical complications due to the immaturity of their body structures and organs, possible exposure to infections and teratogens, and the effects of the medical strategies and the technology required for minimizing illness and sustaining life. In this section, several of the more common medical conditions encountered in the NICU and the medical interventions used to treat them are discussed. The information provided is only a brief overview and the reader is advised to consult neonatal medical texts, care manuals, and the original references cited at the end of this chapter for more in-depth detail.

RESPIRATORY DISTRESS SYNDROME

RDS occurs as a result of pulmonary immaturity and inadequate pulmonary surfactant. Premature infants are predisposed to developing RDS due to structural and physiologic immaturities including poor alveolar capillary development, lack of type II alveolar cells, and insufficient production of surfactant. Surfactant is a substance produced by type II alveolar cells and lines the alveoli and small bronchioles. Decreased surfactant leads to respiratory failure due to increased surface tension, alveolar collapse, diffuse atelectasis, and decreased lung compliance. The preterm infant is further compromised by increased compliance of the chest wall due to the cartilaginous composition of the ribs, decreased type I fatigue-resistant muscle fibers in the diaphragm and intercostal muscles, and instability of neural control of breathing.[175–177]

Identification of RDS is made by prenatal risk factors, assessment of fetal lung immaturity, and postnatal clinical signs. Factors that affect lung maturity and increase predisposition for RDS include prematurity (gestational age less than 34 weeks), maternal diabetes (insulin appears to interfere with surfactant production), genetic factors (Caucasian race, siblings with history of RDS, and male sex), and thoracic malformations with lung hypoplasia.[178] Antenatal steroids are often used to accelerate lung maturity in the fetus and stimulate the production of surfactant. The National Institutes of Health[179] in 2000 recommended that antenatal steroids be given to all pregnant women at 24 to 34 weeks' gestation who are at risk for preterm delivery within 7 days; however, there is a lack of consensus for the type of steroid used and the method of dosing. While a number of studies of antenatal steroid therapy have demonstrated increased surfactant production, decreased length of time on mechanical ventilation, and decreased incidence of IVH,[180] others have shown decreased fetal growth, increased mortality, and poor neurobehavioral outcomes.[181–185]

The diagnosis of RDS is based on history, clinical presentation, blood gas studies, and chest radiography. RDS can develop immediately after birth or within the first hours of life depending on lung immaturity and perinatal events. Clinical signs of RDS include increased respiratory rate, expiratory grunting, sternal and intercostal retractions, nasal flaring, cyanosis, decreased air entry on auscultation, hypoxia, and hypercarbia. The lungs on chest radiography have a reticulogranular or "ground glass" appearance.[178]

Interventions for the premature infant with RDS depend on the severity of the disorder and include oxygen supplementation, assisted ventilation, and surfactant administration. Administration of prophylactic surfactant to intubated infants less than 30 weeks' gestational age has been associated with initial improvement in respiratory status and a decrease in the incidence of RDS, pneumothorax, bronchopulmonary dysplasia, and intraventricular hemorrhage.[186] Current practice is moving away from prophylactic surfactant administration for infants who otherwise do not need to be intubated.[187–189] The Texas Neonatal Research Group[190] recommends that infants greater than or equal to 1250 g with mild to moderate RDS should not be electively intubated solely for the administration of surfactant.

Assisted mechanical ventilation has typically been the intervention of choice for infants with RDS. However, mechanical ventilation can cause airway damage in the form of barotrauma and volutrauma. HFV has been suggested as an alternative to conventional ventilation in order to decrease lung injury.[142–145] Positive pressure ventilation via nasal or nasal–pharyngeal prongs to address respiratory needs while limiting barotrauma from intubation has also been advocated.[139] Studies have shown the combination of early surfactant administration and NCPAP to improve the clinical course of RDS and decrease the need for mechanical ventilation.[191] According to Honrubia and Stark,[178] the use of CPAP with infants with RDS appears to prevent atelectasis, minimize lung injury, and preserve the functional properties of surfactant. The decision of which form of respiratory intervention to use is based on the individual infant's clinical signs and chest radiography.

The prognosis of infants with respiratory distress syndrome varies with the severity of the original lung involvement. Infants who do not require mechanical ventilation are more likely to have resolution of RDS with little or no long-term sequelae. However, the very immature extremely low-birth-weight infants may progress to chronic lung disease or bronchopulmonary dysplasia due to prolonged mechanical ventilation and the associated damage to the lungs. Infants with severe RDS are also at increased risk for intracranial hemorrhage, retinopathy of prematurity, and necrotizing enterocolitis.[178]

In the acute stage of RDS, the infant is considered to be medically unstable and at risk for complications such as apnea, bradycardia, blood pressure variability, and intraventricular hemorrhage. Minimal environmental stimulation in the form of sound, light, and handling is often recommended to decrease infant stress. The physical therapist may perform observational evaluation of the infant using the NIDCAP to provide information to guide the delivery of care. Using this information, the therapist collaborates with the medical team and parents to develop a care plan to support overall growth and development. Suggestions for caregiving may include positioning, comfort, and protective measures.

PATENT DUCTUS ARTERIOSUS

The ductus arteriosus is a structure in the developing fetal heart that allows blood to bypass circulation to the lungs (Fig. 4.12). Since the fetus does not require the lungs to oxygenate blood, the flow from the right ventricle is shunted from the left pulmonary artery to the aorta. The ductus arteriosus typically closes within 10 to 15 hours after birth by constriction of medial smooth muscle. Anatomic closure is complete by 2 to 3 weeks of age and factors that precipitate closure include oxygen, prostaglandin E_2 levels, and maturity.[192]

Oxygen appears to be the strongest stimulus for closure of the ductus. The responsiveness of the smooth muscle to

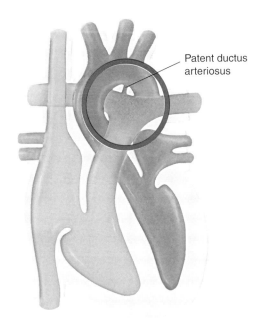

Figure 4.12 ■ *Illustration of patent ductus arteriosus. (From the Anatomical Chart Company.)*

oxygen is related to gestational age. The premature infant has less of a response to oxygen in the environment due to decreased sensitivity to oxygen-induced muscle contractions and high levels of prostaglandin E_2.[193]

When the ductus fails to close, it is termed patent ductus arteriosus. In premature infants the pulmonary vascular smooth muscle is not well developed and there is a more rapid fall in pulmonary vascular resistance than in full-term infants. The blood from the left side of the heart is shunted through the ductus to the right side resulting in hypotension and poor perfusion, and can cause congestive heart failure from cardiovascular overload. Low mean blood pressure, metabolic acidosis, decreased urine output, and worsening jaundice due to poor organ perfusion are systemic consequences of left-to-right shunting.

The clinical signs of PDA include murmur, increased heart rate, and respiratory distress. Other symptoms associated with PDA are failure to gain weight, sepsis, congestive heart failure, and pulmonary edema. Diagnosis is made by chest radiography and echocardiography. Treatment is determined by size of the PDA and clinical presentation. Initially the PDA is treated with increased ventilatory support, fluid restriction, and diuretic therapy.[194] In symptomatic infants indomethacin is used for nonsurgical closure and is effective in approximately 80% of cases.[195,196] The use of indomethacin for prophylaxis in nonsymptomatic infants is controversial as side effects from the medication can occur. Symptomatic infants with a PDA that does not close after the second indomethacin treatment or infants for whom indomethacin is contraindicated undergo surgical ligation after echocardiographic documentation of the PDA.

HYPERBILIRUBINEMIA

Physiologic jaundice or hyperbilirubinemia is the accumulation of excessive amounts of bilirubin in the blood. Bilirubin is one of the breakdown products of hemoglobin from red blood cells. Hyperbilirubinemia commonly occurs in premature infants due to immature hepatic function, increased hemolysis of red blood cells from birth injuries, and possible polycythemia (Fig. 4.13).

The primary concern in the treatment of hyperbilirubinemia is the prevention of kernicterus or the deposition of unconjugated bilirubin in the brain causing neuronal injury. The areas of the brain most commonly affected are the basal ganglia, cranial nerve nuclei, other brainstem nuclei, cerebellar nuclei, hippocampus, and anterior horn cells of the spinal cord.[197,198] Infants with chronic bilirubin encephalopathy can present with athetosis, partial or complete sensorineural hearing loss, limitation of upward gaze, dental dysplasia, and mild mental retardation.

Premature infants are more susceptible to anoxia, hypercarbia, and sepsis, which open the blood–brain barrier, leading to deposition of bilirubin in neural tissue. Bilirubin toxicity in low-birth-weight infants may be more a reflection of their overall clinical status than a function of actual bilirubin levels.[197,199]

Hyperbilirubinemia is diagnosed by serum blood levels of bilirubin and treated with phototherapy or exchange transfusion. There are no consensus guidelines for treatment of low-birth-weight infants with phototherapy or exchange transfusion. Generally, if phototherapy is not effective in reducing serum bilirubin levels or if there is a rapidly increasing bilirubin level, exchange transfusion is done.[200] Phototherapy is used to reduce serum bilirubin levels and is administered by fiberoptic blankets and bank or spot lights. Infants under phototherapy lights are naked except for a diaper and eye patches to protect their eyes in order to provide light exposure to the greatest surface area of skin. Exchange transfusion removes partially hemolyzed and antibody-coated red blood cells and replaces them with donor red blood cells lacking the sensitizing antigen. Bilirubin is removed from the plasma, and extravascular bilirubin binds to the albumin in the exchanged blood. The infant continues under phototherapy after the exchange transfusion.[197,201] Complications of exchange transfusion include hypocalcemia (which can cause cardiac arrhythmias), hypoglycemia, acid–base imbalance, hyperkalemia, cardiovascular problems including perforation of vessels, embolization, vasospasm, thrombosis, infarction, volume overload and cardiac arrest, thrombocytopenia, infection, hemolysis, graft-versus-host disease, hypothermia, hyperthermia, and necrotizing enterocolitis.[197,198,201]

Hyperbilirubinemia tends to decrease levels of arousal and activity. The infant may present with lethargy, hypotonia, and poor sucking ability.[200] Paludetto[201] and Mansi et al.[202] found that infants with moderate levels of hyperbilirubinemia demonstrate transient alterations in visual, auditory, social–interactive, and neuromotor capabilities. These findings are important considerations when performing a developmental assessment on an infant with increased levels of bilirubin.[3] Other issues to consider when assessing and planning treatment are the limitations imposed by phototherapy. When receiving phototherapy the infant is generally positioned so that there is maximal exposure of body surfaces to the lights, limiting the postures available to the infant and preventing the use of some of the positioning devices used for nesting and containment. The therapist will need to assist caregivers in creative ways to promote developmentally supportive postures and comfort without compromising the effectiveness of the phototherapy. Infants under the phototherapy lights need to have their eyes shielded to protect them from damage and to avoid any stress the bright lights may cause. Care must be taken to position eye shields so they are not too tight or too loose as either case can be extremely noxious to the sensitive, high-risk infant.

GASTROESOPHAGEAL REFLUX

Gastroesophageal reflux (GER) has been defined as the movement of gastric contents in a retrograde fashion into the esophagus and above. The gastric contents that reflux are generally acidic gastric fluids, feedings, bile, or even air from crying or distended stomach that can move up to any portion of the esophagus, nasopharynx, or oropharynx, or into the airway.[203,204] While the cause of reflux is still not

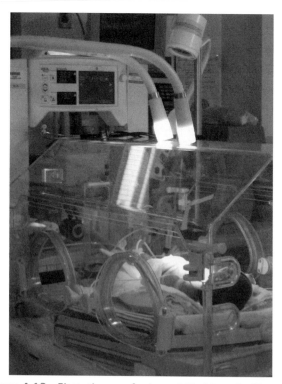

Figure 4.13 ■ Phototherapy for hyperbilirubinemia. Note the motor stress signs demonstrated by the infant because of lack of boundaries.

completely understood, particularly in the high-risk neonate, it is thought to be related to relaxation of the lower esophageal sphincter. The risk factors that have been identified for neonatal GER include prematurity, birth asphyxia, perinatal stress, neonatal stress, delayed gastric emptying, congenital anomalies of the upper gastrointestinal tract, acquired problems of the upper intestinal tract, diaphragmatic defects, respiratory disease, neurodevelopmental delays, ECMO, abdominal surgery, and medications. Acidic fluids can cause esophageal inflammation and further aggravate reflux. Higher risk for GER is associated with premature, stressed infants as well as those with chronic lung disease and congenital anomalies. Tone of the abdominal wall muscles, diaphragmatic activity, esophageal dysmotility, lower esophageal sphincter tone, and the physiologic immaturity of digestive function may be related to the increased incidence in these neonates.[205] Recent studies have demonstrated increased episodes of reflux with the presence of a nasogastric tube as it is an irritant and maintains the patency of the lower esophageal sphincter.[206–208]

All infants have some degree of reflux that is considered to be physiologic or asymptomatic if the infant is thriving well and the reflux resolves with maturation. Infants with asymptomatic GER may demonstrate small episodes of emesis; other infants may reswallow the refluxate without emesis. Infants with physiologic GER tend to grow and gain weight appropriately.[204] When the infant experiences more frequent episodes of GER (pathologic GER), the lining of the esophagus can be injured resulting in inflammation, dysmotility, and pain. This can lead to poor oral feeding patterns, oral aversion, and excessive crying due to pain. Blood loss in the emesis can lead to iron deficiency anemia. The result of severe reflux can be poor oral intake and malnutrition leading to failure to thrive.[209]

Apnea and bradycardia can occur as symptoms of GER. The presence of noxious stimuli in the pharynx due to reflux can trigger apnea as a protective mechanism to prevent aspiration. However, apneic events with or without bradycardia can be life-threatening. Controversy exists as to the association of apnea with GER. The apneic events often appear to be obstructive, suggesting a problem with clearance. Premature infants and term neonates do not cough effectively and therefore lack effective airway clearance.[210] Other respiratory manifestations can present as apnea in the presence of GER. Central apnea can be caused by chemoreceptor stimulation or obstructive apnea due to laryngospasm.

Diagnosis of GER in neonates is by history, clinical evaluation, and studies including esophageal pH probe, fluoroscopy or upper GI series, esophageal manometry, and endoscopy. History and clinical evaluation are important to rule out other conditions.[211] It is important to also identify whether the reflux is physiologic or pathologic, factors that make reflux worse, the mechanism of reflux, and the presence of complications caused by the reflux.

Although there appears to be a lack of consensus, treatment of GER in infancy often includes prone positioning, elevation of the head of the bed, and pharmacologic management. Positioning the infant in supine, right side-lying, and infant seats has been associated with exacerbation of reflux. Prone, elevation of the head of the bed to 30 degrees, and left side-lying have been shown to decrease episodes of reflux.[211–213] Omari et al.[214] found that in healthy preterm infants, right side-lying is associated with increased transient lower esophageal sphincter relaxation and increased GER while at the same time increasing gastric emptying. These researchers also found that in the infants they studied, gastric emptying was not a problem. Other treatment strategies for GER may include changes in the type and delivery of feedings. In their study Heacock et al.[215] found that infants fed with breast milk had less frequent and shorter-duration episodes of reflux than formula-fed infants. This was attributed to increased gastric emptying in breast milk–fed infants. GER has been shown to increase with increased volume of feeds, and giving frequent low-volume feedings may be employed. Removal of nasogastric tubes between feedings has also been advocated in order to allow the sphincter to close and to eliminate irritation caused by the tube. Thickening of feedings with rice cereal has also been used with limited success.[216] Medical pharmacologic treatment includes the use of prokinetics, acid suppression agents, and acid neutralizing agents.

The infant with GER and associated esophagitis may present as an irritable infant with poor state regulation and difficulty consoling. Motor patterns observed may be of increased extension or arching of the head and trunk. Increased muscle tone may be noted in the extremities. Although the medical issues of GER need to be addressed primarily, the therapist in the NICU may be called upon to assist with positioning to minimize reflux and promote comfort. Ongoing neurodevelopmental assessments are required to determine the effect of reflux on behavior and how to adapt interventions to promote appropriate developmental competencies.

NECROTIZING ENTEROCOLITIS

Necrotizing enterocolitis (NEC) is an acute inflammatory disease of the immature intestine that often results in acute intestinal necrosis. Preterm infants are at the highest risk for developing NEC; only 10% of all cases are found in full-term infants. The exact etiology is not known and the disease process appears to result from initial mucosal injury to the immature gastrointestinal tract due to a variety of factors.[217,218] The factors that appear to contribute to the pathogenesis of NEC include intestinal ischemia, infectious agents and toxins, and enteral alimentation. The risk of developing NEC is doubled in infants with prenatal exposure to cocaine due to vasoconstrictive effects on the intestine.

The clinical presentation includes respiratory distress, apnea, bradycardia, temperature instability, decreased peripheral perfusion, and lethargy. Abdominal signs include distension, tenderness, gastric aspirates with residuals of previous feedings, vomiting of bile and/or blood, bloody stools, radiographic evidence of ileus, and intestinal pneumotosis.[219-221] As NEC progresses, the infant may develop intestinal hemorrhage, gangrene, submucosal gas, and in some cases perforation of the intestines, sepsis, and shock.

The most important factor in determining outcome appears to be early diagnosis and treatment. Diagnosis is made by physical examination, laboratory studies, and radiography. Three stages of NEC have been defined. Stage I is defined as suspected NEC and the infant demonstrates suspicious clinical signs and symptoms such as abdominal distention and increased residual feedings. Stage II is definitive NEC and is used when the infant demonstrates clinical signs and symptoms along with pneumatosis on abdominal radiography. In stage III, severe NEC, the infant is critically ill, presenting with advanced clinical signs and symptoms with intestinal pneumatosis and impending or proven bowel perforation.[220,222,223] Infants with stage I or II are treated medically by making them NPO and giving parental alimentation, gastric suction, and antibiotics. Abdominal radiographs are taken every 6 to 8 hours to detect progression of intestinal obstruction or possible perforation. Surgery is indicated when there is evidence of fixed, dilated loops of bowel with abdominal distension. Surgical procedures include intestinal decompression, resection of necrotic bowel, and diversion of the proximal fecal stream by ileostomy, jejunostomy, or colonostomy depending on the location and extent of necrosis (Fig. 4.14).[217,222]

Although enterostomy is a necessary, life-saving procedure, it has also been reported to cause major morbidity in infants. NEC is the most common cause of death in infants undergoing surgery. Complications in surviving infants include failure to thrive, feeding abnormalities,

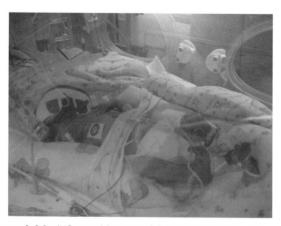

Figure 4.14 ■ Infant with necrotizing enterocolitis with ostomy.

diarrhea, and bowel obstruction due to short gut syndrome and stricture formation.[217,223,224]

The incidence of problems with growth and neurodevelopmental outcome of infants with NEC has been reported in comparison studies with other VLBW infants.[222-225] No growth differences have been found when infants with stage I or uncomplicated NEC were compared to VLBW infants without NEC. Infants with stage II and III NEC had lower head circumference and body length at 12 months and lower weight at 12 to 20 months than age-matched peers without NEC.[225] Neurodevelopmental outcome assessments performed on VLBW infants with stage II and III NEC and age-matched infants without NEC at 12 and 20 months corrected age demonstrated significantly lower general developmental quotients in infants with NEC at both 12 and 20 months. There was a higher incidence of severe psychomotor retardation in infants with stage III NEC and multiple organ involvement.[225]

Infants in the acute stages of NEC are critically ill and therapists must use care in the support of these infants. Protective care in the form of minimizing environmental stimulation and handling is indicated. The therapist should work in coordination with the medical team and family to assess the infant for signs of stress and comfort. Using this information, recommendations for positioning and other comfort measures such as nonnutritive sucking can be implicated. As these infants are at risk for significant developmental delays, it is important that developmental intervention and developmental follow-up continue as their medical status improves and after discharge.

GERMINAL MATRIX-INTRAVENTRICULAR HEMORRHAGE

Germinal matrix-intraventricular hemorrhage (GM-IVH) is the most common type of brain lesion found in premature infants occurring most frequently in infants less than 1500 g and less than 32 weeks' gestation. The incidence of GM-IVH is inversely related to gestational age with the extremely premature being at greatest risk.[226-235] The hemorrhage typically originates in the subependymal layer of the germinal matrix and extends into the intraventricular space between the lateral ventricles (Fig. 4.15). During fetal development this is the site of neuronal proliferation as neuroblasts divide and migrate to the cerebral parenchyma. The neuronal proliferation is complete by 20 weeks, while glial cell proliferation continues until approximately 32 weeks' gestation. The matrix decreases in size from 23 to 24 weeks and nearly complete involution occurs by 36 weeks' gestation.[226-228,235,236] These developmental changes in the brain influence the area and extent of the hemorrhage in the neonate.

A fragile and primitive capillary network supplies blood to this very metabolically active area. It is within this capillary network that periventricular hemorrhage-intraventricular hemorrhage (PVH-IVH) occurs. Intra-

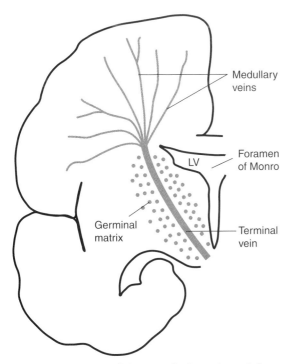

Figure 4.15 ■ Diagram of the germinal matrix and the venous drainage of cerebral white matter. LV, lateral ventricular. (Reprinted with permission from Volpe JJ. Neurology of the Newborn. 4th Ed. Philadelphia: Saunders, 2001:432.)

TABLE 4.6	

Grading of Germinal Matrix-Intraventricular Hemorrhage (GM-IVH)

Grade	Characteristic
I	GMH with absent or minimal IVH
II	IVH occupying 10%–15% of the intraventricular area
III	IVH occupying >50% of ventricular area with ventricular distension
Periventricular hemorrhagic infarction	Intraparenchymal venous hemorrhage

Adapted with permission from Volpe JJ. Neurology of the Newborn. 4th Ed. Philadelphia: Saunders, 2001.

ventricular hemorrhage is thought to be due to hypoxia and/or capillary bleeding resulting from the loss of cerebral autoregulation and an abrupt alteration in blood flow.[226,227,235,237,238] The alteration of cerebral circulation from autoregulation to pressure-passive circulation has been shown to be an important factor in the development of PVH-IVH. Hemorrhage can occur when the pressure-passive circulating pattern is compromised by fluctuations in cerebral blood flow and pressure. Factors associated with the loss of autoregulation are younger gestational age, extremely low birth weight, birth events, asynchrony of spontaneous and mechanical breaths, pneumothorax, rapid volume expansion, seizures, changes in pH, $PaCO_2$, PaO_2, metabolic imbalances, tracheal suctioning, and noxious procedures of caregiving.[226,227,235,239–245]

Intraventricular hemorrhages are diagnosed by cranial ultrasound and classified according to severity.[228,235,246] A four-level grading system was developed by Papile et al.[234] and is still used by many neonatologists, neurologists, and radiologists. Volpe developed a different grading system in 1995 based on neuropathologic and imaging studies. This scale uses three levels to grade intraventricular hemorrhages. Grade I is a germinal matrix hemorrhage with no or minimal intraventricular hemorrhage. Grade II is an intraventricular hemorrhage occupying 10% to 15% of the intraventricular area without distension of the ventricles. Grade III is an intraventricular hemorrhage occupying greater than 50% of ventricular area and usually distends the lateral ventricle (Table 4.6).[226,227]

The neuropathologic complications of IVH include germinal matrix destruction, periventricular hemorrhagic infarction, and posthemorrhagic ventricular dilation.[226,227,232,238] Periventricular leukomalacia is frequently seen in infants with IVH but is not caused by the hemorrhage itself.[227,232,235,247] Germinal matrix destruction and destruction of glial precursor cells is the result of germinal matrix hemorrhage. Destruction of glial precursor cells may negatively influence future development. Neurodevelopmental outcomes for infants with IVH are related to the severity of the hemorrhage. Vohr et al.[238] found that the low-birth-weight infants with intraventricular hemorrhage were more likely to develop cerebral palsy. Spastic diplegic cerebral palsy is most commonly associated with IVH due to the anatomic location of the corticospinal tracts.[227,236,238]

Periventricular hemorrhagic infarction (PHI) was previously considered to be an extension of a large parenchymal hemorrhage or what Papile described as grade IV IVH. Neuropathologic and ultrasound studies have shown that the lesion represents a hemorrhagic venous infarction.[227,238,248] Periventricular hemorrhagic infarctions are generally large unilateral or asymmetric lesions dorsolateral to the lateral ventricle. This lesion is thought to be caused by obstruction of the terminal vein by a large IVH.[226,227,249] PHI generally occurs on the side of the larger IVH and there is generally markedly decreased or absent flow in the terminal vein on that side. Studies have also described the lesion in the distribution of the medullary veins that drain into the terminal vein. Necrosis in this area can develop over time into a single large porencephalic cyst.[226] In the neonatal period, PHI is highly associated with an increased mortality rate as compared to IVH alone. Developmental outcomes associated with PHI are spastic hemiparesis, asymmetric quadriparesis, and cognitive deficits. The lower and upper extremities are equally affected in children with a history of PHI. Lesions due to extensive PHI cause more severe cognitive as well as motor deficits.[227,238]

Posthemorrhagic ventricular dilation (PVD) may occur days to weeks after the original IVH. The progressive ventricular dilation is due to a process that prevents the resorption of cerebrospinal fluid (CSF) and/or obstruction of CSF drainage due to a particulate clot. The injury to the brain from PVD is most likely due to hypoxia–ischemia and distension of the ventricle into the surrounding white matter, which may be more susceptible to additional injury after the effects of the initial hemorrhage.[227] The result of PVD is typically a bilateral cerebral white matter injury.[250] As there is a high incidence of arrest in the progression of ventriculomegaly without intervention, PVD is initially managed with close surveillance of ventricular size, head circumference, and clinical condition. Persistent slow ventricular dilation is treated with serial lumbar punctures to remove large volumes of CSF. Medications such as acetazolamide and furosemide can be used to decrease CSF production.[227,238] Rapidly progressive ventricular dilation with moderate to severe dilation, progressive head growth, and increasing intracranial pressure is managed initially with serial lumbar punctures followed by ventricular drainage of CSF with an external ventricular catheter or tunneled ventricular catheter that is connected to a subcutaneous reservoir.[227,238] Ventricular drainage is generally a temporary measure until a ventriculoperitoneal shunt can be placed. This type of shunt diverts CSF from the lateral ventricles into the peritoneal cavity.[227]

Posthemorrhagic ventricular dilation occurs at a higher incidence in the extremely premature infant with extremely low birth weight as this is the population that is at greater risk for more severe IVH. With each week of increase in gestation the occurrence of PVD decreases. There is an increase in the incidence of PVD with each increase in grade of IVH.[251] Murphy et al. found that the grade of IVH and need for inotropic support, such as dopamine or dobutamine, were significantly related to PVD requiring surgical intervention. Posthemorrhagic ventricular dilation has been associated with neuromotor impairments and pronounced disability.[252–255] Krishnamoorthy et al.[246] demonstrated in their study that ventriculomegaly is an important antecedent of neuromotor sequelae and children with ventriculomegaly had a five times greater risk of developing cerebral palsy independent of the grade of IVH.

While incidence of IVH and PHI has decreased in recent years due to improvements in prenatal and postnatal preventative care, these lesions are still major factors for neurodevelopmental disability in ELBW infants.[227,230,251,256–259] The primary goal of prenatal management is to prevent or delay premature birth. Other strategies focus on providing support during labor and delivery, resuscitation, and plan for neonatal care. Since RDS is highly associated with IVH and PHI, treatments to decrease RDS such as the administration of prenatal steroids are utilized. Postnatal treatment focuses on preventing hypoxia or fluctuations in systemic and blood cerebral pressure. In addition to providing optimal respiratory and medical support, the principles of individualized developmentally supportive care are instituted to minimize stress during caregiving, decrease the potential for loss of physiologic stability, and decrease the risk of IVH.[23,237,260–262]

PERIVENTRICULAR LEUKOMALACIA

Periventricular leukomalacia refers to specific areas of white matter necrosis adjacent to the external angles of the lateral ventricles. These areas involve the frontal horn and body, and optic and acoustic radiations. The incidence of PVL occurs most prominently in infants less than 32 weeks' gestation who have survived more than a few days of postnatal life and have cardiorespiratory compromise.[226,227,263,264] Premature infants of younger gestational ages are at the greatest risk for white matter injury since these areas are poorly vascularized in the immature brain and contain precursors for oligodendrocytes, which are extremely sensitive to ischemia and infection.[226,227,236,263–265]

Focal periventricular necrosis and more diffuse white matter cerebral injury are the pathologic features of PVL. Focal necrosis is related to severe ischemia and occurs most often in infants greater than 26 weeks' gestation.[226,227,249,264] The two main sites of focal injury are near the trigone of the lateral ventricles and the border zones between the terminal arbors of the middle cerebral artery and the posterior cerebral artery or the anterior cerebral artery. Diffuse white matter injury is most apparent in infants less than 26 weeks' gestation who develop atrophy, ventriculomegaly, and cortical underdevelopment with loss of oligodendrocytes and impairment in myelination.[226,227,249,264]

Areas of increased echodensity detected by cranial ultrasound are generally the first evidence of PVL. These echodensities represent areas of focal cellular necrosis due to axonal degeneration. Although echodensities may be transient or radiographic "flares" in some infants, other infants will demonstrate the characteristic evolution of focal PVL with the formation of cavitations that evolve into multiple cysts. This process occurs over the course of 1 to 3 weeks[226,227,237,264] and the diagnosis of PVL will be dependent on the timing and number of cranial ultrasounds performed on the infant. More diffuse lesions less commonly undergo cystic changes and may go undetected by cranial ultrasound. Magnetic resonance imaging (MRI) allows for better definition of brain structures and has been used to document diffuse white matter injury.[249]

The pathogenesis of the white matter destruction seen in PVL has been attributed to the interrelated factors associated with immature circulation and vascular structures of the preterm infant, impaired cerebral autoregulation, and the intrinsic vulnerability of the immature cerebral white matter neuroglia to ischemia–reperfusion.[226,227,247,249,264,266,267] Perinatal infection and the inflammatory response including the release of proinflammatory cytokines have also been shown to play an important role in the pathogenesis of PVL.[236,249,264,267–271] The effect of medications and other therapies used to treat complications of prematurity have been implicated in the pathogenesis of white matter injury.[272]

There is a strong association with mortality and long-term morbidity in infants with PVL. Death in infants with PVL in the neonatal period is usually attributed to the original insult, whether hypoxic, hemorrhagic, or infectious, rather than from PVL. Infants with PVL who survive the neonatal period are at high risk for neurodevelopment problems that affect motor, cognitive, and visual function.[245,255,259,264,269,270,273] Spastic diplegia, with or without hydrocephalus, is the most prominent long-term sequela of PVL. Han et al.[259] found that the presence of PVL was the "strongest and most independent risk factor" for the development of cerebral palsy. The clinical presentation is one of motor disturbance in the lower extremities greater than the upper extremities due to the anatomic location of the descending motor tracts (Fig. 4.16). In larger lesions extending further into the periventricular white matter, the upper extremities and cognitive functions will be more affected. Motor tracts associated with visual, auditory, and somesthetic functions can also be involved.[264,269,270] Extremely premature infants have been found to be at greatest risk for global motor and cognitive impairments.[229,230,247,274]

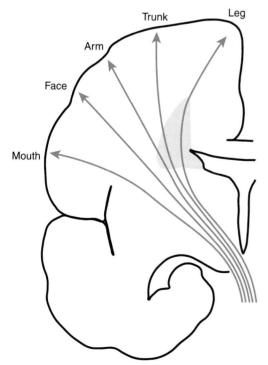

Figure 4.16 ■ *Illustrations of the periventricular area and motor tracts. (Reprinted with permission from Volpe JJ. Neurology of the Newborn. 4th Ed. Philadelphia: Saunders, 2001:432.)*

As with other injuries to the neonatal brain, the primary focus is prevention of prematurity, infection, hypotension, and other associated factors. The initial management after the diagnosis of PVL is treating the primary cause and complications of the insult along with preventing further hypoxic–ischemic damage. Management strategies to prevent or minimize hypoxia, hypotension, acidosis, apnea, bradycardia, and infection are implemented. Developmental care strategies can be implemented to decrease stress and promote development. Serial cranial ultrasounds are done to monitor PVL, possible progression, and hydrocephalus.

RETINOPATHY OF PREMATURITY

Retinopathy is a vasoproliferative disease of the immature retina. Infants at the highest risk are those born less than 30 weeks' gestation and weighing less than 1300 g or infants born at 35 weeks, weighing less than 1800 g, and requiring supplemental oxygen for respiratory distress syndrome. In the past it was thought that increased concentrations of oxygen alone caused retinopathy of prematurity (ROP). Other factors now being investigated as possibly contributing to ROP include hypoxia or anoxia, hypocapnia, acidosis, intraventricular hemorrhage, fluctuation in blood gas tensions, sepsis, respiratory distress syndrome/bronchopulmonary dysplasia, dexamethasone exposure, patent ductus arteriosus, vitamin E deficiency, and precocious exposure to light.[275,276]

The onset of retinopathy is marked by an alteration in the normal development of blood vessels in the eye, which occurs in two stages. In the first stage, severe vascular constriction due to hypoxia, hyperoxia, or hypotension results in decreased circulation to the retina. Stage 2 is marked by the release of growth hormone from the ischemic retina, which stimulates new blood vessel growth through the retina and into the vitreous humor. These blood vessels are atypical in structure and prone to hemorrhage and edema. Extensive growth of these abnormal vessels can form a ring of scar tissue that pulls on the retina and can separate the retina from its attachments.[275–277]

The disease process usually peaks at 34 to 40 weeks' postconceptual age. In the majority of cases there is regression of the disease process with resolution of retinopathy. In severe cases, if the retinal detachment is not corrected, the result will be blindness. Ophthalmology performs regular retinal checks to monitor the progression of ROP starting at 4 to 6 weeks' chronologic age or 31 to 33 weeks' PCA. The AAP recommends that for infants less than 35 weeks' gestational age who receive oxygen treatment, eye exams should occur every 2 to 3 weeks or more frequently when more severe disease is diagnosed. All infants less than 1500 g and 28 weeks or fewer receive early and regular eye exams at the same frequency.[278,279]

ROP is classified by the location, stage, and extent of the pathophysiologic process using the International Classification of Retinopathy of Prematurity.[280,281] The location indicates the distance that the atypically developing retinal blood vessels have traveled. The retina is divided into three concentric circles and these are known as zones (Fig. 4.17). Zone 1 is surrounding the optic nerve extending out to the macula. Zone 2 extends toward the nasal and temporal sides, and Zone 3 extends further to the temporal side. The severity of the disease is classified in stages (Fig. 4.17). In stage 1 there is a thin line of demarcation separating the normal retina from underdeveloped, avascular areas. Stage 2 is when the demarcation becomes a thick, high ridge that protrudes into the vitreous humor. There is extraretinal fibrovascular proliferation along the edge of the ridge extending into the vitreous humor in stage 3. In stage 4, fibrosis and scarring develop, placing traction on the retina and leading to partial detachment. Stage 4 is further subdivided: In 4A the partial detachment does not involve the macula and in 4B the macula is involved. Stage 5 is complete detachment of the retina.[275,280]

Plus disease is a severe form of ROP involving iris vascular engorgement, pupillary rigidity, and vitreous haze. In this form of ROP, the posterior retinal blood vessels become characteristically dilated and tortuous in appearance. This more severe type of ROP tends to progress very rapidly and requires intervention.[275,280]

The extent refers to the location of the disease and is reported in clock hours around the circumference of the zones. The severity for determination of surgery is described in terms of threshold and prethreshold. Threshold refers to conditions of five or more contiguous or eight cumulative clock hours of stage 3 with Plus disease in zone 1 or 2. The risk of blindness is approximately 50% in threshold ROP and surgical intervention is recommended.[275,280]

Prethreshold disease can be any of the following conditions: zone 1 ROP of any stage less than threshold, zone 2 ROP with stage 2 and Plus disease, zone 2 ROP with stage 3 without Plus disease, and zone 2 stage 3 with Plus disease with four sections of stage less than threshold. One in three infants requires surgical intervention with prethreshold ROP. The AAP[279] recommends treatment within 72 hours of the detection of threshold ROP. There is a one in six chance of severe visual impairment if treatment is not done at the time threshold is reached. There is a 1 in 12 chance of severe visual impairment with surgical intervention.[275] Presently there are no proven treatments to prevent ROP. Methods that are used clinically for the prevention of ROP include keeping PaO_2 between 50 to 70 mm Hg, administration of vitamin E, and providing supplemental O_2 to keep SaO_2 at 99%.[275]

Surgical intervention includes cryotherapy, laser surgery, and retinal reattachment. Cryotherapy is used to destroy abnormal blood vessels and has been successful in reducing the risk of extreme visual impairment by 50% in infants with threshold ROP. Laser surgery is applied to the avascular retina to arrest the process of retinal detachment by eliminating abnormal blood vessels and scarring. Outcome studies suggest that laser surgery is more effective than cryotherapy in terms of anatomic and functional visual outcomes.[282–285]

In severe ROP, scleral buckling procedures are used to reattach the retina. Vitrectomy is a procedure that removes the scar tissue, pulling the retina forward. These procedures have had limited success in terms of functional visual outcomes.[275–277,286]

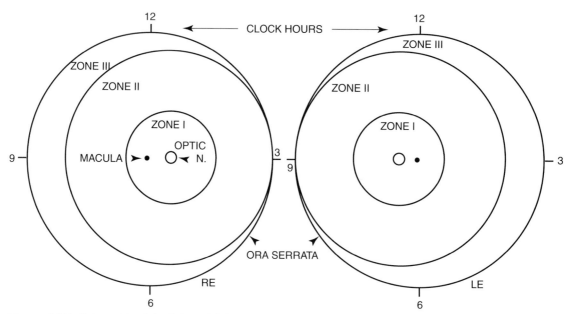

Figure 4.17 ■ Schematic of the left and right eye showing the clock hours and the stages and zones of retinopathy of prematurity (ROP). (Reprinted with permission from Committee for Classification of ROP. An International Classification of Retinopathy of Prematurity. Arch Ophthalmol 1989;102[8]:1131.)

PRENATAL COCAINE EXPOSURE

The deleterious effects of maternal cocaine use during pregnancy have been well documented.[287–291] There is a strong association with prenatal malnutrition and intrauterine growth retardation. Cocaine increases uterine contractility, maternal hypertension, placental vasoconstriction, and decreased uterine blood flow. Other fetal effects include increased rate of premature labor, spontaneous abortion, placental abruption, fetal distress, meconium staining, and low Apgar scores. Congenital anomalies have also been associated with prenatal cocaine exposure. Cardiac anomalies, genitourinary malformations, intestinal atresia, microcephaly, perinatal cerebral infarctions and cystic brain lesions, early onset of NEC, and retinal dysgenesis have been discussed in the literature.[291–293] Alterations in autonomic nervous system development and vagal tone have also been documented.[291,293]

Classic withdrawal signs are not demonstrated in infants with prenatal cocaine exposure. However, abnormal sleep patterns, tremors, poor organizational response, irritability, and inability to be consoled have been described in the literature during the neonatal period. Many of these behaviors are also associated with tobacco use, which is commonly used in combination with cocaine, making it difficult to determine which effects are due solely to cocaine use.[291,293]

When factors associated with poor developmental and growth outcomes such as prematurity, congenital anomalies, cardiac defects, and neurologic insults are ruled out, the literature has not demonstrated major developmental deficits in children exposed to cocaine in utero.[293–296] So-called "minor" deficits such as attention deficits, difficulties with information processing, deficits in language skills, impairments in behavioral regulation, and difficulties with visual–motor skills have been documented in follow-up studies.[291,297,298–302] However, these outcomes are difficult to differentiate from the effects of poor prenatal care, poverty/low socioeconomic status, polysubstance use, and the limited attachment and caregiving abilities associated with drug addiction.[298,299,303,304]

CHORIOAMNIONITIS

Cervicovaginal bacteria that invade the amniotic cavity and cause an inflammatory response in the membranes of the developing fetus cause chorioamnionitis. Chorioamnionitis is the most common cause of preterm labor. Most infants are not septic at birth as the placenta provides an efficient barrier. However, in the cases where there is a fetal inflammatory response in addition to the maternal inflammatory response, babies may be more at risk for BPD, NEC, abnormalities on cranial ultrasound, and long-term neurologic impairment.[305] In addition, there has been evidence of an association between maternal intrauterine infection and the occurrence of fetal brain damage with subsequent neurologic deficits, with the strongest association between chorioamnionitis and PVL.[271,306]

BONE DISEASE OF PREMATURITY/OSTEOPENIA

The third trimester of fetal development is very important for bone formation. Approximately 80% of bone is produced between 24 and 40 weeks' gestation as the fetus accretes large amounts of calcium, phosphorus, and magnesium.[307–313] There is also mechanical stimulation to the bones as the infant actively moves within the fluid-filled environment and pushes against the uterine wall. In addition, further mechanical loading of the skeletal system occurs during the third trimester as the infant is gaining muscle mass and being compressed by the cramped uterine space.[309–311]

Infants who are born prematurely miss out on a portion or all of this period of bone formation and mineral accretion. The more premature, VLBW infants are most at risk for decreased bone density or osteopenia. Other factors that contribute to this bone disease of prematurity include chronic illness, prolonged hyperalimentation, BPD, cholestasis, and NEC. The chronic use of medications such as corticosteroids and diuretics that cause increased mineral excretion are also associated with decreased bone density.[309–313] Infants with osteopenia have fragile bones and are at high risk for fractures and positional deformities such as dolichocephaly.

In the NICU, the prevention and treatment of bone disease in premature infants is addressed through nutritional management. The medical staff carefully monitor the vitamins and minerals they provide the infant through parenteral nutrition, human milk fortifiers, and/or preterm formula.[310–313] Even with carefully managed nutritional programs, cases of osteopenia still occur. There have been some studies suggesting the use of passive range of motion to promote bone formation in preterm infants[309,314–316]; however, these studies had a small number of subjects and did not address the physiologic stress that handling can induce in this very fragile population. Further studies looking at the risks versus benefits of passive range of motion are needed before implementing this practice. Care must be taken when handling premature, VLBW infants in terms of their physiologic vulnerabilities as well as the increased risk of fracturing bone. In addition, attention should be paid to cranial molding with the use of positioning devices and varying postures.

PHYSICAL THERAPY ASSESSMENT AND INTERVENTION: ISSUES OF PREMATURITY

A complete history should include information from the medical chart, nursing and physician staff, and the family. Pertinent information from the medical chart includes prenatal history, birth history, history of the present illness, and family social history. Prenatal history consists of maternal age, circumstances regarding conception (the use of assistive reproductive technology), prenatal care and test results, complications during pregnancy, infections, illnesses, medications taken by the mother (licit and illicit,) interventions such as fetal/maternal surgery, maternal past medical history, and presence/treatment of preterm labor. Birth history includes gestational age at delivery, mode of delivery (spontaneous or induced vaginal delivery, with or without vacuum or forceps assist, or cesarean section), weight, length, head circumference, Apgar scores (Table 4.4), infant's clinical presentation at delivery, necessary resuscitative efforts, and infant's need for ongoing interventions in the delivery room.

History of present illness includes an in-depth review of medical status by systems. A baby requires newborn intensive care because of the immaturity of his or her organs and the fragility of his or her physiologic function. In reviewing the chart the therapist should attend to the baby's level of respiratory support, his or her requirements since birth, and his or her current needs, including modifications to sustain the baby through nursing care or feeding sessions. The therapist should note the frequency and severity of episodes of apnea, bradycardia, and oxygen desaturation, as well as interventions needed. Cardiovascular status is important to understand the health of the baby's other organ systems, in particular the central nervous system (CNS), respiratory system, and gastrointestinal system. The baby's initial means of getting nutrition and how this has been tolerated, modified, regressed, and/or progressed should be understood as it provides a window into the baby's overall health, functioning, and ability to grow. Likewise, the baby's medications can impact his or her functioning and ability to stay alert and sustain a wakeful state. Infants who have required sedatives or narcotics for medical management may display signs and symptoms of withdrawal as the medications are being weaned.

Other medical problems that relate to the infant's current level of functioning and future risk include infections, metabolic issues, hyperbilirubinemia, genetic syndromes, congenital malformations, seizures, intracranial hemorrhages, and surgical issues. After a thorough review of the chart, the therapist should approach the nursing staff with questions to initiate a dialogue about the overall status of the infant. This should be followed by pertinent questions addressing the following: changes in status leading to changes in medical care, tolerance to nursing care, care procedures that lead to distress, and preferred comfort measures. If the family members are present the therapist can seek to establish a relationship with them by initiating a dialogue about their baby. Through this process the therapist can gain insight into the family's overall understanding of the infant's medical problems, their interpretation of the infant's behaviors, and their comfort in interacting with their baby. During this initial visit to the infant's bedside, the therapist is observing environmental information such as bed space location, levels of light

and sound, and how the baby responds to the stresses in his or her immediate environment.

The therapist needs to observe the infant both at rest and during care activities with nursing or other health care professionals. During an observation of nursing or medical care, a baby may demonstrate sensitivity to environmental sounds. The therapist would then recommend strategies to minimize sounds such as encouraging staff to refrain from writing or placing objects on top of the isolette, quietly closing porthole and bedside cart drawers, keeping pagers on vibrate mode, and keeping voices low and conversations to a minimum. Large signs (Fig. 4.18) to keep noise down can be posted indicating that the baby is stressed by sound so that all staff and visitors are aware of the need to keep noise to a minimum. If these measures are not sufficient, the baby's bed may need to be moved to a quieter space away from a sink, a trash can, or a heavily traveled corridor. Similarly, if a baby is sensitive to light, recommendations would be made to shield his or her eyes from bright light. Methods of modifying light include dimming the lights, covering the isolette, tenting the infant's face (by propping a blanket to shade the infant's eyes or draping a sheet over a crib), and cupping a hand over the infant's eyes during care. The physical environment of the NICU should be adapted with individual lighting for each bed space.[317]

A baby may also demonstrate frequent physiologic and motoric stress signs at rest as well as during intervention (Table 4.1). In order to assist the autonomic subsystem and the motor subsystem, the baby may benefit from firm containment through the use of positioning aides. Commercially made products or blanket rolls can be used to provide a nest that simulates the enclosed environment of the womb (Fig. 4.19).

During an observation a baby may demonstrate unsuccessful attempts to self-calm. If the baby is unsuccessful at calming, he or she may become exhausted, limp, and physiologically compromised by the end of the caregiving episode. Suggestions for providing assistance for the baby's self-calming strategies include offering a pacifier, contain-

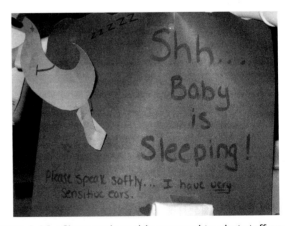

Figure 4.18 ■ Signs such as this are used to alert staff and visitors that the infant is sensitive to sound.

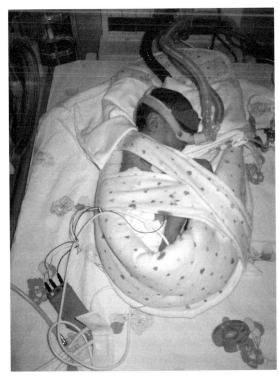

Figure 4.19 ■ Infant positioned in a nest made from a Children's Medical Ventures SnuggleUp.

ing hands near face/mouth, and positioning legs in a tucked position near the baby's trunk. The caregiving may need to be paced to the infant's tolerance, and the infant allowed to rest after particularly disorganizing aspects of care (e.g., diaper change or suctioning). During the rest break the baby should be contained from head to toe by spreading both hands to cover the infant and thus facilitate a tucked position. A blanket wrap can also be used to swaddle the infant and prevent the infant from exhausting him- or herself.[43,318–320]

PARENT EDUCATION

In order for parents to perform the difficult roles of parenting, they need to understand the behaviors of a preterm baby, as well as the course of typical development and what to expect in the future. They need to be able to read their infants and respond supportively to them. When a therapist observes a baby interacting with his or her caregiver during nursing care, the therapist will discover the baby's areas of competence, strength, and vulnerability. Likewise, a NICU therapist, as a developmental specialist, will know the course of development and, therefore, is in a unique role to assist parents as they parent their infants. Parents have benefited in the short term and also in the long term from gaining awareness of their baby's interactive and developmental capabilities and responding appropriately to them.[321–324] The therapist can start the dialogue with the parents by asking, "How do you think your baby is doing?" and then listen to hear their concerns and their

interpretations of the baby's behavior. This will give the therapist a window into the parents' understanding of their baby. The therapist can invite the parents to watch the baby together and the therapist can use that opportunity to point out the baby's unique capabilities, strategies of self-regulation, and sensitivities and vulnerabilities to the environment and medical care. The therapist can provide a synopsis of general components and patterns of infant development and guide the parent with recommendations to focus on the present. For an excellent review of parent teaching strategies, see the Lowman et al.[323] article on using developmental assessments in the NICU to empower families. Parenting is a difficult job at any stage of a child's development, but especially in infancy when children are not capable of articulating their needs and desires.

KANGAROO CARE

Skin-to-skin holding, also known as kangaroo care, is an intervention that supports infant physiologic and behavioral stability and maturation as well as parent–infant interaction and attachment. This practice involves the parent holding the diaper-clad infant underneath his or her clothing, skin to skin, chest to chest,[325] and was initially used with preterm infants in Bogota, Columbia, during a time when there was limited availability of incubators.[326] Skin-to-skin holding has gained wider acceptance in the United States for use in the NICU over the past decade.

The benefits of skin-to-skin holding for the premature infant have been documented in several studies and include improved thermoregulation, improved respiratory patterns and oxygen saturations, decreased apnea and bradycardia, improved behavioral state organization, increased rates of weight gain, as an analgesic during painful procedures, and decreased length of hospitalization.[115,327–333] For parents, the benefits are increased maternal milk production, improved breast feeding, opportunities for more positive interactions with their infant, and an overall more positive view of their infant.[333–335] Feldman and associates[335] found the parents of premature infants who used skin-to-skin holding to be more sensitive to their infant's cues, and to provide a better home environment after discharge. The infants in this study also had improved neurodevelopmental assessments at 6 months as compared to peers who received no skin-to-skin holding.

The initiation of skin-to-skin holding will vary between institutions based on gestational age, weight, and the acuity of the infant. Early in the infant's admission, the physical therapist can help to educate the family as to the benefits of skin-to-skin holding and then encourage the family to engage in the intervention as soon as the medical team approves the practice. The physical therapist can also assist the parents with positioning the infant for comfort and to ensure the most optimal position to promote physiologic stability and behavioral organization.

POSITIONING FOR COMFORT

Preterm infants are more likely to experience muscular fatigue, particularly in the respiratory muscles.[88] Because of the combination of hypotonia, gravitational forces, and loss of uterine constraints, the infant develops postures of extension, leading to discomfort and an imbalance of flexion and extension. In order to support the respiratory and musculoskeletal systems and promote infant comfort, positioning should promote the following components of optimal alignment: neutral head and neck position and, if possible, slight chin tuck, scapular protraction to promote upper extremity flexion and hands midline (Fig. 4.20), flexion of the trunk with posterior pelvic tilt, and flexion of lower extremities with neutral abduction/adduction and rotation of the hips. Supports to assist the infant in maintaining optimal position can be fabricated using blanket rolls or commercially available devices. Children's Medical Ventures and Small Beginnings are two companies that manufacture and sell a variety of positioning products for use in the NICU.

The preterm infant needs to have regular positional changes in order to promote comfort, prevent skin breakdown, promote the development of the musculoskeletal system, promote gaseous exchange in all lung fields, and maintain head shape.[88,336–339] When medically tolerated, preterm infants benefit from prone positioning. Studies have shown that the prone position improves oxygenation and ventilation, improves cerebral venous return and lowers intracranial pressure, promotes self-calming and sleep states, and improves behavioral organization/self-regulation.[340–345] Grenier et al.[345] have found that infants placed in prone, whether nested or unnested, have the fewest stress behaviors compared to infants placed in either side-lying or supine. However, some nurseries have policies discouraging prone for babies who have umbilical lines or are intubated. It is best to know the nursery policy on prone positioning before recommending prone placement for an infant.

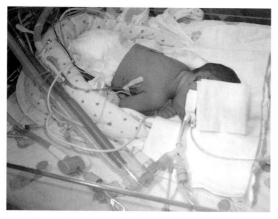

Figure 4.20 ■ Infant positioned in prone position using anterior, midline roll under chest. The nest helps to promote flexion of the trunk, arms, and legs.

The unsupported prone position promotes shoulder retraction, neck hyperextension, truncal flattening, and hip abduction/external rotation, which is uncomfortable and if left uncorrected can interfere with future motor development.[88,339] Infants placed in prone should have a thin roll under their chests to raise their chests from the surface and allow shoulder protraction and a more neutral neck alignment. A roll should be placed under the infant's hips to promote lower extremity flexion and a larger roll around the infant's sides and feet to promote boundaries.

Infants supported in side-lying also demonstrate decreased stress behaviors compared to supine. Other optimal effects of side-lying are symmetry and midline orientation of trunk and extremities, which promotes hands to mouth. In addition, in side-lying the respiratory diaphragm is placed in a gravity-eliminated plane, which lessens the work of breathing. GER is decreased in left side-lying, and gastric emptying is increased in right side-lying.[214,340,346] Blanket rolls are necessary to support infants placed in side-lying in order for side-lying to be beneficial to the infant. Unsupported side-lying has the potential to be stressful for the baby as it provides the least amount of postural support, making the preterm infant maintain body postures and self-organization on his or her own.[340,345,346] In his or her efforts to seek boundaries for postural control, a preterm baby is more likely to extend his or her neck and trunk to end ranges. These hyperextended postures are counterproductive, as tucking, flexion, and hands to face are the postures that promote comfort, calming, and self-regulation.[345]

Supine allows for maximal observation and access to the infant by caregivers. However, when compared to prone or side-lying, supine poses the most challenges for the infant biomechanically, organizationally, and physiologically. In supine the forces of gravity pull the baby into neck extension, trunk extension, scapular retraction, anterior pelvic tilt, external hip rotation, and abduction. In addition, supine assists the baby as he or she actively extends. These postures do not promote calming and self-regulation. Studies of preterm infant positioning have found that infants move more and in a less organized fashion in supine; have shorter and more interrupted sleep periods; have more labored, less coordinated breathing; and have more episodes of GER.[347–349] Since supine is the most challenging position for the preterm infant, infants should be supported with rolls to promote midline symmetric flexion with head and trunk in midline, hands near mouth or face, and legs tucked close to the body with neutral hip position (Fig. 4.21). Benefits of supported supine include the unique potential for weight bearing on the posterior skull. For the older baby, supine allows increased visual exploration of the environment and face-to-face interaction. For the micropreemie during the first few days of life, supine prevents obstruction of cerebral venous drainage and increased cerebral blood flow.[350] In 1992, the American Academy of Pediatrics[351] initiated the "Back-to-Sleep" program, which advocates supine sleeping to

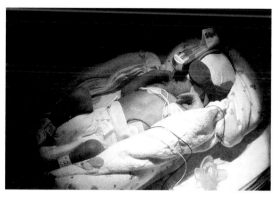

Figure 4.21 ■ An infant positioned in the supine position using a nest made from a Children's Medical Ventures Snuggle Up around the legs and trunk, and a Frederick T. Frog positioning aid around the head and neck to promote midline flexion.

prevent sudden infant death syndrome (SIDS). Preterm infants are more at risk for SIDS and should be transitioned to supine sleeping prior to discharge from the hospital.[351]

The very medically fragile infant may be limited in positioning options due to technologic supports (i.e., chest tubes, umbilical vein [UV]/umbilical artery [UA] lines, and ventilatory support) and medical conditions (i.e., gastroschisis, omphalocele, prior abdominal surgery, and arthrogryposis). Under these circumstances, positioning supports to attain the most optimal alignment available are implemented. The goal is to promote physiologic stability and infant comfort rather than perfect biomechanical alignment. As the infant's condition improves, he or she is assessed for tolerance to positioning in better alignment and other positions.

The musculoskeletal consequences of poor alignment over time in a preterm baby include tightness of neck extensors, shoulder/scapular retractors, low back extensors, and hip abductors. Tight muscles predispose the infant to reinforce certain motor patterns while inhibiting others. The repetitive use of these motor patterns can cause the formation of dominant cerebral motor pathways and the regression of the less frequently used patterns. The effects of these muscle imbalances, malalignment, and dominant motor pathways can prevent the acquisition of developmental skills such as chin tuck and midline head postures, eye–hand regard and reaching, weight shifts, and rolling.[340,352,353] Delays in fine and gross motor development that interfere with play and exploration can delay cognitive development.[352] Research has demonstrated the persistence of an out-toeing gait in children as old as 4 to 6 years and the persistence of toe walking up to 18 months in former preterm infants.[88,354,355]

Positioning can also affect cranial molding and head shape. Preterm infants are more at risk for cranial deformations as their skulls are softer and thinner than full-term infants.[356–358] Head shaping can affect parental perceptions of infant attractiveness and can interfere with the attachment process.[359,360] Due to the forces of gravity and the pressure of the mattress when lying with his or her head to the side, the preterm infant can develop an elongated anterior–posterior diameter of his or her skull. This is known as dolichocephaly and can interfere with the development of midline position of the head in supine. In addition, plagiocephaly or unilateral posterolateral head flattening can occur from prolonged supine positioning with a head preference and lack of head turning to the opposite side. Torticollis, unilateral shortening of the sternocleidomastoid muscle (SCM), can develop as a result of plagiocephaly and is characterized by ipsilateral head tilt and contralateral head rotation. Torticollis may influence the posture of not only the infant's head, but also his or her trunk, and may delay motor skill acquisition as well as prevent the development of binocular vision and visual convergence. To prevent cranial deformities and torticollis, commercially available gel pillows to disperse pressure across the skull can be used.[338,361–364] In addition, regular changes in the head position throughout the day and midline alignment of the head in supine can help to minimize cranial deformities and torticollis.

NEONATAL NEUROLOGIC ASSESSMENT

As physical therapists, we strive to practice under the principle of beneficence—"above all, do no harm" to our patients. When working with the population of high-risk infants, the potential is always present to harm a baby when intervening with him or her. Using careful and skilled observations of the baby's physiologic status allows the therapist to decide on the competence of the infant to withstand an assessment and when to terminate or proceed with handling an infant. A skilled therapist will also collaborate with nursing to understand the baby's current medical status, tolerance to handling, and events of the day before undertaking any direct interaction with the baby. The infant should also be evaluated before, during, and after any assessment or intervention for signs of pain using the neonatal pain assessment approved by the medical facility.

If the results of this preliminary gathering of information show that the baby is easily stressed by the routines of the day, an observational assessment to identify the baby's attempts to regulate and difficulties tolerating care is warranted. The therapist would follow the steps for observational assessment and care as discussed previously in the developmental care section. As the infant demonstrates improving stability, the therapist should continue to weigh the inherent potential costs to the infant with an assessment that involves handling. When the baby can tolerate additional stimulation and is in a sleep state, serial responses to repeated light (flashlight across the eyes) and sound (a soft rattle) are used to assess the baby's ability to filter repetitive stimuli. This provides information regarding the stability of the sleep state and also gives the therapist a chance to determine the readiness for handling. If the baby becomes overly stressed and loses physiologic stability, the therapist should end the evaluation session and provide supports for regulation. However, if the baby is able to transition to an alert state and maintain physiologic stability, the therapist can proceed slowly with assessment that requires gentle handling. The authors do not recommend one standardized assessment tool. See Table 4.7 for a variety of standardized neonatal assessments. Throughout the assessment the therapist needs to assess the baby's state control (i.e., the ability to maintain organized sleep states

TABLE 4.7				
Standardized Neonatal Assessment Tools				
Name/Author	**Purpose**	**Description**	**Psychometrics**	**Training**
Neurologic Assessment of Preterm and Full-Term Infants Authors: Dubowitz V Dubowitz L	To record the functional state of the nervous system and to document preterm infant neurologic maturation and recovery from perinatal insult Age: Preterm and full-term infants	Assessment of behavioral state, neurobehavior, posture, movement, muscle tone, and reflexes with passive manipulation Emphasis on patterns of responses. Test cannot be quantified or compared with normative expectations for age over time. Time to administer: 15 min	No reliability data Sensitivity: 83% Specificity: 84% Discriminates preterm from full-term at 40 wk PCA Correlation between IVH on cranial ultrasound and test items Predictive validity: 81%	Requires minimal training or experience Items within the area of expertise of developmental therapists
Neurobehavioral Assessment of the Preterm Infant (NAPI) Authors: Korner AF Thom VA	To assess infant maturity, monitor progress, and detect lags in development and neurologically suspect performance Age: 32–42 wk PCA	Assessment of state, behavior, reflexes, motor patterns, and tone Most items overlap with other assessments and must be administered from rousing to soothing to alerting. Time to administer: 45 min	Test–retest reliability: .51–.85 Validity: statistically significant age-related changes in performance in preterm infants Acceptable developmental validity	Training video available with manual To be used by any professional caring for or studying preterm infants in the intensive or intermediate care nursery
Neonatal Behavioral Assessment Scale (NBAS) Author: Brazelton TB	To assess the infant's contributions to the interactional process Age: 36 wk gestation to 44 wk	Consists of 28 behavioral items and 18 reflex items Sequence of administration is flexible and examiner seeks to elicit the infant's best performance Time to administer: 30–45 min and scored in 15–20 min	Test–retest reliability: .30 Interrater reliability: .90 Little evidence for long-term predictive validity Describes infant's current behavior and identifies his or her strengths and vulnerabilities	Requires training for reliability in administration and scoring Trainees complete a four-phase process consisting of self-study, skill test, and practice (on 25 babies) before completing certification session
Assessment of Preterm Infant Behavior (APIB) Authors: Als H Lester BM Tronick EZ Brazelton TB	To asses the individual behavioral organizational repertoire of the preterm infant Age: Preterm infants	Based on the BNBAS but focusing on the preterm infant Looks at the preterm infant's physiologic, motor, state, attentional–interactive, and regulatory systems Time to administer: 30–45 min Scoring is labor intensive	Interrater reliability: .90	Requires extensive training in the assessment as well as human development

(continued)

TABLE 4.7

Standardized Neonatal Assessment Tools (Continued)

Name/Author	Purpose	Description	Psychometrics	Training
NICU Network Neurobehavioral Scale (NNNS) Authors: Lester BM Tronick EZ	To assess neurologic integrity and behavioral functioning of infants at high risk Stress scale to document signs of withdrawal Age: 34–46 wk PCA Can be used in term, healthy infants and high-risk infants (substance exposures and preterm infants) Infants <33 wk use just observational items	Draws on NBAS, NAPI, APIB, Neurologic Examination of the Full-term Newborn Infant, and the Neurologic Examination of the Maturity of Newborn Infants Items are grouped in packages, which are presented depending on infant state in a pre-scribed sequence Can be modified for the very preterm, physiologically unstable infant Time to administer: 30 min	Test–rest reliability: .30–.44 across three tests at different GAs Validity: shows differences between substance-exposed groups and substance-exposed and -unexposed infants Normative data for healthy infants as well as some high-risk groups of infants	Requires certification through 2- or 5-day training programs with certified trainers along with practice administering the test to infants in own facility Amount of practice depends on experience, comfort handling infants, and clinical acumen
Assessment of General Movements (GMA) Author: Pretchl HF	To assess for early signs of brain dysfunction using qualitative measure Age: 36 wk PCA to 4 months Can be used with both preterm and full-term infants	Infants are videotaped and observational analysis of movements in terms of variety, fluidity, elegance, and complexity is performed. Video recording and analysis should be done longitudinally Time: 1 hr initial video-tape and 15-min fol-low-up tapes plus time for analysis	Interrater/test–retest reliability: 100% Specificity: 94.8% Sensitivity: 95% for prediction of neurologic outcome at 2 yr Lower in younger infants (earlier months) and increases with age up to 3 mo	Two-day training required for basic principles Practice of ≥100 recordings required to become a skilled observer Training videotape available, which demonstrates qualitative aspects of movement
Test of Infant Motor Performance (TIMP) Authors: Campbell SK Girolami G Oston E Lenke M	To identify motor delay in infants before 4 mo corrected age Age: 34 wk gestation to 4 mo postterm	Consists of 13 observed items focusing on midline alignment, selective control, and quality of movement; 29 elicited items focusing on anti-gravity postural control elicited by handling typically experienced by an infant	Testing at 3 mo predicted 12-mo motor performance Sensitivity: 92% Specificity: 76% Age-related standards for 1200 U.S. infants collected but not yet published	Workshops or self-study instructional CD
Alberta Infant Motor Scale (AIMS) Authors: Piper M Darrah J Pinnell L McGuire T Byrne P	To identify motor delays, monitor individual development, and evaluate intervention Age: 0–18 mo	Observational assessment of 58 transitional gross motor patterns and postures in supine, prone, sitting, and standing	Interrater reliability: .96 Test–rest reliability: .86–.99 until 12 mo Concurrent validity: .85–.99 with PDMS; .84–.97 with BSID	No training requirements specified To be used by any professional with a background in infant motor development

BSID, Bayley Scales of Infant Development; GA, gestational age; IVH, intraventricular hemorrhage; PCA, postconceptual age.
From Pelletier J, Lydic JS. Neurological assessment of the preterm and full-term infant: an analysis. Phys Occupat Ther Pediatr 1986;6(1):93–104.

and demonstrate a range of states; see Table 4.3 for state-related behaviors).

Neuromotor examination, to be accurate, requires a baby to be in a calm, awake state as other states (sleep, crying) can affect muscle tone, range of motion, and active movement. It is generally safe to initiate a neuromotor examination on an infant who is medically stable, on room air, and in an open crib. However, this portion of the assessment can be most stressful to the infant; therefore, the therapist should proceed with caution while maintaining vigilance for signs of tolerance or fatigue. Components of a baseline assessment for a medically stable infant include observation of posture at rest, quality and quantity of active movements, palmar and plantar grasp reflexes, flexor recoil, traction responses, passive range of motion, and French angles (adductor, popliteal, heel to ear, dorsiflexion, and scarf sign angles) (Table 4.7).[391] If the baby is tolerating these procedures, the therapist can move on to more intensive handling items, including pull to sit, slip through, ventral suspension, and prone, side-lying, and sitting placement. During this assessment the therapist should be watching for an optimal time to elicit visual and auditory responses from the infant. This portion of the assessment should also be administered from least stressful to most stressful and unimodal to multimodal stimulation (i.e., inanimate object, blank face, animated face, face coupled with speech). During this time the therapist needs to attend to the baby's responses to touch and movement through space and the baby's strategies to maintain organization in autonomic, state, and motor subsystems and calming strategies. The assessment allows the therapist a window into the baby's functioning at a single point in time; however, the baby's responses are based on his or her own level of maturity as well as contextual factors. Therefore, it is wise to serially examine an infant over time in order to gain an accurate picture of his or her function.

The therapist uses the information from the history, observation, and hands-on examination to determine the baby's strengths and needs and the family's strengths, needs, and expectations. The identified needs are prioritized and a plan of care is developed using interventions that challenge the baby within his or her range of tolerance. Recommendations are made so that the baby is appropriately challenged and supported by his or her family and caregivers throughout the week. For instance, a baby may have shown excessive extensor posturing and tight scapulohumeral and neck extensor musculature. The therapist would then recommend ways to incorporate flexion activities into daily routines and interactions with family and to avoid activities that promote excessive extension. As the baby develops and changes, these recommendations need to be updated.

BRONCHOPULMONARY DYSPLASIA

Bronchopulmonary dysplasia is the most common chronic lung disease (CLD) associated with prematurity and occurs in approximately 3000 to 7000 cases per year in the United States.[392] Infants born less than 32 weeks' gestational age who require supplemental oxygen at 36 weeks or infants born greater than 32 weeks who need additional oxygen after 28 days of postnatal life and have radiographic changes on chest radiographs are considered to have BPD. It has been suggested by experts in the field that the definition of BPD should be updated to be more physiologic as the current definition is imprecise and subjective to individual physicians' philosophy of oxygen use and level of oxygen saturation.[393–396] Although it is most common in ELBW infants because of the degree of lung immaturity, BPD can occur at any gestational age.

The pathogenic process of BPD is not completely understood, but is thought to be multifactorial. Acute lung injury from the combined effects of oxygen toxicity, barotrauma, and volutrauma from mechanical ventilation used to support infants with respiratory distress syndrome has been associated with the development of BPD. Injury to the cells and interstitial tissues of the lungs is due in part to inflammatory responses, which results in the interruption of alveolar development and destruction of the parenchyma leading to pathophysiologic changes. BPD as originally described by Northway et al.[397] in 1967 was characterized by airway injury and inflammatory response, lung parenchymal fibrosis and cellular hypoplasia, and areas of hyperinflation and atelectasis. The end result was thickened and hyperreactive airways, decreased lung compliance due to fibrosis, increased airway resistance, impaired gas exchange with ventilation–perfusion mismatch, and air trapping.[398–401]

Current prenatal and neonatal practices such as the use of antenatal steroids, postnatal surfactant, iNO, and the potential for lower magnitude of mechanical ventilation have changed the pathophysiologic characteristics of the disease.[394,402,403] The lungs of infants with BPD now show less fibrosis and more uniform patterns of inflation; however, decreased alveolar formation and lung vascularization are still major factors in the disease process.[394,395,402,404] In the "new" BPD there are fewer and larger simplified alveoli, fewer airway lesions, variable airway hypoplasia, variable interstitial fibroproliferation, dysmorphic vasculature, and atypical patterns of lung cell proliferation.[404,405]

One of the greatest contributing factors to the development of BPD is the immaturity of the infant's lungs. The lungs are most vulnerable prior to the formation of alveoli, which occurs after 32 weeks' gestation. The preterm infant's lungs are required to develop as they are providing for gas exchange. Injury at this early stage of lung development can interfere with the development of alveoli and pulmonary microvasculature.[395,402,403] Inhibition of vascular growth directly impairs the process of alveolarization.[403] The end result is an arrest in alveolar development, loss of future areas of gas exchange, and the potential for long-term pulmonary complications.[405]

Mechanical ventilation and supplemental oxygen have been shown to interfere with alveolar and vascular development. The use of any type of mechanical ventilation with or without supplemental oxygen can damage the lungs of preterm infants and cause the pathologic changes of BPD.[404,406] CPAP, iNO, and HFV are often utilized in an attempt to decrease trauma to the lungs. Oxygen use alone can interfere with the complex set of genes that mediate lung development and lung healing processes from injury.[403] Premature infants are at greater risk for injury induced by oxygen-free radicals as antioxidant protection does not begin to develop until the third trimester of pregnancy.[402] Defenses against oxidative injury are decreased in the full-term infant as compared to adults and are even lower in the preterm infant. The use of antioxidants such as vitamin A or E has been suggested as protective or therapeutic strategies for BPD.[394,403,407,408]

Intrauterine or perinatal infection may contribute to the development of BPD. Recent studies have shown that *Chlamydia trachomatis* and cytomegalovirus can cause slowly developing pneumonitis. Chorioamnionitis may increase the inflammatory response in premature lungs to injury caused by mechanical ventilation.[395,403,409] Other contributing factors for BPD include early fluid overload and persistent left-to-right shunting through a PDA, undernutrition, familial airway hyperreactivity, genetic influences, and decreased surfactant synthesis.[392,394,395]

Medical treatment strategies are aimed at preventing or limiting the factors that set off the chain of pathogenic sequalae. Respiratory support is used only when necessary and at the lowest peak airway pressure needed to maintain adequate ventilation and decrease barotrauma. Careful fluid and nutrition management are used to provide hydration without overload and to promote growth. Diuretic treatment is used to prevent cor pulmonale, congestive heart failure, and pulmonary edema. Other treatments include infection control with careful monitoring and treatment of bacterial and fungal infections, and steroid treatment to decrease bronchospasm and the inflammatory response. Bronchodilator therapy is also used to decrease bronchospasm.[392,394,395,402]

Complications associated with BPD are systemic hypertension, metabolic imbalance, hearing loss, ROP, nephrocalcinosis, osteoporosis, GER, and early growth failure.[392,399,410,411] Long-term morbidity is associated with BPD due to pulmonary function abnormalities and reactive airways, neurodevelopmental delays, and growth failure.[395,402,412–417] In 1989, Perlman and Volpe[418] described a movement disorder in 2- to 3-month-old infants with BPD that was exacerbated by episodes of respiratory failure and decreased during sleep. Hadders-Algra et al.[419] in 1994 documented a similar movement disorder in another infant with BPD. Movements similar to extrapyramidal disorders or adult dyskinesis were noted in the limbs, neck, trunk, and mouth of these infants. Developmental outcomes vary widely in the literature; however, increased incidence of attention deficits, cognitive deficits, motor coordination dysfunction, and visual–motor functioning have been found in infants with BPD.[227,229,410,415,416,418–421] Mortality occurs in approximately 10% to 20% of infants during the first year of life and is generally related to cardiopulmonary complications. The risk of morbidity and mortality increases with the requirement for prolonged duration of oxygen supplementation and increased level of ventilatory support.[392]

PHYSICAL THERAPY ASSESSMENT AND INTERVENTION: BRONCHOPULMONARY DYSPLASIA

The examination of the infant with BPD/CLD begins with a thorough review of medical history by systems as delineated in the section on prematurity. The therapist needs to gather information as to past and current level of functioning with particular attention to respiratory status and level of respiratory support. It is important for the therapist to know the individual infant's baseline physiologic parameters and recognize that these may differ from age norms. It is imperative to interview the infant's nurse as to which activities the infant tolerates and which activities cause the baby to enter a cycle of respiratory instability. It is also important for the therapist to know the infant's scores on the pain assessment as recorded by nursing and to continue to assess for pain during the assessment. Babies with BPD are known for their ability to desaturate and require prolonged medical intervention to recover physiologic stability. When initiating the observation phase of the assessment, the therapist needs to assess heart rate, respiratory rate and pattern, and oxygen saturation at rest and during care activities. Any blood pressure concerns, edema of the trunk and extremities, and skin integrity issues should be noted. In terms of respiratory status, the infant with BPD/CLD may frequently demonstrate tachypnea, which is defined as a respiratory rate greater than 60 breaths per minute. These babies often exhibit paradoxic breathing and recruit accessory respiratory muscles rather than utilizing the typical pattern of abdominal breathing. The baby should be carefully assessed throughout the evaluation for signs of respiratory distress including retractions of the chest wall, nasal flaring, grunting, and stridor.

A posture and musculoskeletal assessment of the baby provides information relevant to the baby's respiratory function as well as neuromotor development. The baby may develop compensatory motor patterns to assist respiration by opening up the airway and chest and to recruit accessory muscles. Typical posture for a baby with BPD is hyperextension of the head and neck, shoulder elevation and retraction, trunk extension, and anterior pelvic tilt. These postures not only interfere with the development of efficient respiratory function, but they can also interfere with the infant's ability to develop self-calming, feeding, and fine and gross motor skills. Integumentary assessment should include the presence and integrity of scars on the trunk, specifically from PDA ligation, chest tubes, and abdominal surgery. These scars can cause limitations in trunk range of motion and lead to asymmetric trunk postures. Skin color and temperature should be assessed as indicators of perfusion to the trunk and extremities.

A neuromotor assessment as described in the premature infant section should be attempted. Prior to the initiation of a neuromotor examination, the therapist should consider which test items may be unduly stressful for the infant and modify the assessment accordingly. The therapist should pay close attention to the physiologic responses and tolerance to handling. Throughout the assessment, work of breathing and oxygen saturation in the infant should be monitored. Infants with BPD have limited respiratory reserve and the noxious test item may cause the infant to start a cycle of respiratory distress and compromise that requires medical intervention. Another concern is the energy cost and potential fatigue of an assessment even without severe respiratory decompensation.

A neurodevelopmental assessment needs to be completed as the infant's status allows. As with other areas of assessment, the infant with BPD may have decreased tolerance for developmental activities. Items and procedures of standardized assessment tools may need to be modified to accommodate the infant's level of tolerance. The therapist needs to respect the fact that breathing is always the baby's first priority and developmental activities need to be accomplished secondarily.

Intervention for the infant with BPD/CLD is based on the information synthesized from the assessment. The first important consideration is the baby's reserve capacity and tolerance for activity. Timing of the intervention should be done with the knowledge of other activities in the infant's schedule in order to avoid undue stress and fatigue. Infants with BPD often demonstrate episodes of irritability and restlessness due to discomfort and/or hypoxemia. They may have difficulty sleeping due to these factors or disturbance from the environment and caregiving. The therapist may provide suggestions in terms of decreasing environmental stimulation, positioning to support the infant's respiratory status, and assisting the infant in transitioning to deeper sleep states. These activities are not only developmentally appropriate, but they also help to decrease stress and energy expenditure and promote lung healing and growth.

While it is important to consider the posture and alignment, the therapist must consider the baby's ability to tolerate a more optimal postural alignment while maintaining respiratory stability. The therapist may gradually work toward better alignment through gentle handling and mobilization techniques. It may be necessary to start at the pelvis or lower trunk before addressing concerns at the neck and shoulder girdle. One change should be made at a time followed by a period of observation to allow the infant to adjust to the change. It may be necessary to provide scar massage in order to improve the flexibility of the scar tissue and therefore improve the flexibility and alignment of the trunk.

The infant with BPD may have limited reserves for motor activities and social interaction due to the high energy costs of his or her lung disease. It is extremely important that the therapist in the NICU learn to read the infant's cues of distress and availability for interaction. The therapist can assist parents in recognizing their infant's cues so they can provide comfort or social interactions appropriate to the infant's needs and availability. The parents can assist the infant in developing self-calming skills. This in turn helps to foster parental roles and enhances their abilities to care for their infant. The infant benefits from the parental interaction as well as the support to develop behavioral organization skills. Parents benefit from these opportunities to bond with their infant over the course of what can be a long hospitalization.

Activities to promote motor skills and postural control can be built into routines of the day such as feeding, burping, diaper changes, and bathing. Developmental activities should be appropriate to the infant's ability to interact and play. Suggestions for play positions and activities along with precautions should also be provided to the infant's family.

THE BABY WHO REQUIRES SURGERY

CONGENITAL DIAPHRAGMATIC HERNIA

Congenital diaphragmatic hernia (CDH) is a defect in the formation of the respiratory diaphragm during embryogenesis. At the 9th and 10th week of gestation the pleuroperitoneal cavity fails to close and the developing abdominal viscera, as it returns from the umbilical cord where it has migrated during development, may protrude through the opening into the hemithorax. The viscera compress the developing lung on that side, stunting its growth.[422] Because the left hemidiaphragm is larger and closes later than the right, the defect occurs more frequently on the left.[423] The resulting pulmonary hypoplasia on the side of the defect varies in severity and is associated with high neonatal mortality and long-term morbidity. The diagnosis of CDH can be made by prenatal ultrasound demonstrating the presence of abdominal contents in the pleuroperitoneal cavity. Mothers with a prenatal diagnosis of CDH are counseled to deliver in a perinatal center with neonatal/pediatric surgical and ECMO capabilities.[422] Severity of lung hypoplasia is assessed by the lung-to-head ratio and the presence of the left liver lobe in the hemithorax. Once the baby is born, the surgical repair is delayed until after the baby's pulmonary status and pulmonary artery hypertension have stabilized, which can take hours or days. If the baby does not respond to the maximum conventional ventilatory therapy, he or she may be placed on ECMO.

Children with CDH, whether they receive ECMO therapy or not, require close follow-up as there is a high incidence of sensorineural hearing loss, GER, failure to thrive, feeding problems, seizures, developmental delay, pectus excavatum, and scoliosis in these patients.[422]

OMPHALOCELE

An omphalocele results when the fetal midgut fails to return from the umbilical cord where it has migrated during development.[424] The associated abdominal muscles, fascia, and skin are therefore absent but the protruding sac containing the abdominal organs has a membranous covering. Omphalocele occurs in 1 in 5000 to 6000 live births, and is associated with advanced maternal age.[425,426] It occurs more frequently with other congenital anomalies and syndromes such as trisomy 13 and 18, congenital heart defects, diaphragmatic and upper midline defects, malrotation of the intestines, intestinal atresia, and genitourinary anomalies. Almost a third of babies born with omphalocele are born prematurely and males are affected more than females.[425] The defect is associated with a small abdominal cavity.[424,426]

The first priority for a newborn with an omphalocele is respiratory stabilization. The sac also requires sterile dressings to provide pressure to the contents and minimize heat and fluid loss.[426] Surgical repair consists of returning the viscera into the abdominal cavity.[425] The amount of displaced intestine can vary from a small amount hardly distinguishable from an umbilical hernia to a massive amount with the entire midgut and liver present in the umbilical cord.[424] Depending on the size, repair is via a skin flap closure for the former or a staged reduction for a defect greater than 5 cm. When the defect is large the viscera may be suspended above the patient in a silo dressing and require reduction daily over 7 to 10 days before closure.[425] While undergoing this process, the baby is paralyzed with a neuromuscular blockade while the fascial defect and abdominal wall are stretched in order to accommodate the contents of the omphalocele sac. At closure, the surgeons usually perform an appendectomy in order to prevent an atypical presentation of appendicitis later in life and insert a gastrostomy tube for decompression. These babies often require aggressive ventilatory support postoperatively,[425] as the abdominal contents impede diaphragmatic movement and limit lung expansion. Due to the large pressures required to expand the lungs against a large abdominal mass, BPD and CLD are frequent long-term consequences for these babies. In addition, they often also demonstrate feeding difficulties due to the prolonged period of decreased oral stimulation and tachypnea resulting from shallow breathing.[426] They frequently require total parental nutrition and endure long hospitalizations.[425] In addition, the other anomalies

associated with omphalocele have a major impact on the developmental outcome of the baby.[426]

GASTROSCHISIS

Unlike omphalocele, a gastroschisis (Greek for "belly cleft")[427] is a full-thickness abdominal wall defect (usually to the right of the umbilical cord where the wall is thought to be weakened) through which the abdominal contents protrude. The defect is initiated in the sixth gestational week with incomplete closure of the lateral folds of the embryo.[427] The herniated intestines are not covered with skin and become thick, matted, and leathery as a result of contact with the amniotic fluid (chemical peritonitis).[24] Gastroschisis is often associated with prematurity and low birth weight but is infrequently associated with other midline congenital anomalies. It has a higher incidence in mothers less than 24 years of age and is associated with cigarette smoking and delivery in January, February, or March.[427] It occurs in 1 in 30,000 to 50,000 live births. A primary surgical closure is usually not possible due to the chemical peritonitis of the uncovered bowel; therefore, a staged closure is necessary.[425]

TRACHEAL ESOPHAGEAL FISTULA

Between the third and the sixth weeks of gestation, the primitive foregut is in the process of separating into the respiratory and alimentary tracts. When this process fails, a tracheal esophageal fistula (TEF) can occur.[423] A TEF is usually present with varying amounts of esophageal atresia (EA), the most common scenario (80% to 90%) being a blind proximal esophageal pouch with a distal TEF.[424]

A TEF with or without EA occurs in 1 in 4500 live births. Twenty % to 30% of these babies are born prematurely and there are associated abnormalities in 30% to 70%. Fifteen percent are diagnosed with the VACTERL association (*v*ertebral anomalies, *a*nal atresia, *c*ongenital heart defects, *T*EF, *E*A, *r*enal abnormalities, *l*imb deformities). Typical clinical presentation for a baby with TEF and EA includes an accumulation of oral secretions (due to ineffective swallowing), respiratory difficulties, and coughing, choking, and cyanosis with feeds. The medical staff is unable to pass a nasogastric tube and a radiograph may show the tube coiled in the atretic esophagus. Surgical anastomosis of the esophagus and obliteration of the fistula are needed; however, if the distance separating the two ends of the esophagus is great, a staged repair with stretching to promote elongation of the esophagus, circular myotomies of the existing esophagus, or replacing the missing esophagus with a portion of the small or large intestine is required. A gastrostomy tube is placed to allow feeding while the baby heals from surgery. Gastroesophageal reflux is a common complication following TEF repair due to the poor peristalsis and the upward pull on the lower esophageal pouch (Fig. 4.22).[425]

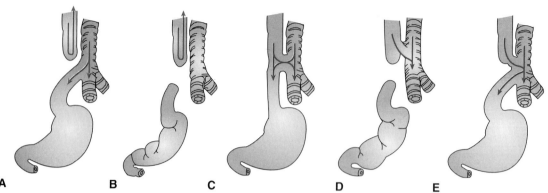

Figure 4.22 ■ *Esophageal atresia and tracheoesophageal fistula. (From Pillitteri A. Maternal and Child Nursing. 4th Ed. Philadelphia: Lippincott Williams & Wilkins, 2003.)*

FETAL SURGERY

With the advances in fetal imaging and diagnostic techniques have come the opportunities to intervene during pregnancy to ameliorate the development of structural problems in the fetus. Fetal surgery has grown out of the understanding of the progression of an untreated condition and which babies might benefit from this early intervention.[428] At present there are three centers in the United States where open procedures involving hysterotomy and direct fetal surgery are performed. These centers provide the multidisciplinary team approach necessary to care for both patients (mother and fetus). The team members include perinatologists, neonatologists, pediatric surgeons, sonographers, anesthesiologists, nurse specialists in surgery and perinatology, nurse coordinators, and social workers. Usually the mother is referred prior to 23 weeks' gestation for surgical evaluation. The mother must relocate to housing near the center in order to be closely monitored after the procedure. She is also placed on bedrest and medications to prevent preterm labor. The baby is delivered by planned cesarean section at 36 weeks in order to prevent the uterus from rupturing during labor. Fetal surgical intervention is available for the following prenatal diagnoses: cystic congenital adenomatoid malformation (CCAM), myelomeningocele (MMC), sacrococcygeal teratoma (SCT), twin-to-twin transfusion syndrome (TTTS), obstructive uropathy, congenital high airway obstruction syndrome (CHAOS), and amniotic band syndrome. Fetoscopic procedures allow the surgery for some of these procedures to be minimally invasive. A National Institutes of Health randomized controlled study is currently under way to determine the efficacy and safety of fetal repair of MMC versus the traditional postnatal repair.[428]

PHYSICAL THERAPY ASSESSMENT AND INTERVENTION FOR THE BABY WHO REQUIRES SURGERY

Although a baby in a NICU who requires surgery may not have been born prematurely, he or she may demon-

strate immaturity and instability in any of the subsystems described in the synactive theory. Babies who require surgery may experience more immobility and pain than other babies in the NICU. It is important that issues of pain be addressed before the therapist proceeds with any direct intervention.

As with any other examination, the therapist starts with a thorough review of the chart, with particular attention to the indications for surgery, the surgical procedure, the outcome of the surgery, and any precautions or contraindications. The nurse should be interviewed to find out how the baby's pain is managed and if the current pain management is adequate for the baby at rest and during nursing care. A baby who requires surgical intervention may also need technological supports such as mechanical ventilation, chest tubes with or without suction, drains, or gastric suctioning devices. These supports can also add to the baby's discomfort as well as limit his or her ability to be positioned and moved. The therapist should assess the surgical incisions for how they are healing and for the presence of scar tissue. The healing process can be delayed by the presence of antibiotic-resistant bacteria and the risk for iatrogenic infections, which can prolong the baby's hospitalization. Prolonged illness, immobilization, and hospitalization can interfere with the baby's acquisition of developmental milestones as well as with his or her socialization and ability to bond, placing him or her at greater risk for delays. Living in a crisis-prone environment disadvantages children who "grow old in the NICU" as they experience multiple caregivers, limited interactions with family, and limited opportunities to move, practice developmental activities, and have typical sensory experiences. In addition, staff may feel challenged to provide the appropriate stimulation in the newborn intensive care setting.[429]

The assessment should also include the impact of the surgical intervention on the infant's respiratory function. The rate and the pattern of the baby's breathing should be examined as it may be influenced by the presence of scarring, thoracic and abdominal pressure changes, anatomic changes, pain, edema, and lack of musculoskeletal support. In addition, the above may also affect the baby's passive and active range of motion. For these patients it is important to assess their developmental skills in an ongoing fashion.

Due to the nature of the illness and intensive care these babies require, they often demonstrate developmental delays and the NICU therapist's role may change from primarily consultative to more traditional "hands on" during the course of the infant's hospitalization.

Interventions for a baby who has had surgery can include positioning, mobilization of soft tissue, facilitation of sensory responses, postural control, and gross and fine motor activities. It is frequent for the initial portions of each therapy session to focus on mobilization techniques for alignment and flexibility prior to handling activities to promote developmental skills. It is not uncommon for babies who have required surgical intervention to their thoracic or abdominal areas to develop asymmetric postures. This may be due to the underlying anatomic lesion or as a result of postsurgical scarring and limitations to positioning. In addition, positioning programs can be developed and caregivers can be shown techniques to incorporate mobilization into daily routines. The therapist should provide developmentally appropriate activity suggestions to family and NICU staff. This can be in the form of direct teaching as well as posting play ideas at the infant's bedside.

THE BABY WITH NEUROLOGIC ISSUES

THE BABY WITH ASPHYXIA

Perinatal asphyxia is a result of a lack of oxygen (hypoxia) and/or a lack of perfusion (ischemia) to various organs.[430] The incidence of asphyxia is 2 to 6 per 1000 births.[255] It is more frequent in preterm infants (60% in VLBW births), where it is usually associated with periventricular/intraventricular hemorrhages,[306] and accounts for 20% of perinatal deaths. Asphyxia is more likely to occur in term infants of diabetic or toxemic mothers and is also associated with IUGR and breech presentation. Ninety percent of asphyxiated births are estimated to occur as a result of placental insufficiency during the antepartum or intrapartum periods.[430] However, cardiopulmonary anomalies of the fetus are also a risk factor for asphyxia.[306] All babies experience hypoxia during normal labor but not to a degree that is damaging. A cord or fetal scalp pH less than 7.0 may indicate substantial intrauterine asphyxia. Other supporting evidence includes the presence of meconium staining, abnormalities in fetal heart rate and rhythm, and an Apgar score less than or equal to 3 for greater than 5 minutes. The organs most susceptible to damage during asphyxia are the kidneys, brain, heart, and lungs, with the most important consequence of perinatal asphyxia being hypoxic–ischemic encephalopathy (HIE).[430] There must be evidence of hypoxia and ischemia to make the diagnosis of HIE, and there may also be an underlying neurologic disturbance predisposing the baby to a hypoxic–ischemic event.[431]

HIE can range from mild to severe. Ten percent to 20% of term asphyxiated infants die and the remainder who survive have a good chance of developing normally even in the presence of seizures in the neonatal period. However, there is a small group of severely asphyxiated infants who, having escaped death, will develop major neurologic sequelae including cerebral palsy, mental retardation, seizure disorder,[430] cortical blindness, hearing impairment, and microcephaly.[255] A baby who has been asphyxiated may develop any of the following five neurologic lesions:

1. Focal or multifocal cortical necrosis
2. Watershed infarcts (occurring in the boundary zones between cerebral and cerebellar arteries where blood flow is reduced with hypotension or hypoperfusion)
3. Selective neuronal necrosis (brainstem nuclei or Purkinje cells in the cerebellum)
4. Status marmoratus (necrosis of the thalamic nuclei and basal ganglia with myelination of astrocytic processes versus neurons)
5. Periventricular leukomalacia[255,306,430]

More extensive lesions occur with more severe asphyxia. Partial episodes of asphyxia result in diffuse cerebral necrosis, while total asphyxia spares the cortex and affects the brainstem, thalamus, and basal ganglia. The Sarnat clinical stages (Table 4.8) are used to estimate the severity of asphyxiation in infants greater than 36 weeks' gestation and are based on clinical presentation and duration of symptoms.[430] Asphyxiation in a preterm infant is more difficult to recognize due to the brain immaturity, hypotonia, and immature reflexes present in preterm infants. Premature infants may be protected from HIE by their immaturity, as the more mature the organism at the time of the asphyxia, the shorter the duration needed to cause brain damage.[306] The most effective intervention is prevention of asphyxia by establishing ventilation and perfusion and minimizing hypotension and hypoxia. Babies should be handled with care with the intention to minimize stress and to avoid fluctuations in blood pressure and sensory overload and to teach parents to do the same (Table 4.8).[255]

THE BABY WITH SEIZURES

Seizures in the neonatal period are difficult to recognize and diagnose because the perinatal brain is functionally and morphologically immature. The electrical discharge underlying a seizure depends on synaptic connections, axonal/dendritic arborization, and myelination, making the well-organized motoric patterns of a seizure in an older infant unlikely in a newborn.[432] The expression of a seizure in a newborn generally manifests as chewing, lip smacking, sucking, apnea, and gaze abnormalities, probably due to

> **TABLE 4.8**
>
> ## Sarnat and Sarnat Stages of Hypoxic–Ischemic Encephalopathy

Stage	Stage 1 (Mild)	Stage 2 (Moderate)	Stage 3 (Severe)
Level of consciousness	Hyperalert: irritable	Lethargic or obtunded	Stuporous, comatose
Neuromuscular control:	Uninhibited, overreactive	Diminished spontaneous movement	Diminished or absent spontaneous movement
Muscle tone	Normal	Mild hypotonia	Flaccid
Posture	Mild distal flexion	Strong distal flexion	Intermittent decerebration
Stretch reflexes	Overactive	Overactive, disinhibited	Decreased or absent
Segmental myoclonus	Present or absent	Present	Absent
Complex reflexes:	Normal	Suppressed	Absent
Suck	Weak	Weak or absent	Absent
Moro	Strong, low threshold	Weak, incomplete high threshold	Absent
Oculovestibular	Normal	Overactive	Weak or absent
Tonic neck	Slight	Strong	Absent
Autonomic function:	Generalized sympathetic	Generalized parasympathetic	Both systems depressed
Pupils	Mydriasis	Miosis	Midposition, often use poor light reflex
Respirations	Spontaneous	Spontaneous; occasional apnea	Periodic; apnea
Heart rate	Tachycardia	Bradycardia	Variable
Bronchial and salivary secretions	Sparse	Profuse	Variable
Gastrointestinal motility	Normal or decreased	Increased diarrhea	Variable
Seizures	None	Common focal or multifocal (6–24 hr of age)	Uncommon (excluding decerebration)
Electroencephalographic findings	Normal (awake)	Early: generalized low voltage, slowing (continuous delta and theta)	Early: periodic pattern with isopotential ph
		Later: periodic pattern (awake): seizures focal or multifocal; 1.0–1.5 Hz spike and wave	Later: totally isopotential
Duration of symptoms	<24 hr	2–14 days	Hours to weeks
Outcome	About 100% normal	80% normal; abnormal if symptoms more than 5–7 days	About 50% die; remainder with severe sequelae

*The stages in this table are a continuum reflecting the spectrum of clinical states of infants over 36 weeks' gestational age.
Source: From Sarnat HB, Sarnat MS. Neonatal encephalopathy following fetal distress: a clinical and electroencephalographic study. Arch Neurol 1976;33:696.
Reprinted with permission from Aurora S, Snyder EY. Perinatal asphyxia. In: Cloherty JP, Eichenwald EC, Stark AR, eds. Manual of Neonatal Care. 5th Ed. Philadelphia: Lippincott Williams & Wilkins, 2004:542–543.

the relative maturity of the limbic structures and their connections to the brainstem.[433] There are five types of seizure patterns:

1. Subtle seizures are the most common in term and preterm infants comprising about 50% of all seizures in this population. They occur most commonly with other seizures. They may not demonstrate electroencephalographic (EEG) correlation and may be refractory to anticonvulsant treatment. They include tonic horizontal deviation of the eyes, oral/buccal/lingual movements, swimming/bicycling movements, apnea, and other autonomic phenomena.[432,433]
2. Focal clonic seizures are characterized by localized clonic jerking with a fast contraction phase and a slower relaxation phase not associated with loss of consciousness. They are usually due to metabolic disturbances, an underlying structural lesion in the contralateral cerebral hemisphere, or focal traumatic injury and have a good prognostic outcome.[432,433]
3. Multifocal clonic seizures consist of random clonic movement of a limb that migrates to other limbs. This is rare in a newborn because of the immaturity of the newborn brain to propagate the discharge throughout the brain.[432,433]
4. Tonic seizures can be focal or generalized and resemble the decerebrate or decorticate posturing of older children involving tonic flexion or extension of the neck, trunk, and upper extremities with tonic lower extremity extension. Prognosis can vary but in general is poor.[432,433]

5. Myoclonic seizures are characterized by twitching of one or several body parts and can include the head and trunk as well. They are distinguished from clonic seizures by their speed and irregular pattern. They are associated with diffuse CNS pathology and carry a poor prognosis.[432,433]

The underlying cause of a seizure in a newborn can be one of several etiologies including CNS trauma, metabolic abnormalities, infection, brain malformation, drugs, polycythemia, and focal infarct, and is unknown in 3% to 25% of cases. Recurrent or continuous seizures can cause biochemical effects leading to brain damage. The goal of medical intervention is to identify and treat the underlying cause of the seizure in addition to controlling the seizure through the administration of anticonvulsants. Prognosis depends on the precipitating condition as well as duration of the seizures and the presence of tonic or myoclonic seizure patterns. Fifteen percent of babies die, 30% have long-term neurologic sequelae, and 55% have a normal outcome.[432,433]

PHYSICAL THERAPY ASSESSMENT AND INTERVENTION FOR THE BABY WITH NEUROLOGIC ISSUES

The therapist should begin the assessment with a thorough chart review as discussed previously. Particular attention should be paid to the neurology consultation, neuroradiographic studies (cranial ultrasound, MRI, computed tomography [CT] scan), and EEGs in terms of the area of lesion(s), size of the lesion(s), and clinical findings. The therapist should be aware of the prognosis made by the physician and whether that information has been communicated to the family. The family members should also be interviewed to ascertain their level of understanding of their infant's condition and prognosis. Attention should also be paid to the medical/surgical intervention such as medications, cerebrospinal fluid tapping, and shunting or ventriculostomy. During examination the therapist should take into consideration the effects of medications such as anticonvulsants that can decrease arousal and muscle tone.

Prior to beginning a hands-on assessment, the therapist should speak to the infant's nurse and family about the events of the infant's day as this may affect the baby's energy level, sleep and awake schedule, and tolerance for the evaluation. The therapist needs to know whether the observed behaviors are typical for the infant. If the infant has seizures, the therapist should inquire as to the typical presentation of seizure activity and if there are triggers for seizures. Other questions for the infant's nurse include timing of administration of seizure medication, presence and quality of aroused states, observed active movement, and atypical posturing.

A crucial part of the assessment focuses on muscle tone; however, infant behavioral state impacts muscle tone and motor behaviors. Infants who have sustained a neurologic insult may present with atypical states that lack variety, lack smooth transitions, and limit interaction. For example, the infant may only display a sleep state or irritable wakeful state. Completing a neurologic assessment in either of these two states would limit the accuracy; however, the therapist can still obtain useful information by observing active movement of trunk and extremities. Active movement should be observed for symmetry, smoothness, variety, complexity, and isolation. The infant should be reassessed in a serial fashion for changes in behavioral state organization and neuromotor status. When appropriate, a neurologic assessment including reflexes, range of motion, and muscle tone should be completed. There are some babies who present with symmetric active movement but may demonstrate asymmetries in elicited responses. Examples include a brisk gallant response, stronger palmar/plantar grasp reflex on one side, and/or asymmetric French angles (Fig. 4.23). These may be subtle signs and should be monitored as they have been predictive of neuromotor outcomes.[434]

Intervention for infants with a neurologic insult should begin with adapting their environment to support their behavioral state. For the infant who is unable to achieve wakeful states, the therapist can suggest strategies to arouse the infant such as unswaddling, using a soothing voice, setting low illumination, tactile stimulation, diaper change, or a sponge bath. An infant who only displays irritability when awake may benefit from modifying the environment to decrease stimulation. These modifications include swaddling, nonnutritive sucking, containment, proprioceptive input, and facilitation of slow transitions to and from awake states. Once state issues have improved, the therapist will want to address neuromotor and musculoskeletal concerns. Due to muscle tone and limited active movement, the infant may demonstrate tightness with range of motion and require interventions such as gentle stretching and splinting. A referral for occupational therapy services may be required to evaluate the need for hand splints. Strategies for positioning and handling to promote symmetric postures and movements should be provided to the family and caregiving staff.

MEDICAL ISSUES OF THE TERM AND NEAR-TERM INFANT

While prematurity and its associated complications represent the concerns of a large number of infants in the NICU, there are a number of conditions specific to near-term and full-term infants that also require intensive care management. These infants are often very critically ill, have extended hospitalizations, and benefit from neonatal physical therapy services. A number of the more common conditions of the near-term and full-term infant and the related interventions are discussed in this section.

Neurologic Development of the High-Risk Infant

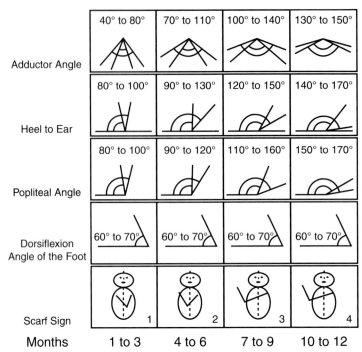

	40° to 80°	70° to 110°	100° to 140°	130° to 150°
Adductor Angle				
	80° to 100°	90° to 130°	120° to 150°	140° to 170°
Heel to Ear				
	80° to 100°	90° to 120°	110° to 160°	150° to 170°
Popliteal Angle				
Dorsiflexion Angle of the Foot	60° to 70°	60° to 70°	60° to 70°	60° to 70°
Scarf Sign	1	2	3	4
Months	1 to 3	4 to 6	7 to 9	10 to 12

Figure 4.23 ▪ Symmetric active movement demonstrating asymmetries in elicited responses, as seen in these French angles. Source: Reprinted with permission from Ellison PH. Neurologic Development of the High-Risk Infant. Clinics in Perinatology11(1):45 and adapted from Amiel-Tison C. A Method for Neurological Evaluation within the First Year of Life. Current Problems in Pediatrics 1976;7(1):45.

MECONIUM ASPIRATION SYNDROME

In the presence of acute or chronic hypoxia the fetus may pass meconium into the amniotic fluid prior to delivery. The act of gasping for the first breath may cause the infant to aspirate the meconium-stained amniotic fluid in the lungs where particles of meconium can obstruct airways, interfere with gas exchange, and result in severe respiratory distress. Approximately 20% to 30% of infants born through meconium-stained amniotic fluid are depressed at birth and require resuscitation.[435–437]

Meconium aspiration rarely occurs in infants less than 37 weeks' gestation and up to 30% of infants with MAS are greater than 42 weeks' gestation at birth.[436,438] Conditions of prolonged fetal compromise predating labor and intrauterine infection have been associated with meconium aspiration. Acute asphyxia may occur during labor due to these processes. The meconium itself can have a direct toxic effect on the lung due to chemical pneumonitis, inflammation, inactivation of surfactant, airway obstruction, and vasoconstriction of the pulmonary vessels.[437] Acute management of infants born through meconium-stained amniotic fluid include amniofusion, suction of airways, surfactant lavage, and antibiotic therapy.[436] Infants with meconium aspiration syndrome may require respiratory management including supplemental oxygen and mechanical ventilation. In more severe cases the respiratory compromise may progress, necessitating more aggressive management such as high-frequency mechanical ventilation and nitric oxide.[436,439] Severely ill infants with meconium aspiration, PPHN, and respiratory failure may require extracorporeal membrane oxygenation.

In the neonatal period, respiratory effects of meconium aspiration include persistent tachypnea and requirement of supplemental oxygen for several weeks. A large number of infants have abnormal pulmonary function and may have symptomatic cough, wheezing, and persistent hyperinflation up to 5 to 10 years of age.[436,440] Neurodevelopmental outcome varies and depends on the injury to the central nervous system due to asphyxia.[440]

PERSISTENT PULMONARY HYPERTENSION OF THE NEWBORN

Persistent pulmonary hypertension of the newborn is most commonly seen in term or postterm infants as the result of disruption in the typical transition of fetal to neonatal circulation. Increased vascular tension leads to right-to-left shunting through the ductus arteriosus and foramen ovale, resulting in severe hypoxemia. Hypoxia and alveolar atelectasis lead to pulmonary vasoconstriction and maintenance of pulmonary hypertension.[441]

Perinatal risk factors for PPHN include meconium-stained amniotic fluid, fever, anemia, and pulmonary disease. Associations have also been made with maternal factors including diabetes, urinary tract infection, aspirin, and nonsteroidal anti-inflammatory use during pregnancy. PPHN is also often associated with CDH. Perinatal asphyxia is the diagnosis most commonly associated with PPHN, followed by respiratory distress syndrome and aspiration syndromes. Pneumonia and/or sepsis, abnormal pulmonary development, myocardial dysfunction, and genetic predisposition also have an association with PPHN.[442]

Diagnosis is made by physical examination, chest radiograph, and electrocardiograph. This is considered a medical emergency and diagnosis and treatment need to be made promptly. Goals of treatment are to reverse hypoxemia and return normal oxygenation. Intervention includes supplemental oxygen, vasodilators, intubation and mechanical ventilation, iNO, ECMO, correction of metabolic acidosis, hemodynamic support, and correction of metabolic abnormalities and polycythemia.[441–444]

The prognosis for infants with PPHN has improved significantly with improved delivery of mechanical ventilation, iNO, and ECMO. However, survivors are at risk for chronic lung disease, intracranial hemorrhage, neurodevelopmental delays, and sensorineural hearing impairment.[442] Significant impairments have been found in survivors of moderately severe and severe PPHN in motor, cognitive, and hearing function.[443]

Therapists working with infants with PPHN need to be aware of potential cardiopulmonary compromise and support development without increasing stress on that system. Family and other caregivers should be provided with suggestions to promote motor, social, and feeding skills while maintaining physiologic stability.[3] Therapists also need to be aware of associated sensory and neurodevelopmental risks and provide appropriate screening, family education, and follow-up services.

INFECTIONS

TORCH is an acronym that stands for *t*oxoplasmosis, *o*ther infections, *r*ubella, *c*ytomegalovirus, and *h*erpes simplex virus. It has represented the congenital and perinatal infections a baby may acquire; however, there are other important agents recognized at this point causing neonatal infections.[445] Several will be considered in this text.

TOXOPLASMOSIS The *Toxoplasma gondii* protozoan parasite, which causes toxoplasmosis, is present throughout the animal kingdom but is transferred to humans through contact with cat feces or undercooked meat. The greatest risk for the baby occurs when a nonimmune mother (primary infection) acquires *T. gondii* during fetal organogenesis. Maternal acute toxoplasmosis is often undetected as the symptoms are mild and may only include enlarged lymph nodes and fatigue without a fever. Diagnosis is

most commonly confirmed by lab titers in the mother and polymerase chain reaction (PCR) in the fetus. Maternal transmission to the fetus increases with gestational age as it appears to correlate with placental blood flow; however, the risk to the fetus is greatest in early gestation. Babies infected in the second and third trimesters have mild disease or are asymptomatic in the newborn period, while babies infected in the first trimester die or present with severe CNS (hydrocephalus, seizures, and intracranial calcifications) and ophthalmic disease (chorioretinitis).[446,447] Eighty percent to 90% of babies with congenital infection may not demonstrate overt signs and symptoms at birth but are at long-term risk for visual impairment, seizures, severe motor and cognitive deficits,[446] and hearing impairment. Treatment for toxoplasmosis infection in the symptomatic and subclinical population of neonates is extended chemotherapy and corticosteroids.[447] Risk factors associated with poor outcome include delayed diagnosis resulting in delayed treatment, prolonged neonatal hypoxemia and hypoglycemia, and prolonged uncorrected hydrocephalus.[446]

RUBELLA Widespread immunization for rubella, a human-specific RNA virus, has existed in the United States since 1969 and has dramatically reduced the incidence of rubella in the United States. The very few cases of congenital rubella syndrome in recent years have occurred in unimmunized immigrants.[445] Like toxoplasmosis, maternal rubella infection may be mild and undetected. Mothers may experience malaise, headache, low-grade fever, and conjunctivitis followed by a macular rash several days later. Diagnosis is confirmed by titers. Transmission to the fetus may occur at any time in gestation but infection after 20 weeks' gestation rarely causes defects in the fetus. Sensorineural hearing loss/impairment, mental retardation, cardiac malformations, and ophthalmic defects are anomalies associated with congenital rubella syndrome. When maternal rubella infection occurs in the first 12 weeks, approximately 20% of fetuses may not become infected. When maternal infection occurs closer to 16 weeks, approximately 45% of fetuses do not become infected; however, antenatal diagnosis is not foolproof or widely available. Diagnosis of congenital rubella syndrome is made via a positive culture for rubella, presence of rubella-specific immunoglobulins in cord blood, or the persistence of titers in the fetus.[445] In the intensive care nursery, treatment is supportive and includes surgical correction of heart defects and cataracts. Signs of congenital rubella infection can continue to appear for 10 to 20 years. Late signs include insulin-dependent diabetes, thyroid abnormalities, hyperadrenalism, hearing loss, and eye damage.[447]

CYTOMEGALOVIRUS A member of the herpes family of viruses, cytomegalovirus (CMV) infection is common, with an estimated 50% to 85% of the population acquiring it some time in their lives.[445] CMV is transmitted via bodily fluids and secretions and results in general malaise, liver involvement, fever, and fatigue.[447] It is typically harmless for a child or adult, but in a neonate it may be severe if not fatal. Primary (first) maternal infection carries the greatest risk for the baby. Reactivation of the disease can occur during pregnancy; however, the baby rarely demonstrates clinical symptoms of CMV infection.[445] CMV can be transmitted to the baby in utero via the placenta, perinatally during transit through the birth canal, through breast milk, or through contact with infected saliva, urine, or blood products. A baby infected as a result of a primary maternal infection may present with prematurity, IUGR, microcephaly, periventricular calcifications, congenital cataracts, hepatosplenomegaly, and jaundice.[447] The babies with multiple system involvement are at higher risk of mortality. Infants who survive are at high risk for developing significant developmental disabilities including profound mental retardation, deafness, blindness, and cerebral palsy. Diagnosis is confirmed by presence of virus in urine, saliva, blood, or respiratory secretions, and if present in the first 2 weeks of life indicates congenital CMV and if present after 4 weeks of life indicates perinatal CMV. Of the term infants who acquire CMV in the perinatal period, most remain asymptomatic with infrequent long-term developmental sequelae. However, preterm infants exposed to CMV during the birth process or postnatally are more frequently symptomatic. All infants with perinatal CMV infection should be followed closely for hearing deficits. Treatment with immunoglobulins provides passive immunity for babies at risk for CMV. For those with proven infections, treatment with ganciclovir or valganciclovir has shown a trend toward improving sensorineural hearing loss.[445,447]

HERPES SIMPLEX VIRUS Herpes simplex virus (HSV) is very common with an 80% incidence for type I (orolabial) and 40% incidence for type II (genital) in the United States. HSV types I and II are distinct viruses; however, they are clinically indistinguishable in the newborn. HSV type II is the predominant cause of disease (95%) in the newborn and transmission occurs primarily during descent through the birth canal. A cesarean section protects an infant from exposure. Mothers with newly acquired HSV during pregnancy transmit the virus to their fetuses at an estimated rate of 50%.[445] If transmission occurs prior to 20 weeks' gestation, the fetus is usually spontaneously aborted. The presenting infection in the newborn can be localized to the skin, eye, and mouth and can involve the CNS (encephalitis) or be disseminated to multiple organs. Infants with localized infection are at risk to develop neurologic complications and should be followed closely. Infants with CNS disease usually present between 10 and 14 days with lethargy, seizures, temperature instability, and hypotonia. Mortality and morbidity are high in this population with long-term sequelae including microcephaly, hydro-

cephaly, porencephalic cysts, cerebral palsy, blindness, chorioretinitis, and cognitive impairments. Babies with disseminated disease have the highest mortality (greater than 50%) and present in the first week of life with respiratory distress, visceral organ involvement, seizures, shock, and disseminated intravascular coagulation (DIC), which results in abnormal clotting, hemorrhaging, and vesicular rash. Forty percent of long-term survivors of disseminated disease have long-term sequelae. Diagnosis is made by isolation of virus from stool, urine, oropharynx, nasopharynx, conjunctivae, and mucocutaneous lesions or by fluorescent antibody detection. Treatment consists of antiviral therapy in the form of acyclovir.[445]

HUMAN IMMUNODEFICIENCY VIRUS Human immunodeficiency virus (HIV) 1 is a cytopathic RNA retrovirus and the principle cause of HIV infection. The principle mode of transmission is heterosexual encounters.[445] The incidence of perinatal HIV in the United States has dropped in the latter half of the 1990s due to the intragestational prophylactic administration of antiretroviral therapy. In the developing world, 40% of women of childbearing age are seropositive for HIV. All HIV-infected infants acquire the disease from their infected mothers. Approximately 20% of the AIDS population in America is women of childbearing age.[445,447] In adults, an asymptomatic phase lasting up to 10 years can occur after initial infection. Transmission to the baby can occur via the placenta in utero, during the intrapartum period through contact with secretions from the birth canal, or through breast milk and is estimated to be between 15% and 40%. Delivery via cesarean section may decrease the risk of transmission to the baby if done before the onset of labor. The majority of pediatric AIDS cases is in infants and young children, through congenitally acquired or perinatally acquired disease. Twenty percent of infected infants die in the first year, while 60% show signs of severe disease by 18 months. It is possible that infected children can remain asymptomatic for 7 to 15 years. Fifty percent demonstrate HIV-related symptoms in the first year with the average age of onset being 9 months. An infant may present clinically with lymphadenopathy, hepatosplenomegaly, poor weight gain, neuromotor abnormalities, and encephalopathy. More infrequently a baby may present with *Pneumocystis carinii* pneumonia (PCP), recurrent bacterial infections, or lymphoid interstitial pneumonitis. During childhood, developmental delays with loss of milestones and cognitive deficits can occur. Diagnosis by serology in infancy is limited, as maternal immunoglobulins having crossed the placenta are maintained into the first year of the infant's life. Therefore, diagnosis is made by HIV culture or viral detection tests generally based on symptomatology and/or specific laboratory findings. There is no cure for HIV; treatment consists of antiretroviral therapy with the goal of suppressing the viral load. Infants with HIV demonstrate high viral loads, which decline as the immune system develops. Infants should be treated in the first year of life to support the development of the immune system.[445]

GROUP B STREPTOCOCCI *Streptococcus agalactiae* (group B streptococci [GBS]) is a bacterium that is found in human genital and gastrointestinal tracts. It can cause urinary tract infections, chorioamnionitis, postpartum endometritis, and bacteremia during pregnancy.[448] In addition, it can cause amnionitis, resulting in premature rupture of membranes or preterm birth.[449] GBS used to be the most common bacterial agent causing sepsis, pneumonia, and meningitis in the newborn in the United States, but recent data show that the incidence of GBS sepsis has decreased with the use of intrapartum antibiotic prophylaxis.[448] Eight percent to 25% of women have asymptomatic vaginal colonization with GBS and the bacteria can be transmitted to the baby by infected amniotic fluid or during transit through the birth canal at an estimated rate of 40% to 70%.[449] Pregnant women are therefore assessed by risk factors and/or cultured at 35 to 37 weeks for GBS. Risk factors for GBS include history of delivering an infant who developed GBS disease, GBS bacteriuria during pregnancy, preterm delivery, rupture of membranes greater than or equal to 18 hours, or fever greater than or equal to 100.4°F during labor and delivery. Women who culture positive for GBS or have a risk factor are given intrapartum antibacterial prophylaxis for GBS. Babies with GBS sepsis present commonly with respiratory distress, vomiting, diarrhea, abdominal distention, ileus, poor feeding, temperature instability, hypotension, hyperglycemia, lethargy, seizures, petechiae, and/or purpura. Babies can also present with fulminant shock and respiratory failure progressing to death. Babies are treated with antibiotics or immunotherapy (immunoglobulins, granulocyte infusions, or exchange transfusions) and may require ECMO if respiratory and circulatory failure occurs despite conventional intensive care.[448] GBS causes the majority of morbidity and mortality in the newborn.[449]

FETAL ALCOHOL SYNDROME

Growth and neurodevelopmental disorders along with dysmorphic physical features have been associated with prenatal alcohol exposure. Fetal alcohol syndrome (FAS) refers to a constellation of physical, behavioral, and cognitive abnormalities; dysmorphic facial characteristics; pre- and postnatal growth deficiencies; and mental retardation (Table 4.9).[227,450–454] First described in detail by Jones and Smith in 1973,[450] FAS is one of the most common causes of mental retardation worldwide. Current research has found that exposure of the fetus to alcohol may result in a variety of less pronounced dysmorphic, cognitive, and behavioral abnormalities rather than the full expression of

TABLE 4.9

Features of Fetal Alcohol Syndrome

Physical Features	Neurodevelopmental Concerns
Prenatal growth deficiencies/IUGR	Developmental delay
Postnatal growth deficiencies	Impaired cognitive function
Microcephaly	Speech impairments
Short palpebral fissures	Conductive hearing loss
Epicanthal folds	Sensorineural hearing loss
Midline facial hypoplasia	Behavioral issues
Short upturned nose	Mental retardation
Hypoplastic long or smooth philtrum	
Thin vermilion of upper lip	
Ear abnormalities	
Optic nerve hypoplasia	
Cardiac defects (ASD, VSD)	
Hydronephrosis	
External genitalia anomalies	
Abnormal palmar creases	
Joint abnormalities (hands, fingers, toes)	
Cutaneous hemangioma	

ASD, atrial septal defect; IUGR, intrauterine growth restriction; VSD, ventral septal defect.

FAS.[227,451,452] The term *fetal alcohol effects* or *fetal alcohol spectrum disorder* has been advocated for use over FAS as a result of these findings.[227,455–458]

The effects of alcohol exposure are related to the amount, timing, and pattern of alcohol consumption by the mother. Alcohol consumption around the time of conception and during the first 2 months of the first trimester has been correlated with fetal alcohol syndrome. Exposure to alcohol during the second and third trimesters has been associated with cognitive and behavioral deficits.[227,456] The hallmark of fetal alcohol exposure is severe growth retardation with length more affected than weight. Growth deficiencies continue postnatally but weight is more affected than length.[227,453]

The most serious feature of fetal alcohol syndrome is disturbance of central nervous system development. Disorders of neuronal proliferation, migration, and midline prosencephalic formation occur as a result of the teratogenic effects of alcohol during the first two trimesters of pregnancy.[227] Microcephaly is present in almost all cases, with delayed neurologic development also present in a majority of cases of children with FAS. Kartin and associates[459] found lower than average developmental performance in preschool children exposed to alcohol and drugs prenatally. Severe mental deficiency has been shown to correlate with severely dysmorphic features, but neurologic deficits can also occur alone. In addition to decreased intellectual functioning, hyperactivity, distractibility, decreased attention span, and impaired speech and language development affect functioning in school. There may also be long-term effects on psychosocial function.[227,454,455,457]

FAS may be difficult to recognize in the neonatal period and may be mistaken for other syndromes. Infants may have no signs of withdrawal if exposed to even moderate amounts of alcohol. Withdrawal signs of jitteriness, sleep disturbance, tremors, hypotonia, or gastrointestinal symptoms may be seen in some infants exposed to very high levels of alcohol.[227,460] The infant may have been exposed to other substances in addition to alcohol and demonstrate more severe withdrawal symptoms due to these substances. Since facial and physical features of FAS may be subtle and the infant may not demonstrate signs of withdrawal, the diagnosis of FAS may not be made until later in the preschool or school-age years when inattention, hyperactivity, and learning problems are more apparent.[457,458] Children with late diagnosis may miss out on early intervention and other services that can address growth and developmental needs. Infants with known prenatal exposure to alcohol or suspected FAS should be referred for developmental follow-up services upon discharge from the hospital.

NEONATAL ABSTINENCE SYNDROME

Prenatal maternal narcotic use can result in fetal dependence on these substances. The drugs associated with dependence and withdrawal most commonly used during pregnancy are heroin, methadone, and prescription pain medicines.[291,461,462] Term infants have more severe withdrawal than preterm infants.[462] There is greater storage of drugs in fat, leading to increased dependency on these substances with increasing gestational age. At birth, when the drugs are no longer being provided, the infant begins the process of withdrawal.

The onset of symptoms for acute narcotic withdrawal can vary from the first hours of life to 2 weeks of age.[463] Symptoms are usually noted within 24 to 48 hours depending on type of drug, length of maternal use, gestational age of the infant, and last maternal dose.[227,291,463] It is not uncommon for infants to be exposed to multiple substances; withdrawal from multiple substances is more severe for infants than withdrawal from methadone or opiates alone.[461–465] Symptoms of withdrawal include irritability, tremors, seizures, apnea, increased muscle tone, inability to sleep, hyperactive deep tendon reflexes, incoordination, hyperactive sucking, inefficient sucking and swallowing, and high-pitched, shrill cry.[291,461–463,465,466]

Treatment for symptomatic infants includes tight swaddling, holding, rocking, decreasing external stimulation of sound and light, and feeding with high-calorie formula as needed. Infants who are unable to respond to these supportive interventions require the addition of medication to their plan of care.[227,291,461–463,466,467] The decision to start pharmacologic intervention is based on objective measurement of symptoms recorded using a neonatal abstinence score. The most commonly used neonatal abstinence score is the system developed by Finnegan.[468,469] The NICU Network Neurobehavioral Scale incorporates features of the Finnegan scale but also assesses maturity, behavioral control, and self-regulation.[378] Decisions in terms of increasing or weaning of medications are also based on abstinence scores.[291,461,462,467] Medications commonly used to treat neonatal abstinence syndrome (NAS) include neonatal morphine solution, neonatal opium solution, paragoric, phenobarbitol, diazepam, methadone, and clonidine.[462,463,466,467]

Infants with NAS may have lower birth weight, height, and head circumference. They often exhibit depressed or inconsistent interactive behaviors and have poor self-calming, which can impact development. In addition, treatment of NAS may require weeks to months of hospitalization, which can interfere with maternal bonding and overall development.[227,461,463,466,467] Developmental follow-up studies of infants with NAS have found a higher incidence of hyperactivity, learning and behavior disorders, and poor social adjustment.[467] Kartin et al.[459] reported that the developmental performance of preschool children with prenatal alcohol and drug exposure was lower than expected for age. It is unclear to what extent environmental factors such as maternal characteristics, tobacco use, polydrug use, poverty, and social factors associated with substance abuse are responsible for these outcomes versus prenatal substance exposure.[227,467] While it is difficult to make a direct link between neonatal substance exposure and developmental outcomes, these children and their families are clearly at risk for social, behavioral, and developmental problems. Therefore, close follow-up and maternal–child services including early intervention are warranted.

PHYSICAL THERAPY ASSESSMENT AND INTERVENTION FOR THE TERM AND NEAR-TERM INFANT

Full-term and near-term infants in the NICU can be very fragile with complex medical conditions. It is important that the physical therapist complete a thorough chart review including maternal/prenatal history, birth history, review of past and present problems by systems, medical test/study findings, medical/surgical interventions, medications, and the infant's response to interventions and medications including neonatal pain assessments. If the infant is withdrawing from substance exposure, neonatal abstinence scores and any change in medical and/or pharmacologic intervention should be noted. Information regarding family psychosocial history and concerns should also be reviewed and discussed with the social worker if appropriate. The therapist should interview the infant's nurse for updated information regarding physiologic status, any changes in care, and the events of the day. A discussion with the family members as to their understanding of the infant's condition and their own concerns for their infant is a helpful starting point in developing a relationship with the family and planning therapy intervention including family education.

The evaluation of the infant should begin with an observation of the type of respiratory support, presence of central or peripheral lines, and presence of feeding tubes, as these are not only indications of the fragility of the infant, but may also limit the infant's positioning and active movement. An observational assessment should include the vital signs, pattern of respiration, behavior state, presence of edema, preferred postures, and active movement. The integumentary system should be assessed for the presence of skin breakdown or scars, which may interfere with alignment, mobility, and function.

Infants recovering from medical conditions such as meconium aspiration syndrome or persistent pulmonary hypertension of the newborn may not tolerate a hands-on assessment if they are still critically ill and requiring large amounts of medical support to promote physiologic function. Infants exposed to prenatal infections may also be very ill and unable to tolerate handling. While withdrawing from substance exposure, infants may not be able to tolerate the stimulation of handling. At this stage in the infant's hospital course the therapist would be primarily consulting with nursing and the family to make suggestions for positional and environmental modifications to promote comfort, physiologic function, and, if possible, positional alignment for future developmental tasks.

The assessment of the stable infant who is able to tolerate handling would include respiratory status and pattern/efficiency of breathing in different positions, integumentary status, behavioral state organization, posture and alignment, passive and active range of motion, muscle tone, presence and symmetry of reflexes, quantity and quality of active movement, postural control, response to sensory stimuli, pain assessment, visual tracking, auditory localization, and social/interaction skills. If appropriate, a standardized developmental assessment may be administered. Physical therapy intervention is then based on the individual infant's strengths and concerns. The concerns may be prioritized according to the infant's medical status and immediate needs in the NICU environment. It is important to be observant of the infant's cardiopulmonary status and behavioral cues when handling the infant and to help the family to understand that the infant may not be able to tolerate as much activity as other infants his or her age.

Infants withdrawing from prenatal substance exposure often require long hospital stays and present with unique needs. Generally older and more physiologically stable, these infants experience significant discomfort and poor behavioral organization. The assessment should include all the elements previously discussed and assessment of neonatal abstinence scores. An emphasis may be placed on assessing and providing comfort measures, particularly early in their withdrawal. Intervention may include bundling and deep pressure during handling and through bed positioning with total containment and environmental modifications to decrease noise and bright light and promote periods of deep sleep. Infant massage using firm strokes may be helpful to some infants and is a good bonding activity for parents. Gentle vestibular input in the form of gentle rocking or swinging can be effective for some infants. It is important to remember that these infants are older and to provide appropriate developmental intervention when they are available and able to tolerate these activities. The therapist should work with the family members to understand the needs of the infant and help them learn calming and appropriate developmental interactions. A priority is to promote attachment and bonding over the course of the hospitalization, which may be weeks to months.

Infants with prenatal alcohol exposure may not demonstrate signs of withdrawal or developmental concerns in the neonatal period. The therapist should perform a full assessment and address any needs or concerns. Whether or not there are specific findings on inpatient assessment, the infant should be referred for developmental follow-up at the time of discharge due to the high risk of long-term developmental concerns.

THE INFANT WITH ORTHOPEDIC ISSUES

The physical therapist practicing in the NICU may be consulted to address orthopedic concerns of preterm and full-term infants. These conditions can include congenital positioning or developmental abnormalities, injury sustained during the birthing process, or positioning deformities occurring over the course of the infant's NICU admission. This section presents a brief overview of some common neonatal orthopedic conditions and interventions. While the physical therapist may not address some of these problems directly in the NICU, it is important that he or she have a good understanding of the conditions, their management, and potential long-term effects in order to help develop a comprehensive plan and make appropriate recommendations.

BRACHIAL PLEXUS INJURY

Injuries to the brachial plexus most commonly result from a difficult birth process during which the nerves may be stretched or avulsed. Factors associated with brachial plexus injury include increased birth weight, prolonged labor, sedated hypotonic infant, sedated mother, traction to the arm in the breech position, maternal gestational diabetes, rotation of the infant's head in a cephalic presentation, difficult cesarean-section extraction, and abnormal uterine position leading to pressure neuropathy.[470–473] Brachial plexus injuries are classified by the level of involvement. Erb's palsy is injury to the upper plexus and involves C-5, C-6, and C-7. Lower plexus injury involving C-7, C-8, and T-1 is referred to as Klumpke's palsy. Whole-arm injury involves the entire plexus, C-5 through T-1. There can be wide variation in injury ranging from mild edema affecting one or two roots to total avulsion of the entire plexus. Involvement is usually unilateral with bilateral brachial plexus injury occurring in 8% to 23% of all of injuries.[474]

Trauma to the brachial plexus is also associated with injury to the facial nerve and mild facial paralysis, fractures of the clavicle or humerus, traction to the cervical spinal cord with upper motor neuron injury signs, subluxation of the shoulder, and torticollis.[470,475,476] Isolated hemiparalysis of the diaphragm can occur due to injury to the phrenic nerve. Congenital anomalies such as cervical rib, abnormal thoracic vertebra, and shortened scalenes may be the cause of lower plexus injury. Damage to the brachial plexus can occur at the level of the nerve rootlet attachment to the spinal cord, anterior or posterior rootlets, or distal to where the rootlets come together to form a mixed nerve root that exits through the canal. A partial or complete rupture can evolve into a neuroma or fibrous tissue mass.

The clinical picture of injury to the upper plexus is the classic "waiter's tip" position of shoulder adduction and internal rotation with elbow extension, pronation of the forearm, and flexion of the wrist and fingers. The arm falls limply to the infant's side with passive abduction. Biceps and radial reflexes are absent, while the grasp reflux is intact. Klumpke's palsy results in weakness of the intrinsic muscles of the hand and long flexors of the wrist and fingers. The biceps reflex is present but grasp is absent. Involvement of the entire plexus results in a flaccid arm without any reflexes.[476] Diagnosis is made by clinical examination, electromyography (EMG) and CT scan or MRI.

Recovery occurs spontaneously within the first 2 months after injury in 80% of cases, and these children typically have normal function of their upper extremity. If the injury is not resolving after 6 months, the infant generally has considerable upper extremity impairment.[477] Residual long-term impairments may include bony deformities, muscle atrophy, joint contractures, impaired growth of the affected limb, weakness of the shoulder girdle, glenohumeral joint deformity, and shoulder subluxation.[472,478]

Treatment initially includes gentle passive range of motion after a period of 7 to 10 days to allow any hemorrhage and edema to resolve.[227,479,480] The therapist should assess the infant for torticollis and promote symmetry of the neck and spine. The family should be taught gentle range-of-motion activities and positioning to support the affected arm prior to leaving the intensive care unit.

The infant with brachial plexus injury should receive follow-up services by a specialist in the management of brachial plexus injury. Ongoing therapy to provide splinting to prevent contracture and promote proper alignment may also be indicated for infants with upper extremity impairment. Activities to promote active movement, motor learning, strengthening, and developmentally appropriate skills may also be provided.

In infants with more severe injury, surgery may be indicated. Total or global injuries require earlier surgical intervention. Microsurgical techniques include reconstruction of nerve ruptures with an interpositional graft, circumvention of nerve root avulsions by nerve transfer, and tendon transfer to stabilize the arm and prevent subluxation. Infants who require surgical interventions often require long-term follow-up and therapy to promote functional use of the extremity.

CONGENITAL HIP DYSPLASIA AND DISLOCATION

In fetal development, the hip joint is fully formed by the 11th week of gestation and from this point forward hip dislocation may occur. The etiology of hip dysplasia and dislocation is multifactorial and involves both genetic and intrauterine environmental factors. Risk factors for congenital hip dysplasia include breech delivery, oligohydramnios, female gender, first born, positive family history or ethnic background, persistent hip asymmetry, torticollis, and lower extremity deformity.[481–483]

Hip dysplasia describes a hip that can be dislocated or one that is dislocated and can be relocated in the acetabulum. A hip that is unreducible is considered to be dislocated and is often associated with secondary adaptive changes such as shortening of the limb, decreased hip abduction, and asymmetry of the gluteal folds.[481,483]

The majority of infants with hip dysplasia or dislocation are diagnosed at birth. The diagnosis is made by physical manipulation of the hip. In typically developed hips, the joint is held tightly together by the surface tension of the synovial fluid and is difficult to dislocate. In congenital hip dysplasia or dislocation, the fit is not tight and the head of the femur can be made to glide in and out of the acetabulum over a ridge of very cellular hyaline cartilage. The palpation of the hip moving over the ridge is considered a positive Ortolani[484] sign (Fig. 4.24). A negative Ortolani sign is when the hip cannot be relocated. Another diagnostic test is the Barlow[485] maneuver (Fig. 4.24). This is performed by flexing and adducting the hip and the femoral head exits the acetabulum partially or completely over the acetabular ridge. This is also known as the click of exit. The click of entry as the femoral head glides back into the acetabulum with abduction is also considered to be a positive Barlow sign. Although some physicians feel that a positive Ortolani sign has greater diagnostic value over the positive Barlow sign,[483] both maneuvers are recommended by the AAP.[481] Despite other medical concerns, the AAP recommends that the hips of preterm infants be examined as part of full physical examination.[481]

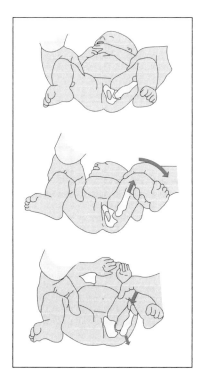
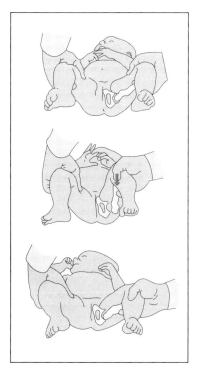

Figure 4.24 ■ Schematic of technique to assess for hip dislocation with Ortolani's and Barlow's signs. (Reprinted with permission from Staheli LT. Fundamental's of Pediatric Orthopedics. 3rd Ed. Philadelphia: Lippincott Williams & Wilkins, 2003:83.)

Hip ultrasonography is used as a screening tool more readily in Europe. In the United States, ultrasounds are used to confirm the diagnosis made by physical examination. The benefits of ultrasound are real-time evaluation and three-dimensional views of the neonatal hip.[481–483] Radiographs have a high false-negative rate and it is difficult to interpret the results due to the lack of calcification of the neonatal femoral head in infants less than 4 months old. While radiographs are rarely used for diagnosis of congenital hip dysplasia or dislocation, they can provide information regarding abnormal development of the acetabulum.[481,486]

All hips diagnosed as unstable are treated early in order to ensure the best developmental outcomes. Most pathologic changes are correctable and there is a 95% success rate using the Pavlik harness. The Pavlik harness is a splint that maintains the hips in flexion and abduction. The Pavlik harness is more likely to fail in cases when there is a negative Ortolani sign or bilateral disease, in males, and if treatment is not initiated until after 7 weeks.[463,487] If congenital hip dysplasia or dislocation is not diagnosed and treated early, it is more difficult to reduce the hip without surgery, formation of a normal acetabulum is less likely, and functional outcomes may be less than optimal.

METATARSUS ADDUCTUS

The most common foot deformity noted at birth is metatarsus adductus (MTA) or metatarsus varus. It is a transverse deformity of the talometatarsal joints with medial deviation of the metatarsals, slight hindfoot valgus, and full dorsiflexion of the ankle. The exact cause of MTA is unknown, but contributing factors include family history of MTA, positioning in utero (increased incidence in the presence of oligohydramnios and breech presentation), and infant sleeping position.[482,486,488] MTA can occur as an isolated deformity or in association with clubfoot. In approximately 2% of cases of MTA there is an association with hip or acetabular dysplasia.[482,488]

MTA can be flexible or rigid and is diagnosed by physical examination. Radiographs may be done in more severe cases. The foot is fully correctable in flexible MTA, while the metatarsals cannot be abducted in rigid MTA. The severity of MTA is graded as mild, moderate, or severe using the system described by Bleck[489] in 1983. Mild cases generally resolve without treatment. Moderate, flexible MTA is treated with prolonged passive stretching, therapeutic taping, corrective shoes, or bracing. Serial casting and surgical intervention may be indicated in cases of severe MTA.[482,486,488]

TALIPES EQUINOVARUS

Congenital clubfoot or talipes equinovarus is a deformity of the foot that involves three or four components. The foot is in equinus, cavus, and varus position, with forefoot adduction.[490] Each deformity has some degree of rigidity limiting the passive correction of the foot. The degree of rigidity varies with each infant and the factors related to the occurrence of clubfoot.[486] The most frequent occurrence of clubfoot is in first-born infants and there is a strong association with oligohydramnios, suggesting the great influence of the intrauterine environment in the evolution of clubfoot. Genetic factors also play a role, as there is an increased risk of having clubfoot when a parent or sibling also has this malformation.[482,486] Clubfoot may also be associated with a syndrome such as arthrogryposis. Infants with neurologic deficits such as myelomeningocele often are born with clubfeet (see Chapter 6).

Treatment is initiated when the infant is physiologically stable enough to tolerate the handling and generally involves serial taping and casting of the foot. If this conservative treatment is not effective, surgical correction may be indicated.[482,488,491]

ARTHROGRYPOSIS

The term *arthrogryposis* means "curved, hooked joint" and is used descriptively (not diagnostically) for a complex of symptoms involving multiple congenital joint contractures. The contractures can have multiple underlying causes[492] and can be a clinical feature in more than 150 known conditions. The contractures are nonprogressive, occur in two or more joints in different body areas,[493] and are thought to be a result of decreased fetal movement. Decreased fetal movement may be due to mechanical limitations (nulliparous mother, multiple fetuses, oligohydramnios, or uterine myomas), fetal myopathy, fetal neuropathy,[494] or abnormal connective tissue in the fetus.[492] Arthrogryposis occurs in 1 in 3000 live births. Isolated joint contractures typically involve the ankle and present as talipes equinovarus or calcaneovalgus deformities.[494] Fatty and fibrous tissues replace muscles in affected areas.[492,495] Prognosis depends on the extent of organ system involvement inasmuch as children with only joint contractures have the most favorable prognosis. Children with visceral organ involvement and CNS involvement have less favorable prognoses.[493]

Amyoplasia, the classic form of arthrogryposis, is the single most common cause of arthrogryposis, accounting for 40% of children with multiple congenital contractures.[492] Babies with amyoplasia present with symmetric involvement of all four limbs with joint involvement increasing from proximal to distal. The extremities are featureless without skin creases and have increased subcutaneous fat and absence or fibrosis of muscles.[492] The etiology is unknown. No identifiable inheritance pattern is recognized; however, the child has a decreased number of anterior horn cells in the spinal cord.[493,495] Physical therapy, for the goal of achieving and maintaining functional range of motion in affected joints,[493] may involve serial casting, splinting, stretching, and parental education in the neonatal period, while surgery may be necessary in early childhood.[495]

PHYSICAL THERAPY ASSESSMENT AND INTERVENTION FOR THE INFANT WITH ORTHOPEDIC ISSUES

The examination of the infant with orthopedic/musculoskeletal concerns begins with a thorough chart review of medical history and present status of all systems. Particular attention should be paid not only to reports by specialists such as orthopedists, neurologists, and radiologists, but also to the physiologic and medical stability of the infant. The nurse at the bedside should be interviewed to update medical information including any new precautions and neonatal pain assessment scores. As with any high-risk infant in the NICU, the first priority is overall safety of the infant and all systems should be assessed. The therapist must determine what level of assessment and intervention the infant is able to tolerate before initiating any tests or measures.

If the infant is too fragile for a hands-on examination, the therapist may gather information through observation of the infant at rest and during care activities. The observation can provide information regarding skin integrity, vascular perfusion, active motion, quality of movement, and symmetry. Based on information from the NICU care team, specialists, the medical record, and the observation, the therapist develops a care plan including suggestions for positioning during rest, caregiving activities, and when being held by parents. The suggestions, along with a plan for re-evaluation and potentially more invasive intervention in the future, should be discussed with the medical care team and the family. Positioning recommendations should be re-evaluated for tolerance and effectiveness. Modifications should be made as appropriate. It is recommended that positioning suggestions with rationale should be written clearly with pictures illustrating the position(s) and be posted at the infant's bedside.

For the more physiologically and medically stable infant, assessment and intervention can include more hands-on procedures. With each maneuver the infant should be carefully assessed for tolerance and/or pain. The evaluation may need to be modified or discontinued based on the infant's responses. Information gathered from hands-on assessment includes skin temperature, integrity of circulation in the extremities, passive movement, bony alignment, flexibility of soft tissue, muscle tone, limb length, and limb circumferences. The therapist must also use caution with each activity to minimize the potential for fracture and dislocation.

Information gathered through indirect and direct assessment measures should be evaluated and the cost–benefit of any intervention carefully weighed. The therapist should consider how musculoskeletal issues impact both present function and the risk for long-term consequences. It is helpful for the therapist to discuss his or her findings with the NICU team and consulting specialists in order to best determine the timing and mode of intervention. The determination should also be made as to which team member will take primary responsibility for the management of the particular musculoskeletal issue(s). Intervention should be specific to the individual infant and his or her physiologic stability, medical priorities, and musculoskeletal concern. Some interventions that may be implemented by physical therapists in the NICU include the following.

RANGE OF MOTION

Gentle passive range of motion is only indicated for stable infants with loss of motion or the potential for loss of motion in situations such as myelomeningocele, arthrogryposis, brachial plexus injury, and loss of mobility due to scar tissue. Response to passive movement should be carefully monitored for physiologic tolerance and pain. Care should be taken to prevent fracture or dislocation. If the infant is physiologically and medically stable, the nursing staff and family should be instructed in safe range-of-motion exercises. Specific instructions with pictures depicting the hand placement, direction of motion, degree of motion, and frequency should be posted at bedside. If these activities are to continue after discharge, the family needs to safely demonstrate each procedure prior to leaving the hospital and home instructions with pictures should be provided.

TAPING

Therapeutic taping with a lightweight porous tape may be implemented to maintain or improve alignment for an infant with wrist drop, foot drop, or congenital malformation such as talipes equinovarus or metatarsus adductus. The therapist should have mentored practice with older, stable infants before using this modality with high-risk infants in the NICU. Taping can be particularly effective in the early neonatal period as there is laxity of the ligaments due to transplacental transmission of relaxin and estrogen from the mother along with the influence of maternal hormones.[7] Taping allows for easy inspection of the skin and vascular integrity. However, the risk for intolerance to the application of the tape, skin irritation or breakdown, fracture, dislocation, joint effusion, and vascular compromise is still a concern with this modality. Taping is not recommended for infants less than 30 to 32 weeks' gestation due to the fragility of the skin.[7] Before initiating a taping program, the therapist should assess integumentary status and perform a patch test to determine any sensitivity to the tape. The therapist should provide the nursing staff and family careful instructions in terms of signs of intolerance and how to safely remove the tape. Careful monitoring must be provided throughout the course of taping.

SPLINTING

Splinting may be indicated for some infants in the NICU with documented or potential alignment and joint motion limitation concerns. As with any of the procedures discussed, the need for splinting must be carefully assessed prior to the fabrication and wearing of the appliance. In addition to the possibility of physiologic intolerance to the fabrication or application, there is the risk of fracture, dislocation, joint effusion, and skin breakdown.[7] Traction on joints and nerves can be a concern due to the weight of the splinting material. Specific instructions for applying, wearing, monitoring, and discontinuing splints should be posted at the infant's bedside and be provided to the family if splint wearing is to continue after discharge. Pictures or photographs are often helpful to provide a visual reference of how splints should be worn. The therapist should make arrangements for postdischarge monitoring of the splints for fit and function.

Casting for infants in the NICU is generally applied by orthopedics to lengthen soft tissue and promote better alignment for infants with congenital talipes equinovarus and metatarsus adductus. This procedure is often deferred until the infant is medically stable and may not be implemented until after discharge. The therapist in the NICU may assist in the positioning of the infant to support the casted limb(s) and promote the most optimal total body alignment. Appliances such as the Pavlik harness for congenital hip dysplasia are usually issued and monitored by orthopedics.

◆ Transition to Home

Normally discharge planning begins on the first day of hospital admission; however, when caring for medically fragile high-risk infants whose survival is not certain, this may be premature. The exact date of discharge may not be predictable, but when an infant begins to demonstrate more consistent physiologic stability, steps can be initiated toward a discharge plan. Infants leaving the NICU often require unique long-term health care follow-up and their families require time to learn their care. Current trends in health care for early discharge mean that families are required to care for younger, less stable infants and therefore families should be included in the discharge process as soon as possible.

A good discharge plan is individually tailored to both the infant and his or her family with clearly identified goals. These goals should be communicated to the family and the medical team, so as to eliminate duplication and fragmentation of family education and follow-up care, to prevent delays in access to health care, to establish links to resources for health and development in the community, and to promote success of the infant and family at home.[496–499] The medical team needs to assess the particular strengths and needs of the infant's family including care-taking capabilities, resource requirements, social supports, and home physical facilities. The AAP[496] recommends that at least two family caregivers are able, available, and committed to learning and providing for the infant(s). Increased risk for attachment disturbances and abuse has been identified for children born prematurely and children with prenatal substance exposure. Family issues that put an infant at risk are lower education level, lack of social support, marital instability, fewer prenatal care visits, substance use, and fewer family visits during hospitalization. Active parent involvement and preparation for posthospital care demonstrate a family's readiness to care for the infant at home.[496,498]

Elements commonly identified as medical requirements for discharge from the NICU include sustained pattern of weight gain, maintenance of normal body temperature in an open environment, a successful mode of feeding (oral or tube feeding), and no episodes of apnea and bradycardia for 5 days.[496,498] Some level II and level III nurseries may have discharge requirements based on gestational age and weight. Feedings and medications need to be streamlined for home routines. Discharge teaching needs to be initiated early to allow the family time to process information and demonstrate proficiency. Families should be provided with blocks of time to provide care for their infant, and "rooming in" (where the parents spend the night in the hospital acting as sole caretakers for their infant) prior to discharge is recommended.[496,498]

The physical therapy regimen should also be modified for home implementation so that parents are able to carry out all of the infant's care without undue exhaustion. The therapist can assist the family in transition to the home environment in terms of positioning and providing appropriate sensory experiences and developmental activities. Positioning supports are common in the NICU; however, the AAP[251] has strongly recommended that the infants should be positioned on their backs for sleeping and the sleep environment should be free of soft or loose bedding materials and stuffed toys or animals that could obstruct infant airways. The therapist can develop a plan to wean the infant of positioning supports and transition to back sleeping as necessary.[500] Positioning supports can be utilized and may be very important for some infants for play and activities while awake. Blanket rolls may be positioned behind the infant's shoulders and along the thighs while he or she is seated in an infant seat to promote symmetry and hands to midline. It is important that the therapist educate the family in safe prone positioning for play when the infant is awake as this may be forgotten in light of the back-to-sleep recommendations. Supervised prone play while the infant is awake offers opportunities to strengthen shoulder, neck, and trunk musculature in preparation for future gross motor skills.

Infants who have required intensive care may continue to have sensitivities to light and sound after discharge to home. In order to help the infant transition successfully to the home environment, the therapist can help the parents to identify the infant's vulnerabilities and make home modifications and recommendations for appropriate settings.

The parents may need to dim or shade bright lights and minimize sound around the infant in order to support regulation and to promote arousal and interaction. The therapist needs to role-model problem solving and ongoing adaptations to the infant's changing cues.

Developmental activities will also change over time as the infant matures. Parents will need to continue to correct the infant's age for prematurity in order to have an accurate framework of expectations, for instance, if the infant's chronologic age at discharge is 4 months, but the adjusted age is 1 month. Toys and play experiences should be targeted at the adjusted age. Activity recommendations should be specific to each infant; however, there are common elements for most babies in early infancy. Many babies who have had high-tech respiratory support, increased work of breathing, and GER; those who have required supine positioning due to medical status; and preterm infants who missed out on the cramping and crowding of the uterine experience may have difficulty initiating flexion of head, trunk, and limbs. Families should be educated in positioning and techniques to facilitate flexion within the infant's tolerance. For example, the parent places the infant on his or her lap, cradled by the thighs, to promote head midline, chin tuck, and shoulder protraction. The infant should be positioned so that his or her legs are flexed against the parent's abdomen. In this position the infant can gaze at the parental face to promote downward convergent gaze and chin tuck (Fig. 4.25). Other activities that fit into families' daily routines can also be provided. For infants whose age or adjusted age is at term or near term, activities should promote symmetry, flexion, and midline orientation.

In addition to providing families with home programs, referrals should be made to community resources such as early intervention. Early intervention services are programs throughout the United States and its territories funded by Federal and local governments that are mandated by the Individuals with Disabilities Education Act (IDEA). Early intervention services provide developmental services

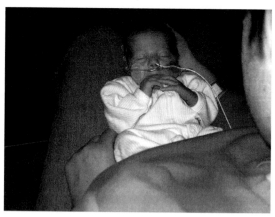

Figure 4.25 ■ Interaction with an infant in the supine position on the parent's lap.

for children and their families. These programs can provide a variety of therapy and educational services for infants at risk for developmental delays or documented delays and their families. However, the time period between referral to the program and initiation of services can be 45 days or longer.[501] Therefore, it may be necessary to set up interim services provided by outpatient or private home-based therapists until early intervention services can start. Interim services are particularly necessary when a child may need frequent monitoring of a splint or peripheral nerve injury such as brachial plexus injury.

 ## Neonatal Follow-up Services

Infants who have required neonatal intensive care are at high risk for both major and minor disabilities. Forty-eighty percent of high-risk infants demonstrate transient neurologic abnormalities consisting of hypotonia or hypertonia, and 10% go on to demonstrate major neurologic sequelae such as cerebral palsy, hydrocephalus, blindness, seizure disorder, and hearing impairment.[254,271,502–507] Minor neurodevelopmental and neurobehavioral impairments include IQ significantly lower than full-term siblings, "temperament problems, language delays, fine motor deficits, visual-motor deficits, sensory integration dysfunction, social incompetence, emotional immaturity, attention deficits, learning disorders, and ultimately diminished school performance."[508] These impairments are prevalent among survivors and become increasingly more apparent with age.[41,229,245,274,416,507–513] In addition, low-birth-weight infants and critically ill term and near-term infants who required intensive care have long-term health issues such as frequent rehospitalization, shunt complications, orthopedic and eye surgeries, chronic lung disease, and failure to thrive.[271,417,502,510,514,515] For these reasons, NICU graduates require specialized long-term follow-up services. The AAP recommends follow-up services for these developmental concerns as well as for organized postdischarge tracking and to provide information regarding outcomes for this population.[496,503]

Most NICUs are associated with neonatal follow-up programs to monitor the outcomes for these high-risk neonates and to determine the effects of NICU interventions on outcomes. In addition, these programs maintain outcome databases, conduct single-center studies, and participate in larger multicentered studies. Tracking information includes growth parameters over time (head circumference, height, and weight), feeding and nutrition, medication use, illnesses and hospitalizations, pain, home technology use (oxygen, apnea monitor, feeding tube/pump), sleep position and sleep patterns, car seat use, follow-up with other specialists, home environment, caretaking plan, parental concerns, and medical and neurologic examinations. Standardized developmental assessments are administered as part of the follow-up program. There

are many from which to choose; the *Bayley Scales of Infant Development* Edition II (BSID II) are the recognized standards for measuring infant development between 0 and 42 months. Many follow-up programs will administer the BSID II in conjunction with other domain-specific assessments for social and emotional development, gross and fine motor development, language and behavior development, and family function.[502,503]

Babies should be seen in the follow-up program (not to be confused with the first pediatrician visit, which should occur the first week from discharge) at 4 months adjusted age unless the discharge team, physical therapist, community pediatrician, home visiting nurse, or caregiver has concerns warranting earlier follow-up. Generally babies who are discharged with technologic supports such as tracheostomy, supplemental oxygen, apnea monitor, and feeding tube are seen within the first month after discharge. The babies return for neonatal follow-up every 3 months for the first year, every 6 months in the second year, and yearly from 3 years adjusted age to school age. However, this schedule can change to more frequent follow-up if more specific concerns are being monitored. For infants who are followed as part of a study, the frequency may be determined as per the protocol for that particular study.

The follow-up team is usually composed of professionals from many disciplines and can include a developmental pediatrician, neonatologist, pediatric nurse practitioner, social worker, psychologist, nutritionist, and physical, occupational, and speech therapists. Administrative support staff includes a clinic coordinator, data manager, and secretary. Due to the multidisciplinary nature of the follow-up clinic, the visits are highly coordinated for efficiency and to address the needs of the high-risk infants and their families. Families often perceive the clinic staff as "experts" in the care of their babies, and will utilize them as a resource and to confirm recommendations made by outside health care providers. Some members of the follow-up team may also have provided care for the infant and his or her family during hospitalization in the NICU, which may provide the family with a level of comfort and familiarity. In this way the family's needs identified during the hospitalization can be more effectively followed, and the family may also feel more at ease to discuss new concerns. The social worker can identify and address financial issues and social risk factors such as poverty, housing, substance abuse, and lack of education, which can pose additional risks for the health and development of the infant. Studies have shown that environmental factors such as maternal years of education and socioeconomic status can mitigate or exacerbate the biologic risk factors typically associated with neonatal intensive care.[41,245,516,517]

Physical therapists bring a unique strength to the follow-up of high-risk infants as their background in kinesiology and development allows them to examine the qualitative aspects of infant movement. Understanding the fundamental components of a movement pattern allows the therapist to determine whether the infant is developing a balanced repertoire of movement patterns needed for the progression of development or is reusing the same maladaptive patterns that prevent this progression. It is helpful for physical therapists to take part in a neonatal follow-up clinic for their own understanding of development and long-term outcomes of high-risk infants. It is important that therapists observe the changes in infants over time as some of the "red flags" seen in the NICU may be transient and may be replaced by more typical movement patterns as the infant develops. It is also a good learning experience, albeit sad, to see babies who have seemingly left the NICU unscathed only to return to a follow-up clinic with atypical neurodevelopmental assessments. Although this is sobering, it can serve to challenge the therapist to seek out other assessment tools and look more closely for subtleties in infant performance. While participating in a follow-up clinic, therapists may also see the responsiveness or limitations of community resources and perhaps learn of new resources that may prove to be effective. In addition, therapists participating in neonatal follow-up programs have the opportunity to see family resilience and the challenges a family may face on the journey that began in the NICU. The experiences of neonatal follow-up care provide the therapist caring for infants in the NICU with a wealth of information, which should be used when intervening with infants in the NICU, providing discharge recommendations, and communicating with families regarding future outcomes.

SUMMARY

The last century has seen the evolution of the subspecialty of neonatology, and as this practice has changed over time, so too has the role of the physical therapist in the NICU. The increasing understanding of preterm infant development and the effects of the environment, neonatal care, and family involvement on the evolving infant systems has led to a unique and specialized opportunity for physical therapists to act as developmental specialists within the setting of the neonatal intensive care unit. In order to effectively and appropriately fulfill this need, therapists require in-depth understanding and knowledge of medical conditions and interventions; fetal and infant behavior and development; family stresses related to pregnancy, childbirth, and transition to parenthood within the NICU; risk factors; and long-term outcomes. In addition, the therapist needs to have a mentored practice within the NICU setting and participate in a neonatal follow-up program. It is also important that the physical therapist be an integrated member of the team providing care for the high-risk baby and his or her family. The physical therapist must take the initiative to keep abreast of the rapidly changing technology and management, and their effects on infant health and development. This requires keeping current with both physical therapy and neonatal literature.

The therapist practicing in the NICU requires the advanced knowledge and skills as outlined previously and the time, training, and mentoring to achieve the highest level of practice in order to provide the sensitive, knowledgeable, and supportive care the babies and their families deserve. To be a physical therapist in the NICU is a meaningful and rewarding role and is well worth the time and training.

CASE STUDIES
CASE STUDY 1

Kayla

Kayla was born at 23 3/7 weeks' gestation with a birth weight of 570 g (1 lb 4 oz) (Fig. 4.26) to a married 30-year-old G2P2 mother who had good prenatal care. Maternal complications included group B streptococcus, bleeding at 22 weeks, and preterm labor at 23 3/7 weeks, at which time she was dilated and contracting. The infant was born via vaginal breech delivery with Apgar scores of 4 at 1 minute and 7 at 5 minutes. Resuscitative efforts in the delivery room included intubation, positive pressure ventilation, and surfactant. Kayla was transported to the NICU where she was placed on conventional ventilator and UA and UV lines were placed. Phototherapy was initiated because of bruising.

Because of worsening respiratory status, Kayla was placed on HFOV, which she received for 33 days before she was able to wean to CMV. She was able to be extubated and placed on CPAP after 2 months on the conventional ventilator. After 2 weeks on CPAP, Kayla was weaned to a nasal cannula but had to be reintubated and placed on mechanical ventilation 2 weeks later because of sepsis. Kayla was extubated and

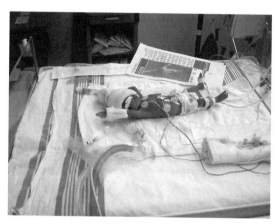

Figure 4.26 ▪ *Kayla being stabilized after birth. Note the size of the infant versus the size of the glove wrapper.*

placed on nasal cannula 2 weeks later. She was finally weaned off all respiratory support at 143 days of life.

Kayla's hospital course was complicated by severe BPD, pulmonary interstitial emphysema, large PDA requiring surgical ligation, hyperbilirubinemia, mild supravalvular pulmonic stenosis, and multiple bouts of sepsis including meningitis, pseudomonas tracheitis, methicillin-resistant *Staphylococcus aureus* (MRSA), and pneumonia.

Pain Management

Pain management was initiated on Kayla's first day of life with the administration of morphine. She continued to receive morphine until day of life 34 when a tapered wean was completed. Morphine was restarted on day of life 120 when she required reintubation and mechanical ventilation. Kayla was weaned off morphine slowly beginning day of life 133 and ending on day of life 143. She tolerated this weaning process well and neonatal abstinence scores were followed closely for any adverse response to withdrawal. Throughout her hospitalization Kayla was assessed for pain by all staff. Pain assessments were also performed by the physical therapist and documented in the chart after each interaction with the therapist.

Physical Therapy Services

Kayla was referred for physical therapy services at 2 weeks of life (25 weeks' postconceptional age). The physical therapist reviewed Kayla's history by thoroughly reading her medical chart and discussing Kayla's status with her nurse. Kayla's nurse reported that she was very restless and became irritable with hands-on care. The physical therapist observed Kayla in her isolette before, during, and after caregiving activities. At this time Kayla was intubated, requiring HFOV, and was under phototherapy. She demonstrated increased extensor posturing of her head, trunk, and extremities and jerky restless movements prior to care. Sensitivity to sound and light were also noted. Kayla had very low tolerance to handling and position changes during care. Her stress signs included color changes, increased heart rate, oxygen desaturation, and motor stress signs of arching of head and trunk and extension of extremities. Kayla was unable to effectively utilize any self-calming behaviors and was difficult to calm with external supports. She did respond to facilitated tucking and firm touch when provided long enough for her to relax and settle into the position. After care she was pale and exhausted.

Physical Therapy Goals

Physical therapy goals at this time were as follows:

1. To decrease environmental stress
2. To promote calming behaviors
3. To promote flexed postures for calming and optimal body alignment for musculoskeletal development
4. To assist family and caregivers in identifying and responding to Kayla's cues

5. To provide education to the family regarding developmentally supportive care

Suggestions included:

1. Minimizing environmental stimulation by covering her isolette and shading her eyes from bright lights, alerting people to keep noise levels down around her bedside with a sign, and education
2. Pacing care activities, providing rest breaks with facilitated tucking, using slow movements and firm touch
3. Positioning in flexion in a deep nest and varying positions between prone, side-lying, and supine as tolerated
4. Allowing for hands to head and grasping, and offering the pacifier for self-calming

Kayla's mother visited every day and the physical therapist was able to meet with her to discuss Kayla's status and suggestions to support her development. Together, they looked at Kayla's cues and discussed strategies for calming and bonding. Kayla's father visited in the evening and her mother shared the suggestions for developmentally supportive care with him.

For the next 2 months Kayla continued to be an extremely fragile, critically ill infant with high respiratory requirements, surgical ligation of her PDA, and episodes of sepsis. Physical therapists continued to observe Kayla and adjust her developmental care plan as appropriate. At 10 weeks of age (33 weeks' PCA), Kayla was able to wean from HFOV to the conventional ventilator. She continued to have low tolerance for handling but was easier to console with the pacifier and firm touch/containment in flexion. She also demonstrated attempts at self-calming with hand-to-head, grasping, and foot-bracing behaviors. The physical therapist continued to work with the nursing staff and Kayla's family to develop care plans to promote self-calming, optimal positioning, and tolerance to caregiving activities. At this time Kayla's parents were practicing kangaroo care and holding Kayla daily (Fig. 4.27). The physical therapist was able to provide suggestions for positioning Kayla during kangaroo care.

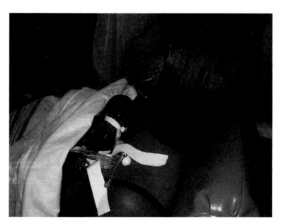

Figure 4.27 ■ Kayla and her mother practicing kangaroo care, or skin-to-skin holding.

Kayla made slow improvements medically and at 36 weeks PCA she still required mechanical ventilation. Her tolerance to handling and position changes was improving. She was able to maintain a quiet, alert state using her pacifier and containment for support. Even with external supports she had limited tolerance for visual or social stimulation. Kayla was very sensitive to light and sound in the environment. Physical therapy examination revealed increased flexor posturing in her lower extremities, with full passive range of motion. She held her upper extremities in scapular retraction, shoulder abduction, and external rotation. Kayla had antigravity movement of her extremities through limited range of motion with jerky, tremulous quality of movement. She still frequently moved into extension rather than flexion. Despite the use of a gel pillow, the time spent on HFOV had left Kayla with flattening of the lateral sides of her head, or dolichocephaly. She held her head in extension with shortening of her capital and neck extensors. Tightness in her thoracic, lumbar, and sacral areas was also noted. Goals for Kayla included:

1. Maintaining quiet alert state for increasing duration of time
2. Improved ability to self-calm
3. Neutral head alignment with decreased tightness in cervical spine
4. Increased flexibility in lumbosacral spine
5. Decreased tightness in scapulae and shoulders
6. Increased antigravity flexion movement

An additional goal was for Kayla's family and caregivers to be independent in positioning and developmentally supportive activities.

The therapist continued to work with Kayla's family and nurses in reading her cues and progressing handling and social interactions to her tolerance. The therapist also provided positioning suggestions to promote midline alignment, flexion, and shoulder protraction. Gentle mobilization to her spine was provided, starting in the lumbosacral area and slowly moving proximally over the course of several weeks, based on Kayla's response.

Over the next month, Kayla was weaned off the ventilator to CPAP and then to nasal cannula. She had one setback in her respiratory stability because of sepsis but was able to be weaned off all support by 43 weeks' PCA. The therapist continued to work on the previously stated goals until time of discharge to home. Concerns at the time of discharge included:

1. Sensitivity to light and sound
2. Limited tolerance to handling
3. Limited range of motion in cervical spine and shoulders
4. Delayed postural responses

Her strengths were robust and defined behavioral states, improved ability to self-calm, and greater availability for social interactions. She was able to visually fix on an object and track

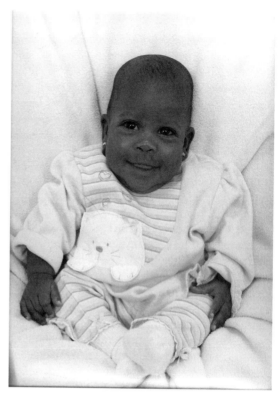

Figure 4.28 ■ Kayla at 7.5 months' chronologic age, or 3.25 months' adjusted age.

it to the left and right. Her parents were able to read Kayla's behavioral cues and respond appropriately. Suggestions for home were provided to her parents, who were able to demonstrate independence in performing these activities. Kayla was discharged to home at 45 weeks' PCA without any respiratory support and taking all feedings by bottle. Follow-up services included ophthalmology, special babies clinic (neonatal follow-up), cardiology, and early intervention services (Fig. 4.28).

CASE STUDY 2

Baby J
HISTORY
Baby boy J was born at 37 2/7 weeks' gestation via spontaneous vaginal delivery to a 24-year-old G4P3A1 AA mother with normal labs. He weighed 3.375 kg, had Apgar scores of $8^1 8^5$, and was taken to the well-baby nursery at the local hospital where he developed respiratory distress without O_2 requirement on day of life 1. Chest radiography was negative. After being fed for 12 hours he developed abdominal distention and was ill appearing. Abdominal radiography showed pneumatosis and baby boy J was transferred to his local children's hospital for surgical evaluation. On day of life 3, he underwent laparoscopic surgery and had ileal cecectomy, with ileostomy and mucous fistula placement. Eleven

centimeters of bowel was resected. Feeds were initiated on day of life 17 and baby J developed abdominal distention and emesis. On day of life 23 upper gastrointestinal series showed possible stoma stenosis. He had a history of fungal line sepsis, treated with amphotericin. Baby J's parents were married and had two preschool-aged siblings; the eldest sibling received speech therapy through early intervention.

PHYSICAL THERAPY EXAMINATION

Baby J was referred for physical therapy at 3.5 weeks of age. At that time his nutrition consisted of 5 mL of Pregestimil by mouth every 3 hours as well as hyperalimentation. His physical therapy examination was limited to the right side-lying position, in an effort to keep the stool from his stoma from draining into his abdominal wound, which had dehisced. He presented in a sleep state throughout the session with mildly distended abdomen, gauze pad over abdomen, colostomy with small amount of yellow seedy stool, and a peripherally inserted central catheter (PICC) line in the left anterior calf. The CRIES pain score was 0–1 throughout examination.

Baby J did not habituate to light over 10 trials and habituated to rattle on sixth stimulus in sleep state. Muscle tone was mildly decreased in sleep state. Initial examination was limited due to positioning precautions and sleep state. Baby J's physical therapy diagnosis was increased risk for developmental delays due to medical status and potential for prolonged hospitalization. He was to be followed by physical therapy two times per week for ongoing assessment, parent education, and developmental stimulation. Initial short-term goals (4 weeks) included alerting for 8 to 10 minutes per session, visually attending to face for 8 to 10 seconds, intact anterior and posterior head righting reactions in upright with support at upper chest, and parents to be independent with positioning baby for comfort. The long-term goal was age-appropriate developmental skills at 15 months. At baby J's second physical therapy session he demonstrated slow state transitions with defined drowsy state and bright-eyed alert periods with visual regard for the therapist, cleared his airway in prone, and demonstrated intact anterior–posterior head righting reactions and symmetric flexor tone of his limbs. His active range of motion (AROM) was jittery with the presence of forearm rotation right to left. He did not demonstrate automatic walking.

PHYSICAL THERAPY COURSE

Baby J's parents were frequently at his bedside with his older siblings. His family decorated his bed space with poems, photographs, and pictures from his siblings and extended family. His parents were receptive to suggested play ideas for baby J, which were explained, demonstrated, and posted at his bedside by his physical therapist. At next re-examination at 1.5 months of age, baby J had missed one session due to fever. He had developed a left head preference and was an animated baby who used yawning or sneezing to regulate intensity of social interactions. He had met all of his short-term goals and new short-term goals (4 weeks) included the following: AROM of head/neck to right 45 to 60 degrees to follow visual cue two times per session, neutral head extension sustained in prone for 8 to 10 seconds, bat at toy in supine once per session, and sustain neutral head extension in upright for 10 to 18 seconds with support at upper trunk. Baby J continued to be seen twice weekly; however, on day of life 56 he underwent laparoscopic surgery for closure of his enterostomy and lysis of adhesions. Postoperatively, baby J developed a fever and was taken back to the operating room for exploratory laparoscopy on day of life 61, where an abscess was discovered; the surgeons drained this abscess and reinforced his reanastomosis. After this latter surgery, physical therapy goals changed as baby J was intubated, irritable, stiff, and colonized with MRSA. The physical therapist provided baby J's parents with suggestions for comforting, handling, and positioning baby J as well as placement of visual stimulation in order to encourage neutral head alignment. New short-term goals (4 weeks) when baby J was 2.5 months old included tolerating prone placement without fussing for 90 to 180 seconds, extending head in prone for 3 to 5 seconds, approximating hands in midline in supine twice per session, and sustaining neutral head in upright for 8 to 10 seconds with support at axilla, and baby J's parents describing two developmentally appropriate activities for baby J. Baby J missed several physical therapy sessions after this latter surgery due to sleep state and critical medical status due to sepsis.

At the next re-examination at 3.5 months, baby J had transferred out of the NICU to an integrated care service to address his ongoing feeding issues. He demonstrated social smiles and could extend his head to 90 degrees in prone with elbows behind shoulders; he demonstrated head righting reaction in prone when the therapist imposed lateral weight shifts; he was able to sustain head in neutral in upright with bobbing. Occupational therapy became involved with him at this time and followed him twice weekly as well. New 4-week short-term goals included taking weight through lower extremities for 8 to 10 seconds in supported standing, sustaining lateral head RR in prone with imposed weight shift for 25 to 40 seconds bilaterally, maintaining 90-degree head extension in prone prop for 40 to 60 seconds with elbows in line with shoulders, and grasping rattle in hand with eye–hand regard two times per session. Baby J was seen twice a week for sensory and developmental stimulation. At 4.5 months of age baby J completed the Test of Infant Motor Performance (TIMP) and performed within the normal limits for his age.

Baby J was discharged home shortly after that on oral feeds. His parents were trained in nasogastric tube placement and use in case baby J was unable to maintain oral feeds. He was to follow up with his pediatrician for developmental and medical monitoring. His parents were given suggestions for developmental activities for the present and upcoming 3 months.

REFERENCES

1. Pressler JL, Turnage-Carrier CS, Kenner C. Developmental care: an overview. In: Kenner C. McGrath JM, eds. Developmental Care of Newborns and Infants. A Guide for Health Professionals. Philadelphia: Elsevier, 2004.
2. Friedrich O. What do babies know? Time August 15, 1983.
3. Vergara ER, Bigsby R. Developmental and Therapeutic Interventions in the NICU. Baltimore: Paul H Brookes Publishing Co, 2004.
4. Brazelton TB. Neonatal Behavioral Assessment Scale. 2nd ed. Philadelphia: JB Lippincott Company, 1984.
5. Sweeney JK. Assessment of the special care nursery environment: effects on the high-risk infant. In: Wilhelm IJ, ed. Physical Therapy Assessment in Early Infancy. New York: Church Livingstone, 1993.
6. Aurora S, Snyder EY. Perinatal asphyxia. In: Cloherty JP, Eichenwald EC, Stark AR, eds. Manual of Neonatal Care. 5th Ed. Philadelphia: Lippincott-Raven, 2004.
7. Sweeney JK, Swanson MW. Low birth weight infants: neonatal care and follow-up. In: Umphred DA, ed. Neurological Rehabilitation. 4th Ed. St. Louis: Mosby, 2001.
8. Campbell SK. Decision Making in Pediatric Neurologic Physical Therapy. Philadelphia: Churchill Livingstone, 1999.
9. Lawhon G. Facilitation of parenting the premature infant within the newborn intensive care unit. J Perinatal Neonatal Nurs 2002;16(1):71–82.
10. Kamm K, Thelen E, Jenson JL. A dynamical systems approach to motor development. Phys Ther 1990;70(12):763–775.
11. Heriza CB. Implications of dynamic systems approach to understanding infant kicking behavior. Phys Ther 1991;71(3): 222–234.
12. Heriza CB. Motor development: traditional and contemporary theories. Contemporary management of motor control problems. Proceedings of the II Step Conference, Foundation of Physical Therapy, Alexandria, 1991.
13. Lockman JS, Thelen E. Developmental biodynamics: brain, body, behavior connections. Child Dev 1993;64:953.
14. Thelen E. Motor development: a new synthesis. Am Psychologist 1995;50(2):79–90.
15. Guiliani CA. Theories of motor control: new concepts for physical therapy. Contemporary management of motor control problems. Proceedings of the II Step Conference, Foundation for Physical Therapy, Alexandria, 1991.
16. Horak FB. Assumptions underlying motor control for neurologic rehabilitation. Contemporary management of motor control problems. Proceedings of the II Step Conference, Foundation for Physical Therapy, Alexandria, 1991.
17. Guide to Physical Therapy Practice. 2nd Ed. Alexandria: American Physical Therapy Association.
18. National Advisory Board of Medical Rehabilitation Research. Research Plan for the National Center for Medical Rehabilitation. Bethesda, MD: National Institutes of Health and Human Development, National Institutes of Health, 1993.
19. World Health Organization. International Classification of Functioning, Disability and Handicaps. Geneva: World Health Organization, 2001.
20. Goldstein DN, Cohn E, Coster W. Enhancing participation for children with disabilities—application of the ICF enablement framework to pediatric physical therapist's practice. Pediatr Phys Ther 2004;16(2):114–120.
21. Palisano RJ, Campbell SK, Harris SR. Decision making in pediatric physical therapy. In: Campbell SK, Vander Linden DW, Palisano RJ, eds. Physical Therapy for Children. Philadelphia: Saunders, 2000.
22. Als H. Infant individuality: Assessing patterns of very early development. In: Call J, Galenson E, Tyson RL, eds. Frontiers of Infant Psychiatry. New York: Basic Books, 1983.
23. Als H. A synactive model of neonatal behavioral organization: framework for the assessment of neurobehavioral development in the premature infant and for support of infants and parents in the neonatal intensive care environment. In: Sweeney JK ed. The High Risk Neonate: Developmental Therapy Perspectives. Phys Occup Ther Pediatr 1986;6:3–55.
24. Als H, Lawhon G, Brown E, et al. Individualized behavioral and environmental care for the very low birth weight preterm infant at high risk for bronchopulmonary dysplasia: neonatal intensive care unit and developmental outcome. Pediatrics 1986;78(6):1123–1132.
25. Als H. Toward a synactive theory of development: promise for the assessment and support of infant individuality. Infant Ment Health J 1982;3(4):229–243.
26. Als H, Lester BM, Brazelton TB. Dynamics of the behavioral organization of the premature infant: a theoretical perspective. In: Field TM, Sostek AM, Goldberg S, et al., eds. Infants Born at Risk. New York: Spectrum, 1979.
27. Als H. Manual for the Naturalistic Observation of Newborn Behavior Newborn Individualized Developmental Care and Assessment Program. Boston: National NIDCAP Training Center, 1995.
28. Lawhon G, Melzar A. developmental care of the very low birth weight infant. J Perinatal Neonatal Nurs 1988;2(1):56–65.
29. Bowden VR, Greenberg CS, Donaldson NE. Developmental care of the newborn. Online J Clin Innovations 2000;3(7):1–77.
30. Gilkerson L, Als H. Role of reflective process in the implementation of developmentally supportive care in the newborn intensive care nursery. Infants Young Child 1995;7(4):20–28.
31. Chappel J. Advancing Clinical Practice and Perspectives of Developmental Care in the NICU. Morristown, NJ:, 2004.
32. Als H, Lawhon G, Duffy FH, et al. Individualized developmental care for the very low-birth-weight preterm infant. JAMA 1994;272(11):853–858.
33. Becker PT, Grunwald PC, Moorman J, et al. Outcomes of developmentally supportive nursing care for very low birth weight infants. Nurs Res 1991;40:150–155.
34. Becker PT, Grunwald PC, Moorman J, et al. Effects of developmental care on behavioral organization in very-low-birth-weight infants. Nurs Res 1993;42(4):214–220.
35. Buehler DM, Als H, Duffy FH, et al. Effectiveness of individualized developmental care for low-risk preterm infants: behavioral and electrophysiologic evidence. Pediatrics 1995; 96(5):923–932.
36. Petryshen P, Stevens B, Hawkins J, et al. Comparing nursing costs for preterm infants receiving conventional vs. developmental care. Nurs Econ 1997;15(3):138–150.
37. Als H, Duffy FH, McAnulty GB, et al. Early experience alters brain function and structure. Pediatrics 2004;113(4):846–857.
38. Symington A, Pinelli J. Distilling the evidence on developmental care: a systematic review. Adv Neonatal Care 2002;2(4): 198–221.
39. Symington A, Pinelli J. Developmental care for promoting development and preventing morbidity in preterm infants (Cochrane Review). Cochrane Database Syst Rev 2002;4.
40. Franck LS, Lawhon G. Environmental and behavioral strategies to prevent and manage neonatal pain. Semin Perinatol 1998;22(5):434–443.
41. Hill S, Engle S, Jorgensen J, et al. Effects of Facilitated Tucking During Routine Care of Infants Born Preterm. Pediatr Phys Ther 2005;17:158–163.
42. Ward-Larson C, Horn RA, Gosnell F. The efficacy of facilitated tucking for relieving procedural pain of endotracheal suctioning in very low birth weight infants. Am J Matern Child Nurs 2004;29(3):151–156.
43. Taquino L, Blackburn S. The effects of containment during suctioning and heelstick on physiological and behavioral responses of preterm infants. Neonatal Nurs 1994;13(7):55.

44. Corff KE, Seideman R, Venkataraman PS, et al. Facilitated tuck-ing: a nonpharmacologic comfort measure for pain in preterm neonates. J Gynecol Neonatal Nurs 1995;24(2):143–147.

45. Corff KE. An effective comfort measure for minor pain and stress in preterm infants: facilitated tucking. Neonatal Netw 1993;12(8):74.

46. Corbo MG, Mansi G, Stagni A, et al. Nonnutritive sucking during heelstick procedures decreases behavioral distress in the newborn infant. Biol Neonate 2000;77:162–167.

47. Field T, Goldson E. Pacifying effects of nonnutritive sucking on term and preterm neonates during heelstick procedures. Pediatrics 1984;74(6):1012–1015.

48. Pinelli J, Symington A. How rewarding can a pacifier be? A sys-tematic review of nonnutritive sucking in preterm infants. Neonatal Netw 2000;19(8):41–48.

49. Kilbride HW, Thorstad K, Daily DK. Preschool outcome of less than 801 grams preterm infants compared with full term siblings. Pediatrics 2004;113(4):742–747.

50. Galvin E, Boyers L, Schwartz PK, et al. Challenging the pre-cepts of family-centered care: testing a philosophy. Pediatr Nurs 2000;26(6):625–632.

51. Harrison H. The principles of family-centered neonatal care. Pediatrics 1993;92(5):643–650.

52. Brazelton TB, Cramer BG. The Earliest Relationship. Reading, MA: Addison-Wesley Publishing Company, Inc., 1990.

53. Lawhon G. Management of stress in premature infants. In: Angelini DJ, Whelan Knapp CM, Gibes RM, eds. Perinatal/Neonatal Nursing: A Clinical Handbook. Boston: Blackwell Scientific Publications, 1986.

54. Mercer RT. Nursing Care for Parents at Risk. Thorofare, NJ: Charles B Slack, Inc, 1977.

55. Bibring GL. Some considerations of the psychological process in pregnancy. Psychoanal Study Child 1959;14:113–121.

56. Bibring GL, Dwyer TF, Huntington DS, et al. A study of the psychological processes in pregnancy and of the earliest mother-child relationship. Psychoanal Study Child 1961;16:9–24.

57. Cowan CP, Cowan PA. When Partners Become Parents. The Big Life Change for Couples. Mahwah, NJ: Lawrence Erlbaum Associates Publishers, 1999.

58. Cowan CP, Cowan PA. Interventions to ease the transition to parenthood. Fam Relations 1995;44:412–423.

59. Cowan CP, Cowan PA, Heming G, et al. Transitions to parent-hood his, hers, and theirs. J Fam Issues 1985;6(4):451–481.

60. Stainton MC, McNeil D, Harvey S. Maternal tasks of uncertain motherhood. Matern Child Nurs J 1992;20(3,4):113–123.

61. Miles MS, Brunssen SH. Psychometric properties of the parental stressor scale: infant hospitalization. Adv Neonatal Care 2003;3(4):189–196.

62. Melnyk BM, Alpert-Gillis LJ, Hensel PB, et al. Helping mothers cope with a critically ill child: a pilot test of the COPE inter-vention. Res Nurs Health 1997;20:3–14.

63. Diagnostic and Statistical Manual of Mental Disorders. 4th Ed. Washington, DC: American Psychiatric Association, 1994.

64. Jotzo M, Poets CF. Helping parents cope with the trauma of premature birth: an evaluation of a trauma-preventive psycho-logical intervention. Pediatrics 2005;115(4):915–919.

65. Holditch-Davis D, Bartlett TR, Blickman AL, et al. Post-traumatic stress symptoms in mothers of premature infants. J Obstet Gynecol Neonatal Nurs 2003;32(2):161–171.

66. Peebles-Kleiger MJ. Pediatric and neonatal intensive care hos-pitalization as traumatic stressor: implications for intervention. Bull Menninger Clin 2000;64(2):257–280.

67. DeMier RL, Hynan MT, Harris HB, et al. Perinatal stressors as predictors of symptoms of posttraumatic stress in mothers of infants at high risk. J Perinatol 1996;16(4):276–280.

68. Affleck G, Tennen H. The effect of newborn intensive care on parents' psychological well-being. Child Health Care 1991;20(1):6–14.

69. Sydnor-Greenberg N, Dokken D, Ahmann E. Coping and car-ing in different ways: understanding and meaningful involve-ment. Pediatr Nurs 2000;26(2):185–190.

70. Clubb RL. Chronic sorrow: adaptation patterns of parents with chronically ill children. Pediatr Nurs 1991;17(5):461–466.

71. Pohlman S. Fathers role in the NICU care: evidence-based prac-tice. In: Kenner C, McGrath JM, eds. Developmental Care of Newborns and Infants: A Guide for Health Professionals. St. Louis: Mosby, 2004.

72. Kaplan S, Bolender DL. Embryology. In: Polin RA, Fox WW, Abman SH, eds. Fetal and Neonatal Physiology. 2nd Ed. Philadelphia: WB Saunders Co, 1998.

73. Graham EM, Morgan MA. Growth before term. In: Batshaw MA, ed. Children with Disabilities. 4th Ed. Baltimore: Paul Brooks Publishing Company, 1997.

74. Walker JM. Musculoskeletal development: a review. Phys Ther 1991;71(12):878–889.

75. Wilkens-Haug L, Heffner LJ. Fetal assessment and prenatal diagnosis. In: Cloherty JP, Eichenwald EC, Stark AR, eds. Manual of Neonatal Care. 5th Ed. Philadelphia: Lippincott Williams & Wilkins, 2004.

76. Comparetti AM. Pattern analysis of normal and abnormal development: the fetus, the newborn, the child. In: Slaton DS, ed. Development of Movement in Infancy. Chapel Hill, NC: UNC, 1980.

77. Dipietro JA. Fetal neurobehavioral assessment. In: Singer LT, Zeskind PS, eds. Biobehavioral Assessment of the Infant. New York: The Guilford Press, 2001.

78. Rivkees SA, Mirmiran M, Ariagno RL. Circadian rhythms in infants. NeoReviews 2003;4(11):298–303.

79. Prechtl H, Beintema D. The Neurological Examination of the Newborn Infant. Clinics in Developmental Medicine, 12. London: Heinemann Educational Books, 1964.

80. Lester BM, Tronick EZ. History and description of the neonatal intensive care unit network neuro-behavioral scale. Pediatrics 2004;113(3):634–640.

81. Glass P. Development of the visual system and implications for early intervention. Infants Young Child 2002;15(1):1–10.

82. Morrissey K. Seminar in Pediatric Physical Therapy: Infant Development and Therapeutic Interventions. Fall Semester 1994. Hahnemann University Program in Pediatric Physical Therapy.

83. Brazelton TB. Neonatal Behavioral Assessment Scale. 2nd Ed. Philadelphia: Lippincott, 1984.

84. Yoos L. Applying research in practice: parenting the premature infant. Appl Nurs Res 1989;2(1):30–34.

85. Hunter JG. Neonatal intensive care unit. In: Case-Smith, J, ed. Occupational Therapy for Children. 4th Ed. Philadelphia: Mosby, 2001.

86. Allen MC, Capute AJ. Tone and reflex development before term. Pediatrics 1990;85:393–399.

87. Dargassies SSA. Neurological Development in the Full-Term and Premature Neonate. Amsterdam: Exerpta Medica, 1977.

88. Sweeney JK, Gutierrez T. Musculoskeletal implications of preterm infant positioning in the NICU. J Perinatal Neonatal Nurs 2002;16(1):58–70.

89. Palmer PG, Dubowitz LMS, Verghote M, et al. Neurological and neurobehavioral differences between preterm infants at term and full-term newborn infants. Neuropediatrics 1982;13: 183–189

90. Mercuri E, Guzzetta A, Laroche S, et al. Neurologic examina-tion of preterm infants at term age: comparison with term infants. J Pediatr 2003;142:647–655.

91. Duffy FH, Als H, McNulty, GB. Behavioral and electrophysi-ological evidence for gestational age effects in healthy preterm and fullterm infants studied two weeks after expected due date. Child Dev 1990;61:1271–1286.

92. Huppi PS, Schuknecht B, Boesch C, et al. Structural and neuro-behavioral delay in postnatal brain development of preterm infants. Pediatr Res 1996;39(5):895–901.

93. Mouradian LE, Als H, Coster WJ. Neurobehavioral functioning of healthy preterm infants of varying gestational ages. Dev Behav Pediatr 2000;21(6):408–416.

94. Graven SN. Sound and the developing infant in the NICU: conclusions and recommendations for care. J Perinatol 2000; 20:S88–S93.

95. McGrath JM. Neurologic development. In: Kenner C, McGrath JM, eds. Developmental Care of Newborns and Infants: A Guide for Health Professionals. St. Louis: Mosby, 2004.

96. Lutes LM, Graves CD, Jorgensen KM. The NICU experience and its relationship to sensory integration. In: Kenner C, McGrath JM, eds. Developmental Care of Newborns and Infants. A Guide for Health Professionals. Philadelphia: Elsevier, 2004.

97. American Academy of Pediatrics Committee on Fetus and Newborn, Committee on Drugs, Section on Anesthesiology, Section on Surgery. Canadian Paediatric Society Fetus and Newborn Committee. Prevention and management of pain and stress in the neonate. Pediatrics 2000;105(2):454–461.

98. Porter FL, Wolf CM, Gold J, et al. Pain and Pain management in newborn infants: a survey of physicians and nurses. Pediatrics 1997;100:626–632.

99. Anand KJS, International Evidence-Based Group for Neonatal Pain. Consensus statement for the prevention and management of pain in the newborn. Arch Pediatr Adolesc Med 2001;155:173–180.

100. Harrison LH, Lotas MJ, Jorgensen KM. Environmental issues. In: Kenner C, McGrath JM, eds. Developmental Care of Newborns and Infants. A Guide for Health Professionals. Philadelphia: Elsevier, 2004.

101. Syman A, Cunningham S. Handling premature neonates. Nurs Times 1995;91(17):35–37.

102. Blackburn S, Barnard K. Analysis of caregiving events relating to preterm infants in the special care unit. In: Gottfried AW, Gaiter JL, eds. Infants Under Stress: Environmental Neonatology. Baltimore: University Park, 1985.

103. Werner NP, Conway AE. Caregiver contacts experienced by premature infants in the neonatal intensive care unit. Matern Child Nurs J 1990;19:21–43.

104. Gottfried AW, Hodgman JE, Brown KW. How intensive is intensive care? An environmental analysis. Pediatrics 1984;74: 292–294.

105. Franck LS, Miaskowski C. Measurement of neonatal responses to painful stimuli: a research review. J Pain Symptom Manage 1997;14(6):343–378.

106. Stevens B, Johnston C, Franck L, et al. The efficacy of developmentally sensitive behavioral interventions and sucrose for relieving procedural pain in very low birth weight neonate. Nurs Res 1999;48:35–43.

107. Stevens B, Gibbins S, Franck LS. Treatment of pain in the neonatal intensive care unit. Pediatr Clin North Am 2000; 47(3):633–650.

108. Johnston CC, Stevens BJ, Yang F, et al. Differential response to pain by very premature neonates. Pain 1995;61:471–479.

109. Johnston CC, Stevens BJ, Franck LS, et al. Factors explaining lack of response to heel stick in preterm infants. J Obstet Gynecol Neonatal Nurs 2004;33(2):246–255

110. Craig KD, Whitfield MF, Grunau RV, et al. Pain in the preterm neonate: behavioral and physiological indices. Pain 1993;52: 287–299.

111. Joint Commission on Accreditation of Healthcare Organizations. Joint Commission Hospital Quality Report. Available at: www.jcaho.org.

112. Hatch DJ. Analgesia in the neonate. BMJ 1987;294:920.

113. Stevens B, Johnston C, Franck L, et al. The efficacy of developmentally sensitive behavioral interventions and sucrose for relieving procedural pain in very low birth weight neonate. Nurs Res 1999;48(1):35–43.

114. Franck L. Some pain some gain reflections on the past two decades of neonatal pain research and treatment. Neonatal Netw 2002;21(5):37–41.

115. Gray L, Watt L, Blass EM. Skin-to-skin contact is analgesic in healthy newborns. Pediatrics 2000;105(1):4–19.

116. Stevens B, Yamada J, Ohlsson A. Sucrose for analgesia in newborn infants undergoing painful procedures. Cochrane Database Syst Rev 2004;3.

117. Turnage-Carrier CS. Caregiving and the environment. In: Kenner C, McGrath JM, eds. Developmental Care of Newborns and Infants. A Guide for Health Professionals. Philadelphia: Elsevier, 2004

118. American Academy of Pediatrics Committee on Environmental Health. Noise: a hazard for the fetus and newborn. Pediatrics 1997;100(4):724–727.

119. Philbin MK. Planning the acoustic environment of a neonatal intensive care unit. Clin Perinatol 2004;31:331–352.

120. Chang YJ, Lin CH, Lin LH. Noise and related events in a neonatal intensive care unit. Acta Paediatr. 2001;42:212–217.

121. Evans JB, Philbin MK. The acoustic environment of hospital nurseries. J Perinatol 2000;20(8):S105–S112.

122. White RD. Recommended standards for newborn ICU design. J Perinatol 2003;23(1):5–21.

123. Philbin MK. Some implications of early auditory development for the environment of hospitalized preterm infants. Neonatal Netw 1996;15(7):71–73.

124. Philbin MK, Evans JB. Noise levels, spectra and operational function of an occupied newborn intensive care unit built to meet recommended permissible noise criteria. J Acoustic Soc Ame 2003;114(4 part 2):2326 (#2aNS2).

125. Morante A, Dubowitz LMS, Levene M, et al. The development of visual function in normal and abnormal preterm and fullterm infants. Dev Med Child Neurol 1982;24:771–784.

126. Prechtl HFR, Fargel JW, Weinmann HM, et al. Postures and respiration of low-risk pre-term infants. Dev Med Child Neurol 1979;21:3–27.

127. Brazelton TB, Nugent JK. The Neonatal Behavioral Assessment Scale. 3rd Ed. London: MacKeith Press, 1995.

128. Als H. Reading the premature infant. In: Goldson E, ed. Nurturing the Premature Infant Developmental Intervention in the Neonatal Intensive Care Nursery. New York: Oxford University Press, 1999.

129. Pompa KM, Zaichkin J. The NICU baby. In: Zaichkin J, ed. Newborn Intensive Care. What Every Parent Needs to Know. Santa Rosa, CA: NICU Ink Book Publishers, 2002.

130. Lee, KG, Cloherty JP. Identifying the high risk newborn and evaluating gestational age, prematurity, post maturity, large for gestational age, and small for gestational age. In: Cloherty JP, Eichenwald EC, Stark AR, eds. Manual of Neonatal Care. 5th Ed. Philadelphia: Lippincott Williams & Wilkins, 2004.

131. Gregory S. Homeward bound. In: Zaichkin J, ed. Newborn Intensive Care. What Every Parent Needs to Know. 2nd Ed. Santa Rosa, CA: NICU Ink Book Publishers, 2002.

132. Apgar V. A proposal for a new method of evaluation of the newborn infant. Curr Res Anesth Analg 1953;32(4):260–267.

133. Ringer SA. Resuscitation in the delivery room. In: Clouherty JP, Eichenwald EC, Stark AR, eds. Manual of Neonatal Care. 5th Ed. Philadelphia: Lippincott Williams & Wilkins, 2004.

134. American Academy of Pediatrics Committee on Fetus & Newborn, American College of Obstetricians & Gynecologists & Committee on Obstetric Practice. The apgar score. Pediatrics 2006;117(4):1444–1447.

135. Eichenwald EC. Mechanical ventilation. In: Cloherty JP, Eichenwald EC, Stark AR, eds. Manual of Neonatal Care. 5th Ed. Philadelphia: Lippincott Williams & Wilkins, 2004.

136. Cameron J, Haines J. Management of respiratory disorders. In: Boxwell G. Neonatal Intensive Care Nursing. New York: Routledge, 2000.

137. Wiswell TE, Pinchi S. Continuous positive airway pressure. In: Goldsmith JP, Karotin EH, eds. Assisted Ventilation of the Neonate. 4th Ed. Philadelphia: Saunders, 2003.

138. Czervinske MP. Continuous positive airway pressure. In: Czervinske MP, Barnhart SC, eds. Perinatal and Pediatric Respiratory Care. 2nd Ed. Philadelphia: Saunders, 2003.

139. Lee KS, Dunn MS, Fenwick M. A comparison of underwater bubble continuous positive airway pressure with ventilator derived continuous positive airway pressure in premature infants ready for extubation. Biol Neonate 1998;73(2):69–75.

140. Spitzer AR, Greenspan JS, Fox WW. Positive-pressure ventilation-pressure-limited and time cycled ventilation. In: Goldsmith JP, Karotin EH, eds. Assisted Ventilation of the Neonate. 4th Ed. Philadelphia: Saunders, 2003.

141. Schwartz JE. New technologies applied to management of the respiratory system. In: Kenner C, Lott JW, eds. Comprehensive Neonatal Nursing: A Physiologic Perspective. 3rd Ed. Philadelphia: Saunders, 2003.

142. Meredith KS. High frequency ventilation. In: Czervinske MP, Barnhart SC, eds. Perinatal and Pediatric Respiratory Care. 2nd Ed. Philadelphia: Saunders, 2003.

143. Mammel MC. Mechanical ventilation of the newborn. Arch Dis Child Fetal Neonatal Ed 2000;83(3):F224.

144. Mammel MC. High frequency ventilation. In: Goldsmith JP, Karotin EH, eds. Assisted Ventilation of the Neonate. 4th Ed. Philadelphia: Saunders, 2003.

145. Keszler M, Derand DJ. Neonatal high frequency ventilation: past, present, future. Clin Perinatol 2001;28(3):579–607.

146. MacIntyre NR. High frequency jet ventilation. Respir Care Clin N Am 2001;7(4):599–610.

147. Bouchet JC, Goddard J, Claris O. High frequency oscillatory ventilation. Anesthesiology 2004;100:1007–1012.

148. Moriette G, Paris-Llado J, Walti H, et al. Prospective randomized multicenter comparison of high frequency oscillatory ventilation and conventional ventilation in preterm infants of less than 30 weeks with respiratory distress syndrome. Pediatrics 2001;107(2):363–372.

149. Osborn DA, Evans N. Randomized trial of high frequency oscillatory ventilation versus conventional ventilation: effect on systemic blood flow in very premature infants. J Pediatr 2003;143(2):192–202.

150. Sreenan C, Lemke RP, Hudson-Mason A, et al. High-flow nasal cannulae in the management of apnea of prematurity: a comparison with conventional nasal continuous positive airway pressure. Pediatrics 2001;107(5):1081–1083.

151. Locke RG, Wolfson MR, Shaffer TH, et al. Inadvertent administration of positive-end-distending pressure during nasal cannula flow. Pediatrics 1993;91(1):135–138.

152. Saslow JG, Aghar ZH, Nakhla TA, et al. Work of breathing using high flow nasal cannula in preterm infants. J Perinatol 2006;26(8):476–480.

153. Walsh B. Comparison of Vapotherm 2000i with a bubble humidifier humidifying flow through a nasal cannula. Respir Care 2003;48(18).

154. Kopelman AE, Holbert D. Use of oxygen cannulas in extremely low birthweight infants. J Perinatol 2003;23:94–97.

155. Vapotherm. Available at: http://www.vtherm.com/forclinicians/lowflow.asp. Accessed 7/21/05.

156. Woodhead DD, Lambert DK, Clark JM, et al. Comparing two methods of delivering high-flow gas therapy by nasal cannula following endotracheal extubation: a prospective, randomized, masked, crossover trial. J Perinatol 2006;26(8):481–485.

157. Waugh JB, Granger WM. An evaluation of two new devices for nasal high flow gas therapy. Respir Care 2004;49(8):902–906.

158. Panitch HB, Wolfson MR, Shaffer TH. Epithelial modulation of preterm airway smooth muscle contraction. J Pediatr 1993;74(3):1437–1443.

159. Cullen AB, Wolfson MR, Shaffer TH. The maturation of airway structure and function. American Academy of Pediatrics. NeoReviews 2002;3(7):e125–e130.

160. Williams LJ, Shaffer TH, Greenspan JS. Inhaled nitric oxide therapy in the nearly term or term infant with hypoxic respiratory failure. Neonatal Netw 2004;23(1):5–13.

161. Neonatal Inhaled Nitric Oxide Study Group (NINOS). Inhaled nitric oxide in full-term and nearly term infants with hypoxic respiratory failure. N Engl J Med 1997;336:597–604.

162. Neonatal Inhaled Nitric Oxide Study Group (NINOS). Inhaled nitric oxide in term and nearly term infants: neurodevelopmental follow-up of the neonatal inhaled nitric oxide study group (NINOS). J Pediatr 2000;136(5):611–617.

163. Ellington M, O'Reilly D, Allred EN, et al. Child health status, neurodevelopmental outcome, and parent satisfaction in a randomized, controlled trial of nitric oxide for persistent pulmonary hypertension of the newborn. Pediatrics 2001;107(6):1351–1356.

164. American Academy of Pediatrics, Committee on Fetus and Newborn. Use of inhaled nitric oxide. Pediatrics 2000;106(2 part 1):344–345.

165. Ballard RH, Truog WE, Cnaan A, et al. Inhaled nitric oxide in preterm infants undergoing mechanical ventilation. N Engl J Med 2006;355(4):343–353.

166. Kinsella JP, Cutter GR, Walsh WF, et al. Early inspired nitric oxide therapy in premature newborns with respiratory failure. N Engl J Med 2006;355(4):354–364.

167. Ford JW. Neonatal ECMO: current controversies and trends. Neonatal Netw 2006;25(4):229–238.

168. Rais-Bahrami K, Short BL. The current status of neonatal extracorporeal membrane oxygenation. Semin Perinatol 2000;24(6):406–417.

169. Jaillard S, Pierrat V, Truffert P, et al. Two years' follow-up of newborn infants after extracorporeal membrane oxygenation. Eur J Cardiothorac Surg 2000;18(3):328–333.

170. Kim ES, Stolar CJ. ECMO in the newborn. Am J Perinatol 2000;17(7):345–356.

171. Nield TA, Langenbacher D, Poulsen MK, et al. Neurodevelopmental outcome at 3.5 years of age in children treated with extra corporeal life support: relationship to primary diagnosis. J Pediatr 2000;136(3):338–344.

172. Rais-Bahrami K, Wagner AE, Coffman C, et al. Neurodevelopmental outcome in ECMO vs near-miss ECMO patients at 5 years of age. Clin Pediatr 2000;39(3):145–152.

173. Tappero EP. NICU technology. In: Zaichkin J, ed. Newborn Intensive Care. What Every Parent Needs to Know. 2nd Ed. Santa Rosa, CA: NICU Ink Book Publishers, 2002.

174. Cooper M, Arnold J. Extracorporeal membrane oxygenation. In: Cloherty JP, Eichenwald EC, Stark AR, eds. Manual of Neonatal Care. 5th Ed. Philadelphia: Lippincott Williams & Wilkins, 2004.

175. Massery M. Chest development as a component of normal motor development: implications for treatment for pediatric physical therapists. Pediatr Phys Ther 1991;3(1):3–8.

176. Make BJ, Hill NS, Goldberg AI, et al. Mechanical ventilation beyond the intensive care unit: report of a consensus conference of the American College of Chest Physicians. Chest 1998;113(5):289S–344S.

177. Vohr BR, Cashore WJ, Bigsby R. Stresses & interventions in the neonatal intensive care unit. In: Levine MD, Carey WB, Crocker AC, eds. Developmental-Behavioral Pediatrics. 3rd Ed. Philadelphia: Saunders, 1999.

178. Honrubia D, Stark AR. Respiratory distress syndrome. In: Cloherty JP, Eichenwald EC, Stark AR, ed. Manual of Neonatal Care. 5th Ed. Philadelphia: Lippincott Williams & Wilkins, 2004.

179. National Institutes of Health. Report of the Consensus Development Conference on Anti-natal Corticosteroids Revisited: Repeat Courses. Bethesda, MD: National Institute of Child Health and Human Development, 2000.

180. Baud O. Antenatal glucocorticoid treatment and cystic periventricular leukomalacia in very preterm infants. N Engl J Med 1999;341(16):1190–1196.

181. Banks BA, Cnaan A, Morgan MA, et al. Multiple courses of antenatal corticosteroids and outcome of premature neonates. Am J Obstet Gynecol 1999;181:709–717.

182. Banks BA, Macones G, Cnaan A, et al. Multiple courses of antenatal corticosteroids are associated with early severe lung disease in preterm neonates. J Perinatol 2002;22:101–107.

183. Jobe AH, Ikegami M. Biology of surfactant. Clin Perinatol 2001;28:671–694.

184. Egerman RS, Mercer BM, Doss JL, et al. A randomized controlled trial of oral and intramuscular dexamethasone in the prevention of neonatal respiratory distress syndrome. Am J Obstet Gynecol 1998;179(5):1120–1123.

185. Hack MF, Minisch N, Fanaroff A. Antenatal steroids have not improved the outcomes of surviving extremely low birth weight (ELBW) infants [< 750 grams]. Pediatr Res 1998;43(2):214A.

186. Soll RF. Surfactant treatment of the very premature infant. Biol Neonate 1998;74(suppl 1):35–42.

187. Suresh GK. Current surfactant use in premature infants. Clin Perinatol 2001;28:671–694.

188. Escobedo MB, Gunkel JH, Kennedy RA, et al. Texas Neonatal Research Group. Early surfactant for neonates with mild to moderate RDS: a multicenter randomized trial. J Pediatr 2004;144(6):804–808.

189. Jobe AH. Surfactant for RDS: when and why? J Pediatr 2004;144(6):A2.

190. Dani C, Bertini G, Pezzati M, et al. Early extubation and nasal continuous positive airway pressure after surfactant treatment for respiratory distress syndrome among preterm infants <30 weeks gestation. Pediatrics 2004;113(6):e560–e563.

191. Park MK. Pediatric Cardiology for Practitioners. 4th Ed. St Louis: Mosby, 2002.

192. Heyman MA, Teitel DF, Liebman J. The heart. In: Klaus MH, Fanaroff AA, eds. Care of the High-Risk Neonate. 4th Ed. Philadelphia: Saunders, 1993.

193. Wechsler SB, Wernovsky G. Cardiac disorders. In: Cloherty JP, Eichenwald EC, Stark AR, eds. Manual of Neonatal Care. 5th Ed. Philadelphia: Lippincott Williams & Wilkins, 2004.

194. Gersony WM, Peckham GJ, Ellison RC, et al. Effects of indomethacine in premature infants with patent ductus arteriosus: results of a national collaborative study. J Pediatr 1984;102(6):895–906.

195. Gersony WM. Patent ductus arteriosus. Pediatr Clin North Am 1986;33(3):545–560.

196. Martin CR, Cloherty JP. Neonatal hyperbilirubinemia. In: Cloherty JR, Eichenwald EC, Stark AR, eds. Manual of Neonatal Care. 5th Ed. Philadelphia: Lippincott Williams & Wilkins, 2004.

197. Dennery PA, Seidman DS, Stevenson DK. Neonatal hyperbilirubinemia. N Engl J Med 2001;334:581–590.

198. Poland RL, Ostrea EM. Neonatal hyperbilirubinemia. In: Klaus MH, Fanaroff AA, eds. Care of the High Risk Neonate. Philadelphia: Saunders, 1993.

199. AAP Subcommittee on Neonatal Hyperbilirubinemia. Neonatal jaundice and kernicterus. Pediatrics 2001;108(3):763–765.

200. Patra K, Storfer-Isser A, Siner B, et al. Adverse events associated with neonatal exchange transfusion in the 1990's. J Pediatr 2004;144:626–631.

201. Paludetto R, Mansi G, Raimondi F, et al. Moderate hyperbilirubinemia induces a transient alteration of neonatal behavior. Pediatrics 2002;110(4):e50.

202. Mansi G, De Maio C, Araimo G, et al. "Safe" hyperbilirubinemia is associated with altered neonatal behavior. Biol Neonate 2003;83(1):19–21.

203. Jadcherla SR. Gastroesophageal reflux in the neonate. Clin Perinatol 2002;29(1):135–158.

204. Noviski N, Yehuda YB, Yorum B, et al. Does the size of nasogastric tube affect gastroesophageal reflux in children. J Pediatr Gastroenterol Nutr 1999;29:448–451.

205. Hammer D. Gastroesophageal reflux and prokinetic agents. Neonatal Netw 2005;24(2):51–58.

206. Peter CS, Sprodowski N, Bohnhorst B, et al. Gastroesophageal reflux and apnea of prematurity. No temporal relationship. Pediatrics 2002;109(8):8–11.

207. Poets CF. Gastroesophageal reflux: a critical review of its role in preterm infants. Pediatrics 2004;113(2):e128–e132.

208. Krishnamoorthy M, Muntz A, Liem T, et al. Diagnosis and treatment of respiratory symptoms of initially unsuspected gastroesophageal reflux in infants. Am Surg 1994;60:783–785.

209. Menon AP, Schefft GL, Thach BT. Apnea associated with regurgitation in infants. J Pediatr 1985;106(4):625–629.

210. Orenstein SR. Gastroesophageal reflux. Curr Probl Pediatr 1991;21(5):193–241.

211. Orenstein SR, Whittington PF. Positioning for prevention of infant gastroesophageal reflux. J Pediatr 1983;103:534–537.

212. Tobin JM, McCloud P, Cameron DJS. Posture and gastroesophageal reflux: a case for left lateral positioning. Arch Dis Child 1997;76:254–258.

213. Ewer AK, James ME, Tobin JM. Prone and lateral position reduce gastroesophageal reflux in premature infants. Arch Dis Child 1999;81:F201–F205.

214. Omari T, Rommel N, Staunton E, et al. Paradoxical impact of body positioning on gastroesophageal reflux and gastric emptying in the premature infant. J Pediatr 2004;145:194–200.

215. Heacock HJ, Jeffrey HE, Baker JL, et al. Influence of breast versus formula milk in physiological gastroesophageal reflux in healthy newborn infants. J Pediatr Gastroenterol Nutr 1992;14:41–46.

216. Huang RC, Forbes DA, Davies MW. Feed thickener for newborn infants with gastro-esophageal reflux. [Software. Research. Systematic Review.] The Cochrane Library (Oxford) 2004;(2):ID# CD003211.

217. McAlmon KR. Necrotizing enterocolitis. In: Cloherty JP, Eichenwald EC, Stark AR, eds. Manual of Neonatal Care. 5th Ed. Philadelphia: Lippincott Williams & Wilkins, 2004.

218. Reber KM, Nankervis CA. Necrotizing enterocolitis: preventative strategies. Clin Perinatol 2004;31(1):157–167.

219. Kleigman RM, Walsh MC. Neonatal necrotizing enterocolitis: pathogenesis, classification, and spectrum of illness. Curr Probl Pediatr 1987;17:213–288.

220. Kanto WP, Hunter JE, Stoll BJ. Recognition and medical management of necrotizing enterocolitis. Clin Perinatol 1994;21:335–346.

221. Stoll BJ, Kliegman RM. Necrotizing Enterocolitis. Clinics in Perinatology. Philadelphia: Saunders, 1994.

222. Walsh MC, Kliegman RM. Necrotizing enterocolitis: treatment based on a staging criteria. Pediatr Clin North Am 1986;33:179–201.

223. Kleigman RM. Necrotizing enterocolitis: bridging the basic science with the clinical disease. J Pediatr 1990;117(5):833–835.

224. Cikrit D, Mastandrea J, West KW, et al. Necrotizing enterocolitis: factors affecting mortality in 101 surgical cases. Surgery 1984;96:648–665.

225. Sonntag J, Grimner I, Scholtz T, et al. Growth and neuro-developmental outcome of very low birth weight infants with necrotizing enterocolitis. Acta Paediatr 2004;89:528–532.

226. Volpe JJ. Brain injury in the preterm infant. Clin Perinatol 1997;24(3):567–583.

227. Volpe JJ. Neurology of the Newborn. 4th Ed. Philadelphia: Saunders, 2001.

228. Vohr B, Allen WC, Scott DT, et al. Early onset intra-ventricular hemorrhage in preterm neonates: incidence of neurodevelopmental handicap. Semin Perinatol 1999;23(3):212–217.

229. Vohr B, Wright LL, Dusick AM, et al. Neurodevelopmental and functional outcomes for extremely low birth weight infants in the National Institutes of Child Health and Human Development Neonatal Research Network, 1993–1994. Pediatrics 2000;105(6):1216–1226.

230. Vohr B, Allan WC, Westerveld M, et al. School-age outcomes of very low birth weight infants in the indomethacin intraventricular hemorrhage prevention trial. Pediatrics 2003;111(4):e340–e346.

231. Larroque B, Morret S, Ancel PY, et al. White matter damage and intraventricular hemorrhage in very preterm infants: the EPIPAGE study. J Pediatr 2003;(143):477–483.

232. Vohr B, Ment LR. Intraventricular hemorrhage in the preterm infant. Early Human Dev 1996;44(1):1–16.

233. Lucey JF, Rowan CA, Shiono P, et al. Fetal infants: the fate of 4172 infants with birth weights of 410 to 500 grams-The Vermont Oxford Network experience (1996–2000). Pediatrics 2004;113(4):1559–1566.

234. Papile LA, Burstein J, Burston R. Incidence and evolution of subependymal and intraventricular hemorrhage: a study of infants with birthweights less than 1500 grams. J Perinatol 1978;92:529–534.

235. Papile LA. Periventricular-Intraventricular hemorrhage. In: Fanaroff AA, Martin RJ, eds. Neonatal-Perinatal Medicine: Diseases of the Fetus and Infant. 5th Ed. Philadelphia: Mosby, 1992.

236. Shalik L, Perlman JM. Hemorrhagic-ischemic cerebral injury in the preterm infant: clinical concepts. Clin Perinatol 2002;29:745–763.

237. Cullens V. Brain injury in the premature infant. InL Boxwell, G, ed. Neonatal Intensive Care Nursing. New York: Routledge, 2000.

238. Soul JS. Intracranial hemorrhage. In: Cloherty JS, Eichenwald EC, Stark AR, eds. Manual of Neonatal Care. 5th Ed. Philadelphia: Lippincott Williams & Wilkins, 2004.

239. Bada HS, Korones SB, Perry EH, et al. Frequent handling in the neonatal intensive care unit and intraventricular hemorrhage. J Pediatr 1990;117(1 part 1):126–131.

240. Bada HS, Korones SB, Perry EH, et al. Mean arterial blood pressure changes in premature infants and those at risk for intraventricular hemorrhage. J Pediatr 1990;117(4):607–614.

241. Perlman JM, Thach B. Respiratory origins of fluctuations in arterial blood pressure in premature infants with respiratory distress syndrome. Pediatrics 1988;81(3):399–403.

242. Perlman JM, McMenamin JB, Volpe JJ. Fluctuating cerebral blood velocity in respiratory distress syndrome: relationship to subsequent development of intraventricular hemorrhage. N Engl J Med 1983;309(4):204–209.

243. Fanconi S, Duc G. Intratracheal suctioning in sick preterm infants: prevention of intracranial hemorrhage and cerebral hypofusion by muscle paralysis. Pediatrics 1987;79:583–543.

244. Bregman J, Kimberlin LVS. Developmental outcomes in extremely premature infants. Pediatr Clin North Am 1993;40(5):937–950.

245. Perlman JM. Cognitive and behavioral deficits in premature graduates of intensive care. Clin Perinatol 2002;29(4):779–797.

246. Krishnamoorthy KS, Kuban KC, Leviton A, et al. Periventricular-intraventricular hemorrhage, sonographic localization, phenobarbital, and motor abnormalities in low birth weight infants. Pediatrics 1990;85(6):1027–1033.

247. Zach T, Brown JC. Periventricular leukomalacia. Emedicine J 2003. Accessed April 9, 2003.

248. Shankaran S. Hemorrhagic lesions of the central nervous system. In: Stevenson DK, Benitz WE, Sunshine P, eds. Fetal and Neonatal Brain Injury. 3rd Ed. New York: Cambridge University Press, 1997.

249. Inder TE, Weels SJ, Mogride NB, et al. Defining the nature of cerebral abnormalities in the premature infant: a qualitative magnetic resonance imaging study. J Pediatr 2003;143(2):171–179.

250. Scher MS. Fetal and neonatal neurologic consultations and identifying brain disorders in the context of fetal-maternal-perinatal disease. Semin Pediatr Neurol 2001;8(2):55–75.

251. Murphy BP, Inder TE, Rooks V, et al. Posthemorrhagic ventricular dilation in the premature infant: natural history and predictors of outcome. Arch Dis Child 2002;87:F37–F41.

252. Anonymous. Randomised trial of early tapping neonatal post hemorrhagic ventricular dilatation results at 30 months. Arch Dis Child Fetal Neonatal Ed 1994;70(2):F129–136.

253. Allan WC, Sobel DB. Neonatal intensive care neurology. Semin Pediatr Neurol 2004;11(2):119–128.

254. Peterson BS, Vohr B, Staib LH, et al. Regional brain volume abnormalities and longterm cognitive outcome in preterm infants. JAMA 2000;284(15):1939–1947.

255. Blackburn ST. Assessment and management of the neurologic system. In: Comprehensive Neonatal Nursing: A Physiologic Perspective. 3rd Ed. Philadelphia: Saunders, 2003.

256. Jones MW, Bass WT. Perinatal brain injury in the premature infant. Neonatal Netw 2003;22(1):61–67.

257. Schmidt B, Davis P, Moddemann D, et al. Long-term effects of indomethacin prophylaxis in extremely-low-birth-weight infants. N Engl J Med 2001;344(26):1966–1972.

258. Ment LK, Vohr B, Allen W, et al. Change in cognitive function over time in very low-birth-weight infants. JAMA 2003;289(6):705–711.

259. Han TR, Bang MS, Yoon BH, et al. Risk factors for cerebral palsy in preterm infants. Am J Phys Med Rehabil 2002;81:297–303.

260. Als H, Lawhon G, Duffy FH, et al. Individualized developmental care for the very low birth weight preterm infant: medical and neurofunctional effects. JAMA 1994;272(11):853–858.

261. Westrup B, Bohm B, Lagercrantz H, et al. Preschool outcomes in children born very prematurely. Acta Paediatr 2004;93:498–507.

262. Sizan, J, Ratynski N, Boussard C. Humane neonatal care initiative: NIDCAP and family centered neonatal care. Neonatal individualized developmental care and assessment program. Acta Paediatr 1999;88(10):1172.

263. Zupan V, Gonzalez P, Laaze-Masmonteil T, et al. Periventricular leukomalacia: risk factors revisited. Dev Med Child Neurol 1996;38(12):1061–1067.

264. Volpe JJ. Neurobiology of periventricular leukomalacia in the preterm infant. Pediatr Res 2001;50(5):553–562.

265. Larroque B, Marret S, Ancel P-Y, et al. White matter damage and intraventricular hemorrhage in very preterm infants. The EPIPAGE study. J Pediatr 2003;143:477–503.

266. Blumenthal I. Periventricular leukomalacia: a review. Eur J Pediatr 2004;163:435–442.

267. Batten D, Kirtley X, Swails T. Unexpected versus anticipated cystic periventricular leukomalacia. Am J Perinatol 2003;20(1):33–40.

268. Kadhim H, Tabarki B, Verellen G, et al. Inflammatory cytokines in the pathogenesis of periventricular leukomalacia. Neurology 2001;56:1278–1284.

269. Dammann O, Kuban KC, Leviton A. Perinatal infection, fetal inflammatory response, white matter damage and cognitive limitations in children born preterm. Ment Retard Dev Disabil Res Rev 2002;8(1):46–50.

270. Dammann O, Leviton A. Infection remote from the brain, neonatal white matter damage and cerebral palsy in the preterm infant. Semin Pediatr Neurol 1998;5:190–201.

271. Wilson-Costello D, Borawski E, Freidman H, et al. Perinatal correlates of cerebral palsy and other neurologic impairment among very low birth weight children. Pediatrics 1998;102(2): 315–322.

272. Gressens P, Rogido M, Paindaveine S, et al. The impact of neonatal intensive care practices on the developing brain. J Pediatr 2002;140:646–653.

273. Perrott S, Dodds L, Vincer M. A population-based study of prognostic factors in very preterm survivors. J Perinatol 2003; 23(2):111–116.

274. Lemons JA, Bauer CR, Oh W, et al. Very low birth weight out-comes of the national institute of child health and human development neonatal research network, January 1995 through December 1996. Pediatrics 2001;107(1):E1–8.

275. Zuparncic JAF, Stewart JE. Retinopathy of prematurity. In: Cloherty JP, Eichenwald EC, Stark AR, eds. Manual of Neonatal Care. 5th Ed. Philadelphia: Lippincott Williams & Wilkins, 2004.

276. Stout AU, Stout JT. Retinopathy of prematurity. Pediatr Clin North Am 2003;50(1):77–87.

277. Ertzbischoff LM. A systematic review of anatomical and visual outcomes in preterm infants after scleral buckle and vitrectomy for retinal detachment. Adv Neonatal Care 2004;4(1):10–19.

278. Lee S. Retinopathy of prematurity in the 1990's. Neonatal Netw 1999;18(2):32.

279. Screening Examination of Premature Infants for Retinopathy of Prematurity. Policy Statement American Academy of Pediatrics. Pediatrics 2001;108(3):809–811.

280. Committee for the Classification of ROP. An international classification of retinopathy of prematurity. Arch Ophthalmol 1989;102(8):1130–1134.

281. Anderson CL, Stewart JE. Retinopathy of prematurity. In: Cloherty JP, Stark AR, eds. Manual of Neonatal Care. 4th Ed. Philadelphia: Lippincott Williams & Wilkins, 1997.

282. Paysse EA, Miller A, Brady-McCreery KM, et al. Acquired cataracts after diode laser photocoagulation for threshold retinopathy of prematurity. Ophthalmology 2002;109(9): 1662–1665.

283. Kellner JC, Heimann H, Foerster MH. Comparison of anatomical and functional outcome after laser or cryotherapy for retinopathy of prematurity. Ophthalmologie 2004;101(6).

284. Azad RV, Pasumala L, Kumar H, et al. Prospective random-ized evaluation of diode laser and cryotherapy in prethreshold retinopathy of prematurity. Clin Exper Ophthalmol 2004; 32(3):251–254.

285. Ng EY, Connelly BP, McNamara JA, et al. A comparison of laser photocoagulation with cryotherapy for threshold retinopathy of prematurity at 10 years. Part 1. Visual function and structural outcome. Ophthalmology 2002;109(5):928–934.

286. Quinn GE, Dobson V, Barr CC. Visual acuity in infants after vit-rectomy for severe retinopathy of prematurity. Ophthalmology 1991;98(1):5–13.

287. D'Harlingue AE, Durand DJ. Recognition, stabilization, and transport of the high-risk newborn. In: Klaus MK, Fanaroff AA, eds. Care of the High-Risk Neonate. 4th Ed. Philadelphia: Saunders, 1993.

288. Martinez A, Partridge JC, Bean X, et al. Perinatal substance abuse. In: Taeusch HW, Ballard RA, eds. Avery's Diseases of the Newborn. 7th Ed. Philadelphia: Saunders, 1998.

289. Mayes LC. Developing brain and in utero cocaine exposure: effects on neural ontogeny. Dev Psychol 1999;11:685–714.

290. Smeriglio VL, Wilson HC. Prenatal drug exposure and child outcome. Clin Perinatol 1999;26(1):1–16.

291. Schechner S. Drug abuse and withdrawal. In: Cloherty JP, Eichenwald EC, Stark AR, eds. Manual of Neonatal Care. 5th Ed. Philadelphia: Lippincott Williams & Wilkins, 2004.

292. Smith LM. Prenatal cocaine exposure and cranial sonographic findings in preterm infants. J Clin Ultrasound 2001;29(2): 72–77.

293. Viadeff AC, Mastrobattista JM. In utero cocaine exposure: a thorny mix of science and mythology. Am J Perinatol 2003;20(4):165–172.

294. Mehta SK, Super DM, Connick D, et al. Autonomic alter-ations in cocaine exposed infants. Am Heart J 2002;144(6): 1109–1115.

295. Richardson GA., Hamel SC, Goldschmidt L, et al. The effects of prenatal cocaine use on neonatal neurobehavioral status. Neurotoxicol Teratol 1996;18: 519–528.

296. Hurt H. Are there neurologic correlates of in utero cocaine exposure at age 6 years? J Pediatr 2001;138(6):911–913.

297. Frank DA, Augustyn M, Knight WG, et al. Growth, develop-ment, and behavior in early childhood following prenatal cocaine use: a systematic review. J Pediatr 2001;139(3): 1613–1625.

298. Singer LT. Cognitive and motor outcomes of cocaine exposed infants. JAMA 2002;287:1952–1960.

299. Mayes LC, Cicchetti D, Acharyya S, et al. Developmental tra-jectories of cocaine-and-other-drug-exposed and noncocaine exposed children. J Dev Behav Pediatr 2003;24(3):323–335.

300. Bandstra ES. Severity of prenatal cocaine exposure and child language functioning through age seven years: a longitudinal latent growth curve analysis. Subst Use Misuse 2004;39(1): 25–59.

301. Heffelfinger AK, Craft S, White DA, et al. Visual attention in pre-school children prenatally exposed to cocaine: implications for behavioral regulation. J Int Neuropsychol Soc 2002;8(1):12–21.

302. Schroder MD, Snyder PJ, Sielski I, et al. Impaired performance of children exposed in utero to cocaine on a novel test of visuo-motor working memory. Brain Cogn 2004;55(2):409–412.

303. Hurt H, Malmud E, Betancourt LM, et al. A prospective com-parison of developmental outcome of children with in utero cocaine exposure and controls using the battelle developmen-tal inventory. J Dev Behav Pediatr 2001;22(1):27–34.

304. Lester B, LaGasse L, Seifer R, et al. Maternal lifestyle study: effects of prenatal cocaine and/or opiate exposure on auditory brain response at one month. J Pediatr 2003;142(3):279–285.

305. Redline RW. Placental pathology. In: Fanaroff AA, Martin RJ, eds. Neonatal-Perinatal Medicine Diseases of the Fetus and Infant. 7th Ed. St. Louis: Mosby, 2002.

306. Vannucci RC, Palmer C. Hypoxia-ischemia: neuropathology, pathogenesis, and management. In: Fanaroff AA, Martin RJ, eds. Neonatal-Perinatal Medicine Diseases of the Fetus and Infant. 7th Ed. St. Louis: Mosby, 2002.

307. Demari S. Calcium and phophorus nutrition in preterm infants. Acta Paediatr Supp 2005;94(449):87–92.

308. Huttner KM. Metabolic bone disease of prematurity. In: Cloherty JP, Eichenwald EC, Stark AR, eds. Manual of Neonatal Care. 5th Ed. Philadelphia: Lippincott Williams & Wilkins, 2004.

309. Miller M. The bone disease of preterm birth: a biomechanical perspective. Pediatr Res 2003;53(1):10–15.

310. Krug SK. Osteopenia of prematurity. In: Groh-Wargo S, Thompson M, Cox J, eds. Nutritional Care for High-Risk Newborns. Rev. 3rd Ed. Chicago: Precept Press, Inc, 2000.

311. Rauch F, Schoenau E. Skeletal development in premature infants: a review of bone physiology beyond nutritional aspects. Arch Dis Child Fetal Neonatal Ed 2002;86:F82–F85.

312. Rigo J, DeCurtis M, Pieltain C, et al. Bone mineral metabolism in the micropremie. Clin Perinatol 2000;27:147–170.

313. Rigo J, Senterre J. Nutritional needs of premature infants: current issues. J Pediatr 2006;149(3 supp):S80–S88.

314. Eliakim A, Nemet D. Osteopenia of prematurity-the role of exercise in the prevention and treatment. Pediatr Endocrinol Rev 2005;2(4):675–682.

315. Moyer-Mileur LJ, Brunstetter V, McNaught TP, et al. Daily physical activity program increases bone mineralization and growth in preterm very low birth weight infants. Pediatrics 2000;106(5):1088–1092.

316. Litmanovitz I, Dolfin T, Friedland O, et al. Early physical activity intervention prevents decrease of bone strength in very low birth weight infants. Pediatrics 2003;112(1):15–19.

317. Browne J, Cicco R, Erikson D, et al. Recommended Standards for Newborn ICU Design. Available at: http://www.nd.edu/~kkolberg/frmain.htm. Accessed January 13, 2005.

318. Vanden Berg KA. Basic principles of developmental caregiving. Neonatal Netw 1997;16(7):69–71.

319. Lawhon G. Providing developmentally supportive care in the neonatal intensive care unit: an evolving challenge. J Perinatal Neonatal Nurs 1997;10(4):48–61.

320. Ohgi S, Akiyama T, Arisawa K, et al. Randomized controlled trial of swaddling versus massage in the management of excessive crying in infants with cerebral injuries. Arch Dis Child 2004;89(3):212–216.

321. Eiden RD, Reifman A. Effects of Brazelton demonstrations on later parenting: a meta-analysis. J Pediatr Psychol 1996;21(6):857–868.

322. Culp RE, Culp AM, Harmon RJ. A tool for educating parents about their premature infants. Birth 1989;16(1):23–26.

323. Lowman LB, Stone LL, Cole JG. Using developmental assessments in the NICU to empower families. Neonatal Netw 2006;25(3):177–186.

324. Loo KK, Espinosa M, Tyler R, et al. Using knowledge to cope with stress in the NICU: how parents integrate learning to read the physiologic and behavioral cues of the infant. Neonatal Netw 2003;22(1):31–37.

325. Gale G, VandenBerg KA. Kangaroo care. Neonatal Netw 1998;17(5):69–71.

326. Sloan N, Camacho LWI, Rojas EP. Kangaroo mother method: randomized controlled trial of an alternative method of care for stabilized low-birth-weight infants. Lancet 1994;344:782–785.

327. Acolet D, Sleath K, Whitelaw A. Oxygenation, heart rate and temperature in very low birthweight infants during skin-to-skin contact with their mothers. Acta Paediatr 1989;78:189–193.

328. Fohe K, Kropf S, Avenarius S. Skin-to-skin contact improved gas exchange in premature infants. J Perinatol 2000;20:311–315.

329. Feldman R, Eidelman AI. Skin-to-skin contact (kangaroo care) accelerates autonomic and neurobehavioral maturation in preterm infants. Dev Med Child Neurol 2003;45:274–281.

330. Lundington-Hoe SM, Anderson GC, Swine JY, et al. A randomized control of kangaroo care and cardiorespiratory and thermal effects on healthy preterm infants. Neonatal Netw 2004;23(3):39–48.

331. Johnston CC, Stevens B, Pinelli J, et al. Kangaroo care is effective in diminishing pain response in preterm neonates. Arch Pediatr Adolesc Med 2003;157(11):1084–1088.

332. Bier JA, Ferguson AE, Morales Y, et al. Comparison of skin-to-skin contact with standard contact in low birth weight infants who are breast fed. Arch Pediatr Adolesc Med 1996;150(12):1265–1269.

333. Anderson G. Kangaroo care and breastfeeding for preterm infants. Breastfeeding Abstracts 1989;9(2):7.

334. Feldman R, Weller A, Sirota L, et al. Testing a family intervention hypothesis: the contribution of mother-infant skin-to-skin contact (kangaroo care) to family interaction, proximity, and touch. J Fam Psychol 2003;17(11):94–107.

335. Feldman R, Eidelman AI, Sirota L, et al. Comparison of skin-to-skin (kangaroo) and traditional care: parenting outcomes and preterm infant development. Pediatrics 2002;110(1):16–26.

336. Hemingway M, Oliver S. Water bed therapy and cranial molding of the sick preterm infant. Neonatal Netw 1991;10(3):53–56.

337. Hemingway M, Oliver S. Bilateral head flattening in hospitalized premature infants. Neonatal Intens Care 2000;13(6):18–22.

338. Hemingway M. Preterm infant positioning. Neonatal Intens Care 2000;13(6):18–22.

339. Vaivre-Douret L, Ennouri K, Jrad I, et al. Effect of positioning on the incidence of abnormalities of muscle tone in low-risk, preterm infants. Eur J Pediatr Neurol 2004;8:21–34.

340. Hallsworth M. Positioning the pre-term infant. Clin Neonatal Nurs 1995;7(1):18–20.

341. Chang YJ, Anderson GC, Lin CH. Effects of prone and supine positions on sleep state and stress responses in mechanically ventilated preterm infants during the first postnatal week. J Adv Nurs 2002;40(2):161–169.

342. Wolfson MR, Greenspan JS, Deoras KS, et al. Effect of positioning on the mechanical interaction between the rib cage and abdomen in preterm infants. J Appl Physiol 1992;72(3):1032–1038.

343. Bjornson K, Deitz J, Blackburn S, et al. The effect of body position on the oxygen saturation of ventilated preterm infants. Pediatr Phys Ther 1992;4(3):109–115.

344. Goldberg RN, Joshi A, Moscoso P, et al. the effect of head position on intracranial pressure in the neonate. Crit Care Med 1983;11:428–430.

345. Grenier IR, Bigsby R, Vergara ER, et al. Comparison of motor self-regulatory and stress behaviors of preterm infants across body positions. Am J Occupat Ther 2003;57(3):289–297.

346. Vohr BR, Cashore WJ, Bigsby R. Stresses and interventions in the neonatal intensive care unit. In: Levine MD, Carey WB, Crocker AC, eds. Developmental-Behavioral Pediatrics. Philadelphia: Saunders, 1999.

347. Hashimoto T, Hiurs K, Endo S, et al. Postural effects on behavioral states of newborn infants: a sleep polygraphic study. Brain Dev 1983;5:286–291.

348. Hadders-Algra M, Prechtl HFR. Developmental course of general movements in early infancy. I. Descriptive analysis of change in form. Early Human Dev 1992;201–213.

349. Adams JA, Zabaleta, Sackner MA. Comparison of supine and prone noninvasive measurements of breathing patterns in full-term newborns. Pediatr Pulmonol 1994;18:8–12.

350. Pellicier A, Gaya F, Madero R, et al. Noninvasive continuous monitoring of the effects of head position on brain hemodynamics in ventilated infants. Pediatrics 2002;109(3):434–440.

351. American Academy of Pediatrics Task Force on Infant Sleep Position and Sudden Death Syndrome. Changing concepts of sudden death syndrome: implications for infant sleeping environment and sleep position. Pediatrics 2000;105(3):650–656.

352. van Heijst JJ, Touwen BCL, Vos JE. Implications of a neural network model of sensori-motor development for the field of developmental neurology. Early Human Dev 1999;55(1):77–95.

353. de Groot L. Posture and motility in preterm infants. Dev Med Child Neurol 2000;42:65–68.

354. Fay MJ. The positive effects of positioning. Neonatal Netw 1988;23–28.

355. Monterososso L, Kristjanson L, Cole J. Neuromotor development and the physiologic effects of positioning in very low birthweight infants. J Obstet Gynecol Neonatal Nurs 2002;31(2):138–146.

356. Shaw JC. Growth and nutrition of the preterm infant. Br Med Bull 1988;44(4):984–1009.

357. Clarren SK, Smith DW, Hanson JW. Helmet treatment for plagiocephaly and congenital muscular torticollis. J Pediatr 1979;94(1):43–46.

358. Kriewell TJ. Structural, mechanical, and material properties of fetal cranial bone. Am J Obstet Gynecol 1982;143(6):707–714.

359. Budreau GK. The perceived attractiveness of preterm infants with caranial molding. J Obstet Gynecol Neonatal Nurs 1989; 18(1):38–44.

360. Budreau GK. Postnatal cranial molding and infant attractiveness: implications for nursing. Neonatal Netw 1987;5(5):13–19.

361. Schwirian PM, Eesley T, Cuellar L. Use of water pillows in reducing head shape distortion in preterm infants. Res Nurs Health 1986;9(3):203–207.

362. Geerdink JJ, Hopkins B, Hoeksma JB. The development of head positioning preference in preterm infants beyond term age. Dev Psychobiol 1994;27(3):253–268.

363. Cartlidge PH, Rutter N. Reduction of head flattening in preterm infants. Arch Dis Child 1988;63(7):755–757.

364. Chan JS, Kelley MC, Khan J. The effects of a pressure relief mattress on postnatal head molding in very low birth weight infants. Neonatal Netw 1993;12(5):19–22.

365. Pelletier J, Lydic JS. Neurological assessment of the preterm and full-term infant: an analysis. Phys Occupat Ther Pediatr 1986;6(1):93–104.

366. Korner AF, Stevenson DK, Kraemer HC, et al. Prediction of the development of low birth weight preterm infants by a new neonatal medical index. J Dev Behav Pediatr 1993;14(2): 106–111.

367. Korner AF, Constantinou J, Dimiceli S, et al. Establishing the reliability and developmental validity of a neurobehavioral assessment for preterm infants: a methodological process. Child Dev 1991;62:1200–1208.

368. Korner AF, Kraemer HC, Reade EP, et al. A methodological approach to developing an assessment procedure for testing the neurobehavioral maturity of preterm infants. Child Dev 1987; 58(6):1478–1487.

369. Korner AF, Thom VA. Neurobehavioral Assessment of the Preterm Infant (NAPI). San Antonio TX: The Psychological Corporation, 1990.

370. Available at: http://www-med.stanford.edu/school/pediatrics/NAPI. Accessed 7/21/05.

371. Ferrari F, Cioni G, Einspieler C, et al. Cramped synchronized general movements in preterm infants as an early marker for cerebral palsy. Arch Pediatr Adolesc Med 2002;156(5):460–467.

372. Einspieler C, Prechtl HFR, Ferrari F, et al. The qualitative assessment of general movements in preterm, term, and young infants-review of the methodology. Early Human Dev 1997; 50:47–60.

373. Hadders-Algra M, Klip-Van den Nieuwendijk AWJ, Martijn A, et al. Assessment of general movements: towards a better understanding of a sensitive method to evaluate brain function in young infant. Dev Med Child Neurol 1997;39:89–99.

374. Zuk L, Harel S, Leitner Y, et al. Neonatal general movements: an early predictor for neurodevelopmental outcome in infants with intrauterine growth retardation. J Child Neurol 2004; 19:14–18.

375. Hadders-Algra M. Evaluation of motor function in young infants by assessment of general movements. Pediatr Phys Ther 2001;13(1):27–37.

376. Available at: http://www-ang.kfunigraz.ac.at/~gmtrust. Accessed 7/21/05.

377. Boukydis CFZ, Bigsby R, Lester B. Clinical use of the neonatal care unit network neurobehavioral scale. Pediatrics 2004; 113(3):679–689.

378. Lester BM, Tronick EZ. The neonatal intensive care unit network neurobehavioral scale procedures. Pediatrics 2004; 113(3):641–667.

379. Available at: http://www.infantdevelopment.org/trainingand education. htm. Accessed 7/21/05.

380. Vohr B. The quest for the ideal neurologic assessment for infants and young children. J Pediatr 1999;135(2, Part 1):140–142.

381. Dubowitz L, Dubowitz V. The Neurological Assessment of the Preterm and Full-Term Newborn Infant. Clinics in Developmental Medicine. No. 12. Philadelphia: Lippincott, 1981.

382. Dubowitz LMS, Dubowitz V, Palmer PG, et al. Correlation of neurologic assessment of preterm neonate-developmental outcome. J Pediatr 1984;105(3):452–456.

383. Dubowitz V, Dubowitz LMS. Gestational Age of the Newborn: A Clinical Manual. Reading, MA: Addison-Wesley, 1977.

384. Available at: http://www.paclac.org/manuals_Guidelines/Gestational. Accessed 7/21/05.

385. Lester BM, Tronick EZ. Behavioral assessment scales. In: Singer LT, Zeskind PS, eds. Biobehavioral Assessment of the Infant. New York: The Guilford Press, 2001.

386. Available at: www.Brazelton-Institute.com. Accessed 7/21/05.

387. Case-Smith J, Bigsby R. Motor assessment. In: Singer LT, Zeskind PS, eds. Biobehavioral Assessment of the Infant. New York: The Guilford Press, 2001.

388. Available at: www.TheTIMP.com. Accessed 7/21/05.

389. Campbell SK. The infant at risk for developmental disability. In: Campbell SK, ed. Decision Making in Pediatric Neurologic Physical Therapy. Philadelphia: Church Livingstone, 1999.

390. Long TM, Cintas HL. Handbook of Pediatric Physical Therapy. Baltimore: Williams & Wilkins, 1995.

391. Ellison PH. Neurologic Development of the high-risk infant. Clin Perinatol 11(1):45, and adapted from Amiel-Tison C. A method for neurological evaluation within the first year of life. Curr Probl Pediatr 1976;7(1):45.

392. Parad RB. Bronchopulmonary dysplasia/chronic lung disease. In: Cloherty JP, Eichenwald EC, Stark AR, eds. Manual of Neonatal Care. 5th Ed. Philadelphia: Lippincott Williams & Wilkins, 2004.

393. Walsh MC, Wilson-Costello D, Zadell A, et al. Safety, reliability, validity of a physiologic definition of bronchopulmonary dysplasia. J Perinatol 2003;23:45145–45146.

394. Ambalavanan N, Carlo WA. Bronchopulmonary dysplasia: new insights. Clin Perinatol 2004;31:613–628.

395. Jobe AH, Bancalari E. Bronchopulmonary dysplasia. Am J Respir Crit Care Med 2001;63(7):1723–1729.

396. Bancalari E. Neonatal chronic lung disease. In: Fanaroff AA, Martin RJ, eds. Neonatal-Perinatal Medicine: Diseases of the Fetus and Infant. St. Louis: Mosby, 2002.

397. Northway WH, Rosan RC, Porter DY. Pulmonary disease following respirator therapy of hyaline-membrane disease: bronchopulmonary dysplasia. N Engl J Med 1967;16(276): 357–368.

398. Goetzman BW. Understanding bronchopulmonary dysplasia. Am J Dis Child 1986;40:332–334.

399. Abman S, Groothius J. Pathophysiology and treatment of bronchopulmonary dysplasia. Respir Med 1994;41:277–307.

400. Jobe AH, Ikegam M. Mechanisms initiating lung injury in the preterm infant. Early Human Dev 1998;53:91–94.

401. Parad RB, Berger TM. Chronic lung disease. In: Cloherty JP, Stark AR, eds. Manual of Neonatal Care. 4th Ed. Philadelphia: Lippincott Williams & Wilkins, 1997.

402. Clark RH, Gerstmann DR, Jobe AH, et al. Lung injuries in neonate: causes, strategies for prevention, and long-term consequences. J Pediatr 2001;239(4):478–484.

403. Jobe AH. An unknown. Lung growth and development after very preterm birth. Am J Respir Crit Care Med 2001;166: 1529–1530.

404. Coalson JJ. Pathology of new bronchopulmonary dysplasia. Semin Neonatol 2003;8(1):73–81.

405. Husain AN, Siddiqui NH, Stocker JT. Pathology of arrested acinar development in post surfactant bronchopulmonary dysplasia. Human Pathol 1998;29(7):710–717.

406. Naik A, Kallapur S, Bachurski CJ, et al. Effects of different styles of ventilation on cytokine expression in the preterm lamb lung. Pediatr Res 2000;47:370A.

407. Welty SE. Antioxidants and oxidations in bronchopulmonary dysplasia: there is no easy answer. J Pediatr 2003;143(6): 697–698.

408. Mentro AM. Vitamin A and bronchopulmonary dysplasia: research, issues, and clinical practice. Neonatal Netw 2004; 23(4):19–23.

409. Speer CP. Inflammation & bronchopulmonary dysplasia. Semin Neonatol 2003;8(1):29–38.

410. Lewis BA, Singer LT, Fulton S, et al. Speech and language outcomes of children with bronchopulmonary dysplasia. J Commun Disord 2002;35(5):393–406.

411. Holditch-Davis D, Docherty S, Miles MS, et al. Developmental outcomes of infants with bronchopulmonary dysplasia: comparison with other medically fragile infants. Res Nurs Health 2001;24:181–193.

412. Meisels SJ, Plunkett JW, Roloff DW, et al. Growth and development of preterm infants with RDS and BPD. Pediatrics 1986;77:345–352.

413. Farel AM, Hooper SR, Teplin SW, et al. Very-low-birthweight infants at 7 years: an assessment of the health and neurodevelopmental risk conveyed by chronic lung disease. J Learn Disabil 1998;31(2):118–126.

414. Kilbride HW, Gelatt MC, Sabath RJ. Pulmonary function and exercise capacity of ELBW survivors in preadolescence: effect of neonatal chronic lung disease. J Pediatr 2003;143(4): 488–493.

415. Bohm B, Katz-Salamon M. Cognitive development at 5.5 years of children with chronic lung disease of prematurity. Arch Dis Child Fetal Neonatal Ed 2003;88(2):F101(5).

416. McGrath M, Sullivan M. Birthweight, neonatal morbidities, and school age outcomes in fullterm and preterm infants. Issues Compr Pediatr Nurs 2002;25(4):231–254.

417. Korhonen P, Laitmen J, Hyodymaa E, et al. Respiratory outcome in school aged, very-low-birth-weight children in the surfactant era. Acta Paediatr 2004;93:316–321.

418. Perlman JM, Volpe JJ. Movement disorder of premature infants with severe bronchopulmonary dysplasia: a new syndrome. Pediatrics 1989;84(2):215–218.

419. Hadders-Algra M, Bos AF, Martijn A, et al. Infantile chorea in an infant with severe bronchopulmonary dysplasia: an EMG study. Dev Med Child Neurol 1994;36(2):177–182.

420. Hack MF, Fanaroff A. Outcomes of children of extremely low birthweight and gestational age in the 1990's. Early Human Dev 1998;53:193–218.

421. Hack M, Friedman H, Fanaroff AA. Outcomes of extremely low-birth-weight infants. Pediatrics 1996;98:931–937.

422. Bianchi DW, Crumbleholme TM, D'Alton ME. Diaphragmatic hernia. In: Fetology Diagnosis and Management of the Fetal Patient. New York: McGraw-Hill, 2000.

423. West SE. Normal and abnormal structural development of the lung. In: Polin RA, Fox WW, Abman SH, eds. Fetal and Neonatal Physiology. 2nd Ed. Philadelphia: WB Saunders Co, 1998.

424. Ross AJ. Organogenesis, innervation and histologic development of the gastrointestinal tract. In: Polin RA, Fox WW, Abman SH, eds. Fetal and Neonatal Physiology. 2nd Ed. Philadelphia: WB Saunders Co, 1998.

425. Thigpen TL, Kenner C. Assessment and management of the gastrointestinal system. In: Kenner C, Lott JW, eds. Comprehensive Neonatal Nursing: A Physiologic Perspective. 3rd Ed. Philadelphia: Saunders, 2003.

426. Bianchi DW, Crumbleholme, TM, D'Alton ME. Omphalocele. In: Fetology Diagnosis and Management of the Fetal Patient. New York: McGraw-Hill, 2000.

427. Bianchi DW, Crumbleholme TM, D'Alton ME. Gastroschisis. In: Fetology Diagnosis and Management of the Fetal Patient. New York: McGraw-Hill, 2000.

428. Bianchi DW, Crumbleholme TM, D'Alton ME. Invasive fetal therapy and fetal surgery. In: Fetology Diagnosis and Management of the Fetal Patient. New York: McGraw-Hill, 2000.

429. Jones MW, McMurray JL, Englestad D. The "geriatric" NICU patient. Neonatal Netw 2002;21(6):49–58.

430. Aurora S, Snyder EY. Perinatal asphyxia. In: Cloherty JP, Eichenwald EC, Stark AR, eds. Manual of Neonatal Care. 5th Ed. Philadelphia: Lippincott-Raven, 2004.

431. Kuban KCK, Philiano J. Neonatal seizures. In: Fanaroff AA, Martin RJ, eds. Neonatal-Perinatal Medicine Diseases of the Fetus and Infant. 4th Ed. St. Louis: Mosby, 1998.

432. Yager JY, Vannucci RC. Seizures in neonates. In: Fanaroff AA, Martin RJ, eds. Neonatal-Perinatal Medicine Diseases of the Fetus and Infant. 7th Ed. St. Louis: Mosby, 2002.

433. du Plessis AJ. Neonatal seizures. In: Cloherty JP, Eichenwald EC, Stark AR, eds. Manual of Neonatal Care. 5th Ed. Philadelphia: Lippincott-Raven, 2004.

434. Lekskulchai R, Cole J. The relationship between the scarf ratio and subsequent motor performance in infants born preterm. Pediatr Phys Ther 2000;12:150–157.

435. Shankaran S. The postnatal management of the asphyxiated term infant. Clin Perinatol 2002;29(4):675–692.

436. Lee JS, Stark AR. Meconium aspiration. In: Cloherty JP, Eichenwald EC, Stark AR, eds. Manual of Neonatal Care. 5th Ed. Philadelphia: Lippincott Williams & Wilkins, 2004.

437. Gelfand SL, Fanroff JM, Walsh MC. Controversies in the treatment of meconium aspiration syndrome. Clin Perinatol 2004;31:445–452.

438. Martin RJ, Fanaroff AA, Klaus MH. Respiratory problems. In: Klaus MH, Fanaroff AA, eds. Care of the High-Risk Neonate. 4th Ed. Philadelphia: Saunders, 1993.

439. Wiswell TE. Advances in the treatment of the meconium aspiration syndrome. Acta Paediatr Suppl 2001;90(436):28–30.

440. Stoll BJ, Kliegman RM. Respiratory tract disorders. In: Berhman RE, Kliegman RM, Jenson HB, eds. Nelson's Textbook of Pediatrics. 17th Ed. Philadelphia: Saunders, 2004.

441. Konduri GG. New approaches for persistent pulmonary hypertension of the newborn. Clin Perinatol 2004;31:591–611.

442. VanMarter LJ. Persistent pulmonary hypertension of the newborn. In: Cloherty JP, Eichenwald EC, Stark AR, eds. Manual of Neonatal Care. 5th Ed. Philadelphia: Lippincott Williams & Wilkins, 2004.

443. Lipkin PH, Davidson D, Spivak L, et al. Neurodevelopmental and medical outcomes of persistent pulmonary hypertension of the newborn in term neonates treated with nitric oxide. J Pediatr 2002;140(3):306–310.

444. Walsh MC, Stark ER. Persistent pulmonary hypertension of the newborn. Rational therapy based on pathophysiology. Clin Perinatol 2001;28(3):609–627.

445. Burchett SK. Viral infections. In: Cloherty JP, Eichenwald EC, Stark AR, eds. Manual of Neonatal Care. 5th Ed. Philadelphia: Lippincott Williams & Wilkins, 2004.

446. Guerina NG. Toxoplasmosis. In: Cloherty JP, Eichenwald EC, Stark AR, eds. Manual of Neonatal Care. 5th Ed. Philadelphia: Lippincott Williams & Wilkins, 2004

447. Lott JW, Kenner K. Assessment and management of the immune system. In: Kenner C, Lott JW, eds. Comprehensive Neonatal Nursing; A Physiologic Perspective. 3rd Ed. Philadelphia: Saunders, 2003.

448. Puopolo KM. Bacterial and fungal Infections. In: Cloherty JP, Eichenwald EC, Stark AR, eds. Manual of Neonatal Care. 5th Ed. Philadelphia: Lippincott Williams & Wilkins, 2004.

449. Cowles TA, Gonik B. Perinatal infections. In: Fanaroff AA, Martin RJ, eds. Neonatal-Perinatal Medicine Diseases of the Fetus and Infant. 7th Ed. St. Louis: Mosby, 2002.

450. Jones KL, Smith DW. Recognition of the fetal alcohol syndrome in early infancy. Lancet 1973;2:9.

451. Jones KL. Smith's Recognizable Patterns of Human Malformation. 5th Ed. Philadelphia: Saunders, 1997.

452. AAP Committee on Substance Abuse 1999–2000. Fetal alcohol syndrome & alcohol related neurodevelopmental disorders. Pediatrics 2000;106(2):358–361.

453. Jobe AR. Alcohol as a fetal neurotoxin. J Pediatr 2004; 194(3):338.

454. Mukherjee RAS, Hollins S, Turk J. Fetal alcohol spectrum disorder: an overview. J Roy Soc Med 2006;99:298–302.

455. Jones MW, Bass WT. Fetal alcohol syndrome. Neonatal Netw 2003;22(3):63–70.

456. Day NL, Jasperse D, Richardson G, et al. Prenatal exposure to alcohol: effect of growth & morphologic characteristics. Pediatrics 1989;84(3):536–541.

457. Sokol RJ, Delaney-Black V, Norstrom B. Fetal alcohol spectrum disorder. JAMA 2003;290(22):2996–2999.

458. Koren G, Nulman I, Chudley AE, et al. Fetal alcohol spectrum disorder. Can Med Assoc J 2003;169(11):1181–1185.

459. Kartin D, Grant TM, Streissguth AP, et al. Three-year developmental outcomes in children with prenatal alcohol and drug exposure. Pediatr Phys Ther 2002;14(3):145–153.

460. Gardner J. Fetal alcohol syndrome: recognition and intervention. J Matern Child Nurs 1997;22(6):318–322.

461. Johnson K, Gerada C, Greenough A. Treatment of neonatal abstinence syndrome. Arch Dis Child 2002;F2–F5.

462. AAP Committee on Drugs. Neonatal drug withdrawal. Pediatrics 1998;10:1079–1088.

463. Akera C, Ro S. Medical concerns in the neonatal period. Clin Fam Pract 5(2):265.

464. Wright ML, Robinson MJ. Neonatal abstinence syndrome. Arch Dis Child Fetal Neonatal Ed 1995;73:F122.

465. Bada HS, Bauer CR, Shankaran S, et al. Central and autonomic systems signs with in utero drug exposure. Arch Dis Child Fetal Neonatal Ed 2002;F106–F112.

466. Fike DL. Assessment and management of the substance-exposed infant. In: Kenner C, Lott JW, eds. Comprehensive Neonatal Nursing: A Physiologic Perspective. 3rd Ed. Philadelphia: Saunders, 2003.

467. D'Apolito K. Substance abuse: infant and childhood outcomes. J Pediatr Nurs 1998;13(5):307–316.

468. Finnegan LP, Connaughton JF, Kron RE, et al. Neonatal abstinence syndrome: assessment and management. Addict Dis 1975;2(1–2):141–158.

469. Finnegan LP. Neonatal abstinence syndrome: assessment and pharmacotherapy. In: Rubatelli FF, Granati B, eds. Neonatal Therapy: An Update. New York: Exerpta Medica, 1986.

470. Gilbert WM, Nesbitt TS, Danielsen B. Associated factors in 1611 cases of brachial plexus injury. Obstet Gynecol 1999; 93(4):536–540.

471. Gilbert A, Tassin JC. Obstetrical palsy: clinical, pathologic, and surgical review. In: Terzis JK. ed. Microreconstruction of Nerve Injuries. Philadelphia: WB Saunders, 1987.

472. Kozin SH. Brachial plexus palsy: evaluation & management. Lecture. Philadelphia: Shriner's Hospital for Children, 2001.

473. Kozin SH. Injuries of the brachial plexus. In: Iannotti JP, Williams GR, eds. Disorders of the Shoulder: Diagnosis and Management. Philadelphia: Lippincott Williams & Wilkins, 1999.

474. Piatt JH. Birth injuries of the brachial plexus. Pediatr Clin North Am 2004;51(2):421–440.

475. Eng GD, Koch B, Smokvina MD. Brachial plexus palsy in neonates and children. Arch Phys Med Rehabil 1978;59(10):458–464.

476. Uhing MR. Management of birth injuries. Pediatr Clin North Am 2004;51:1169–1186.

477. Waters PM. Comparison of the natural history, the outcome of microsurgical repair, and the outcome of operative reconstruction in brachial plexus birth palsy. J Bone Joint Surg 1999;81-A:649–659.

478. Donn SM, Fairfax RG. Long-term prognosis for the infant with severe birth trauma. Clin Perinatol 1983;10(2):507–520.

479. Shepard RB. Brachial plexus injury. In: Campbell SK, ed. Decision Making in Pediatric Neurologic Physical Therapy. 2nd Ed. Philadelphia: Church Livingstone, 1999.

480. Norton ES. Development of muscular torticollis and brachial plexus injury. In: Campbell SK, Vander Linden DW, Palisano RJ, eds. Physical Therapy for Children. Philadelphia: Saunders, 2000.

481. American Academy of Pediatrics Committee on Quality Improvement, Subcommittee on Developmental Hip Dysplasia. Clinical practice guidelines: early detection of developmental dysplasia of the hip. Pediatrics 2000;105:896–905.

482. Beaty JH. Congenital anomalies of the lower extremity. In: Canale ST. Campbell's Operative Orthopedics. 10th Ed. St. Louis: Mosby, 2002.

483. Weinstein SL, Mubarak SJ, Wenger DR. Developmental hip dysplasia and dislocation: part I. AAOS Instruct Course Lectures 2004;53:525–530.

484. Ortolani M. Congenital hip dysplasia in the light of early and very early diagnosis. Clin Orthop 1976;11(9):6–10.

485. Barlow TG. Early diagnosis and treatment of congenital dislocation of the hip. J Bone Joint Surg 1962;44B:292–301.

486. Kasser JR. Orthopedic problems. In: Cloherty JP, Eichenwald EC, Stark AR, eds. Manual of Neonatal Care. 5th Ed. Philadelphia: Lippincott Williams & Wilkins, 2004.

487. Guillle JT, Pizzutullo PD, MacEwen GD. Developmental dysplasia of the hip from birth to six months. J Am Acad Orthop Surg 1999;8:232–242.

488. Staheli LT. Fundamentals of Pediatric Orthopedics. 3rd Ed. Philadelphia: Lippincott Williams & Wilkins, 2003.

489. Bleck EE. Metatarsus adductus: classification and relationship to outcomes of treatment. J Pediatr Orthop 1983;3(1):2–9.

490. Bleck EE. Clubfoot. Dev Med Child Neurol 1993;35(10): 927–931.

491. Leach J. Orthopedic conditions. In: Campbell SK, Vander Linden DW, Palisano RJ, eds. Physical Therapy for Children. 2nd Ed. Philadelphia: Saunders, 2000.

492. Bianchi DW, Crumbleholme TM, D'Alton ME. Arthrogryposis. In: Fetology Diagnosis and Management of the Fetal Patient. New York: McGraw-Hill, 2000.

493. Butler J. Assessment and management of the musculoskeletal system. In: Kenner C, Lott JW, eds. Comprehensive Neonatal Nursing: A Physiologic Perspective. 3rd Ed. Philadelphia: Saunders, 2003.

494. Hudgins L, Cassidy SB. Congenital anomalies. In: Fanaroff AA, Martin RJ, eds. Neonatal-Perinatal Medicine Diseases of the Fetus and Infant. 7th Ed. St. Louis: Mosby, 2002.

495. Cooperman DR, Thompson GH. Congenital abnormalities of upper and lower extremities and spine. In: Fanaroff AA, Martin RJ, eds. Neonatal-Perinatal Medicine Diseases of the Fetus and Infant. 7th Ed. St. Louis: Mosby, 2002.

496. American Academy of Pediatrics Committee on Fetus and Newborn. Hospital discharge of the high risk neonate-proposed guidelines. Pediatrics 1998;102(2):411–417.

497. Kenner C, Bagwell GA, Torok LS. Transition to home. In: Kenner C, Lott JW, ed. Comprehensive Neonatal Nursing: A Physiologic Perspective. 3rd Ed. Philadelphia: Saunders, 2003.

498. Zaccagnini L. Discharge planning. In: Cloherty JP, Eichenwald EC, Stark AR, eds. Manual of Neonatal Care. 5th Ed. Philadelphia: Lippincott Williams & Wilkins, 2004.

499. Hack M. The outcomes of neonatal intensive care. In: Klaus MH, Fanaroff AA, eds. Care of the High-Risk Neonate. 5th Ed. Philadelphia: Saunders, 2001.

500. Lockridge T, Taquino LT, Knight A. Back to sleep: is there room in that crib for both AAP recommendations and developmentally supportive care? Neonatal Netw 1999;18(5):29–33.

501. Bailey DB, Hebbeler K, Scarborough A, et al. First experiences with early intervention: a national perspective. Pediatrics 2004;113(4):887–896.

502. Hack MB, Wilson-Costello D, Friedman H, et al. Neurodevelopmental predictors of outcomes of children with birth weight of less than 1000 grams: 1992–1995. Arch Pediatr Adolesc Med 2000;154(7):725–751.

503. Vohr BR, O'Shea M, Wright LL. Longitudinal multicenter follow-up of high-risk infants: why, who, when, and what to assess. Semin Perinatol 2003;27(4):333–342.

504. Vohr B. Overview of infants and children with hearing loss. Part 1. Ment Retard Dev Disabil Res Rev 2003;9(2):62–64.

505. Vohr B. Infants and children with hearing loss. Part 2. Overview. Ment Retard Dev Disabil Res Rev 2003;9(4):218–219.

506. Bear LM. Early identification of infants at risk for developmental disabilities. Pediatr Clin North Am 2004;51:685–701.

507. Wood NS, Marlow N, Costloe K, et al. Neurologic and developmental disability after extremely premature birth. N Engl J Med 2000;343(6):378–384.

508. Bennett FC. Perspective: low birth weight infants: accomplishments, risks, and interventions. Infants Young Child 2002;15(1):vi–ix.

509. Wolf MJ, Koldewijn K, Beelen A, et al. Neurobehavioral and developmental profile of very low birthweight preterm infants in early infancy. Acta Paediatr 2002;91:930–938.

510. Stewart JE. Follow-up of very-low-birth-weight infants. In: Cloherty JP, Eichenwald EC, Stark AR. Manual Neonatal Care. 5th Ed. Philadelphia: Lippincott Williams & Wilkins, 2004.

511. Davis DW. Cognitive outcomes in school-age children born prematurely. Neonatal Netw 2003;22(3):27–38.

512. Foulder-Hughes LA, Cooke RW. Motor, cognitive, and behavioral disorders in children born very preterm. Dev Med Child Neurol 2003;45(2):97–103.

513. Pinto-Martin J, Whitaker A, Feldman J, et al. Special education services and school performance in a regional cohort of low-birthweight infants at age nine. Pediatr Perinatal Epidemiol 2004;18:120–129.

514. Latal-Hajnal B, von Siebenthal K, Kovari H, et al. Postnatal growth in VLBW infants: significant association with neurodevelopmental outcome. J Pediatr 2003;143(2):163–170.

515. Smith VC, Zupanicic JA, McCormick MC, et al. Rehospitalization in the first year of life among infants with bronchopulmonary dysplasia. J Pediatr 2004;144(6):799–803.

516. McCormick MC. The outcomes of very low birth weight infants: are we asking the right questions? Pediatrics 1997;99(6):869–875.

517. Weisglas-Kuperus N, Baerts W, Smrkovsky M, et al. Effects of biological and social development of very low birth weight children. Pediatrics 1993;92(5):658–665.

RECOMMENDED READINGS

Brazelton TB, Nugent JK. Neonatal Behavioral Assessment Scale. 3rd Ed. London: Mac Keith Press, 1995.

Cloherty JP, Eichenwald EC, Stark AR, eds. Manual of Neonatal Care. 5th Ed. Philadelphia: Lippincott Williams & Wilkins, 2004.

Goldson E. Nurturing the Premature Infant. London: Oxford University Press, 1999.

Hunter JG. Neonatal intensive care unit. In: Case-Smith J, ed. Occupational Therapy for Children. 4th Ed. St. Louis: Mosby, 2001.

Kenner C, Lott JW, eds. Comprehensive Neonatal Nursing A Physiologic Perspective. 3rd Ed. Philadelphia: Saunders, 2003.

Kenner C, McGrath JM, eds. Developmental Care of Newborns and Infants A Guide for Health Professionals. Philadelphia: Elsevier, 2004.

Mercer RT. Nursing Care for Parents at Risk. Thorofare, NJ: Charles B. Slack Inc, 1977.

Sweeney J. Practice guidelines for the physical therapist in the neonatal intensive care unit (NICU). Pediatr Phys Ther 1999;11(3):119–132.

Sweeney JK, Swanson MW. Low birth weight infants: neonatal care and follow-up. In: Umphred DA, ed. Neurological Rehabilitation. 4th Ed. St. Louis: Mosby, 2001.

Vergara ER, Bigsby R. Developmental and Therapeutic Interventions in the NICU. Baltimore: Paul H Brookes Publishing Co, 2004.

Volpe JJ. Neurology of the Newborn. 4th Ed. Philadelphia: Saunders, 2001.

Zaichkin J. Newborn Intensive Care What Every Parent Needs to Know. 2nd Ed. Santa Rosa, CA: NICU Ink Book Publishers, 2002.

Common Abbreviations

A	Apnea
ABG	Arterial blood gas
AGA	Appropriate for gestational age
AOP	Apnea of prematurity
APIB	Assessment of Preterm Infant Behavior
AROM	Artificial rupture of membranes
B	Bradycardia
BAER	Brainstem auditory-evoked potentials
BPD	Bronchopulmonary dysplasia
BPI	Brachial plexus injury
BW	Birth weight
CDH	Congenital diaphragmatic hernia
CHD	Congenital heart disease
CHD	Congenital hip dysplasia
CLD	Chronic lung disease
CMV	Conventional mechanical ventilation
CMV	Cytomegalovirus
CPAP	Continuous positive airway pressure
CS	Cesarean section
D	Desaturation
DOL	Day of life
ECMO	Extracorporeal membrane oxygenation
EGA	Estimated gestational age
ELBW	Extremely low birth weight
FAS	Fetal alcohol syndrome
FiO_2	Fraction of inspired oxygen
FT	Full term
G	Gravida
GA	Gestational age
GBS	Group B streptococcus
GER	Gastroesophageal reflux
GM	Germinal matrix
GMA	General Movement Assessment
HAL	Hyperalimentation
HC	Head circumference
HFFI	High-frequency flow interruption
HFJV	High-frequency jet ventilation

HFOV	High-frequency oscillatory ventilation
HFV	High-frequency ventilation
HIE	Hypoxic–ischemic encephalopathy
HMD	Hyaline membrane disease
HR	Heart rate
ICH	Intracranial hemorrhage
ICN	Intensive care nursery
IDVA	Intravenous drug abuse
IMD	Infant of diabetic mother
IMV	Intermittent mandatory ventilation
iNO	Inspired nitric oxide
IVH	Intraventricular hemorrhage
IUGR	Intrauterine growth retardation
LBW	Low birth weight
LGA	Large for gestational age
MAS	Meconium aspiration syndrome
MCA	Multiple congenital anomalies
MV	Mechanical ventilation
NAPI	Neurobehavioral Assessment of the Preterm Infant
NAS	Neonatal abstinence syndrome/neonatal abstinence scale
NBAS	Neonatal Neurobehavioral Assessment Scale
NC	Nasal cannula
NEC	Necrotizing enterocolitis
NICU	Neonatal intensive care unit
NIDCAP	Newborn Individualized Developmental Care and Assessment Program
NNNS	Neonatal Intensive Care Network Neurobehavioral Scale
NJ	Nasal gastric
NO	Nitric oxide
NP	Nasal prongs
OC	Open crib
OD	Right eye
OG	Oral gastric
OS	Left eye
P	Para
PCA	Postconceptual age

PDA	Patent ductus arteriosus
PEEP	Positive end-expiratory pressure
PHI	Periventricular hemorrhage infarction
PIE	Pulmonary interstitial emphysema
PO	By mouth
PPHN	Persistent pulmonary hypertension of the newborn
PPV	Positive pressure ventilation
PROM	Premature rupture of membranes
PT	Preterm
PTL	Preterm labor
PVD	Posthemorrhagic ventricular dilation
PVL	Periventricular leukomalacia
RDS	Respiratory distress syndrome

ROM	Rupture of membranes
ROP	Retinopathy of prematurity
RR	Respiratory rate
SaO_2	Oxygen saturation
SGA	Small for gestational age
SIMV	Synchronized intermittent mechanical ventilation
TORCH	Congenital viral infections (toxoplasmosis, other infections, rubella, cytomegalovirus, herpes)
TPF	Toxoplasmosis fetalis
TPN	Total parental nutrition
TTN	Transient tachypnea of the newborn
UAC	Umbilical arterial catheter
US	Ultrasound
UVC	Umbilical venous catheter
VLBW	Very low birth weight

Equipment Resources

Children's Medical Ventures
275 Longwater Drive
Norwell, MA 02061
888-766-8443 (Parents)
800-345-6443 (Hospitals)
866-866-6750 (Education)
www.childmed.com

Small Beginnings Inc.
17525 Alder Street
Suite #28
Hesperia, CA 92345
800-676-0462
www.small-beginnings.com

The Infant and Child with Cerebral Palsy

Jane Styer-Acevedo

Definition

Various authors agree that cerebral palsy is an umbrella term covering a group of nonprogressive but often changing motor impairment syndromes that may or may not involve sensory deficits, that are caused by a nonprogressive defect, lesion, or anomaly of the developing brain, and that can be in part a developmental diagnosis.[1–4]

Incidence

The U.S. Collaborative Perinatal Project conducted by the National Institute of Neurologic and Communicative Disorders and Stroke is known as a landmark study and is still referred to in studies done today.[5] It was a study of 54,000 pregnant women from 12 urban teaching hospitals in the United States between 1959 and 1966. Of the women in the study, 46% were white, 46% were black, and most of the rest were Puerto Rican. The socioeconomic status of the sample was lower than that of the general population. The children born to these women had a regular schedule of examinations, including a general physical examination and a neurologic examination at both 1 and 7 years of age. Among the 38,533 children whose outcome was known at 7 years of age, 202 met criteria for cerebral palsy (CP). Of the 202 children, 24 (12%) children had an acquired motor deficit secondary to a variety of factors in the early developing years, rather than congenital motor deficits occurring as a result of in utero factors or events at the time of labor and delivery. Infectious meningitis and trauma were the most common causes of acquired CP. In addition to the 202 children with CP who were alive at 7 years of age, 24 children with CP, most commonly with spastic quadriplegia, had died before 7 years of age. The following figures indicate the prevalence of CP based on the National Collaborative Perinatal Project:

5.2:1000—diagnosed as having CP
4.6:1000—when acquired cases of CP are excluded
2.6:1000—excluding mildly afflicted children (This figure more closely represents the prevalence of handicapping congenital CP.)

Further study of the population in the U.S. Collaborative Perinatal Project indicated that there are "relatively low risks for cerebral palsy (1.3 to 2.9 per 1000) among children who had no abnormal signs, whether or not they had seizures in the nursery period."[6]

The more recent studies on the incidence of cerebral palsy prove it to be 2 to 2.5 per 1000 live births in the United States, the United Kingdom, Western Australia, and Sweden.[1,4,7] The survival of infants has improved over time but the prevalence of cerebral palsy has remained the same with little change over the past 40 years. This is thought to be due to the increase in cerebral palsy within the population of preterm and very preterm infants.[1,7,8] The reported prevalence rate in twins is said to be 15 per 1000 live births, in triplets it is 80 per 1000 live births, and in quadruplets it is 43 per 1000 live births.[8] In a British survey, it was shown that 100% of children noted to have cerebral palsy in 1970 were still alive 10 years later, an increase in the numbers from the first survey done in 1958.[1]

Etiology

There has been no evidence of increased duration of survival of infants since the 1950s despite advances in medical care.[1] More than 100 years ago, Freud recognized that problems in prenatal development might lead to perinatal distress.[2] There is no one specific cause of the constellation of symptoms known as cerebral palsy. Rather, the potential causes of cerebral palsy are known to occur in the antenatal or prenatal stage of development and are also grouped with congenital problems in the perinatal or neonatal time period, and in the postnatal or postneonatal time period.[7,8]

Miller lists several possible congenital problems that can result in the infant and child with cerebral palsy. These include schizencephaly, a segmental defect that causes a cleft in the brain; lissencephaly, a defect in the neuronal migration that normally goes toward the periphery of the brain but which then results in a smooth brain, also known as decreased cerebral gyri; microcephaly and megalocephaly; cortical dysgenesis, a disorder of brain cortex formation; and defects in the normal formation and remodeling of synapses.[8] According to Hadders-Algra, approximately

half of the created neurons die off (apoptosis), in particular during midgestation. Axons and synapses are also eliminated during normal development for the first decade or more. This shaping of the nervous system is guided by neurochemical processes and neural activity. The neural elements that best persist are those that fit the environment.[9] Therefore, when there are changes in the formation of the developing nervous system, the result can be an infant with cerebral palsy. However, the immature brain has much more plasticity or equipotentiality, terms used to define the greater ability of the uninjured part to assume the function of the injured part of the brain.[8] Therefore, the response to injury is much different and makes diagnosis and prognosis difficult.

Prenatal events are thought to be responsible for about 75% of all cerebral palsy. Perinatal asphyxia is thought to cause 6% to 8% of cerebral palsy, with the underlying causes being unpreventable. And 10% to 18% of cerebral palsy is thought to be caused postnatally.[7] The cause of cerebral palsy in the majority of infants born at term in developing countries is found to be due to prenatal influences and is not associated with significant neonatal encephalopathy.[3] For a more complete list of the antenatal causes of cerebral palsy, refer to Display 5.1; for the perinatal causes, refer to Display 5.2; and for the postneonatally acquired causes, refer to Display 5.3.

Typically, one may see risk factors present in the infant or fetus (via medical testing) that may indicate a potential problem. Risk factors can be present before or during pregnancy, during labor and birthing, and in the period shortly after the birth of the infant.[7] Refer to Displays 5.4 through 5.8 for comprehensive lists of these risk factors.

Diagnosis and Prognosis

Predicting the long-term outcome of infants in the neonatal period continues to be difficult based on the available testing and data and the knowledge that developing brains are more plastic than mature brains and may change unexpectedly during growth and development. Physicians tend to be very cautious in their diagnosis of cerebral palsy and usually wait until the infant reaches at least 12 months of

---

⟩⟩ DISPLAY 5.1

Antenatal Causes of Cerebral Palsy

Vascular events such as a middle cerebral artery infarct

Maternal infections during the first and second trimesters such as rubella, cytomegalovirus, and toxoplasmosis

Less common: metabolic disorders, maternal ingestion of toxins, and rare genetic syndromes

Perinatal Causes of Cerebral Palsy

Problems During Labor and Delivery
Obstructed labor
Antepartum hemorrhage
Cord prolapse

These require that essential criteria be fulfilled for this diagnosis including neonatal encephalopathy

Other Neonatal Causes
Hypoxic–ischemic encephalopathy
Neonatal stroke, usually of the middle cerebral artery
Severe hypoglycemia
Untreated jaundice
Severe neonatal infection

Risk Factors Present Before Pregnancy

Maternal Factors
Delayed onset of menstruation
Irregular menstruation
Long intermenstrual intervals
Unusually short or long interval between pregnancies
Low social class in children with normal birth weight
Parity of three or more in preterm infants
Relationship with previous fetal deaths

Medical Conditions
Intellectual disability
Seizures
Thyroid disease

Paternal and Sibling Factors
Advanced paternal age (seen more frequently in those with athetoid dystonic cerebral palsy)
Motor deficit in sibling

age before making a definitive diagnosis. When possible, neurologic testing and neuroimaging studies are used to enhance the understanding of the infant's movements or lack of movements and the possible prognosis. Seventy percent to 90% of children with cerebral palsy have been found to have abnormalities on a brain magnetic resonance image (MRI).[2] Term infants studied between days 2 and 8 of life who were found to have abnormalities of the basal ganglia and thalamus on MRI showed strong association with adverse outcomes including the diagnosis of cerebral palsy.[3]

The most extensively studied neuroimaging modality today is cranial ultrasound, especially for the high-risk preterm infant.[2,3] Ultrasound studies are done via the anterior fontanelle and can therefore be used until the fontanelle closes, generally until the infant reaches about 1 year of age. Hemorrhages occur in the ventricles and periventricular white matter of the brain, as can be viewed through the anterior fontanelle. Hemorrhages are labeled as intraventricular hemorrhage (IVH), bleeding into the ventricles; germinal matrix hemorrhage (GMH), bleeding into the tissue around the ventricles; periventricular intraventricular hemorrhage (PIVH), bleeding into both areas; and periventricular cyst (PVC), which form in these same areas as the acute hemorrhage resolves.[8] There are some known risk factors for developing hemorrhages, which include an infant of younger gestational age and an infant requiring mechanical ventilation.[8] Hemorrhages are graded I through IV, IV being the most severe bleed. It is generally believed that grades I through IV bleeds do not have good predictive values for the development of cerebral palsy.[8] Palmer indicated that cranial ultrasound should be used for low-birth-weight infants to detect grades III and IV hemorrhages,

Postneonatally Acquired Cerebral Palsy

Metabolic Encephalopathy
Storage disorders
Intermedullary metabolism disorders
Metabolic metabolism
Miscellaneous disorders
Toxicity such as alcohol

Infections
Meningitis
Septicemia
Malaria (in developing countries)

Injuries
Cerebrovascular accident
Following surgery for congenital malformations
Near-drowning
Trauma
Motor vehicle accident
Child abuse such as shaken baby syndrome

Risk Factors During Pregnancy

Pre-eclampsia in term infants but not in preterm infants
Multiple pregnancies associated with:
    Preterm delivery
    Poor intrauterine growth
    Birth defects
    Intrapartum complications

IVH, cystic periventricular leukomalacia (PVL), and ventricular enlargement as these can be indicative of future problems.[3] At term age, cranial ultrasound is used to identify cystic PVL and ventriculomegaly, which are associated with subsequent development of cerebral palsy.[3,7] This is suggestive of an adverse event occurring well before delivery.[7] Infants and children with white matter injury, primarily PVL, can demonstrate mild to severe neurologic dysfunction. Often spastic diplegia is noted with lower extremity spasticity, truncal hypotonia, and upper extremity athetosis or dystonia.[2]

It is understood that a neurologic examination alone is insufficiently sensitive enough or specific enough for early detection of cerebral palsy.[3] Doctors and researchers are looking at the quality of an infant's "general movements" (GMs) to evaluate brain function.[3,9] A study done by Ferrari et al. included 84 preterm infants studied at 16 to 20 weeks'

postterm age and found abnormalities in the GMs. When there was a predominance of cramped synchronous GMs and absence of normal fidgety movements of limbs, neck, and trunk, it was predictive of CP at 2 to 3 years of age with a sensitivity of 100% and a specificity of 92.5% to 100%.[3] The presence of definitely abnormal GMs at the fidgety age (2 to 4 months postterm) implies a total absence of the elegant, dancing complexity of fidgety movements and predicts CP with an accuracy of 85% to 98%.[9] GMs can be predictive of later cerebral palsy and are the best expression of functional motor development. They are analogous to later functional motor milestones and may also predict severity, as the earlier the abnormality is recognized, the more severe the later limitations in motor function.[3] According to these observations and clinical testing, it warrants referral for therapeutic intervention to improve the infant's later function.[9]

Miller has found that children who are walking at age of 7 years should continue to walk equally well after their completion of growth. Therefore, he encourages one to look at the child walking and not at the child's reflexes to predict the child's future function.[8]

Others have found cognitive abilities to be linked with the severity of the cerebral palsy and to be predictive of many outcomes.[1,10] Katz reported on a study of the Australian registry of 2014 children with cerebral palsy completed by Blaire et al. in 2001, which indicated that intellectual disability was the single strongest predictor of survival of the child with cerebral palsy (profoundly mentally retarded children with CP do not live into adulthood) and that the second most important factor impacting life expectancy was the severity of the physical impairments.[1] Katz researched the life expectancy of children with cerebral palsy and found, from multiple sources, that the causes of mortality related most commonly to the respiratory and circulatory systems, certain cancers, and neurologic complications, specifically surgery and hydrocephalus.[1]

Classification

There are multiple ways to classify infants and children with cerebral palsy, including topography, what body parts are affected; types, describing the predominant characteristics of the motor findings; severity; pathology; and cerebral imaging techniques.[11,12] The classification that tends to be most useful to the physical therapist is the classification of type, describing the predominant characteristics of the motor findings. This author will present here the type of cerebral palsy and then further classify the types according to what body parts are affected by the particular characteristic.

The usual classification of types includes spastic, dyskinetic and movement disorders, ataxic, and hypotonic.[1,2,8,10,12] Most authors agree that the predominant type of cerebral palsy is of the spastic classification, making up about 70% of all children with cerebral palsy.[1,12] The second most common type of cerebral palsy is athetosis or the dyskinetic form, involving about 20% of children with cerebral palsy. Ataxic cerebral palsy makes up the remaining 10% of the population with cerebral palsy. There are many children with mixed types of cerebral palsy who do not fit clearly into one of these classifications but rather have characteristics of more than one type of cerebral palsy.[1,10,12]

Within the type known as spastic, one finds classifications known as diplegic CP, where both legs are affected and are more affected than both the arms; hemiplegic CP, where one side of the body (either the arm may be more involved than the leg on the same side or the leg may be more involved than the arm on the same side) is more affected than the other side; and quadriplegic CP (less frequently referred to as tetraplegia), where all four limbs are affected.[1,2,8,10,12] The combination of diplegic, hemiplegic, and quadriplegic CP makes up about 75% of all children with cerebral palsy.[12] A correlation between clinical findings and neuroanatomy is possible to a limited degree. According to Howle, a white matter infarct in the periventricular areas caused by hypoxia can lead to spastic diplegic CP. Periventricular atrophy is the most common abnormality found in preterm infants who develop hemiplegic CP, as noted by Howle.[12] Some clinicians use the topography classification of double hemiplegia to describe a child whose four limbs are involved but who clearly has one side of the body more involved than the other side.[8,12] One might also find the characteristics of monoplegia (one extremity only involved) and triplegia (three extremities involved), but this is not common.

Dyskinesia and movement disorders are a group of disorders where the movement is generally uncontrolled and involuntary and includes athetosis, rigidity, tremor, dystonia, ballismus, and choreoathetosis.[1,2,8,10,12] Athetosis always has involuntary movements that are slow and writhing; abnormal in timing, direction, and spatial characteristics; and usually are large motions of the more proximal joints.[1,8,12] Rigidity is much less common and is felt as resistance to both active and passive movement and is not velocity dependent.[12] Tremor, a rhythmic movement of small magnitude, usually of the smaller joints, rarely occurs as an isolated type in CP but rather in combination with athetosis or ataxia.[8,12] Dystonia is a slow motion with a torsional element that may involve one limb or the entire body and in which the pattern itself may change over time.[8] Ballismus is the most rare movement disorder and involves random motion in large, fast patterns usually of a single limb.[8] Choreoathetosis involves jerky movement, commonly of the digits and varying in the range of motion.[8,10]

Ataxic CP is primarily a disorder of balance and control in the timing of coordinated movements along with weakness, incoordination, a wide-based gait, and a noted tremor.[1,12] This type of CP results from deficits in the cerebellum and often occurs in combination with spasticity and athetosis.[12]

Hypotonic CP can be permanent but is more often transient in the evolution of athetosis or spasticity and might not represent a specific type of CP.[12] Hypotonia has not been correlated with a particular neural lesion.

Classifying an infant or child according to the severity of the cerebral palsy can be helpful when looking at prognosis. The Gross Motor Function Classification System (GMFCS) was developed to fill the need to have a standardized system to measure the "severity of movement disability" in children with cerebral palsy.[8,13] There are five levels in the test. Level I describes the child with the most independent function, where he or she can perform all the activities of his or her age-matched peers, albeit with some difficulty with speed, coordination, and balance. Level V describes the child who has difficulty controlling his or her head and trunk posture in most positions and in achieving any voluntary control of movement.[12,13] According to Howle, Beckung and Hagberg[12] described a Bimanual Fine Motor Function Classification System (BFMFCS), which is similar to the GMFCS and has a five-level scale. There is a strong correlation between the GMFCS and the BFMFCS, indicating that the severity of gross and fine motor function runs in parallel.[12]

Associated Problems

Frequently the child with cerebral palsy will have a sensory processing dysfunction. Three sites of central nervous system damage result in primary sensory processing dysfunctions and are often associated with CP.[14]

1. The cerebellum is a major sensory processing center, and when impaired, it will result in ataxia.
2. The cortical–basal ganglia–thalamic loop is a sensory and motor feedforward and feedback circuit and when impaired, results in athetosis.

3. The cerebral cortex and pyramidal tracts, when impaired, result in spasticity as the pyramidal system plays an important role in regulating sensory information.

The sensory deficits in infants and children with cerebral palsy may be primary or secondary and should always be addressed in the treatment program. Cooper et al.[15] found significant bilateral sensory deficits in children, with hemiplegia with stereognosis and proprioception the chief modalities affected bilaterally.[15]

Beckung and Hagberg[16] evaluated children between the ages of 5 and 8 years who had cerebral palsy. They found that 40% of the children had mental retardation, which, when combined with the slow learners and persons with learning disabilities, increased to 75% (refer to Display 5.9 for the categories of intellectual disability/mental retardation); epilepsy occurred in 35% of the population; visual impairment in 20%; and hydrocephalus in 9%. Thirteen percent of the children had a combination of two impairments and 15% had a combination of three impairments.[16] Additional associated problems include difficulty with speech in 25% and hearing impairments in 25%.[4] Stiller et al.[4] found an increased frequency of visual impairments, as high as 40% to 50% in children with cerebral palsy.

Liptak and Accardo[10] referred to studies done by Goodman (1996) and Graham and Goodman (1998), which looked at the specific impairments relating to the child with hemiplegia. These include emotional disorders in 25%, conduct disorders in 24%, pervasive hyperactivity in 10%, and situational hyperactivity in 13%.[10] He also referred to secondary conditions in associated problems as nonmedical outcomes, listing lack of mobility, incontinence, and relative social isolation.[10]

Older individuals with athetoid CP are at risk for acquiring devastating neurologic deficits owing to disc degeneration and instability in their cervical spines. After radiologic study of 180 patients, Harada and associates found that disc degeneration occurred earlier and progressed more rapidly in subjects with athetoid CP than in those without CP. Advanced disc degeneration was found in 51% of those studied, which is eight times the typical frequency.[17] Individuals with athetosis typically initiate and attempt control of movement with the jaw and head. This eventually causes the musculoskeletal changes noted on radiographic studies.

Assessment of the Infant and Child with Cerebral Palsy

There is disagreement in the literature and in practice regarding how early an infant can be diagnosed with cerebral palsy. Burns and colleagues believe that a diagnosis of very mild cerebral palsy should be possible at 8 months of age.[18] Identification depends on a combination of suspicious and abnormal signs revealed during comprehensive assessment of motor attainments, neurologic signs, primitive reflexes, and postural reactions.

Infants and children with persistent subtle or mild signs should be monitored closely until the possible outcome is clear.[18] Harris, using the Movement Assessment in Infants (MAI), found that certain items can help distinguish the infant with cerebral palsy from the nonhandicapped infant at 4 months of age.[19] Items of diagnostic value include neck hyperextension and shoulder retraction, ability to bear weight on the forearms while prone, ability to maintain a stable head position in supported or independent sitting, and the infant's ability to flex the hips actively against gravity.[19,20] Seven of the 17 MAI items that Harris found to be highly significant predictors are observational items. Both Harris and Milani-Comparetti found that watching the infant move against gravity is of greater diagnostic value than intrusive handling or attempts to stimulate a response.[19,20] Harris compared the diagnostic value of the MAI with the Bayley Scales in infants at 4 months of age and found that the MAI was more sensitive than the Bayley Scales.[19] However, the Bayley Motor Scale was extremely sensitive at 1 year of age. Rose-Jacobs et al. evaluated whether the MAI predicted 2-year cognitive and motor development status measured by the Mental and Psychomotor Scales of the Bayley Scales of Infant Development.[21] They found that the MAI appears to be valid for use with infants born at term who are at risk of developmental delay. This test may be a useful tool to help clinicians make decisions about the provision of intervention services. Nelson and Ellenberg[22] studied children who were diagnosed with CP at 1 year of age who subsequently "outgrew the cerebral palsy." They found that children with mild motor impairment at 1 year of age and those thought to have CP were all free of CP by the age of 7. However, all who were diagnosed with severe CP, and many with moderate CP, still carried the same diagnosis at the age of 7. Those who "outgrew" the CP were likely to have neurologic problems, such as mental retardation, nonfebrile seizures, or difficulty with speech articulation.[22] These findings substantiate the fact that any infant or child who demonstrates neurologic or behavioral abnormalities should undergo follow-up until early school age.

In order to understand the atypical movement and motor control that occurs in children with cerebral palsy, the therapist must understand the acquisition of motor control against gravity, the development of postural control, and

Nutrition for the Child with Cerebral Palsy

Susan Boyden, MS, RD, LDN
Clinical Dietitian
The Children's Hospital of Philadelphia

Nutrition-Related Problems	Interventions
GASTROINTESTINAL (GI) ISSUES/RISKS	
• Constipation	Ensure adequate fiber and fluids
• Gastroesophageal reflux	Small frequent feedings
	May require concentrated formula or calorie additives
	May require medication
• Aspiration	Tube feedings
	Thickened liquids
	Mechanically altered diet
Drug–nutrient interaction	Dietary assessment for adequacy of vitamins D, K, C, B$_{12}$, folate,
• Anticonvulsant therapy	calcium intake. If long-term use consider dual-energy X-ray absorptiometry (DEXA) scan to assess bone density
FEEDING DIFFICULTIES	
• Inadequate oral motor skills	Oral motor evaluation
• Chewing	Feeding team referral (if available)*
• Sucking	Nutrition evaluation for adequacy of diet/fluids
• Swallowing	
• Tongue thrust	
• Sucking/breathing coordination	
• Excessive drooling	
• Paresis	
• Poor dentition	Dental evaluation
• Extended meal times	Limit meals to 30 minutes
	Calorie-dense foods
	Nutritional supplements
• Feeding refusals/aversions	Feeding team referral (if available)*
INADEQUATE NEUROMOTOR/MUSCULAR SKILLS	
• Eye–hand coordination	Occupational therapy referral
• Head, trunk control	Adaptive feeding equipment
• Positioning	Physical therapy evaluation
INADEQUATE GROWTH	
• Inadequate calorie intake	Nutrition evaluation and intervention
• Increased calorie requirements	Calorie-dense foods
• Athetosis	Nutritional supplements
• Hypertonicity	Tube feedings
• Infections	
• Pressure sores	May require increased protein, vitamins A, C, zinc
• GI issues/risks	(See above)
• Mental retardation	Speech therapy referral
• Unable to communicate food preferences/requests	
• Pain issues	Medication
• Recent surgery	Child life therapy
	Music therapy

(continued)

> ## Nutrition for the Child with Cerebral Palsy (Continued)
>
> | Nutrition Related Problems | Interventions |
> |---|---|
> | **OBESITY** | |
> | • Decreased mobility | Physical therapy program |
> | | Limit juice/soda |
> | | Decrease high-fat/calorie foods |
> | | Increase intake of fruits, vegetables |
>
> *Feeding teams provide interdisciplinary evaluations for children with feeding and swallowing disorders. Specially trained team members may include physicians, nurses, dietitians, speech/language pathologists, physical therapists, occupational therapists, social workers, case managers, and psychologists.
>
> ### SUGGESTED READINGS
> Cloud HH. Developmental disabilities. In: Samour PQ, Helm KK, Lang CE, eds. Handbook of Pediatric Nutrition. 2nd Ed. New York: Aspen Publishers, Inc., 1999:293–313.
> Ekvall SW. Pediatric nutrition in chronic diseases and developmental disorders. In: Bandini L, Patterson B, Ekvall SW, eds. Cerebral Palsy. New York: Oxford University Press, 1993:93–98.
> Mascarenhas MR, et al. Nutritional assessment in pediatrics. Nutrition 1998;14:105–115.

the musculoskeletal development in typically developing children. This information can be found in Chapter 2. Atypical development has been described by multiple authors, including sources cited in this chapter.[23–26]

The purpose of the assessment is to discover the functional abilities and strengths of the child, determine the primary and secondary impairments (compensations used because of the primary impairments), and discover the desired functional and participation outcomes of the child and/or family. The therapist must use an organized approach to the observation of, interaction with, and handling of the child in order to get an accurate baseline of the child's functional abilities. Display 5.10 is a suggested organization for an assessment according to the Neuro-Developmental Treatment Association Instructor's Group to document the assessment findings and plan of care.[12]

ASSESSMENT OF MOVEMENT

Much of the information about an infant or child's movement and posture can be gathered by observing the child when he or she enters the treatment area. The infant and child can also be observed while taking a history and discussing with the parents the various concerns that have brought them to a habilitation or rehabilitation program.

Observation of the baby or young child being held in the arms or lap of the parent or caregiver can reveal important information. The following questions may be answered through observation:

1. How does the mother hold the baby? Does she support the head and trunk, or does she hold the baby at the pelvis?
2. Are the baby's head and trunk rotated or collapsed consistently to one side?
3. Do the baby's arms come forward to hold the mother or play with a toy in midline? Are the arms held behind the body with the scapulae adducted, or are the arms flexed and adducted against the trunk?
4. While being held, does the baby thrust backward into trunk extension or collapse forward into trunk flexion?
5. How are the lower extremities held: Are they adducted tightly in extension or are they floppy in flexion and abduction?
6. Is there isolated movement at the toes or ankles, or are the ankles held in plantar flexion or dorsiflexion? Is the foot everted or inverted, and are the toes held loosely or tightly curled?

This type of observational analysis is not limited to the child held in the parent's arms. When the child comes at the physical therapist in a wheelchair, there are additional questions that may add to the baseline information.

1. Did the child independently propel the wheelchair, or did someone help him or her?
2. In addition to mobility, does the wheelchair provide total postural support for major segments of the body? If the segments are free of support from the wheelchair, are those segments of the body in good postural alignment and do they move freely?
3. Does the child tend to thrust backward in the chair into trunk extension? Is the pelvis positioned in a posterior or an anterior tilt? If the child does posture him- or herself in this manner, is there similar thrusting and tightness in the extremities?

DISPLAY 5.10

Organization for an Assessment of the Infant and Child with Cerebral Palsy (based on the Neurodevelopmental Treatment Approach Model of Assessment)

Data Collection

Date of birth

Date of assessment

Chronologic age/adjusted age

Reason for referral

Relevant medical history

Overview of function (a few sentences)

Family and environmental characteristics

Contextual factors (conditions and restraints on function)
  Assistive technology/adaptive equipment

Examination

Morphology

Functional skills and the capacity for change
  Gross motor control
  Communications
  Fine motor control
  Social skills/control of behavior

Objective test results

Observation of posture and movement

Individual system review related to function
  Neuromuscular
  Musculoskeletal
  Sensory
  Respiratory

Cardiovascular
Integumentary
Gastrointestinal
Perceptual/cognitive
Regulatory

Evaluation

List client's competencies

Areas of concern
  System impairments
  Ineffective posture and movement
  Functional limitations
  Barriers to participation

Analyze each level and how they interrelate, creating the functional limitations of the client

Analyze the potential for change according to the findings

Plan of Care

Specify the anticipated goals and expected outcomes (long term and short term)

Specify frequency and duration of intervention

Strategies of intervention

Role of client, family, and other medical and educational professionals

Client-centered programs as appropriate

Measures to promote health, wellness, and fitness

Schedule for re-examination

---

4. Is the child seated in a reasonably symmetric position or are there significant asymmetries in the posture?
5. Does the child seem comfortable in the chair?

Children with less severe movement disorders may ambulate into the department. The following group of questions will be helpful in assessing the quality of movement of the ambulatory child.

1. Did the child ambulate with or without an assistive device, such as a walker, cane, or crutches?
2. Did the child need physical assistance from another person while ambulating?
3. Is the child's gait pattern stable, and is the child safe?
4. When assessing spatial and temporal parameters such as length of step, stance time, swing time, or base of support, is the gait pattern generally symmetric or asymmetric?
5. Does the child's trunk collapse into lateral flexion on weight bearing on one or both legs, or is the trunk maintained in proper antigravity extension?

6. Does the child have a heel–toe gait pattern? Does the child stand on the balls of the feet?
7. Are the hips and knees locked or stuck in extension during stance phase, or are they falling into gravity or pulled into flexion with the child in a crouched position?

In addition to the gross observational assessment described, the therapist should examine individual aspects of motor function as part of the overall evaluation of the child. The therapist should begin with the level of function appropriate to the child's age and functional ability. The following list of positions provides a guideline by which to assess functional antigravity control:

- Supine
- Prone
- Side-lying
- Sitting—short sit, long sit, side sit, ring sit
- Quadruped
- Kneeling

- Half-kneeling
- Standing
- Walking

If the child possesses higher level skills, the evaluation should be extended to include the following:

- Climbing stairs
- Navigating ramps or curbs
- Unilateral stance
- Running
- Jumping
- Hopping
- Galloping
- Skipping

The child who functions from a wheelchair should be evaluated via observation in terms of the following parameters:

- Alignment and mobility of body
- Shifting of weight
- Propulsion of wheelchair
- Management of wheelchair and its parts
- Transfer to and from wheelchair

ASSESSMENT OF POSTURAL CONTROL

Historically, posture was defined through reflex terminology and facilitated through controlled sensory feedback.[27] Infants were evaluated for the presence or absence of and the strength of primitive reflexes. The reflexes were thought to "integrate" as the infant developed. Therapists utilized stimulation of and feedback from optical righting, labyrinthine righting, neck righting, body righting on the head, and body righting on the body to facilitate normal righting and equilibrium responses in the clients.[27] In treatment, lower level reflexes were inhibited to decrease the abnormal sensory feedback and facilitate the emergence and integration of the righting and equilibrium responses.

According to more recent motor science studies, the human system is no longer thought to function via a hierarchical model. Various systems models are used currently to describe the organization and functions of the nervous system.[27]

In assessing postural control of the infant and child with cerebral palsy, it is important to understand several concepts. Postural activity is noted when the child has muscle activation against the supporting surface.[28] An example would be the infant, at 7 to 9 months of age, who has just learned how to gain stability in sitting by pushing his or her legs into the floor. The arms and hands are now free to explore toys and play, as they are no longer needed for propping. Postural preparations are strategies that the child uses well before a functional movement and increase stability by changing the base of support or increasing muscle activation around joints.[28] These changes are in anticipation of a specific task that has been learned previously. The child received sensory input (feedback) from having completed the task previously and makes the necessary postural adjustments to complete the task in the most efficient, effective way. For example, the infant, sitting on the floor, sees a toy to the side and tries reaching for it. If it is too far outside the base of support, the infant may fall in attempting to grab the toy. On the next try, the infant will make adjustments to the base of support and/or muscle activation in the attempt to grasp the toy without falling over.

Feedforward is identified in postural preparations for movement. It occurs as a result of learning through experience.[27] Postural setting is the muscles getting active around a joint or joints, without obvious movement, in anticipation of the task. Current motor sciences endorse the importance of anticipation (feedforward) in movement and postural control.[28] Feedforward is learned through trial-and-error practice as the example illustrates and must be client generated and be goal or task oriented. Postural control is learned specific to a task and in a variety of environmental conditions.[28] Motor learning occurs when the child is actively involved in the session and advances from using only the feedback responses to feedforward control.[27] For example, the child experiences the tactile and proprioceptive properties of objects (feedback) when handling and playing with toys. This helps in preshaping of the hand in preparation for more refined reach and grasp tasks in the future.

When assessing the infant/child's postural control, find answers to the following questions:

- Does the child have a variety of ways to transition between postures or only stereotypic choices?
- Does the child actively push into the supporting surface with the pelvis or extremities?
- Is the child able to repeat movements or tasks and make small changes in his or her motor performance?

ASSESSMENT OF POSTURAL TONE

The clinical term *tone* describes the impairments of spasticity and abnormal extensibility. Abnormally high tone may be caused by spasticity, a velocity-dependent overactivity that is proportional to the imposed velocity of limb movement.[29]

Clinicians tend to use the word *tone* to describe how a muscle or group of muscles feels under their hands when the joints of a body part are moved through a particular range. The sense of abnormally high tone can result from hypoextensibility of the muscle because of abnormal mechanical characteristics.[29] These same muscles can have increased stiffness if they require greater force to produce an expected change in length than is typically expected. Some clinicians use the terms *tone* and *stiffness* interchangeably. Here, the word *stiffness* describes the resistance to movement felt when a limb or the trunk is moved in space.

In assessing the child's stiffness, it is necessary to describe the relative amounts of stiffness in the head, neck, trunk, and extremities. For example, the child with classic spastic diplegia will typically demonstrate hypotonia through the neck and trunk while having increased stiffness in both legs. Frequently, one can observe stiffness of the limbs while watching a child play. However, for detailed and accurate information, it is necessary to "feel" the child transition between postures and move the limbs through space. The clinician may feel the change in the level of stiffness while working with and assisting the child to move through space. This response is typical as the child expends greater effort to perform a task or as the child brings his or her center of mass higher off the support surface. The child may also exhibit an increase in the level of stiffness in particular limbs, frequently in the legs, with an increase in the level of excitement of the activity or the transition.

It is necessary to distinguish between stiffness that is a primary impairment (a loss or abnormality at the organ or organ system level of the body)[30] and stiffness that is compensatory (used by the child to compensate for a primary impairment). Treatment is most effective when aimed at changing the primary impairments, as the secondary compensations may be reduced or eliminated in this situation.

It is important to identify compensatory stiffness. Focusing on the child with spastic diplegia again, the level of stiffness may increase in the upper extremities when the child is seated on a bench secondary to the hypotonia noted in the trunk and the child seeking greater stability as the body is moved higher against gravity. The child may elevate the shoulders and attempt to use the scapulae in adduction with the arms in humeral hyperextension and elbow flexion as an assist to sitting erect because he or she cannot push the hips and thighs into the base of support for stability. The increased stiffness noted in the arms and shoulder girdles is considered compensatory stiffness. Treatment therefore needs to be aimed at treating the hypotonia in the trunk while teaching the child how to push into his or her base of support to gain stability. This is a more effective and efficient means of treatment as the child learns new methods of acquiring postural stability and the need for compensatory stiffness is eliminated.

Signs of increased stiffness include distal fixing (toe curling or fisting), difficulty moving a body segment through a range, asymmetric posture, retracted lips and tongue, and so on. Signs of decreased stiffness include excessive collapse of body segments, loss of postural alignment, and inability to sustain a posture against gravity. A child may also have fluctuating levels of stiffness, which is noted as signs of both increased and decreased levels of stiffness. Two more commonly known types of cerebral palsy exhibiting fluctuating levels of stiffness are athetosis and ataxia.

MUSCULOSKELETAL ASSESSMENT

Persistent shortening of a muscle or group of muscles without adequate activation of antagonists—resulting from spasticity, increased or decreased stiffness, weakness, or static positioning—places the child at risk for soft tissue contractures and, over time, bony deformity. With an awareness of the sequence usually seen in atypical motor development and with knowledge of the postural and movement consequences, the therapist must be alert for areas at risk for contracture and deformity.

GONIOMETRIC MEASUREMENTS

Range of motion (ROM) should be measured with a goniometer at joints with limited motion. The results should be documented clearly for later comparison. Muscles whose influence is exerted across two joints should be examined and elongated over both joints when measurements are taken. Move the child's limb slowly through the range to avoid eliciting a stretch reflex. The first "catch" or tightening of the muscle is the child's functional range for tasks. It is the range that the child can access for function. Therapists can slowly and carefully stretch muscles beyond this point to the second "catch" or what is called the absolute range. This is the actual length of the muscle, but the child cannot actively access the muscle beyond the functional range. The therapist must work with the child and caregivers to bring the two values closer together, approximating the functional range to the absolute range.

EVALUATION OF THE SPINE

Mobility of the spine in all planes is necessary for correct alignment; for smooth, symmetric movements of the spine; and for full ROM of the extremities. Evaluation of the child's passive and active movement of the trunk is an essential part of the evaluation. Passive spinal flexion can be evaluated with the child in supine by rounding the spine and putting the child's knees up to his or her chest. Look for the spinous processes to be showing evenly down the child's spine. This is smooth flexion of the spinal column. If an area is flattened—without the spinous processes showing or showing less—it is indicative of a decrease in spinal flexion. Spinal extension, lateral flexion, and rotation are most easily assessed in sitting. The pelvis must be stabilized by the therapist and the trunk taken through the various movements. Note the smoothness of the movement, the end range and end feel, the symmetry in the trunk, and the amount of movement at each joint in the spinal column. Infants and children with cerebral palsy often have tightness and limitation in length of the capital extensor muscles and lumbar extensor muscles. Movement into thoracic extension can be limited by shortened rectus abdominus and intercostal muscles.

The therapist must document any deviation from normal in the spinal curves. Note scoliosis and excessive kyphosis and lordosis, and whether the curves are structural or functional.

THORACIC MOVEMENT

An area of special concern for the child with cerebral palsy is the coordinated motion of the thorax that occurs during the breathing cycle. In typically developing babies younger than 6 months of age, there is an approximate 90-degree angle between the ribs and the spine. As control of the head and trunk develops typically, and as the baby begins to develop a more upright posture, there is a change in this 90-degree relationship. Owing to both gravity and the forces of the axial musculature in resisting gravity, there is a posterior to anterior downward slant to the ribs. As a result of this slant, there is an increased ability to expand the diameter of the thorax in both an anterior–posterior (pump-handle motion) and lateral direction (bucket-handle motion). In addition to this ability to change the inspired volume, the thoracic (external intercostal) and abdominal (obliques) muscles act to fix the ribcage. This fixation facilitates more complete contraction of the diaphragm, thus increasing lung volume. Most children with cerebral palsy tend to have low levels of stiffness proximally. They also tend to have decreased active balance of trunk flexors and extensors when in an upright position with difficulty sustaining their postural muscles. As a result, there are differences in motion of the chest wall during inspiration. First, the downward slant of the ribs never fully develops, thus minimizing the mechanical advantage of the pump-handle and bucket-handle motions of inspiration. Second, without the muscle tone necessary to stabilize the ribcage, the diaphragmatic fibers, particularly the sternal fibers, serve an almost paradoxic function; that is, they cause depression of the xiphoid process and the sternum during inspiration. The lack of thoracic expansion, in conjunction with the sternal depression, causes shallow respiratory efforts. Vocalizations will be of short duration and will be low in intensity because of poor breath support. Examination of the respiratory excursion of the thorax is a critical portion of the motor assessment for the child with cerebral palsy. Respiratory function should be assessed with the child in various functional positions. The therapist should develop interventions aimed at increasing postural control throughout the trunk. The therapist must specifically facilitate the postural system muscles, both axial extensor and flexor muscles, particularly the oblique abdominal muscles that aid in the forceful expiration needed for coughing and sneezing.

EVALUATIONS OF THE SHOULDER GIRDLE AND UPPER EXTREMITY

The child with cerebral palsy with excessive axial extension and poor activation of capital flexors and abdominal muscles will likely demonstrate tightness and limitation of the shoulder girdle. Tightness of the pectoralis major muscle persists from infancy as the infant never attains adequate upper extremity weight bearing in prone to lengthen the pectoralis from birth. Dynamic scapular stability fails to develop, and the scapulae become fixed in downward rotation and a forward-tipped position. These fixed positions will restrict motion at the sternoclavicular and acromioclavicular joints.[25] The child with cerebral palsy is likely to be limited in passive flexion, abduction, and external rotation of the shoulder. Elevation of the shoulder, which is used to stabilize the head, as well as excessive thoracic spine kyphosis, may produce limitations in scapulothoracic movement needed for depression of the shoulder. Moving distally, the therapist often finds limitations in extension of the elbow, supination of the forearm, and extension of the wrist and fingers.

EXAMINATION OF THE HIP AND PELVIS

The child with cerebral palsy, typically with spastic diplegia or quadriplegia, commonly has tightness in the hip flexors, adductors, and internal rotators with resultant limitation in hip extension, abduction, and external rotation. The Thomas test is used to identify a flexion contracture of the hip. Abduction and adduction of the hip should be assessed with the hip and knee extended. Internal and external rotation of the hip should be measured while the infant or child is prone with the hips extended and the knees flexed.

Subluxed or dislocated hips can occur in children with very tight hip flexion, adduction, and internal rotation. The subluxed or dislocated hip has limited abduction. The Ortolani click test is used to help determine whether a hip is congenitally dislocated. The infant/child is supine, and both hips are flexed to 90 degrees. The hips are abducted and externally rotated, with the examiner's first two fingers placed over the lateral hip and the infant's knees in the examiner's palms. If the hip is dislocated, the femoral head can slide over the acetabular rim, reducing the hip and producing a palpable and sometimes audible click.[31] An older child in the same position will be evaluated by the apparent length of the femur. A subluxed or dislocated hip is suggested by a relatively shorter femoral length.

FEMORAL ANTEVERSION

Femoral anteversion is a torsion or internal rotation of the femoral shaft on the femoral neck. Other terms that may be synonymous with femoral anteversion include fetal femoral torsion and persistent fetal alignment of the hip.

At birth, an infant has approximately 40 degrees of femoral anteversion, as measured by the angle between the transcondylar axis of the femur and the femoral axis of the neck. The neonate also has 25 degrees of flexion contracture of the hip owing to intrauterine positioning and physiologic flexor tone. In the progression of typical development, hip flexors lengthen as the result of gravitational pull while the child is lying in either a prone or supine position. Active extension and external rotation of the hip tighten the anterior capsule of the hip joint, thus producing a torque or torsional stress that decreases the anteversion that is present from birth.[32] In addition to the effects of the tightened hip capsule, the hip extensors and external rotators insert near the proximal femoral growth plate.

When activated, the extensors and external rotators pull on the plate and help decrease the torsion on the femur. The result of the various forces is that the adult value of 15 degrees of femoral anteversion is reached by 16 years of age.[33,34] Femoral anteversion is determined by biplane roentgenograms. Anteversion may be suspected on the basis of a simple clinical test. Internal and external rotation of the hip are tested with the hip in a position of extension (i.e., with the child in a prone position with knees flexed). Femoral anteversion may be suspected when external rotation at the hip is substantially less than internal rotation.

The infant or child with cerebral palsy often has overactivity and shortening of the flexors of the hip and poor control of extensors and of external rotators of the hip. Beals,[35] in 1969, studied 40 children with CP and found that the degree of femoral anteversion was normal at birth. However, this study also revealed that the amount of anteversion did not decrease over the first few years of life, as occurs with typically developing children. After 3 years of age, there was no significant change in anteversion with either age or ambulation status. The sample of children with CP had a mean of 14 degrees greater anteversion than the children without CP.[35]

Staheli and associates[36] found greater angles of anteversion of the femur in the involved lower extremity of a group of children with CP than was found in their uninvolved limb. Children with hemiplegia also commonly show poor activation of extensors and external rotators of the hip, with or without flexion contractures of the hip.

EXAMINATION OF THE KNEE

The child with cerebral palsy may have limited knee flexion or extension as a result of inadequate length of the quadriceps or hamstrings. Length of the medial and lateral hamstrings and the rectus femoris, all of which cross two joints, should be assessed elongating the muscle over the knee and the hip. Passive straight leg raising or measurement of the popliteal angle will indicate the degree of hamstring tightness. If hamstring tightness is excessive, the child may be unable to sit on the ischium with 90-degree of flexion of the hip, and stride length may be limited during ambulation.

Tightness of the quadriceps, which limits flexion of the knee, can be identified by looking for a patella that is located more superiorly than typical and by assessing the degree of flexion of the knee with the child in a prone position.

TIBIAL TORSION

Tibial torsion (tibial version) describes a twist of the tibia along its long axis so that the leg is rotated internally or externally. The specific angle of torsion is determined by the intersection of a line drawn vertically from the tibial tubercle and a line drawn through the malleoli.

Like the femur, the tibia undergoes developmental torsional changes. The malleoli are parallel in the frontal plane at birth. During infancy and early childhood, the tibia rotates externally, which places the lateral malleolus in a posterior position relative to the medial malleolus.

The "unwinding" of the tibia, or the progression from relative internal to external tibial torsion, is attributable to changes in force on the tibia arising from the decrease in femoral anteversion that occurs as the child grows.

EXAMINATION OF THE FOOT

Dorsiflexion of the ankle is often limited in the child with cerebral palsy and must be assessed with the subtalar joint maintained in a neutral position. Neutral alignment will prevent hypermobility of the forefoot while ensuring excursion of the hindfoot.[37]

Midtarsal movement can be assessed stabilizing the hindfoot with one hand while passively supinating and pronating the forefoot with the other. Toes should be straight and mobile with approximately 90 degrees of extension available at the first metatarsophalangeal joint.

With the child standing, the calcaneus should be vertical or slightly inverted in relation to the lower one-third of the leg. Children should begin to show a longitudinal arch at 3.5 to 4 years of age. Depression of the medial longitudinal arch is caused by adduction and plantar flexion of the talus with relative eversion of the calcaneus. This alignment is also associated with internal rotation of the lower extremity. Another mechanism for malalignment during standing occurs in children who have stiffness into extension, including plantar flexion. Their calcaneus is often maintained in some degree of plantar flexion and does not truly participate in weight bearing. The talus stays plantar flexed with "apparent full weight bearing," with pronation achieved through hypermobility into extension through the midtarsal joint.[37,38] These two mechanisms must be examined carefully when considering an orthosis for standing or ambulating.

DISCREPANCY IN LEG LENGTH

Measurement of leg length should be done in supine with the pelvis level in all planes, the hips in neutral rotation and abduction or adduction, and the knees fully extended. Measurements are taken from the anterosuperior iliac spine to the distal aspect of the medial malleolus.

Staheli and associates studied the inequality in the leg lengths in 50 children with spastic hemiparesis.[36] Of the 16 children who were older than 11 years of age, 70% had a significant discrepancy in leg length. Ten children had a discrepancy of 1 cm or more, and two children had discrepancies of greater than 2 cm between the involved and uninvolved limbs.

Correction of a discrepancy in the leg length by using a shoe lift is not advocated by some sources.[32] However, children with cerebral palsy who have asymmetry in tone, muscle activation, posture, and movement are placed at even greater risk for muscle shortening and scoliosis when a discrepancy in leg length exists. Such a child will try to equalize the length by ambulating with the shortened limb in plantar flexion with the heel off the floor, thus maintaining a continually shortened position of the ankle plantar flexors. Leg length in vertical weight bearing should be equalized as early as possible to facilitate equal growth of the child's long bones. When a full-length shoe lift is used to correct the discrepancy in length, the child should be assessed in a standing posture for symmetry of the posterior iliac spines, anterior superior iliac spines, and the iliac crests. When the child wears an orthosis, the shoe lift thickness must take the thickness of the orthosis into account when determining the necessary thickness of the lift. Shoe lifts can be placed inside the shoe or applied to the shoe sole relatively inexpensively.

EVALUATION OF GAIT

A baby prepares for ambulation by acquiring antigravity movement components of the neck, trunk, and extremities while in prone, supine, and side-lying positions. These movement components are also practiced by the baby in higher level positions against gravity (i.e., sitting, quadruped, kneeling, and standing). Stability of the joints increases as strength is gained in the surrounding musculature. Weight shifting through the body has been practiced by the baby and is mastered in all directions.

From the onset of independent ambulation until approximately 3 years of age, the young child's gait pattern will continue to change with the acquisition of mature components in gait. An early, immature gait pattern is characterized by the following:

- Uneven step length
- Excessive flexion of the hip and knee during swing phase
- Immobility of the pelvis without pelvic tilting or rotation
- Abduction and external rotation of the hips throughout swing phase
- Base of support that is wider than the lateral dimensions of the trunk
- Pronation of the foot as a consequence of the wide base
- Contact with the floor that is made with the foot flat
- Hyperextension of the knee throughout stance phase
- Upper extremities in a high-, medium-, or low-guard position[39]

Sutherland and colleagues[40] described five kinematic gait characteristics that change in typical childhood development during the ages of 1 to 7 years:

1. The duration of single-limb stance increases with age (especially up to the age of 2.5 years).
2. Walking velocity increases steadily (especially up to the age of 3.5 years).

3. Cadence (and its variability) decreases with age.
4. Step length increases (especially until the age of 2.5 years).
5. The ratio of body width to stride width (computed from the "pelvic span," which is measured from the level of the anterosuperior iliac spines, and the "ankle spread," which is the distance between left and right ankle centers during double-limb support) increases rapidly until the age of 2.5 years. It then increases more slowly until the age of 3.5 years, and then plateaus.

To gain the stability not yet available at the trunk and pelvis, an early ambulator maintains a certain degree of scapular adduction, either bilaterally or unilaterally. The high-guard position (Fig. 5.1) consists of adduction of the scapulae; extension, abduction, and external rotation of the shoulder; and flexion of the elbow. This position affords the greatest stability by maintaining maximal scapular adduction, leading to strong extension of the trunk with an anterior, immobile pelvis. A medium-guard position reduces the degree of scapular adduction. Shoulders

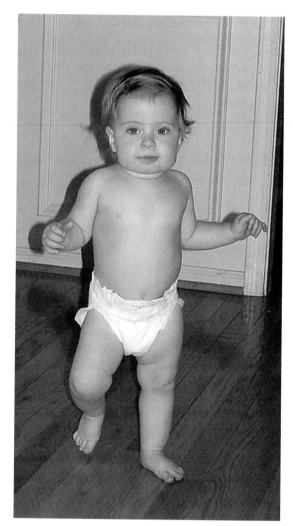

Figure 5.1 ■ High guard position: infant using a high guard position during early ambulation (courtesy of C. Tecklin).

continue to be held in extension, abduction, and external rotation, and elbows are flexed with forearms pronated. The low-guard position consists of scapular adduction with the arms at the sides.

The mature components of gait provide a useful framework for evaluating the gait of a child with cerebral palsy.[41]

1. *Pelvic tilt.* A downward tilt of the pelvis from the horizontal plane occurs on the non–weight-bearing side. This tilt allows the center of gravity to be lowered as the body passes over the stance limb, thus reducing vertical oscillations of the body.
2. *Pelvic rotation.* Transverse rotation of the pelvis in an anterior direction occurs with internal rotation of the lower extremity at the end of the swing phase. This rotation contributes to a narrowing of the base of support and changes the distribution of weight during stance phase to the lateral border of the foot.
3. *Knee flexion at midstance.* This position permits a more fluid, smoother gait pattern.
4. *Heel strike.* Ankle dorsiflexion near the end of the swing phase readies the foot for contact with the floor made at the heel.
5. *Mature mechanism of the foot and knee.* These mechanisms consist of an extension of the knee just before or at heel strike, flexion of the knee in a midstance position, and extension of the knee at heel-off.
6. *Mature base of support.* The base of support narrows to within the lateral dimensions of the trunk.
7. *Synchronous movement of the upper extremities.* Arm swing achieves a reciprocating movement with the lower extremities. Movements of the upper extremities balance out the leg advance and pelvic rotation that produce angular momentum to the lower body.[41]

GAIT IN CEREBRAL PALSY

One of the most frequently asked questions from parents and caregivers upon being told their child has cerebral palsy is, "When will my child walk?" This prediction can be very difficult and should be approached with caution. To answer that question, it is extremely helpful to understand typical gait and how the movement components in the child with cerebral palsy influence his or her ability to ambulate, either positively or negatively. Miller presented typical gait as well as the gait of the child with cerebral palsy and the possible intervention.[42] In 1987, Bleck reviewed 423 patients with cerebral palsy and found 66% to fit in the classification of spastic diplegia. Of those, 79% were independent ambulators, 19% ambulated with external assistance, and 2% were nonambulators.[43] Rosenbaum et al. used the GMFCS to assist clinicians and caregivers to look at the infant/child and make predictions based on the findings of the GMFCS.[44] They plotted the patterns of motor development based on longitudinal observations of 657 children with cerebral palsy and felt that the findings will help parents understand the outlook for their child's gross motor function based on age and the GMFCS level.[44]

There are several classic gait patterns that are characteristic of the different types of cerebral palsy. Variations do exist within each type, however. The classic gait patterns are described in the following section.

Many children with spastic diplegia have limited mobility in their lumbar spine, pelvis, and hip joints and show limited asymmetric pelvic tilt or pelvic rotation during gait.[45] In an effort to compensate for the lack of mobility of the lower body, these children shift their weight and maintain balance by using excessive mobility through the head, neck, upper trunk, and upper extremities. Their hips stay flexed during stance, and full extension of the hip is never achieved. Excessive adduction and internal rotation of the hip are frequently found; in severe cases, the medial aspect of the knees may approximate. Depending on the function of the pelvic, lumbar, and ankle musculature, the knees may be either flexed or hyperextended during stance. The feet may be in valgus outside the lateral dimensions of the trunk, or they may be close together in a narrow base of support in plantar flexion with the heels off of the floor. There can be concern and confusion regarding the differentiation between idiopathic toe walking and spastic diplegic cerebral palsy. Hicks et al.[46] found that idiopathic toe walkers typically have heel cord contracture but minimal or no hamstring tightness, along with increased knee extension in stance and increased external rotation of the foot with increased plantar flexion. Conversely, they found that children with cerebral palsy had an essentially normal gait pattern with the exception of sustained knee flexion at terminal stance and initial contact.[46] Although children with more severe involvement may require an assistive device for ambulation, many children ambulate without any devices, or with only a shoe insert or orthosis. Generally, children with spastic diplegic cerebral palsy ambulate at about half the speed of children without cerebral palsy, and the self-selected velocity is usually the most efficient rate of ambulation.[47]

Asymmetry is the most obvious feature of the gait of a child with hemiplegia, with most of the body weight borne on the uninvolved lower extremity. Shifting of weight to the involved side is brief and incomplete. Limbs on the involved side are retracted or rotated posteriorly, when compared with the shoulder and pelvis on the contralateral side. Arm swing occurs only on the uninvolved side, with the involved upper extremity typically held in shoulder hyperextension and elbow flexion. The lower extremity can vary between stiffness in extension to greater mobility with flexion. Almost all children with spastic hemiplegia ambulate without assistive devices, but many use a shoe insert or an orthosis.

Children with milder cases of athetosis have underlying low postural tone that fluctuates to high levels of stiffness. The gait pattern in the lower extremity is poorly graded and in total patterns of movement. The lower extremity is usually lifted high into flexion and placed down in stance into extension with adduction, internal rotation, and plantar flexion. The hips stay slightly flexed, the lumbar spine is hyperextended, and the thoracic spine is excessively rounded with capital hyperextension, flexion, and rotation of the cervical spine with the jaw jutting forward and rotated to one side.

ASSESSMENT OF FINE MOTOR AND ADAPTIVE SKILLS

Assessment of the fine motor and adaptive skills of the infant and child with cerebral palsy is traditionally one of the main areas of concern for the occupational therapist, as well as for the physical therapist. If a treatment center or a school does not have an occupational therapist available, the physical therapist should have the basic skills to assess this area of motor skills and development. Questions to the parents, caregivers, or teachers that may alert the therapist to the need for intervention relate to the infant/child's functional abilities during feeding, dressing, toileting, bathing, and prehensile and manipulation skills for play and school function. Additional firsthand information may be obtained by having the child undress and dress (including shoes, socks, and shirt) independently before and after the assessment session. As the child moves to perform these tasks, the therapist can evaluate sitting balance, mobility and control of the head and trunk, weight shifting through the pelvis, and use and mobility of the limbs. Other parameters that can be evaluated as the child removes clothes include the ability to reach as well as various modes of grasp—depending on the object, the ability to release an object, and bimanual skills, such as managing fasteners. During the evaluation process, the therapist should ascertain the following:

1. How the particular skill is accomplished
2. The degree of assistance required
3. At what point in the task assistance was necessary
4. Why the assistance was necessary
5. Whether the child accomplishes the task using compensatory movement that will lead to structural changes and potential deformity

CONSIDERATION OF SPEECH AND LANGUAGE ABILITIES

A comprehensive assessment of speech and language is not within the scope of practice of the physical therapist. However, the physical therapist can offer important information to the speech and language pathologist regarding the speech and language abilities and quality of respiration of the infant and child based on observations made during physical therapy assessment and treatment. In obtaining this information, the physical therapist should consider the following questions:

- Did the infant/child hear your voice or other environmental sounds as noted by becoming quiet or looking in the direction of the stimulus?

- Did the child understand questions asked during the evaluation, and did he or she follow step-by-step directional commands?
- Did the infant/child vocalize or verbalize during the assessment? What types of sounds were made? Did the infant/child repeat or stutter speech sounds?
- If the child was verbal, were the words intelligible? Was breath support adequate for speech, or was the child able to speak in only one- or two-word utterances owing to poor control of respiration? Are the expressive language skills delayed for the infant/child's chronologic age?
- If the child was nonvocal, was there another means of communication used (i.e., gestures, sign language, manual language board, electronic communication system)? Did the child use eye localization, pointing, or another means within this alternate system?
- Was the infant/child's communication at a functional level?

The therapist should also ask if the parents/caregivers or teachers have noted any problems with the infant or child's speech or related functional areas, such as difficulty sucking, swallowing, chewing, feeding, or drinking.

These observations and questions can assist in making a referral to a speech and language pathologist who will perform a more detailed assessment. As appropriate, the speech and language pathologist can institute a therapeutic program that can be augmented during physical therapy sessions.

A comprehensive assessment of the mobility and control of the thorax is essential and will assist the speech and language pathologist in attaining the outcomes established for the child. The mobility of the vertebral column and the ribcage has a great impact on the effectiveness of respiration and breath support for vocalization. It also has an impact on pulmonary hygiene, as improved ribcage mobility and deeper respirations help air to flow in the lungs and can prevent or help cure pneumonia. Ribcage mobility and abdominal support provide a good basis for speech control and voice quality. Cotreatment with the speech and language pathologist can be very beneficial to the child, often resulting in more rapid progress. Addressing the child's musculoskeletal problems will assist the speech and language pathologist in planning therapy for communication and respiration issues.

◆ Establishing Functional Outcomes

All physical therapy intervention should be aimed at the achievement of a function or functions that have been identified by the child, the infant or child's parents/caregivers, or specific members of the infant/child's team. Successful achievement of the functional outcome is enhanced when the infant or child is motivated by the outcome that has been identified. An example of an outcome may be that the infant will reach for and grasp a toy that is suspended in front of him or her. Therefore, the toy must be one that is interesting to the infant to encourage the act of reaching with or without facilitation. Perhaps a child is interested in kicking a soccer ball so that he or she may join the local soccer team. The child will be more motivated to participate in therapy if he or she realizes that the outcome has potential to make him or her a better soccer player. "Outcomes" must be functional in nature and should be identified as short-term and long-term outcomes with the appropriately stated time periods. Each treatment session should be guided by an established treatment session outcome. This outcome will usually be related to the previously identified short-term and long-term outcomes. There will be some sessions where the identified session outcome will not be related to the short-term or long-term outcomes because the infant or child comes to the session with an immediate problem that the physical therapist can remedy. An example might be that the child's family is leaving on vacation in 2 days and the family was just told that there are two steps to enter their rental house. You must teach the child and family a strategy to get the child into and out of the house given physical assist as necessary so the family vacation can be successful. These identified session outcomes will guide the therapist in the selection and sequencing of appropriate treatment strategies for the particular treatment session.

Goals are aimed at changing the impairments of the infant or child and are not, in themselves, functional in nature. A few examples of treatment strategy goals are lengthening of the hamstrings, strengthening of a particular muscle or group of muscles, deeper respirations, improved circulation to a body part, symmetric smile, etc. The therapist will have many treatment goals within a single treatment session that are all aimed toward the successful achievement of the identified session functional outcome. They will address single systems, will merge systems, and should prepare the systems and the client for the accomplishment of the outcome.

Stamer[48] has stated clearly the requirements for writing acceptable outcomes in a variety of situations. Each outcome must be observable and measurable. The following items should be part of every outcome:

1. Subject
2. An observable action verb
3. An observable functional performance with a beginning and an end point
4. Conditions under which the performance will be met (conditions describe the circumstances and environment)
5. Criteria, or how well the client performs this function[48]

The time frame for achievement of the stated long-term and short-term outcomes will vary with each facility in which a therapist functions. Long-term outcomes might be written for achievement at the end of a school year, for a 6-month review within the early intervention system, at the end of an admission to the hospital or rehabilitation setting, or perhaps for a 1-month period of time at an outpatient clinic setting as possible examples. Short-term outcome time frames may be for a 3-month review within the school system, for a quarterly review (3 months) within the early intervention system, for 1 week within the hospital or rehabilitation setting, or perhaps for accomplishment within two or three sessions at an outpatient clinic. Short-term outcomes may be directly related to the long-term outcome, as when the child will successfully kick a soccer ball rolled to him or her from a distance of 5 feet away and make the goal in two of five trials for the short-term outcome but in five of five trials for the long-term outcome. In other cases, the short-term outcomes may not be related to a specified long-term outcome.

Displays 5.11 through 5.13 list examples of acceptable long-term and short-term outcomes for various infants and children and their situations.

 Therapeutic Intervention

The therapeutic team should consist of the infant or child and the family, medical staff, allied health professionals and paraprofessionals, and educational team based on the child's functional abilities and needs (both in the medical model and the school system). The infant/child and family are the core of the team, with the emphasis placed on function in the home as well as in the community (including school, church, recreation, etc.).

The therapeutic intervention must be guided by the functional outcomes and/or the participation outcomes

---

>> **DISPLAY 5.11**

Functional Outcomes: Mary, 8 Years Old with Spastic Diplegia

Long-Term Outcome (6 months)
Mary will ascend 10 of the 13 8-inch rise steps in the household staircase leading to the second floor using a step-to pattern and leading with either leg while her right hand is on the railing and the left hand at her side; she will require standby supervision only and complete this task in four of five trials in a 1-week period of time.

Short-Term Outcome (2 months)
1. Mary will safely ascend and descend a 6-inch curb from her sidewalk to the street using forearm crutches and require standby assist only for five of five trials.
2. Mary will walk independently without assistive device and carrying a plastic cup, while wearing her articulating molded ankle–foot orthoses, for 4 feet between the kitchen cupboard and the refrigerator, keeping her head and trunk erect over her vertical pelvis and her other arm free to assist in balance in three out of five trials.

DISPLAY 5.12

Functional Outcomes: Emily, 10 Months Old with a Diagnosis of Moderately Severe Spastic Quadriplegia

Long-Term Outcome (6 months)
Emily will sit in a ring on the carpeted floor with her head in midline with a chin tuck and an erect spine over a vertical pelvis, her eyes looking downward to the toy held in her two hands, given full support at her pelvis for 30 to 45 seconds, in two of three trials in a single treatment session.

Short-Term Outcomes (2 months)
1. Emily will prop on her extended arms with hands open and wrists in at least 45-degree extension when placed in prone on the floor, keep her head in a vertical position in relationship to the floor to visually scan the environment, and hold the position for 15 to 30 seconds given minimal assistance for stability through her pelvis in two out of three trials.
2. Emily will sit in an adapted chair with tray in place in the therapy room with her hips, knees, and ankles at 90 degrees; her feet touching the surface; head erect over her shoulders; and both arms on the tray for swiping at a cause–effect toy placed in midline on the tray, and sustain postural control for 1 to 2 minutes, twice, by the end of the therapy session.

---

that the child and family have identified upon seeking physical therapy intervention. With the outcome(s) identified, the physical therapist must analyze the function or task that is desired and compare the task analysis to the completed assessment of the infant or child. Answers to the following questions should assist the therapist in selecting and sequencing the appropriate treatment strategies to meet the needs of the client and be successful in the function or task:

- What strengths/competencies does the client possess that will provide a foundation upon which to build toward the functional outcome?
- Which posture and movement behaviors interfere with the successful completion of the functional outcome?
- Which identified impairments are critical to the successful completion of the functional outcome?
- How should these impairments be prioritized with regard to the functional outcome? Place the impairment that most greatly impacts the task first on a list of five or six impairments and continue to place the other four or five impairments in order of importance to the identified outcome.
- What treatment strategies can be utilized to address each of the prioritized impairments?

- Do any of the identified treatment strategies address more than a single impairment? Can they be combined?
- Which of the impairments must be treated in preparation to address any of the other identified impairments?
- In what order must the strategies be sequenced to be most successful?
- How many repetitions are necessary for the client to "own" the task at the end of the treatment session?
- How much assistance is necessary to achieve the desired outcome? Can this be decreased within the treatment session?

Once the session is completed, the therapist should analyze the results of the session and make notes about any necessary changes in treatment strategies, sequencing, amount of assistance or facilitation required, a change in a device used for assistance, or the number of repetitions used within the session. These notes will assist the therapist in planning for the following session if the outcome has not been achieved, or if the outcome has been successfully achieved, what the next step should be toward the short-term outcome. Tieman et al. looked at the capability and performance of mobility in children with cerebral palsy across the settings of home, school, and outdoors/community that must be taken into account when writing

---

DISPLAY 5.13

Functional Outcomes: Teddy, 6 Years Old with a Diagnosis of Athetoid Cerebral Palsy of Minimal to Moderate Severity

Long-Term Outcome (6 months)
Teddy will cruise to both sides along a support surface of 36 inches in height and 8 feet in length, using bilateral hand support on the surface, keeping his head in neutral extension/flexion position with active rotation to scan the environment, with abduction of the advancing leg in the coronal plane, in his classroom of peers given stand by supervision at least two times per day, 5 out of 5 days.

Short-Term Outcome (2 months)
Teddy will independently raise his left hand to 80 degrees of shoulder flexion, hand toward the ceiling in 90-degree external rotation, shifting his base of support through his pelvis, while sitting in his classroom chair with his legs in 90-degree hip and knee flexion, both feet flat on the floor with his head, neck, and trunk held in balanced flexion and extension, in response to the teacher's question, two out of three trials.

and determining successful completion of the identified functional outcomes.[49] They found that capability and performance of mobility of the children varied across settings. They tended to perform less well in the higher demand settings such as school or the community. Since much of the testing in physical therapy occurs in the clinical setting, one must be cautious in determining when an outcome is completed successfully and use child and parent or school staff reporting to be accurate.

Documenting and quantifying outcomes for the client is critical to physical therapy. Several authors discuss the need for outcome research and efficacy studies.[50–52] The Gross Motor Function Measure (GMFM) and the Gross Motor Function Classification System (GMFCS) have been identified as useful standardized tools to document current status and functional change with intervention provided for children with cerebral palsy.[11–13] Chapter 3 in this book identifies a variety of assessments and tests of motor development that can prove helpful in quantifying change and functional outcomes in the provision of physical therapy to infants, young children, and older children with cerebral palsy.

Children with cerebral palsy face a lifetime of functional challenges that can intermittently be ameliorated with physical therapy. The nervous system of the infant and child with cerebral palsy is impaired in some way (by definition) and it is not possible to make that child "normal."[53] Therapists should never allow parents to misunderstand or misinterpret the intent of physical therapy. In general, it is to allow the infant or child to become the most independent possible in performing functional tasks throughout his or her lifetime. The provision of physical therapy should change in frequency and duration as the infant or child grows and develops, with periods of time when the child does not receive formal physical therapy intervention. Therefore, it is paramount that we identify the times that are most critical to receive formal therapy, the times when therapy can be supplemented or replaced with adjunctive therapies, and the times when the child, adolescent, or young adult can take a hiatus from formal therapy and continue an independent program for health and wellness with identified points for reassessment by the physical therapist. As an example, physical therapy can minimize the need for or postpone orthopedic surgery, thereby reducing the number of surgeries a child may need.[54,55] Prepubescence and puberty are time periods when the adolescent should be in active physical therapy, as the long bones grow faster than the muscles can accommodate. The result is that the child/young adult will potentially develop poor posture, pain, and movement compensations, which will result in a decrease in his or her current functional abilities. Considering other times when physical therapy is the most beneficial, it is necessary to look at the infant or child in terms of his or her current function, prognosis for acquiring new functional skills, "windows of opportunity" when he or she may make the greatest gains in the shortest period of time, his or her growth spurts, recent surgery,

the family's ability to manage a home program at each level of the infant or child's progress, and the infant or child's level of comfort in terms of pain and deformity. A burst of physical therapy is essential after neurosurgery and orthopedic surgery, after growth spurts that impact the bio-mechanics of the movement, and whenever there is a "window of opportunity." Intensive therapy may be required for shorter periods of time to accomplish specific tasks.[12] According to Fetters, we need a new way to look at treatment, and we need ecologically valid movement goals to guide treatment of motor dysfunction, as well as research in motor control.[56]

Treatment from a dynamic systems approach considers the outcome of treatment to be working on the system when it is in transition.[12,57] According to this approach, the therapist would complete an assessment, then attempt to predict under what conditions and how clients will change. The therapist would also anticipate systemwide responses to small changes in a control parameter. For example, placing an orthotic device in a shoe may alter the pattern of weight bearing, thus influencing the posture of the knee, hip, pelvis, and trunk. "When patients are able to explore and use the limits of postures to actively engage in tasks, they are adaptive and independent."[57]

Discussions and explanations are presented in this chapter as to various methods of treatment intervention, including therapeutic exercise, neurodevelopmental treatment (Bobath), sensory integration (SI), electrical stimulation (ES), alternative interventions, equipment uses and considerations, neuromedical and neurosurgical interventions, orthopedic surgical interventions, and orthotics (bracing) of the lower extremities. There is no singular recommended intervention for any specific category of cerebral palsy as each infant and child presents a unique array of functional competencies, desired outcomes, functional limitations, and impairments. It would be a great disservice to the reader to be limited to one or two ways to treat an individual. It is common and necessary to use various principles from a variety of treatment approaches for an effective and efficacious treatment. The therapist must determine the array of methods useful for client. Displays 5.14 through 5.17 present the "typical" impairments in four major types of cerebral palsy. They are meant to be used as references only and not as the "true picture" of every infant or child in that type. Frequently, infants and children will demonstrate impairments that cross two or more types of cerebral palsy. For example, an infant or child may have spastic quadriplegia with an athetoid component that involves the upper extremities more than the lower extremities. The information included in these tables is derived from numerous sources.[12,24,58–60]

THERAPEUTIC EXERCISE

Therapeutic exercise plays an important role in the habilitation/rehabilitation of the infant or child with cerebral palsy. The exercise program should be developed

---

DISPLAY 5.14

"Typical" Impairments of the Infant and Child with Hypertonia

Neuromotor System

Decreased stiffness in neck and trunk

Increased stiffness in extremities, distal > proximal; varies with type, extent, and location of the lesion

Difficulty grading between coactivation (CA) and reciprocal inhibition (RI), times with excessive amounts of either CA or RI

Difficulty initiating certain muscle groups (i.e., hip extensors and triceps)

Difficulty sustaining certain muscle groups (i.e., thoracic extensors and abdominals)

Difficulty terminating certain muscle groups (i.e., hip flexors, adductors, and internal rotators)

Activation of muscles tends to be in small ranges

Difficulty with eccentric control (i.e., quadriceps)

Musculoskeletal System

Limited range of motion of certain muscles (soft tissue shortening)

Other muscles are overlengthened (the antagonists)

Decreased ability to generate force in certain muscles, also in spastic muscles

Strength of poor grade

High risk for scoliosis

At risk for hip subluxation and/or dislocation

Sensory/Perceptual System

Decreased tactile and proprioceptive awareness

Difficulty discriminating different kinds of touch

Decreased kinesthesia throughout the body

Decreased vestibular registration

Decreased body awareness

Vision used more in an upward gaze, sometimes asymmetrically

Cardiovascular and Respiratory Systems

Poor cardiovascular fitness due to decreased mobility

Reduced breath support with flared ribs and tight rectus abdominus

Gross Motor Impairments

Limited independent mobility on the floor or in vertical

May use assistive device for mobility

Poor sitting balance with spastic quadriplegia

Poor higher level balance skills

Fine Motor Impairments

Decreased use of hands due to use for stability and for assistive device for mobility

Poor grasp and release and decreased in hand manipulation with spastic quadriplegia

Oral Motor Impairments

Usually noted more with spastic quadriplegia

May have drooling, poor articulation

May have difficulty feeding

---

in relation to the assessment of the infant/child, the identified long- and short-term functional outcomes, the functional abilities, and the impairment goals of the infant/child. It is understood that individuals with cerebral palsy have poor recruitment of muscle unit activity, inconsistent maintenance of maximal efforts, and considerable weakness, even under the muscles that are spastic. Current research and understanding of motor control and motor learning make it possible, even mandatory, to promote a strengthening program with children of all ages who have cerebral palsy. Strength training has been shown to improve identified parameters of gait and improve muscle performance.[61,62] According to Damiano, strengthening is justifiable to improve a motor skill or function and can be accomplished when the child has at least some voluntary control in a muscle group. When utilized along with invasive procedures such as dorsal rhizotomy, intrathecal baclofen pump, soft tissue and bony surgeries, and Botox injections, strength training may prolong the outcomes of these procedures and the strengthening may be more effective.[53]

To have an effective strength-training program, the child must:

1. comprehend the process;
2. consistently produce a maximal or near-maximal effort;
3. be motivated and be able to attend to the task; and
4. have a family that can support the program and the child.[53]

A strength-training program can be used with children as young as 4 to 5 years of age who can fulfill the above-mentioned requirements. For the therapist to develop a training program, the child must be able to lift a load two to three times before fatigue in order to strengthen the muscle. To promote strengthening, one must use high loads with a low number of repetitions (three to eight) arranged in multiple sets with a rest between each set. To improve on muscle endurance, the child should lift less of a load but for more repetitions (8 to 20) before resting. With improvement, the therapist can increase the load or the number of repetitions. When strengthening particular

---

>> **DISPLAY 5.15**

"Typical" Impairments of the Infant and Child with Hypotonia

Neuromotor System
Decreased stiffness throughout the trunk and extremities

Inability to grade the level of stiffness necessary for functional activities

Extension favored over flexion for function

Difficulty coactivating for stability in trunk and in the extremities in horizontal and vertical positions

Muscle activity is initiated in phasic bursts for functional activity

Great difficulty sustaining most muscle groups, especially abdominals and gluteals for proximal stability

Muscles tend to terminate passively

Poor eccentric control of certain muscles (i.e., quadriceps)

Musculoskeletal System
Joints tend to be hypermobile so the child relies on ligaments for stability

Stability gained through end-range positioning

Contractures develop secondary to positioning of the arms and legs (i.e., pectorals, tensor fascia latae, flexors of the hips and elbows)

Ribcage at risk to become flat/ovoid due to gravity in supine and prone positions

Difficulty generating force throughout the body

Sensory/Perceptual System
Difficulty with tactile and proprioceptive awareness (requires greater input for the sensory information to register)

Decreased kinesthesia and body awareness

May seek increased sensory input, sometimes in unsafe situations

Decreased ability to use both sides together as a wide base is used for stability

Cardiovascular and Respiratory Systems
Decreased breath support and shallow breathing with weak abdominals and diaphragm

Poor cough

Decreased cardiovascular fitness

Gross Motor Impairments
Developmental milestones achieved later

May skip creeping on hands and knees

Uses "W" sitting for stability

Lacks higher level balance skills

Uses end-range stability without midrange control

Fine Motor Impairments
Lacks shoulder girdle stability and therefore distal strength

Hands without arches

Decreased bimanual skill and in-hand manipulation

Decreased success with independent activities of daily living

Oral Motor Impairments
Decreased strength of oral motor muscles

Breathy voice and short utterances

Decreased rotary chew ability with inability to handle variety of textures

Stuffs mouth due to decreased proprioception

---

muscle groups in children with cerebral palsy, it is imperative that the therapist promote a balance of muscle activity across a joint and not exercise the same muscle or muscle group on consecutive days.[53a] Damiano further presents multiple references that show improvement in scores on the GMFM, gait, and self-perception.[53a] Centers across the United States have instituted strength-training programs in their clinics with anecdotal results showing improvement in function and participation with peers.

One can achieve a strengthening program without the use of weights by carefully selecting the activities that require the use of specified muscle groups to be successful. This allows the therapist to develop programs for infants and children who are too young to comprehend a strength-training program or who lack the cognitive ability to follow the necessary directions. Careful documentation of the activity or position utilized will allow the therapist to design a strengthening progression by changing the activ-

ity or position required. When the infant or child is too weak or has too little postural control or ability to sustain postural control to utilize resistance of weights or even of his or her own body weight as resistance, the therapist can position the infant or child to eliminate gravity or to provide the handling and assistance necessary for the infant or child to complete the motion against gravity. An example of progression against gravity is demonstrated with the infant or child who has poor head control. Begin with the infant or child in a supported vertical position, head aligned over the shoulders so that the infant or child has to balance the head in vertical. Progression will be taking the infant or child slightly off vertical alignment and requiring him or her to return the head to vertical and maintain it there. As strength is increased, he or she will show improvement in the ability to return the head to vertical and maintain it with eyes parallel to the horizon while the body is taken further toward horizontal. This could happen within a few

>> **DISPLAY 5.16**

"Typical" Impairments of the Infant and Child with Athetosis

Neuromotor System
Profound global decrease in stiffness, proximal > distal

Poor damping, see high-amplitude and low-frequency oscillations

Difficulty with coactivation, reciprocal inhibition noted much more frequently

Inability to grade initiation or sustaining of muscle activation

Muscle termination tends to be passive

Difficulty with eccentric control of muscles

Musculoskeletal System
Significant asymmetry of the spine and hips

Joints may be hypermobile due to excessive reciprocal inhibition

Significant hypermobility at C-1 and C-6 to C-7 with increasing age, resulting in possible spinal subluxation

Frequent temporomandibular joint problems

Poor ability to generate force

Sensory/Perceptual System
Vision used in upward gaze

Decreased proprioception, tends to be worse in the upper extremities than the lower extremities

Poor body awareness

Poor kinesthesia

Cardiovascular and Respiratory Systems
Respiration fluctuates in rate and rhythm

Poor breath support

Gross Motor Impairments
Developmental milestones achieved later

Limited floor mobility with great difficulty sitting on the floor

Delayed acquisition of ambulation skills

Use of "W" sitting for stability

Fine Motor Impairments
Difficulty using hands for tasks as they are used for stability in vertical and on the floor

Decreased bimanual skill and in-hand manipulation

Decreased success with independent activities of daily living

Oral Motor Impairments
Poor articulation

Breathy voice and short utterances

Prone to temporomandibular joint impairments due to asymmetric use of the facial muscles

Frequent drooling with poor lip closure

---

treatment sessions or over several months or several years, depending on the severity of the cerebral palsy.

EXTERNAL SUPPORT

The therapist's hands or a piece of equipment may be used to provide initial support to decrease the infant or child's recruitment of excessive stiffness, maintain alignment, initiate a weight shift, support a movement, or aid smooth transitions of movement. This external support should be altered intermittently to provide the infant or child with an opportunity to practice the movement independently.

Support of the body to decrease compensatory stiffness in the absence of proximal stability and to facilitate movement can be moved from a proximal point such as the trunk, shoulder, or pelvis, which provides a greater amount of support, to a more distal point along any of the limbs. By moving the point of support more distally, the therapist expects that the client will assume a greater degree of control over the movement at the unsupported joints.

SENSORY SYSTEMS

It is necessary to address the infant or child's sensory systems as they specifically affect motor performance and functional activities. The infant or child with cerebral palsy has difficulty receiving and interpreting sensory information accurately, and is therefore at a disadvantage to respond to the information with appropriate motor output. The therapist must provide the infant or child with sensory information and movement experiences that will help to correctly interpret sensory information and then select a motor output that is functional. When the sensory information or "diet" is supplied throughout the infant or child's day, he or she will more quickly and accurately be able to apply the information in a functional way. It is necessary to educate parents and teachers in ways that will assist the infant or child in learning about sensory information and how it relates to his or her body. Some examples include:

- Use firm pressure when toweling dry after the bath.
- Provide a swinging motion to the infant or child every time you pick him or her up.
- "Dance" with the infant or young child on your shoulder or in your arms when passing between rooms.
- Encourage floor play with rolling over, pushing up, moving the extremities, etc.
- Propose play activities requiring use and strength of the hands such as play dough, silly putty, playing in wet sand, etc.
- Provide opportunities for "heavy" work such as pushing a laundry basket of clothes or books, pushing the grocery cart or carrying selected "heavier" groceries

"Typical" Impairments of the Infant and Child with Ataxia

Neuromotor System

Tends to have slight decrease in stiffness in trunk, sometimes in the limbs as well

Poor grading of stiffness

Poor damping, oscillations are of high frequency and low amplitude

Difficulty timing and sequencing initiating, sustaining, and terminating muscle activation

Decreased ability to grade coactivation and reciprocal inhibition

Poor coactivation of trunk, hips, and shoulder girdles

Musculoskeletal System

Difficulty generating force

Tends to rest in end range and rely on ligaments for stability

Sensory/Perceptual System (very significant sensory deficits, which are as restricting as the motor deficits)

Relies on vision for balance and postural alignment; therefore, not free to scan the environment

Visual system with severe nystagmus

Decreased visual perception

Decreased proprioception throughout the body

Increased latency in processing sensory information

Severe postural insecurity; very fearful of movement

Poor vestibular system

Tends to be tactilely defensive with poor discrimination; never gets sustained input

Difficulty generalizing sensory and motor information to perform novel tasks

Cardiovascular and Respiratory Systems

Often fluctuating with poor proximal stability

Limited mobility impacts ribcage development, especially in thoracic expansion

Poor cardiovascular fitness

Shallow and rapid breathing

Gross Motor Impairments

Uses a very wide base to move on the floor independently

Keeps legs flexed in vertical to lower the center of gravity

Pace of development tends to be slower due to poor balance in upright

Fine Motor Impairments

Poor skills due to an inability to grade precise movements

Difficulty with activities requiring dissociation of the arms

Oral Motor Impairments

Wide range of movement

Difficulty with a variety of textures and tastes

---

into the house or pantry, pushing the chair under the classroom table, replacing the toys that are heavier during classroom clean-up time, etc.

• Select equipment on the playground that provides movement to the child such as sliding boards, see-saws, merry-go-rounds, jungle gyms, etc., according to his or her capabilities and available safety features.

This is presented as a small list of ideas that one can use in the treatment program and within the infant or child's day to promote increased function. There are multiple books available to therapists, teachers, and families that can provide wonderful ideas for incorporating sensory play and a sensory diet into the daily activities of the infant or child.[14,63,64] When the child's primary impairment is sensory based, it is helpful to refer the child to an occupational therapist who has acquired special training in the sensory systems and perhaps in sensory integration.[14]

SECONDARY MUSCULOSKELETAL CHANGES

A child's difficulty in performing functional tasks may be attributable to changes within the musculoskeletal system. An assessment should identify which muscles are shortened, which soft tissue is shortened, and where the fascia has thickened over time owing to injury or stress of move-

ment. These areas should be addressed so that smoothly coordinated motor tasks can be accomplished. It is beyond the scope of this chapter to address myofascial release; however, once learned, it can be quite beneficial in treatment of the pediatric client.

OTHER CONSIDERATIONS

The therapist should avoid prolonged holding in static positions during treatment. Smoothly graded transitions in movement with brief holding of midline or neutral alignment are more desirable than extended periods in static postures. Facilitated weight shifts and transitional movements should be varied, both in speed and range, so the infant or child cannot anticipate rhythmic displacements. Initiation of weight shifts and transitions in movement are important parts of treatment with the therapist continually looking to increase the variability of the postures and movements and the choices that the infant or child can make in order to achieve fluid, independent movement. It is imperative that the infant or child use active movement as much as possible, supported and/or assisted by the therapist, and that opportunities are provided for repetition of a task or skill in order for the infant or child to learn it. Tables 5.1 through 5.3 and Figures 5.2 through 5.5

TABLE 5.1

Activities for Treatment Sequence—Example 1

Placement of Infant/Child or Stimulus	Response
1. Infant/small child placed in side-lying across the therapist's legs with the leg under the infant's head raised slightly above the other leg. Therapist's hand reaches between the infant/child's legs to place the hand on the abdominals while assisting the top leg into flexion for dissociation. The cephalad hand is prepared to assist the head as needed. The infant/child may be holding a toy with both hands.	1. The infant's head should be in line with the trunk with capital flexion to look at the toy in his or her hands. Eyes should be in a downward gaze. Trunk is activating with balanced flexion and extension to maintain the side-lying position.
2. Using the hand on the abdominals, provide a weight shift that is caudal and diagonal so the infant rolls posterior into a supine reclined position, pushing his or her weight onto the ischial tuberosities.	2. Infant/child should maintain the head in line with the trunk during the roll and keep the head in midline with a chin tuck once in supine. Provides midline orientation of the body.
3. Once in midline, the therapist should assist the infant/child to reach hands to knees and hands to feet. This assist may be in the form of rounding the buttocks off the surface or assisting in upper extremity extension to reach the knees and then the feet. a. Right hand to right foot and left hand to left foot b. Both hands to one foot	3. Lower abdominal activation and strengthening, activation of shoulder flexion with elbow extension, exploration of lower body with the hands, and increasing sensory awareness of the lower body. a. Symmetric activation of upper abdominals to bring upper trunk forward b. Activation of obliques with diagonal weight shift
4. Begin in side-lying position as described in #1 above. Therapist's imposed weight shift is now anterior and caudal so the infant/child's upper extremities bear weight on the floor beside the therapist's leg or on the therapist's leg itself.	4. Infant/child should maintain the head in line with the trunk during the assisted roll and keep the head in midline. Infant/child should maintain a chin tuck to look at a toy on the floor or use capital and cervical extension to look forward.
5. Prop on forearms with the elbows below the shoulders on the therapist's leg, scapulae stable on the thoracic wall. Place the caudal hand over the gluteals and provide a posterolateral weight shift. Assist the weight shift by placing the hand over the gluteals and providing pressure into the base of support. Repeat to the opposite side, passing slowly across midline. Therapist may need to assist the hip into neutral adduction and rotation (in line with the trunk) to the side to which the infant/child is rolling.	5. Coactivation of serratus anterior and pectorals on the weight-bearing side as the infant/child maintains a stable position. Head and neck will laterally flex slightly to maintain eyes horizontal to the horizon. Abdominals will activate synergistically with the pectoral and serratus anterior muscles. Weight-bearing hip will internally rotate and extend while the opposite leg will shift slightly into abduction, flexion, and external rotation.
6. Assist infant/child to extend elbows and place the hands on the floor next to the therapist's leg. Provide weight shift as described in #5 above. Therapist may need to lift the leg under the infant/child's chest to lessen the amount of weight bearing in order to be successful.	6. Similar response as described in #5 above but now with more strength and intralimb coordination required with shoulders in flexion and elbows in extension. Hips and legs should respond as described in #5.
7. When increased strength and coordination are noted, therapist can entice the infant/child to shift onto one arm/hand in order to reach for a toy placed down and in front of him or her. Assist the weight shift by placing the hand over the gluteals and providing pressure into the base of support.	7. The upper extremity of the unweighted side should reach toward the toy. The shoulder girdle on the weighted side is coactivating (serratus anterior and pectorals) along with the abdominals and hip extensors. Spinal lateral flexion should occur with upper and lower extremity dissociation.

TABLE 5.2

Activities for Treatment Sequence—Example 2

Placement of Child or Stimulus	Response
1. Prone in a jogger's stretch position on top of a large ball (one leg flexed under the trunk and the other leg in line with the lateral trunk but in full hip and knee extension with ankle plantar flexion), arms in full shoulder flexion with elbow extension and propped on the ball.	1. Neck and trunk extension balanced with abdominal flexion for midline alignment with lower extremity dissociation. Latissimus dorsi lengthened bilaterally with scapulae stabilized on the thoracic wall.

2. With therapist's hands on the lateral hips, encourage child to "push the legs into the ball" and gently lower the side of the extended hip until it touches the ball.	2. Abdominal activation and strengthening with eccentric control through the trunk and hips.
	    Spinal lateral flexion with trunk flexion rotation.
	    Lower extremity strengthening.

3. Keep hands on the lateral sides of the child's hips assisting to push the legs into the ball as you instruct the child to raise the hips toward midline and lower the hips to the opposite side.	3. Same response as #2 but to the opposite side.
4. Child's hands now placed on the ball in front of the knee for upper extremity weight bearing in shoulder flexion and elbow extension. Assist the child on the calf below the flexed knee to push that knee into the ball while the therapist holds the opposite leg in the air in hip and knee extension.	4. Arms used in bilateral symmetric fashion to balance the upper body on the ball with coactive shoulder girdles (pectorals with serratus anterior and scapular stabilizers) while the weight-bearing hip is coactive (hip flexors and extensors with the abductors and adductors) in pushing into the surface.
5. Therapist provides slow and gentle cephalocaudal weight shift through the extended hip and leg. Tell the child, "Don't let the wind blow you over! Can you find . . . ?" and name an object for the child to find.	5. Pelvic and shoulder girdles active in maintaining stable position on the moving surface as in #4. Head stable on shoulders and looking around the room in response to the therapist's question of "Can you find . . . ?" This will promote spinal lateral flexion.
6. Assist child in placing both knees onto the ball and assuming a quadruped position. Place hands on the calves just below the knees, telling the child to stay on top of the ball. Impose very gentle shifts of the ball in all directions.	6. Shoulder and pelvic girdles continue to activate to remain stable on the ball. The trunk will lengthen on the side that is bearing more weight and slight spinal flexion may be seen.
7. Maintain the same hold and keep contact with the ball when the limb is providing stability for forward progression. Tell the child to "walk the ball across the room." Verbal cues can be given such as which hand or knee to move and to push into the ball. By pushing the ball forward, forward progression across the room will be noted.	7. Full body activation with increased control and coordination of all limbs required. Child will move one limb at a time; it can be either two arms followed by both legs, or it may be alternate arm and leg, arm and leg. Latissimus dorsi lengthening with eccentric control, balanced pectorals with serratus anterior, unilateral hip extensor concentric activation with balanced adductors and abductors while the opposite leg is stabilizing the lower body in weight bearing.
8. Have the child stabilize in a symmetric quadruped position. Assist him or her to shift the ball forward and lateral.	8. Transition of movement into side sit, causing hip flexion bilaterally, internal rotation of the "top" hip and external rotation of the weight-bearing hip, and lateral spinal flexion.
9. Shift weight into a symmetric seated position near the top of the ball, therapist's hands on both lower legs. Shift the ball anterior so the child will shift pelvis posteriorly and laterally. Hands may hold onto a toy or be used for balance.	9. Activation of neck and abdominals (obliques with posterolateral weight shift) with gluteals activating against the base of support. Child may dissociate the legs while shifting the weight lateral and posterior.

Figure 5.2 demonstrates the position as described in #1 above, Figure 5.3 demonstrates the position as described in #4 above, and Figure 5.4 demonstrates the response as described in #9 above.

TABLE 5.3 ▶▶▶▶▶▶▶▶▶▶
Activities for Treatment Sequence—Example 3

Placement of Child or Stimulus	Response
1. Standing at a table higher than waist level or with both hands on the wall about shoulder height, place objects of interest to the child to either side.	1. Child will cruise to the side using abduction and adduction of the hips with extension; therapist assisting at the gluteus medius and maximus as needed.
2. With the child standing with as little external support as necessary, place toys to both sides of the child on a shorter surface and on the floor.	2a. Play activities will require concentric and eccentric use of the lower extremity muscles through their full range to retrieve the toys (flexion and extension, adduction and abduction, internal and external rotation).
	2b. Child may go down to a squat position to play and transition into and out of kneeling and half-kneeling with greater dissociation of the lower extremities.
3. Have the child return to the original position, placing a ball against the wall on which he or she places both hands. The child should weight shift onto the forward leg with hands pushing into the ball that is stabilized against the vertical surface.	3a. Slight hip and knee flexion of the forward leg with ankle dorsiflexion as child pushes the arms into the ball, stabilizing it so the ball does not roll away, he or she brings the hips forward over the foot and moves the limb into full hip and knee extension.
	3b. Posterior leg with full hip extension and soft knee extension as child pushes off the ball of the foot with mobility through the metatarsal-phalangeal joints allowing for dissociation of the toes from the foot (preparation for push-off in gait).
	3c. With hands on the ball, the child should roll the ball sideways with the hands and arms while side-stepping to facilitate symmetric use of the trunk, midline orientation, and strengthening of the hip abductors.

Figure 5.5 demonstrates the response as described in #3 above.

provide examples of activities for treatment sequences within treatment sessions. These are to be used as guides only—not prescribed activities for a particular infant or child with cerebral palsy. There may be different responses noted with a given activity. The treatment session is limited only by the therapist's experience and creativity and the abilities of the infant or child.

NEURODEVELOPMENTAL (BOBATH) TREATMENT

Neurodevelopmental treatment (also known originally as the Bobath approach) was developed by the Bobaths in England in the early 1940s for the treatment of individuals with pathophysiology of the central nervous system

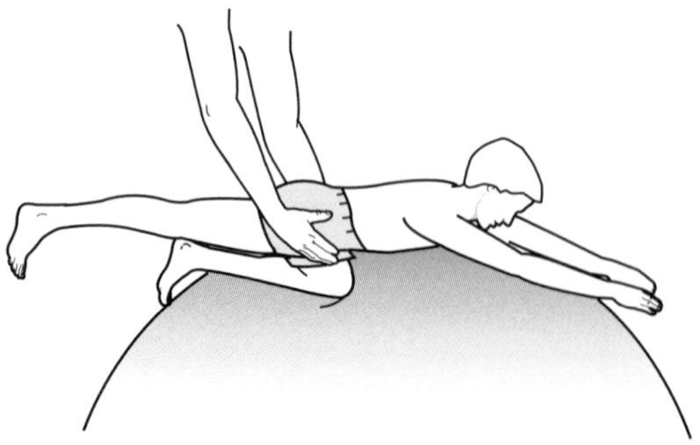

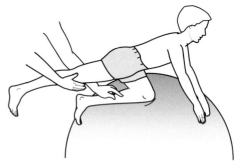

Figure 5.2 ▪ Jogger's stretch on the ball: prone in a jogger's stretch position on top of a large ball, arms in full shoulder flexion with elbow extension and propped on the ball.

Figure 5.3 ▪ Maintaining three point on the ball: arms used in bilateral symmetric fashion to balance the upper body on the ball with coactive shoulder girdles while the weight-bearing hip is coactive in pushing into the surface.

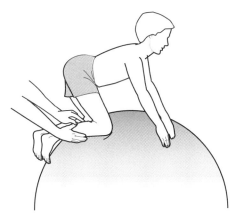

Figure 5.4 ■ Balancing on the ball: activation of neck and abdominals (obliques with posterolateral weight shift) with gluteals activating against the base of support.

(CNS), specifically children with cerebral palsy and adults with hemiplegia.[65] Dr. and Mrs. Bobath described neurodevelopmental treatment as a "living concept," and as such, it has continued to evolve over the years. "The Neuro-Developmental Treatment approach is not a set of techniques but more an understanding of the developmental process of motor control and the motor components which make up functional motor tasks."[60] The goal is to have effective carryover from the treatment session to real life and the following treatment sessions. Carryover is actually

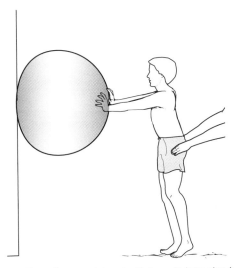

Figure 5.5 ■ Standing pushing both hands into the ball: slight hip and knee flexion of the forward leg with ankle dorsiflexion as child pushes the arms into the ball, stabilizing it so the ball does not roll away, he brings the hips forward over the foot and moves the limb into full hip and knee extension; posterior leg with full hip extension and soft knee extension as child pushes off the ball of the foot with mobility through the metatarsal-phalangeal joints allowing for dissociation of the toes from the foot (preparation for push-off in gait).

motor learning, "a relatively permanent change in the capability for responding."[27]

The ultimate goal of neurodevelopmental treatment is for the infant or child to have the most independent function possible according to his or her age and abilities. Treatment sessions are directed toward a functional outcome and include as much client-initiated movement as possible. The therapist plans for the necessary preparatory work (e.g., muscle elongation) to enable the client to perform the task and will facilitate and guide the movement as needed to decrease or prevent posture and movement behaviors that would interfere with the functional abilities of the infant or child. Feedforward is developed as the child practices the skill or task with the therapist's guidance. The therapist provides less guidance and assistance as the infant or child takes over and anticipates postural and motor requirements.[27]

The following is a brief synopsis of current key theoretical statements that neurodevelopmental treatment–trained therapists subscribe to:

- Neurodevelopmental treatment is a problem-solving approach to treating infants, children, and adults with central nervous system deficits for the most independent functional outcomes that are age appropriate and appropriate for the cognitive level.
- Examination and evaluation are integral to the process in prioritizing the impairments and limitations and are continuous throughout the treatment process.
- The functional limitations are changeable with intervention strategies targeting specific impairments within contexts that are meaningful to the client.
- Treatment is directed toward functional outcomes and is active, with the therapist providing the necessary "handling" to guide the movement and assist as necessary toward successful achievement of the identified outcome.
- Handling is used carefully to establish or re-establish the postures and movements that the client needs to become functional in a meaningful way.
- Active carryover by the client and caregivers is essential to successful outcomes.
- Understanding how typical development occurs and how atypical development is a departure from that enables the therapist to anticipate and prevent undesirable postural changes and subsequent decrease in functional abilities.
- Movement and sensory processing are linked. Therapists must address both systems in treatment of the client with CNS dysfunction.
- Neurodevelopmental treatment provides therapists with flexible guidelines for selecting treatment strategies to manage the client according to their individual field of therapy.

The neuroscientific basis that explains the work of this approach has changed since its beginnings with Dr. and

Mrs. Bobath given a great deal of study and clinical observation and treatment. Today, the approach uses the Neuronal Group Selection Theory (NGST) to explain how the systems can respond in particular ways and why there is the possibility of change given the treatment intervention.[12] This theory extends the dynamic theory and offers a balance between maturation and interactive physical systems, looking at selection matching motor commands to constraints imposed by neural and body structures and the environment. Therefore, it is critical that the infant/child engage in activities as much as possible in functionally and developmentally appropriate contexts to generate movement to meet task requirements.[12]

For a more full understanding of the current philosophy and concepts of the neurodevelopmental treatment approach, it is suggested that you read Janet Howle's book, *Neuro-Developmental Treatment Approach, Theoretical Foundations and Principles of Clinical Practice*, published in 2002.[12]

SENSORY INTEGRATION

Sensory integration (SI) focuses on sensory aspects and their impact on motivation, attention, movement, and socioemotional well-being.[14,63] "Sensory Integration (SI) is the primary treatment approach with children who have learning disorders, attention deficits, and autism."[14] The principles of SI treatment include:

1. Providing the opportunity to experience a variety of controlled sensory input to encourage the production of an adaptive response that includes motor behaviors, social interactions, or cognitive skills
2. Encouraging the child to utilize intrinsic motivation
3. Promoting purposeful behaviors within a meaningful activity[14]

SI can be used to obtain an optimal state of arousal and to affect the child's motivation, initiation, and purposeful interaction with the environment. This is frequently helpful for the child with low levels of arousal who is difficult to encourage interacting with peers in the classroom or in a treatment session. Utilizing the techniques of SI intervention in the early part of the treatment session as well as interspersed throughout the treatment session will prepare the child for more active participation in the session, which is necessary for carryover and learning.

As noted previously, feedforward is a vital part of functional movement. "Feedforward needs to be treated from both a sensory and motor planning point of view, as it requires sensory input to organize the actions and it requires the ability to volitionally organize the movement."[14] Many infants and children with cerebral palsy experience difficulty in processing sensory input and therefore have even greater difficulty producing a desired motor output.

Some pediatric therapists will use a combination of SI and neurodevelopmental treatment with infants and chil-

dren who require both interventions. SI focuses primarily on the sensory processing aspect of the motor act, whereas neurodevelopmental treatment focuses primarily on the motor response to the sensory input.[14] The same therapist can provide the intervention, or two separate therapists can provide the intervention in which each is skilled. Excellent communication is mandatory for the most efficient and effective functional outcomes. Be diligent in your observations when using SI with a child who has increased stiffness as a primary or secondary impairment. There can be an increase in the compensatory postures and movements as the linear vestibular input provided through the SI approach increases extensor tone. The use of the techniques must be well graded when used with infants or children with cerebral palsy. They often lack independent mobility in their environment, and therefore a pure SI approach is difficult and inappropriate.[14]

ELECTRICAL STIMULATION

Interest in using electrical stimulation in the population with cerebral palsy has been growing over time. Damiano mentioned its use as a possibility with children who are unable to comprehend or follow a muscle-strengthening program or who are too weak to do strengthening of the muscles in isolation.[53a] The two methods that have been researched and most extensively used are neuromuscular electrical stimulation (NMES) and threshold electrical stimulation (TES).[66,67] NMES is the application of stimulation of an electrical current of sufficient intensity to elicit muscle contraction resulting in greater muscle strength. When this is used in a task-specific manner in which a muscle is stimulated when it should be contracting during a functional activity, it is referred to as functional electrical stimulation (FES).[66] Daichman et al. found that NMES was effective in strengthening the quadriceps of a 13-year-old adolescent with spastic diplegic cerebral palsy for the development of new skills such as stair climbing.[68] TES is described as a low-level, subcontraction electrical stimulus applied at home during sleep, proposed by Pape originally to increase the blood flow during a time of heightened trophic hormone secretion resulting in increased muscle bulk.[66,69,70] TES is intended to be used as an assist to the total management of the child, not to replace primary therapeutic intervention.[70] Pape's research has shown that the child demonstrates results faster when it is used in conjunction with hands-on therapy.[69] To ready the increased muscle bulk for functional use, it must be strengthened and integrated into the child's daily activities. Research that has been completed on these two methods was compiled and reviewed in the article by Kerr et al. stating that the scarcity of well-controlled trials makes it difficult to support definitively or discard the use of electrical stimulation in the pediatric population with cerebral palsy.[66] There appears to be more evidence to support the use of NMES than TES, but the findings must be interpreted with caution due to the lack of insufficient statistical power to provide conclusive evidence for or against these modalities. "The age and type of patient most likely to benefit from this intervention and optimal treatment parameters are as yet unknown."[66]

CONDUCTIVE EDUCATION

Conductive education is a pedagogic approach created by Dr. Andreas Peto in the 1940s in Hungary that addresses all aspects of development (motor, cognitive, communication, psychosocial, and activities of daily living) in a classroom setting with the overall goal to improve the child's "orthofunction"—the capacity of individuals to respond to biologic and social demands made upon them.[71,72] It was designed specifically for children with motor disorders who are not blind or deaf, do not have uncontrolled seizures, and do not have a mental impairment precluding following instructions. The program is run by a specially trained "conductor" (a sort of combination teacher, physiotherapist, occupational therapist, and nurse) using highly structured activities broken into a series of steps aimed toward the independence of the child. Rhyme and song are used to provide background rhythm. The only equipment utilized are wooden slatted beds and ladder-back chairs because assistive devices are frowned upon, and physical assist to the child is minimal.[4,71,72] A typical program meets 5 days per week, 6 hours per day, with the length of the program varying between 5 weeks to 1 year. Common features across programs include:

- Group work using a highly structured framework
- The use of a task series
- The use of rhythmic intention
- The use of specific equipment[71]

The American Academy for Cerebral Palsy and Developmental Medicine (AACPDM) has as an objective to provide the biomedical research and clinical practice communities with the current state of evidence about various interventions for the management of developmental disabilities. With this objective in mind, evidence reports on conductive education were compiled and evaluated. Along with two other authors not associated with the AACPDM, they found that there was no conclusive evidence to support anecdotal claims to the effectiveness of conductive education over other programs to improve the functional motor activities of children with cerebral palsy.[4,71,72] There was also no evidence to indicate that conductive education is harmful in any way.[71]

ALTERNATIVE INTERVENTIONS

Formal physical therapy should be supplemented in early adolescence and adulthood in those with mild to moderate impairment by alternative activities such as recreational pursuits.[54,73] With the child's age, functional abilities, level of participation, family support, and contextual factors in mind, consider alternatives to traditional physical therapy, either to replace the physical therapy intervention for a specified period of time or to augment the physical therapy sessions in a specified manner or for an identified functional outcome. The following suggested alternative interventions can be pursued in a group to enhance the client's ability for participation in a peer group or with the family as well as in an individual pursuit. These suggestions may be perceived as "nontherapy" by a child tired of going to therapy sessions routinely and therefore will elicit greater cooperation and motivation. Self-esteem rises when the child feels that he or she has accomplished that which friends are doing and he or she can join in the fun. All of the following listed alternative interventions need more research to identify that which is most effective in achieving functional outcomes. Anecdotal evidence is available, but little high-level research has been done to date.

Therapeutic aquatics has been used for centuries for medicinal purposes and is currently pursued for habilitation, rehabilitation, health and wellness, and general fitness. The physical properties of water are used to address specified impairments and functional limitations of clients in pursuit of successful achievement of functional outcomes.[53,74] It can be pursued on a participatory level as in swimming at a local pool, as competitive swimming with Special Olympics, or as an individual pursuit. Therapeutic aquatics should be distinguished from adaptive aquatics. In therapeutic aquatics, the therapist examines and analyzes the abilities and limitations of the client, noting the identified goals and functional outcomes. Activities, movements, and exercises can be used in the water to address the identified impairments and limitations and/or a swimming stroke can be taught that will encourage the client to work to ameliorate the impairments and strive toward the identified functional outcome. Adaptive aquatics addresses the client's current abilities and matches the abilities to a stroke for successful swimming. Here is an example of a child who has a diagnosis of hemiplegic cerebral palsy. The stroke of choice by the child will be a side stroke, utilizing the strong side under the body to pull him- or herself through the water. The therapeutic stroke of choice would be a breast stroke so that both arms would be used underwater simultaneously, looking toward independence and successful use of both arms in the future. In this example, the therapist will need to facilitate the stroke for its successful completion by assisting the child until the weaker arm has adequate strength to take over the arm pull, more closely resembling the strong arm's pull.[74]

Hippotherapy is the use of a horse for habilitation or rehabilitation of an individual as distinguished from therapeutic riding, which focuses on recreation or riding skills for disabled riders.[53,75,76] Hippotherapy has been defined by the North American Riding for the Handicapped Association (NARHA) as the use of a horse as a tool to address impairments, functional limitations, and disabilities in patients with neuromusculoskeletal dysfunction.[53] It is found to be useful to decrease identified impairments in the pursuit of functional outcomes while utilizing the tri-planar movement of the horse, which closely resembles the human pelvic motion during gait. The mobile surface of the horse is utilized to promote relaxation, increased range of motion, strengthening, proximal control, etc., toward a functional outcome. It is usually provided without a saddle, but rather on a blanket for the warmth of the horse to reach the child. Certain contraindications exist, which should be reviewed before selecting this alternative approach.[53] Some stables include the care of the horse and the work of the stable in the routine of the therapy, thereby encouraging cognition, following commands, sequencing activities, memory, and psychosocial elements as well as the sensory-motor elements inherent in the activity. The therapist providing this intervention needs special training, clinical experience, and expertise to help the child with cerebral palsy realize his or her identified functional outcomes.[76]

Other alternative interventions that should be considered include yoga, karate, dance classes, tumbling, and music lessons to enhance the child's current abilities and to build on his or her strengths toward new functional skills or enhanced current functional abilities. These alternatives can be very powerful motivators for many children as they perceive that it is only "fun" and not therapy. They can be pursued in regular classes or classes designed specifically for children with special needs, or on an individual basis dependent on the child's abilities and the local or regional options.

 Equipment Uses and Considerations

Equipment may be used as an aid to therapeutic intervention and handling. The therapist may use equipment to place the infant or child in a position to enhance movement, inhibit undesirable responses, introduce instability into the context of movement, assist in controlling the amount of instability and the degrees of freedom,[57] or assist in the handling and movement of larger clients. The positions and movements available to the therapist are limited only by the therapist's creativity, experience, and handling skills.

MATS

A firm mat provides a good working surface on the floor against which the infant or child can push or work in attempting to attain specific postures, complete transitions, or perform movements against gravity. The mat provides proprioceptive and tactile feedback so that the infant or child receives better sensory information regarding movement. A softer mat will challenge the infant or child's balance while he or she moves across the surface and can add resistance to the movement.

BENCHES

Benches of various heights can be used for short-sitting, tabletop activities, transitioning up from the floor, stepping, climbing, stair climbing, cruising, role playing (as in sneaking through a jungle and crossing the bridge), and so on. One bench can be adjustable in height, or the therapist may wish to have several benches of graduated height to accommodate the tabletop and climbing activities.

BALLS AND BOLSTERS

Firm balls and bolsters provide mobile surfaces that can aid the therapist in facilitating postural control and postural preparations of the infant or child. The direction in which the ball is moved and the position of the infant or child on the ball can be varied to facilitate movement of the head and trunk into flexion, extension, lateral flexion, and/or rotation. It is essential to remember that the ball has a curved surface so that lateral displacement of the ball when a child is sitting on the ball will result in weight bearing through the child's ischium that is on top of the ball (the shortened side of the trunk). The therapist must handle the child, elevating the opposite side of the pelvis and the "downhill" leg, to gain length on the weight-bearing side of the trunk (see Fig. 5.3). Using the mobile surface will frequently be more motivational for a child to work the trunk and work against gravity than when he or she is sitting on the solid, immobile surface of the floor. Varied use of the ball and its infinite possibilities for movement allow the therapist to control the degree to which the movement is assisted by or performed against gravity. Figures 5.2 through 5.4 give visual examples of ways in which one can utilize a ball in therapy.

ADAPTIVE EQUIPMENT

Adaptive equipment is often a necessary and useful adjunct to treatment of the infant or child with cerebral palsy. Equipment may be provided to offer postural support to the infant or child, or it may aid functional skills and mobility.[53] Any equipment used should be "family friendly" (functional for the family), comfortable, safe, easy to use, and attractive. Adaptive equipment and its use should coincide with and reinforce functional outcomes for the child. The equipment should be reassessed frequently and adapted as necessary based on the infant or child's current requirements and growth.

A brief description of common items used for infants or children with cerebral palsy will be presented here. Chapter 11 deals exclusively with adaptive equipment and environmental aids for children with disabilities and should be consulted for detailed information, including information on the appropriate use of and ordering of wheelchairs.

EQUIPMENT TO AID POSITIONING

Infants or children with cerebral palsy may lack the necessary postural control and coordination to function in a variety of positions unless they are given support or assistance. All infants and children should have a variety of positions to choose from in which they can function, travel, and rest. Adaptive seating systems and systems that are used to promote and support standing are the more common items used by infants and children in the home environment and in the classroom to optimize their function; their ability to explore the environment and toys; and their opportunity to interact with siblings, caregivers, and classmates. Other equipment found to be helpful in the home for improved function and safety includes adapted high chairs, tub seats, adapted potty chairs, and car seats.

Side-lying is used to promote eye–hand coordination and bilateral play skills as well as to encourage more typical development of the ribcage and the alignment of the spine and pelvis. Prolonged supine and prone positioning with weak trunk musculature and immobility contributes to abnormal shaping of the ribcage with a decrease in the anterior–posterior diameter. Side-lying can be achieved with a towel or blanket rolls in front of and behind the infant or child. Individuals have found that putting rice or dry beans into the legs of pantyhose assists in positioning the infant in side-lying as the rice or beans can easily be shifted from one leg to the other and more closely shaped against the infant for a secure position, placing the fabric itself between the legs. There are also a variety of side-lyers on the market for purchase. Side-lying should be considered as a positioning option for infants and children with spinal malalignment, pelvic obliquity due to a scoliosis, and asymmetry of the head and neck. In an infant with a shortened sternocleidomastoid muscle, the infant can be laid with the longer side of the neck down so that gravity can assist in bringing the head toward midline, thereby lengthening the neck musculature. For a flexible scoliosis, lay the child on the side of the convexity with a pillow under the ribs leading to the spinal column where you find the apex of the scoliosis. Gravity will assist in bringing the head and shoulders down toward midline as well as the pelvis and lower body. Be sure to position the downward shoulder forward to allow the child to use both hands for play and exploration. Frequently, one of the quadratus lumborum is shortened in children with spastic athetosis (on the side of the concavity). Use myofascial release, transfriction massage, or gentle deep pressure to decrease the stiffness and add length to the muscle before positioning the child on his or her side.

When assessing an infant or child for adaptive seating, you must first complete your assessment out of the chair. Here are some questions that can assist the therapist, family, and teacher in making wise choices:

- What is the intent or the intended purpose of the chair? In other words, how is the parent/caregiver/teacher expecting the infant or child to function once positioned in the chair?
- Can the older infant or child sit independently without external support?
- Can the infant or child sit by propping on his or her arms, or is he or she dependent on external support to maintain an upright posture?
- How can the pelvis be maintained in neutral alignment with the trunk and head held in proper alignment?
- How does the infant or child need to be positioned in space for his or her optimal function?
- Is the infant or child's posture fixed or flexible?

The more severely involved child may require 90 degrees of hip and knee flexion but may also need to be tilted back in space so the head has support and will not fall forward onto the chest, thereby overlengthening the posterior neck muscles. The older infant or child may function best in a simple corner chair, a commercially available adaptive chair, or a bolster seat, all with an attached tray. There are also numerous commercial options offering an adjustable system to allow for high chair seating at the table and positioning to be used at floor level. Many systems also have detachable trays for hand use and play. The best option is generally the one the family finds most functional for use in the home or the teacher finds most adaptable for the children in the classroom. Carryover to the home and classroom is improved if the family and teacher respectively find the equipment easy to use and aesthetically pleasing.

Infants and children with cerebral palsy often have atypical methods of standing and bearing weight. The following are some typical lower extremity postures:

1. Asymmetric weight bearing with an oblique or retracted pelvis, one short leg, or one leg weaker than the other
2. Hip flexion, adduction, and internal rotation with knee flexion, ankles in excessive dorsiflexion with feet pronated and forefoot abducted (crouched gait)
3. Knees held in full extension with hips flexed, adducted, and internally rotated, ankles in equinovarus (heels off floor)
4. Hips flexed with knees hyperextended and ankles plantar flexed (heels on floor) with pronation

For older infants or children who are unable to stand independently or for whom sustained standing in proper alignment is indicated, standing systems should be used for external support.[53] The child can be placed in various positions from supine or prone toward vertical, or in vertical standing, dependent on his or her neuromotor control and coordination. Many standers adjust to the exact position needed for good alignment. Stuberg indicated that standing is thought to reduce or prevent secondary impairments by maintaining lower extremity extensibility, by maintaining or increasing bone mineral density, and by promoting optimal musculoskeletal development.[77] Stuberg further recommended positioning in standing for 45 minutes two or three times a day to control lower extremity flexor contractures, and for 60 minutes four or five times per week to facilitate bone development.[77]

ASSISTIVE DEVICES TO AID AMBULATION

Several devices are available to assist a child in ambulation and to make ambulation as functional, energy efficient, and least cumbersome as possible. A study by Rose et al. documented a linear relationship between oxygen uptake and heart rate throughout a wide range of walking speeds for children with and children without CP.[78] They suggested that heart rate be used to evaluate the child's fitness and to measure energy expenditure. This may be a good method to aid in the decision about which assistive device should be used for the child.

WALKERS A thorough assessment of the child and his or her functional capabilities in vertical must be completed before deciding what aid to walking the child will need to function at his or her most independent level. Communicate with the child's team in its entirety so that the child's routines, necessary transitions through the day, and distances to be traveled are all known. What transfers does the child do? Are the transfers independent, assisted, or dependent? When and how will the child be expected to walk using the walker?[53] Historically, children's walkers were forward walkers, sometimes known as rollator walkers. However, posterior walkers have proven to be more energy efficient, and have resulted in improved upright posture.[79,80] The shoulders are held in greater depression with humeral extension, the scapulae tend to be more adducted, and therefore greater thoracic extension is noted. The posterior walker may have either two or four wheels. Logan and associates found that the posterior walker with two wheels increased stride length by 41% and decreased double limb support by 39% over anterior walkers.[79] However, Levangie and colleagues, in their comparison of posterior walkers with four wheels, posterior walkers with two wheels, and anterior walkers, found that the four-wheel posterior walker was more efficient and allowed more significant increases in the child's velocity, right and left stride length, and left step length.[80] The results obtained with anterior walkers and posterior walkers with two wheels were similar.[80]

It should be remembered that each child's ambulation abilities and deficits are unique and should be evaluated on an individual basis when determining which walker affords the greatest stability and safety while providing for the most energy-efficient gait pattern.

CRUTCHES AND QUAD CANES Young children who have been diagnosed with diplegic cerebral palsy have good upper body strength and use and tend to rely on the arms to do much of the weight-bearing work of the legs. As an example, the infant with diplegia may learn to creep on all four limbs but will bear the majority of the weight on the two arms and less weight will be distributed to the two knees. When this child is taught to ambulate with a rolling posterior walker, he or she will frequently rely on his or her arms for much of the weight bearing and simply do toe touch in stance phase or drag the legs behind him or her. This results in functional mobility for this child and can be extremely useful. However, forearm crutches or quad canes may be assistive devices of choice for the child with fair balance, good proximal strength, and good motivation. The child tends to be more successful if this gait pattern is taught before using a posterior walker. Initially, the child will need assistance as he or she must rely on the legs for weight bearing and balance while moving the crutches or canes forward. Typically, a four-point gait is taught for maximal stability so that there are always three points in contact with the floor. As the child learns more about his or her own sensory system, strengthens the legs and postural muscles, and learns about balance, he or she can use the crutches or quad canes more independently or at specified times during the day. In the older child who needs relatively little assistance for balance, falls occasionally, and has difficulty with longer community distances or uneven surfaces, the crutches or canes may be the device of choice. The child may choose to use the device when in the community and around larger groups of people, attending school to prevent falls, or when planning to go on uneven terrain so that he or she can join peers in social activities. Different styles, grips, and tips are available to customize the cane and crutches to each individual. The older child may also choose to learn to walk with forearm crutches as the crutches allow for more freedom of movement in the community with less architectural barriers than when walking with a posterior walker.

EXERSAUCERS AND INFANT WALKERS Historically, there was great controversy over the use of infant walkers for any infant, owing to the accidents associated with their use. The Canadian Medical Association had requested that their government ban the sale of walkers. They believed that their use is too risky, recognizing that two of five children (30% to 45%) who use walkers have mishaps ranging from finger entrapment to falls down stairs.[81] Mechanical errors during gait and adversely affected muscle development, cognitive development, and coordination were all documented in the literature before the fabrication and sale of infant walkers was stopped.[82,83] Manufacturers then changed their equipment and began producing what has been named the "exersaucer." Infants cannot move them across the floor, thereby eliminating the danger of falling down steps and entrapping fingers. The relative seat height can be changed by adjusting the legs of the exersaucer to put the infant or young child's feet flat on the floor with some hip and knee flexion, thereby allowing the infant/young child to stand and bounce in this supported environment. There is a large variety of toys that are manufactured and placed on the tray of the exersaucer, which will help to teach the infant about cause and effect and perhaps practice hand skills and manipulation of toys. The elimination of the traditional infant walker has been good for health and safety reasons. The advent of the exersaucer has proven to be helpful to some children who have fair trunk, neck, and head control. Each infant and child must be carefully assessed before being positioned in the exersaucer and deciding whether the alignment and support of the device is adequate for the individual. It may be used as a vertical stander for some infants by adding towel rolls around the infant according to his or her size and stability within this particular piece of equipment, thereby reserving the need for a large piece of equipment until the infant or young child grows a bit taller, and the equipment (such as a stander) will provide service to the child while he or she is growing bigger and taller.

EQUIPMENT FOR MOBILITY

Typically, infants and children have a strong desire to move through the environment. This movement allows them to explore the surroundings, to retrieve a toy lost during play, and to interact with others for comfort and play. The infant or child with cerebral palsy may lack independent mobility, may have poor endurance in whatever means of mobility may exist, or may exert such effort as to produce an increase in stiffness that may limit other body functions, such as upper extremity use or vocalization. Adaptive equipment, either manual or power, may expand the world of the infant or child with cerebral palsy and may foster independence not only in mobility, but also in other areas of function. Mobility, which offers a level of control over oneself and the environment, will improve self-image and lead to other positive behavioral changes.

MOVE (Mobility Opportunities Via Education) Curriculum is an activity-based curriculum developed to teach basic functional motor skills that are needed for adult life. It is a six-step program developed by Linda Bidabe, founder and author of the MOVE curriculum, that uses the Top-Down Motor Milestone Test to evaluate 16 basic motor skills (not within the developmental sequence) to develop an individualized program for each child.[83a] It combines functional body movements with an instructional process designed to help people acquire increasing amounts of independence in sitting, standing, and walking. Equipment is used as a support to make the instruction possible.[83a] It can be used for any age child or adult, regardless of their current motor or cognitive status, as long as there are no contraindications such as osteogenesis imperfecta; bone and joint deformities that would worsen with sitting, standing, or walking; pain or discomfort; or inability to hold the head up unless there can be external support provided.[83a] The John G. Leach School, the nation's first model site, completed a pilot study in 1998. Eleven students aged 4 to 18 years with a variety of severe disabilities were included in this pilot study. After 5 months of instruction, gains were noted in sitting, standing, and walking as well as in communication, alertness, and overall health.[83a]

Since that time, the MOVE curriculum has spread to other parts of the country where schools and facilities utilize the method to encourage increased mobility in their clients of varying abilities.

The necessary equipment to complete the curriculum now comes in a variety of forms. One type is known as the Gait Trainer or Pacer that is manufactured by Rifton Equipment. A picture of the Pacer as well as a mechanical lift walker can be seen in the work of Capone et al. as they present an introduction to the MOVE curriculum.[83a] Many other types of mobile devices are now available to provide support to the child who has moderate to severe functional limitations so that he or she may explore the environment, join peers when leaving the classroom or home, and gain more independence in life. Tricycles, big wheels, and scooters of different types can provide mobility, and their use should be considered early in the habilitative effort for the older infant or child who needs more independent mobility. Of course, this mobility also affords the opportunity for the infant or child with cerebral palsy to get into the same kinds of trouble and predicaments encountered by peers with typical motor abilities. It is essential that the adult monitor the child closely to allow for safe exploration and discovery without injury to him- or herself or to others.

Neurologic Interventions for Infants and Children with Cerebral Palsy

NEUROMEDICAL INTERVENTIONS

MUSCLE RELAXANTS

Oral medications have been used for children with cerebral palsy who have spasticity, for the dampening of excessive motor activity. Black et al. indicated that there are different types of motor control problems that result from brain injury. They fall into the following categories: spasticity, 60%; dyskinesia, 20%; ataxia, 1%; and about 20% have a combination of the preceding with one of the movement disorders being dominant.[84] Pranzatelli labels the movement disorders slightly differently as dystonia, hyperkinesias choreoathetosis, and myoclonus.[85] Commonly used oral muscle relaxant drugs include diazepam, dantrolene, and baclofen. There has been little study of the functional effects of these drugs in children, and little is known about optimal dosing, safety, and side effects.[84] McManus adds tizanidine and clonidine to this list and indicates that the sedating effects of these oral drugs are not well tolerated in children.[85a] In particular, Black et al. list baclofen as a drug to be used with caution, and the *Physician's Desk Reference* (Medical Economics, Montrale, NJ) does not recommend its use for cerebral palsy or for children under the age of 12 years.

NEUROMUSCULAR BLOCKS

Infants and children with cerebral palsy have difficulty balancing the agonist against the antagonist muscle group for smooth, coordinated, efficient motor function. Instead, they frequently overuse one muscle, the agonist, and have great difficulty activating its antagonist, which may cause muscle shortening, contractures, and eventually deformity. The physical therapist must assess the joint and the muscles crossing the joint or joints carefully to determine whether a deformity is dynamic or fixed. According to Sutherland et al., a dynamic deformity results from dominance of certain agonist muscles over antagonist muscles. This muscle imbalance results in abnormal motion and function.[86] Dynamic deformity will frequently become fixed over time. The goal is to manage a dynamic deformity carefully to delay the need for surgical intervention, which is often required with a fixed deformity. A dynamic deformity offers options to the child, family, and team. Sutherland says that the ideal treatment must:

1. prevent fixed deformity;
2. be painless;
3. be cost effective; and
4. not result in any serious complications.[86]

It is well known that children with cerebral palsy have spasticity that presents itself in typical patterns for a specific type of cerebral palsy but in its own unique way in each child. This spasticity can interfere with function in multiple arenas including motor skills, self-care, communication, and fine motor activities. One method of reducing spasticity in certain muscles is to do neuromuscular blocks.

Historically, phenol was used as it is low cost and long lasting, but it has some disadvantages: It is necessary to locate the individual neuromuscular junction, and in a mixed nerve, it is essential to avoid the sensory branch to avoid neurolysis; it is generally painful; and it can result in dysesthesias.[87]

Since 1993, botulinum toxin A injections have been used to treat children with cerebral palsy with spasticity that interferes with their function. It is an injection into the dominant agonist muscle at the nerve terminals to cause temporary paralysis of the muscle lasting 3 to 6 months. Botulinum A toxin blocks the release of acetylcholine by the synaptic vesicles. Recovery occurs by terminal sprouting of the nerves.[86,88] Because axonal innervation of the neuromuscular junction is eventually re-established, multiple sessions are usually required. The sessions need to be separated by at least 12 weeks to decrease the risk of developing neutralizing antibodies.[89] It has fewer clinical complications, is easy to use, is more pain free, can be administered without sedation, and diffuses readily into the muscle; however, it is high cost with possible short-term effects.[87] Kinnett reviewed and analyzed articles on the actual injections of botulinum toxin A in children and found that there is a range of dosing and injection techniques in the literature. The total amount of botulinum toxin A has increased in the past 10 years without any adverse systemic events reported.[90]

According to Pidcock, the clinical goals for treating a child with botulinum toxin A include the following:

1. Improve function
2. Prevent or treat musculoskeletal complications
3. Increase comfort
4. Facilitate ease of care
5. Improve appearance[89]

The use of injections must be in combination with a therapeutic program of stretching, bracing, and functional exercises to ultimately assist the child's functional improvements to his or her maximal level of function.[86,88,89,91] Studies of the use of botulinum toxin A have shown improvements in children with cerebral palsy, such as delay of orthopedic surgery, improvement in gait variables, achievement of independent ambulation, improvement in the functional performance in standing and walking, and a decrease in spasticity.[87,89,92] Currently, medical teams are pairing botulinum toxin A injections with a period of serial casting to the limb for various lengths of time. This combination may prevent deformities, thereby potentially avoiding orthopedic surgeries later in life, and may achieve the range-of-motion goals in less time than with casting alone and prevent the subsequent decrease in ambulation status that sometimes happens with surgical release of the gastrocnemius.[92,93]

O'Neil et al. studied the changes in the provision of physical therapy services to the children who received botulinum toxin A injections and agreed that changes are made at the impairment level as well as the functional level skills. However, she proposed that the botulinum toxin A injections are actually an adjunct to the physical therapy services and not the reverse, which is commonly accepted. She stated that the injections enable the therapist to provide more impairment and functional level strategies so that goals and outcomes are more successful. Her study helps to identify strategies useful in achieving the goals and improving outcomes.[91] Fragala et al. studied children's achievements after botulinum toxin A injections based on their level of function according to the GMFCS and found that the children who had higher functional levels at baseline (level I and level II) and had injections in one muscle group versus multiple groups made improvements in disability and the satisfaction level was higher.[88]

Some medical centers are also using a combination of phenol and botulinum toxin A in order to treat more muscles in a single anesthesia. Using a retrospective study, Gooch and Patton found that an average of 14 muscles were injected when using the combination. They agreed with the findings above that injections lower the tone of the muscles in the short run. They concluded that further studies are needed to determine optimal dosages and injection sites for both phenol and botulinum toxin A.[94]

NEUROSURGICAL INTERVENTIONS

SELECTIVE DORSAL RHIZOTOMY

Selective dorsal rhizotomy (SDR), otherwise known as selective posterior rhizotomy (SPR), is not a new surgical approach to the treatment of children with cerebral palsy but has been a poorly understood procedure aimed at reducing the spasticity of children with cerebral palsy.[95–98] Oppenheim et al. have provided a current explanation for the effectiveness of this intervention: ". . . it focuses on the spinal reflex arc and its modulation at the level of the anterior horn cell by supraspinal and segmental influences. Selective division of posterior spinal nerve rootlets is believed to balance the decrease of normal inhibitory influences on the motoneurons."[99] Simply removing the spasticity does not, however, produce improved motor control. The team approach is absolutely vital to this procedure, both before and after surgery.[43,99] Patient selection is critical to a good outcome as only two types of patients are appropriate candidates. The first group includes patients who are functionally limited by spasticity but who have sufficient underlying voluntary power to maintain and eventually improve their functional abilities. Keen intelligence and motivation are also helpful. The second group includes nonambulatory patients whose spasticity interferes with sitting, bathing, positioning, perineal care, classroom activities, and so on.[97,98] The surgery is typically completed across segments L-2 to S-2[95,97] or L-2 to S-1[98] and only a selected number of dorsal rootlets are sacrificed—those that appear to have the greatest influence on the spasticity and produce abnormal movement patterns.

Research from the 1990s has shown that patients who have undergone SPR have been very positive about the outcome and that the quality of life has been enhanced.[100,101] This surgical intervention had delayed orthopedic surgery by improving both passive and dynamic ROM in children, specifically in the hip adductors, hamstrings, and heel cords, and preventing lateral migration of the femoral head in children with spastic quadriplegia.[102–105]

Research published in 2004 indicates that there are longer term sequelae that must be considered when determining whether a child is a good candidate for the spinal dorsal rhizotomy. Of significance is the increase in spinal deformity at long-term follow-up consisting of lumbar hyperlordosis (50%), grade I spondylolisthesis (18%), and scoliosis (24%).[106,107] A positive change in the child's functional status after dorsal rhizotomy is inconclusive at this time. Evidence suggests that hip adductor spasticity is reduced and that strength may or may not be decreased in these same muscles,[108,109] while the ambulatory status of the children may or may not change, especially when compared to a population of children with spastic diplegic cerebral palsy who received only intensive physical therapy services.[110,111] This is again in direct conflict with the findings published in the 1990s.[95–98]

In light of the inconclusive evidence on the functional changes after spinal dorsal rhizotomy, it is imperative that the medical team look very closely at all candidates for this neurosurgical procedure and compare the potential outcomes and child and family desired outcomes to other forms of intervention.

INTRATHECAL BACLOFEN PUMP

Another method of managing spasticity in the child with cerebral palsy is by insertion of an intrathecal baclofen pump. Baclofen has been used orally for over a decade in the management of spasticity. As noted previously, however, there are potential drawbacks making it less likely to be used with children with cerebral palsy.[84,85a] The effectiveness of oral baclofen is limited by its inability to cross into the central nervous system.[112] Doctors are now able to implant a pump into the abdomen of an older (and somewhat larger) child with cerebral palsy and insert a catheter directly into the intrathecal space. Concentrations of baclofen have been found to be 10 times higher in the cerebrospinal fluid with the intrathecal pump than when using oral baclofen and to have a gradient from the lumbar spine to the cervical region of four to one.[85a] McManus indicated that the effectiveness of this method is as good as a rhizotomy but may be preferable as it is not ablative and is reversible. The criteria used for patient selection includes a client with *moderately severe* spasticity of spinal and cerebral origin as can be found in some cases with cerebral palsy, trauma, anoxic brain injury, stroke, or dystonia.[85a,113] The other requirements include the following:

- The client must have sufficient body mass to maintain the pump.
- The patient and the family must understand and accept the cosmesis of the pump.
- There must be appropriate goals of the client, family, and team.
- The family and team must be committed to the necessary follow-up.
- Patients must be free of infection and medically stable.[85a,113]

Clients with minimal or moderate functional limitations are not candidates for insertion of the intrathecal baclofen pump. Once the client has been chosen with the entire medical team and family, he or she must go through a trial of baclofen injected into the intrathecal space during a hospitalization prior to implanting the pump. This is done with 50, 75, or 100 µg of baclofen, during which time the client must be monitored very closely and under strict protocols.[85a]

The three most common goals stated for choosing the baclofen pump are to decrease pain/improve comfort, prevent worsening of deformity or function, and improve ease of care.[85a,113] Gooch et al. reviewed multiple studies of clients who have received the pump. Findings included a significant reduction in tone, improvement in function, reported improved upper extremity function, caregivers report of increased ease of care, and improvement in gait in a few.[112]

It should be noted that the amount of baclofen may need to be altered according to the results noted by the client and caregiver and that the pump must be refilled once every 1 to 3 months depending on the size of the reservoir and the amount of baclofen utilized. Some clients have experienced too great a reduction in their tone, which resulted in losing function as they achieved their prior function through use of their stiffness and spasticity.[112]

The role of the physical therapist is to help to identify clients appropriate for the baclofen pump, assist in the evaluation process to distinguish between spasticity that interferes with function and that which the client is using to function, document change with the trial of baclofen and the change after implantation, assist in setting realistic outcomes, and while in the hospital, assist the family and client to become acquainted with bodies that feel and move differently from presurgery. Postoperatively, the physical therapist plays a key role in assessing equipment needs, rehabilitation service needs, and documentation of outcomes as well as strengthening, improving motor control, and monitoring skin integrity.[113] Not all clients will require therapy services. Those with desired outcomes of increased ease of care and decreased pain will not likely need much intervention. The client whose desired outcomes include functional changes will need intervention, the frequency of which the physical therapist can help to determine, but the client may need to wait about a month before therapy services begin. Safety is of paramount importance as all functions will "feel" different to the client initially.[113]

◆ Orthopedic Surgery for Infants and Children with Cerebral Palsy

As in the neurosurgical intervention presented in this chapter, the discussion will be limited to children with cerebral palsy, and not infants diagnosed with cerebral palsy, as most procedures are best done as late as possible to prevent the need to do a repeat surgery once the child has grown more. Orthopedic management for children with cerebral palsy is best accomplished with a team approach, including the child, family, and medical team and with specific ongoing care. Problems such as severe contracture, joint deformity, and scoliosis interfere with the basic requirement of comfortable seating.[114] The goal of orthopedic management is to help each individual reach optimal functional ability and prevent deformity through detection at an early stage when simple and more effective treatment options may be instituted.[55,115,116] The goals of surgical intervention are to improve function, decrease discomfort, and prevent structural changes that may become disabling.[115]

An understanding of atypical development and movement compensations is critical for determining how surgery will likely impact the child's future function. As Green said in the 1980s:

> ". . . treating one problem without consideration of the others will result in unnecessary additional hospitalizations for subsequent operations. In addition, since each joint is intimately linked to another, surgical treatment of one joint problem may lead to worsening of an adjacent joint deformity unless it too is addressed. Thus, the surgical care of the lower extremities in spastic cerebral palsy requires that the entire patient be evaluated and all necessary surgical procedures be coordinated."[117]

The more common orthopedic problems that involve the lower extremities will be addressed in the following sections. General physical therapy interventions are also discussed. However, many surgeons have established their own postoperative protocols, including the prescribed period of immobilization. Therefore, the information presented here should be used only as a guide in planning and implementing a therapeutic program.

THE SPINE

Management of the spine is noted more frequently in the child with severe functional limitations, who is confined to a wheelchair most of the time, and who has limited mobility. Indications for a posterior spinal fusion with a unit rod is a curve approaching 90 degrees when the child is sitting and has difficulty side bending back toward the midline.[118] An anterior spinal release is done in conjunction with the posterior spinal fusion with unit rod when the curve exceeds 100 degrees, or for severe kyphosis or lordosis.[118] It is preferable to delay any spinal fusion until the child reaches puberty and/or has achieved most of his or her growth since the trunk will not be able to grow any taller once the fusion is completed.

The therapist, family, and teacher must look at all seating devices that the child has been using as the alteration in alignment can result in skin breakdown and sores if alterations are not completed in a timely manner. Look for changes in respiration and vocalization and improvements in respiratory hygiene as the lungs will generally have more room for air exchange and expansion after the spinal surgery. Work toward these changes once the child is back in the therapy setting. It is highly recommended that therapy be performed in preparation for any spinal surgeries. The length of operation and the period in recovery can be shortened when the spinal column is more flexible/less rigid through mobility techniques performed in therapy.

THE HIP

SUBLUXATION/DISLOCATION

Hips migrate laterally or sublux as a result of the lack of pelvic femoral alignment changes and femoral shape changes that take place through normal growth and development, the lack of lower extremity weight bearing in multiple positions, and muscular imbalance across the hip joint. The hip adductors are more active than the abductors, diminishing the possibility of biomechanical changes to occur as needed. Instead, the angle of inclination remains too great and the hip can migrate laterally with the excessive pull of the adductors, unopposed by the abductors. When left untreated, the hip may continue the migration until it is dislocated. Gamble and coworkers maintain that this process occurs over a 6-year period and that there is a strong correlation between the stability of the hip and the ambulatory status of the patient.[119] Other causes of hip dislocation include acetabular dysplasia and flexion-adduction contractures.[119]

Conservative treatment options for the subluxated hip include passive muscle stretching of the adductors and hip flexors and splinting of the hips in abduction (generally overnight while the child sleeps). Some progress may be made with proper positioning during the day, especially if the child has adaptive seating in which the knees can be maintained wider than the hips. With progression of the subluxation, surgery may become necessary, in which case tenotomies or myotomies are the treatments of choice. The effectiveness of muscle transfer is controversial.[119]

Dislocated hips are a more serious problem for the child, as the hip(s) may become painful, sitting may become more difficult, decubitus ulcers may be caused by asymmetric weight bearing, care of the child may be made more difficult, and fractures are possible.[120] Ultimately, surgical intervention may be appropriate. The following is a list of surgeries in order of increasing complexity:

1. Soft tissue transfer and/or releases involving the adductors, iliopsoas muscle, and/or proximal hamstring[80,82–84,116,118,121–123]
2. Femoral osteotomy[80,82,83,118,119,121,124,125]
3. Pelvic osteotomy (iliac, Chiari, Salter, Steel, Pemberton type)[119,126]
4. Combined femoral osteotomy and pelvic osteotomy (with and without soft tissue release)[118,124,127–130]
5. Resection of the femoral head and neck[118,119,130,131]
6. Arthrodesis and arthroplasty[118,119]

Treatment of each child must be individualized, and should be done with consultation to all team members and clear understanding of what the desired functional outcome is. Miller's postoperative regimen indicates that immobilization is not necessary and the physical therapist begins range-of-motion exercises within the first day or two after surgery with weight bearing to tolerance for numbers one through four listed above. The client remains non–weight bearing after arthroplasty until maximal pain relief is acquired, which will take between 6 and 18 months.[118]

Postoperative management should also include strengthening of the muscles in an effort to achieve improved muscle balance around the hips, proper positioning to prevent recurrence of the malalignment, and teaching the child new ways to move in order to increase function and prevent the need for further surgery in the future. Miller's statistics from the A.I. duPont Hospital for Children in Wilmington, DE, indicate that when hip surgeries are completed on "younger" children (in prevention of increased deformity), 70% have not needed bony hip surgery as a 10- to 12-year-old.[55]

ADDUCTION TIGHTNESS

Indications for management of the hip adductors are:

- prevention of hip subluxation as mentioned in the previous paragraphs;
- improvement in a scissored gait; and
- improved care of the perineum.

Conservative management is attempted first such as botulinum toxin A injections discussed earlier in this chapter, stretching and positioning, and strengthening of the hip abductors to promote muscle balance across the hip joint. When the migratory percentage is 25% to 60% in spastic hip disease and the child is between the ages of 2 and 8 years, it is necessary to perform surgical lengthening according to Miller.[118] Soft tissue releases tend to be ineffective when the child is older as there is too much bony deformity. The hip adductors can be lengthened in isolation or the iliopsoas can be lengthened as well, dependent on the presentation of the child.

There is no period of immobilization postoperatively and range of motion can be started immediately according to Miller.[118] Physical therapy must also include stretching, strengthening of the muscles around the hips in order to achieve improved muscular balance between the hip abductors and adductors, and functional training, returning to ambulation and teaching new ways to move to prevent recurrence of the tightened adductors.

FLEXION TIGHTNESS

Hip flexion contractures interfere with function in a standing position because full hip extension becomes impossible. Compensation occurs typically with excessive extension at the thoracolumbar junction and the knees remain flexed so that body orientation in space remains vertical. It is generally difficult to stretch the hip flexors because the pelvis rocks forward into anterior tilt while extension occurs at the thoracolumbar junction. For passive stretching to be effective, the pelvis must be stabilized in either a supine or prone position. Conservative management includes positioning, typically in prone for activities while gravity can assist in pulling the pelvis down toward the floor; standing in a standing, supine, prone, or vertical frame dependent on the child's competencies; and activation and strengthening of the hip extensors, seeking muscle balance across the hip joint.

Surgical intervention involves lengthening of the iliopsoas muscle.[118] It is rarely done in isolation but rather as one part of multiple surgical sites in a child with greater functional limitations.

Physical therapy after surgery should include prone lying to maximize the lengthening into hip extension and strengthening of the hip extensors and abductors. Facilitation of functional skills should continue, with care taken to prevent a return to the child's previous compensatory patterns of movement.

INTERNAL ROTATION DEFORMITY

Femoral anteversion, rather than muscular action, is a consistent deformity associated with exaggerated internal rotation during gait. Anteversion interferes with functional ambulation by tripping the child when the toe of one shoe gets caught behind the heel of the opposite shoe. A femoral derotation osteotomy, which may include medial hamstring release, is the standard surgery performed for this deformity.[117,118,125] Miller indicates that a peri-ilial pelvic osteotomy is almost always done with a femoral varus and shortening osteotomy to correct posterior–superior acetabular dysplasia.[118]

Postsurgical management does not include any cast immobilization, and physical therapy begins passive range of motion on day 1 or 2 postsurgery, getting the client out of bed and into a wheelchair by day 2. Full weight bearing and assisted ambulation is expected by discharge, which occurs between day 4 and 7 postsurgery.[118] Again, rehabilitation is directed toward increasing ROM and strengthening the muscles around the hips for improvement in muscle balance. Functional training must occur for the child to learn new ways of moving with the new alignment and possible motor control. Improvement to presurgical status and beyond can be expected for up to 1 year postsurgery.[118] Unilateral hip surgery may result in leg length discrepancy, which must be considered during treatment and in consultation with the surgeon.

THE KNEE

Knee flexion deformity is often related to spastic, shortened hamstrings and may be secondary to a hip flexion contracture. Persistent flexion of the knee can lead to a contracture of the knee joint capsule and shortening of the sciatic nerve. Botulinum toxin A injection is a conservative approach being used to treat increased stiffness in the hamstrings with some success (addressed earlier in this chapter). Another conservative measure is the use of soft knee immobilizers. They can be used at various times during the day or while the child is sleeping. Providing the child with a standing regime can help to prevent knee flexion contracture and may help to gain length when there is not excessive tightness.

Indications for surgical lengthening of the hamstrings include:

- Kyphotic seating due to shortened hamstrings
- Fixed knee flexion contractures
- Popliteal angle of greater than 40 to 45 degrees or straight leg raise less than 45 degrees
- Knee flexion of 20 to 30 degrees at foot contact during gait
- Knee flexion during midstance of 20 to 30 degrees[118,131,132]

Variations on lengthening of the hamstrings have been developed, with the medial transfer of the distal rectus femoris tendon to the sartorius or gracilis being the more successful.[118,122,132] In extreme cases of harmful spasticity, selective neurotomies have been performed on the hamstring branches of the sciatic trunk.[133] Posterior capsulotomy is indicated when there is a fixed knee flexion contracture of 10 to 30 degrees and is done in conjunction with a hamstring lengthening.[118]

Root's goals of distal hamstring lengthening include the following:

1. Eliminate or diminish inefficient crouched gait pattern
2. Improve stride length
3. Decrease compensatory ankle equinus and hip flexion
4. Minimize internal rotation in gait
5. Improve sitting balance and posture
6. Decrease abnormal pull that can cause hip dislocation[131]

Postoperative management includes the use of knee immobilizers for 8 to 12 hours per day and at night time, which is weaned down to only night time wear for 3 months.[118] Physical therapists must provide range-of-motion and active exercise into knee extension and strengthening of both knee extensors and flexors for improved balance across the joint. Because the hamstrings cross the knee and hip joints, the therapist must also emphasize ROM and strengthening exercises for the hip musculature. Functional training must assist the child in learning new ways of moving and using full knee extension appropriately.

THE ANKLE AND FOOT

EQUINUS DEFORMITY

Equinus, a very common foot deformity in children with cerebral palsy, results from a muscular imbalance between the plantar flexors and dorsiflexors. It can be manifested as toe walking in the ambulatory child, as premature heel rise during gait, or as premature ankle plantar flexion moment during gait.[118] Children with more severe involvement may have difficulty with foot placement on the pedals of the wheelchair, assisted stand-pivot transfers, and donning of shoes. Conservative management includes passive stretching, with care taken to "lock" the subtalar joint before stretching toward dorsiflexion; night time splinting into a neutral or slightly dorsiflexed ankle; and strengthening of the dorsiflexors. A molded ankle–foot orthosis (MAFO) can help maintain a neutral position at the ankle but will not stretch the muscle group nor allow for any strengthening of the dorsiflexors. Lengthening of the gastrocnemius muscle is the more conservative approach in surgery. This is indicated if there is dorsiflexion to neutral when the knee is flexed but less than neutral when the knee is extended.[118] The soleus muscle is noted to be shortened as well when there is greater than −10-degree dorsiflexion with the knee flexed. This represents a severe contracture. This is commonly seen in children with hemiplegic or quadriplegic cerebral palsy. Achilles tendon lengthening (both the gastrocnemius and the soleus are lengthened) is the most frequent surgical intervention for equinus deformity.[117,118,134]

Rosenthal and Simon have had success with young children as well and indicate that if the procedure is done at 6 years of age or younger, a repeat procedure can be anticipated in 6 to 7 years. In the younger patient, the recurrence rate is 14%; in children older than 6 years of age, the recurrence rate drops to 1%.[135] Overlengthening is the most common complication of surgery, and it results in a calcaneal gait or an increase in dorsiflexion during stance. This gait is crouched in nature, with increased energy demands and subsequent shortening of the muscles in the hips and knees.[118]

Postoperative care requires that a short leg cast be worn for about 4 weeks, set in neutral dorsiflexion. If only the gastrocnemius muscle is lengthened, the cast will be set in 10 degrees of dorsiflexion. After removal of the cast, the child's ankle will be quite weak due to the surgery and the immobilization. It is critical to strengthen the ankle and to facilitate as much use of the dorsiflexors as possible. Some clinicians use NMES or FES (discussed previously in this chapter) to activate the dorsiflexors at the appropriate time. Do not have a child wear a splint throughout the day. The splint will only hold the position that was achieved surgically but will not allow any strengthening to take place. Each child should have an individualized schedule for wearing splints and using the ankle actively while the therapist facilitates functional skill development and strengthening.

PES VALGUS

Pes valgus is a deformity that includes eversion, plantar flexion, and inclination of the calcaneus with abduction of the forefoot. These positions cause a medial prominence of the talus, which is commonly accompanied by callous formation on the skin. This deformity is usually flexible and can be corrected by reducing the subtalar joint and forefoot to a neutral position with the ankle plantar flexed. Three situations contribute to the deformity: (1) spastic peroneal muscles that change the axis of rotation of the subtalar joint to a more horizontal alignment and abduct the midfoot and forefoot; (2) gastrocnemius/soleus contracture causing plantar flexion of the calcaneus; and (3) persistent fetal medial deviation of the neck of the talus.[32]

Conservative measures used to treat pes valgus include stretching and strengthening the foot and ankle and posi-

tioning in a splint for partial-day or night time use. It is critical that the young child's foot and ankle be well positioned during growth and development, including weight bearing so the bones and joints will grow with good alignment. When that is not possible, surgery is indicated. The foot deformity can be of highly varied severity and therefore require different approaches in surgery. The most common of the later procedures that are performed include the (1) Grice extra-articular subtalar arthrodesis,[117] (2) triple arthrodesis for rigid deformities,[117,118] and (3) Grice-Schede procedure.[136]

Postoperative immobilization with a short leg cast will last about 4 weeks with weight bearing to tolerance. An orthotic will sometimes be used depending on the results of the surgery and whether the joint(s) require further stability.[118] Motion will either be significantly limited or eliminated in most of the procedures noted above. Long after surgery, the therapist may note joint hypermobility at sites proximal and distal to the fusion, in which case orthotics may be required.

VARUS DEFORMITY

Varus deformity is less common in children with cerebral palsy and seen mostly in the population with hemiplegia and diplegia. It results from imbalance between weak peroneal muscles and spastic posterior or anterior tibialis muscles.[117]

It is best to delay surgery until about 8 years of age and manage the foot with positioning, splinting, stretching, and strengthening until that time. The indication for surgery is a foot that is in varus in stance phase of gait or during swing phase of gait. The varus foot is very unstable and it is easy to acquire a strain or sprain on it.

A variety of surgical procedures are performed for this deformity, including lengthening or splitting and transferring of either the posterior or anterior tibialis muscle.[117,118,137–139]

Therapeutic intervention should emphasize muscle re-education, particularly when a muscle has been transferred; ROM exercise; strengthening; and facilitation of functional activities for which foot alignment is important (e.g., standing and gait).

 Lower Extremity Orthoses

The decision to use an orthosis and the choice of which orthosis to use should be a collaborative decision between the family, orthopedic surgeon, physiatrist, client, and therapist. The physical therapist's contribution must include assessment of available range of motion, passive and active; foot alignment and flexibility both in weight bearing and non–weight bearing (structural vs. functional deformity); voluntary control of movement in the leg, ankle, and foot; current functional abilities; and the desired functional and participatory outcomes of the infant or child and family. Because the foot is used both for stability and mobility, the effects of an orthosis on both functions must be considered carefully. It is critical to remember that an orthosis will provide stability but will also limit the available movement and therefore any opportunity to strengthen the muscles across the joint that is being stabilized. The need to provide an orthosis for an infant is rare unless the young infant has a structural deformity that can be influenced by bracing. It is usually when an infant should begin weight bearing in vertical that a lower extremity orthosis may be considered to manage how the foot contacts the surface and therefore the alignment of the entire lower body. Therefore, the term "child" will be used during the remainder of this discussion, understanding that there may be some exceptions according to age, size, and unique needs. When a child is provided with an orthotic, the family should be given a specific wearing schedule to avoid the atrophy that occurs when a joint or limb is immobilized over an extended period of time. Recognizing the weakness of the gastrocnemius/soleus group after a short leg cast is removed 4 to 6 weeks after surgery will give you a better understanding of the negative consequences of wearing an orthotic for too many hours a day. The child must have time to use the muscles that cross the joint actively, even if the limb is not in the preferred alignment, to avoid possible atrophy from immobilization.

If the ankle and foot cannot be brought into a neutral position with the knee in extension in a non–weight-bearing position, it indicates that the child will not be able to stand with his or her heels on the ground and will need to compensate in some manner. This can be seen as standing on the toes or bringing the knee posterior to the ankle. When a foot and ankle are forced into an orthosis set at 90 degrees with a shortened Achilles tendon, there will be breakdown on the heel or the foot will become hypermobile in joints distal to the calcaneus, therefore becoming unstable. A conservative method to manage a shortened Achilles tendon is via serial casting,[86,93,140] with or without botulinum toxin A injections (see previous discussion). There are a variety of protocols to complete a regimen of serial casting across a joint. Typically, a cast is placed for 1 week with the joint set in the greatest range that does not produce discomfort. The cast should be removed and the child encouraged to play using the mobility at the joint for at least 24 to 48 hours to prevent atrophy of the muscles around the joint and encourage strengthening in the new muscle length that was achieved. The next cast is placed for another week in the new end range that is comfortable for the child. The number of casts utilized will vary, however; typically the trial of casting does not last longer than 2 to 6 weeks. Care must be exercised to lock the subtalar joint while applying the cast to gain dorsiflexion of the ankle, to ensure stretching of the gastrocnemius/soleus group, and to prevent hypermobility of the subtalar joint. Some of the orthoses commonly used for children with

cerebral palsy and their specific benefits are described in the following section.

INHIBITIVE CASTS

Historically, inhibitive casts were used frequently to manage the feet and lower extremities of children with cerebral palsy who exhibited stiffness during gait and with the effort of standing and attempted walking. In 1997, Radtka et al. wrote that the inhibitive casts were purported to decrease spasticity by prolonged stretch and pressure on the tendons of the triceps surae muscle and toe flexors and to inhibit or decrease abnormal reflexes in the lower extremity by protecting the foot from tactile-induced reflexes.[141]

> ". . . the inhibitive casts are reported to prevent excessive ankle plantar flexion, improve lower-extremity muscle timing, and normalize movements of the trunk, pelvis, and lower extremity in standing and during gait. Studies have shown changes in the stretch sensitivities of the ankle plantar flexors, increased ambulation ability, improved passive ankle dorsiflexion and foot-floor contact during gait and improved stride length. . . ."[141]

They were initially constructed of plaster and later of a fiberglass wrap, which was preferable due to the decreased weight of the casts. Inhibitive casts had been developed over the years and come to a point of improved fabrication and aesthetic quality. However, low-temperature plastics came onto the market, which physical therapists began learning to use in a similar manner to the inhibitive casts. Orthotists began to use high-temperature plastics to make inhibitive ankle–foot orthoses (AFO) that were intended for the same use as the inhibitive casts. Therefore, inhibitive casts are no longer used as they were known in the past. In its place, the inhibitive AFO is lightweight, flexible, and easily worn with regular shoes.[141] One type of inhibitive AFO is the dynamic ankle–foot orthosis (DAFO) with a plantar flexion stop and high tibial support with proximal strap to prevent ankle joint movement into dorsiflexion or plantar flexion (Fig. 5.6).

DYNAMIC ANKLE–FOOT ORTHOSIS

Radtka et al. described the construction of the DAFO.[141] The footplate is a custom-contoured plate similar to the inhibitive cast. It has built-up areas under the toes, lateral and medial longitudinal arches, and a transverse metatarsal arch with recessed areas under the metatarsal and calcaneal pad areas. These features provide support and stabilization to the arches of the foot and position the midtarsal and subtalar joints in a neutral position.[141] "The footplate is designed to reduce abnormal muscle activity and to effect biomechanical changes, including decreased excessive ankle plantar flexion and improved motions of the lower extremity, pelvis, and trunk during standing and gait."[141] The DAFO provides total contact to the ankle and foot when

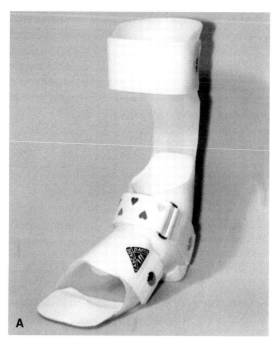
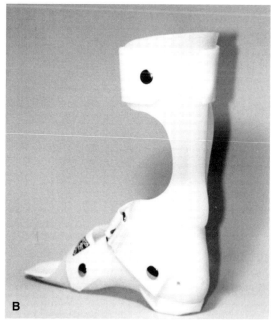

Figure 5.6 ■ Dynamic ankle–foot orthosis with a plantar flexion stop. **(A)** Front view. **(B)** Rear view. (Courtesy of Cascade DAFO, Inc., Bellingham, WA.)

it has a plantar flexion stop. A toe loop stabilizes the first digit while there is a forefoot strap and an ankle strap. The DAFO with a plantar flexion stop is thinner, more flexible, and shorter than the conventional MAFO (Fig. 5.7).

Use of a DAFO is indicated for the following:

- Control of excessive stiffness into plantar flexion from hypertonus of the gastrocnemius/soleus group
- Medial–lateral stability of the ankle joint

- Fixed ankle joint to prevent free dorsiflexion or plantar flexion (achieved with a high posterior wall)
- Improved alignment and stability of the lower extremities and pelvis
- Control of genu recurvatum during stance phase
- Management of the forefoot for neutral positioning

Therapists might also make a low-temperature plastic DAFO by molding the plastic over the child's lower leg and

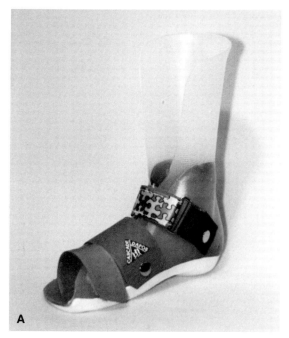
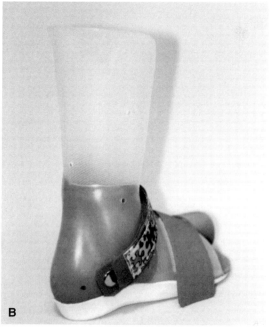

Figure 5.7 ■ Dynamic ankle–foot orthosis with a great toe loop, forefoot strap, and ankle strap. **(A)** Front view. **(B)** Rear view. (Courtesy of Cascade DAFO, Inc., Bellingham, WA.)

foot once the ankles and foot have been padded properly. This is indicated when the exact orthosis is not yet known and a trial brace is warranted or when the child is quite small and is just beginning weight-bearing activities and early ambulation and the feet are likely to grow quickly in the next 6 months. These braces can be carefully modified according to the child's needs by using a heat gun. Continuing education courses are essential to learn proper technique to fabricate this brace.

Radtka et al. studied the effects on the gait of children with cerebral palsy of DAFOs with a plantar flexion stop, MAFOs (an AFO without a dynamic footplate), and no AFOs.[141] Both orthoses increased stride length, decreased cadence, and reduced excessive ankle plantar flexion when compared with no orthoses. There were no differences in the gait variables when comparing the two orthoses. However, "parents, subjects, and their physical therapists commented that the DAFO was lighter and more cosmetically appealing, but slightly more difficult for the children to initially learn to independently don and doff as compared with the solid AFO."[141] Therefore, each child should be considered on an individual basis when deciding on an orthotic intervention.

ARTICULATING ANKLE–FOOT ORTHOSIS

An articulating AFO is quite similar to a DAFO but it includes an ankle articulation, allowing free dorsiflexion with a plantar flexion stop (Fig. 5.8). Significant biomechanical changes were found such as more natural ankle motion during stance and greater symmetry of segmental lower extremity motion when the ankle was given freedom to move.[142,143] These orthoses inhibit plantar flexion hypertonus while permitting free dorsiflexion, thus allowing the child increased ease in rising to stand, negotiating stairs, and ambulating. They may also help strengthen the muscles crossing the ankle.

Use of an articulating AFO with a plantar flexion stop is indicated for the following:

- Control of excessive stiffness into plantar flexion from hypertonus of the gastrocnemius/soleus group
- Medial–lateral stability of the ankle joint (slightly less than with the DAFO)
- Improved alignment and stability of the lower extremities and pelvis
- Control of genu recurvatum in stance phase
- Management of the forefoot for neutral positioning

Night splinting can be used to increase the length of the gastrocnemius/soleus group by maintaining a prolonged stretch into dorsiflexion (Fig. 5.9). By using an ankle articulation with an adjustable strap attached to the footplate by the toes, one can alter the degree of dorsiflexion while the child is wearing the orthosis.

FLOOR REACTION ORTHOSIS

Some children with cerebral palsy walk with a crouched gait, with increased hip and knee flexion and increased dorsiflex-

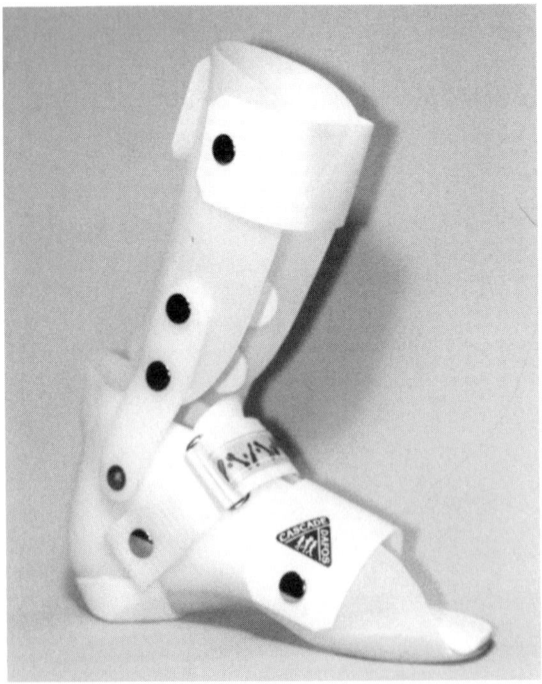

Figure 5.8 ■ *Articulating ankle–foot orthosis allows free dorsiflexion with a plantar flexion stop. (Courtesy of Cascade DAFO, Inc., Bellingham, WA.)*

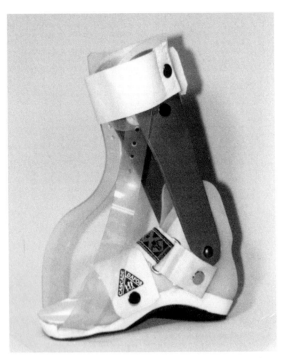

Figure 5.9 ■ *Night splint to provide prolonged stretch into dorsiflexion. Uses an adjustable strap with an ankle articulation. (Courtesy of Cascade DAFO, Inc., Bellingham, WA.)*

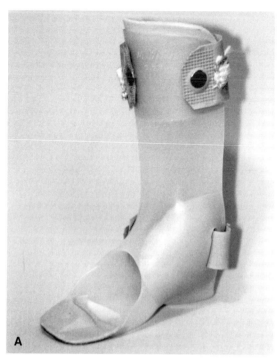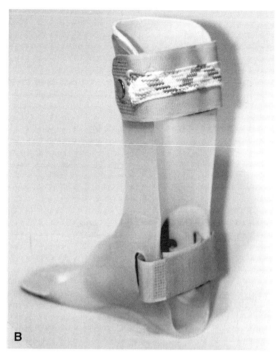

Figure 5.10 ■ Floor reaction orthosis. **(A)** Front view. **(B)** Rear view. (Courtesy of Cascade DAFO, Inc., Bellingham, WA.)

ion. This may be due to weakness of the extensor postural muscles or to stiffness in the hamstrings pulling the child down into more flexion. Clinically, the physical therapist notes a child who cannot get tall against gravity and maintain the postural system against gravity. A floor reaction brace such as seen in Figure 5.10 covers the anterior surface of the lower leg while leaving the posterior aspect open for donning and doffing, provides medial–lateral stability, and uses a dynamic footplate to control any atypical hypertonus. To benefit from this type of orthosis, the child cannot have any fixed contracture of the hamstrings, which would prevent passive full knee extension in standing; otherwise, the center of gravity would be taken posterior to the foot due to the knee flexion with the ankle held in neutral.

Use of a floor reaction orthosis is indicated for the following:

- Control of excessive knee flexion in stance phase
- Medial–lateral stability of the ankle joint
- Improved alignment and stability of the lower extremities and pelvis
- Management of the forefoot for neutral positioning

SUPRAMALLEOLAR ORTHOSIS

An orthotic progression utilized once the child with cerebral palsy has gained more control through the lower limbs and less external stability is required is the supramalleolar orthosis (SMO). The trim lines are cut anterior and superior to the malleoli providing the necessary medial–lateral stability for the ankle joint as noted in Figure 5.11.

Use of a supramalleolar orthosis is indicated for the following:

- Medial–lateral stability of the ankle joint
- Control of tibial motion, allowing free dorsiflexion and plantar flexion
- Improved alignment and stability of the lower extremities and pelvis
- Management of the forefoot for neutral positioning

SHOE INSERTS

When the child with cerebral palsy has control of the ankle joint but still requires external support when the foot comes in contact with the floor, a shoe insert is desirable. Dynamic control of the knee and ankle during stance and gait is required for the child to function successfully. Trim lines can be anterior or inferior to either the medial or lateral malleoli, and the foot plate can be proximal or distal to the metatarsal heads, dependent on each child's unique needs. Shoe inserts can be made of low-temperature plastic as well as purchased commercially from a variety of sources such as Cascade in Bellingham, WA, and Birkenstock (Fig. 5.12). They are sold under various names and are particularly popular with athletes. It is essential to look at the alignment of the entire foot, the hindfoot as well as the forefoot, to decide on the correct shoe insert.

Use of a shoe insert is indicated for the following:

- Control of the calcaneus, subtalar, and midtarsal joints
- Improved alignment and stability of the lower extremities and pelvis
- Management of the forefoot for neutral positioning

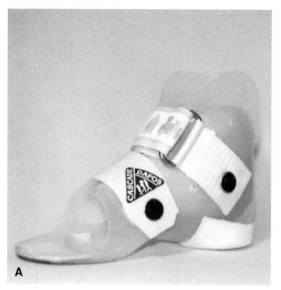 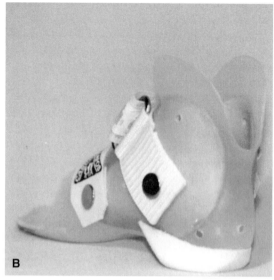

Figure 5.11 ■ *Supramalleolar orthosis. Provides medial–lateral ankle support with free dorsiflexion and plantar flexion.* **(A)** *Front view.* **(B)** *Rear view. (Courtesy of Cascade DAFO, Inc., Bellingham, WA.)*

◆ The Adolescent with Cerebral Palsy

During adolescence, children become more interested in school activities and community life opportunities. It is a time of increased peer pressure and transition into a period of growth and development when one is expected to be more self-sufficient and independent. This period may be difficult for some adolescents with cerebral palsy as they become more aware of limitations and the impact of their disability on themselves, their family, and their friends.

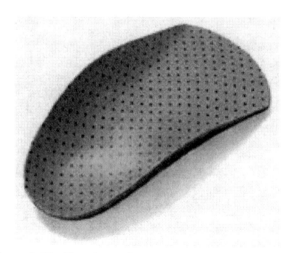

Figure 5.12 ■ *Shoe insert: This particular shoe insert is known as Birkobalance. It has a breathable leather lining and assists in controlling the medial–lateral alignment of the hind foot in weight bearing. (Courtesy of Birkenstock, Novato, CA.)*

Awareness of their own sexuality is developing, as well as potential interest in the opposite sex.

Growth spurts are expected during adolescence and can create difficulty for the adolescent with cerebral palsy. Bones grow more quickly than muscles and therefore muscle shortening, contractures, and discomfort are possibilities. As their bodies grow taller and bigger, one can find that they have decreased endurance for aerobic activities and daily routines. Typical disabilities at this time include a lack of independent mobility and continued difficulty and slowness with self-care and hygiene skills at a time when personal privacy is increasingly important.[144] Goals for the adolescent, in response to the growth, may be to maintain or increase the level of function and work toward more independence in life skills. It is necessary to anticipate musculoskeletal changes before they occur in order to prevent the secondary impairments of contractures and decreased endurance for ambulation and other activities.

When the child encounters a larger physical space in middle school and high school, the physical therapist may need to consider alternate modes for mobility. A manual or power wheelchair may be appropriate. As the child grows, there is often more physical stress on the family members and continued family teaching is necessary, including body mechanics, lifting, performing assisted or dependent transfers, aiding mobility, and assisting in general self-care and hygiene.

The adolescent may not have the typical opportunities in the community or to socialize with peers, which may limit the social–emotional development that typically takes place at this time. "Therapists should strive to foster self-esteem and assertiveness in children and adolescents by emphasizing their abilities, finding areas in which they can excel, and helping them to acknowledge their difficulties with a view toward identifying appropriate compensations."[144]

Magill-Evans and Restall conducted a longitudinal study of self-esteem in 22 adolescents with cerebral palsy and 22 nondisabled peers. They found that as adolescents, only girls with cerebral palsy scored lower on physical, social, and personal self-esteem. This difference with the other groups disappeared as adults.[145] This indicates that we, as professionals, need to be diligent in our support of these children and adolescents and foster their self-esteem and independence.

Strength-training research in individuals with cerebral palsy has typically been with adolescents and teenagers. It has generally been thought that strength training has improved the self-esteem and self-confidence of individuals, especially when the program takes place in a fitness center or school gym.[62] However, Dodd found a decrease in self-concept in the domains of scholastic competence and social acceptance compared to the control group when the individuals performed their 6-week program in their homes; however, after the intervention, the self-concept remained positive.[146] It appears that environmental context may play a significant role in the successful outcome of a strength-training program in children and adolescents.

The Adult with Cerebral Palsy

With medical advances in the past several decades, clients with cerebral palsy are now living into adulthood, with a full range of functional abilities, as well as severity of functional limitations and participation restrictions. Liptak did a survey in 2003 that showed that 40% of adults with cerebral palsy were employed and that only 6% of children with special health care needs received support for their transition between adolescence and adulthood and found a high prevalence of comorbid conditions of adult women with cerebral palsy living in the community. They consisted of:

- seizures (40%);
- mental retardation (34%); and
- learning disabilities (26%).

Conditions found to be secondary to the cerebral palsy along with their prevalence included:

- significant pain (84%);
- hip and back deformities (59%);
- bowel problems (56%);
- urinary problems (49%);
- poor dental health (43%);
- increased spasticity during menses (35%); and
- gastroesophageal reflux symptoms (28%).

Liptak included a list of other complications, which were fatigue, malnutrition, osteoporosis, cervical spinal arthritis with neurologic changes and Barrett esophagitis.[10] In analyzing this list, it is noted that the musculoskeletal changes

that occurred by adulthood may be addressed by physical therapists during the aging process and perhaps sooner. It is clear that attention must be paid to the alignment and movement options of the older child, adolescent, and young adult with cerebral palsy so that pain and deformity can be minimized. This topic cannot be addressed within the realm of this chapter but should not be ignored by the physical therapist.

Home Management

A home management program is an essential part of the overall treatment plan for the infant or child with cerebral palsy as the ultimate outcome is the most independent function the infant or child can possibly attain over time. The home program should be designed to reinforce movements, positions, and skills that have been practiced in the physical therapy sessions, and to assist in preparing the infant or child for the next session. The therapist must consider the daily routine of the infant/child and family when planning activities for the home and family and the obligations that are inherent in running the household. Perhaps there are siblings, extended family members, and/or multiple generations living in the household who can be facilitators to progress or sometimes barriers, dependent on the demands of the remainder of the household. Siblings can be very valuable in assisting with the home program and incorporating activities and movement into an established routine. "The unique, spontaneous and competitive interaction of siblings offers increased incentives for functional independence."[147]

The household demands will change over time as will the infant's or child's needs, making it mandatory to review and upgrade the home program during each therapy session. Movements, positions, and skills that are incorporated into the activities of daily living and play of the infant/child are more likely to be carried out than a separate, formal exercise regimen. The therapist must also realistically consider the other non–child-related demands placed on the parents/caregivers.

Tetreault et al. studied the compliance of 41 families of children with global developmental delay that were given home activity programs. The activities given to the parents addressed caring for their child in the home and the actual physical care of the child. It was recommended that the activities be imbedded in the daily routine to promote more practice opportunities and facilitate generalization. They found a compliance rate of 75.6% after 7.5 to 8.5 months.[148]

They attribute this high rate to five factors:

1. Support from the therapist
2. Type of clientele studied
3. Family size
4. Age of the child
5. Marital stability of participants[148]

This study supports the need to imbed activities into a family's daily and weekly routine to enhance the ability of the family to comply with the activities in the program.

Therapeutic movement and activity for the infant can be easily incorporated into daily care activities. Therapeutic handling aimed at increasing movement can be done during routine activities, such as diapering, dressing, feeding, bathing, carrying, and lifting the baby from a supported position. A simple way to carry over positioning and hip range of motion for an infant or young child is to teach the parents/caregivers specific ways to carry him or her that will add range of motion and dissociation of the hips every time the infant is carried! Another idea is to have the young child stand (with or without support) every time the pants are managed, as in dressing, undressing, potty training, and toileting. This reinforces weight bearing through the legs, proprioception, and perception of self as a vertical being. To reinforce proximal strength and balance via routine, the child can be encouraged to sit on a stool or the side of the bed and don a shirt as independently as possible. An ambulatory child should be encouraged to walk to a household event or task such as coming to the dinner table or walking to the bathroom whenever the opportunity presents itself. Ideas such as these are more likely to be maintained as a home program than would be a 30-minute period of passive range of motion and exercise on a daily basis. These are examples only and are not meant to be a child's home program. Each infant or child is a unique entity along with the caregivers and household and must therefore be treated individually with creativity and understanding. There will be events in the child's life that require a more intensive home program such as postsurgery or during a growth spurt. If the family can manage the routine activities on a regular basis, the times for increased intervention may be less stressful.

For the child who has an interest in other activities, a therapist might recommend taking up a musical instrument, therapeutic horseback riding, therapeutic aquatics, or any other activity that coincides with and reinforces the desired functional outcomes of the child. Please refer to the section in this chapter addressing alternative interventions.

 ## Consultation with the School

Communication between the therapist and the child's teacher is essential for appropriate and effective management and education of the child in the classroom. The therapist should obtain information from the teacher regarding the child's daily routine at school. With that information, joint planning for the child can result in an effective and efficient educational program.

The therapist must emphasize correct alignment while the child is sitting. Optimal height of a desk will contribute to postural control and, thus, to a greater degree of success with desktop activities. The result of keeping the child in a sitting position too long will likely be flexion contractures at the hip and knee. Periodic opportunity for movement throughout the day, such as standing, walking between activity centers in the classroom, or participating in physical education class, will provide relief from the sitting position. There should be a sharing of the responsibility, assistance, and supervision required between the classroom staff and the child for quality of movement and safety. The physical education teacher should be informed of joint movement goals and specific types or patterns of movement that may either be deleterious or beneficial for the child. There should also be a review conducted with teachers for the purpose of and proper use of splints, orthotics, and other assistive or adaptive devices. For full details of enhancing the child's function in the school system, please refer to Chapter 19 in this book.

The occupational therapist will share information about the child's fine motor, visual motor, visual perception, visual discrimination, and manipulation skills; attention span; cognition; sensory system modulation; emotional level; and adaptive self-help skills. The speech pathologist will inform the team about the child's speech and language capabilities. This information, along with specific suggestions, should facilitate learning for the child.

Therapists should not expect teachers to handle children therapeutically for the purpose of obtaining postural control. A more realistic expectation would be maintenance of correct alignment, relief from sitting, use of adaptive or assistive devices, and attention to issues regarding safety. The therapist must recognize the teacher as an important ally in the therapeutic arena.

 ## Other Disciplines Involved in the Care of Infants and Children with Cerebral Palsy

Because cerebral palsy is a developmental disability, it affects not only the infant or child's posture, movement, and acquisition of motor skills, but also the development of perceptual skills, language and cognition, and social–emotional growth. The infant or child with cerebral palsy must have a treatment program that considers the child as a "whole" person, not merely a combination of systems[12] (see the Case Studies).

In addition to the child's individual needs, the child must be seen as a member of a family unit. The impact of a disabled child on parents, siblings, and the extended family must be considered in treatment planning. Although families are expected to carry out specific home programs, professionals must recognize that family members may need periodic relief or respite from the burden of care.

There must be a coordinated effort among the disciplines involved in treating the infant or child with cerebral palsy. Medical care may include the services of a general pediatrician, neurologist, orthopedic surgeon, podiatrist, ophthalmologist, physiatrist, and other specialists as the medical complications indicate such as gastroenterologists, ear-nose-throat specialists, nutritionists, homeopaths, psychiatrists or psychologists, and neonatologists. Allied health professionals may include any one or all of the following: physical therapist, physical therapy assistant, occupational therapist, certified occupational therapy assistant, speech and language pathologist, and speech and language assistant. If the infant or child is in early intervention, there may also be a special instructor on the team. Nurses are sometimes included in early intervention programs when the child is termed as being medically fragile or at risk. Communication among the team members and family is vital to the infant or child's well-being and ultimate success.

The occupational therapist works with postural control and movement primarily as a prerequisite for transitional skills and fine motor skills as they relate to self-help activities—feeding, dressing, bathing, and play. During the child's adolescent and teenage years, the occupational therapist becomes more involved with prevocational testing and training and graphomotor skills.

The speech and language pathologist is also involved with the acquisition of postural control and movement against gravity. Specific attention should be paid to alignment of the head, trunk, and pelvis in order to promote optimal respiration in support of speech. The coordination of breathing with oral motor skills is necessary for feeding and, on a more differentiated level, for speech. A manual or electronic communication board may be indicated if oral speech is not a possibility. Manual sign language can be appropriate for children with cerebral palsy if they have the fine finger control to sign successfully. A system of signs and gestures can be used successively and appropriately in the home and classroom. In addition to motor deficits, the child's acquisition of language concepts may be delayed.

The psychologist may be involved in formal psychological testing of the child with cerebral palsy to identify cognitive strengths and deficits. The psychologist will then make recommendations for appropriate educational placement to best meet the child's needs. Psychological therapy may be indicated if behavioral or emotional problems interfere with the social and emotional growth of the child and the family.

The recreational therapist may be involved in identifying leisure interests and may work with the child and family in the selection and pursuit of leisure activities. Identification of toys appropriate for the infant or child's developmental level and movement capabilities may allow independent play for him or her, and is among the responsibilities of the recreational therapist. Some commonly used toys may be converted so they can be operated by battery and remote control. A joystick or press plate control may be used depending on the child's level of fine motor skill. Specially adapted access switches can be made or purchased for particular toys. Computer programs can be used for fun and academic pursuits for the child. It is important to work with an individual knowledgeable about the available hardware and software and how adaptations can be made for your child. Refer to Chapter 11 in this text for specific information.

A social worker may assist the family in locating services for the disabled child. The social worker can also play an important role in guiding and teaching family members to be advocates for the disabled family member. The disabled child, as a member of a larger family unit, will have a significant impact on that unit. The social worker can provide counseling and support for the family to help resolve issues of concern.

SUMMARY

Infants and children with cerebral palsy present with a wide range of neuromuscular, sensory/perceptual, and cognitive concerns. To be effective in the assessment, evaluation, and treatment of the infant and child, an interdisciplinary team must have excellent communication skills with the child, the family/caregiver, and one another. This chapter presents physical therapy intervention as a problem-solving approach necessary to treat each infant or child as an individual with unique needs and desired functional outcomes. The ultimate outcome is for the infant or child to reach his or her potential independence as a functioning member of the family and community.

CASE STUDIES
CASE STUDY 1

Elsa

Elsa is a 13-year-old girl, born with multiple cranial neuropathies. A computed axial tomography (CAT) scan after birth revealed no definitive findings. A repeat CAT scan at 10 years of age revealed a migrational defect (lack of migration of some of the gray matter during the development of the brain). By 8 months of age, Elsa was diagnosed with right hemiplegia and a movement disorder. The movement disorder has been labeled myoclonus or hemiballismus at different stages in her life. Elsa had six surgeries on her eyes before 1 year of age. A trial of bilateral serial casting was completed at 3 years of age for her shortened gastrocnemius/soleus groups and hamstrings. She required surgical heel cord lengthening at 5 years of age and bone graft in her left foot at 11 years of age to correct severe pronation. Elsa was initially medicated with phenobarbital for the movement disorder without any success at decreasing the hemiballistic movements. She was changed to a regimen of valproic acid, then to a dopamine agent. She is now receiving valproic acid, which has afforded the most control over the hemiballistic movements.

At 11 months of age, Elsa began therapy consisting of 1-hour sessions per week, each of physical, occupational, and speech therapies. Initially in therapy, Elsa demonstrated severe hypotonia and was unable to lift her head off the surface when she was placed in a prone position. Physical therapy concentrated on increasing her function toward independent mobility on the floor, independent sitting and transitions between postures, and eventually, ambulation with assistive devices. These services remained in place until after she entered kindergarten, when physical, occupational, and speech services began twice weekly in the school system and continued in the outpatient medical model for several years. Outpatient medical-based physical therapy changed to a consultative role by the time Elsa was 8 years old. At 13 years of age, she continues to receive physical and occupational therapy in school and monthly consultative medical, physical therapy services.

Academically, Elsa can read and write her work on the computer. At 13 years of age, she is changing her school placement from an academic program to a life skills program to place more emphasis on gaining independence in self-care skills. The services in the school system have focused on her ability to learn information and improve the mobility required in the school buildings and community. Services included adaptive seating in the classroom, augmentative communication in her early school experience, and using a computer for all her school work. Elsa now uses verbal communication to interact but continues to do all her school work on the computer, using her left hand on the keyboard and a trackball.

Physical therapy has emphasized independent mobility both on the floor and vertical throughout her life. Elsa started walking with a walker by the age of 3 years and progressed to a quad cane used interchangeably with a walker until 10 years of age, when Elsa required the stability of a walker full time for ambulation. She has always required orthotics and has used articulating orthotics since age 6. She has consistently required assisted ambulation to a minimum of standby supervision because of the hemiballistic movement. Elsa has great difficulty regaining her balance quickly enough to prevent a fall when she experiences the involuntary movements. At 12 years of age, Elsa changed to a posterior walker with a right forearm platform, which has afforded her more independence in the house for up to a distance of 30 feet.

For assisted mobility, Elsa began using a tricycle at 3 years of age and now uses an adult-size model. She received a manual wheelchair for long distances on entering kindergarten and has remained dependent on its use because of her inability to use her right arm for propulsion. When Elsa turned 11, she was measured and fitted for a power wheelchair, which offers her independence in the school and the surrounding community, although supervision for safety is required.

Elsa has had the benefit of recreational and therapeutic activities throughout her life. She has participated in hippotherapy since 4 years of age, attended dance classes for spe-

cial needs children for 1 year at the same age, and attended therapeutic aquatics from ages 4 through 8. She goes to summer camp with an attendant and enjoys the pool there on a daily basis.

Elsa's family has been intimately involved in all intervention decisions and has advocated for all her needs. She has benefited from a variety of interventions at home, in the medical model, in school, and in the community. Elsa has achieved a level of independence with which she is very happy and enjoys the associated interactions. She should continue to make progress toward a productive, full life with her family and friends, given the therapeutic and mechanical supports necessary for her mobility in her environment.

CASE STUDY 2

M.B. is a 12.5-month-old female born with a diagnosis of branchiooculofacial syndrome. Her medical history includes a prolonged hospitalization due to medical complications and the necessity for a tracheostomy and ventilation. Her hearing and vision are impaired but it is not clear how much she can see or hear at this point. Associated diagnoses include cleft lip and palate, vocal cord paralysis, hypoplastic aortic arch, chronic respiratory failure, gastroesophageal reflux, absent/poor suck and swallow, urinary complications, and global developmental delay with torticollis with M.B.'s head laterally tilting to the left. M.B. underwent multiple surgeries within the first year of life to correct the physical facial deformities and has had multiple hospitalizations. She lives at home with her parents and a brother and has nursing services 16 hours per day for her medical care so that she could live at home with the ventilator.

M.B. has been in the early intervention system since 6 months of age and has been receiving vision services twice a month for 1 hour, hearing services weekly for 1 hour, and physical therapy services weekly for 1 hour.

The parents' identified functional outcome for physical therapy was that M.B. would be able to hold herself upright and begin to move to enable her to participate in the life of the family and explore her environment with assistance. The short-term outcomes identified include that M.B. will keep her head upright, in neutral, in supported sitting for 1 to 2 minutes by the end of the session and that M.B. will roll from her stomach to her back, by herself, in three of four trials.

Initially, M.B. presented with significant hypotonia throughout her neck and trunk and was unhappy when asked to do the antigravity work of supported sitting or fully supported standing. Intervention and family activities revolved around the provision of movement to arouse M.B. to become interested in her surroundings as well as exploration of her small world in the crib, in her adapted seat, and on the floor. After bouncing M.B. on the ball or on the adult's legs, M.B. would begin to smile and attempted to sit erect with support through her ribcage and trunk. The initial attempts were quite short but sweet. The family purchased a large ball and soon M.B. was bouncing in sitting on the ball several times a day and enjoying the interaction. The family and nursing staff also carried over a "sensory diet" where M.B. could touch and play with a variety of textures several times a day and begin to accept more and varied touch.

The physical therapist began a supported standing program within the first 2 months of service (by 8 to 9 months of age) using the ball or the physical therapist's body for full support. This required preparation of her legs and feet from a sensory perspective first, so that she could tolerate having her feet in full contact with a surface. This was accomplished by the family putting dried beans in a Tupperware container into which her hands or her feet could be placed. She began to enjoy the experience and to seek it herself when the environment was set up for her. After about 2 months, M.B. was able to stand in a supported standing position, propped in her infant walker with towel rolls around her trunk. The height is set so that her hips and knees are slightly bent and she can push into the surface. By her 1-year birthday, M.B. could stand, once placed, in the standing device for up to 45 minutes, using both of her arms to play with toys on the tray that make music and have bright lights. She understands cause-and-effect toys and repeats the motions for play for 45 to 60 minutes.

By 11¼ months, M.B. was propping herself in sitting by putting her two arms down on the surface. By report, M.B. can do this for up to 2 minutes, depending on her focus at the time. Within the therapy session, the physical therapist observes M.B. sitting independently for up to 4 to 5 seconds before toppling over. She is able to hold her head in midline for up to 1 minute in supported sitting and attends to people and things in her immediate environment.

In the early intervention system, M.B. will have quarterly reviews of her identified functional outcomes and revision of same as necessary. Once she turns 3 years of age, she will progress to the next stage of early intervention, that which is typically offered in a center-based program. M.B. has great potential to make functional gross motor gains and to learn to support herself in vertical and to move/walk with assistance as needed. She will make progress as her medical condition allows and with her parents, sibling, and nurses supporting her growth and development through the coming years.

ACKNOWLEDGMENTS

I would like to thank my husband and son who have unfailingly supported my growth as a physical therapist, teacher, and writer. I extend my thanks to my friend Denita for her continued support and encouragement and also to Margo as a friend and colleague for caring, sharing, and giving so much of herself and her knowledge. I extend my gratitude to Kim for her friendship and encouragement and her review of the occupational therapy content of this edition.

REFERENCES

1. Katz RT. Life expectancy for children with cerebral palsy and mental retardation: implications for life care planning. NeuroRehabilitation 2003;18:261–270.
2. Accardo J, Kammann H, Hoon AH Jr. Neuroimaging in cerebral palsy. J Pediatr 2004;145(2 Suppl):S19–27.
3. Ferrari F, Cioni G, Einspieler C, et al. Cramped synchronized general movements in preterm infants as an early marker for cerebral palsy. Arch Pediatr Adolesc Med. 2002 May;156(5): 460–7.
4. Stiller C, Marcoux BC, Olson RE. The effect of conductive education, intensive therapy, and special education services on motor skills in children with cerebral palsy. Phys Occup Ther Pediatr 2003;23(3):31–50.
5. Niswander KR, Gordon M. The Collaborative Perinatal Project. In: The Women and Their Pregnancies. DHEW Publication no. 73-379, 1972.
6. Ellenberg JH, Nelson KB. Cluster of perinatal events identifying infants at high risk for death or disability. J Pediatr 1988;113: 546–552.
7. Reddihough DS, Collins KJ. The epidemiology and causes of cerebral palsy. Aust J Physiother 2003;49(1):7–12.
8. Miller F. Etiology, epidemiology, pathology, and diagnosis. In: Miller F, ed. Cerebral Palsy. New York: Springer-Verlag, Inc., 2004.
9. Hadders-Algra M. General movements: a window for early identification of children at high risk for developmental disorders. J Pediatr 2004;145(2 Suppl):S12–18.
10. Liptak GS, Accardo PJ. Health and social outcomes of children with cerebral palsy. J Pediatr 2004;145(2 Suppl):S36–41.
11. Gorter JW, Rosenbaum PL, Hanna SE, et al. Limb distribution, motor impairment, and functional classification of cerebral palsy. Dev Med Child Neurol 2004;46(7):461–467.
12. Howle JM. Neuro-Developmental Treatment Approach Theoretical Foundations and Principles of Clinical Practice. Laguna Beach, CA: The North American Neuro-Developmental Treatment Association, 2002.
13. Morris C, Bartlett D. Gross Motor Function Classification System: impact and utility. Dev Med Child Neurol 2004;46(1): 60–65.
14. Blanche EI, Botticelli TM, Hallway MK. Combining Neurodevelopment Treatment and Sensory Integration Principles: An Approach to Pediatric Therapy. Tucson, AZ: Therapy Skill Builders, 1995.
15. Cooper J, Majnemer, A, Rosenbaltt B, et al. The determination of sensory deficits in children with hemiplegic cerebral palsy. J Child Neurol 1995;10(4):300–309.
16. Beckung E, Hagberg G. Neuroimpairments, activity limitations and participation restrictions in children with cerebral palsy. Dev Med Child Neurol 2002:44(5):309–316.
17. Harada T, Erada S, Anwar MM, et al. The cervical spine in athetoid cerebral palsy. A radiological study of 180 patients. J Bone Joint Surg Br 1996;78(4):613–619.
18. Burns YR, O'Callaghan M, Tudehope DI. Early identification of cerebral palsy in high risk infants. Aust Pediatr J 1989;25: 215–219.
19. Harris SR. Early neuromotor predictors of cerebral palsy in low birthweight infants. Dev Med Child Neurol 1987;29: 508–519.
20. Harris SR. Movement analysis—an aid to diagnosis of cerebral palsy. Phys Ther 1991;71:215–221.
21. Rose-Jacobs R, Cabral H, Beeghly M, et al. The Movement Assessment of Infants (MAI) as a predictor of two-year neurodevelopmental outcome for infants born at term who are at social risk. Pediatr Phys Ther 2004;16(4):212–221.
22. Nelson KB, Ellenberg JH. Children who "outgrew" cerebral palsy. Pediatrics 1982;69:529–535.

23. Bly L. Motor Skills Acquisition in the First Year, An Illustrated Guide to Normal Development. Tucson, AZ: Therapy Skill Builders, 1994.

24. Bly L. Abnormal motor development. In: Slaton DS, ed. Proceedings of a Conference on Development of Movement in Infancy offered by the Division of Physical Therapy, University North Carolina at Chapel Hill, May 18–22, 1980.

25. Cochrane CD. Joint mobilization principles: considerations for use in the child with central nervous system dysfunction. Phys Ther 1987;67:1105–1109.

26. Illingworth RS. The Development of the Infant and Young Child. 8th Ed. New York: Churchill Livingstone, 1983.

27. Bly L. What is the role of sensation in motor learning? What is the role of feedback and feedforward? NDTA Netw 1996;1–7.

28. Cupps B. Postural control: a current view. NDTA Netw 1997; 1–7.

29. Olney SJ, Wright MJ. Cerebral palsy. In: Suzann Campbell, ed. Physical Therapy for Children. Philadelphia: WB Saunders, 1994.

30. Research Plan for the National Center for Medical Rehabilitation Research. NIH Publication No. 93-3509, March 1993.

31. Hoppenfeld S. Physical Examination of the Spine and Extremities. Norwalk, CT: Appleton-Century-Crofts, 1976.

32. Bleck EE. Orthopedic Management of Cerebral Palsy. Philadelphia: WB Saunders, 1979.

33. Shands AR, Steele MK. Torsion of the femur. J Bone Joint Surg 1958;40A:803–816.

34. Michele AA. Iliopsoas. Springfield, IL: Charles C Thomas, 1962.

35. Beals RK. Developmental changes in the femur and acetabulum in spastic paraplegia and diplegia. Dev Med Child Neurol 1969;11:303–313.

36. Staheli LT, Duncan WR, Schaefer E. Growth alterations in the hemiplegic child. Clin Orthop 1968;60:205–212.

37. Jordan P. Evaluation and Treatment of Foot Disorders. Presentation at the Neurodevelopmental Treatment Association Regional Conference, New York, May, 1984.

38. Calliet R. Foot and Ankle Pain. Philadelphia: FA Davis, 1970.

39. Burnett CN, Johnson EQ. Development of gait in childhood. Parts 1 and 2. Dev Med Child Neurol 1971;13:196–215.

40. Sutherland D, Olshen R, Cooper L, et al. The development of mature gait. J Bone Joint Surg 1980;62A:336–353.

41. Saunders JB, Inman VT, Eberhart HD. The major determinants in normal and pathological gait. J Bone Joint Surg 1953; 35A:543–558.

42. Miller F. Gait. In: Miller F, ed. Cerebral Palsy. New York: Springer-Verlag, Inc., 2004.

43. Dias LS, Marty GR. Selective posterior rhizotomy. In: Sussman MD, ed. The Diplegic Child: Evaluation and Management. Rosemont, IL: American Academy of Orthopaedic Surgeons, 1992.

44. Rosenbaum PL, Walter SD, Hanna SE, et al. Prognosis for gross motor function in cerebral palsy. JAMA 2002;288(11): 1357–1363.

45. Bobath B, Bobath K. An analysis of the development of standing and walking patterns in patients with cerebral palsy. Physiotherapy 1962;48:3.

46. Hicks R, Durinick N, Gage JR. Differentiation of idiopathic toe-walking and cerebral palsy. J Pediatr Orthop 1988;8: 160–163.

47. Mossberg KA, Linton KA, Fricke K. Ankle-foot orthoses: effect on energy expenditure of gait in spastic diplegic children. Arch Phys Med Rehab 1990;71:490–494.

48. Stamer M. Functional Documentation. Tucson, AZ: Therapy Skill Builders, 1995.

49. Tieman BL, Palisano RJ, Gracely EJ, et al. Gross motor capability and performance of mobility in children with cerebral palsy: a comparison across home, school, and outdoors/community settings. Phys Ther 2004;84(5):419–429.

50. Campbell SK. Quantifying the effects of interventions for movement disorders resulting from cerebral palsy. J Child Neurol 1996;11(Suppl 1):561–570.

51. Harris SR, Atwater SW, Crowe TK. Accepted and controversial neuromotor therapies for infants at high risk for cerebral palsy. J Perinatol 1988;8(1):3–13.

52. Palisano RJ, Kolobe TH, Haley SM, et al. Validity of the Peabody Developmental Gross Motor Scale as an evaluative measure of infants receiving physical therapy. Phys Ther 1995; 75(11):939–948.

53. Miller F. Rehabilitation techniques. In: Miller F, ed. Cerebral Palsy. New York: Springer-Verlag, Inc., 2004.

53a. Damiano D. Strengthening Exercises. In Miller F. ed. Cerebral Palsy. New York: Springer-Verlag, Inc., 2004.

54. Binder H, Eng GD. Rehabilitation management of children with spastic diplegic cerebral palsy. Arch Phys Med Rehabil 1989;70:482–489.

55. Lecture by Dr. Freeman Miller, MD, on Orthopedic Surgeries for the Child with Cerebral Palsy, at A.I. duPont Hospital for Children, Wilmington, DE, October 28, 2004.

56. Fetters L. Measurement and treatment in cerebral palsy: an argument for a new approach (review). Phys Ther 1991;71: 244–247.

57. Kamm K, Thelen E, Jensen J. A dynamical systems approach to motor development. Phys Ther 1990;70:763–775.

58. Bobath B, Bobath K. Motor Development in the Different Types of Cerebral Palsy. London: William Heineman Medical Books, 1982.

59. Finnie NR. Handling the Young Cerebral Palsied Child at Home. 2nd Ed. New York: Dalton Publications, 1975.

60. Davis S. Neurodevelopmental Treatment/Bobath Eight Week Course in the Treatment of Children with Cerebral Palsy. Lecture notes, June–July 1997.

61. Pippenger WS, Scalzitti DA. Evidence in practice, what are the effects, if any of lower extremity strength training on gait in children with cerebral palsy? Phys Ther 2004;84(9):849–858.

62. Eagleton M, Iams A, McDowell J, et al. The effects of strength training on gait in adolescents with cerebral palsy. Pediatr Phys Ther 2004;16(1):22–30.

63. Fisher AG, Murray EA, Bundy AC. Sensory Integration, Theory and Practice. Philadelphia: F. A. Davis, 1991.

64. Ayres AJ. Sensory Integration and the Child. Los Angeles: Western Psychological Services, 1979.

65. Birkmeier K. Curriculum and theoretical base committee update. NDTA Netw 1997;6:4;1–7.

66. Kerr C, McDowell B, McDonuough S. Electrical stimulation in cerebral palsy: a review of effects on strength and motor function. Dev Med Child Neurol 2004;46:205–213.

67. Pape KE, Chipman ML. Electrotherapy in rehabilitation. In: Delisa BM, Gans NE, Walsh NE, et al. eds. Physical Medicine and Rehabilitation: Principles and Practice. Baltimore: Lippincott Williams & Wilkins, 2004.

68. Daichman J, Johnson TE, Evans K, et al. The effects of neuromuscular electrical stimulation home program on impairments and functional skills of a child with spastic diplegic cerebral palsy: a case report. Pediatr Phys Ther 2003;15(3):153–158.

69. Pape KE. Therapeutic electrical stimulation the past, the present, the future. NDTA Netw 1996;1–7.

70. Pape KE, Kirsch SE. Technology-assisted self-care in the treatment of spastic diplegia. In: Sussman MD, ed. The Diplegic Child: Evaluation and Management. Rosemont, IL: American Academy of Orthopaedic Surgeons, 1992.

71. Darrah J, Watkins B, Chen L, et al. Conductive education intervention for children with cerebral palsy: an AACPDM evidence report. Dev Med Child Neurol 2004;46:187–203.

72. Liberty K. Developmental gains in early intervention based on conductive education by young children with motor disorders. Int J Rehab Res 2004;27(1):17–25.

73. Molnar GE. Rehabilitation in cerebral palsy. West J Med 1991;154:569–572.

74. Styer-Acevedo JL. Aquatic rehabilitation in pediatrics. In: Ruoti RG, Morris DM, Cole PJ, eds. Aquatic Rehabilitation. Philadelphia: Lippincott-Raven, 1997.

75. McCloskey S. Notes from Lecture on Hippotherapy at Arcadia University, April 28, 2004.

76. Casady RL, Nichols-Larsen DS. The effect of hippotherapy on ten children with cerebral palsy. Pediatr Phys Ther 2004;16(3): 165–172.

77. Stuberg WA. Considerations related to weight-bearing programs in children with developmental disabilities. Phys Ther 1992;72:35–40.

78. Rose J, Gamble JG, Medeiras J, et al. Energy cost of walking in normal children and in those with cerebral palsy: comparison of heart rate and oxygen uptake. J Pediatr Orthop 1989;9: 276–279.

79. Logan L, Byers-Hinkley K, Ciccone CD. Anterior versus posterior walkers: a gait analysis study. Dev Med Child Neurol 1990;32:1044–1048.

80. Levangie PK, Chimera M, Johnston M, et al. The effects of posterior rolling walkers on gait characteristics of children with spastic cerebral palsy. Phys Occup Ther Pediatr 1989;9:1–17.

81. Canadian Medical Association. Editorial. Can Med Assoc J 1987;136:57.

82. Kauffman IB, Ridenour M. Influence of an infant walker on onset and quality of walking pattern of locomotion: an electromyographic investigation. Percept Mot Skills 1977;45: 1323–1329.

83. Mothering 46, Winter 1988.

83a. Capone K, Hoopes D, Kiser D, and Rolph B. M.O.V.E.™ (Mobility Opportunities via Education) Curriculum. In Miller F. ed. Cerebral Palsy. New York: Springer-Verlag, Inc., 2004.

84. Black JA, Reed MD, Roberts CD. Muscle relaxant drugs for children with cerebral palsy. In: Sussman MD, ed. The Diplegic Child: Evaluation and Management. Rosemont, IL: American Academy of Orthopaedic Surgeons, 1992.

85. Pranzatelli MR. Oral pharmacotherapy for the movement disorders of cerebral palsy. J Child Neurol 1996;11(Suppl 1): S13–22.

85a. McManus M. Intrathecal Baclofen Pumps. In Miller F. ed. Cerebral Palsy. New York: Springer-Verlag, Inc., 2004.

86. Sutherland DH, Kaufman KR, Wyatt MP, Chambers MG, et al. Injection of botulinum A toxin into the gastrocnemius muscle of patients with cerebral palsy: a 3 dimensional motion analysis study. Gait Posture 1996;4:269–279.

87. Wong AMK, Chen CL, Chen CPC, et al. Clinical effects of botulinum toxin A and phenol block on gait in children with cerebral palsy. Am J Phys Med Rehabil 2004;83(4):284–291.

88. Fragala MA, O'Neil ME, Russo KJ, et al. Impairment, disability, and satisfaction outcomes after lower extremity botulinum toxin A injections for children with cerebral palsy. Pediatr Phys Ther 2002;14(3):132–144.

89. Pidcock FS. The emerging role of therapeutic botulinum toxin in the treatment of cerebral palsy. J Pediatr 2004;145(2 Suppl): S33–S35.

90. Kinnette DK. Botulinum toxin A injections in children: technique and dosing issues. Am J Phys Med Rehabil 2004;83 (10 Suppl):S59–S64.

91. O'Neil ME, Fragala MA, Dumas HM. Physical therapy intervention for children with cerebral palsy who receive botulinum toxin A injections. Pediatr Phys Ther 2003;15(4):204–215.

92. Bottos M, Benedetti MG, Salucci P, et al. Botulinum toxin with and without casting in ambulant children with spastic diplegia:

a clinical and functional assessment. Dev Med Child Neurol 2003;45(11):758–762.

93. Booth MY, Yates CC, Edgar TS, et al. Serial casting vs combined intervention with botulinum toxin A and serial casting in the treatment of spastic equinus in children. Pediatr Phys Ther 2003;15(4):216–220.

94. Gooch JL, Patton CP. Combining botulinum toxin and phenol to manage spasticity in children. Arch Phys Med Rehabil 2004;85(7):1121–1124.

95. Peacock WJ, Stoudt LA. Functional outcomes following selective posterior rhizotomy in children with cerebral palsy. J Neurosurg 1991;74:380–385.

96. Guiliani CA. Dorsal rhizotomy for children with cerebral palsy: support for concept of motor control. Phys Ther 1991;71: 248–259.

97. Abbott R, Forem SL, Johann M. Selective posterior rhizotomy for the treatment of spasticity: a review. Child Nerv Syst 1989;5: 337–346.

98. Oppenheim W. Selective posterior rhizotomy for spastic cerebral palsy. A review. Clin Orthop Rel Res 1990;253:20–29.

99. Oppenheim WL, Staudt LA, Peacock WJ. The rationale for rhizotomy. In: Sussman MD, ed. The Diplegic Child: Evaluation and Management. Rosemont, IL: American Academy of Orthopaedic Surgeons, 1992.

100. Peter JC, Arens LJ. Selective posterior lumbosacral rhizotomy in teenagers and young adults with spastic cerebral palsy. Br J Neurosurg 1994;8(2):135–139.

101. Bloom KK, Nazar GB. Functional assessment following selective posterior rhizotomy in spastic cerebral palsy. Childs Nerv Sys 1994;10(2):84–86.

102. Thomas SS, Aiona MD, Pierce R, et al. Gait changes in children with spastic diplegia after selective dorsal rhizotomy. J Pediatr Orthop 1996;16(6):747–752.

103. Chicoine MR, Park TS, Kaufman BA. Selective dorsal rhizotomy and rates of orthopedic surgery in children with spastic cerebral palsy. J Neurosurg 1997;86(1):34–39.

104. Hendricks-Ferguson VL, Ortman MR. Selective dorsal rhizotomy to decrease spasticity in cerebral palsy. AORN J 1995; 61(3):514–518, 521–552.

105. Heim RC, Rark TS, Vogler GP, et al. Changes in hip migration after selective dorsal rhizotomy for spastic quadriplegia in cerebral palsy. J Neurosurg 1995;82(4):567–571.

106. Johnson MB, Goldstein L, Thomas SS, et al. Spinal deformity after selective dorsal rhizotomy in ambulatory patients with cerebral palsy. J Pediatr Orthop 2004;24(5):529–536.

107. Spiegel DA, Loder RT, Alley KA, et al. Spinal deformity following selective dorsal rhizotomy. J Pediatr Orthop 2004; 24(1):30–36.

108. Engsberg JR, Ross SA, Wagner JM, et al. Changes in hip spasticity and strength following selective dorsal rhizotomy and physical therapy for spastic cerebral palsy. Dev Med Child Neurol 2002;44(4):220–226.

109. Ross SA, Engsberg JR, Olree KS, et al. Quadriceps and hamstring strength changes as a function of selective dorsal rhizotomy surgery and rehabilitation. Pediatr Phys Ther 2001;13(1):2–9.

110. Graubert C, Song KM, McLaughlin JF, et al. Changes in gait at one year post-selective dorsal rhizotomy: results of a prospective randomized study. J Pediatr Orthop 2000;20(4):496–500.

111. Steinbok P, McLeod K. Comparison of motor outcomes after selective dorsal rhizotomy with and without preoperative intensified physiotherapy in children with spastic diplegic cerebral palsy. Pediatr Neurosurg 2002;36(1):142–147.

112. Gooch JL, Oberg WA, Grams B, et al. Care provider assessment of intrathecal baclofen in children. Dev Med Child Neurol 2004;46(8):548–552.

113. Barry MJ, Albright AL, Shultz BL. Intrathecal baclofen therapy and the role of the physical therapist. Pediatr Phys Ther 2000;12:77–86.

114. DeLuca PA. The musculoskeletal management of children with cerebral palsy. Pediatr Clin North Am 1996;43(5): 1135–1150.

115. Sprague JB. Surgical management of cerebral palsy. Orthop Nurs 1992;11(4):11–19.

116. Dormans JP. Orthopedic management of children with cerebral palsy. Pediatr Clin North Am 1993;40(3):645–657.

117. Green NE. The orthopedic management of the ankle, foot, and knee in patients with cerebral palsy. Neuromuscular disease and deformities. Instr Course Lect 1987;36:253–256.

118. Miller F. Surgical techniques. In: Miller F, ed. Cerebral Palsy. New York: Springer-Verlag, Inc., 2004.

119. Gamble JG, Rinsky LA, Bleck EE. Established hip dislocations in children with cerebral palsy. Clin Orthop Rel Res 1990;253: 90–99.

120. Pritchett JW. Treated and untreated unstable hips in severe cerebral palsy. Dev Med Child Neurol 1990;32:3–6.

121. Pronsati M. Baby walkers-considering full price of convenience. Adv Phys Ther 1992;7.

122. Patrick JH. Techniques of psoas tenotomy and rectus femoris transfer: "new" operations for cerebral palsy diplegia—a description. J Pediatr Orthop B 1996;5(4):242–246.

123. Moreau M, Cook PC, Ashton B. Adductor and psoas release for subluxation of the hip in children with spastic cerebral palsy. J Pediatr Orthop 1995;15(5):672–676.

124. Atar D, Grant AD, Mirsky E, Lehman WB, et al. Femoral varus derotational osteotomy in cerebral palsy. Am J Orthop 1995; 24(4):337–341.

125. Moens P, Lammens J, Molenaers G, et al. Femoral derotation for increased hip anteversion. A new surgical technique with a modified Ilizarov frame. J Bone Joint Surg Br 1995;77(1): 107–109.

126. Pope DF, Bueff HU, DeLuca PA. Pelvic osteotomies for subluxation of the hip in cerebral palsy. J Pediatr Orthop 1994; 14(6):724–730.

127. Root L, Laplasa FJ, Brourman SN, et al. The severely unstable hip in cerebral palsy. Treatment with open reduction, pelvic osteotomy, and femoral osteotomy with shortening. J Bone Joint Surg Am 1995;77(5):703–712.

128. Brunner R, Baumann JU. Clinical benefit of reconstruction of dislocated or subluxated hip joints in patients with spastic cerebral palsy. J Pediatr Orthop 1994;14(3):290–294.

129. Atar D, Grant AD, Bash J, et al. Combined hip surgery in cerebral palsy patients. Am J Orthop 1995;24(1):52–55.

130. Barrie JL, Galasko CS. Surgery for unstable hips in cerebral palsy. J Pediatr Orthop B 1996;5(4):225–231.

131. Root L. Distal hamstring surgery in cerebral palsy. In: Sussman MD, ed. The Diplegic Child Evaluation and Management. Rosemont, IL: American Academy of Orthopaedic Surgeons, 1992.

132. Gage JR. Distal hamstring lengthening/release and rectus femoris transfer. In: Sussman MD, ed. The Diplegic Child Evaluation and Management. Rosemont, IL: American Academy of Orthopaedic Surgeons, 1992.

133. Abdennebi B, Bougatene B. Selective neurotomies for relief of spasticity focalized to the foot and to the knee flexors. Results in a series of 58 patients. Acta Neurochir Wien 1996;138(8): 917–920.

134. Yngve DA, Chambers C. Vulpius and Z-lengthening. J Pediatr Orthop 1996;16(6):759–764.

135. Rosenthal RK, Simon SR. The Vulpius gastrocnemius-soleus lengthening. In: Sussman MD, ed. The Diplegic Child Evaluation and Management. Rosemont, IL: American Academy of Orthopaedic Surgeons, 1992.

136. Hamel J, Kissling C, Heimkes B, Stutz S, et al. A combined bony and soft-tissue tarsal stabilization procedure (Grice-Schede) for hindfoot valgus in children with cerebral palsy. Arch Orthop Trauma Surg 1994;113(5):237–243.

137. Kagaya H, Yamada S, Nagasawa T, et al. Split posterior tibial tendon transfer for varus deformity of hindfoot. Clin Orthop 1996;323:254–260.

138. Roehr B, Lyne ED. Split anterior tibial tendon transfer. In: Sussman MD, ed. The Diplegic Child: Evaluation and Management. Rosemont, IL: American Academy of Orthopaedic Surgeons, 1992.

139. Green NE. Split posterior tibial tendon transfer: the universal procedure. In: Sussman MD, ed. The Diplegic Child: Evaluation and Management. Rosemont, IL: American Academy of Orthopaedic Surgeons, 1992.

140. Mazur JM, Shanks DE. Nonsurgical treatment of tight Achilles tendon. In: Sussman MD, ed. The Diplegic Child: Evaluation and Management. Rosemont, IL: American Academy of Orthopaedic Surgeons, 1992.

141. Radtka SA. A comparison of gait with solid, dynamic, and no ankle-foot orthoses in children with spastic cerebral palsy. Phys Ther 1997;77(4):395–409.

142. Middleton EA, Hurley GR, McIlwain JS. The role of rigid and hinged polypropylene ankle-foot orthoses in the management of cerebral palsy: a case study. Prosthet Orthot Int 1988;12: 129–135.

143. Carmick J. Managing equinus in a child with cerebral palsy: merits of hinged ankle-foot orthoses. Dev Med Child Neurol 1995;37(11):1006–1010.

144. Olney SJ, Wright MJ. Cerebral palsy. In: Campbell SK, ed. Physical Therapy for Children. Philadelphia: W. B. Saunders, 1994.

145. Magill-Evans JE, Restall G. Self-esteem of persons with cerebral palsy: from adolescence to adulthood. Am S Occup Ther 1991;45(9):819–825.

146. Dodd KJ, Taylor NF, Graham HK. Strength training can have unexpected effects on the self concept of children with cerebral palsy. Pediatr Phys Ther 2004;16(2):99–105.

147. Craft MJ, Lakin JA, Oppliger RA, et al. Siblings as change agents for promoting the functional status of children with cerebral palsy. Dev Med Child Neurol 1990;32:1049, 1057.

148. Tetreault S, Parrot A, Trahan J. Home activity programs in families with children presenting with global developmental delays: evaluation and parental perceptions. Int J Rehabil Res 2003;26(3):165–173.

Spina Bifida

Elena Tappit-Emas

Incidence and Etiology

Spina bifida is one type of neural tube birth defect causing neuromuscular dysfunction. The occurrence of spina bifida approaches 1 in every 1000 live births, making it the second most common birth defect after Down syndrome. Studies examining the possible causes of spina bifida have evaluated genetic, environmental, and dietary factors that might affect its occurrence. However, no definitive cause, including chromosomal abnormalities, has yet been identified.[1,2]

Many factors contribute to a baby being born with spina bifida. The presence of a genetic predisposition may be enhanced by numerous environmental influences. Low levels of maternal folic acid prior to conception have been implicated in several studies. One study by Duff et al. found a significant though temporary increase of children born with all types of neural tube defects on the island of Jamaica who were conceived during the several months immediately following Hurricane Gilbert in September of 1988. The normal diet of this island is rich in folic acid from fresh fruit and vegetables. The hurricane destroyed much of the island's crops, and for a temporary period, fresh produce was scarce.[3] This study as well as an annotation by Seller proposed a need to fortify commonly eaten foods with folic acid such as orange juice, cereals, flour, rice, and salt.[4]

In 1992, the U.S. Public Health Service made the recommendation that all women should receive 400 µg of folic acid daily during the months prior to conception and 600 µg through the first trimester of pregnancy. With improved education and the support of the medical community, this level of folic acid can be reached through improved diet, dietary supplements, and fortified foods. Folic acid is abundant in green leafy vegetables, cooked dry beans, nuts and seeds, enriched grains, pasta, bread, and rice.[5] In 1998, the health departments of both the United States and Canada recommended that all cereal grains be fortified with folic acid to enable women to more easily reach this daily requirement. The U.S. Department of Health and Human Services has set a national objective to reduce by 50% the number of children born with spina bifida by the year 2010.[5–8] It appears that the ability of folic acid to reduce the incidence of spina bifida has made the genes involved with folic acid metabolism and transport the target of further intensive investigation.[9,10]

Maternal use of valproic acid, an anticonvulsant, is also known to increase the potential for spina bifida. It appears that the developing nervous system is especially sensitive to disruption after exposure to this drug.[10] Maternal hyperthermia caused by saunas, hot tub and electric blanket use, and maternal fevers during the first trimester of pregnancy were also studied. Only the use of hot tubs showed any tendency to increase the risk of spina bifida.[11] But it appears in more recent investigations that this cause has not attracted wide concern.

A higher occurrence, as much as 4.5 per 1000 births, is seen in families of Irish and Celtic heritage. Japanese families have a low occurrence with only 0.3 per 1000 births. A changing pattern of births has also been noted in the United States with an increase in the incidence of spina bifida in Hispanic and African-American families, perhaps owing to environmental factors and pollution as populations have shifted to industrialized urban areas in the past decades.[12] A dramatic change in diet as these two populations have moved from rural farms and small towns is also thought to be a potential influence. For families in which spina bifida is already present, there is a 2% to 5% greater chance than in the general population of having a second child born with the defect.

 Prognosis

In previous generations, long-term survival of children with spina bifida was reported to range from as low as 1% without treatment to 50% with treatment. A survival rate of more than 90% is now expected when aggressive treatment is provided to the spinal defect and its associated problems. This chapter presents the primary problems for this population of children, including hydrocephalus, motor and sensory deficits in the lower extremities, and urologic impairment as well as the secondary issues that are of clinical significance.

The use of antibiotics to limit infection in the open spine, starting in 1947, and the surgical insertion of ventricular shunts in 1960 to limit hydrocephalus were major advances in the treatment of spina bifida. Early and consistent use of clean, intermittent catheterization to completely empty the bladder has also dramatically improved the survival rate by controlling urinary tract infection and renal deterioration, both of which have been major causes of mortality. These measures, along with the practice of early back closure, continue to improve the chances of survival of children with spina bifida. As the survival rate improved, an increased awareness evolved for the associated problems that were neither evident nor a priority for treatment in the past. The number of severely affected children who have survived has increased. Additionally, there is an increased number of less severely involved individuals who would not have lived with earlier, less aggressive treatment protocols. Therefore, the full spectrum and complexity of this disability can now be appreciated. Clinicians have the opportunity, unavailable in previous eras, to work with and learn a great deal from this heterogeneous group.[13,14]

 Definitions

The terms myelomeningocele, meningomyelocele, spina bifida, spina bifida aperta, spina bifida cystica, spinal dysraphism, and myelodysplasia are all synonymous. Spina bifida is a spinal defect usually diagnosed at birth by the presence of an external sac on the infant's back (Fig. 6.1). The sac contains meninges and spinal cord tissue protruding through a dorsal defect in the vertebrae. This defect may occur at any point along the spine but is most commonly located in the lumbar region. The sac may be covered by a transparent membrane with neural tissue attached to its inner surface, or the sac may be open with the neural tissue exposed. The lateral borders of the sac have bony protrusions formed by the unfused neural arches of the vertebrae. The defect may be large, with many vertebrae involved, or it may be small, involving only one or two segments. The size of the lesion is not by itself predictive of the child's functional deficit.[12,14,15]

There are several other congenital spinal defects that should be mentioned here. Spina bifida occulta and myelocele are less severe anomalies associated with spina bifida. *Spina bifida occulta* is a condition involving nonfusion of

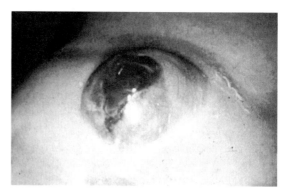

Figure 6.1 ▪ Spina bifida defect in a newborn infant before surgical repair.

the halves of the vertebral arches, but without disturbance of the underlying neural tissue. This lesion is most commonly located in the lumbar or sacral spine and is often an incidental finding when radiographs are taken for unrelated reasons. Spina bifida occulta may be distinguished externally by a midline tuft of hair, with or without an area of pigmentation on the overlying skin. Between 21% and 26% of parents who have children with spina bifida cystica have been found to have an occulta defect. Otherwise, spina bifida occulta has only a 4.5% to 8% incidence in the general population.[12,14,16] Neurologic and muscular dysfunction were previously thought to be absent in individuals with spina bifida occulta. However, a high incidence of tethered cord, its associated neurologic problems, and urinary tract disorders in these individuals have been found.[17–19]

A *myelocele* is a protruding sac containing meninges and cerebrospinal fluid (CSF), but the nerve roots and spinal cord remain intact and in their normal positions. There are no motor or sensory deficits, associated hydrocephalus, or other central nervous system (CNS) problems typically associated with a myelocele.[15]

Lipomeningocele is a superficial fatty mass in the low lumbar or sacral level of the spinal cord and is usually included in this group of diagnoses. Significant neurologic deficits and hydrocephalus are not expected in patients with a lipomeningocele. However, a high incidence of bowel and bladder dysfunction resulting from a tethered spinal cord has been noted in this population as well as subtle changes in distal leg and foot function.[20,21] Refer to additional information regarding tethered cord later in this chapter.

 Embryology

Spina bifida cystica, one of several neural tube defects, occurs early in the embryologic development of the CNS. Cells of the neural plate, which forms by day 18 of gestation, differentiate to create the neural tube and neural crest. The neural crest becomes the peripheral nervous system, including the cranial nerves, spinal nerves, autonomic nerves, and ganglia. The neural tube, which becomes the CNS, the brain, and the spinal cord, is open at both the cranial and caudal ends. Over a period of 2 to 4 days the cranial end begins to close and this process is completed on approximately the 24th day of gestation.[10] Failure to close results in anencephaly, a fatal condition. The caudal end of the neural tube closes on approximately day 26 of gestation. Failure of the neural tube to close at any point along the caudal border initiates the defect of spina bifida cystica or myelomeningocele. Common clinical signs of spina bifida cystica include absence of motor and sensory function (usually bilateral) below the level of the spinal defect and loss of neural control of bowel and bladder function. Unilateral motor and sensory loss has been reported and the pattern of loss may also be asymmetric, with a higher motor

or sensory level on one side compared to the other. The functional deficits may be partial or complete, but they are almost always permanent.[14,22,23]

 Hydrocephalus and the Chiari II Malformation

Hydrocephalus and the Arnold-Chiari malformation are CNS abnormalities that are closely associated with spina bifida. *Hydrocephalus* is an abnormal accumulation of CSF in the cranial vault. In individuals without spina bifida, hydrocephalus may be caused by overproduction of CSF, a failure in absorption of CSF fluid, or an obstruction in the normal flow of CSF through the brain structures and spinal cord. Obstruction by the Arnold-Chiari malformation is considered to be the primary cause of hydrocephalus in most children with spina bifida. This malformation, also known as the *Chiari II malformation*, is a deformity of the cerebellum, medulla, and cervical spinal cord. The posterior cerebellum is herniated downward through the foramen magnum, with brainstem structures also displaced in a caudal direction. The CSF released from the fourth ventricle is obstructed by these abnormally situated structures, and its flow through the foramen magnum is disrupted. Traction on the lower cranial nerves occurs and is associated with the malformation. Studies using magnetic resonance imaging (MRI) have shown that most children with spina bifida have the Chiari II malformation. Among those with this malformation, the likelihood of hydrocephalus developing is greater than 90%.[24–27]

Theories related to the development of the Chiari II malformation are of interest. At one time it was thought that the primary spinal defect acted as an anchor on the spinal cord, preventing it from sliding proximally within the spinal canal as the fetus grew. It was believed that this traction on the cord pulled down the attached brainstem structures into an abnormally low position. Hydrocephalus was thought to result solely from the hydrodynamic consequence of this blockage.[28] In 1989, a study by McLone and Knepper more closely linked the occurrence of spina bifida, the Chiari II malformation, and hydrocephalus.[29] These researchers postulated that a series of interrelated, time-dependent defects occur during the embryonic development of the primitive ventricular system, causing the Chiari II malformation first and then hydrocephalus.[30] Their findings indicate that most affected children have a small posterior fossa that is unable to accommodate the hindbrain and brainstem structures and this influences the abnormal positioning. Significantly, McLone and Knepper found that more than 25% of the neonates with spina bifida that they examined had head circumferences measuring below the fifth percentile. Therefore, neither downward traction from the spinal defect nor downward pressure from hydrocephalus causes the malformation. These researchers postulated that spina bifida results from mistimed steps in the development of the ventricular system initiated by the failure of the neural tube to close. This explanation has received widespread acceptance among both neuro-anatomists and neurosurgeons and should be of interest to physical therapists who have speculated about the cause of the CNS dysfunction they have observed in children with spina bifida. These children differ greatly from those children who only have hydrocephalus and not spina bifida, with whom they are often compared. The McLone and Knepper theory begins to offer an anatomic rationale for the CNS abnormalities seen in many patients, and offers a viable basis for future investigation.[29]

Approximately 2% to 3% of children with spina bifida show significant impairment from the Chiari II malformation (Display 6.1).[30] Tracheostomy and gastrostomy may be life-saving measures for the symptoms, which are reported to resolve as the child grows and the brain matures. In severe cases, upper extremity weakness or opisthotonic postures may be seen. Posterior fossa decompression and cervical laminectomy to relieve pressure on the brainstem and cervical spinal structures are accepted courses of treatment but are associated with varying degrees of success. It is of interest that no correlation has been found between the severity of the Chiari II symptoms and the degree of hydrocephalus seen in the infant; nor has a correlation been found between the child's motor level and these CNS findings. Therefore, attempts to predict which children will experience significant CNS difficulties resulting from the Chiari II malformation have been unsuccessful. Examination by MRI has revealed severe abnormalities in some children who present as asymptomatic. There is speculation that brainstem auditory-evoked potentials may provide some diagnostic assistance in the future. Physicians also believe that there is much to learn at the microscopic level about this abnormality.[12,14,31–34]

>> **DISPLAY 6.1**

Symptoms Associated with Chiari II Malformation

Stridor—especially with inspiration
Apnea—when crying, or at night
Gastroesophageal reflux
Paralysis of vocal cords
Swallowing difficulty
Bronchial aspiration
Tongue fasciculations
Facial palsy
Poor feeding
Ataxia
Hypotonia
Upper extremity weakness
Seizures
Abnormal extraocular movements
Nystagmus

◆ Prenatal Testing and Diagnosis

Increasingly sophisticated and more widely available prenatal testing has allowed the early diagnosis of spina bifida. Such testing provides information that allows families to make informed decisions about the pregnancy. As prenatal testing has become more the routine than the exception, a significant number of pregnancies are terminated each year when the results have indicated a high likelihood of the fetus having a neural tube defect.[6,35,36] For the family that chooses to bring their baby to term, appropriate and coordinated medical care can be arranged in anticipation of the birth.

α-Fetoprotein (AFP) is normally present in the developing fetus and is found in the amniotic fluid. AFP levels reach their peak levels in the fetal serum and in the amniotic fluid from the sixth to the 14th week of gestation. In the presence of spina bifida, after the 14th week AFP continues to leak into the amniotic fluid through the exposed vascularity of the open spine. Abnormally high levels of AFP in the amniotic fluid provide strong diagnostic evidence for the presence of a neural tube defect. Testing for AFP by amniocentesis and, more recently, in maternal blood samples has been responsible for the detection of approximately 89% of neural tube defects. Unfortunately, the tests have the potential for both false-positive and false-negative results. Therefore, AFP results are routinely compared clinically with the results of ultrasound imaging before a definitive diagnosis is made.[14,24]

Improved ultrasound equipment and experienced technicians have enabled obstetricians to observe and document several cranial abnormalities that have a high correlation with the presence of spina bifida in the developing fetus. Because a small back lesion can be difficult or impossible to detect, clinicians use the presence of the cranial signs as an indication that the fetus may have spina bifida. The frontal bones of the fetal skull lose their normal convex shape and appear flattened when spina bifida is present, similar to the shape of a lemon. The "Lemon sign" can be detected before 24 weeks of gestation. It disappears as the fetus matures and the skull becomes stronger or as hydrocephalus develops and pushes on the flattened skull, reversing its shape into the normal configuration.[37] The detection of the Lemon sign can then be followed by additional ultrasound studies specifically for the purpose of locating the back lesion.[38,39]

There has been speculation regarding the best method of obstetric delivery when spina bifida is detected. A cesarean section may have a protective effect on the sensitive neural tissue of the neonatal back, thus possibly improving the child's ultimate functional status. Cesarean section reduces the trauma to the exposed nerves of the back that might occur during a vaginal delivery. Moreover, a cesarean delivery avoids the bacterial contamination of the neonate's open lesion associated with passage through the vaginal canal, thereby reducing the risk of the baby contracting meningitis. A cesarean section also avoids trauma to the back in the case of a breech presentation, which could also affect the infant's neurologic function. Finally, arrangements for back closure can be planned and accomplished more rapidly following a scheduled cesarean section than after an unscheduled vaginal delivery.[40-44]

In recent years, there have been efforts in several institutions to perform fetal surgery to repair the spinal defect prior to the birth of the infant. As early as 1998, a study by Johnson et al. performing prenatal surgery, between 20 and 25 weeks' gestation, saw a survival rate of 94% with significant reversals in hindbrain herniation, a significant decrease in the need for shunting of hydrocephalus, and improvement in lower extremity function.[45] Two other studies by Sutton et al. and Buner et al. also demonstrated an improvement in hindbrain herniation, a decrease in the need for shunting, and an older median age for the insertion of the first shunt for those infants who did develop hydrocephalus. In these studies there was no indication that lower extremity motor function was changed with this surgical intervention.[46,47] The studies did point out several risk factors for prenatal back surgery that include an increase in premature births, lowered birth weights, and increased morbidity. But the authors are optimistic that there are significant benefits to be gained by prenatal surgery and over time the risk factors can be addressed and the negative effects diminished.[46,47]

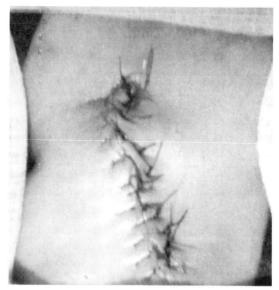

Figure 6.2 ■ The same defect shown in Figure 6.1, after surgical repair.

Management of the Neonate

GENERAL PHILOSOPHY OF TREATMENT

Philosophies of treatment for the neonate with spina bifida vary throughout the world as well as within the United States. Because the back lesion was not universally thought to be life threatening, hospitals developed their own protocols for the timing and intensity of treatment for these infants. However, comparing the results of studies in which various initial treatment regimens were used supports the efficacy of early medical intervention. Immediate sterile care of the lesion to prevent infection is essential, and surgical closure of the back within 72 hours of birth is now the accepted goal in most institutions.[12,14,48]

The objective of back surgery is to place the neural tissue into the vertebral canal, cover the spinal defect, and achieve a flat, watertight closure of the sac (Fig. 6.2). The open spine provides direct access for infection to the spinal cord and brain. By preventing infection and its associated brain damage, the child's level of function, both physical and cognitive, can be preserved. McLone and associates have shown that babies who suffer Gram-negative ventriculitis are less adept intellectually than babies who had no infec-

tion. This study is significant in that intellectual function was otherwise not negatively affected by either the presence of hydrocephalus or the level of lower limb paralysis.[12,48-50]

In many institutions children with spina bifida are treated aggressively with immediate back closure and rapid management of hydrocephalus. Other institutions practice selective treatment. That is, more aggressive management is offered to those children who appear to be less physically involved. In these institutions, the care of the neonate with spina bifida will vary depending on the level of lower extremity paralysis and the presence of other factors. Some of the factors that influence treatment decisions include accompanying abnormalities, such as hydrocephalus, kyphoscoliosis, and renal problems. Still other institutions attempt to educate parents regarding their child's status and the implications spina bifida will have on all of their lives. The parents may then act in a thoughtful manner in combination with the medical staff to choose a mutually acceptable course of action. During this period of education, which may last several hours or several weeks, the infant is usually treated to maintain a stable condition and prevent infection.

Regardless of the treatment protocols, this early period provides time for the medical staff to gather information about the child's condition. Discussions can begin about the management of hydrocephalus or orthopedic deformities that are present and which may require more involved care. It is important to note that an accurate prediction of the child's potential is difficult in these early days. A vast number of variables will influence the child's condition and function in the coming years, so clinicians must be wary about presenting long-term prognostic information about the child's future. The exception to this may be in the case of a severely impaired child who presents with

Nutrition and Spina Bifida in Pediatrics
Rebecca Thomas, RD, LDN
Clinical Dietitian
Children's Hospital of Philadelphia

Nutrition-Related Problems	Considerations/Interventions
OBESITY	
After six years of age, 50% of people with SB are overweight	Consistent eating pattern/meal schedule
Children with spina bifida have a higher percentage of body fat, lower total energy expenditure, and reduced physical activity	Decrease high fat/calorie foods Limit juice/soda Increase intake of fruits/vegetables
• Increased risk of decubitus ulcers	Encourage lean meats, low-fat dairy products
• Increased difficulty with mobility	Increase physical activity/physical therapy program
• Decreased social acceptance	Decubitus ulcers/wound healing 　High-protein diet 　Additional ascorbic acid and zinc 　Monitor visceral protein stores 　Increase physical activity
	Bone health 　Encourage weight-bearing activity 　Encourage low-fat dairy products 　Ensure adequacy of calcium, Vitamin D intake
MALNUTRITION	
Caused by limited variability in intake: limited fruits and vegetables, inconsistent eating patterns, overconsumption of foods/beverages with low nutritional value	Encourage varied, balanced diet Encourage calorie-dense foods, nutritional supplements if underweight Daily multivitamin
Abnormal or stunted growth	
Due to poor vertebral growth, atrophy of the muscles in the lower extremities; deformities of the spine, hips, and knees; hydrocephalus; renal disease; prolonged hospitalizations	
• Decreased weight-bearing activity	
• Decreased bone mineralization	
BOWEL CONTINENCE/INCONTINENCE	
Due to inadequate fiber and fluid in diet and decreased physical activity	Consistent eating pattern/meal schedule Ensure adequate fiber intake via fruits, vegetables, whole grains, nuts/seeds Ensure adequate fluid intake Encourage physical activity

SUGGESTED READINGS

Leibold S, Ekmark E, Adams RC. Decision-making for a successful bowel continence program. European Journal of Pediatric Surgery.2000 Dec;10 Suppl 1:26–30

Littlewood RA, Trocki O, Shephard RW, Shephard K, Davies PSW. Resting energy expenditure and body composition in children with myelomeningocele. Pediatric Rehabilitation. 2003 Feb vol. 6 No. 1 31–37.

Nevin-Folino NL. (Ed.). (2003). Pediatric Manual of Clinical Dietetics.

Pediatric Nutrition Practice Group, American Dietetic Association., 2nd ed.

multiple congenital anomalies as well as spina bifida whose outcome is apparently bleak.[51–53]

PREOPERATIVE ASSESSMENT

In many centers, the preoperative assessment is done by one physician experienced in the overall care of children with spina bifida. Consults are then requested as needed for specialty services. In other centers, a team of experts will each evaluate the baby and monitor him or her throughout the course of the hospitalization within their individual area of expertise. These professionals may also comprise the team that will be involved in the long-term care of the child after discharge, in the clinic setting.

The neurosurgeon is concerned initially with the location and extent of the infant's back lesion. Skin grafting may be necessary to gain adequate coverage over a large lesion. Kyphoscoliosis presents a complication that may lead to impaired wound healing because of excessive pressure over the suture site. Congenital scoliosis with accompanying fused ribs at the level of the back lesion may be present and usually predicts a rapid progression of the scoliosis during the growth periods of childhood. The resultant effect of progressive scoliosis on cardiopulmonary function may ultimately be life threatening, even with spinal bracing and surgical intervention. This anomaly is important to note.

A pediatrician or neonatologist may be consulted to assess the general health of the baby and to identify other congenital defects or cardiopulmonary dysfunction that may be present. The urologist can request urodynamic testing during the early neonatal period. Goals of the urologist include minimizing the effects of a neurogenic bladder on the upper urinary tract and producing urinary continence without compromising the urinary tract. Clean intermittent catheterization is widely accepted as the protocol to follow for the above goals, and though immediate attention may not be indicated until after back closure, it is understood that families will better accept intermittent catheterization as a management strategy if it is discussed and begun early rather than later in the infant's life. Intermittent catheterization is recognized as a method to preserve kidney function and prevent deterioration that can begin as early as 3 years of age in the population of children with spina bifida.[54,55]

A comprehensive orthopedic evaluation may not be imperative at this early stage, but an assessment can offer insight into the severity of any orthopedic problems that are present at birth. The need for surgery, splinting, or casting and its timing can be discussed, providing additional valuable information and education to the family and medical team. Following the evaluation of the lower extremities and spinal alignment, a plan of orthopedic care can be established for the baby's first months of life. This plan may in turn activate other staff, such as the physical therapist, to begin their role in the baby's intervention.[12,14,53–56]

MANAGEMENT OF HYDROCEPHALUS

After surgery for back closure, 10% of the infants recover, have their sutures removed, and leave the hospital without further complication. The remaining 90% will begin to develop hydrocephalus. Preoperatively, the open back lesion may act as a natural drain for CSF and when it is closed the CSF pressure begins to rise in the cranium. Of the 90% of the infants who develop hydrocephalus, approximately 25% are born with evidence of hydrocephalus and need immediate shunt insertion. Studies show that an additional 55% will develop hydrocephalus within several days of birth. The remaining babies will need shunting within 6 months. The neurosurgeon carefully monitors changes in the baby's head circumference, and studies such as ultrasound, computed tomography, or MRI provide baseline information regarding the size of the lateral ventricles. Later comparisons can assist in determining the appropriate time for insertion of a shunt.

Changes in the baby's state often indicate increasing intracranial pressure. As the enlarging ventricles cause the brain to expand within the flexible cranial vault, symptoms of hydrocephalus may be seen singularly or in combination. The most common symptoms are "sunsetting," a downward deviation of the eyes, and separation of the cranial sutures with a bulging anterior fontanelle.

The increasing fluid pressure may stabilize without surgery in some individuals, but it is impossible to predict when this will occur, how great the pressure will become, or how large the head will expand. Vital signs become depressed and respiratory arrest can occur when pressure on the brainstem structures becomes too great. Some individuals may survive without treatment but they may be severely impaired as a result.[12,13,53]

Surgical insertion of a shunt will relieve the signs and symptoms associated with increased intracranial pressure. The shunt is a thin, flexible tube that diverts CSF away from the lateral ventricles. It is secured at the proximal and distal ends and is radiopaque for easy location. The ventriculoatrial (VA) shunt moves excess CSF from one lateral ventricle to the right atrium of the heart. Because infections of the system can lead to septicemia, ventriculitis, superior vena cava occlusion, and pulmonary emboli, this type of shunt is not used as commonly used as it once was. The ventriculoperitoneal (VP) shunt is currently the preferred treatment for hydrocephalus. Although occlusion of this type of shunt may occur more easily than with the VA shunt, complications associated with the VP shunt are far less severe. As it exits the lateral ventricle, the shunt can be palpated running distally down the neck, under the clavicle, and down the anterior chest wall, just below the superficial fascia. The shunt inserts into the peritoneum, where CSF is reabsorbed and the excess excreted (Fig. 6.3).[56,57]

Although shunt insertion is a commonly performed operation for the neurosurgical team, it is yet another event for the infant who has already had back surgery. In

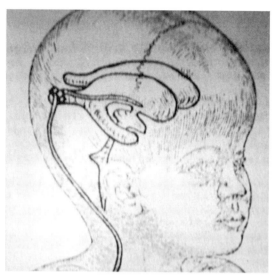

Figure 6.3 ■ *Location of the lateral ventricles and placement of ventriculoperitoneal shunt.*

order to spare the infant a second anesthesia, several centers perform simultaneous back closure and shunt insertion. Advocates of this approach believe that healing of the back wound from the inside is compromised when the CSF pressure is permitted to build internally. Therefore, more rapid healing of the back wound is expected and neither negative sequelae nor increased postoperative complications have been reported by performing the double procedure.[58,59]

After surgery, a plan for physical therapy, based on the infant's condition, can be developed. The priority is for rapid healing, an uneventful recovery, and a speedy discharge to home. Therefore, it is appropriate to wait at least 24 to 48 hours postoperatively before initiating physical therapy. In many cases, the extent of hydrocephalus prior to surgery will affect the timing of when the baby may receive oral feedings, position changes, range-of-motion exercises, and normal handling in the upright position. Premature aggressive handling after surgery is not safe, particularly for the baby who had significant hydrocephalus. Intracranial pressure can drop dramatically after shunt insertion, and vascular insult can occur if the baby is held upright too quickly.[53]

 Physical Therapy for the Infant with Spina Bifida

OVERVIEW

The role of the physical therapist can begin in the early preoperative period before back closure with an assessment of the neonate's active lower extremity movement. Ideally, the therapist who provides this preoperative evaluation is able to continue treating the baby throughout the hospi-

talization. It is also helpful if this same therapist can provide long-term monitoring and parent education as the baby graduates to the outpatient department or specialty clinic. This staffing approach provides consistent support for parents during a stressful period. Also, the importance of staff continuity becomes increasingly important as the child grows. When changes in function are suspected, the therapist who is familiar with the infant and has a good baseline of observations and documentation can be a valuable resource for the medical team. When a therapist has monitored the baby through the early period of care, the ability to detect even subtle changes is greatly enhanced.[53]

MANUAL MUSCLE TESTING

A manual muscle test performed by the physical therapist can provide objective information regarding the presence of active movement and the quantity of muscle power present in the baby's lower extremities (Display 6.2). Manual muscle testing should be performed before back surgery whenever possible. It is suggested that testing be repeated approximately 10 days after surgery, then at 6 months, and yearly thereafter unless a problem arises indicating a more frequent schedule. The goal of these early testing sessions is to assist the medical staff to identify the level of the back lesion by assessing the lower extremity movement or lack thereof.[53]

Consideration must be given when positioning the baby for this muscle test. Depending on the status of the back lesion or surgical site and to protect the involved area, the infant may be limited to prone or side-lying. But careful observation and palpation should still allow for identification of most major muscle groups (Figs. 6.4 and 6.5).

A motor level is assigned according to the last intact nerve root found. Lindseth has defined the motor level as the lowest level at which the child is able to perform antigravity movement through the available range.[60] While this level of certainty may not be possible when testing the infant, preliminary identification of the motor level encour-

> ## DISPLAY 6.2

Information Provided by Early Manual Muscle Testing for Children with Spina Bifida

Baseline analysis for long-term comparisons

Assessment of existing muscle function

Evaluation of muscular imbalance at each joint

Establishing the degree and character of existing deformity

Preliminary prediction of potential for future deformity

Assistance in determining the need for early splinting

Assistance in determining need for early surgery

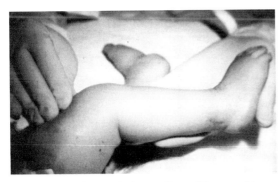

Figure 6.4 ■ Palpation and observation of the quadriceps muscle during a preoperative assessment of the active movement in the lower extremities.

ages consistency of communication among professionals involved with the baby. However, keep in mind that children assigned the same motor level will vary widely in their muscle function, so it is wise to locate and grade the individual muscle groups as soon as it becomes feasible.

Several factors may influence movement ability during the infant's first hours of life. The effects of maternal anesthesia, increased cerebral pressure from hydrocephalus, and general lethargy and fatigue from a difficult or long labor may depress spontaneous movements. Conversely, these same factors may render the baby hyperirritable to stimulation. The therapist should tickle or stroke the baby above the level of the lesion or around the neck and face as a stimulus to keep the baby awake and moving. Movement of the legs can be observed and contractions palpated by stabilizing the limb proximally. Proper limb stabilization is necessary to avoid misinterpreting the origin of a movement. The principles for muscle testing in the infant population are much the same as those for the older patient; gentle resistance to movement at one part of the leg may help increase the strength of a movement at a distal part of the limb, and allowing movement to occur at only one joint at a time will assist in a more accurate interpretation. For example, holding the hip and knee firmly in either

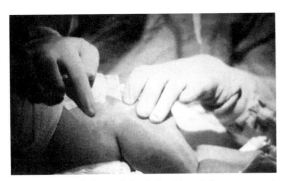

Figure 6.5 ■ Stimulation of the infant to elicit movement and palpation during manual muscle testing for the gluteus medius and maximus muscles.

partial flexion or extension and preventing movement at those joints will enable the therapist to detect weak ankle motion that might otherwise go unnoticed. After locating each movement, the therapist must then assess the strength of the responsible muscle group. Above all, practice, experience, patience, and ingenuity will improve the accuracy of this measure of the baby's motor ability.[53,61]

The therapist should note whether or not muscles are functioning, which muscles are strong and can move a joint through its entire range, and which are weak and can move the joint only partially. This distinction will help make determination of the motor level more precise. The ability to distinguish between active and reflexive movement, although sometimes difficult during this early period, will provide a more accurate identification of the lesion level.[61]

Reflex movement is common in infants with thoracic paralysis. In these patients, there is usually no activity at the hip joint, but movement is noted distally at the knee or ankle. This movement, which looks like fasciculations of the muscle belly with a weak continuous movement of the joint, may be seen when the baby is sleeping or at rest when the other joints of that limb are not moving. Reflex movement is often observed as flexion of the knee or may be seen at the ankle in the form of either dorsiflexion or plantar flexion. Reflex movement represents sparing of the local reflex arc though cortical control of the movement has been interrupted by the spinal defect. This reflex movement is of concern due to its involuntary nature and because it is usually unopposed by an active antagonist at the same joint. Therefore, this unchecked reflex activity can be a deforming force that often requires intervention. The movement is often misleading to both staff and family who may interpret the movement as functional motion. However, because the motion is not cortically initiated, it seldom has any functional value.[53]

Manual muscle testing grades can be modified until the child can be positioned appropriately for gravity and gravity-eliminated responses. Modification is also suggested until the child is older and can follow verbal cues and be tested with resistance to increase the consistency and reliability of the results. One successful method developed at Children's Memorial Hospital in Chicago uses an "X" to indicate the presence of a strong movement, an "O" for an absent response, a "T" for trace movement when a contraction is palpated but movement cannot be seen, and an "R" to indicate reflex movement. This scheme of grading, when combined with the existing scale of 0 through 5, or "absent" through "normal" classification, provides significant information about the lower extremities even in these very young patients.

Early manual muscle testing can deduce muscle imbalance around a joint and its potential for deformity. If a deformity is already present, muscle testing can help ascertain whether the cause of the limitation is passive, as a result of positioning in utero, or active, from unopposed muscle movement in one direction at a joint. Distinguishing the cause of joint deformity is helpful for the orthopedic surgeon who may want to consider early surgery to the lower extremities. The surgeon will want to spare potentially useful muscle function while eliminating movement that will be deforming in nature. Conversely, if the origin of the movement is uncertain, the surgeon may wisely choose to wait until the child is older and a more accurate evaluation is possible before deciding on the type of surgery to perform. Some centers have attempted to use electromyography (EMG) to evaluate lower extremity innervation. EMG studies are interesting from an academic standpoint but have offered little functional information and are not widely used.

It is also of interest that poor correlation exists between early manual muscle testing and the child's ultimate level of gross motor function, so predictions regarding the child's future based on these early assessments must be made carefully. Future function depends on the strength of the lower extremity musculature; the child's CNS status, motivation, and intellectual capacity; and the family's commitment for long-term compliance, support, and interest. These variables are only a few of the many factors that can influence the functional outcome of the child with spina bifida. Some of these concerns are addressed in greater detail in subsequent sections of this chapter.[62,63]

Results of early manual muscle tests should be compared with later tests in order to monitor the child's neuromuscular stability. It is a pleasant surprise to find increased movement or strength after back closure, but if a decrease in movement is noted the neurosurgeon must be alerted. Deterioration of lower extremity motor function may indicate a problem and should be brought to the physician's attention.[64]

RANGE-OF-MOTION ASSESSMENT

Preliminary assessment of range of motion (ROM) of the lower extremities can also be performed prior to back closure. Typical neonates have flexion contractures of up to 30 degrees at the hips and 10 to 20 degrees at the knees, and ankle dorsiflexion of up to 40 or 50 degrees.[65–67] Limitations of ROM in the baby with spina bifida should not be considered an indication for immediate and aggressive stretching. Early limitations of range require a safe plan of management executed over several weeks or months. When it becomes apparent that limitations will be both severe and long lasting, a long-term plan can be developed that will likely include splinting and/or surgical correction.[69,70]

Several common limitations are seen in the neonate with spina bifida. Extreme tightness of the hip flexors may be evident in the child with motor level involvement at L-2 to L-3 or L-3 to L-4 owing to the presence of a strong iliopsoas with no opposing force offered from weak or absent hip extensors. Hamstrings, which exert a secondary hip extension force, may also be weak or absent. Adductor

tightness may be seen as a result of innervation of the adductors with the absence of the antagonist, the gluteus medius. If the baby has insufficient range of hip extension to tolerate prone positioning, the neurosurgeon and nursing staff must be informed in an effort to prevent possible fractures of the femur when placing the baby in prone. Adapted prone positioning for the operating room may be indicated during back closure. One suggested position is to elevate the baby's body on a small raised platform or stack of towels so both hips can remain safely flexed while the body is supported. Postoperatively, this modified prone position or side-lying will be the safest postures for the baby with limited hip extension. The physical therapist may be the first to note the need for this special positioning during the preoperative assessment.[50]

Extreme dorsiflexion or a calcaneus deformity at the ankle is another common contracture seen at birth. The child with an L-5 innervation has strong ankle dorsiflexion, provided by the anterior tibialis and toe extensors, but weak or absent toe flexors and lack of plantar flexion from the gastrocnemius/soleus group. Plans may call for serial splinting of the ankle to bring it down to 90 degrees, and in addition to splinting, gentle passive exercise often helps reduce this deformity within a short period of time.

Provided that the baby is medically stable and the physician agrees, daily ROM exercise for the lower extremities can begin at bedside as early as the day after back closure. Although positioning options are limited after surgery, the prone and side-lying positions are adequate to perform all lower extremity motions at this time.[12,53]

POSTOPERATIVE PHYSICAL THERAPY

In order for the physical therapist to develop a comprehensive and appropriate program for the infant who has undergone back closure and shunt insertion, consideration must be given to both the neurologic and orthopedic findings, and to be most effective, the therapist should also be sensitive to the state of the family members, who will be more available as they begin to visit their baby on a regular basis.

COMMUNICATION WITH TEAM MEMBERS AND PARENTS

In most cases, the parents of an infant born with spina bifida will experience a very different and more difficult postpartum period than had been anticipated. Their baby was probably transferred to another facility shortly after birth so he or she can receive specialty care. Often, the needs of the recovering mother are superseded by the needs of the baby, so it might be difficult for the father and other family members to be as attentive to her as they focus on the infant. Inaccurate information about spina bifida, in general, and their child, in particular, may further compromise family coping skills during this physically and emotionally difficult time. It has been reported that parents are often told by hospital staff that their child will be mentally retarded, will never walk, and will require institutionalization. These professionals, although well intentioned, may not be experienced in current methods of evaluation and treatment of children with spina bifida and may only recall information from a previous era in which a bleak outlook for these babies was the norm rather than the exception. This misinformation causes many parents to become confused and frustrated, especially if the specialty team, after assessing the infant, presents what seems to be conflicting information. Therefore, close communication between the therapist and other team members is important. All persons working with the infant should know and understand each other's findings so contradiction does not occur. Information should be provided to the family by the appropriate personnel in an open and honest manner, but it should also be presented in a sensitive manner.

One objective for the physical therapist should be to reflect a positive and caring attitude during treatment sessions. This approach can help begin to normalize the family members' involvement with their infant. Teaching portions of a home program to the family can begin immediately. This is a constructive way for the therapist to begin interacting with family members and to facilitate interaction with their infant. The therapist can encourage the family members to observe and participate in the infant's care during the hospitalization in order to prepare them for providing care at home. Waiting to educate the family until discharge places increased stress on the family members, who will have much to learn from many people in a short period of time. An unexpectedly quick discharge may also leave little time for family education, which could have been spread over the entire period of hospitalization and completed by discharge. After discharge, follow-up sessions can be scheduled during outpatient or clinic visits to help reinforce this teaching and progress the program as feasible. Frequent follow-up appointments that inconvenience a family may not be as valuable as periodic sessions scheduled over a longer period of time.

RANGE-OF-MOTION EXERCISES

Daily sessions for lower extremity ROM exercises can begin after back closure and taught to parents as soon as feasible. Passive ROM exercises should be brief and performed only two or three times each day. It is also suggested that parents fit the exercises into a daily routine with their infant, such as during diaper changes, when the baby's legs are normally exposed. The therapist can combine individual leg movements into patterns of movement so the family only needs to learn three or four patterns for their home program. An example would be to combine flexion of the hip and knee of one leg, while holding the opposite leg in full extension. With the baby supine, both hips can be abducted at the same time, leaving only the foot and ankle to be done individually (Figs. 6.6 and 6.7).[53]

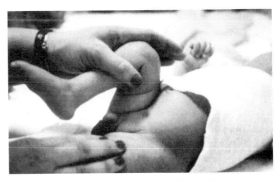

Figure 6.6 ■ Exercises for range of motion of the lower extremities. Full flexion of one hip and knee is combined with extension of the opposite extremity.

These ROM exercises are performed gently with the hands placed close to the joint being moved in order to use a short lever arm, which prevents unnecessary stress to soft tissue and joint structures. Several repetitions of each pattern, holding the joint briefly at the end of the range, will maintain and may increase ROM in joints with mild or moderate limitations. If severe limitations exist, exercise at that joint may require additional time and repetitions. But aggressive stretching should be avoided, regardless of the severity of the joint limitation.

By participating in the exercise program during these early days, parents are encouraged to touch and move their baby's legs while being observed by the therapist. Opportunities to handle their baby with supervision can help alleviate anxiety that many families express about injuring their infant. With the therapist's comforting and supportive words and demonstrations, the exercise program offers a valuable opportunity for positive parent–child interaction.

Passive ROM exercises must continue throughout the child's life. The goal is that the child will ultimately learn to perform the exercises independently. Passive exercise

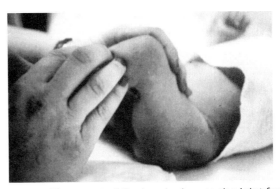

Figure 6.7 ■ Placement of the hands close to the joint for range-of-motion exercise of the knee. Note the use of a short lever arm.

is often forgotten by both therapists and parents as the child becomes more active and the focus of therapy shifts to concentrate on gross motor activities and gait training. Although one may think these activities are adequate for maintaining joint flexibility, they are not. Regardless of how active the child is, only the innervated portions of the limb are being moved, in only some planes of motion, and through only part of the full range of the joint. Therefore, if ROM exercises are discontinued, contractures will develop. For some children, it may take years to note tightening, but for others, range is lost in a short time. Whenever there is loss of flexibility, function will be compromised.[12,14,24,53]

POSITIONING AND HANDLING

The physical therapist often assumes responsibility for developing a program of positioning and handling for the hospitalized baby that will be taught to the parents prior to discharge. Although many positioning options are available as discharge nears, options during the first few postoperative days may be limited to prone or side-lying. As the child's medical status stabilizes and tolerance to movement improves, it is advisable to avoid leaving the child immobile for long periods of time. Handling and carrying strategies can be practiced by the therapist and then recommended to the parents. Finding a comfortable chair is most important, and once seated, the therapist or family member can hold the child prone over their lap, rocking or swaying slowly side to side. This position is restful for the parent and provides novel movement for the infant. The baby may also enjoy a slow walk around the hospital floor while being held up and slightly over the parent's shoulder. This position gives the infant an opportunity to attempt to raise his or her head and look around. If the supine position is contraindicated, parents may gently cradle the infant prone across one forearm as they walk or sit. These few position options will provide the family members with a repertoire of acceptable handling strategies when they come to visit their baby. These positions are also safe for the infant, who needs time to recover and who may not respond well to aggressive movement and handling. One must remember that the primary postoperative goals for the infant is an uncomplicated healing of the back wound, speedy recovery from shunt insertion, and discharge from the hospital.[53]

In most cases, with medical clearance, short periods of supine and supported upright sitting in the therapist's arms should not affect the course of healing of the back wound and may be added to the handling repertoire after a few days. A variety of positions helps normalize the baby's experiences during waking hours, while eating, or quietly observing the surroundings. These short periods are also useful for the therapist, to note the baby's responses to gravity in these positions; feel for changes in muscle tone, particularly through the shoulders and neck; and observe

any significant asymmetries. Documenting this information will provide a useful baseline against which to compare later developmental findings.[24,53]

Families should first watch, then try to duplicate, the activities recommended for their baby. Be aware that most parents show some hesitation or anxiety on first handling their baby. If they do not it may indicate a poor understanding of the baby's medical condition and may contribute to subsequent poor judgment in other areas of care. Even for families with experience raising older children, some initial level of anxiety can be a healthy sign.

The therapist can begin to "role release," delegating to the parents some ROM and handling activities, as these teaching sessions proceed. As this change in roles occurs, the therapist can concentrate on other areas of the child's plan of care. At many hospitals, the therapist is asked to repeat the lower extremity manual muscle test prior to the infant's discharge.

The therapist can also observe the baby's state, noting changes secondary to hydrocephalus and shunt insertion; gathering this additional information may help identify a later shunt malfunction. When a shunt malfunction begins to occur, in addition to the signs and symptoms presented in Table 6.1, a change in the baby's tone, reaction to movement, and increased irritability during movement may also be noted.

TABLE 6.1
Signs and Symptoms of Shunt Malfunction

Infants
  Bulging fontanelle
  Vomiting
  Change in appetite
  "Sunset" sign of eyes
  Edema, redness along shunt tract
Toddlers
  Vomiting
  Irritability
  Headaches
  Edema, redness along shunt tract
School-Aged Children
  Headaches
  Lethargy
  Irritability
  Edema, redness along shunt tract
  Handwriting changes
  High-pitched cry
  Seizures
  Rapid growth of head circumference
  Thinning of skin over scalp
  Newly noted nystagmus
  Newly noted eye squint
  Vomiting
  Decreased school performance
  Personality changes
  Memory changes

The family members should also be encouraged to be active in gathering information about their infant. They should be encouraged to play with and observe their baby, not only to foster positive interaction but also to aid the medical staff in assessing the infant's function. Interaction with the medical team becomes less frequent as the child becomes more medically stable. Therefore, observations by parents can help identify problems at an early stage so that appropriate medical care can be sought.

SENSORY ASSESSMENT

The physical therapist should perform a sensory assessment on the neonate with spina bifida, to ascertain areas of the infant's lower extremities that are sensitive or insensitive to touch. By mapping this sensory information, along with the results of muscle testing, the level of the spinal lesion can be more accurately established. This assessment can also identify the areas of intact sensation on the baby's trunk and legs so stimulation at those areas will make the baby move. It is the novice clinician who strokes the plantar surface of the foot, expecting to make the child react. This technique is successful only when the infant has intact sensation at the sacral nerve roots. Most infants with spina bifida have a higher level of insensitivity and need to be stimulated on the thigh or somewhere on the trunk. The therapist may also find that the level of motor function and sensation may not be similar in both legs. Be aware that early results of sensory testing may be inaccurate, depending on the state of the infant. In addition, it is difficult to accurately assess all sensory modalities at this time: light touch, deep pressure, and temperature. A more comprehensive assessment will be indicated when the baby is older.

As sensory findings become more stable and reproducible, the information should be shared with the family members, who must become educated about their child's skin anesthesia. Educating parents about skin care for the baby is often the shared responsibility of the nursing and therapy staffs. It is sometimes difficult for parents to understand the concept that their baby has areas of the lower body and legs that are insensitive to touch. The therapist can help the family discover this information on their own. Using a gentle touch, caress, or tickle, a family member can map out areas of responsiveness when the infant is awake but quiet. The therapist should not use a pin or other sharp object during testing or when demonstrating to parents. The baby's response to a pinprick is no more valid than its response to a gentle touch, and further, seeing staff using a sharp object on their baby may add to the parent's anxieties and concern.

Insensitive areas of the lower extremities will require protection because the child will be unaware of injury at these areas of denervation. For example, families must always test the temperature of bath water prior to immersing the child. They cannot rely on the child's reaction to judge if the temperature is correct. They must be cautious and not allow their child to play with the faucets and inadvertently add hot water. Open space heaters or radiators need covering or relocation to keep babies from resting too close and suffering serious burns. Prior to placing the infant on the floor to play, a search for hidden objects in the carpet may prevent an accidental injury from loose carpet tacks or a small sharp toy. The infant's legs and feet should always be protected when crawling on the floor. Wearing socks or booties will also help prevent problems when children begin to reach for, mouth, and even bite at their toes, at the age of 6 to 8 months.

Skin insensitivity will continue to be a concern throughout the child's life. Application of new shoes or braces, for example, requires vigilance to avoid pressure areas, sores, and abrasions. Normal sensation keeps the typical person from sitting immobile for long periods of time. Intact sensory feedback causes individuals to shift around frequently and change their weight distribution, relieving pressure and discomfort. Persons with areas of insensitivity, however, tend to develop skin problems secondary to prolonged sitting because they do not feel the discomfort and therefore do not shift their weight, change their position, and relieve pressure. Similarly, when people with typical sensation feel pressure from an ill-fitting shoe, they are able to readjust their gait to avoid continued abrasion until they can get off their feet or change shoes. For the child without full sensation, such readjustments will not occur, as areas of pressure are not perceived. It is important to gradually introduce any new orthotics. The brace should be worn for only a few hours at a time, and the skin should be inspected carefully to determine whether there are any pressure areas. When areas of redness last for longer than 30 minutes, an adjustment to the orthosis is indicated. The child should not be permitted to keep wearing the orthosis in the hopes that the skin will toughen. The plan for accommodation to a new brace is best implemented over a weekend or in the evenings, when the child is at home, unless this schedule can be successfully implemented at school. It is not wise to have the child wear a new device for a full day until proper fit and good skin tolerance are ensured. If these issues are not initially addressed and the child experiences skin breakdown, it will lead to extended periods of time out of bracing, serious infection, and possibly hospitalization.[14,24,53]

 ## Care of the Young Child

ONGOING CONCERNS AND ISSUES

As the initial medical intervention for the baby with spina bifida comes to an end, a plan for long-term care should be developed. Various approaches to the delivery of medical care are seen and in most cases it is delivered by specialists located in one institution. There are instances where a pediatrician may follow the child and choose to refer the child to additional specialists as specific needs are identified. Professionals in the child's community who are affiliated with early intervention programs or private offices may provide care, but when care is divided among several institutions, a new role emerges for the parents. They are forced to become the case managers for their child to facilitate continuity of care and communication between the professionals. This added responsibility may present a burden for many families and may result in less-than-optimal care for their child. It appears that, because of the multiple specialty areas needed by the child with spina bifida, care may best be delivered by experienced professionals who work together as a coordinated team. That is why many pediatric facilities attempt to organize an interdisciplinary clinic for children with spina bifida, where several primary specialists can see the child and preferably on the same day. Families are encouraged to continue their child's care at one of these spina bifida clinics if possible. With a team of specialists working together to complement one another, both the child and parents benefit. Communication is facilitated and expedited among the professionals. Information can be more easily shared to increase learning and maintain a current outlook. If problems are detected, the necessary personnel are often nearby to address the concern without the need for a return appointment. With consistency and coordination, trust in the professional staff can develop, thereby enabling the family members to be less stressed and potentially better able to cope with and focus on their child's needs.[14,24,53,51]

The child may have to return frequently to the clinic during the first year of life for ongoing follow-up by the various specialists. The neurosurgeon will monitor the status of the back closure, look for the presence of hydrocephalus, and check shunt function (Display 6.3).[12,56] The orthopedic surgeon will evaluate limb flexibility, strength,

---

DISPLAY 6.3

Goals of Neurosurgical Care for Patients with Spina Bifida

Coordinate early care prior to back closure

Assess location and size of the back defect

Perform closure of the back defect

Assess extent of lower extremity paralysis

Assess and treat hydrocephalus

Monitor function of ventricular shunt

Monitor patient for acute and chronic central nervous system (CNS) abnormalities

Monitor the patient for CNS deterioration, tethered cord, and hydromyelia

Provide support/collaboration to clinical team

DISPLAY 6.4

Goals of Orthopedic Care for Patients with Spina Bifida

Provide pertinent information to family: current and projected issues

Prevent fixed joint contractures

Correct musculoskeletal deformities

Prevent skin breakdown from structural malalignment

Provide resources to achieve best mobility

Monitor for scoliosis

Monitor the patient for central nervous system deterioration, tethered cord, and hydromyelia

Provide support/collaboration to clinical team

---

and joint integrity. Plans for splints and surgery are made to prepare the child for standing (Display 6.4).[14,53] The urologist will monitor bowel and bladder function, assess renal status at regular intervals, and plan a course of care that includes intermittent catheterization and possibly pharmacologic management (Display 6.5).[53] At the appropriate time, a bowel program to attain fecal continence should be implemented that may involve scheduled toileting, diet, medication, biofeedback, and behavior modification.

As the child's status stabilizes in each of the specialty areas, visits to the clinic will become less frequent. It is not unusual for the child to be seen at 6-month intervals over several years and then yearly if there are no ongoing problems or major concerns. However, more frequent visits are necessary when a chronic problem requires close monitoring or treatment.

DEVELOPMENTAL ISSUES

As stated earlier in this chapter, the survival of a greater number of infants born with spina bifida has permitted the clinician, working with these children, to gain experience

---

DISPLAY 6.5

Goals of Urologic Care for Patients with Spina Bifida

Assess and preserve renal function

Provide for adequate bladder emptying

Provide for urinary continence

Provide resources for bowel management

Monitor the patient for central nervous system deterioration, tethered cord, and hydromyelia

Provide support/collaboration to clinical team

and insight into the full scope of the disability and all of its primary and secondary issues. It has become apparent that a significant number of children with spina bifida exhibit CNS deficits and for some, the effect of these deficits can be more detrimental to the child's function than the lower extremity paralysis. These deficits have a negative impact on the child's gross motor, fine motor, perceptual motor, and cognitive functioning, and it is critical that the physical therapist understand and address the problems.

The Chiari II malformation was identified and studied for a long time but only recently have there been discussions regarding this malformation as it relates to the CNS dysfunction seen in the child with spina bifida. Using MRI studies, the structural abnormalities have been identified and can be visualized.[21] However, from these studies, as previously noted, predicting the clinical presentation of a particular child cannot be made with any consistency. But it has been observed that up to 85% of children with spina bifida have low tone, with minimal to moderate developmental delay. The most common difficulties are delayed and/or abnormal development of head and trunk control and delayed and/or abnormal acquisition of righting and equilibrium responses. Interestingly, children who do not have spina bifida and only have hydrocephalus do not exhibit the same movement problems with the frequency or severity as the population of children with spina bifida and hydrocephalus. So as physical therapists we begin working with the babies, combining a knowledge of early gross motor development and keen observation skills, and can only postulate that the Chiari II malformation is a contributor to the movement difficulties we may be seeing.[14,24,53,55–58] The earliest problem noted in many infants is prolonged instability of the head and upper body with delayed or weak acquisition of balance and equilibrium responses.

For the typical baby, parents carry, lift, and move their infant, and compensate for the lack of head and neck stability by supporting the baby's head in a protective manner. It is an automatic reaction, and if the parent does not protect the head, a startle response is elicited and the baby is visibly upset. But as the baby begins to gain some head and neck stability, this support is removed and the infant actually improves very quickly in strength as valuable experience is gained holding his or her head up many times during the normal routines of the day.

The child with poor neck stability may retain the startle response longer than a typical infant and parents respond by continuing to provide needed head support well past the time the baby would hold his or her head up independently. This begins an abnormal cycle in which the support provided by the parent's hands actually limits the experiences and opportunities the baby receives to practice and develop better head control and so the delay is prolonged.

The typical baby spends time in various positions from the beginning of life and experiences the effects of gravity on the head and body in all positions. Typical infants will first begin to stabilize their head over their shoulders in the supported upright position. This early stability is seen well before the baby can lift his or her head up from a prone or supine position. As the baby's head becomes progressively more stable, parents find new ways to carry and handle their baby. This parent–child feedback is most apparent when the baby is held upright in the parent's arms while being carried. At first, the parent's hand is placed behind the baby's head to prevent it from falling backward. Several weeks later, we see this supporting hand only when parents raise or lower the baby from a crib or changing table or if the baby is asleep. In just a few months, no guarding of the head is required at all when the baby is upright as the parent has responded to the baby's new skills accordingly.

For the infant with typical tone, there is physiologic stability of the head and neck. Typical joint proprioception through the cervical spine and the normal stretch reflexes of the soft tissue structures of the neck permit the baby's head to fall slowly into gravity, with movement or a position change, but only to a small degree. The head is held reasonably steady without much active participation.

For the infant with low tone, the proprioceptive responses to gravity may be slow and weak, permitting the head to fall forward or to the side much farther before these stabilizing responses occur. A mechanical disadvantage compounds the problem as the baby grows and the head becomes larger and heavier so the task of head righting is made more difficult by the additional weight and relatively weak musculature.

When the infant with spina bifida is placed in various positions and makes attempts to stabilize his or her head, compensatory patterns of movement can often be seen. Elevation of the shoulders is one pattern noted. This is developmentally immature alignment for the infant who should have head stability in upright by 4 months of age. Stabilizing the head with this shoulder pattern interferes with the further development of righting skills and also limits the free movement and use of the upper extremities. The upper arms may be held stiffly to provide neck stability at a time when the infant should be experiencing and practicing increased freedom of movement and skills of the upper extremities.

As this scenario progresses, months later, the child with insufficient trunk strength and stability to maintain the body upright against gravity may consistently use the upper extremities to prop when placed in sitting and there the child remains stuck, unable to move into or out of the position except in stereotyped ways. To change positions, the child may eventually develop strategies to move but these strategies are usually passive, involving little muscle activity or control from the neck and trunk, and thus do not help to further improve the strength and coordination of the body. The child may lower his or her head to one side and collapse down to the floor, or may lean forward and crawl out of the sitting position. Getting into and out of sitting from one side or the other requires balance, control, and strength of the head and trunk that the child lacks. So, assuming the "W" sitting position is usually easiest. The child merely pushes his or her body straight backward till the buttock reaches the surface, in between the knees.

Compensatory patterns of overusing the arms are also seen when the baby attempts to lift his or her head and look around while in a prone position. Proper side-to-side weight shifting over the hands and arms will not occur easily. When the child lifts an arm to reach for a toy, the prop is removed, stability is lost, and the head and upper chest drops. Even with experience and practice, this pattern does not improve without appropriate intervention. The child may tilt his or her head to one side for a weight shift and let it hang there to free one arm to reach for a desired object. The head cannot be maintained upright against gravity without leaning on the arms.

When a typical baby lifts an arm to reach for an object while in prone, a weight shift to one side occurs that activates the neck, trunk, hip, and leg musculature to balance and stabilize the baby's position. The baby does not depend on upper extremity support to lift the head and can therefore reach without the head dropping. During typical weight shifting and movement in a prone position, the upper arms become more externally rotated while the forearms rotate into supination with pressure shifting across from the radial to the ulnar surface of the hands. Increased and varied weight bearing and tactile stimulation across the hands help reduce the sensitivity of the grasp response. Also, the typical upper extremity weight-bearing progression aids in opening the baby's flexed fingers and hands. Experiences in the prone position provide considerable proprioception through the joints of the upper extremities that increases both control and strength.

The child with spina bifida needs coordination and strength of the upper extremities to use assistive devices for ambulation, to perform activities of daily living, and to manipulate paper and pencil for tasks in school. But using the upper extremities in lieu of head and trunk support limits the motor experiences of the arms and hands. The shoulders remain elevated to continue providing stability for the head. Arms tend to be held in internal rotation with scapular protraction. The forearms are pronated and wrist and hand flexion may also be seen. Weight bearing on the hands may also be limited to the radial aspect.

Paralysis of the lower extremities decreases the total amount of tactile, proprioceptive, and vestibular input that the child is receiving. The degree to which this loss affects the individual depends on the remaining movement and sensation available in the legs, the function of the upper body, and the child's CNS status. If a child is able to explore the environment actively and independently, he or she gains direct knowledge about his or her body in relation to the environment. A typical baby has a vast number of movement experiences, many occurring at the same time, and learning is gleaned from many sensory modalities. When movement and exploration are limited, learning is affected.

Lower extremity paralysis, in combination with low tone and poor head control, makes gross motor movements more difficult for many children with spina bifida, and that can also affect the child's motivation to move. When movement is more difficult, it can become a negative experience and learning more sophisticated motor skills can be hampered.

Therapists need to appreciate the impact of these impediments on learning motor skills for children with spina bifida and use this information to facilitate and encourage early handling strategies for parents that will enhance their baby's development and encourage the acquisition of more typical movement patterns.[72–81]

Handling Strategies for Parents

As mentioned earlier, instruction sessions with parents should begin before the child is discharged from the hospital and should continue until the parents are comfortable with their handling or acceptable movement and function of the child is observed. Parents should be aggressive in their approach but tempered by the medical status and age of their baby. Teaching sessions should include verbal instruction as well as many opportunities for the parents to observe the therapist handling their baby.

Parents often focus on the most conspicuous deficit, the lower extremity paralysis. But the physical therapist has the responsibility of also incorporating into the instructional program information that will promote the family's understanding of gross, fine, and perceptual motor abilities above the waist. The pace of instruction should be based on the status of the infant and the capacity of the family. Frequent gentle reminders can be given in early treatment sessions about the developmental delays seen in some children. The family can be warned of potential problems, especially the child's possible difficulty in developing control of the head and neck.

The presence of hypotonus may cause a delay in acquisition of antigravity head control in all directions. Parents should not permit the baby to be held or positioned with the head at severe angles to the body. These positions allow overstretching of muscles and other soft tissue structures. In the supine position, the infant who lacks active neck flexion will appear the most asymmetric and may exhibit difficulty turning the head from side to side from the effects of gravity. Abnormal compensatory patterns of movement may be seen when the baby tries to turn his or her head in supine. The prone position, while a position that promotes greater symmetry, may lead to frustration if neck and upper trunk extensor strength is poor and the baby cannot easily lift and turn his or her head. As the infant tires of keeping the head to one side in either prone or supine, he or she may begin to cry. In response, the parent may lift the baby or roll it into a different position. By responding in this manner, the parent unknowingly assumes responsibility for a motor skill that the child should be mastering. Parents should be educated that their good intentions may actually interfere with appropriate muscle development that is needed for their baby to move more correctly.

Extensive literature is available describing early motor development of the typical child. From this information, we learn that infants acquire head and neck stability in supported upright postures before they can lift their heads from prone or maintain midline control in supine. Gaining the ability to stabilize the head while upright facilitates strengthening of the musculature needed to lift and control the head in the other positions (Figs. 6.8 and 6.9). With these thoughts in mind, the therapist can recommend that parents offer their baby with spina bifida experiences in all positions, but with a strong emphasis on upright postures.[24,74–79]

Parents can be taught to carry their awake, alert child with the head unsupported to facilitate development of head control, but without allowing the head to fall suddenly in an uncontrolled manner, thereby eliciting a startle response. Holding the baby high on the parent's shoulder rather than at the chest level is one position that can be tried (Fig. 6.10). Another useful strategy is for the parent to sit at a table and hold the baby sitting on the table, facing them and at eye level. The parents can encourage visual play with their child and can provide experiences for practicing independent head control. The infant can be

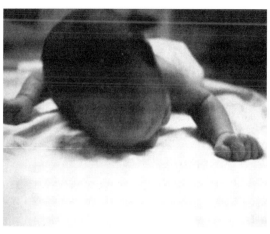

Figure 6.9 ■ The same infant as shown in Figure 6.8, barely able to elevate his head to turn it side to side in a prone position.

held around the shoulders at first and then lower, at chest level, as head control develops.

Parents should be instructed to observe the infant for prolonged asymmetries. But the therapist does not have to wait until these asymmetries are seen to demonstrate appropriate, symmetric alignment of the baby in various positions that the parent can practice during their normal routines of the day: diaper changes, dressing, meal time, rest, and play (Fig. 6.11). Another position that encourages a more symmetric alignment is with the parent sitting comfortably in a soft chair or sofa with legs partially flexed up and the baby nestled supine, on the parent's legs.

Children with spina bifida may require long-term therapeutic intervention that may be unavailable or inconvenient in the hospital setting. This is especially true for those babies in whom CNS deficits are seen and a more frequent or

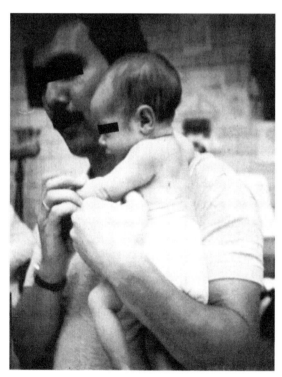

Figure 6.8 ■ Typical infant at 6 weeks of age. The infant is stabilizing his head while in an upright position. Note the erect alignment of the thoracic spine in an infant with normal muscle tone.

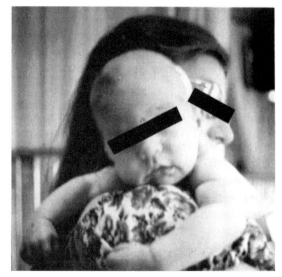

Figure 6.10 ■ Infant is being carried high on the adult's shoulder to allow independent movement of the head and an improved position of the upper extremities.

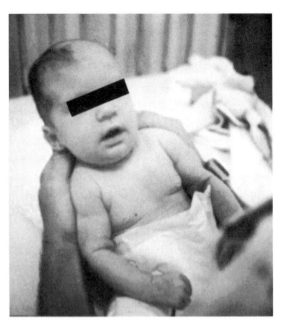

Figure 6.11 ▪ A suggested position for handling an infant in supine. Note hand placement of the parent to provide a symmetric midline posture while stimulating the baby in face-to-face play.

intense program is indicated. Multidiscipline, early intervention programs in the community are recommended if the program is able to provide the needed therapy services. Ideally, the community program should also provide supportive services for the family as well. The family often needs ongoing support and assistance once they leave the secure environment of the hospital and take their baby home.

The support, assistance, and teaching provided by a 0-to-3 program may be necessary for families in which there are other children as well as for first-time parents. This author finds it interesting to note that some parents who have older children are accustomed to seeing the varying rates of typical development and may deny or minimize the developmental delays of their child with spina bifida regardless of the information they are receiving to the contrary. Consistent input by the clinician is required to help parents develop a critical eye and an effective approach to address the needs of the child. This can be provided in any number of settings, and it is inappropriate to wait until significant delays or abnormalities are seen before referring a child.

Physical Therapy for the Growing Child

DEVELOPMENTAL CONCERNS

A long-range plan of care should be developed by the physical therapist that is acceptable to the neurosurgeon, orthopedic surgeon, and family. The plan for the young child with spina bifida is based largely on the objective findings from the physical therapist's evaluations as well as the concerns of the other specialists. Repeated manual muscle tests and careful observation of the child's development enables the therapist to identify the child's strengths and weaknesses. Intervention can then be directed at the specific needs of the lower extremities and gross motor development (Display 6.6).

Children with spina bifida need to practice activities that will improve righting and equilibrium responses of the head and trunk. When the therapist addresses these needs and sees improvement, there is an important secondary benefit. While stimulating the child's automatic balance responses against gravity in all positions, overflow in the form of active movement in the trunk and lower extremities can be seen. So, these balance responses should become an important part of the child's home exercise program.[53]

Sitting stimulates the child's balance, improves control of the head and trunk, increases the child's visual field, and provides an opportunity for many eye–hand experiences. Head-righting and equilibrium responses in sitting can be tested and improved by holding the child at the shoulders and slowly tilting him or her backward. Beginning conservatively at 20 to 30 degrees, the infant should respond by holding the head steady and then returning the head forward depending on the baby's age and skill level. Next, the therapist brings the infant's body back to midline and repeats the activity to one side, the other side, forward, and to the diagonal directions. If no response occurs in any direction and the child's head hangs, or if the child

---

>> **DISPLAY 6.6**

Goals of Physical Therapy for Patients with Spina Bifida

Establish preliminary motor level by manual muscle test

Provide medical team with accurate information regarding lower limb movement

Perform periodic manual muscle testing for comparison purposes

Provide instruction to family for a long-term home program to prevent lower extremity deformity

Provide home program instruction to facilitate motor development as close to chronologic age as is possible

Assist in determining appropriate orthosis

Facilitate mobility program for ambulation and wheelchair use, where indicated

Provide information regarding the patient's neurologic function to treating physicians

Monitor the patient for central nervous system deterioration, tethered cord, and hydromyelia

Provide support/collaboration to clinical team

becomes upset with the activity, the movement may have been too rapid or the baby was tilted too far. A slower and less challenging movement is used until a response is noted. Changing the position of the supporting hands may also enable a child to react in the direction that was weaker. With the baby positioned on the lap of the handler, gentle bouncing to stimulate and approximate the joint surfaces of the cervical spine may assist the baby as well. As the child's responses to the tilting become more brisk and strong, the angle of the tilting can be increased. Over time as the child improves, support can be moved to the chest and then to the waist, but the activity continues. During this balance and equilibrium routine, especially when the baby is tilted to the diagonal directions, the oblique abdominals and lower extremity musculature will contract to stabilize the body in response to shifts in the baby's center of gravity and in an attempt to return the body back to midline. As equilibrium responses strengthen, active hip flexion, hip adduction and abduction, knee extension, and ankle and foot movement can be elicited. It is interesting to note that there have been instances when this author has worked with children who had limited head and upper body control and significant improvement was seen in leg strengths secondary to the righting and equilibrium activities. Also, using these automatic balance reactions to directly work on strengthening the legs is a strategy that can be used for young children who do not understand and cannot follow verbal directions.

When asymmetries in the baby's skill are noted to one or more directions, those directions can be repeated more frequently, but the stronger responses should still be included and not forgotten. For the young child it is recommended that these sessions of tilting last only about 5 to 10 minutes. But several opportunities should be found during the child's daily routine to repeat the activity so the responses can strengthen more quickly (Fig. 6.12).

In the prone position, neck extension and thoracic extensor strengthening is achieved as the child attempts and becomes successful at maintaining the head and thorax up against gravity without the use of his or her upper extremities. Low back extensors, gluteals, quadriceps, and plantar flexors will be activated during these prone extension patterns of movement, provided of course that the muscles are innervated. During routine carrying of the infant in the prone position or during face-to-face play with a family member while both are laying on the floor, the child can be tilted slowly from prone to one side then the other with visual stimulation to stimulate the baby to maintain the head erect. As this balance reaction becomes stronger and the baby can maintain his or her head erect while being shifted, strengthening of the neck, trunk, and lower extremities occurs.

As mentioned earlier, in the supine position the effects of gravity may cause the child to look the most asymmetric. Strengthening of active neck flexion during the sitting balance activities will improve the child's active head con-

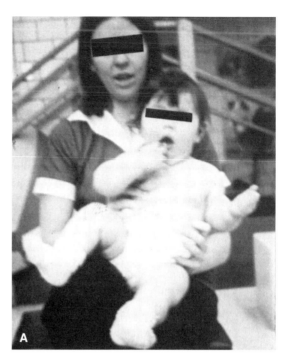

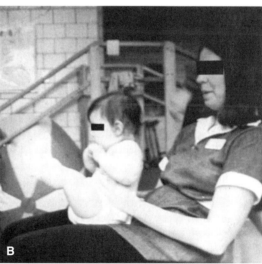

Figure 6.12 ■ **(A,B)** *Challenging the child's balance responses to elicit more sophisticated and stronger upper body reactions and strengthening of the lower extremities as they respond.*

trol in midline when supine, thus decreasing much of the asymmetry. Spending time in supine is an important position that facilitates beginning eye–hand coordination and bilateral upper extremity play for the typical child. But if the child with spina bifida remains asymmetric with the head turned to a preferred side, then development of these skills can be hampered. Supine also facilitates disassociation of body parts as the child moves into and out of the position or merely remains in supine, active and at play. Through rotation of the thorax on the lumbar spine, the lumbar spine on the pelvis, and the lower extremities on the pelvis, a great deal of strengthening and control of these body parts is gained. When the child holds his or her legs up in supine, extending them to kick and play against gravity, neck and abdominal musculature are strengthening as well as the muscles of the lower extremities. It is important to note that the neck and trunk flexors combine with the extensors to provide for good spinal alignment in sitting.

A typical infant, as early as 2 months of age, will bear weight on the lower extremities as a result of the positive support reaction. When this novel response is discovered by parents, it is quickly included in the repertoire of positions parents use to play with their child. Proprioceptive input is provided by this weight bearing. Also, extension is stimulated by gravity acting on the joint surfaces through the neck, trunk, and lower extremities. This sensory input is important for body awareness and perception of body in space. Standing also provides the baby with a new perspective of his or her relationship to the surroundings. During this early weight bearing, contact between the femoral head and acetabulum, together with muscle contractions around the hip joint, help to stimulate acetabular development. As the child grows, practice in this position evolves from being reflexive to being voluntary. Upright weight bearing continues to challenge and improve body control and balance against gravity and stimulate available muscles in the trunk and lower extremities that will assist with independent stance.

Families can be taught to assist their young child with spina bifida to perform brief periods of standing several times each day until the child can stand with less assistance, or until a first standing device or bracing is provided for longer periods in upright (Fig. 6.13).[24,53]

If the child learns to push and pull with his or her arms to compensate for weakness in the trunk and neck, it may allow the child to roll, attain the four-point position, and, perhaps, pull to a stand if lower extremity function is adequate. But this progression, with increased reliance on the arms, and poor truncal strength will ultimately lead to the child requiring a higher level of bracing than the level the back lesion might indicate, and the child will also require a more supportive assistive device during gait than would otherwise have been predicted. Therefore, during assessment and treatment of the child with spina bifida, it is not sufficient merely to identify that a developmental milestone has occurred. Rather, it is important to assess the movement qualitatively, including such considerations as the child's ability to perform the movement against gravity, whether the movement is typical in appearance, or whether compensatory or abnormal patterns have developed. One can then identify the patterns of movement to be enhanced and strengthened as foundations for future skills, as well as the movements that should be avoided or changed.[53]

Intervention for the areas of concern can be addressed in a safe and appropriate therapeutic regimen. The physical therapy plan can include activities performed in all positions, the use of gravity to challenge the child, and varied and changing movement stimuli to facilitate motor development. By providing these opportunities and experiences,

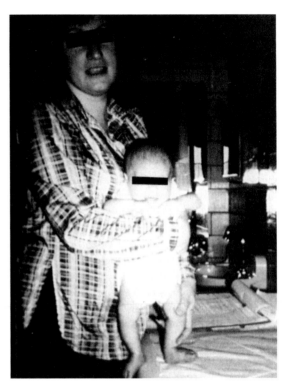

Figure 6.13 ■ Brief periods of standing throughout the day will help provide for well-aligned weight bearing in the child without fully innervated musculature of the lower extremities.

there is an increased likelihood that the child's gross, fine, and perceptual motor abilities will be less negatively affected, and the child's gross motor skills will be commensurate with the motor level of the lower extremities.[72–82]

INFANT DEVICES

The issue of using infant seats and various baby devices always arises during conversations with parents and should be addressed as soon as possible by the therapist. The available literature is consistent in its insistence that all infants need to be active to acquire the strength and motor control necessary to move against gravity, attain erect sitting and standing postures, and walk. The infant must receive and integrate vast amounts of sensory and motor information to build a foundation of knowledge about his or her body and to develop the ability to function effectively within the environment. Infant walkers, jumper seats, swings, bouncer chairs, and the excessive use of infant car seats can have a negative impact on motor development and sensorimotor learning. The use of these devices may further retard the development of the baby with spina bifida who is already at risk for motor delay. (Several of these concerns are explored in greater detail in Chapter 11.)

All infants must experience the upright sitting position because of its influence for mastering many skills. This position gives the child a new visual perspective of his or her surroundings and provides the first sensation of the effects of gravity, the weight of the head, and the work necessary to stabilize the head over the shoulders. However, to practice and gain confidence in these early skills, the infant must be stimulated by movement, for example, while being carried in a parent's arms. The experiences of random and varied weight shifting and tilting as the parent moves and walks are physiologically important. Bobbing and jerking movements of the head stimulate the stretch reflexes in the joint receptors of the neck, producing muscle contractions that mark the infant's beginning attempts at head control. This stimulation is essential. However, most infant seating devices offer total support. This degree of support is unwise for the infant with spina bifida who may be slow to develop head control. Infants with spina bifida need frequent sessions of activities that challenge the head, neck, and trunk. The infant should be actively moving and turning to see his or her surroundings and to appreciate gravity acting on the body in different planes. To be passively entertained in seating devices allows little or no active participation in movement or in the learning process. The device allows the infant to be passively entertained without offering any developmental benefits. When the infant wants to move in a seated device, it is common to see an arching or hyperextending of the neck against the back of the device, a pattern that is not conducive to further acquisition of desired skills.

Now consider the child who has sufficient lower extremity function to successfully move around the room in an infant walker. The child is often seen with poor alignment, possibly tilted to one side in the walker. Coordinated reciprocal movements of the legs are not necessary to gain momentum in this device, and weight bearing through the legs is often momentary and sporadic. Only a quick, thrusting pattern is necessary to propel the device. It is inappropriate to facilitate and strengthen these patterns because they have no carryover for developing coordinated movements of or providing stability to the lower extremities and trunk, both of which are vital components for independent standing and ambulation. Rather, infants should bear weight on their lower extremities while maintaining appropriate, erect alignment of the trunk and upper body. Parents who are concerned about the "weak" legs of their infant with spina bifida must be guided and encouraged to provide standing experiences that require more active participation from the child's whole body. Typically, when moving and playing, children use many parts of their body at once. A child who is excited by a bright object will move his or her arms while also lifting and kicking his or her legs. These movements help strengthen the musculature of the legs while the child is also learning motor control. It is more beneficial to hold the infant in a standing position while offering adequate but not total support. This will promote control of the legs and upper body while offering unique sensory stimulation.

Parents often initially plan to use these devices for only short periods of time. But since most parents strive to keep their children happy and content, the time the infant spends in these devices often increases insidiously, further reducing the time the baby spends moving actively around on the floor. In assessing the use of such devices and the type of instruction a therapist may give a parent, one must consider the lifestyle of the family. Many parents spend long periods of time in the car each day, traveling to appointments, a supermarket, shopping center, or other destinations where the infant will then be placed in a supported position in a stroller or shopping cart. Add this to the time the infant spends sleeping and eating, and it becomes apparent that little time is left for the more beneficial positions and activities. However radical this approach may seem, the therapist may find it best to totally discourage the use of these devices except, of course, for the use of a car safety seat while traveling. Then, if parents must use an infant seat for brief periods of time during feeding, for example, they will be conscientious and the baby will more likely be removed as soon as possible.[24,53,72,74,76–78,83]

Orthotics

INTRODUCTION TO BRACING

A discussion of orthotics for the young child with spina bifida is most logically approached by grouping together children who share motor levels that require similar orthopedic and orthotic management. In this chapter, we consider the children with thoracic level lesions in one group, those with high lumbar L-1 to L-3 lesions in a second group, children with low lumbar L-4 to L-5 lesions in a third group, and those with sacral lesions in a fourth final group. Early splinting, standing devices, and bracing for initial ambulation will be discussed for each of the groups. One should be aware that within each group children will have very different patterns of active movement, strengths, and upright function. Thus, the clinician should remember that each child must be evaluated individually and, depending on the findings, a management plan can be developed with the information in this section serving as a guide.

PHILOSOPHIES OF BRACING

Some clinics follow a bracing philosophy that establishes a plateau of maximum function for children based on their lesion level and general gross motor ability. In addition, several publications have supported the concept that a predictable level of mobility exists for children at each motor level. Such a philosophy advocates establishing reasonable expectations for each child because much time, effort, and expense can be spent on orthotic management and physical therapy services to teach gait training. This philosophy of bracing is thought, by some, to be an efficient, cost-effective method that supports the concept that later functional outcome can be predicted primarily by the child's motor level. Institutions that follow this model are often reluctant to brace a child with a thoracic or high lumbar lesion after the early childhood years, as the literature indicates that most adolescents with high-level lesions are mobile only from a wheelchair and have discarded the possibility of ambulation by their teen years. However, there is research acknowledging that a number of variables affect the ultimate level of performance of the child, of which lower extremity function is only one factor. Family interest and participation and the child's CNS function, motivation, learning capacity, and the desire for movement are just a few of the factors that should be considered when deciding whether to proceed with or terminate an ambulation program. A recent article from a major clinic in Australia identified that the later the child began to ambulate, the earlier he or she was to abandon it. But the article also pointed to rapid growth and weight gain, the need for frequent brace adjustments, and other medical problems as interfering factors that stop a child from ambulation even earlier than would have been expected.[84] A recent editorial by Dr. Malcolm Menelaus stated that early ambulation is important even if it is abandoned later in the individual's life.[85] Finally, from an ethical standpoint, one might question whether discontinuing a gait program should be determined by anyone other than the patient as evidenced by his or her abilities.

The Children's Memorial Hospital in Chicago follows a unique plan of action in which all children and their families that are seen through their myelomeningocele clinic begin a program of early standing and gait training and as the child grows the medical staff, parents, school personnel, and the child communicate and share their impressions and experiences so a plan can be established for continued bracing and ambulation training for as long as it seems reasonable. Even if a patient is considered a household ambulatory and uses a wheelchair for primary mobility out of the home, this level of gait is supported and encouraged by the clinic staff. Adopting this approach means that more time must be spent in communication between various institutions and individuals so that everyone is aware of the ambulation goal and is working toward the same end. Because the patient's needs and abilities are constantly changing, the goals established for mobility also have to be flexible. Changes in medical care for children with spina bifida, as well as advances in orthotics technology and materials, warrant an active and creative approach toward bracing and gait. The goal is to help each child attain his or her optimal level of performance, regardless of his or her motor level, and to assist the child to maintain this level for as long as is feasible.[24,53,67]

GENERAL PRINCIPLES OF ORTHOTICS

Any discussion of bracing raises the fundamental question of whether the child should be braced high, with levels of bracing removed as motor control is mastered, or whether the child should be braced low, with sections added as

the need dictates. Unfortunately, orthotic prescription can be imprecise and only becomes more refined with clinical experience. A brace that is prescribed for a moving, growing, changing child can only be correct for the brief period of time that the child remains exactly as he or she was when evaluated. That period of time may be shorter for the 3- to 5-year-old child than for the teenager at 14 to 16 years. This means that the younger child who is growing rapidly and is very active may require more frequent brace re-evaluations, revisions, and repairs. This is not an indication to become frustrated and to revise or give up on the ambulation plan, but rather to be diligent and committed to supporting the ambulation process so the patient and family are not negatively affected.

In order to make an appropriate brace selection, the CNS function and the effects of CNS dysfunction on the child's ability to move must be considered as well as the motor level of the lower extremities. The orthopedic surgeon, physical therapist, and family should try to gather as much objective information about the child as possible prior to beginning an orthotics program. The physical therapist, having spent time with the child, should have a good impression of the child's motor capabilities. Asking parents to share their perceptions of their child's motor function can identify any differences between home and clinic performance. Parents can be asked to describe the ways in which their child likes to play, their child's favorite positions, responses to the upright position, degree of assistance needed to change positions, and the method the child uses to move on the floor. The answers to these questions can give the therapist valuable information. There have been families who, though excited about the prospects of beginning a bracing and gait program with their child, were able to verbalize that their child did not seem ready to be upright, follow directions, and walk with braces and an assistive device. Changes to a bracing program can often be based on sound observations and recommendations from parents, who are living with and working with their child each day.

Regardless of the brace that is ordered, families must be made aware of whom to call and what action must be taken if the brace is inadequate or does not produce the desired result. They must also understand that the failure of or problems with the brace do not mean that they or their child are failures or are somehow inadequate. Selecting and fitting the appropriate brace for a child is an ongoing process that may take time to perfect.

Once a brace is fabricated for a child, the family should be shown proper donning and doffing of the brace and appropriate leg coverings should be suggested to protect the child's skin. This therapist recommends a long, boys' tube sock for leg protection, or thin, nontextured tights for both girls and boys. Parents should be alerted to look for improper fit of a brace and when brace modification would be indicated due to poor fit. Parents should be aware of the plan to change, add, or subtract sections of the brace based on their child's progression or if problems are encountered.

With this knowledge, parents can directly contact the therapist, clinic coordinator, or orthotist with their needs so that direction can be given and necessary appointments can be made. Families should not have their child's braces sitting in a closet for several months, unused, while awaiting a routine clinic appointment to discuss a problem with the therapist or orthopedic surgeon. Likewise, a poorly fitting brace causing skin damage should not be worn because the parents are blindly compliant with their home program instructions. Changes to a brace that require increased support should not be construed as the child's failure, regression, or lack of progress. Rather, it should be handled as a matter of course for an oftentimes difficult decision that is based on both objective and subjective findings.

Decisions to change the bracing level, unlock joints, or change an assistive device should be made in a thoughtful and considered manner. The child's attitude toward and readiness for gait training plays a large part in the timeliness of these decisions. Generally the aim is for safe and functional ambulation by 5 or 6 years of age in preparation for mobility in school, but given the numerous tasks and skills to be mastered, this is not a great deal of time in which to prepare. Parents and therapists may feel rushed when the child is nearing school age, but sufficient time must be allowed for mastery of skills at one stage before progressing to the next. Some families are assertive when expressing their desire to have their child standing and ambulating as soon as possible. This should not rush the clinician into making a premature decision that might have a negative effect on the child's outcome. The responsible method of practice is to pace the progression of skills slowly to achieve the safest, most secure, and least stressful result for the child and family. In keeping with this measured approach, only one change at a time should be made to an orthosis or an assistive device. Otherwise, diagnosing a problem that may arise becomes more difficult.

A well-defined orthotic program should begin as early as the child's first days of life after the initial evaluations are concluded. The physical therapist and orthopedic surgeon can discuss the deformities that are present and those that may likely occur secondary to muscle imbalance or bony deformity around a joint. The therapist and surgeon can then develop a plan of care, including the necessary splinting and bracing, to address the current and/or anticipated problems. Orthopedic surgery and an early orthotics program can then be coordinated to prepare the child for upright positioning at as close to the typical age as possible.[14,53,68]

CHILDREN WITH THORACIC-LEVEL PARALYSIS

The child with no motor control below the thorax has flaccid lower extremities and is at risk for developing a frog-legged deformity. This posture is commonly seen in the immobile infant who remains in supine for long periods of time. The legs are abducted, externally rotated, and flexed at the hips and knees with the feet in plantar flexion. There is no active leg motion to counteract the effects of gravity and reverse this position. Muscle and other soft tissue structures become increasingly tight over time without proper attention. Prone positioning and daily ROM exercises are advised. Also, gentle nighttime wrapping of the legs in extension and adduction with an elastic bandage can prevent the deformity. Flexibility can be gained using these intervention strategies when minimal to moderate tightness already exists, but trying to avoid the problem before it occurs should be the primary goal. As the child grows, a total body splint may be used during naps and through the night to prevent loss of joint range. This device may also be known as a total contact or "A frame" orthosis. Proper fit of the orthosis will prevent limb movement within the brace that can lead to abrasions. Because the child may also need to work on control of the head and trunk, this first orthosis, adapted with wedged rubber soles, can be used for brief periods of standing. During these sessions of standing, the child can practice and become proficient in balance and equilibrium reaction activities of increasing difficulty (Fig. 6.14). Prone lying in the splint is recommended to help avoid pressure over the bony prominences, such as the ischial tuberosity, sacrum, and calcaneus. Skin breakdown at these sites is common with persistent supine positioning. Inspection of the skin is also essential after each session with the orthosis, and any red marks that do

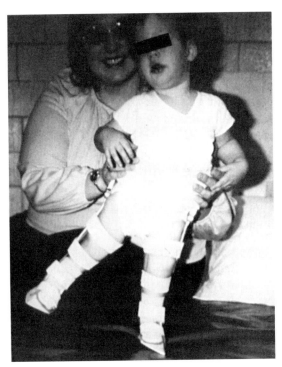

Figure 6.14 ■ A total contact orthosis to be worn at night fitted with wedged soles for periods of standing and weight-shifting activities.

not fade should be brought to the attention of the orthotist for splint adjustment.

If the child has moderate to severe limitations in ROM, it is inappropriate to use an orthosis to force the limbs into better alignment. This is dangerous and can result in skin breakdown and/or a fracture. Significant limitations in flexibility are managed best by surgical release of the tight soft tissue structures, including the iliotibial band, hip external rotators, and knee flexors. The orthosis then can be used following surgery to maintain the desired position.

The total-contact orthosis should always include a thoracolumbar section to stabilize the pelvis and lumbar spine. Without this section, the child can laterally flex the trunk, causing malalignment of the lower extremities with adduction of one hip and abduction of the other hip relative to the pelvis. Contractures at the foot will make later brace and shoe fit difficult, so the total body orthosis should include a lower leg section to hold the ankle in a neutral or plantigrade position.

For the older child or adolescent with a high thoracic lesion who is no longer ambulatory, the total body orthosis may be appropriate to use at night, to decrease contractures that can easily develop in individuals who are sitting all day. In addition, a lightweight, foot splint or ankle–foot orthosis (AFO) can be fabricated for use during the day to maintain good positioning, thus allowing proper shoe fit.[14,53]

CHILDREN WITH HIGH LUMBAR PARALYSIS

Children with a motor level from L-1 to L-3 will usually exhibit some amount of active hip flexion and adduction but no other strong movements at the hips or knees are present. Weak quadriceps may be noted in those children with an L-3 motor level. To prevent flexion/adduction contractures at the hips, the child with a high lumbar lesion will also benefit from the use of the total contact orthosis. The splint can maintain hip and knee extension with moderate abduction (approximately 30 degrees) and be worn during sleep. It can also serve as the child's first standing device.

Children with high lumbar paralysis will require a high level of bracing to stand and walk. Bracing is necessary to stabilize the knees and ankles and to provide medial–lateral control at the hips and pelvis. A number of children with this level of paralysis who have strong truncal musculature, good sitting balance, and intact CNS function may be able to control the medial/lateral planes of hip movement and ambulate without orthotic control at the hips, but they will still require bracing above the knees, as well as some type of assistive device such as a walker or crutches.

Hip subluxation and dislocation are common in children with high lumbar paralysis owing to the significant muscle imbalance around the hip. When hip dislocation is detected, therapists and parents should continue passive ROM exercises to ensure that there will be no additional loss of joint flexibility or related muscle shortening. There is often fear that damage will occur with ROM exercises, but this is not the case. Rather, more harm is done by discontinuing the exercises. There has been much discussion and debate regarding the optimal surgical approach to the hip in patients with this level of paralysis. The current consensus is that surgery to relocate the hip is not always indicated. This approach avoids many postoperative complications, including a frozen, immobile joint, which may result from an open reduction procedure. An immobile hip joint will compromise sitting and standing alignment, and often requires additional surgery if it can be corrected at all. Redislocation is also common, owing to the lack of dynamic forces around the hip to provide joint stability. Simple surgical release of soft tissue structures may be decided if the active and unopposed hip flexors and adductors have tightened to the point of restricting range without addressing the hip joint at all. In the case of a unilateral dislocation, an asymmetric pelvis can result if the involved hip becomes tight. This asymmetric posture creates an uneven foundation for sitting and standing and interferes with proper fit and alignment of braces. Again, addressing the limitation of range of motion and achieving a level pelvis without hip surgery is more important than relocating the hip joint. Evaluation for a shoe lift will be necessary for the child with a unilateral hip dislocation in order to equalize leg lengths when the child is upright. Even a small leg length difference may affect standing alignment and stability of the young patient.

When hip surgery will be performed, it is appropriate for the physical therapist to be involved with the patient and family for home program instruction when the child leaves with a cast as well as after the cast is removed.[14,53,90,91,101]

ORTHOTICS FOR CHILDREN WITH THORACIC AND HIGH LUMBAR PARALYSIS

When children with T-12 to L-3 motor levels are almost 12 months old and exhibit adequate head control to be positioned upright, they should be considered for the "A frame," also known as the Toronto standing frame. This frame can be used for multiple, short standing sessions during the day in an attempt to duplicate the activities of typical children who pull to stand for short periods of time but are still predominantly mobile on the floor (Fig. 6.15). The device is easy to don and doff and a schedule of upright positioning for 20 to 30 minutes four or five times each day seems manageable for most parents. The device is freestanding and represents the child's first opportunity to be upright for play without having hands-on assistance from a parent or using the upper extremities for support. Engaging the child for self-feeding and fine motor activities is ideal during this standing time. Additionally, parents can

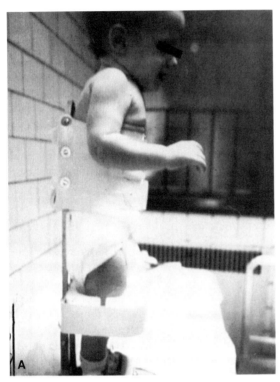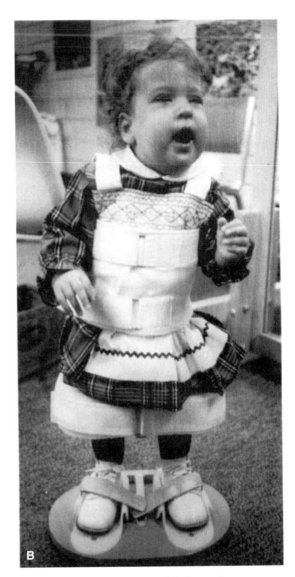

Figure 6.15 ▪ Toronto A frame showing good alignment for standing. **(A)** Side view. **(B)** Front view.

be instructed to further challenge their child during these standing periods by working on head-righting and balance skills. A recommended activity is to slowly tilt the frame in one direction, watching for the child's righting response of the head and trunk. The frame is returned to midline and then tilted in another direction, waiting again for the child's balance response. The frame should be tilted slowly and at a small angle, and all directions should be performed: forward, back, right and left sides, and to the diagonals. This routine is recommended for the first 5 to 10 minutes of each standing session. Based on the child's success, further strengthening of the responses and the musculature involved can be achieved by increasing the angle of the tilt. Again, as mentioned earlier, if asymmetry is seen in the quality of the child's responses, then tilting can be performed more frequently to specific directions to strengthen the weaker reactions. Placing the child to passively stand in front of the television is not recommended, and unsuper-

vised standing is not advisable because the child's wiggling body may topple the device, causing injury.[24,53] As the child progresses in developmental activities, such as rolling, getting into and out of a sitting position, and attempting to crawl, the child may no longer tolerate the immobility of the standing frame. This may indicate a readiness for bracing and ambulation training.

Children with moderate to severe CNS deficits and delayed head control and upper extremity function may continue to use the standing frame until they are too tall to properly fit into the frame (at about 6 years of age, depending on the child's height). As the child outgrows the frame, the parapodium or the Orlau swivel walker may be considered. These are two orthotic options that will provide continued and valuable time in an upright posture while providing adequate support of the upper body to meet the needs of the child with significant motor delay. Both are easy to don and doff, they are simple to size and fit well, and they are also free standing. Regardless of the device chosen, the child should continue an exercise program that includes developmental and preambulation skills to improve function in the neck, trunk, arms, and upper body. While in either device, the child can practice weight-shift activities as described above. For the child using a parapodium, a walker or forearm crutches can be introduced at some point to teach forward mobility, if the child has coordinated and strong upper extremities. The Orlau swivel walker has a ball-bearing plate at its base that causes a forward progression on a level surface without the use of assistive devices. Movement of the Orlau requires the child to move the shoulders, upper trunk, and head in a side-to-side movement that causes the device to unweight on one side and swivel forward. As skills improve, children can progress to another, less supportive/restrictive orthosis.[53]

For a long time, the standard hip–knee–ankle–foot orthosis (HKAFO) was the only option for the child with a high level of paralysis who was ready to ambulate. A thoracic extension could be added to the HKAFO for the child with limited trunk control, but this could result in an extremely immobile child and limit his or her potential to only walk as an exercise or household ambulator. Another option, the Louisiana State University Reciprocating Gait Orthosis (RGO), was developed. The RGO uses a system of cables with a dual-action hip joint that flexes one hip while maintaining the opposite hip in locked extension for a stable one-legged stance and a reciprocating pattern of gait. A properly fitted RGO maintains extension at all lower extremity joints and aligns and supports the trunk and pelvis over the legs with a thoracic portion. Many children who have used the RGO and an assistive device have progressed to a more energy-efficient and safer gait pattern than was possible with the HKAFO. As a child's upper trunk stability improves, the RGO can be modified without decreasing the child's ability. By retaining the cables and dual-action hip joints but removing the chest strap and thoracic uprights, the child can still use the brace mechanism for an assisted reciprocating gait, but with less restriction to the upper body.[92-95]

The isocentric RGO is yet another device that eliminates the posterior cable system but maintains the same functional properties as the original RGO. Patients and families accustomed to using the original RGO can be switched to the isocentric model when the child grows and a new brace is required or it can be prescribed as the child's first brace.[93]

With hip and knee joints locked, the child ambulating with either of these reciprocating braces and an assistive device performs a lateral weight shift onto one leg and leans slightly back at the shoulders to facilitate the forward flexion of the unweighted leg. Repeating the weight shift and leaning to the other side and back produces forward flexion of the opposite lower extremity. This gait pattern requires no active motor function in the lower extremities, but if active hip flexion is present, it can be utilized to flex the limb (Figs. 6.16 to 6.18).[93-95]

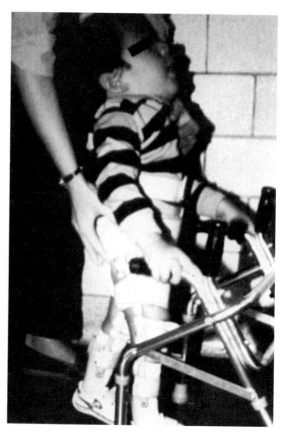

Figure 6.16 ■ Gait training with a reciprocating gait orthosis. A lateral weight shift with a slight tilt backward causes the unweighted leg to swing forward.

When using the standard HKAFO with pelvic band, locked hip and knee joints, and solid ankle joints, the child can learn either a hop-to or swivel pattern of gait using a walker, later mastering the swing-through pattern with crutches as arm strength increases and control improves. The child with active hip flexors can attempt to walk with one or both hip joints unlocked, using a reciprocating gait pattern. In the absence of functional low back extensors or gluteals when both hips are unlocked, the child will tend to fall forward. To maintain an erect posture, the child must hyperextend at the lumbar spine to shift the center of gravity posterior. The child must also use both upper extremities to remain erect by pushing on the walker or crutch handles (Fig. 6.19). When unlocking the hip joints of the HKAFO, the pelvic band provides control of abduction/adduction and medial/lateral rotation of the lower extremities, motion the child is unable to actively control. For some children with a high lumbar lesion and an intact CNS, the pelvic band may at some point be removed to allow further freedom for transfers and to permit a faster swing-through gait pattern, if the child progresses to using crutches. Adequate arm strength, trunk stability, and the ability to hyperextend the lumbar spine are essential for a stable stance, and when these skills are present the child more closely resembles a

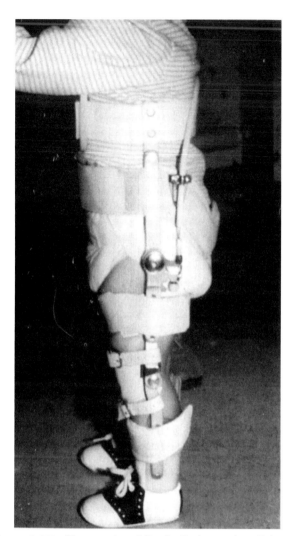

Figure 6.17 ■ Alignment and fit of a Reciprocating Gait Orthosis with a thoracic strap and uprights, cable, and dual-action hip joints. Note use of patellar pad to maintain true knee extension.

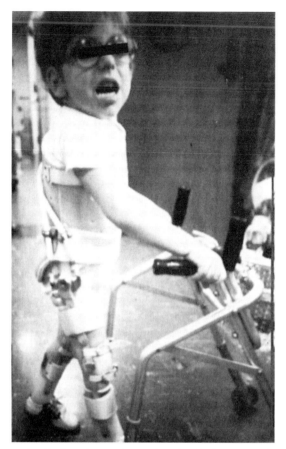

Figure 6.18 ■ A reciprocating gait orthosis, fit over a plastic body jacket, to manage scoliosis. Note the erect alignment in this child with paralysis at the T-10 level.

patient with acquired, traumatic paraplegia than one with a congenital disability.[93,94]

Regardless of the orthosis, most young children and their therapists find that the rollator walker is the most effective assistive device to begin gait training. With four points of stability and two front wheels, this walker provides good support and the child does not have to lift the walker to advance it. For this reason, the standard walker is almost never used any longer with this population. If possible, the use of parallel bars should be avoided during initial gait training because they provide too much stability and the child may develop patterns of pulling and leaning on the bars that will be dangerous when making the transition to a walker. Exceptions may be made in cases where a child has extreme difficulty learning to use a walker or is very fearful. In this case, one should first check that the level of bracing is appropriate and that the child was not braced too low and should have additional support (Table 6.2).

The decision to progress the child to either axillary or forearm crutches will depend on the child's ability. A typical timeline for progression cannot be easily predicted or plotted, and a degree of experimentation is always necessary. A child wearing a body jacket due to scoliosis may find axillary crutches difficult to use. They can slip and be difficult to stabilize. But axillary crutches encourage a more upright posture and they are best used for the child who will walk with a reciprocating gait or the hop-to patterns. The swing-to and swing-through patterns are most safely and efficiently accomplished with forearm crutches. However, the child using forearm crutches over several years may easily develop a tendency to lean forward onto the crutches, and this habitual pattern can lead to an upper thoracic kyphosis and tight pectoral muscles that cause protraction of the shoulders with elevated and protracted scapulae. If these postural malalignments begin to develop, the therapist and family should work together with the child to maintain a flexible, erect thoracic spine and well-aligned shoulders. Prone lifts and exercises for shoulder external rotation and depression, in sitting, prone, and supine, will help strengthen the rhomboids and lower trapezius muscles and stretch the pectorals, which will reduce the severity of this problem.

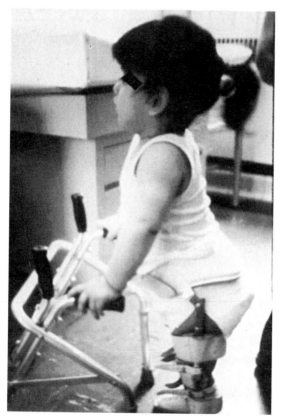

Figure 6.19 ■ Hip–knee–ankle–foot orthosis (HKAFO) with hip joints unlocked. The child with an L-4/L-5 motor level maintains balance with a hyperextended lumbar spine and upper extremity support on the walker. The HKAFO is needed to control medial–lateral instability at the hips due to muscle imbalance.

By the time the child with high-level paralysis approaches adolescence, he or she may have already chosen to use a wheelchair as the primary form of mobility to achieve more competitive function with peers. As transition to a wheelchair occurs, children and families may discard the idea of

bracing, standing, and walking. The growth spurts and weight gains that are typical of all adolescents make brace management more of a problem for the child with spina bifida. Braces may require more frequent adjustment, repair, and/or replacement. The child might be spending little or no time standing and walking during the school day so the value of the braces is greatly reduced. But spending a full day in a wheelchair increases the likelihood of hip and knee flexion contractures and foot deformity. These are common in the nonambulatory adolescent and can also impact the child's wheelchair and transfer skills. Therefore, when wheelchair mobility is chosen, if at all possible, children should also maintain a program of positioning and physical activity aimed at avoiding joint contractures and musculoskeletal deterioration. Prone positioning, standers, parapodiums, or braces can be used during prescribed therapy sessions and for periods of time through the week, both at home and at school. Swimming, wheelchair sports, wheelchair aerobics, and other activities that help control weight gain and improve cardiovascular function can be a part of the child's activity regimen. Maintaining and increasing trunk and arm strength and coordination is important for the older child/adolescent so that during times of growth and weight gain no loss of function is experienced.[14,84–86,89,90]

ORTHOTICS FOR CHILDREN WITH LOW LUMBAR PARALYSIS

Children with L-4 or L-5 motor function usually have strong hip flexors and adductors. Gluteus medius and tensor fascia lata may be present to contribute to hip abduction, although the strength of these muscles can vary from a "poor" to "good" grade. Hip extension from the gluteus maximus is usually absent. Children at this level are at risk for flexion contractures as well as early hip dislocation or later progressive subluxation, depending on the relative

---

TABLE 6.2

Ambulation Sequence: T-12 to L-3 Motor Level

	CNS Status		
	Typical → Mild Deficit	Mild → Moderate	Moderate → Severe
Preambulation orthosis	Toronto A Frame	Toronto A Frame	Toronto A Frame
Assess	Ambulation bracing at 15–24 mo	Ambulation bracing at 15–24 mo	Continue with A Frame
↓			
Ambulation orthosis	HKAFO; locked hips; rollator walker	RGO; thoracic uprights; rollator walker	Orlau swivel walker; no assistive device
↓			
Progress	As above, hips unlocked	RGO; remove uprights; rollator walker	RGO; thoracic uprights; rollator walker
↓			
Progress	As above, crutches	As above, crutches	
↓			
Progress	KAFO, pelvic band removed; crutches	Assess for further changes; consider standard HKAFO or KAFO	Assess for further changes

CNS, central nervous system; HKAFO, hip–knee–ankle–foot orthosis; KAFO, knee–ankle–foot orthosis; RGO, reciprocating gait orthosis.

strengths of the muscles surrounding the hip joint. Inherent ligamentous laxity in the child with low tone also contributes to hip joint instability.

Manual muscle testing around the knee usually shows strong quadriceps and medial hamstrings (semitendinosus and semimembranosus) but absent lateral hamstring function. Kicking and crawling during the early childhood years can produce an internal tibial torsion deformity from the unopposed stimulation of the tibia by the medial hamstrings. This imbalance in forces causes a toeing-in posture during standing and gait, which is first seen as the child pulls to stand and begins to cruise.

Careful manual muscle testing is crucial in children with lower level lesions because there is often great variation of motor ability at the ankle and foot (Display 6.7). The anterior and posterior tibialis muscles, long and short toe extensors, peroneus longus and brevis muscles, and toe flexors may be functional, but the strengths in these muscle groups may vary greatly. If significant imbalance in strength is found, patients may need to be splinted at night to prevent a progressive loss of flexibility.

With strong dorsiflexors and absent plantar flexors, a calcaneus deformity may have been present at birth, or it may develop through early childhood. An exceptionally high arch, a pes cavus deformity, is caused by the unopposed action of the anterior tibialis, and results in a foot with a dangerously reduced weight-bearing surface. The distribution of body weight is limited to the heel and ball of the foot and pressure problems can develop when the child begins to walk. Bracing and shoe fit can be difficult, and surgery is often indicated to weaken or eliminate the deforming forces, realign the bones, and provide a greater weight-bearing surface over the entire sole of the foot.

A calcaneovarus or calcaneovalgus foot may be seen in children with this level of paralysis when there is an absence of the plantar flexor (gastrocnemius/soleus) muscle group. Other combinations of strengths and weaknesses of the intrinsic musculature in the foot and ankle can produce additional abnormal foot and toe alignment and abnormality of the weight-bearing surfaces of the foot. The orthopedic surgeon may consider muscle-lengthening procedures and tendon transfers in an attempt to balance the dynamic forces around the joints or excise the tendons if active muscle balance cannot be reached. The goal is to attain a flat foot that is easy to fit with bracing and shoes.[97] Torosian and Dias stated that deformities of the foot are the most common lower limb problem in the spina bifida population. Foot deformities cause pain, interfere with shoe and brace fit, and negatively affect the child's ability to walk.[98] They addressed the management of severe hindfoot valgus, but the principles are universal to all foot malalignment. A mild deformity may be accommodated by a brace, but if it is severe, the insensate foot requires surgical correction because it is vulnerable to pressure sores and ulceration.

The clubfoot deformity (talipes equinovarus) is the most common foot deformity in children with spina bifida at the L-4 or L-5 motor level (Fig. 6.20). The diagnosis and management of clubfoot has prompted extensive discussion by orthopedic surgeons. Many now follow a protocol that includes gentle manipulation and taping as early as the baby's first weeks of life, followed by application of a well-padded splint, rather than serial casting. Casts had been used extensively in recent years, and this change of approach is a response to the problems that were seen from pressure over bony prominences and the associated skin irritation and breakdown that were seen. The clubfoot is often very resistant to conservative treatment and surgical correction is inevitable. Recurrence of a clubfoot deformity secondary to incomplete surgical correction is not uncommon, and may lead to skin problems from a poorly fitting brace or shoe. Gentle passive stretching exercises to maintain flexibility and a well-padded, properly fitting brace are important, although additional surgery to fully correct the deformity will be indicated. It is reported that when tendon lengthening is used in lieu of excision of the tendons, the deformity is more likely to recur. Since children with this level of motor paralysis will most always need bracing to stabilize the ankle for gait, tendon excision has no functional impact on the child's level of bracing or ambulation

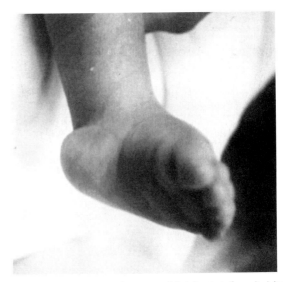

Figure 6.20 ■ *Talipes equinovarus (clubfoot deformity) in a neonate. She will be treated with serial taping to gently stretch soft tissue structures into a more neutral position followed by surgery.*

> **DISPLAY 6.7**

Common Foot Deformities in Patients with Spina Bifida

Pes calcaneus, calcaneovarus, calcaneovalgus

Talipes equinovarus or clubfoot

Pes equines or flatfoot

Convex pes valgus or rocker-bottom foot with vertical talus

Pes cavus, high arch with toe clawing

Ankle valgus, at the mid- or hindfoot

potential. The midfoot of this deformity has a prominent crease and the forefoot is adducted. With surgery the foot lengthens as it becomes better aligned. Prior to surgery, parents can be instructed to perform frequent but gentle stretching of the skin and soft tissue structures of the medial aspect of the foot. This has been found to help prevent wound dehiscence, a common complication following surgery, when the skin is stretched thin and taut to cover the longer, corrected foot.[14,53,99,100]

Debate continues regarding surgery for the child with a unilateral or bilateral hip dislocation and an L-4 or L-5 motor level. When deciding on a course of management, the surgeon must consider the child's total function, including lower extremity strength and developmental skills. Surgical correction may not be indicated if bracing to the hips and/or assistive devices will always be indicated for mobility, based on the pattern of lower extremity innervation or the presence of significant CNS involvement. On the other hand, surgical correction may be indicated for the child with good motor control of the trunk and strong quadriceps. This child may eventually be able to walk with an AFO or an unlocked KAFO. In addition, active gluteus medius musculature may indicate the child's potential for future ambulation with no assistive device. Therefore, a surgeon may choose to relocate the child's hip(s) to prevent or correct significant gait deviations that would hamper the child's unassisted walking. Surgery might also prevent later degenerative changes in the unstable hip that could cause pain in the joint for the child with intact sensation.

However, other surgeons contend that bilateral hip dislocations should never be surgically repaired for fear that postoperative complications could be harmful, diminishing the child's potential for gait, and the gains would be minimal. A unilateral dislocation is usually corrected in the child with intact CNS function who has the potential for ambulation with short bracing and no assistive device.[14,53,101]

It is apparent from this section as it is from the literature that the management of hip dislocations is a confusing and controversial subject for the child with a low lumbar lesion. The therapist can play a role in assisting the physician to identify the child's muscle strengths and weaknesses, skills in the upright position, trunk and pelvic alignment, and overall gross motor ability. This information may then enable the physician to better evaluate the treatment options and choose accordingly. Function, not x-ray findings, should guide this important decision.

Children with L-4 to L-5 paralysis who have significant CNS deficits may not be able to control the trunk in upright positions or move their legs well. This lack of movement often conveys the impression that a higher level of paralysis exists. The therapist and the family should continue their attempts to remediate the effects of the CNS deficit, by improving coordination of the head, shoulders, and trunk. The child can begin with a Toronto standing frame and progress to the RGO for gait training. Both devices offer a psychological and motivational boost for the family and the child who has been slow to acquire gross motor skills. If gait training is performed in a patient and thoughtful manner, some measure of success can be realized. In error, a child with poor trunk stability but a low lumbar paralysis might be fitted for bracing that is too low, based solely on the lower extremity movements. These inappropriate orthotics and the ineffective attempts at gait training result in great frustration for children, parents, and therapists alike. To avoid these situations, use of the RGO seems to provide significant benefits for this group of children who can then be progressed to a lower brace level at some point in the future, as their skills indicate.[93,100]

Children who have a lesion level at L-4 to L-5 and without any apparent CNS deficit can be provided with bracing according to their lower extremity function (Table 6.3). Many children at this level are attempting to stand or are already able to pull to stand by 10 to 12 months of age, and will not require a standing frame. If the child can control his or her knees while upright, one can go directly to an AFO (Fig. 6.21). Though some children at this motor level will be able to stand and begin to walk without foot support, the AFO will provide leg stability for stance and gait and assist in normalizing gait parameters, increasing ambulation speed, increasing stride length, decreasing double support time, and decreasing oxygen consumption. The orthosis will also help to control the subtalar joint, preventing heel valgus, and control forefoot adduction/abduction.[14,53,102] "Twister" cables, which provide a rotatory force, may be added later if leg rotation needs correction. Internal rotation, emanating from unequal forces at the hip or behind the knee, is very common at this lesion level (Fig. 6.22). However, external rotation of both legs, or a combination of internal rotation of one leg and external rotation of the other leg, may also be seen. Twister cables can be adjusted to control any of these combinations, and are valuable in aligning the lower leg for a safer and more cosmetic gait. Twister cables should always be attached to both AFOs. They cannot be attached unilaterally. If one leg does not require correction, then the cable on that side can be set at neutral. Twisters can also reduce some of the stance-phase varus or valgus deviations at the knee that are seen in the limb with excessive torsion. Twisters may prevent overstretching of the loose ligamentous structures at the knee if the child were to continue walking with the legs malaligned. Over time, the child may learn to control minimal rotational deviations with the help of the twister cables and avoid surgical correction, but ultimately surgery to derotate the legs will be indicated for most children. Surgery is usually recommended at approximately the age of 6 years. The procedure should correct the bony malalignment at the femur or tibia, depending on the source of the rotation. If rotation is at the lower leg, tendon transfer of the active medial hamstrings to a more midline orientation behind the knee is performed, so that deformity of the tibia does not recur.[53]

TABLE 6.3		
Orthotic Management for L-4 to L-5 and Sacral Motor Lesions		

	L-4 to L-5	**Sacral**
Muscles present	Hip flexors and adductors Quadriceps Medial hamstrings Anterior tibialis Some gluteus medius Some foot intrinsics	All, with possible exception of gluteus maximus, gastrocnemius/soleus group, and foot intrinsics
Preambulation orthotics	Toronto standing frame (some children may pull to stand, bypassing the frame, and begin with bracing*)	Usually none needed*
Ambulation bracing	RGO; if CNS deficits present KAFO with weak quadriceps AFO with good truncal balance, with or without "twisters" if torsion is present*	AFO with weak gastrocnemius/soleus or crouched gait. Some need no bracing, but shoe insert may help maintain proper foot alignment
Assistive devices	Start with rollator walker and progress to crutches. An independent gait is possible for some, usually with a gluteus medius lurch and lumbar lordosis	Possibly a walker early on; most progress to an independent gait*
Expected functional level	Ambulatory in life unless increased body weight; flexion contractures; poor CNS status; further complications may reduce ambulatory status	Independent gait with moderate to minimal deviations based on patterns of weakness

*Control of upper body and CNS status may modify these levels.

AFO, ankle–foot orthosis; CNS, central nervous system; KAFO, knee–ankle–foot orthosis; RGO, reciprocating gait orthosis.

A KAFO may be used for a child with weak quadriceps who has difficulty maintaining either unilateral or bilateral knee extension when upright. Many braces that incorporate the knee joint are fabricated with straps across the thigh and lower leg. This author has found that adding a

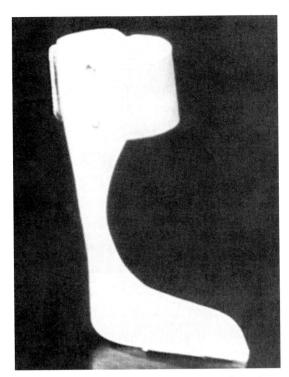

Figure 6.21 ■ A plastic ankle–foot orthosis is aligned at 90 degrees or at a neutral position.

knee/patellar pad will help maintain better knee extension while reducing the pressure exerted across the thigh and tibial straps of the KAFO. This reduction in pressure decreases the probability of skin breakdown at those sites. Although a pad at the knee adds to the time spent donning and doffing the brace, it appears to be a valuable component that ensures true knee extension that the more proximal and distal straps alone will not offer. In some children, a posterior displacement of the tibia relative to the femur can occur when excessive force is exerted into the tibial strap during standing. The patellar pad prevents this from occurring. Also, if knee flexion is noted on one side when the child stands and walks, prior to considering the KAFO, a possible leg length discrepancy should be ruled out, which would cause the longer leg to flex.[14,53]

Some clinics have used a "floor reaction" or "anticrouch" orthosis for children who have difficulty attaining knee extension. This orthosis is a standard AFO with an anterior shell that should facilitate knee extension at heel strike. The orthosis is theoretically sound and has been used successfully with other disabilities. But problems with excessive pressure across the anterior tibia and skin breakdown have caused some centers to avoid using this brace with children who have spina bifida.

A recent study presented by Hunt et al. explored the use of a hinged AFO that limited mobility at the ankle from 5 degrees of dorsiflexion to 10 degrees of plantar flexion rather than the typical solid ankle. It demonstrated a positive influence on walking velocity; therefore, this brace may warrant further investigation.[103] Dorsiflexion at the ankle that produces consistent knee flexion may have to

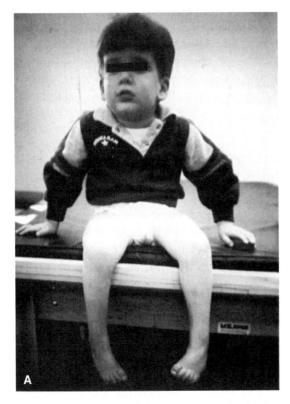

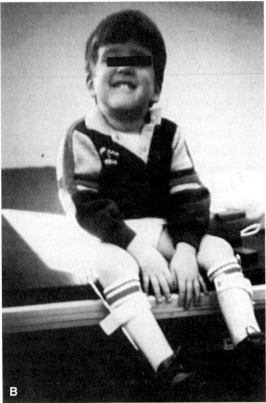

Figure 6.22 ■ **(A,B)** A child with an L-4 to L-5 motor level and significant in-toeing is portrayed. Twister cables are attached to an ankle–foot orthosis to control rotation or torsion until surgery is indicated.

be evaluated at more frequent intervals by the clinician to avoid contractures that will limit a child's gait skills. Regardless of the orthosis chosen, a careful assessment of the resulting gait pattern will indicate the likelihood of success or failure of a particular device and the need for revision or replacement.

The child with an L-4 or L-5 motor level is often able to begin ambulation after one or two sessions of gait training with a rollator walker. The family can continue working with the child at home after only a brief demonstration in the clinic. Crutch training for the young child is often more involved and lengthy, and many clinicians believe that crutches are ill-advised until the child is 4 or 5 years old and has reached a reasonable level of skill and self-confidence in the upright position. The child must also have a sufficient attention span to benefit, without stress to the child or the instructor, from the crutch training sessions and be safe. Some children with L-4 to L-5 paralysis will attempt independent, unassisted ambulation. The gait pattern usually includes a hyperlordotic lumbar spine and a side-to-side gluteus medius lurch that can be quite severe. The degree of these deviations depends on the strength of the hip extensors and abductors relative to the flexors and adductors as well as the stability and control of the trunk. Gait will improve when good back and abdominal strength can assist with better alignment of the lumbar spine and pelvis, but deviation will always be seen when there is weakness and/or muscle imbalance around the hip joints. For this reason, therapists should support the continued use of an assistive device through adolescence to prevent over-stretching of soft tissue structures and arthritic changes to the joints with accompanying pain. Prevention of these future problems is imperative.

Despite the high degree of activity demonstrated by children with a low lumbar lesion, ROM exercises remain important. A prone positioning program is useful to counteract the hyperlordotic posture of the spine and flexion of the hips that is seen during ambulation. Prone positioning for prescribed periods during the day such as for TV time or reading, as well as through the night, can minimize development of hip flexion contractures. Moderate to severe hip flexion contractures are the single most influential factor leading to the deterioration of ambulation skills in these children. Hip flexion contractures of 20 degrees or more for the child using AFOs and crutches can diminish gait velocity by as much as 65%. Activities to maintain spinal mobility, to prevent a fixed lordotic spine, along with supine and sitting activities to address abdominal muscle strength are also recommended for a long-term program at school and in the home.[63,67,53,91,97,100]

ORTHOTICS FOR CHILDREN WITH SACRAL-LEVEL PARALYSIS

The child with a sacral-level lesion will have a greater degree of muscle function throughout the lower extremities than a child with any other motor level. But, as with the other motor levels, there remains a great degree of variation among the children in this group as well. Muscle forces around the hips and knees are in better balance, with full or partial innervation of the major muscle groups. At the S-1 and S-2 motor levels, strong knee flexors and gluteus medius are expected, while gluteus maximus and gastrocnemius/soleus are present but may be weak. Children with S-2 to S-3 motor levels have all musculature of the hips, knees, and ankles present and good strengths can be expected.

The incidence of hip subluxation and dislocation is lower in this population than at other motor levels. Significant hip flexion contractures should not develop, and abnormal torsions of the femur and tibia are not as prevalent as with higher level lesions. Because of the additional musculature available at the proximal joints, through the trunk, hips, and knees, the gait pattern of the child with sacral innervation will more closely resemble a typical gait, although deviations will still be seen.

Manual muscle testing demonstrates that variation in this population is greatest at the foot and ankle with weakness seen in the gastrocnemius/soleus muscle group. Toe flexors may be present and may provide some secondary ankle plantar flexion, but they are usually not strong enough to totally compensate for a weak gastrocnemius/soleus and stabilize the ankle during stance and gait. As a result, AFOs will be indicated for these children. If strong plantar flexors are present, external support may not be necessary while the child is young but close observation is necessary especially during periods of rapid growth and weight gain. The gastrocnemius/soleus may be strong enough to adequately stabilize the tibia of a small child for standing and walking alignment over short distances but may not be strong enough for the older, taller, and heavier child. Gait deviations may begin to emerge. As the child grows and the lever arm for the muscle lengthens, a decrease in muscle efficiency may result. The loss of mechanical advantage means that additional strength is needed for stabilization, not available in a partially innervated muscle. The gastrocnemius/soleus controls the forward movement of the tibia over the foot as the stance phase of gait progresses from heel strike. When strength is inadequate, a crouched gait may develop. Because the tibia is permitted to roll too far forward and too rapidly into dorsiflexion, secondary hip and knee flexion will occur. Therefore, the child should always be observed both in static stance postures and dynamic gait during each physical therapy or clinic appointment. Flexion contractures, though not expected in children with sacral-level lesions, can develop if this flexed posture is not remediated. The added energy expense of walking with a deformity may also reduce ambulation capacity. Surgical lengthening of tight hamstrings is unusual but might be necessary as a result of these changes in gait, and a once independent ambulator may need an assistive device for support. But the crouched gait and its associated prob-

lems can be prevented simply by using an AFO as soon as the child demonstrates a need. The child whose posture is maintained by an orthosis will then be free to go for short periods of time without bracing, to attend a party or special event, without compromising future potential.[53] The child with a sacral motor level is not as intact as was once thought and the issues and problems that can develop are not benign.

As our profession becomes more experienced in addressing foot and ankle problems, the child with a sacral-level lesion may benefit from having molded shoe orthotics placed within the typically prescribed AFO. This arrangement may prevent many of the hindfoot and midfoot malalignments that can arise as the child grows and imbalances of the intrinsic muscles of the foot become more pronounced. AFOs with articulating ankle joints or an AFO fabricated from a more flexible material that permits some limited dorsiflexion and plantar flexion may be indicated for specific children who will benefit from the opportunity to have a more dynamic gait, allowing them to utilize their active musculature at the ankle and foot.[103,104]

Compared to the child with a higher motor paralysis, the child with a sacral paralysis may not appear to need therapeutic intervention. But many children with a sacral-level innervation will exhibit some mild gait deviation. Benefits can be gained from a therapeutic program to "fine-tune" the child's gait, and this program can be delivered by occasional sessions over a long period of time, with short periods of more intense intervention, when changes are seen, especially after a growth spurt that may negatively affect the child's alignment and gait. Abdominal strengthening, especially the oblique abdominals as well as the rectus abdominus, and strengthening to the extensors of the trunk and limbs, is recommended. The child should also practice correct alignment of the shoulders, trunk, pelvis, and limbs during standing and ambulation. Tactile, verbal, and visual reinforcement can all be used to help the child learn and maintain proper posture for progressively longer periods of time. Children involved in a long-term program like this may still exhibit their abnormal gait pattern most of the time, when they are not thinking about how they look. But, as the child matures, he or she may desire to walk with a more typical pattern. The child will then have the skill and muscle strength to do so. It is a pleasure to work with a child who can reach high levels of motor function. The process of working with a child like this is also an educational opportunity for the clinician. The therapist learns to observe more closely, analyze subtle gait deviations, and determine the areas of trunk and limb weakness that contribute to the deviations, so an appropriate intervention plan can be made. The development of careful and critical observational skills ultimately benefits all patients, not only those with spina bifida (Fig. 6.23).

Compared to children with higher levels of paralysis, fewer children with sacral lesions have hydrocephalus that require a shunt, and fewer exhibit hypotonicity that is pathologic and that affects their gross motor function.

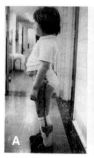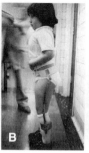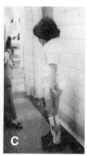

Figure 6.23 ■ *Nine-year-old girl with an S-1 motor level. (A) An independent gait has been achieved with ankle–foot orthoses and twisters. Note the poor alignment and low tone of the trunk, as well as the anterior pelvic tilt with hip flexion. (B) Following a long-term program of active exercises for problem areas, she works hard to align the thorax and lumbar spine cortically and improve pelvic alignment. (C) Increasing success with correct posture, holding during gait, is next.*

Many of the CNS, biomechanical, and neuromuscular factors that negatively influence the acquisition of mobility skills are not as prevalent in children with sacral paralysis. As a result, children with sacral paralysis who present with hip instability or other joint deviations are treated aggressively to preserve their potential for lifelong functional ambulation.[14,53]

The use of a preambulation or standing device may not be necessary for the child at the sacral level if the child is developing strong balance responses in the trunk and a good quality of movement. The child may already be pulling up to stand at 10 to 15 months of age, as expected of a typical child. A foot splint, commonly fabricated to be worn at night to maintain alignment, may also be used during the day to stabilize a weak ankle, enabling the child to stand while awaiting definitive bracing.

For the child who does experience CNS difficulties, one can follow the same course of intervention that would be prescribed for a child with a higher level lesion. The program should include activities that address flexion and extension strength against gravity through the head and trunk, as well as balance and equilibrium reactions in all positions. The program should also include passive and active exercises for the lower extremities to prevent joint contractures and an orthotics program based on the skill level of the child.[53,75–79]

THREE-DIMENSIONAL GAIT ANALYSIS

The development of increasingly more sophisticated and more readily available gait analysis technology is providing objective information that enables therapists, orthotists, and orthopedic surgeons to visualize and more accurately understand the gait parameters and deviations of the patient with spina bifida. Widely held beliefs and treatment protocols that were developed based solely on subjective or anecdotal evidence may now be validated or discarded by utilizing the three-dimensional information provided by gait analysis. Orthotic prescriptions can be better tailored to the specific needs of the child when the effects of the orthosis can be understood, especially in the sagittal plane kinematics, walking speed, and progression of ground reaction forces across the foot, and on the three planes of motion of the pelvis, hips, and knees. Vankoski et al. at the gait lab at Children's Memorial Hospital in Chicago have found that comparing the gait studies of children with spina bifida to the gait parameters of typical individuals has not provided the most meaningful information to guide and evaluate treatment plans.[105,106] Rather, children with spina bifida at a given lesion level demonstrate characteristic gait patterns that are reasonably homogenous. These identifiable patterns then become the baseline from which comparisons can be drawn, enabling the clinician to focus on realistic goals for the patient based on his or her motor level and to evaluate more fairly the result of interventions, either conservative or surgical. In one study it was found that in the absence of the gluteus medius, gluteus maximus, and ankle plantar flexors, certain compensatory movements at the pelvis and hip were consistently noted to enable children to maintain ambulation without an assistive device. This gait pattern of the child with a lumbosacral-level lesion is characterized by exaggerated movement at the pelvis and pelvic obliquity, increased stance-phase hip abduction, increased stance-phase knee flexion, knee valgus, and increased ankle dorsiflexion.[107,108] In another study, Williams et al. reported a 24% incidence of late knee pain in ambulatory patients with a lumbosacral level lesion. Knee valgus, causing the discomfort, was found to be a result of a combination of internal pelvic and hip rotation and stance-phase knee flexion.[109] The use of gait analysis for early detection of these abnormal knee movements can direct the clinician toward the most appropriate treatment—either a surgical intervention such as a tibial derotation osteotomy or the use of KAFOs—to assist the patient to support the knee in extension and avoid pain and deterioration during gait. The continued use of crutches was also found to be an important deterrent to later arthritic joint changes and pain in this population. Even though the children were able to walk unaided at an early age, continued use of crutches reduced the exaggerated range of movements and joint stress through the lumbar spine, pelvis, hips, and knees, helping to decrease pain in those areas.[104–106] Analysis of the effects of an AFO on gait found that in many of the children examined there was less stress placed on the knee without the brace than was noted with it. This was especially true for the children with L-4 to sacral-level lesions.[110] This type of analysis may lead to the development of new orthotics that will control the ankle as needed while avoiding negative influences on the more proximal joints. This study is certainly not an indication to stop using a brace in a child with a lumbar- or sacral-level paralysis, because the gait deviations that would arise could be far more disastrous.

Finally, it is interesting to note that most gait labs incorporate the results of manual muscle testing and gross motor assessments provided by the physical therapist when evaluating the child's movement skills and developing a treatment plan for intervention.

Casting Following Orthopedic Surgery

Earlier in this chapter, various deformities commonly associated with different motor levels were mentioned, as were some of the surgical procedures to correct them. After most of these procedures, the child must be immobilized in a cast for a period of time to allow the surgical site to heal undisturbed. The period of time can vary from 2 to 3 weeks following soft tissue surgery, 6 to 8 weeks for a bony procedure such as a pelvic osteotomy, and even longer. Casts and the associated immobilization should never be considered a benign treatment modality for the child with spina bifida. Pressure and irritation to insensitive skin are always a risk. Fractures, loss of joint flexibility, and loss of gross motor skills are also complications. Children with minimal or no CNS deficits may exhibit a loss of postural security and antigravity muscle strength following a period of immobilization. Children with significant CNS problems may regress even more. It is troublesome to see children lose skills that they have struggled a long time to gain.

Most surgeons agree that children with spina bifida should be casted for the shortest possible time needed for adequate healing.[111] Because of problems related to immobility and to minimize the number of hospitalizations and anesthesia, some surgeons will try to perform several procedures at the same time so the child is casted only once. The therapist can assist the child and family to make this period less problematic while supporting the fact that surgery and the subsequent casting period are important parts of the orthopedic program to reduce deformity and ultimately maintain or gain function.[53] Returning the child as quickly as possible to his or her preoperative status, or to an improved status, should be the objective. Recommendations to manage the child in a cast should be discussed with the family prior to surgery whenever possible so the child's needs are understood and adequate preparation can be made for the postoperative period. A child undergoing surgery creates added stress to the normal routine of family life. Important questions are often forgotten and the therapist may have to anticipate and address the issues families will have to face during the time their child will be immobile.

Many children will be in a hip spica cast following pelvic or hip surgery. If unilateral surgery is performed, the full hip spica may still be used to stabilize the pelvis and opposite limb, thereby preventing movement at the surgical site. With the surgeon's approval, prone positioning will help prevent skin breakdown at bony sites, the calcaneus, sacrum, and ischial tuberosity, and will challenge the child to lift and extend his or her head to watch television, read, or play. Prone positioning in a reclining wheelchair or scooter board can provide mobility if the child can use his or her upper extremities for self-propulsion. This mobility will also reduce the amount of carrying by family members. Similarly, prone positioning on a padded wagon for long walks outdoors may help the family survive this period with less anxiety and frustration because the child is occupied and happy. After several days, the physician may permit the child to stand, a position that can be easily maintained for long periods, especially during mealtime and play. One clever family adapted a hand truck to safely stand and move its older, heavier adolescent while she was in a hip spica cast (Fig. 6.24). If the cast is asymmetric, towels propped under one foot will help to level the child. To ensure the child's safety, it will be necessary to lean the child forward onto a heavy chair, table, or sofa that will not move. Depending on the child's age and reliability, it may be necessary for a family member to always remain with the child to prevent falling. Families living in multilevel homes may have to prepare a temporary bedroom for the child on the first floor. An old crib mattress or a few thick blankets

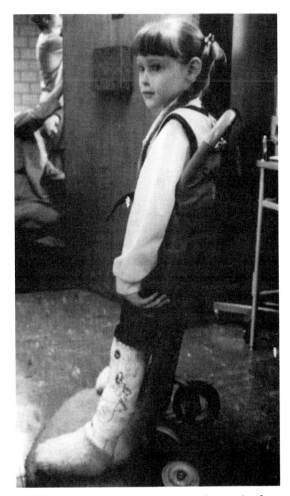

Figure 6.24 ■ A parent finds an imaginative and safe way of standing and moving the older child in a hip spica by adapting a commercially available hand truck.

on the floor can be comfortable. Care should be taken to avoid abrasion to the toes when the child is prone by allowing the feet to hang over the end of the mattress. Instruction should be given to family members for safe lifting and turning of the child using good body mechanics while also considering the alignment of the child. Even plans to get the child home from the hospital and through the front door of the house may be a chore.

Regardless of the age of the child in a spica cast, daily exercise periods are important to prevent loss of neck and trunk strength and to maintain the automatic balance responses that will be important when the cast is removed and the child resumes his or her daily activities. Several times each day the child should perform a routine of exercises with a family member for 15 to 20 minutes that includes prone lifts for neck and back extensors, supine head lifting and partial sit-ups for neck and trunk flexors, and standing with tilting in all directions. As the child attempts these activities, muscles are contracting within the cast as well as those muscles above the cast level. These activities place stress on the bones of the lower extremities, thereby reducing bone demineralization and, possibly, the risk of a fracture when the cast is removed. Postural insecurity will also be reduced as vestibular and proprioceptive stimulation are provided by these challenging antigravity activities (Fig. 6.25). Families should be warned to avoid having the child propped in a half-sitting position for long periods of time that will cause pressure at the bony prominences as mentioned earlier and can contribute to a kyphotic upper back.

In some institutions, the child is admitted for a brief period of intensive therapy once the cast is removed. But whether therapy is provided as an inpatient or outpatient, the goal should be to ensure the child's rapid return to function following cast removal. Lower extremity ROM and strength, especially at the surgical site, are the immediate concerns, along with improvement in balance and equilibrium responses of the neck and upper body. A return to former function can be achieved in a short period of time if the therapist targets all of the child's needs, not only the lower extremity range of motion.

If the child has a high-level lesion, surgery might have been performed to gain passive flexibility for better limb alignment and brace fit. For this child, a review of ROM exercises with the parents, an orthotic evaluation, and a review of activities to further improve upper body control may be all that is needed after cast removal. The child may then be monitored, until adequate function is achieved, through an outpatient clinic, community facility, or school-based physical therapy program.[38]

The child with a high-level lesion who demonstrates a significant loss of motion at the hip or knee is at risk for fracture. A brief hospitalization may be indicated to regain lost mobility. The child may also be sent home in a bivalved cast to be worn most of the time and removed for a program of frequent ROM exercises and sedentary activities until range is regained, if the family is able to comply.

Some children are immobilized in their HKAFOs instead of a cast following soft tissue lengthening or tendon excision to allow parents to gently range the legs and stand their child during the healing process. Procedures to relocate or stabilize the hip joint in children with L-4 to L-5 lesions include simple tendon lengthening, femoral or pelvic osteotomy, or the more complex Lindseth procedure, which involves a muscle transfer of the external obliques. Candidates for this procedure are those children with the potential for unassisted gait and an intact CNS. Admission to the hospital after cast removal following a Lindseth procedure may be necessary to ensure that joint mobility and balance skills are again safe and acceptable, and that the child is working toward ambulation without an assistive device. Concentration on trunk strengthening activities helps the transferred muscles regain their role of stabilizing the trunk and pelvis and eliminating the excessive lateral trunk flexion seen prior to surgery when the child walked unaided.

Reduced mobility in the lumbar spine and the lower extremities is common after a longer casting period. After cast removal it is often difficult for the child to achieve 90 degrees of flexion at the hips for good sitting alignment because of adapted shortening of the hamstrings and hip extensors. Hip and low back tightness causes the pelvis to be rocked posteriorly, with a secondary thoracic kyphosis that requires remediation. Gentle activities are

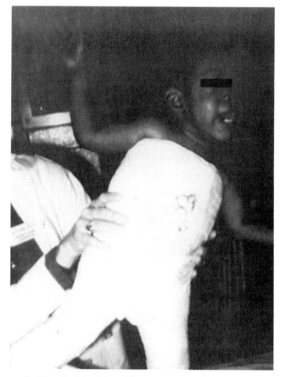

Figure 6.25 ■ *Child with a hip spica cast after hip reduction surgery. Note how the child is both standing and being tilted. Standing, when the surgeon approves, about 10 days after surgery, is one aspect of the home care program.*

indicated to increase pelvic and hip mobility and strength. Active thoracic extension with active hip flexion and use of abdominal muscles will help the child attain and hold a 90-degree alignment. It is safer to help the child work on actively holding a more erect sitting position than to only move the limbs passively and possibly push too hard on a fragile bone. Care should also be taken to avoid allowing the child to sit with this rounded posture for extended periods of time.

Parents should also be warned to initially prohibit their child from crawling after a spica cast is removed. Crawling requires hip and knee flexion exceeding 90 degrees. Hip rotation is also required as the child moves into and out of sitting and the four-point position. If the necessary flexibility is not present for these motions when the cast is removed, fractures can occur.[38]

Following surgery at the knee or ankle, children will have either one or two long or short leg casts and the family will require instructions to avoid excessive time in supine or sitting for these children as well. Besides contributing to skin breakdown, development of flexion contractures is always a major concern. Excessive sitting, crawling, and knee walking with short leg casts will increase tightness of the hip and knee flexors. Information regarding alternative positions should be offered to avoid positions that encourage flexion. Prone lying is the preferred position, with standing and ambulation the preferred activities, when feasible. Ambulation in the cast(s) is achieved quickly when a walker, rather than crutches, is used as an assistive device for this temporary period. Crutch training is difficult for a young child due to the additional weight of the cast, potential lack of adequate balance, poor proprioception, and possibly malaligned casts. By comparison, instruction with a walker is usually a faster and safer choice. Strengthening exercises can be taught for back, hip, and knee extensors, along with exercises for the trunk to help keep the child mobile during the casting period. With such a multifaceted program, the child will be more likely to rapidly return to the previous or an improved level of function, once the cast is removed.[14,24,53,111–115]

Central Nervous System Deterioration

Throughout life, individuals with spina bifida, their family members, and the clinicians involved with their care should be vigilant for any deterioration in function that could indicate hydromyelia or a tethered spinal cord. These neurologic conditions can affect the patient's mobility and gross motor function, urologic function, fine motor skills, and activities of daily living (ADLs). If diagnosed and treated in a timely fashion, the effects can be temporary. If left untreated, the symptoms can worsen and their effects will be permanent. Therapists must be knowledgeable about these problems because they are often discovered by the clinician during routine appointments, evaluations, manual muscle testing, or conversations with parents.[14,24,53]

HYDROMYELIA

Hall et al. conducted a study of patients with spina bifida who exhibited rapidly progressive scoliosis and found that CSF had migrated into the spinal cord.[116] Excess CSF was seen collecting in pockets down the spinal cord that created areas of pressure and necrosis of the surrounding peripheral nerves, causing the scoliosis. Other symptoms found to be associated with hydromyelia include progressive upper extremity weakness and hypertonus. One point to note: Initial examination of the lateral ventricles showed no enlargement and did not indicate that the shunt was malfunctioning. However, revision of the VP shunt produced improvement in the symptoms for those children in which the diagnosis was made in a timely fashion.

Some children required a shunt placed at the level of the fluid pockets in the spine to ensure that the excess CSF and its accompanying pressure would be completely eliminated. Lindseth, though an orthopedic surgeon, is a strong advocate for close investigation in all cases of rapidly progressive scoliosis. He states that it is important to always consider the possibility of CNS complications and not treat scoliosis as a purely musculoskeletal phenomenon. Left untreated, the fluid continues to collect along the spinal cord causing continued deterioration in both upper and lower extremity function.[14,24,53,116,117]

TETHERED SPINAL CORD

At approximately 10 weeks' gestation, the vertebral column and spinal cord of the fetus are the same length and the spinal nerves exit horizontally at their corresponding vertebrae. By 5 months' gestation, the vertebral column has grown more rapidly than the spinal cord, which now ends at S-1. At birth, the cord is at L-3, and by adulthood, the cord is at the L-1 to L-2 vertebral level.

A tethered spinal cord occurs when adhesions anchor the spinal cord at the site of the original back lesion. The child is growing rapidly, but the cord is not free to slide upward and reposition as it should, instead remaining bound at the level of the back defect. Excessive stretch to the spinal cord causes metabolic changes and ischemia of the neural tissue, with associated degeneration in muscle function. Rapidly progressive scoliosis, hypertonus at one or several sites in the lower extremities, changes in gait pattern, and changes in urologic function may be attributed to this tethering of the spinal cord. Occurrences of increased tone on passive ROM, asymmetric changes in manual muscle testing results, areas of decreasing strength, or discomfort in the back or buttocks should alert the examiner to consider the presence of a tethered cord.[117,118] Close periodic examination by professionals and alert parents can identify early functional changes associated with this complication so appropriate medical management can be considered (Display 6.8). Petersen suggests, based on his study population, that those children with repaired lesions at levels above L-3 will begin to exhibit symptoms of a tethered cord before age 6 and those with lesion levels below L-4 tend to become symptomatic after age 6. He also found that children with unrepaired back defects exhibit symptoms much earlier, regardless of the location of their lesion level.[119] When tethering is suspected, myelography may be utilized to confirm the diagnosis and subsequent neurosurgical release can free the cord. After release, the cord may not migrate to its appropriate position, but further growth of the child may proceed without recurrence of the symptoms or further degeneration in function. If the release is performed in a timely manner, permanent neurologic damage can usually be prevented. However, it is becoming clear that total correction of all the symptoms following surgery cannot be assumed.[53] McClone et al. conducted a study of 30 children who exhibited scoliosis as a symptom of cord tethering and who received surgical intervention to release the spinal cord. The children who exhibited the greatest improvement of their scoliosis were those who had spinal curves of less than 50 degrees. During a 2- to 7-year follow-up, 38% of the children began to show progression of their curves owing to the spine retethering, but the remaining children showed a stabilized or improved spinal alignment.[120]

The child who has a thoracic-level paralysis does not have the full complement of active trunk musculature to provide adequate antigravity strength to maintain an erect posture and is always at risk for scoliosis. However, a child with a lumbar or sacral lesion with full innervation of trunk musculature should be evaluated when any curvature develops, especially when it develops over a short period of time. Hydromyelia and tethered cord should always be suspected if scoliosis occurs in a child with a motor level below T-12. Clinics that aggressively treat hydromyelia and tethered cord by surgical correction report a reduction in the overall occurrence of scoliosis that will require spinal fusion.[121–125]

SCOLIOSIS

The development of a spinal deformity is serious for the child with spina bifida. When scoliosis occurs and trunk alignment is compromised, the child will require additional support to remain erect in upright postures. If the child leans on his or her upper extremities to stay up, this compensation directly impacts the child's freedom of movement and increases the energy expense for all activities. Propelling a wheelchair becomes more strenuous, as the child must work both to maintain the upright posture as well as to move the chair. In sitting, a moderate to severe scoliosis creates pelvic obliquity that changes the surface area for weight bearing causing areas of increased pressure that can quickly lead to skin breakdown. The posterior aspects of the thighs and bony prominences of the ischial tuberosity, greater trochanter, sacrum, and coccyx are especially vulnerable.

Gait can become more unstable as truncal alignment and balance are affected by a spinal deformity. Pelvic and trunk asymmetry will affect the fit of the HKAFO and RGO bracing. When braces do not fit and gait is made more difficult, the orthotics may not be worn as frequently as they should. This can lead to further deterioration of the child's mobility skills.

The use of spinal braces or body jackets can be useful for the child without trunk stability or to assist in slowing the progression of the curve, but surgical fusion is inevitable for many children. There are numerous methods for and preferred approaches to spinal fusion, and the periods of immobility and restrictions on daily activity vary with each. The type of instrumentation employed and the area and extent of the fusion will also influence the child's functional parameters.

If the fusion extends to the sacrum, pelvic mobility will diminish and ambulatory ability will be directly affected. Gait analysis has shown greater excursion of movement at the pelvis in ambulatory children with spina bifida than in typical children. Given this information, surgeons have been reluctant to fuse down to the sacral area of an ambulatory child if this can be avoided. Upper extremity and trunk movement are also necessary for successful and efficient wheelchair propulsion. If flexibility of the distal spine is diminished or absent, an individual can lose his or her independent mobility in a wheelchair, and this should also be a consideration when surgery is planned.

Maintaining flexibility and strength in all extremities and preventing skin problems during the period of immobility should be addressed immediately after surgery. When a return to full activity is permitted, it is important to reassess

---

►► DISPLAY 6.8

Clinical Findings That May Lead to Diagnosis of Tethered Cord

Spasticity in muscles with sacral nerve roots

Increased tone in legs with resistance to passive range of motion

Sudden increase in lumbar lordosis

Back or buttock pain

Development of scoliosis at a young age

Rapidly progressing scoliosis

Scoliosis above level of paralysis

Change in urologic function

Change in gait pattern

Progressive weakening in leg musculature

the patient to determine whether functional skills have been lost. The physical therapist should be concerned with the patient's postoperative activity level and assist with resumption of mobility. Spinal fusion may influence the performance of many ADLs, so adaptive strategies may also need to be developed.[14,24,53]

 ## Latex Allergy

Allergic reaction to latex by individuals with spina bifida has become a relatively recent concern. Latex is a natural rubber used in a wide variety of products that come into contact with human skin and other body surfaces. In the health field, a vast number of commonly used items contain or are made exclusively from latex. Latex has been depended on for its impermeable qualities and strength while still providing sensitivity to touch. This makes it an excellent material for use in sterile gloves, where it provides protection and prevents the spread of illness. It is durable as well as elastic, which accounts for its popularity and wide usage for various types of flexible tubing and in the toy industry (Display 6.9).

>> ## DISPLAY 6.9

Partial List of Commonly Used Products Containing Latex

Balloons
Pacifiers
Chewing gum
Dental dam
Rubber bands
Elastic in clothing
Beach toys
Koosh balls
Some types of disposable diapers
Glue
Paints
Erasers
Some brands of adhesive bandages
Bulb syringes
Ready-to-use enemas
Ostomy pouches
Oxygen masks
Pulse oximeters
Reflex hammers
Stethoscope tubing
Suction tubing
Vascular stockings
Crutch axillary pads, tips, and hand grips
Kitchen cleaning gloves
Swim goggles
Wheelchair tires
Some wheelchair cushions
Zippered food storage bags

Although it is believed that only 1% of the general population is allergic to latex, the results of various studies point out that 18% to 37% of patients with spina bifida exhibit a significant sensitivity to latex. It was also found that 7% to 10% of health care workers exhibit a latex sensitivity. Allergic reactions may appear as watery and itchy eyes, sneezing, coughing, hives, and a rash in the area of contact. More serious reactions may produce swelling of the trachea, and changes in blood pressure and circulation, resulting in anaphylactic shock. Diagnosis of latex sensitivity is based on a clinical history, observation of a reaction, and immunologic findings following a skin prick allergy test. The cause, to date, is not known, but it is theorized that early, intense, and consistent exposure to latex products results in the development of the sensitivity in many individuals. Some of the more severe symptoms were believed to be a result of inhalation of the powder contained in most sterile latex gloves. The powder makes the gloves easy to don and doff, and it can become airborne upon removal of the gloves. However, further investigation found this was not a consistent irritant.

The Food and Drug Administration and the Centers for Disease Control and Prevention continue to investigate the problem and support efforts to find the components of latex that are responsible for the allergy, develop methods of producing safe nonallergenic rubber, and conspicuously label products that have a latex content. There has been evidence that the latex allergy is also related to sensitivity to bananas, chestnuts, avocados, and kiwi fruit in some patients and this relationship is also being investigated. A blood test has been developed that is being used during pre-employment testing for health care workers and for patients with spina bifida.

It is thought that children with spina bifida develop a latex allergy because of their high level of exposure to materials containing latex right from birth. One study points out that the presence of spina bifida should be considered a risk factor for a latex allergy.[126] One method employed to prevent latex sensitivity is to practice primary prevention right from the first day of life and create a latex-free environment for the children. In one study employing this strategy for 6 years, the percentage of sensitive children dropped from 26.7% to 4.5%.[127]

Valuable information regarding patient safety and education was obtained from ELASTIC (Education for Latex Allergy/Support Team Information Coalition). They recommend that parents, older patients, or their caregivers carry an auto-injectable type of epinephrine that is easy to use, in case a patient experiences a serious allergic reaction.

All sensitive individuals should wear a Medic Alert bracelet, necklace, or dog tags. Neighborhood paramedic teams, the fire department, and local Emergency Medical Services who might respond to an emergency call should be alerted to the patient's sensitivities. Keeping a set of nonlatex gloves near the front door for use by emergency personnel is also encouraged. Families and patients are encouraged to also become familiar with products that must be avoided. A complete list of latex products and alternative nonlatex products is available from the Spina Bifida Association of America. Refer to the end of this chapter for sources of latex information and latex-free products, and resources.[128–136]

Perceptual Motor and Cognitive Performance

The population of children with spina bifida represents a group of children that are diverse across many domains. Their strengths and limitations are varied, and besides the motor and CNS problems that have already been discussed throughout this chapter, therapists should be aware of possible difficulties that may affect the learning styles and cognitive potential of their patients. This section provides only a brief overview of the vast amount of information that is available regarding perceptual and cognitive performance with this group.

Great interest and concern has been expressed regarding the intellectual, sensory, and perceptual motor function of children with spina bifida. Studies have shown that the overall intelligence of the population is unrelated to motor level, severity of hydrocephalus prior to shunt insertion, or the number of shunt revisions. The factors that do influence cognition include untimely treatment of hydrocephalus, episodes of cerebral infection, and the presence of other CNS abnormalities.[48–50]

Intelligence testing for children with spina bifida places them within the normal range for most tests but below the population mean. Willis and associates found the test scores of their subjects to be particularly low in performance IQ, arithmetic achievement, and visual motor integration.[137] When the same children were retested at an older age, their arithmetic achievement and visual motor integration scores declined even further, but reading and spelling abilities did not decline. One conclusion of this study was that a visual–perceptual–organizational deficit was found that influenced the child's ability to solve mathematic and visual–spatial problems.[138] These deficits then become relatively more severe as the child ages when greater accomplishment in math is expected. If early foundation skills are not strong, the development of more advanced, intuitive math processes is limited. Test scoring reflects the expectation that acquisition of skills will increase with age and therefore the results declined in the group that was studied.

Other research has noted a high degree of attention deficit or distractibility in some children with spina bifida; these problems were especially profound in children who showed poor language development. These same children had poor development of auditory figure-ground, which allows a child to recognize and attend to relevant features in the auditory environment. A child with difficulty in this area may not be able to identify the primary auditory input such as a teacher speaking and giving directions, nor can the child dismiss the irrelevant input such as noise from a truck passing by an open window. Therefore, in a rich auditory environment, extraneous sounds easily distract the child from his or her assigned task. These children may perform better in a quiet, secluded testing situation, but classroom performance for similar tasks can be poor.

Horn et al. found limited development of language comprehension in many of the children tested.[138] Individual vocabulary comprehension was normal, but comprehension of a story was poor. The children had difficulty identifying and retaining the relevant features of a story while ignoring the unimportant facts. Difficulty learning and memorizing lists of unrelated words has also been noted. However, memory for related facts was better, such as when answering questions about a short story that was recently read aloud.[138–140]

In all the studies that are cited, little information was available regarding the early medical treatment of the subjects. Methods and timeliness of intervention for hydrocephalus, possible ventricular infections, or other complications were not delineated. Additional factors that might have influenced sensorimotor learning and testing outcome, including level of mobility and sensation in the trunk and lower extremity, were not mentioned. Therefore, it is difficult to hypothesize which factors may have been responsible for the problems. Decreased opportunity to develop manual skills has been thought to be a factor.[139] Other negative influences on the learning processes might be the limitations of early mobility that affect the child's experiences: exploring the environment, moving his or her body relative to stationary objects, and manipulating and moving those objects. Theoretical rationales for dysfunction include potential cerebellar damage from the Chiari II malformation that would influence the range, direction, force, and rate of voluntary movements of the body and the manner in which movement is interpreted. But, regardless of the cause, the learning difficulties that result are important to note as they will affect many aspects of the child's function and may be a limiting factor for the child's ultimate successes in school and throughout life.

Any discussion of perceptual problems in the spina bifida population should also address issues with ocular function. When compared to the typical population, strabismus occurs six to eight times more frequently in children with spina bifida. The lack of conjugate gaze influences spatial relationships, constancy of size, and development of normal visual perception. Visual–spatial problems during manipulation activities have been noted in some children with spina bifida. Other, more frequent ocular problems include nystagmus, poor ocular motility, and other convergence defects. These abnormalities have been attributed to brainstem dysfunction, although there has been no correlation of the severity of the Chiari II malformation with these ocular defects.[141–143]

The consensus seems to be that children with spina bifida need a broad range of movement and learning experiences during their early years. Increased experiences in many areas may help to decrease the impact of any specific limitation. Testing with age-appropriate materials and in an environment where the child can focus on the task is critically important. Also, eliminating test items that include a motor component may afford a more accurate and valid result (Fig. 6.26).[137–145]

Wheelchair Mobility

Much of this chapter has been devoted to bracing and preparing the child for ambulation, but some type of seated mobility must also be considered for the children for whom this is appropriate and necessary. Any decision to use one of the many devices that are available should include input from the patient when it is appropriate, family members, and the professional staff involved with the child. A discussion might first determine the need for and proposed uses of seated mobility. Questions to consider might be, Is the device for recreation and peer group interaction, for indoor and/or outdoor use, for use at school or preschool, for long family outings, or primarily for family convenience and transport?

A first device might be a hand-propelled caster cart or "star car" ordered through a medical supply company or often found in a local toy store. Many commercially available electric cars or motorcycles can be modified with a hand switch rather than the usual foot pedal. These devices are inexpensive and low to the ground, facilitating easy transition to the floor or to a standing position. They are cosmetically appealing and are acceptable to both disabled and typical children alike. They can be fast and safe when used in the proper environment, and they provide beneficial stimulation and opportunities for recreation and socialization. The child's perceptual skills, upper extremity abilities, and the presence of abnormal tone can guide the therapist in selecting whether the manual or battery-operated device is more appropriate. Excessive upper extremity exertion to propel and maneuver a device may frustrate the child and produce unacceptable changes in tone if CNS dysfunction is present. One study of interest examined young children with otherwise poor independent mobility skills who received instruction in using a motorized wheelchair. Most of the children did very well and the benefits that were noted included increased curiosity, initiative, motivation, communication, exploration, and interaction with objects in the environment. There were also significant decreases in dependency and in demanding and hostile behaviors.[146]

Families that require a wheelchair so their child can be included on trips out-of-doors can use a stroller until the child is 5 or 6 years of age. Strollers are available in larger sizes, and can be used in combination with ambulation. It is not unusual for a typical child of that age to alternate walking and riding in a stroller for periods of time during a long family outing, but care must be taken not to increase the child's dependency on others for mobility as he or she gets older. Some seated mobility is helpful for the child who is not ready to ambulate all day in school because of limitations in balance or endurance. It is helpful to know which strollers, travel chairs, or wheelchairs can be safely secured on a bus and what the local regulations are for appropriate school transport (Fig. 6.27). A standard wheelchair can be obtained prior to the child starting school if boarding, exiting, and safe transportation on the school bus is an issue. Other indications for a wheelchair might include the child's lack of efficient community mobility, marginally functional or unsafe ambulation, speed of ambulation that is inadequate to maintain a level consistent with peers and/or family, and the child's need for increased recreational activities that would be unavailable with ambulation. The child who is ambulatory but small in size and weight

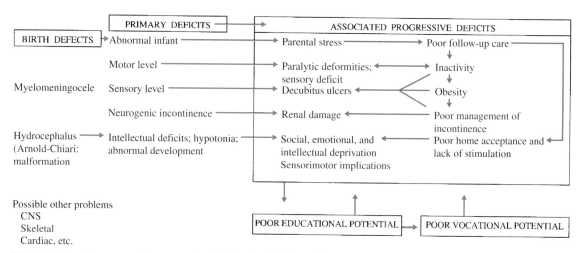

Figure 6.26 ■ *Primary and progressive deficits in children with spina bifida. (Adapted from Syllabus of Instructional Courses, American Academy for Cerebral Palsy, 1974.)*

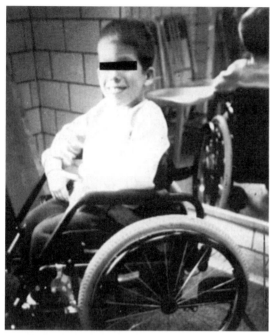

Figure 6.27 ▪ A lightweight wheelchair is selected for long-distance use in the school and community. This child also uses a reciprocating gait orthosis for shorter distances in the home and school.

can be carried onto the bus and secured in a car seat or a regular bus seat with a safety belt and/or harness. The child would then be required to ambulate upon arrival at school.

The therapist should remember the increased risks for the child in a wheelchair. Scheduling time to use the chair and time out of the chair should be considered. The chance of abandonment of a gait program by a child who may have the potential of reaching a high level of efficient ambulation is always a risk when introducing wheelchair use. Flexion contractures of the hips and knees, skin and pressure problems, and spinal deformity are other issues common to the seated child that will impact the potential for gait.[115] Therefore, the child should spend time both out of the wheelchair and out of the seated position every day. Prone positioning, standing at a standing table or in a prone or supine stander with bracing, and exercise periods of ambulation are options that should be made available to the child.

As the child matures and mobility needs change, a power wheelchair or electric scooter can provide added speed and efficiency. A motorized device, which will conserve energy, may be very important for the individual facing a long and hectic day at school or work. In some instances the device may remain at school if the demands for gait are the greatest at that location. Accessibility issues may prevent a powered device from going home as well. In the area of wheeled mobility, as in many other aspects of care, the skills, imagination, and problem-solving abilities of the therapist can be extremely helpful to the individual with

spina bifida and his or her family. Developing trusting relationships with dependable vendors and equipment representatives will enable the therapist to remain current in the latest devices that are available, and therefore the child's life will be enhanced.

Adding a wheelchair cushion should also be included for the individual with spina bifida. Various wheelchair cushions may prevent or reduce the development of pressure sores. Several materials are available, including high-density foam and inflatable types, which can be modified for more even weight distribution when the child exhibits asymmetry. But, regardless of the cushion chosen, activities for pressure relief are still the best means of preventing skin breakdown on the posterior thighs and buttocks and should be performed diligently throughout the day. Frequent wheelchair push-ups, side-to-side weight shifting, and out-of-chair time should be incorporated into the child's daily schedule to provide for regular pressure relief. Also, many methods should be explored that will assist the child to become independent in performing these important activities including the use of a wristwatch alarm, talking clock, or beeper.[53,147,148]

 ## Recreation and Leisure Activities: Aquatics

As the child reaches school age, the time available for extended periods of play and movement on the floor is greatly reduced. Generally speaking, a full-time academic curriculum in an integrated or regular education setting provides little chance for consistent recreation. Gym class with an instructor who is imaginative and motivated and willing to collaborate with a physical therapist is the ideal. Strategies can be developed to include the student with spina bifida into the regular array of activities the rest of the class is performing. Giving the child the opportunity to participate in the regular physical education curriculum, with adaptations or accommodations, may assist the child to find activities in which he or she is able to participate and those which he or she might also enjoy when out of school. It should never be assumed that the child with spina bifida enrolled in a regular educational program will be excused from physical education or not be expected to participate in at least some portion of the activities and skills expected of the typical group of students. The physical therapist can collaborate with the physical education teacher to develop a modified grading system as well.

The child enrolled in special education may have periods of physical education as well as additional sessions scheduled into the school day for the development of recreation and leisure skills as part of his or her educational curriculum. Once again, having an innovative and motivated staff will help to expose the child to many experiences that he or she might otherwise have no exposure to and that may become a lifelong hobby or interest.

But, as is true with the population of typical children, children with spina bifida are dependent on the knowledge and resources of family and friends to provide them with experiences in new, novel, and consistent recreational pursuits after the school day ends. Identifying activities that can be learned and pursued throughout one's life should be considered an important part of the total care plan for the individual with spina bifida. The physical therapist has a valuable role in assisting the patient and his or her family to find appropriate programs that offer wheelchair games and sports or adaptive programs for the child who is ambulatory, such as "T-ball" instead of traditional little league baseball. There are also increasing numbers of special needs teams being formed each season throughout the country, to which the child and family can be referred. The child with spina bifida should be encouraged to regularly participate in activities that provide an appropriate cardiovascular challenge, muscle strengthening, improved eye–hand coordination, wheelchair maneuvering skills, and sportsmanship from which all children can benefit. It is not uncommon for the therapist to be asked for an opinion or a recommendation regarding adapted bicycles and other home exercise or recreation equipment. Helping to keep the child active, by providing professional advice, is an important contribution.

The inclusion and expansion of aquatics within the physical therapy profession has resulted in a significant increase in the body of research and information available for the therapist who has the opportunity to add aquatics to his or her clinical repertoire. The interest in health and fitness within the general population has resulted in the building of many more pools that are handicapped accessible and available for both recreation and therapeutic purposes. Providing opportunities to explore and enjoy the benefits of moving in water may assist the child with spina bifida to participate in this recreational activity that is also physically beneficial. Learning water safety and basic swimming skills can be taught to the young child and utilized throughout his or her lifetime. Water competency with or without the use of flotation devices can enable the person with spina bifida to experience a level of independent freedom of movement otherwise unavailable on land. More advanced aquatic skills can also be incorporated into a multifaceted therapeutic program that can be designed for the individual, taught and monitored by the physical therapist who has access to a pool facility. By utilizing the natural properties of resistance and buoyancy of the water, strengthening of the body, increasing cardiovascular efficiency, and fun can result.

This therapist has found that providing physical therapy sessions in the pool can also be a useful tool in the rehabilitation program of the child following orthopedic surgery. Children who are already comfortable in the water are easily motivated to work hard in an exercise program with the excitement and novelty of this environment. Mobilizing a child who has been in a cast or in bed recovering from surgery has been achieved more rapidly in the water. Brief free swim periods can be the rest time that is given in between therapeutic activities or they can be the reward for a child who did a good job. When working on a mat program in therapy, taking a rest break usually means the patient is not moving, but the child will continue to move when in the water. Lap swims, races, and in-pool team games such as underwater search and retrieve, basketball, volleyball, or tag are just a few of the many possibilities that will have the child moving significantly more than he or she would in a traditional therapy session. But, as in all merging of recreation and therapy, the therapist must not compromise the child's goals that must be addressed just to have the child happy and playing. Specific exercise routines should be developed, as they would be for a mat program, so intervention is truly targeting the appropriate areas (Display 6.10).

 ## The Adult with Spina Bifida

Our concerns regarding the population with spina bifida should not end when the patient moves to an adult facility for his or her medical care. Being aware of the problems that

---

>> **DISPLAY 6.10**

Examples of Therapeutic Strategies That Can Be Utilized in a Pool Setting

Provides strengthening to innervated lower extremity musculature, upper extremities, and trunk:

1. Movement of legs in all directions, all planes, with combination patterns of movement not feasible on a two-dimensional gym mat. Can be passive range of motion, active, active assistive, and resistive, depending on need
2. Use of flotation device in deep water with legs in the water, kicking in place against water's resistance
3. Pushing off from side of pool or therapist's hands while prone or supine on water surface to strengthen extension musculature and enjoy the sudden propulsion through the water
4. Swimming laps with only leg motions while holding kick board or in an inner tube if necessary
5. Lap swims using webbed gloves for added propulsion and resistance and a variety of strokes to address all muscles of shoulders (flotation cuffs can be used around ankles if necessary to prevent legs from dragging on pool floor and provide extension if active gluteal musculature is not present)
6. Resistive swimming with therapist holding legs and preventing forward movement prone or supine
7. Supine, within flotation ring, lifting legs out of water and twisting them side to side for work on all abdominals
8. Ball toss and catch, basketball, newcomb, or volleyball in various water depths depending on children's ages and abilities

adults with spina bifida face is also helpful for the clinician specializing in pediatrics. By being knowledgeable about the aging process and its effect on patients with this disability, the therapist can gain a perspective that will influence the care provided to the younger patient. Understanding the long-term effects of surgical and therapeutic decisions and interventions can provide insight and can help improve the approach to care by modifying existing management protocols utilized with the pediatric patient.[149]

Selber and Dias looked at a population of young adults with sacral-level spina bifida who had been followed at the same medical clinic and by the same staff since they were young children. They were treated aggressively for any symptoms of tethered cord or lower limb deformity. There were several complications that many of these individuals shared, including episodes of osteomyelitis, scoliosis, amputations, and a decrease in ambulation function. Most of the group maintained their community ambulation status but some experienced significant knee pain and returned to using orthotics and crutches to stabilize their gait and reduce joint stress.[150]

In a study conducted through Riley Children's Hospital in Indiana, the parents of adolescents with spina bifida voiced concerns that centered on lifelong issues affecting their children, such as accessibility, transportation in the community, and independence. The teens were more concerned with their immediate needs of finances, medical issues, communication and socialization with friends, and peer acceptance. The study concluded that coordinated programs for the adolescent and young adult are important to help transition the individuals into independent adults. Based on their findings, attention should be given to social integration, vocational training, and sexual counseling.[151]

In a study of patients with spina bifida, Dias et al. found that 80% of their subjects lived with their parents or other relatives.[152] Half of those individuals were older than 30 years of age. Eighty-two percent had achieved some level of independence, whereas 6% were totally dependent. Seventeen patients had married and were living away from family members. Interestingly, the individual's degree of independence was not related to their lesion level or the level of ambulation they had achieved.[152]

Dunne and Shurtleff identified some common complaints from adults with spina bifida that included obesity, incontinence, recurrent urinary tract infections, chronic decubiti, joint pain, hypertension, neurologic deterioration, and depression.[153] Urinary incontinence was a central issue in a self-rating survey completed by a group of adolescent boys and girls with spina bifida.

In general, the girls rated themselves lower in physical appearance, athleticism, and global self-worth than the boys. But both the girls and the boys who were continent rated themselves higher than the children who were incontinent. It appeared from this study that urinary continence was more important than gait for many of these young adults.[154]

Urinary tract infection is the most frequently reported cause of morbidity in the adult population. Patients are also concerned with urinary incontinence, and a variety of methods are employed to try and keep this population dry and infection free. Urinary diversion, a surgical procedure resulting in urine emptying from a stoma in the abdomen into a collecting bag, was a preferred solution for many patients who did not want to wear diapers or perform intermittent catheterization. But if residual urine remains in the bladder, with this approach it becomes a reservoir for bacteria, resulting in a high rate of infection and potential renal damage. Regardless of this fact, many patients preferred the diversion to other forms of bladder management. An indwelling Foley catheter was used for some patients but resulted in a high rate of infection. Other external collecting devices, Valsalva voiding, and diapers were methods commonly tried as well and with varying results. It appears that intermittent catheterization performed diligently and on schedule remains the most successful method for adult management of urinary incontinence and was also associated with the lowest risk of infection or renal damage.[155,156] McClone cited still other problem areas affecting the adult with spina bifida including lack of job training, lack of viable employment, and the desire to achieve psychological and physical independence from family.[157]

In two studies, when multifaceted neuropsychological testing was performed on young adults with spina bifida, with and without hydrocephalus, the subjects scored low in areas of verbal learning, verbal recall, and sequencing of complex tasks and exhibited a high rate of attention deficit. It appeared that the subjects were performing in the average range for delayed memory, spatial memory, and visual recognition memory. Almost 50% of the subjects with hydrocephalus in one of the studies exhibited some type of impairment even though their full IQ fell within the normal range.[158,159]

It appears clear that the adult population has multiple and varied needs in many areas of concern that may best be met by a comprehensive multidisciplinary team approach that can efficiently test, identify, and address their issues and make referrals to specialists as indicated, similar to the approach with the pediatric population.

SUMMARY

There are many approaches for the physical therapist to consider when treating children with spina bifida. Often the role the therapist defines when providing care is determined by the venue. The disability is a complex one that requires an understanding of the many systems that are affected. The information presented in this chapter provides a background for a better understanding of this birth defect. Depending on the setting in which the physical therapist is employed, certain sections of the chapter may be more or less relevant than others. Concerns and strategies for intervention suggested throughout this chapter reflect a general philosophy that physical therapists must be knowledgeable about the neurologic, orthopedic, and developmental issues common to spina bifida and the trends and protocols being applied to their care. The therapist should also always be sensitive to the concerns of the other professionals treating the child and to the families. The true challenge to the physical therapist is to integrate these various perspectives into a creative treatment plan that produces the best result for each child. Beginning with a strong basis in anatomy and neurology combined with experimentation and exploration, the therapist will discover new ideas for treatment that will advance the clinician to a more sophisticated manner of intervention and, more importantly, help the child progress to his or her most productive and functional ability.

CASE STUDY

Crystal, 9 years old

SIGNIFICANT HISTORY

Crystal's back was closed when she was 3 days old and a VP shunt was inserted to control hydrocephalus at 12 days. She was discharged home and had no further complications. She lives with her grandparents and a younger brother. She attended an early intervention program from 3 to 5 years of age where she received occupational therapy, physical therapy, and speech services. Crystal entered school 3 years ago and came in her personal manual wheelchair, with no bracing. She has had only one shunt revision.

PRESENT FINDINGS

She has moderate limitations in expressive and receptive language and cognition. She is in a full-time special education classroom for children with similar learning difficulties. She is the only student in the class with a physical disability. Her gross and fine motor skills are her strength.

GROSS MOTOR SKILLS

She is able to transfer from her wheelchair to a desk chair and back with close supervision for safety. She is impulsive and can forget to lock her chair or may be careless moving her legs. Crystal is able to propel her chair well and steer it without assistance in multiple environments.

PASSIVE RANGE OF MOTION

Passive range of motion is full in both legs except for her knees, where she lacked 40-degree extension (R) and 20-degree extension (L). Last year she had hamstring releases and was in bilateral long leg casts for 6 weeks. When the casts were removed, she remained with a 15-degree knee flexion contracture on the right but the left knee extended to neutral.

UPRIGHT MOBILITY

She was fitted with an HKAFO, butterfly pelvic band to maintain hip extension, and drop locks on the hips and knees. The ankles are solid and set at 90 degrees. She was taught to perform a hop-to pattern with all joints locked, using a posterior walker. Her grandparents were instructed in brace use at the local children's hospital where she receives her medical care. For 1 year she has been coming to school with her braces and sneakers in a bag to be donned in school for ambulation training. Multiple calls to her family have produced no change in this routine. She is not in her braces at home either in the evenings or on the weekends. Crystal's grandmother expresses that donning the brace in the morning is difficult for her. It is not reasonable to request that the classroom staff place her in her braces. The school nurse was willing to doff and don them for Crystal's AM and PM catheterization, but she is resentful of the responsibility to put Crystal in her braces each day.

Crystal receives a weekly physical therapy session in school and her program consists of gait training/practice walking and a strengthening program for her trunk and upper extremities. She is consistently able to ambulate with close guarding for a distance of approximately 500 yards before becoming tired. She likes to walk to the school nurse for a visit before returning to her class. Crystal's greatest difficulty is her right knee flexion contracture causing that leg to be relatively shorter than the left. This creates instability when she is upright because her weight bearing is predominantly on the left leg. She must overuse her arms for additional support.

MANUAL MUSCLE TESTING

She has the following bilateral active muscle function: fair hip flexion and adduction; poor knee extension; poor knee flexion; and trace ankle dorsiflexion.

ACTION TAKEN

A conference call was held between the school-based physical therapist, the physical therapist staffing the spina bifida clinic, and the clinic orthopedic surgeon. We decided to experiment and the pelvic band of the brace was removed. The orthotist also added a 2-inch wedged shoe lift under the right shoe to compensate for her knee flexion and to equalize the leg lengths, giving her a flat surface for standing on the right. Crystal's grandmother was brought into the clinic and again taught how to place Crystal in the braces, and she was instructed to have Crystal wear them daily. She expressed that the long leg braces were much easier for her to don. Additional information was given to alert her that Crystal is nearing adolescence, the time when she will be less likely to gain new upright skills unless her functional walking significantly improves. Crystal's grandmother left that appointment with renewed commitment.

RESULTS

Crystal is presently coming to school wearing her braces each day. She sits in class with both knees locked to stretch her knee flexors on the right and to prevent further tightening on the left. She is walking with the therapist each week, and standing has been added to her program. She is positioned upright by the classroom staff in a standing box for up to 1 hour each day. The staff also walks with her from her seat to the standing table and back. Because she has weak hip flexors, she is able to use a reciprocating pattern of leg movement without excessive use of her arms that would impact her endurance. She is able to maintain her trunk erect over her hips and does not flex forward. It is planned that the staff will expand her walking program and she will leave the classroom for longer distances, as they feel more comfortable.

The removal of the pelvic band has not impacted her speed, endurance, or pattern of movement in a negative way. She is an exercise ambulatory, and for weight control; leg, trunk, and arm strengthening; and cardiovascular function, this plan has been successful. If her walking skills improve and additional distances and time upright are feasible, they can be added to the sessions with the classroom staff. Also, continued efforts will be made to have someone walk her at home at least on the weekends and during extended holiday and summer vacations.

REFERENCES

1. Morrisey RT. Spina bifida: a new rehabilitation problem. Orthop Clin North Am 1978;9:379–389.
2. Myers GJ. Myelomeningocele: the medical aspects. Pediatr Clin North Am 1984;31:165–175.
3. Duff WE, Nutr M, Cooper ES. Neural tube defects in Jamaica following Hurricane Gilbert. Am J Public Health 1994;84(3):473–476.
4. Seller M. Risks in spina bifida: annotation. Dev Med Child Neurol 1994;36:1021–1025.
5. Share with women: folic acid—what's it all about. J Midwifery Womens Health 2003;48(5):365–366.
6. MMWR Editorial Note. Center for Disease Control and Prevention. 2004;53(17):362–365.
7. Ray JG, Meier C, Vermeulen MJ, et al. Association of neural tube defects and folic acid food fortification in Canada. Lancet 2002;360(9350):2047–2048.
8. Frey L, Hauser WA. Epidemiology of neural tube defects. Epilepsia 2003;44(Suppl 3):4–13.
9. Finnell RH, Gould A, Spiegelstein O. Pathobiology and genetics of neural tube defects. Epilepsia 2003;44(Suppl 3):14–23.
10. Dias MS, Partington M. Embryology of myelomeningocele and anencephaly. Neurosurg Focus 2004;16(2).
11. Lunsky AM, Ulcicus M, Rothman KJ, et al. Maternal heat exposure and neural tube defects. JAMA 1992;268:882–885.
12. McClone D. Neurosurgical management and operative closure for myelomeningocele. Presented at the Annual Myelomeningocele Seminar, Chicago, 1982.
13. Scarff TB, Fronczak S. Myelomeningocele: a review and update. Rehab Lit 1981;42:143–147.
14. Tachdjian MO. Pediatric Orthopedics. 2nd Ed. Vol 3. Philadelphia: WB Saunders, 1990:1773–1880.
15. Behrman RC, Vaughn VC, eds. Nelson's Textbook of Pediatrics. 11th Ed. Philadelphia: WB Saunders, 1979.
16. Wolraich M. The association of spina bifida occulta and myelomeningocele. Presented at the 2nd Symposium on Spina Bifida, Cincinnati, OH, 1984.
17. Fidas A, MacDonald HL, Elton RA, et al. Prevalence of spina bifida occulta in patients with functional disorders of the lower urinary tract and its relation to urodynamics and neurophysiological measurements. BMJ 1989;298:357–359.
18. Warder DE. Tethered Cord Syndrome and Occult Spinal Dysraphism American Association of Neurological Surgeons. Neurosurg Focus 2001;10(1).
19. Tubbs RS, Wellons III JC, Grabb PA, et al. Chiari II malformation and occult spinal dysraphism. Case reports and a review of the literature. Pediatr Neurosurg 2003;7:39(2):104–107.
20. D'Agasta SD, Banta JV, Gahm N. The fate of patients with lipomeningocele. Presented at the American Academy of Cerebral Palsy and Developmental Medicine (ACPDM), Boston, 1987.
21. Kanev PM, Lemire RJ, Loeser JD, et al. Management and long-term follow-up review of children with lipomyelomeningocele. J Neurosurg 1990;73:48–52.
22. Moore KL. The Developing Human: Clinically Oriented Embryology. Philadelphia: WB Saunders, 1974.
23. Robbins SL. Pathologic Basis of Disease. Philadelphia: WB Saunders, 1974.
24. Umphred DA. Neurological Rehabilitation. St. Louis: CV Mosby, 1985.
25. Sharrard WJ. Neuromotor evaluation of the newborn. In: Symposium on Myelomeningocele. St. Louis: CV Mosby, 1972.
26. Peach B. The Arnold-Chiari malformation. Arch Neurol 1965;12:165.
27. Peach B. The Arnold-Chiari malformation. Arch Neurol 1965;12:109.
28. McCullough DC. Arnold-Chiari malformation—theories of development. Presented at the 2nd Symposium on Myelomeningocele, Cincinnati, OH, 1984.
29. McLone DG, Knepper PA. The cause of Chiari II malformation: a unified theory. Pediatr Neurosci 1989;15:1–12.
30. Mclone DG, Dias MS. The Chiari II malformation: cause and impact. Childs Nerv Syst 2003;19(7–8):540–550.
31. Lutschg J, Meyer E, Jeanneret-Iseli C, et al. Brainstem auditory evoked potential in myelomeningocele. Neuropediatrics 1985;16:202–204.
32. Hesz N, Wolraich M. Vocal cord paralysis and brainstem dysfunction in children with spina bifida. Dev Med Child Neurol 1985;27:528–531.
33. Hoffman HJ, Hendrick EB, Humphreys RP, et al. Manifestations and management of Arnold-Chiari malformation in patients with myelomeningocele. Childs Brain 1975;1:255–259.
34. Staal MJ, Melhuizen-de Regt MJ, Hess J. Sudden death in hydrocephalic spina bifida aperta patients. Pediatr Neurosci 1987;13:13–18.
35. Biggio JR, Wenstrom KD, Owen J. Fetal open spina bifida: a natural history of disease progression in utero. Prenat Diagn 2004;24(4):287–289.
36. Palomaki GE, Williams JR, Haddow JE. Prenatal screening for open neural-tube defects in Maine. N Engl J Med 1999;340(13):1049–1050.
37. Thomas M. The lemon sign. Radiology 2003;228(1):206–207.
38. Pilu G, Romero R, Reece A, et al. Subnormal cerebellum in fetuses with spina bifida. Am J Obstet Gynecol 1988;158:1052–1056.
39. Benacerraf BR, Stryker J, Frigotto FD. Abnormal ultrasound appearance of the cerebellum (banana sign): indirect sign of spina bifida. Pediatr Radiol 1989;171:151–153.
40. Thiagarajah S, Henke J, Hogge WA, et al. Early diagnosis of spina bifida: the value of cranial ultrasound markers. Obstet Gynecol 1990;76:54–57.
41. Bensen J, Dillard RG, Burton BK. Open spina bifida: does cesarean section delivery improve prognosis? Obstet Gynecol 1988;71:532–534.
42. Luthy DA, Wardinsky T, Shurtleff DB, et al. Cesarean section before the onset of labor and subsequent motor function in infants with myelomeningocele diagnosed antenatally. N Engl J Med 1991;324:662–666.

43. Shurtleff DB, Luthy DA, Benedetti TJ, et al. Perinatal management, cesarean section and outcome in fetal spina bifida. Presented at the American Academy of Cerebral Palsy and Developmental Medicine, Boston, 1987.

44. Hogge WA, Dungan JS, Brooks MP, et al. Diagnosis and management of prenatally detected myelomeningocele: a preliminary report. Am J Obstet Gynecol 1990;163:1061–1064.

45. Johnson MP, Sutton LN, Rintol N, et al. Fetal myelomeningocele repair: short term clinical outcomes. Am J Obstet Gynecol 2003;189(2):482–487.

46. Sutton LN, Adzick NS, Bilaniuk LT, et al. Improvement in hindbrain herniation demonstrated by serial fetal magnetic resonance imaging following fetal surgery for myelomeningocele. JAMA 1999;282(19):1826–1831.

47. Buner JP, Tulipan N, Paschall RL, et al. Fetal surgery for myelomeningocele & the incidence of shunt-dependent hydrocephalus. JAMA 1999;282(19):1819–1825.

48. Raimondi AJ, Soare P. Intellectual development in shunted hydrocephalic children. Am J Dis Child 1974;127:664–671.

49. McLone DG, Czyzewski D, Raimondi AJ, et al. Central nervous system infections as a limiting factor in the intelligence of children with myelomeningocele. Pediatrics 1982;70:338–342.

50. Ellenbogen RG, Goldmann DA, Winston KW. Group B streptococcal infections of the central nervous system in infants with myelomeningocele. Surg Neurol 1988;29:237–242.

51. Banta J. Long-term ambulation in spina bifida. Presented at the American Academy of Cerebral Palsy and Developmental Medicine, Chicago, 1983.

52. Murdoch A. How valuable is muscle charting? Physiotherapy 1980;66:221–223.

53. Schafer M, Dias L. Myelomeningocele: Orthopedic Treatment. Baltimore: Williams & Wilkins, 1983.

54. Kaplan G. Editorial: with apologies to Shakespeare. J Urol 1999;161:933.

55. Tanaka H, Katizaki H, Kobayashi S, et al. The relevance of urethral resistance in children with myelodysplasia: its impact on upper urinary tract deterioration and the outcome of conservative management. J Urol 1999;161:929–932.

56. An Introduction to Hydrocephalus. Chicago: Children's Memorial Hospital, 1982.

57. Raimondi AJ. Complications of ventriculoperitoneal shunting and a critical comparison of the 3-piece and 1-piece systems. Childs Brain 1977;3:321–342.

58. Bell WO, Sumner TE, Volberg FM. The significance of ventriculomegaly in the newborn with myelodysplasia. Childs Nerv Syst 1987;3:239–241.

59. Bell WO, Arbit E, Fraser R. One-stage myelomeningocele closure and ventriculo-peritoneal shunt placement. Surg Neurol 1987;27:233–236.

60. Lindseth RE. Treatment of the lower extremities in children paralyzed by myelomeningocele (birth to 18 months). Am Acad Orthop Surg Inst Course Lec 1976;25:76–82.

61. Daniels L, Williams M, Worthingham C. Muscle Testing: Techniques of Manual Examination. Philadelphia: WB Saunders, 1956.

62. Strach EH. Orthopedic care of children with myelomeningocele: a modern program of rehabilitation. BMJ 1967;3:791–794.

63. Asher M, Olson J. Factors affecting the ambulatory status of patients with spina bifida cystica. J Bone Joint Surg 1983;65A:350–356.

64. Bunch W. Progressive neurological loss in myelomeningocele patients. Presented at the American Academy of Cerebral Palsy and Developmental Medicine Conference, San Diego, 1982.

65. Coon V, Donato G, Houser C, et al. Normal ranges of hip motion in infants. Clin Orthop 1975;110:256–260.

66. Haas S. Normal ranges of hip motion in the newborn. Clin Orthop Rel Res 1973;91:114–118.

67. Dias L. Hip contractures in the child with spina bifida. Presented at the 2nd Symposium on Spina Bifida, Cincinnati, OH, 1984.

68. Banta JV, Lin R, Peterson M, et al. The team approach in the care of the child with myelomeningocele. J Prosthet Orthot 1989;2:263–273.

69. Lie HR, Lagergren J, Rasmussen F, et al. Bowel and bladder control of children with myelomeningocele: a Nordic study. Dev Med Child Neurol 1991;33:1053–1061.

70. Brem AS, Martin D, Callaghan J, et al. Long-term renal risk factors in children with myelomeningocele. J Pediatr 1987;110:51–55.

71. Anagnostopoulos D, Joannides E, Kotsianos K. The urological management of patients with myelodysplasia. Pediatr Surg Int 1988;3:347–350.

72. Wolf LS. Early motor development in children with myelomeningocele. Presented at the American Academy of Cerebral Palsy and Developmental Medicine, Washington, DC, 1984.

73. Mazur JM. Hand function in patients with spina bifida cystica. J Pediatr Orthop 1986;6:442–447.

74. Anderson P. Impairment of a motor skill in children with spina bifida cystica and hydrocephalus: an exploratory study. Br J Psychol 1977;68:61–70.

75. Dahl M, Ahlsten G, Carlson H, et al. Neurological dysfunction above cele level in children with spina bifida cystica: a prospective study to 3 years. Dev Med Child Neurol 1995;37:30–40.

76. Bobath B. Motor development, its effect on general development and application to the treatment of cerebral palsy. Physiotherapy 1971;57:526–532.

77. Bobath B. The treatment of neuromuscular disorders by improving patterns of coordination. Physiotherapy 1969;55:18–22.

78. Bobath B. The very early treatment of cerebral palsy. Dev Med Child Neurol 1967;9:373–390.

79. Caplan F. The First Twelve Months of Life. New York: Grosset and Dunlap, 1973.

80. Turner A. Upper-limb function in children with myelomeningocele. Dev Med Child Neurol 1986;28:790–798.

81. Turner A. Hand function in children with myelomeningocele. J Bone Joint Surg Br 1985;67:268–272.

82. Agness PJ. Learning disabilities and the person with spina bifida. Presented at the Spina Bifida Association of America Meeting, Chicago, 1980.

83. Cronchman M. The effects of babywalkers on early locomotor development. Dev Med Child Neurol 1986;28:757–761.

84. Williams EN, Broughton NS, Menelaus MB. Age-related walking in children with spina bifida. Dev Med Child Neurol 1999;41(7):446–449.

85. Menelaus M. The evolution of orthopedic management of myelomeningocele. J Pediatr Orthop 1999;18:421–422.

86. Charney EB, Melchionni JB, Smith DR. Community ambulation by children with myelomeningocele and high level paralysis. Presented at the American Academy of Cerebral Palsy and Developmental Medicine, San Francisco, 1989.

87. Beaty JH, Canale ST. Current concepts review. Orthopedic aspects of myelomeningocele. J Bone Joint Surg Am 1990;72:626–630.

88. Dias L. Orthopedic care in spina bifida: past, present, and future. Dev Med Child Neurol 2004;46(9):579.

89. Menelaus M. Hip dislocation: concepts of treatment. Presented at the 2nd Symposium on Spina Bifida, Cincinnati, OH, 1984.

90. Stauffer ES, Hoffer M. Ambulation in thoracic paraplegia [Abstract]. J Bone Joint Surg 1972;54A:1336.

91. Hoffer MM, Feiwell EE, Perry R, et al. Functional ambulation in patients with myelomeningocele. J Bone Joint Surg 1973;55A:137–148.

92. Yngve D, Douglas R, Roberts JM. The reciprocating gait orthosis in myelomeningocele. J Pediatr Orthop 1984;4:304–310.

93. Dias L, Tappit-Emas E, Boot E. The reciprocating gait orthosis: the Children's Memorial experience. Presented at the American Academy of Developmental Medicine and Child Neurology, Washington, DC, 1984.

94. Douglas R, Larson PF, D'Ambrosia R, et al. The LSU reciprocating gait orthosis. Orthopedics 1983;6:834–839.

95. Center for Orthotics Design, Inc. www.centerfororthotics design.com. Accessed 5/7/07.

96. Williams L. Energy cost of walking and of wheelchair propulsion by children with myelodysplasia. Dev Med Child Neurol 1983;25:617–624.

97. McDonald CM, Jaffe KM, Mosca VS, et al. Ambulatory outcome of children with myelomeningocele: effect of lower extremity muscle strength. Dev Med Child Neurol 1991; 33:482–490.

98. Torosian CM, Dias LS. Surgical treatment of severe hindfoot valgus by medial displacement osteotomy of the os calsis in children with myelomeningocele. J Pediatr Orthop 2000;20(2): 226–229.

99. Neto J, Dias L, Gabriel A. Congenital talipes equinovarus in spina bifida: treatment and results. J Pediatr Orthop 1996;16: 782–785.

100. Schopler SA, Menelaus MB. Significance of the strength of the quadriceps muscles in children with myelomeningocele. J Pediatr Orthop 1987;7:507–512.

101. Sherk HH, Uppal GS, Lane G, et al. Treatment versus non-treatment of hip dislocations in ambulatory patients with myelomeningocele. Dev Med Child Neurol 1991;33:491–494.

102. Duffy CM, Graham HK, Cosgrove AP. The influence of ankle-foot orthosis on gait and energy expenditure in spina bifida. J Pediatr Orthop 2000;20(3):356–361.

103. Hunt, et al. The effects of fixed and hinged ankle-foot orthoses on gait myoelectric activity in children with myelomeningocele. Meeting Highlights of AACPDM. J Pediatr Orthop 1994;14(2):269.

104. Knutson LM, Clark DE. Orthotic devices for ambulation in children with cerebral palsy and myelomeningocele. Phys Ther 1991;71:947–960.

105. Vankoski S, Dias L. Children with spina bifida benefit from gait analysis. Vicon Motion Systems. The Standard 1997;1:4–5.

106. Vankoski S, Sarwark J, Moore C, et al. Characteristic pelvis, hip and knee kinematic patterns in children with lumbosacral myelomeningocele. Gait Posture 1995;3:1:51–57.

107. Ounpuu S, Davis R, Bell K, et al. Gait analysis in the treatment decision making process in patients with myelomeningocele. 8th Annual East Coast Gait Laboratories Conference. Rochester, MN, May 5-8, 1993.

108. Duffy C, Hill A, Cosgrove A, et al. Three-dimensional gait analysis in spina bifida. J Pediatr Orthop 1996;16:786–791.

109. Williams J, Graham G, Dunne K, et al. Late knee problems in myelomeningocele. J Pediatr Orthop 1993;13:701–703.

110. Thompson JD, Ounpuu S, Davis RB, et al. The effects of ankle-foot orthosis on the ankle and knee in persons with myelomeningocele: an evaluation using three dimensional gait analysis. J Pediatr Orthop 1999;19(1):27–33.

111. Porsch K. Origin and treatment of fractures in spina bifida. Eur J Pediatr Surg 1991;1(5):298–305.

112. Drummond D. Post-operative fractures in patients with myelomeningocele. Dev Med Child Neurol 1981;23:147–150.

113. Rosenstein BD, Greene WB, Herrington RT, et al. Bone density in myelomeningocele: the effects of ambulatory status and other factors. Dev Med Child Neurol 1987;29:486–494.

114. Lock TR, Aronson DD. Fractures in patients who have myelomeningocele. J Bone Joint Surg Am 1989;71:1153–1157.

115. Bartonek A, Saraste H, Samuelson L, et al. Ambulation in patients with myelomeningocele: a 12 year follow-up. J Pediatr Orthop 1999;19(2):202–206.

116. Hall P, Lindseth R, Campbell R, et al. Scoliosis and hydrocephalus in myelomeningocele patients: the effect of ventricular shunting. J Neurosurg 1979;50:174–178.

117. Mazur JM, Menelaus MB. Neurologic status of spina bifida patients and the orthopedic surgeon. Clin Orthop Rel Res 1991;264:54–64.

118. Jeelani NO, Jaspan T, Punt J. Tethered cord syndrome after myelomeningocele repair. BMJ 1999;318:516–517.

119. Petersen M. Tethered cord syndrome in myelodysplasia: correlation between level of lesion and height at time of presentation. Dev Med Child Neurol 1992;34:604–610.

120. McClone D, Herman J, Gabriele A, et al. Tethered cord as a cause of scoliosis in children with a myelomeningocele. Pediatr Neurosurg 1990;91(16):8–13.

121. Banta J. The tethered cord in myelomeningocele: should it be untethered? Dev Med Child Neurol 1991;33:167–176.

122. Mazur J, Stillwell A, Menelaus M. The significance of spasticity on the upper and lower limbs in myelomeningocele. J Bone Joint Surg Br 1986;68:213–217.

123. Flanagan RC, Russell DP, Walsh JW. Urologic aspects of tethered cord. Urology 1989;33:80–82.

124. Kaplan WE, McLone DG, Richards I. The urological manifestation of the tethered spinal cord. J Urol 1988;140:1285–1288.

125. Grief L, Stalmasek V. Tethered cord syndrome: a pediatric case study. J Neurosci Nurs 1989;21:86–91.

126. Hochleiter BW, Menardi G, Haussler B, et al. Spina bifida as an independent risk factor for sensitivization to latex. J Urol 2001;166(6):2370–2373.

127. Nieto A, Mazon A, Pamies R, et al. Efficacy of latex avoidance for primary prevention of latex sensitization in children with spina bifida. J Pediatr 2002;140(3):370–372.

128. Centers for Disease Control. Anaphylactic reaction during general anesthesia among pediatric patients, United States. Jan 1990–Jan 1991. MMWR Morb Mortal Wkly Rep 1991;40: 437–443.

129. Allergic Reactions to Latex-Containing Medical Devices: FDA Medical Alert. Food and Drug Administration. March 29, 1991.

130. Meeropol E, Frost J, Pugh L, et al. Latex allergy in children with myelomeningocele. J Pediatr Orthop 1993;13:1–4.

131. D'Astous J, Drouin M, Rhine E. Intraoperative anaphylaxis secondary to allergy to latex in children who have spina bifida. J Bone Joint Surg 1992;74-A:1084–1086.

132. Meehan P, Galina M, Daftari T. Intraoperative anaphylaxis due to allergy to latex. J Bone Joint Surg 1992;74-A:1103–1109.

133. Lu L, Kurup V, Hoffman D, et al. Characterization of a major latex allergen associated with hypersensitivity in spina bifida patients. J Immunol 1995;155:2721–2728.

134. Medical Sciences Bulletin. Available at: http://pharminfo.com/pub/msb/latex.html. Accessed 1/03.

135. Good Latex Allergy Survival Skills. Available at: http://www.netcom.com/~ecbdmd/Glass.html. Accessed 1/03.

136. Latex Allergy. Available at: http://www.Waisman.Wisc.Edu/~rowley/sbkids/Sb_latex.html. Accessed 1/03.

137. Willis KE, Holmbeck GN, Dillon K, et al. Intelligence and achievement in children with myelomeningocele. J Pediatr Psychol 1990;15:161–176.

138. Horn DG, Pugzles Lorch E, Lorch RF, et al. Distractibility and vocabulary deficits in children with spina bifida and hydrocephalus. Dev Med Child Neurol 1985;27:713–720.

139. Wolfe GA, Kennedy D, Brewer K, et al. Visual perception and upper extremity function in children with spina bifida. Presented at the American Academy of Cerebral Palsy and Developmental Medicine, San Francisco, 1989.

140. Cull C, Wyke MA. Memory function of children with spina bifida and shunted hydrocephalus. Dev Med Child Neurol 1984;26:177–183.

141. Mauk JE, Charney EB, Nambiar R, et al. Strabis-mus and spina bifida. Presented at the American Academy of Cerebral Palsy and Developmental Medicine, 1987, Portland, OR.
142. Lennerstrand G, Gallo JE. Neuro-ophthalmological evaluation of patients with myelomeningocele and Chiari malformations. Dev Med Child Neurol 1990;32:415–422.
143. Rothstein TB, Romano PE, Shoch D. Meningomyelocele. Am J Ophthalmol 1974;77:690–693.
144. Horn DG, Lorch EP, Lorch RF, et al. Distractibility and vocabulary deficits in children with spina bifida and hydro-cephalus. Dev Med Child Neurol 1985;27:713–720.
145. Ruff HA. The development of perception and recognition of objects. Child Dev 1980;51:981–992.
146. Butler C. Effects of powered mobility on self-initiated behaviors of very young children with locomotor disability. Dev Med Child Neurol 1986; 28:325–332.
147. DeLateur B, Berni R, Hangladarom T, et al. Wheelchair cushions designed to prevent pressure sores. Arch Phys Med Rehabil 1976;57:129–135.
148. Fiewell E. Seating and cushions for spina bifida. Presented at the 2nd Symposium on Spina Bifida, Cincinnati, OH, 1984.
149. Borjeson MC, Lagergren JL. Life conditions of adolescents with myelomeningocele. Dev Med Child Neurol 1990;32:698–706.
150. Selber P, Dias L. Sacral level myelomeningocele: long term outcome in adults. J Pediatr Orthop 1998;18:423–427.
151. Buran CF, McDaniel AM, Brej TJ. Needs assessment in a spina bifida program: a comparison of the perceptions of adolescents with spina bifida and their parents. Clin Nurse Spec 2002; 16(5):256–262.
152. Dias LS, Fernandez AC, Swank M. Adults with spina bifida: a review of seventy-one patients. Presented at the American Academy of Cerebral Palsy and Developmental Medicine, Boston, 1987.
153. Dunne KB, Shurtleff DB. The medical status of adults with spina bifida. Presented at the American Academy of Cerebral Palsy and Developmental Medicine, 1987, Washington, DC
154. Moore C, Kogan BA, Parekh A. Impact of urinary incontinence on self-concept in children with spina bifida. J Urol 2004; 171(4):1659–1662.
155. Lobby NJ, Ginsburg C, Harkaway RC, et al. Urinary tract infections in adult spina bifida. Infect Urol 1999;12(2):51–55.
156. Campbell JB, Moore KN, Voaklander DC, et al. Complications associated with clean intermittent catheterization in children with spina bifida. J Urol 2004;171(6 Pt 1):2420–2422.
157. McClone DG. Spina bifida today: problems adult face. Semin Neurol 1989;9:169–175.
158. Iddon JL, Morgan DJR, Loveday C, et al. Neuropsychological profile of young adults with spina bifida with or without hydro-cephalus. J Neurol Neursurg Psychiatry 2004;75:112–118.
159. Barf HA, Verhoef M, Jennekens-Schinkel A, et al. Cognitive status of young adults with spina bifida. Dev Med Child Neurol 2003;45(12):813–820.

ADDITIONAL RESOURCES

Scherzer A, Tscharnuter I. Early Diagnosis and Therapy in Cerebral Palsy. New York: Marcel Dekker, 1982 (handling strategies for young children).

Williamson GG. Children with Spina Bifida: Early Intervention and Pre-School Programming. Baltimore: Brooks Publishers, 1987 (family concerns and PT/OT interventional strategies).

OTHER SOURCES FOR LATEX INFORMATION

Food and Drug Administration Latex Hotline, Tel. 301-594-3060.

Spina Bifida Association of America, Tel. 800-621-3141.

Latex-free products can be ordered from the following:

Alternative Resource Catalog, Tel. 708-503-8298.

NO LATEX Industries, Tel. 800-296-9185.

Relia Care Express, Tel. 888-225-1941.

Traumatic Injury to the Central Nervous System: Brain Injury

Amy Both

Definition

Traumatic brain injury (TBI),[1] a frequent cause of morbidity and mortality in the pediatric population, occurs when an external, mechanical force either accidentally or intentionally impacts the head. TBI is characterized by a period of diminished or altered consciousness that ranges from brief lethargy to prolonged unconsciousness or even brain death.[2] According to the *Guide for Physical Therapist Practice,*[3] pediatric TBI falls into one of three preferred practice patterns (see Table 7.1). Symptoms vary greatly depending on the location of the lesion and the extent of underlying brain injury. TBI is not associated with congenital injury or degenerative insult. It is also referred to as brain injury, head injury, or closed head injury. Many children with TBI recover uneventfully.

TABLE 7.1
Preferred Practice Patterns— *Guide to Physical Therapist Practice, Second Edition*
5C   Impaired Motor Function and Sensory Integrity Associated with Nonprogressive Disorders of the Central Nervous System: Congenital Origin or Acquired in Infancy or Childhood
5D   Impaired Motor Function and Sensory Integrity Associated with Nonprogressive Disorders of the Central Nervous System: Congenital Origin or Acquired in Adolescence or Adulthood
5I   Impaired Arousal, Range of Motion, and Motor Control Associated With Coma, Near Coma, or Vegetative State

From Guide to physical therapist practice. 2nd edition. Phys Ther 2001;81(1):1–768.

Others, however, are left with partial or total functional disability and/or psychosocial impairment.

Incidence

Each year there are up to 250,000 new cases of children who sustain TBI in the United States.[4–7] Of the approximately 100,000 who are hospitalized, approximately 7000 die and at least 29,000 experience permanent physical, intellectual, communication, psychosocial, and behavioral deficits.[4–7] Brain injury is the leading cause of death and disability in children between 1 and 19 years of age.[7–10] It is also the third leading cause of death in children less than 1 year of age. However, the survival rate of children with TBI is better in children than in similarly injured adults.[11] There are two peak periods of incidence of TBI in children. The first occurs in early childhood (less than 5 years of age) and the second occurs during mid-to late adolescence.[12,13] The incidence of TBI is 2.8 times greater in boys than girls.[4,5,7] Premorbid personality and behavior have been found to predispose children to brain injury.[14] Children who are aggressive, fearless, and hyperactive and who have difficulty with discipline are at an increased risk of injury.[15,16] In addition, there is evidence that once a child sustains a TBI, even a mild TBI, the likelihood of reinjury increases.[17]

Brain injury and death rates vary considerably by race and socioeconomic status.[4,18] TBI-associated mortality rates are highest in African Americans, followed by Caucasians and then other races.[4,18] For all races, death rates are inversely related to socioeconomic status.[18] Thus, children of families with low incomes have higher death rates than children of families with upper and middle incomes.

Causes of Injury

FALLS

Falls account for 35% of all pediatric TBIs that require hospitalization or result in death.[18] Two-thirds of the trauma injuries in infants are caused by falls from heights or stairs, but of these, only 8% result in severe injury.[19] However, because of the high center of gravity in younger children and the tendency to fall head first, infants and preschool-age children are more susceptible to severe injury from falls of less than 4 feet than older children.[18,20] Among preschoolers, 51% of the trauma injuries occur from falls, including falls from playground equipment, of which only 6% are serious.[18] Older children usually escape severe injury in falls from heights of less than 10 feet.[18,20] Although many falls occur accidentally, falls of less than 10 feet bear investigation for potential child abuse.[18,20]

MOTOR VEHICLE ACCIDENTS

Motor vehicle accidents (MVAs) account for approximately 25% of all pediatric TBIs and are the most common cause of trauma death in children 5 to 9 years old.[2,18] MVAs cause the vast majority of serious injuries with multiple trauma in children, and approximately 70% of the children injured in an MVA will be in a coma for some period of time.[2,10] The incidence of TBI resulting from MVAs progressively increases with age, from 20% in children 0 to 4 years old up to 66% in adolescents.[12,13]

Between 4 and 14 years of age, the majority of injuries occur when the child is a bicyclist or pedestrian.[12,13,21] MVAs are the most common cause of trauma death in children 5 to 9 years old.[18] In contrast, the majority of motor vehicle injuries sustained during adolescence occur when the adolescent is an unprotected occupant in the automobile.[12,13] The shift in cause of TBI is associated with obtaining a driving license and driving and drinking among teenagers.[18] A number of studies indicate that up to 40% of adolescents are intoxicated at the time of a motor vehicle crash.[22,23]

GUNSHOT WOUNDS

Firearm injuries occur from accidental gun discharges, homicides, and suicides and rank second only to MVAs as the leading cause of trauma death in school-age children and adolescents.[22] The incidence of gunshot wounds among male inner city youth is extremely alarming, as the children are often both the victims and the perpetrators.[24] More than twice as many children survive their injuries as die, with approximately 25% having permanent sequelae.[25]

ABUSE/ASSAULT

Physical abuse in infants and young children is prevalent in children 0 to 4 years old.[12,13] Approximately 24% of the

Nutrition for the Child with Traumatic Brain Injury

Susan Boyden, MS, RD, LDN

Clinical Dietitian

The Children's Hospital of Philadelphia

Nutrition-Related Problems	Interventions
UNABLE TO EAT BY MOUTH:	Alternate means of nutrition:
• Impaired gastrointestinal system	Parenteral nutrition
• Comatose/vegetative state	Tube feedings
• Respiratory failure	
• Aspiration risk	
UNABLE TO CONSUME ADEQUATE NUTRITION:	
• Impaired oral motor skills	Dietary modifications:
• Chewing	Modification of food texture/consistency
• Pocketing	Thickened liquids
• Swallowing	High-calorie supplements
• Drooling/leakage	Tube feedings
• Sensory and communication deficits:	
• Unable to see food offered	Ophthalmology evaluation
• Unable to communicate when hungry	Speech therapy referral
• Difficulty communicating at mealtime	Occupational therapist
due to hearing loss	Audiology evaluation
• Depression	Psychology referral
• Pain issues	Medication
	Music therapy
	Child life therapy
INCREASED CALORIE/NUTRIENT NEEDS:	
• Metabolic stress	Nutritional supplements
• Fractures	Tube feedings
• Wound healing	Vitamins/minerals
• Involuntary movements	Parenteral nutrition
Constipation	Adequate fiber and fluids
	Bowel program
	Medications
Gastroesophageal reflux	Small frequent feedings
	Nutrient-dense meals/snacks/formula
	Medication
OBESITY	
• Decreased mobility	Physical therapy program
• Insatiable appetite related to	Reduce fat/calories in diet
injury to appetite control center	Food diary
	Consistent meal schedule

SUGGESTED READINGS

Ekvall SW. Pediatric nutrition in chronic diseases and developmental disorders. In: Cloud H, ed. Feeding Problems of the Child with Special Health Care Needs. New York: Oxford University Press, 1993:203—217.

Loan T. Metabolic/nutritional alterations of traumatic brain injury. Nutrition 1999;15:809–812.

children who are abused require hospital admission[26] and approximately 80% of the head trauma deaths in children under 2 years of age are due to physical abuse.[12,13,26] Abuse frequently results in head injury owing to the vulnerability of the immature brain and the weak supporting neck musculature. Abuse resulting in TBI is characterized by a marked discrepancy between the explanation of how the injury occurred and the nature and severity of the injury. Early identification of abuse is critical to prevent repeated or progressive injury.

SPORTS/RECREATIONAL ACTIVITIES

Sports and recreational causes account for approximately 21% of the brain injuries to school-age children and adolescents.[18] High-risk contact sports, such as football and boxing, result in up to half of the injuries.[18] TBI is also seen in other recreation activities when head protection is either not used or forgotten, including diving, baseball, cycling, horseback riding, and rugby.

 Mechanisms of Injury

IMPRESSION INJURIES

Impression injuries occur when a solid object, such as a rock or a blunt object, impacts a stationary head. Impression injuries produce skull fracture and a focal lesion at the site of the impact. The presence of skull fracture is associated with an increased risk of intracranial injury; however, the absence of skull fracture does not reliably exclude a significant intracranial injury.[27,28]

ACCELERATION–DECELERATION INJURIES

Acceleration–deceleration injuries are caused when a moving head hits a relatively fixed object, such as the ground or a windshield. The young infant is particularly

susceptible to acceleration–deceleration injuries, as there is less restraint of motion in the neck.[29] Therefore, acceleration–deceleration injury in infancy may result in greater differential displacement of the skull and cranial contents.[29] The direction of acceleration injuries may be translational (linear) or rotational (angular). Most TBIs are a result of a combination of both translational and rotational injuries.

TRANSLATIONAL INJURY

In translational injury, the head in motion strikes a stationary object and responds with lateral displacement of both the skull and the brain. The injury that results from the initial impact of the skull on the brain is known as *coup*. The lesion that occurs in the direction opposite of the initial force is termed *contrecoup*. Contrecoup occurs as the brain decelerates against the bony structures of the skull.

ROTATIONAL INJURY

Rotational injury occurs when the skull rotates as the brain remains stationary. The effect is angular forces on the brain, surface contusions, lacerations, and shearing trauma.[30] Rotational injury can result in either focal or diffuse brain damage.

 Primary Brain Damage from Trauma

Primary brain damage (Table 7.2)[29–31] from trauma is a direct result of the forces that occur to the head at the time of initial impact.

CONCUSSION

Concussion is a clinical state characterized by altered awareness and loss of memory immediately following trauma. Impaired consciousness can last a few seconds to several

---

TABLE 7.2

Damage from Head Trauma

Primary Head Injury	Secondary Head Injury	Other Consequences
Immediate impact/concussion	Cerebral edema	Hydrocephalus
Skull fracture	Increased intracranial pressure	Seizures
Cerebral contusion	Herniation syndromes	Infection
Intracranial hemorrhage: epidural, subdural	Ischemic/hypoxic damage	Endocrine disorders
Diffuse axonal injury	Neurochemical events	

From Kaufman BA, Dacey RG. Acute care management of closed head injury in childhood. Pediatr Ann 1994;23:18–28; Pang D. Pathophysiologic correlates of neurobehavioral syndromes following closed head injury. In: Ylviasaker M, ed. Head Injury Rehabilitation. Austin, TX: Pro-Ed, 1985:3–70; and Griffith ER, Rosenthal M, Bond MR, et al., eds. Rehabilitation of the Child and Adult with Traumatic Brain Injury. 2nd Ed. Philadelphia: FA Davis, 1990.

hours and is related to the transmission of stretching forces to the brainstem as the brain is thrown back and forth in the cranial vault.[32] Concussion can be seen without obvious pathologic changes to the brain; however, it may also be caused by mild diffuse white matter lesions or neurochemical injury.[32] Following concussion, a child may exhibit clinging behavior, disturbances in sleep, irritability, or more distractibility than usual. These behavior changes can last a few days to a few months.[32]

CONTUSION

A contusion is a bruising or hemorrhage of the crests or gyri in the cerebral hemispheres. Contusion can be seen following a crush injury or blunt trauma, or during an inertial load injury, such as acceleration–deceleration of the brain within the skull.[29] Contusions occur most commonly in the frontal and temporal lobes of the brain because of bony irregularities in the cranial vault.[32]

SKULL FRACTURES

Skull fractures are seen in both closed head injuries and open, compound head injuries. Brain injury can occur both with and without the presence of skull fracture.[27,28,33] Linear comminuted fractures result from impact with low-velocity objects and depressed fractures generally result from impact with higher velocity objects. Linear fractures can produce contusions, hemorrhage, and cranial nerve damage.[29] Depressed skull fractures of greater than 5 mm are considered significant.[29] Depressed fractures can produce herniation syndromes, contusions, lacerations, and cranial nerve damage.[29]

INTRACRANIAL HEMORRHAGES

Intracranial injury can occur with or without immediate loss of consciousness or skull fracture.[27,28] Two types of intracranial hemorrhage frequently seen following pediatric TBI are extradural and intradural hematomas. Intracranial hemorrhage may not appear initially on clinical examination.[28,29] The rate of blood collection and the location of the hematoma are related to severity and outcome.[34] Intracranial hemorrhage is a common cause of clinical deterioration and death in patients who have experienced a lucid interval after injury.

EXTRADURAL HEMATOMAS

Extradural or epidural hematomas develop because of the tearing of an artery in the brain, primarily the middle meningeal artery and its branches. In children, epidural hematomas usually follow skull fracture or bending of the skull into the brain.[34] With unilateral epidural hematoma, there is often herniation of the temporal lobe.[35] Coma may ensue and cardiorespiratory arrest is possible.

INTRADURAL HEMATOMAS

Intradural hematomas include subdural and intracerebral hematomas. Acute subdural hematomas occur secondary to injury to veins in the subdural space. Subsequent recovery depends on both the time before hemorrhage evacuation and the extent of damage to underlying brain tissue.[34] Subdural hematomas are frequently seen with inertial injuries and occur commonly in the temporal and frontal lobes.[32] Subdural hematomas are associated with higher mortality rates and poorer functional outcomes. Intracranial hematomas can result from trauma or rupture of a congenital vascular abnormality.[36] Very severe injuries may cause large intracerebral hematomas that can rupture into the ventricles, causing intraventricular hemorrhage.[32]

DIFFUSE AXONAL INJURY

Diffuse axonal injury (DAI) is a microscopic phenomenon not commonly visible on computed tomography (CT) scan. DAI is seen following rotational injury within the cranial vault.[29] The shearing trauma results in diffuse disturbance of cellular structures following TBI. DAI is associated with much of the significant brain damage seen in TBI, including sudden loss of consciousness, extensor rigidity of bilateral extremities, and autonomic dysfunction.[32]

 ## Secondary Brain Damage from Trauma

Secondary brain damage from trauma (see Table 7.2)[29–31] evolves as a result of the pathophysiologic changes initiated by the primary trauma. Research suggests that secondary brain damage from trauma develops over a period of several hours or days.[32] Secondary injuries account for a significant amount of the overall damage that occurs in TBI and prevention of secondary brain damage is a major goal of the acute management of the child with TBI.[34]

CEREBRAL EDEMA

Perhaps the most frequently occurring cause of secondary injuries is cerebral edema. Unchecked cerebral edema accompanied by an increase in intracranial pressure can lead to multiple cerebral infarctions, brain herniation, brainstem necrosis, and irreversible coma.[35] Control of brain swelling is often difficult and may require the use of a combination of the following techniques: narcotic sedation, diuretics, barbiturates, systemic neuromuscular paralysis, or hyperventilation.[34,35]

INTRACRANIAL PRESSURE

When a mass, such as a hematoma or cerebral edema, is present following TBI, intracranial pressure (ICP) increases in response to the pressure exerted on the brain. Initial increases in ICP are accommodated by the mechanisms of the ventricular system.[35] However, when the compensatory mechanisms are no longer effective, ICP rises.

In infancy, increases in ICP will cause bulging of the fontanels and separation of the sutures. In children older than 5 years of age, as ICP rises, the contents of the cranial vault are forced downward through the foramen magnum. This causes brainstem compression and may lead to difficulty breathing and even cardiorespiratory arrest.[29] Prolonged increased ICP may lead to the development of posttraumatic hydrocephalus.[29]

HERNIATION SYNDROMES

Herniation syndromes result from displacement of the brain by an expanding lesion and cerebral edema. Depending on the location of the lesion, herniation can cause obstructive hydrocephalus, brain shift past midline, or brainstem compression.[32] Herniation can lead to neurologic deterioration of a grave nature, with resultant decreasing levels of consciousness, altered respiration, hypertonicity, hemiparesis, and decorticate posturing.[32]

HYPOXIC–ISCHEMIC INJURY

The supply of oxygen and nutrients to the brain is dependent on adequate cerebral perfusion. Alterations of cerebral perfusion, raised ICP, or lack of oxygen to the brain may result in hypoxic–ischemic brain damage.[32] Ischemia frequently occurs in the tissue surrounding cerebral contusions or hematomas and ultimately leads to further brain damage. Severe hypoxic injury and diffuse axonal injuries are most likely to cause severe disabilities, including prolonged postcoma unawareness.[32,37]

NEUROCHEMICAL EVENTS

When trauma occurs to the brain, there is a disruption of the blood–brain barrier and a release of excitatory neurotransmitters and oxygen-free radicals into the blood system.[32] Oxygen-free radicals have an extremely toxic effect on the brain and are damaging to cell membranes and vessel walls.[38] The damage from oxygen-free radicals causes internal disruption of neuronal functioning and further brain damage.[38]

 Other Consequences from Brain Damage

HYDROCEPHALUS

Hydrocephalus can be differentiated as either communicating or noncommunicating types. In communicating hydrocephalus, all components of the ventricular system are enlarged and ICP may only be intermittently elevated. Communicating hydrocephalus is seen in the vast major-

ity of posttraumatic cases.[39] Noncommunicating hydrocephalus refers to enlargement of the ventricles of the brain owing to an obstruction of the flow and impaired absorption of cerebrospinal fluid. Children with hydrocephalus may present with changes in mental status, lethargy, nausea/vomiting, headache, gait ataxia, and urinary incontinence.[39] Neurosurgical ventriculoperitoneal shunting procedures are performed in children with hydrocephalus to improve the flow and absorption of cerebrospinal fluid.[39]

SEIZURES

The occurrence of early posttraumatic seizures is more common in children than adults, with an incidence of approximately 10%.[40,41] Early posttraumatic seizures in children are frequently of a generalized onset type, such as grand mal and tonic-clonic seizures.[40,41] Partial or focal seizures and seizures of late onset are uncommon in children.[40,41] The development of early seizures has been found to be associated with more severe injury, diffuse cerebral edema, acute subdural hematoma, and open, depressed skull fractures with damage to the brain.[42] The frequency of seizure activity within the first year after TBI may be predictive of further recurrence.[41] Thus, children who do not experience seizure within the first year following injury are unlikely to develop seizures at a later time.

INFECTIONS

Penetrating injuries, such as gunshot wounds and depressed skull fractures, carry inherent risk of brain infection. In addition, neurosurgical procedures to insert ICP monitors and shunts for increased cerebrospinal fluid also carry risk of brain infection. Two common infections following penetrating wounds are meningitis and brain abscess.[39] The physical therapist can assist the medical team by monitoring for signs of infection, such as fever, headache, confusion, neck stiffness, and increased ICP.

ENDOCRINE DISORDERS

Although rare, hypopituitarism and precocious puberty are both reported in children following TBI.[41,43] Linear growth and weight are closely followed so that the need for medical intervention may be determined. The physical therapist should report any concerns of increased weight gain or the development of secondary sexual characteristics to the child's physician.

Predictors of Injury Severity and Outcome

Clinical rating scales are used to standardize the description of patients with TBI, monitor progress, determine a general plan for appropriate medical intervention, predict outcome, and assist with clinical outcomes research.

Predicting recovery and outcome in children with TBI is complex. The rate of recovery following TBI is most rapid in the first few months and continues throughout the first year after the accident.[44] In children with severe injury, some improvement is also noted in the second and third years following TBI.[41]

Outcome is affected by a number of factors, including location and morphologic characteristics of the injury, complications that occur during the initial stabilization of the injury, the age of the child at the time of injury, the length of coma, the duration of posttraumatic amnesia (PTA), the severity of the injury, premorbid psychological and cognitive adjustment, and the family response to the injury.[45–47] Of all the factors listed, the duration of coma appears to be the single most consistent predictor of outcome.[45,46]

COMA SCALES

Coma is defined as a complete state of unconsciousness in which the child does not open his or her eyes, follow commands, speak, or react to painful stimuli.[48] To assist with determining the level of unconsciousness, Glasgow neurosurgeons Teasdale and Jennett developed a coma assessment scale known as the Glasgow Coma Scale (GCS).[48] It is a standardized tool for assessing the neurologic status of a trauma victim and is based on the patient's best response to three categories: motor activity, verbal responses, and eye opening.

Two variations of the GCS, the Children's Coma Scale (CCS)[49] and the Pediatric Coma Scale (PCS),[50] have been found useful in assessment of outcome in children (Table 7.3). The CCS is commonly used in children under 36 months of age, whereas the PCS is used in children 9 to 72 months of age.[51] In addition, the PCS developed interpretive norms for several age groups between birth

and 5 years (Table 7.4). Children whose coma scores were below the norm for age tended to have poorer outcomes.

DURATION OF COMA

The duration of coma is directly related to outcome.[52,53] Thus, the longer the coma is, the worse the outcome.[52,53] For children with loss of consciousness for 1 night or less and mild TBI, the results on long-term outcome measures of cognition, achievement, and behavior are indistinguishable from those of uninjured children.[44,47]

In contrast, children with coma lasting more than a few days and moderate to severe TBI experience a variety of physical, cognitive, language, and psychological sequelae that may improve following the injury or remain permanent.[54] In addition, significant school problems were present in 59% of the children and adolescents with a coma duration between 15 minutes and 1 week.[45]

For children less than 15 years of age with TBI who had a coma with a duration of 1 week or more and survived, it should be noted that a return to regular education was not possible. Rarely do young children stay in a persistent state of coma. Ninety percent have been shown to recover to be moderately disabled or better over a 3-year period.[41]

DEPTH OF COMA

In addition to the duration of coma, the depth of coma, as measured by the CCS, is easy to assess and correlates well with prognosis and functional outcome.[49] Using the Children's Coma Scale, a coma score of 3 or 4 is predictive of a poor outcome, while a score of 7 or greater is predictive of a good outcome.[49,55]

Most children who sustain mild brain injury, as determined by the coma scales, are expected to experience a

---

TABLE 7.3

Comparison of Glasgow Coma Scale and Adelaide Pediatric Coma Scale

	Glasgow Coma Scale (Adults)	Adelaide Pediatric Coma Scale
Eyes open	Spontaneously 4 To speech 3 To pain 2 None 1	As in adults
Best motor response	Obeys commands 6 Localizes pain 5 Withdraws 4 Flexion to pain 3 Extension to pain 2 None 1	Obeys commands 5 Localizes to pain 4 Flexion to pain 3 Extension to pain 2 None 1
Best verbal response	Oriented 5 Confused 4 Words 3 Sounds 2 None 1	Oriented 5 Words 4 Vocal sounds 3 Cries 2 None 1

From Kaufman BA, Dacey RG. Acute care management of closed head injury in childhood. Pediatr Ann 1994;23:18–28.

TABLE 7.4	
Age Norms*	
0–6 mo	= 9
6–12 mo	= 11
12–24 mo	= 12
2–5 yr	= 13
>5 yr	= 14

*For the Adelaide Pediatric Coma Scale Score (from Kaufman BA, Dacey RG. Acute care management of closed head injury in childhood. Pediatr Ann 1994;23:18–28.)

full recovery within several weeks. However, new evidence suggests that following even a mild TBI, problems with balance, response speed, and running agility can persist at discharge.[56] For children who are moderately and severely injured, the degree of initial impairment on a coma scale is related to both the degree of recovery and residual deficit.[47] Strong correlations of depth of coma and outcome severity have been noted, especially in the areas of intelligence, academic performance, and motor performance.[47]

ORIENTATION AND AMNESIA ASSESSMENT

Posttraumatic amnesia is defined as the interval between injury and the moment at which an individual can recall a continuous memory of what is happening around him or her.[45] Evaluation of PTA in children is challenging, as traditional assessment methods rely on the subject's verbal response. Because standard orientation questions are inappropriate for children owing to their limited cognitive and language skills, the Children's Orientation and Amnesia Test (COAT)[57] was developed. The COAT is reliable for children between the ages of 4 and 15 years.[57] Although the COAT is useful in the age range established, a reliable method of assessing PTA in children under 4 years of age has not been established.[58]

DURATION OF POSTTRAUMATIC AMNESIA

In children, the duration of PTA has been found to be more predictive of future memory function than coma scales.[57] The length of PTA has been used to classify the severity of TBI. Severity of injury is mild if PTA lasts less than 1 hour, moderate if PTA lasts between 1 and 24 hours, and severe if PTA lasts longer than 1 day.[59] As a further refinement, severity is very mild if PTA lasts 5 minutes or less, very severe if PTA lasts over 7 days, and extremely severe if PTA lasts longer than 4 weeks.[59] In children with PTA of more than 3 weeks' duration, verbal and nonverbal memory was found to be significantly impaired at both 6 months and 12 months postinjury.[59]

RANCHO LOS AMIGOS LEVELS OF COGNITIVE FUNCTIONING

The Rancho Los Amigos Levels of Cognitive Function Scale (Rancho Scale)[60] is a descriptive scale of cognitive and behavioral functioning. It is used primarily during inpatient rehabilitation. The Rancho Scale summarizes neurobehavioral function and serves to enhance communication between staff. The Rancho Scale is also useful as a framework for the physical therapist to identify probable treatment issues and to develop treatment strategies based on the current level of cognitive function. The main limitation of the Rancho Scale is that there are poor correlations between the "phases of recovery" and prediction of discharge functional ratings.[61] In addition, cognitive function and behavior may fluctuate depending on the environment as well as fatigue or stress (see Display 7.1).

In a group of children admitted with Rancho scores between levels I and III, significant improvement was noted within the first year of recovery.[62] At 1 year postinjury, only 17% of the children were still at Rancho levels of less than IV. Seventy-one percent of the children with TBI returned home, 10% were admitted to a nursing home, and the others were in institutions. Functional mobility was noted to significantly improve as 79% of the group achieved independence, including the 46% that did not need to use an assistive device. At 1 year postinjury, 40% of the children were at a Rancho level of VIII. At 2 years postinjury, 61% of the children were at a Rancho level of VIII, and by 3 years postinjury, 67% of the children were at a Rancho level of VIII.[62]

PEDIATRIC RANCHO SCALE

The Pediatric Rancho Scale[63] is an adapted version of the Rancho Los Amigos Scale that can be used to evaluate young children between the ages of infancy and 7 years of age. Like the Rancho Scale, the Pediatric Rancho Scale serves to enhance communication of recovery among staff and to assist with developing a framework for treatment management based on cognitive level (see Display 7.2).

AGE

The capacity of the brain to guard against and respond to trauma changes with age.[21] Although at one time young children were thought to be spared greater dysfunction following TBI, newer research has demonstrated an increased vulnerability of the young child to the effects of TBI.[29,64] In infants, the skull is thin and easily deformable, thus increasing the susceptibility to injury from trauma.[29,65] In addition, immature myelination in the cerebral hemispheres places the child at risk for injury, as the younger child's brain is soft and compressible.[65]

The age of the child at the time of injury also appears to correlate with increased risk for specific impairments.

>> **DISPLAY 7.1**

Rancho Los Amigos Levels of Cognitive Functioning

I. *No response:* Patient appears to be in a deep sleep and is completely unresponsive to any stimuli.

II. *Generalized response:* Patient reacts inconsistently and nonpurposefully to stimuli in a nonspecific manner regardless of stimulus presented. Responses may be physiologic changes, gross body movements, and/or vocalization and are often limited and delayed. Often, the earliest response is to deep pain.

III. *Localized response:* Patient reacts specifically but inconsistently to stimuli. Responses are directly related to type of stimulus presented. May withdraw an extremity and/or vocalize when presented with a painful stimulus. May follow simple commands such as closing eyes or squeezing hand in an inconsistent, delayed manner. May also show vague awareness of self-discomfort by pulling at nasogastric tube, catheter, or resisting restraints. May show a bias responding to familiar persons. Once external stimuli are removed, may lie quietly.

IV. *Confused-agitated:* Patient is in a heightened state of activity, and agitation is generally in response to own internal confusion. Behavior is bizarre and nonpurposeful relative to immediate environment. Verbalizations frequently are incoherent and/or inappropriate to the environment. May cry or scream out of proportion to stimuli and even after removal, show aggressive behavior, attempt to remove restraints or tubes, or crawl out of bed. Gross attention to environment is very brief; selective attention is often nonexistent. Patient lacks any recall. Severely decreased ability to process information and does not discriminate among persons or objects; is unable to cooperate directly with treatment efforts. Unable to perform self-care without maximal assistance. May have difficulty performing motor activities such as sitting, reaching, and ambulating on request.

V. *Confused-inappropriate:* Patient is able to respond to simple commands fairly consistently. However, with increased complexity of commands or lack of any external structure, responses are nonpurposeful, random, or fragmented. Demonstrates gross attention to the environment but is highly distractible and lacks ability to focus attention on a specific task. With structure, may be able to converse on an automatic level for short periods of time. Verbalization is often inappropriate and confabulatory. Memory is severely impaired; often shows inappropriate use of objects; and may perform previously learned tasks with structure but is unable to learn new information. Responds best to self, body, comfort, and family members. May show agitated behavior in response to discomfort or unpleasant stimuli. Can usually perform self-care activities with assistance. May wander off, either randomly or with vague intentions of "going home."

VI. *Confused-appropriate:* Patient shows goal-directed behavior but is dependent on external input or direction. Response to discomfort is appropriate and is able to tolerate unpleasant stimuli when need is explained. Follows simple directions consistently and shows carryover for relearned/newly learned tasks such as self-care. Responses may be incorrect owing to memory problems, but they are appropriate to the situation. Past memories show more depth and detail than recent memory. No longer wanders and is inconsistently oriented to time and place. Selective attention to tasks may be impaired. May have vague recognition of staff; has increased awareness of self, family, and basic needs.

VII. *Automatic-appropriate:* Patient appears appropriate and oriented within the hospital and home settings; goes through daily routine automatically but frequently robot-like. Patient shows minimal to no confusion and has shallow recall of activities. Shows increased awareness of self, body, family, food, people, and interaction in the environment. Has superficial awareness of but lacks insight into condition; decreased judgment and problem solving. Lacks realistic ideas/plans for the future. Shows carryover for new learning but at a decreased rate. Requires supervision for learning and safety purposes. With structure is able to initiate social or recreational activities.

VIII. *Purposeful-appropriate:* Patient is able to recall and integrate past and recent events and is aware of and responsive to environment. Shows carryover for new learning and needs no supervision once activities are learned. May continue to show a decreased ability relative to premorbid activities, abstract reasoning, tolerance for stress, and judgment in emergencies or unusual circumstances. Social, emotional, and intellectual capacities may continue to be at a decreased level but functional in society.

From Hagen C, Makmus D, Durham P, et al. Levels of cognitive functioning. In: Rehabilitation of the Head-Injured Adult: Comprehensive Physical Management. Downey, CA: Professional Staff of Rancho Los Amigos Hospital; 1979:87–90.

Young children are more vulnerable to the effects of diffuse injury on memory than older children. Children that experience TBI before the age of 5 years exhibit more profound language deficits than those injured later in childhood.[66] In addition, children who are severely injured between the ages of 15 and 21 years are at higher risk than older adult patients for late behavioral and emotional sequelae.[67]

Although the plasticity of the developing brain can allow for dramatic recovery of function, the effects of a diffuse insult produced by TBI may ultimately result in greater cognitive impairment in the developing brain than in the mature brain.[64] Moreover, deficits may remain hidden until a time in which the child needs to participate in higher level academic activities. Clearly, the young child is vulnerable to brain injury.

Pediatric Rancho Scale

V. *No response to stimuli:* Complete absence or observable change in behavior to visual, auditory, or painful stimuli.

IV. *Generalized response to sensory stimulation:* Reacts to stimuli in a nonspecific manner; reactions are inconsistent, limited in nature, and often the same regardless of stimulus present. Responses may be delayed. Responses noted include physiologic changes, gross body movement, or vocalizations. First responses are often to pain. Gives generalized startle to loud sounds. Responds to repeated auditory stimulation with increased or decreased activity. Gives generalized reflex response to painful stimuli.

III. *Localized response to sensory stimuli:* Reacts specifically to stimulus. Responses are directly related to type of stimuli presented. Responses include blinking when strong light crosses field of vision, following moving object passed within visual field, and turning toward or away from loud sound or withdrawing from painful stimuli. Reactions can be inconsistent and delayed. May inconsistently follow simple commands such as close eyes, move an arm. May show vague awareness of self by pulling at tubes or restraints. May show a bias by responding to family and not others.

II. *Responsive to environment:* Appears alert and responds to name. Recognizes parents or other family members. Imitates examiner's gestures or facial expressions. Participates in simple age-appropriate vocal play/vocalizations. Gross attention but highly distractible. Needs frequent redirection to focus on task. Follows commands in an age-appropriate manner and is able to perform previously learned tasks with structure. Without external structure, responses may be random or nonpurposeful. May be agitated by external stimuli. Increased awareness of self, family, and basic needs.

I. *Patient is oriented to self and surroundings:* Shows active interest in environment and initiates social contact. Can provide accurate information about self, surroundings, orientation, and present situation as age-appropriate.

Staff from Denver Child's Hospital. Notes from Pediatric Rehab: Traumatic Brain Injury. Denver CO, 1989.

FUNCTION

Functional limitations and impairments following TBI impact outcome and often persist for a period of time postinjury. Even children with mild TBI have shown problems with balance on the Bruininks Pediatric Clinical Test of Sensory Integration for Balance and the Postural Stress Test at 12 weeks postinjury.[68] Such information should be taken into consideration when predicting a return to physical activities that require refined balance skills. When the problems with balance are combined with lower extremity fractures, the physical therapist can anticipate even further limitations in functional mobility.[69] In spite of improvement in function over time, children with TBI persist in exhibiting lasting differences in gait velocity, stride length, cadence, and balance when compared with healthy peers.[70] In addition, hand motor skills generally improve less than gait.[70]

Functional limitations and impairments may also be used to predict discharge status for children with TBI. During admission to a rehabilitation unit, the recovery of walking is a primary goal for children with TBI.[71,72] Knowing whether the patient can ambulate by discharge impacts decisions regarding the discharge environment and the equipment needs at discharge. Four factors associated with a nonambulatory status at discharge include prolonged loss of consciousness, lower extremity injury, impaired responsiveness, and presence of lower extremity spasticity.[72] In addition, low scores on the Pediatric Evaluation of Disability Inventory (PEDI) Mobility Functional Skills scale and a long length of stay were also associated with nonambulation at discharge.[72]

ENVIRONMENTAL INFLUENCES

Children with TBI may be particularly vulnerable to the influence of the family dynamics. In families of children between the ages of 6 and 12 years, it has been shown that greater parental distress and burden was associated with poorer fine motor dexterity, behavioral control, and academic performance.[73] The negative consequences of the TBI combined with high levels of family dysfunction make it more difficult for the family to support the child's recovery. Physical therapists need to consider the influence of the home environment on the prognosis for improvement in the child with TBI.[71,73]

OTHER FACTORS

It has been difficult to use early physiologic markers as predictors of outcome in children with TBI, as they are generally unreliable.[49] Large percentages of children with hypertension, seizures, fixed and dilated pupils, flaccidity, or prolonged forceful posturing have been reported to have good long-term outcomes.[74]

◆ **Physical Therapy Examination of the Child with Traumatic Brain Injury**

When a child with TBI is referred for treatment, a thorough physical therapy examination is necessary to ensure appropriate physical therapy management. The examination (Display 7.3) should contain, but may not be limited to, inclusion of information on past medical history, social

>> **DISPLAY 7.3**

Physical Therapy Evaluation/Assessment Format

Medical History
Onset and mechanism of injury
Diagnostic test results (CT scan, MRI, radiographs)
Medical precautions
Vital signs
Autonomic nervous system function

Skin integrity
Respiratory status
Bowel and bladder status
Dysphagia status
Medications

Social History and Living Environment
Family and support system
Educational/prevocational status

Cultural issues
Discharge environment

Cognitive/Behavioral Status
Level of arousal
Orientation
Attention
Behavior/affect

Memory
Language/communication
Executive functions
Neuropsychological or psychological assessments

Basic Sensorimotor Status
Hearing/auditory processing
Vision, perception, and visuospatial ability
Sensation
Range of motion
Strength
Muscle tone
Abnormal movement patterns, posture, and reflexes
Balance and balance strategies
Praxis and coordination
Speed of movement
Endurance

Functional Status
Bed/floor mobility
Transfers/transitions
Sitting and standing skills
Ambulation on level surfaces
Stair ascension/descension
Ambulation outside/rough terrain
Advanced gross motor skills/sports
Generalization of functional abilities

---

history and living environment, cognitive/behavioral status, basic sensorimotor status, and functional status. While performing the examination, consideration should be given to the child's tolerance level and attention span, as deficits in either area may limit the physical therapist's ability to complete the examination in one session. The physical therapist may also need to incorporate play into the assessment in an effort to enhance cooperation and obtain a more accurate picture of the child with TBI.

SUBJECTIVE EXAMINATION: PATIENT HISTORY

MEDICAL HISTORY

The therapist must thoroughly review the child's past medical/surgical and current condition prior to initiating the physical examination. Information should be gathered regarding the mechanism of the injury, severity of damage, and significant changes in the clinical picture over time. Particular attention should be given to reports from CT scans, magnetic resonance imaging (MRI) scans, radiographs, and other diagnostic tests.

SOCIAL HISTORY AND LIVING ENVIRONMENT

Interviewing the parents, siblings, and/or caregivers of the child with TBI is imperative, as successful therapeutic intervention should be family and child centered.[75] The family members are the experts in knowing their child and often can give helpful advice to the therapist regarding the best way to motivate the child in therapy. In addition, information can be gained regarding the conditions and limitations of the home environment. Families should be encouraged to collaborate with the rehabilitation team in the development of an appropriate plan of care and the identification of equipment needs upon discharge. Family or psychosocial information may also be gained by talking to the social worker.

SYSTEMS REVIEW

A thorough review of all body systems helps the physical therapist decide which systems will require further testing and often directs the selection of subsequent tests (see Display 7.4). During this review information that was not noted in the initial history may be obtained.

OBJECTIVE EXAMINATION: TESTS AND MEASURES

Children who sustain TBI may experience a complex array of impairments and functional limitations in physical abilities, emotional development, and cognitive/behavioral functioning (Display 7.5).[73]

COGNITIVE/BEHAVIORAL STATUS

A comprehensive cognitive examination is beyond the scope of practice of the physical therapist. However, cognition should be grossly assessed by the physical therapist to assist in determining realistic treatment goals and appropriate interventions. Physical therapy examination of cognition should include the following areas: arousal/orientation, attention span and focus, behavior/affect, memory, communication, mental flexibility, problem solving, judgment, and insight.

LEVEL OF AROUSAL/ORIENTATION Trauma that damages the frontal lobe and brainstem may result in impair-

ment of arousal and orientation of the child with TBI. In addition, medications used to diminish spasticity, seizures, or pain may decrease arousal.[36] Impairment in arousal may be expressed as lethargy, drowsiness, or even coma. Decreased levels of arousal will interfere with the child's ability to attend to pertinent stimuli, follow commands, and benefit from feedback in therapy.

ATTENTION Trauma to the frontal lobe may impair attention in the child with TBI. Impairment in attention may affect both the ability to attend to a specific stimulus and the ability to sustain attention over time. Children with TBI who have problems with attention often have difficulty following commands and relearning motor tasks; thus, the impairment may be expressed as distractibility or inattention. This is especially noted when therapy is conducted in busy environments with many distractions. Care must be taken to structure the environment and remove extraneous stimuli as appropriate.

BEHAVIOR/AFFECT After TBI, children may display a wide array of problems in behavior and affect (see Display 7.5).[76] Two common changes in behavior noted during the time of rehabilitation are agitation and confusion. Agitation is characterized by a heightened state of activity and a severely decreased ability to process stimuli from the environment in a useful manner. The child who is agitated may be restless, irritable, and combative. Impulsivity and unsafe behavior may be observed as the child acts before thinking. Fortunately, agitation in children with TBI does not last as long as the agitated phase of recovery for adults with TBI.[65]

Confusion is characterized by general disorientation and inability to make sense out of the surrounding environment. Confusion may persist through most of the rehabilitative process. Children with TBI who are confused may interact either appropriately or inappropriately.

When problems with behavior persist and interfere with participation in therapy, it is important for the brain injury rehabilitation team to work together and implement a behavior modification program. Initially, the team must identify the unwanted behaviors and any precipitating factors, including environmental factors, that contribute to the behavior problem. Agitation may be precipitated by factors such as pain, occult fractures, restraints, urinary tract infections, constipation, and overstimulation by staff, family, and friends. Precipitating factors should be addressed prior to the implementation of the behavior modification program and be removed when possible.

Then, rewards and reinforcements for desired behavior and a reward schedule must be determined. The patient's family may be very helpful in identifying rewards that are both motivating and satisfying. The reward schedule must be agreed on by the rehabilitation team to maximize compliance and promote the desired behavior. Once the rewards and schedule have been addressed, the team then moves

---

>> **DISPLAY 7.4**

Sample System Review Questions: Yes/No Answers to a Series of Questions

Is your patient experiencing any of the following?

General: Fatigue, sleep disturbance, appetite change

Cardiopulmonary: Irregular heart rate or rhythm, blood pressure fluctuations, edema, dyspnea, ventilator use, sputum production

Integumentary: Color changes, abrasion, bruising, decubitus ulcer, infection

Musculoskeletal: Pain, stiffness, swelling, joint limitation

Neuromuscular: Headache, seizures, spasticity, weakness, tremor, gait disturbance, balance loss

Communication, language, affect, and cognition: Inability to make needs known, altered consciousness, disorientation, memory loss, affect changes, behavioral changes

>> **DISPLAY 7.5**

Common Clinical Impairments and Functional Limitations

Physical	Emotional	Cognitive/Behavioral	Functional
Headaches	Mood swings	Decreased arousal	Limited bed mobility
Dizziness	Denial	Disorientation	Limited transfers
Visual disturbance	Anxiety	Distractibility	Poor sitting control
Visuospatial impairment	Depression	Inattention	Poor standing control
Hearing loss	Irritability	Impaired concentration	Gait impairment
Sensory loss	Guilt/self-blame	Confusion	Impaired hygiene skills
Cranial nerve injury	Emotional lability	Agitation	Impaired dressing skills
Spasticity	Low self-esteem	Memory deficits/amnesia	Impaired feeding skills
Ataxia/incoordination	Egocentricity	Sequencing difficulty	Fine motor impairment
Balance impairment	Lability	Slowed processing	Sexual dysfunction
Fatigue	Apathy	Impaired judgment	Sleep disorders
Seizures	Impaired problem solving	Speech/language problems	Decreased academic skills

From Koch L, Merz MA, Lynch RT. Screening for mild traumatic brain injury: a guide for rehabilitation counselors. J Rehabil 1995;61:50–56.

toward redirecting the child to appropriate actions by praising approximations of desired actions. As the team works together to address the behavior problem in a consistent manner, the incidence of inappropriate actions slowly decreases. Keep in mind that in some cases the environment cannot be modified and behavior management is ineffective. In that case, the managing physician will consider pharmacologic management.

MEMORY Memory impairment is the most common cognitive impairment in children with TBI.[77] Trauma to the temporal lobe commonly affects memory in children with TBI. Memory includes the ability to learn and recall new information as well as the ability to recall previously learned information. The presence of memory loss, or amnesia, is an indication that a concussion has occurred. The amnesia may be retrograde, involving a period of time prior to the accident, or anterograde, extending from the incident forward in time.

Retrograde amnesia may be temporary and may cover events that occurred several months or years prior to the injury. Memory for most past events will usually return over several hours or days.[78] However, permanent retrograde amnesia may exist for the brief period of time preceding the accident.[78] Anterograde amnesia is problematic during the rehabilitation process and may interfere with new learning. Anterograde amnesia is rarely permanent.[78]

Memory deficits involve verbal recall and visual recognition. They may appear as the inability to remember the sequence of motor tasks from one treatment to another or as unsafe performance of functional skills. The omission of safety-related behaviors when performing functional motor skills, such as transfers and ambulation, can limit independence.

Memory with respect to a child's ability to learn new material is of particular interest to the physical therapist. Although retention of information learned prior to the TBI may remain unharmed, the memory for learning new information may be problematic. The results of a neuropsychological evaluation of a child's memory skills and capacity for new learning will be helpful in the establishment of realistic functional goals and the development of an appropriate rehabilitation program.[36] Working jointly with the child's family and psychologist, the physical therapist may help determine the need for compensatory strategies, assistance, and environmental modification in the rehabilitation setting.

LANGUAGE Language deficits in the child with TBI are addressed in depth by speech and language pathologists. Damage to the temporal lobe may result in expressive or receptive language deficits that will impede communication between the physical therapist and child, thus complicating therapy sessions. For example, receptive language deficits will impair a child's ability to understand verbal instructions for the performance of a gross motor task. When a receptive language impairment exists, determination of the best means of communication will decrease frustration for the child and the therapist.

Expressive language disorders impair a child's ability to communicate with others. Although the child with an expressive language disorder may be able to fully comprehend verbally communicated information and form an appropriate response mentally, a breakdown occurs between the formulation of the response and the verbal or gestural execution of what was intended. Once again, the physical therapist's knowledge of the child's most effective mode of communication may lessen the frustration related to the inability to communicate thoughts and feelings.[34]

EXECUTIVE FUNCTIONS Trauma to the prefrontal regions of the frontal lobes results in impairment of executive functions. Executive functions refer to the ability to show initiative, plan activities, change conceptual sets, solve problems, regulate behavior in social settings, and use feedback to initiate behavioral change and monitor success.[34,76]

Deficits in executive functioning may be demonstrated by impulsive behavior, resulting in failure to observe safety precautions or the inability to recognize when behavior is socially inappropriate.[34] Mental inflexibility may be demonstrated as perseveration on a task or the inability to change activities without becoming disorganized.[34] Difficulty switching conceptual sets may also influence the ability to perform tasks with alternating patterns or reciprocal movements.

SENSORIMOTOR STATUS

ABNORMAL TONE

Spasticity　Because of damage to the cerebral cortex, children with TBI may present with spasticity. The degree of spasticity may range from mild to severe, with distribution that may be either unilateral or bilateral. Children who present with unilateral involvement display motor impairment and dysfunction similar to that of children with hemiplegic cerebral palsy. Children who present with bilateral involvement often have asymmetric distribution and movements dominated by primitive reflex activity.

Children with spasticity may also present with abnormal posturing of the extremities or the whole body. The upper extremities typically present with flexor synergy posturing. Flexor synergy posturing interferes with hygiene and functional use of the upper extremity for play, schoolwork, and self-care. The lower extremities commonly present with extensor synergy posturing. Extensor synergy posturing interferes with bed mobility, transfers, and ambulation.

Children with TBI who are severely involved may present with whole body posturing. Whole body posturing can be decorticate (flexion of the upper extremities and extension of the lower extremities) or decerebrate (extension in all extremities) in nature and is frequently seen in the early stages of recovery. As the child improves, whole body posturing is often replaced with more volitional movement, including movement utilizing abnormal synergistic patterns.

Ataxia　Because of damage to the cerebellum and basal ganglia, children with TBI may experience ataxia and motor incoordination. The distribution of ataxia can also be unilateral or bilateral. Ataxia may initially be masked by spasticity in the early recovery period. Timing and execution of movement may be difficult, and intention may or may not be present. Gait in children with ataxia is characterized by a wide base of support and difficulty maintaining static stance. Ataxia is generally not associated with loss of range of motion unless combined with spasticity.

MUSCLE PERFORMANCE IMPAIRMENT

STRENGTH LOSS After TBI and loss of consciousness, children may remain in bed for a prolonged period of time. During that time, weakness due to disuse atrophy may be expected. Weakness is also seen in both the agonist and antagonist muscle groups of a spastic extremity. Standardized manual muscle testing may be difficult to perform, as the child with TBI is unable to follow instructions for testing. Therefore, the physical therapist must observe active movement and judge the child's ability to move against gravity and sustain weight.

IMPAIRED ENDURANCE Children with TBI often present with an overall state of lethargy, which is common in TBI. Fatigue for a child with TBI may be due to both physical activity and mental activity associated with motor planning. Both impair the child's ability to participate in activities of functional mobility and self-care. Rest breaks within sessions and rest between therapies may help the child with TBI to sustain participation and build endurance.

RANGE-OF-MOTION LOSS Because of the poverty of movement and stereotypic abnormal movement patterns used, children with TBI who present with spasticity are at risk for loss of active range of motion and contracture development. Joints particularly at risk include the elbows, wrists, fingers, knees, and ankle–foot complex. Range-of-motion loss can occur quickly and early management is the key to effective prevention.

BALANCE LOSS After TBI, a loss of balance is present in most children. Research has shown that even in children with mild TBI, a loss of balance that prohibits safe participation in preinjury activities persists for 12 weeks or more postinjury.[69] Care must be taken to thoroughly re-evaluate a child for postural control and tolerance of perturbations before allowing the child to safely return to activity.

SENSORY DEFICITS

HEARING Hearing loss is also common in pediatric TBI.[79] All children with moderate to severe traumatic brain injuries should have a thorough audiologic evaluation to determine the presence of hearing loss. When hearing loss is present, hearing aids, an FM transmitter, or preferential classroom seating may be indicated.[58]

VISION Visual disturbances in children with TBI are common. These deficits may include decreased visual acuity, disturbances of visual pursuit and accommodation, field cuts, reduced depth perception, diplopia, transient cortical blindness, and retinal hemorrhages.[58] When visual problems exist, eye patching, glasses, or preferential classroom seating may help alleviate the difficulty.[58]

Transient cortical blindness lasting no longer than 30 days has been associated with nearly complete recovery of vision.[58,80] However, cortical blindness lasting more than 30 days generally carries a grave prognosis for children with TBI. Retinal hemorrhages in young children with TBI are strongly suggestive of child abuse.[78,81,82]

VISUOSPATIAL SKILLS Problems with vision are also associated with problems of perception and visuospatial function. Such deficits are frequently associated with lesions in the temporal or occipital lobes of the brain. Visuospatial and perceptual deficits may impair gross motor performance and functional mobility skills, thus limiting the potential for functional independence in a child. A figure-ground deficit, or the inability to distinguish a given form from the background, may make noting a change in terrain depth during gait training more difficult. Visuospatial deficits may make activities of daily living, such as donning an orthosis, more difficult. A child with deficits in visuospatial memory may demonstrate difficulty developing a mental map of his or her environment and consequently may have difficulty moving independently from place to place in the home, school, or community.[34]

ORTHOPEDIC COMPLICATIONS

HETEROTOPIC OSSIFICATION Heterotopic ossification (HO), the formation of mature lamellar bone in soft tissue, can occur in children and adolescents following TBI.[83] The risk of incidence of HO is reported to be 14% and identified risk factors include age greater than 11 years and a longer duration of coma.[83] HO commonly occurs at the elbow, shoulder, hip, and knee. Early signs of HO include decreased joint range of motion and pain with testing, swelling, erythema, and increased warmth near the involved joint.

The use of physical therapy in the treatment of HO is controversial. Some studies have associated physical therapy and aggressive range-of-motion exercises with HO as a result of local microtrauma and hemorrhage to the tissue.[84] In general, gentle but persistent range-of-motion exercises and management of spasticity with medications or nerve blocks are imperative.[84] When HO results in significant functional impairment, surgical excision of the bone from the soft tissue is indicated. HO rarely results in functional impairment in younger children.[83,85] HO in older children and adults is associated with a poorer functional outcome.[86]

FRACTURES Fractures in the pelvis and lower extremities are commonly associated with the traumatic events causing pediatric TBI. Up to one-third of children sustaining a severe TBI have skeletal fractures in the long bones, clavicle, or spine.[87,88] Surgical repair of fractures may be delayed until the child is neurologically and medically stable. Postsurgical care may be complicated by the decreased cognitive status of the child, especially when the child is alert and confused. Therefore, the child must be closely monitored to ensure that proper alignment and weight-bearing status are maintained during functional activities.

Although radiographs identify major trauma to the extremities, care should be exercised in evaluating additional musculoskeletal complaints, as there is potential for minor trauma and occult fractures to be present in the acute recovery phase. Particular attention should be given to persistent complaints and activities that are poorly tolerated. In addition, children may have complaints of soft tissue injuries that would not be detected by radiography.

FUNCTIONAL MEASURES

Early examination of function is difficult because of the compromised cognitive status of the child with TBI. As the child is more alert and appropriate in interactions in the clinic, the use of standardized measures, especially those that have shown sensitivity in measuring functional change, may be helpful.

The WeeFIM (Functional Independence Measure)[89] has been useful for assessing and tracking the development of functional independence in children with disabilities between the ages of 6 months and 7 years. The adult FIM can be used with older children. The WeeFIM measures six domains of function: self-care, sphincter control, mobility, locomotion, communication, and social cognition. In addition, it measures the level of function within those domains.

The PEDI[90] has also been developed as a functional assessment tool for children. It measures both capability and performance in the domains of self-care, mobility, and social function. The PEDI can be used in children between the ages of 6 months and 7.5 years. Recent research has examined the sensitivity of Acquired Brain Injury (ABI)–Specific PEDI subscales in measuring functional change in patients with TBI. The ABI-specific PEDI subscales were constructed from the mobility, self-care, and caregiver assistance scales of the PEDI. Initial results revealed that the Caregiver Assistance Self-Care subscale was more sensitive to measuring change than the generic PEDI, but further research is needed to determine the usefulness of the adapted tool.[91]

The Bruininks-Oseretsky Test of Motor Proficiency[92] is also used to assess gross and fine motor functioning. It is standardized for children from 4.5 years to 14.5 years. Each of these assessment tools is more fully described in Chapter 3.

Evaluation, Diagnosis, Prognosis, and Plan of Care

EVALUATION

After the examination is complete, the physical therapist must consider all of the data collected and make judgments that will lead to the development of a plan of care. The therapist must weigh the evidence of observed impairments and functional limitations with the knowledge of the pathophysiology of brain injury and other physiologic processes associated with trauma to better understand the patient's prognosis for expected improvement. In addition, the therapist should consider the patient's social support and the home environment. Evidence supports the notion that good family support can positively impact recovery and outcome.[60,74] Finally, the physical therapist should consider the amount of time that has passed since the injury, any interventions received, and progress made during recovery and treatment.

DIAGNOSIS AND PROGNOSIS

Using the *Guide to Physical Therapist Practice*[3] as a resource, a physical therapy diagnosis can be determined for the child with TBI. This diagnosis, while not a medical diagnosis, will align the child with a preferred practice pattern and assist with decision making (see Table 7.1). The prognosis of the patient will be affected by predictors associated with severity and outcome as well as complicating factors experienced during the course of recovery. The physical therapist must consider these factors and the anticipated response to intervention while formulating the prognosis. According to the *Guide,* the expected range of number of visits per episode of care for a child or adolescent with TBI or coma ranges from five to 90 sessions.[3]

PLAN OF CARE

Based on the physical therapy diagnosis, the physical therapist should determine a plan of care for the child with TBI. The plan of care includes not only the prescribed treatment interventions, but also specific long-and short-term goals designed to help the patient achieve the desired outcomes prior to discharge. Goals should be written based on identified system impairments, qualitative movement deficits, and functional limitations. Goals should be measurable and expressed in behavioral terms. Each short-term goal should be written as a component that leads to the accomplishment of the long-term goal. Time frames in which goals will be achieved are dependent on the setting in which the child is seen as well as consideration of the child's cognitive and behavioral status.

Coordination of services through a case manager may assist with the identification of a projected length of stay and the resources available to achieve the child's goals in physical therapy. When establishing goals, the physical therapist should also consider the proposed discharge environment so that the goals are correlated with where the child is going to once discharged from the rehabilitation setting.[93]

 Management/Interventions

Rehabilitation of children with TBI is different from adults with TBI in that children are still completing the process of typical development. Intervention, then, must take into consideration both the typical developmental progression and the recovery from the neurologic insult.[93,94] Therefore, when planning therapeutic interventions, the physical therapist must design programs that incorporate age-appropriate gross motor challenges at the appropriate level of cognitive function. Although the efficacy of various rehabilitation programs is not known, research is indicative of a positive trend in the benefit of rehabilitative services.[95]

ACUTE MEDICAL MANAGEMENT

Early medical management of the child with TBI focuses on preservation of life, determination of injury severity, and prevention of secondary brain damage.[32] Once vital signs are stabilized, the child will undergo a general assessment for potential injuries and a neurologic examination. These tests may include radiographic examination of the skull and cervical spine, CT scan of the head, and the use of the GCS.

Acute medical intervention for children with TBI may include emergency surgery, the use of mechanical ventilation, and the use of pharmacologic agents. If a subdural or intracerebral hematoma is present, immediate neurosurgery is indicated.[32] A delay in performing the surgery can be life threatening, as it helps decrease intracranial pressure and reduce pressure-related secondary brain injuries.[32]

Mechanically assisted ventilation at a rate greater than normal or hyperventilation is used to temporarily reduce intracranial pressure.[34] In addition to hyperventilation, pharmacologic agents are also used to decrease cerebral edema and minimize secondary brain damage. Drugs commonly used in the management of edema include mannitol and corticosteroids.[34] Medications may also be used to induce paralysis when the child's body movements interfere with the stability of vital signs and the administration of further medical interventions.[34]

Physical therapy in the acute stage may be deferred to a time in which the child is less medically fragile. Once the child is stable, the physical therapist may use the child's current level of cognitive functioning as a guide in planning interventions. It is important for the physical therapist to remember that the cognitive levels of recovery serve only as a general guideline for recovery. Not all children will experience each level of cognitive recovery or progress through recovery in a strict hierarchical sequence. Either the Rancho Scale or the Pediatric Rancho Scale may assist with identification of current cognitive status and potential concerns for the various stages.

ACUTE PHYSICAL THERAPY MANAGEMENT: PREVENTION

Physical therapy management for children with TBI functioning at low cognitive levels is aimed at the prevention of complications from prolonged inactivity and sensory deprivation. Common complications of prolonged inactivity may include skin breakdown, respiratory complications, and contracture development.

POSITIONING

A positioning program will assist with improving pulmonary hygiene, maintaining skin integrity, preventing contractures, and providing support for body alignment and movement. Positioning should be implemented with the assistance of the nursing staff and the family. Changes in position for the child confined in bed should be made every 2 hours. When the child is sitting, pressure relief procedures should be performed every 30 minutes. Pressure relief is accomplished by having the child recline on a mat in side-lying or by tilting the wheelchair backward to a semi-supine position.

When designing a positioning program, the physical therapist should take into consideration any orthopedic and neurologic positioning precautions as well as the influence of abnormal tone and primitive reflexes on posture. Positioning in side-lying (Fig. 7.1) may be preferred to positioning in supine or prone as it is helpful to decrease the influence of abnormal primitive reflexes. Positioning in supine should incorporate strategies to reduce the influence of the tonic labyrinthine reflex and extensor tone. Positioning in prone, although allowable, will seldom be carried out at this phase of recovery as it interferes with accessibility for adequately monitoring the child's vital signs and medical status.

Upright positioning even at an early stage of recovery may be achieved with the use of an adapted wheelchair (Figs. 7.2 and 7.3). The adapted wheelchair should incorporate either a tilt-in-space or reclining seating system with postural support to assist the child in safely achieving upright while preventing overfatigue. A removable headrest can be used to encourage head control when the child is alert and allow for rest when the child is fatigued.

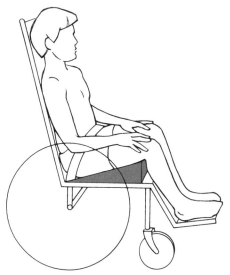

Figure 7.2 ■ Child is supported in a wheelchair with a tall back and a seat wedge to maintain hip flexion. The back may be designed to either recline or tilt in space to accommodate fatigue in the child.

CONTRACTURE MANAGEMENT

The importance of preventing soft tissue contractures in the acute recovery phase cannot be overemphasized. Development of contractures will delay functional independence and lead to the need for additional therapy or even surgery later in the rehabilitative phase. In addition to the use of a positioning program, range of motion and the application of splints and casts may help improve lower extremity function and prevent soft tissue contractures.[96]

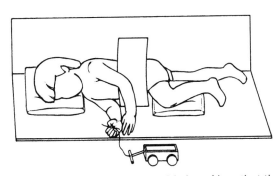

Figure 7.1 ■ Child positioned in a side-lyer. Note that the head is maintained in line with the trunk, the upper extremities are in midline, and the lower extremities are dissociated. Gravity is eliminated, and the influence of primitive reflexes is minimized.

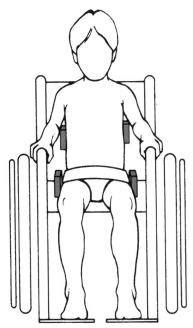

Figure 7.3 ■ Child is sitting in a wheelchair with hip blocks and lateral trunk supports for assistance with postural control.

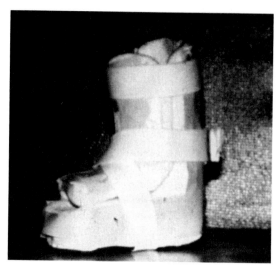

Figure 7.4 ■ An example of a bivalved inhibitive cast.

Contractures in prepubertal children who are not forcefully posturing often may be successfully managed with positioning and splinting alone because of the child's smaller size and relative weakness.[57] Coordination of a wearing schedule is a key to enhancing the effectiveness of splinting. Wearing tolerance may be gradual, and the child must be monitored for signs of skin breakdown. In a larger child who is not forcefully posturing, serial casting followed by bivalved fiberglass cast splints may be used to manage contractures.

For children with severe extensor posturing who do not respond to a positioning program, splints, or bivalved casts, serial casts are warranted (Fig. 7.4).[57] These casts must be changed initially every 3 to 5 days to prevent skin breakdown. Once it is determined that the child will tolerate the casts without skin breakdown, the casts can be worn for up to 2-week intervals until posturing diminishes and volitional control increases. Bivalved fiberglass cast splints may then be used at night to maintain range of motion. Continuous use of serial casts in a child who is alert and moving actively should not exceed 2 months.

Serial casts may be used in conjunction with oral or injectable medications to manage spasticity. Oral medication, such as dantrolene (Dantrium), although useful in decreasing spasticity, is often undesirable because of its sedating properties.[57] Diazepam (Valium) can also be used for treating spasticity but may be associated with increased agitation in children who are emerging from coma.[57] As an alternative, nerve and motor point blocks, such as phenol and Botox injections, may be more desirable in the management of spasticity in children, as there are no sedating and cognitive side effects.[57] Recent work on the use of Botox injections in children is promising. Effects of the injectable medications can last up to 3 to 6 months.[57]

LOW COGNITIVE LEVEL PHYSICAL THERAPY MANAGEMENT: STIMULATION

COMA STIMULATION PROGRAM

Coma stimulation programs were developed on the premise that structured stimulation could prevent sensory deprivation and accelerate recovery.[97] However, controversy exists regarding the amount of stimulation that can be safely used early in the care of a comatose child.[98] Sensory input may be provided through the vestibular, visual, tactile, auditory, and olfactory systems (Display 7.6).[99] The rehabilitation team should involve the family in selection of meaningful items to be used for stimulation. An emphasis should be placed on selecting items that reflect the child's culture, personality, likes/dislikes, hobbies, significant relationships, and pets. In addition, items that are selected should be re-evaluated periodically so those ineffective stimuli can be eliminated.

The next step in program development is to determine an appropriate schedule for stimulation. The physical therapist needs to determine the time of day at which alertness is optimal to conduct therapy and modify the child's schedule as necessary. In the event that this is not possible, the physical therapist will need to modify the treatment goals within a given session and attempt to

---

>> **DISPLAY 7.6**

Sources of Sensory Stimulation

Auditory	Visual	Olfactory	Tactile	Vestibular
Verbal orientation	Photographs	Vinegar	Hand holding	Turning
Music	Penlight	Spices	Rubbing lotion	Range of motion
Bells	Familiar objects	Perfume	Heat/cold	Sitting in chair
Familiar voice	Faces	Potpourri	Cotton balls	Tilt table
Tuning fork	Flashcards	Orange/lemon	Rough surfaces	
Clapping	Picture books		Familiar objects	

From Sosnowski C, Ustik M. Early intervention: coma stimulation in the intensive care unit. J Neurosci Nurs 1994;26:336–341.

engage the child at the current level of arousal and attention.[34] Again, the family can assist by describing what a typical day was like for the child prior to injury. This information can later be used to individualize the child's program. A schedule of the coma stimulation program and the materials to be used may be kept in a box in the child's room for convenience.

Prior to implementation, the physical therapist will need to educate the family on the provision of appropriate levels of sensory stimulation, including the amount of environmental stimulation being provided. Care should be taken to create an environment that is stimulating but not overstimulating or noxious. Decreasing extraneous auditory and visual activity in the child's room or treatment area may help the child focus on commands and elicit a response related to specific treatment stimuli.

At the beginning of the coma stimulation session, the physical therapist should orient the child with TBI to his or her surroundings, who is interacting with him or her, and the current date and time. Stimulation should be brief, not lasting for more than 15 minutes, and occur frequently, eight to 10 times a day, in order to avoid habituation. Stimulation should be implemented in an organized fashion, orienting the child to the stimulation prior to use, using one or two sensory modalities at a time and slowly presenting meaningful items. The therapist needs to be patient and allow time for the child to respond, as processing of sensory input may be delayed. A variety of responses may occur depending on the stimulation used (Display 7.7).[99] Precautions should be taken to prevent overstimulation of the child and to ensure that the child's medical status remains stable following stimulation. Unfavorable responses to stimulation include the development of seizure activity and sustained increases in heart rate, blood pressure, and respiratory rate.[99]

For the child who is generally unresponsive or responds only to pain, the initial goal of input is to elicit any type of response to stimuli. Once again, care should be taken to monitor the child for signs of overstimulation or poor tolerance of stimulation. However, as the child becomes more alert, the therapist should focus on increasing the consistency, duration, and quality of the child's response.

All team members and the family should be encouraged to document the stimuli utilized and the child's response to note progress and assist with carryover.

As the child begins to attend to therapy and follow one-step motor commands, the physical therapist can begin facilitation of movement with emphasis on head and trunk control and upper extremity movement patterns. The therapist should continue to monitor the patient for physiologic signs of sensory overload during treatment and make adjustments accordingly. As a more specific response to stimulation occurs, the physical therapist should try to improve the variety and consistency of the response and decrease delays in responding. Response should then be channeled into purposeful activity and functional skills. At this time, the physical therapist should also begin family education about future recovery phases and possible treatment techniques.

MIDCOGNITIVE LEVEL PHYSICAL THERAPY MANAGEMENT: STRUCTURE

When the child has emerged from coma and begins to participate in functional activities, other cognitive deficits may become evident. Selection of appropriate activities by the physical therapist should be based on cognitive as well as physical demands. However, the therapist will need to remember that the progression of cognitive and physical function can proceed at different rates.

THE AGITATED PATIENT

Initially, agitation is in response to poor regulation of stimulation and internal confusion. Factors that may contribute to agitation include overstimulation by staff, parents, and friends; restraints; occult fractures; pain; constipation; and urinary tract infections. Agitation may be expressed as bizarre or aggressive behaviors. Clinicians should take care in determining what extraneous stimuli increase agitation and attempt to reduce or eliminate the stimuli when possible. A child in a confused and agitated state requires the use of a highly structured environment to decrease the number of behavioral outbursts and prevent

---

>> **DISPLAY 7.7**

Common Responses to Stimulation

Auditory	Visual	Olfactory	Tactile	Vestibular
Startle reaction	Eye blink	Grimacing	Posturing	Spasticity/movement
Localization	Visual localization	Tearing	Withdrawal	Assisted range of motion
Turn toward sound	Visual tracking	Head turning	Localization	Head righting
Follow commands	Visual attention	Sniffing	General response	

From Sosnowski C, Ustik M. Early intervention: coma stimulation in the intensive care unit. J Neurosci Nurs 1994;26:336–341.

overstimulation. The physical therapist may need to give verbal reassurance to the child with TBI as some agitated behaviors can be related to fear. If precipitating factors cannot be successfully reduced or eliminated, then pharmacologic management should be considered.

In the management of agitation, it is important to utilize a team approach that includes the family. Common management strategies include having a quiet room with no television or telephone, limited visitors, and planned rest periods as needed. The child's family may resist suggestions to decrease visitors and stimuli, believing that talking loudly and turning on lights, television, and radio can help to increase the child's alertness and speed recovery.[52] Staff should reinforce appropriate levels of stimulation during family education.

It is important to protect the child who is agitated from potential injury. Restraints should be removed when possible as they may further agitation. If the unrestrained child is at risk for falling out of bed, it may be necessary to modify the room by placing the mattress on the floor or switch to an enclosed protective bed. Other protective devices include alarm devices, such as sensitized doormats and monitor bracelets used for a child or adolescent who is ambulatory and may wander away from supervision.

During the agitated phase, treatment should be modified to include activities that are familiar to the child and well liked to enhance participation and cooperation. Although the child may be able to perform familiar motor activities, the physical therapist should anticipate behavior that is essentially nonpurposeful. Appropriate tasks and activities include range-of-motion exercises to the child's tolerance and functional gross motor activities such as rolling, coming to sit, coming to stand, and walking. It is important for the physical therapist to work within the child's tolerance level on previously learned skills and to expect no carryover for new learning during this phase of recovery.

The child with TBI is often very unpredictable during the agitated phase, so the therapist should be prepared with numerous activity options. Choices of activities should be offered to the child when possible. When the child is uncooperative with familiar or routine activities, the physical therapist should first try to redirect the child to another therapeutic activity. If unsuccessful, the physical therapist may need to resort to involving the child in any activity in which he or she is willing to participate. Therapy of this nature is still beneficial to the child with TBI as it serves to increase attention span.

For the child who is extremely difficult to manage, co-treatment with other team members and shortened therapy sessions may be necessary until the child tolerates longer interactions. As attention span gradually increases, the physical therapist reinforces longer periods of attention and directs the child with TBI back to more challenging tasks.

THE CONFUSED PATIENT

Although no longer internally agitated, the child with TBI who is confused will require continued behavior management and structure during the therapy session to perform optimally. Structure may include decreasing the complexity of instructions, simplifying the environment, or breaking a motor task down into smaller components (Figs. 7.5 and 7.6). The primary goal of therapy during the confused phase of recovery is to enhance successful participation in functional tasks.

Initially, it will be necessary to keep the environment as distraction free as possible as the child may become agitated with external stimuli. In addition, the physical therapist should give the child as much structure and assistance for functional activities as necessary to allow for success. In patients with serious deficits, partial weight-bearing locomotion shows promise for retraining the patient during the early stages of gait training.[100] As performance improves, structure can be decreased and the child can be challenged to function in a more distracting environment.

When the child is confused, it is helpful to work on familiar activities so that the need for verbal instruction is reduced. When giving verbal instruction, the therapist should speak slowly and keep directions simple to allow for delays in processing verbal instructions. In addition,

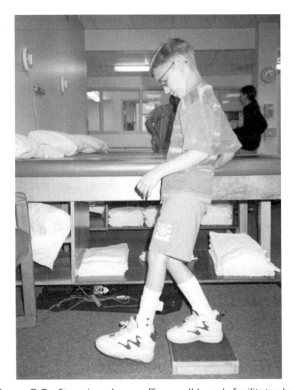

Figure 7.5 ■ Stepping down off a small bench facilitates heel strike with knee extension and improved eccentric control of the lower extremity. This component should later be practiced within the context of gait.

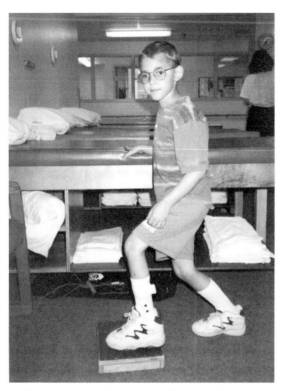

Figure 7.6 ■ Lunges on the involved lower extremity enhance weight shifts and may help improve hip and knee control.

the physical therapist may need to demonstrate new tasks instead of providing the child with verbal explanations to enhance understanding.

Orientation is very important during the confused phase of recovery. The physical therapist should remember to orient the child to his or her surroundings frequently and establish a familiar routine. The child's routine should allow for the same team members to see the child at the same times of the day in the same places. Thus, the child may begin to work on recall skills and begin to anticipate what is going to happen next in the day. Familiarity and routine are calming and reassuring and may assist with behavior management as well. Items such as a calendar, clock, and a schedule card may assist with orientation in an older child. In addition, the therapist may need to assist the child with topical orientation to his or her surroundings.

Encouraging the child to rely on his or her own memory for sequencing of movement or safety rules will challenge the child to become more independent. The use of a therapy journal or verbal rehearsal may help improve the child's memory. However, the therapist should be careful not to frustrate the child who has difficulty remembering. Instead of a continued open line of questioning, the therapist may offer choices and see if the child can recognize the right response. For example, a child who is learning to transfer from a wheelchair may be asked if he or she should scoot forward in the chair or lock the brakes first.

Although new learning is still limited, the physical therapist can begin to integrate principles of motor control and motor learning with principles of neurofacilitation to treat various focal deficits, impairments, and functional limitations. It is the physical therapist's responsibility to select developmentally appropriate functional skills that are motivating and challenging with the correct spatial and temporal demands for the child's abilities. The physical therapist should also focus on selecting functional activities that incorporate the use of both cognitive and physical skills. For example, an activity involving maneuvering a walker through an obstacle course addresses memory for verbal commands, motor planning, and mobility skills.

An essential element in motor learning is the opportunity for practice. The child with TBI should be allowed to experience movement with assistance as necessary, make mistakes, and make corrections as his or her ability levels dictate. Practice should encourage active participation in a meaningful play activity within the current capabilities of the child. Repeated practice will be necessary for the child to learn new or previously mastered gross motor tasks. The physical therapist will have to determine a practice schedule that is related to the expectations established in the plan of care. The therapist should be aware during practice that children with TBI may display reduced endurance and increased fatigue. The therapist may need to provide rest breaks for the child both within the therapy session and in between therapies.

Determining the type of feedback to be used during therapy is another important consideration in promoting learning. The physical therapist must make choices regarding the timing, precision, and frequency of feedback. In addition, the child's cognitive and sensory function will provide a guideline for determining the appropriate feedback mode. If a child is not aware of one side of his or her body, kinesthetic feedback may not be helpful to enhance learning, and visual and verbal feedback may be more appropriate (Fig. 7.7). Likewise, if a child is aphasic, the therapist will need to facilitate learning using visual and kinesthetic information.

As the child with TBI improves, the physical therapist must modify the task and the environment in order to continue to engage the child actively in therapy. If persistent behavioral problems exist, it may be necessary for the physical therapist to continue to use behavior modification techniques in order to increase compliance in therapy. At this stage of recovery, the child's judgment will be impaired, so it will be important to continue to protect the child from injury.

During both the agitated and the confused phases of recovery, the physical therapist should continue the use of positioning, resting splints, and casting as needed. Dynamic splints and orthotics for standing and gait activities may also assist with the management of spasticity. Tone-reducing ankle–foot orthoses (AFOs) with a footplate that supports

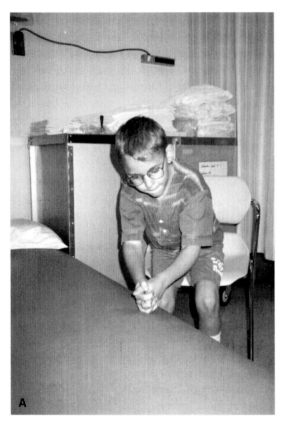
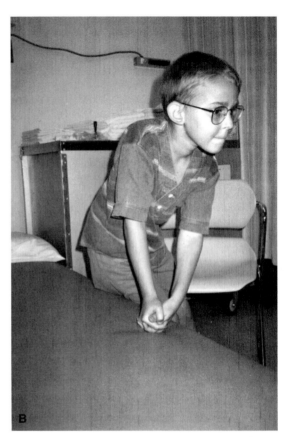

Figure 7.7 ■ (A, B) Verbal cues to use hands in midline during transfers may enhance the awareness of the involved side and improve safety during movement.

the longitudinal as well as the transverse arches have been found to be useful in reducing lower extremity spasticity and improving gait.[101–103] The disadvantages of braces are that they are more difficult to apply and need to be replaced more frequently than standard AFOs.[57]

HIGHER COGNITIVE LEVEL PHYSICAL THERAPY MANAGEMENT: SCHOOL/COMMUNITY REINTEGRATION

It is important for the physical therapist to remember that not all children will reach a high level of cognitive function and have complete physical recovery. Toward the end of the rehabilitation phase, permanent losses of cognitive and physical function become more apparent and plans must be made to reintegrate the child with TBI back into the home and/or school setting. The family, medical rehabilitation team, and school must work together and jointly plan for re-entry into the school setting. The physical therapist may re-evaluate the child for orthotics, assistive devices, and mobility devices necessary for function in the child's home and at school. In addition, the physical therapist may assist with recommendations regarding any environmental modifications to the child's home or school.

For the child with TBI who does reach the higher stages of cognitive recovery, the physical therapist will begin to wean the child from the cognitive cues and structure previously used in order to enhance further independence at home and/or school. Owing to the tendency of TBI to affect vision and hearing, memory, concentration, impulse control, and organizational skills, the classroom environment may be particularly difficult for the child with TBI.[57] Care should be taken to not remove the structure too early as memory retention and generalization of learning to new settings occurs at slower rates.

The physical therapist should also continue to focus on treating any residual motor deficits that interfere with functional independence at home or in school. For some children, this will mean continued training with assistive devices and physical assistance for basic motor skills, such as transfers and gait (Figs. 7.8 and 7.9). Constraint-induced movement therapy may show promise for improving the amount of use and the quality of movement in an impaired upper extremity.[104] For other children who may experience only subtle problems with balance and the speed, coordination, timing, and rhythm of movement, it will mean participation in more challenging physical activities, such as walking carrying objects, running, jumping, hopping, skipping, or exercise on the balance board and therapy ball (Figs. 7.10 and 7.11).

In addition to the problems of motor control and function, children who have experienced moderate or

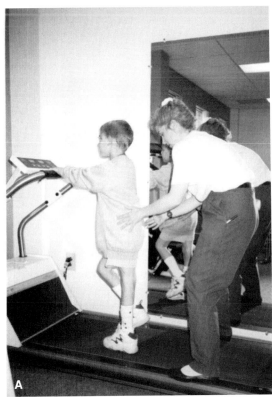
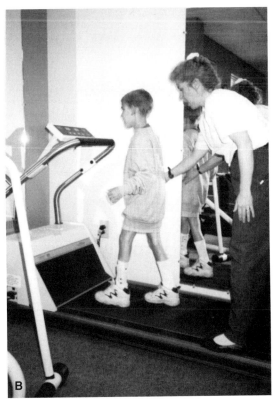

Figure 7.8 ■ The use of a treadmill in gait training may facilitate control at various speeds. Training may be performed both with **(A)** and without **(B)** upper extremity support to challenge balance on a dynamic surface.

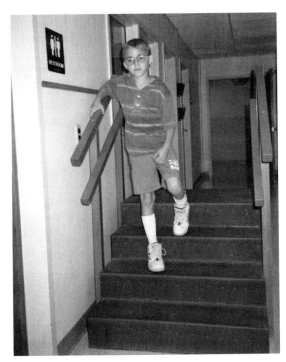

Figure 7.9 ■ In gait training on the stairs, note the increased support at the right forearm and the mild internal rotation of the right hip used to stabilize balance during descent. Verbal cues for trunk alignment and upper extremity support combined with leading with the left lower extremity may improve skill.

severe brain injury often have difficulty maintaining an appropriate level of fitness (Figs. 7.12 and 7.13). The physical therapist should design a fitness program that can be continued after contact with therapy as exercise may decrease feelings of depression and poor health.[105] The physical therapist can work also with the physical education teacher in designing an adapted physical education program for the child with TBI (Fig. 7.14).

SCHOOL ISSUES

Before 1990, the education system had no formal identification or tracking system for children with TBI. With the reauthorization of Public Law 94-142 in Public Law 101-476, the Individuals with Disabilities Education Act, the law now recognizes "brain injury" as a separate category of impairment in children.[57] Programs must be adapted for children with TBI. In addition to modifying the educational services the child receives, it is also reasonable to expect the school to provide physical assistance for activities of daily living, mobility, and motoric tasks, such as writing, in order to assist the child with achieving academic success. In turn, rehabilitation specialists, including physical therapists, are being called on to educate and train the existing teaching staff.[57]

Although the child with TBI may perform at a nearly age-appropriate level on achievement tests examining

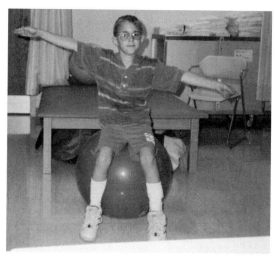

Figure 7.10 ■ The therapy ball can be used to challenge dynamic sitting balance and coordination. In addition to moving his arms to the side, the child could also practice alternating forward placement of his feet or move arms and legs in reciprocal, rhythmic patterns.

previously learned material, cognitive skills for future academic achievement are frequently impaired.[106] Often, the higher the preinjury IQ, the greater the IQ point loss following TBI.[107] Learning is frequently disrupted by complex information processing demands, distractions,

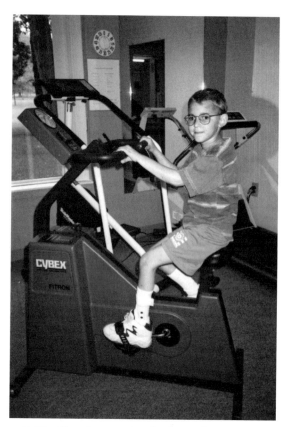

Figure 7.12 ■ Bicycling on standard exercise equipment can be used to promote aerobic exercise. It can also be done as part of training before returning to riding a standard child's bike.

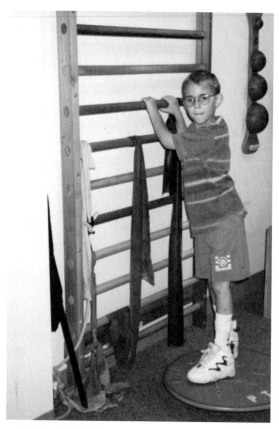

Figure 7.11 ■ A BAPS board can be used to enhance balance and coordination of the lower extremities.

and stress from lack of success.[47] In addition, although some children with TBI may physically appear normal, high social and academic expectations may cause the child to become frustrated and depressed. Without program modification, the child with TBI may develop significant academic and social problems during the pre-adolescent years.

To assist with the potential for academic success, the child with TBI will need modifications to his or her academic program. In his research, Telzrow identified 10 educational modifications that can be used to enhance the education of moderately to severely involved children with TBI.[106] These modifications include gradual reintegration into the general classroom; behavioral programming; integration of rehabilitation therapies; low pupil-to-teacher ratios; repetition and multimodality presentation of academic material; cueing and shadowing for vocational training; emphasis on process and not volume of material; simulations for generalization of skills to real life; readjustment counseling; and home–school liaison. In addition to these adaptations, the child with TBI may also benefit from an extended school year and additional tutoring, as the prolonged summer vacation may cause some students with TBI to lose headway in academic achievement.[57] A complete discussion of physical therapy in the school system is found in Chapter 19.

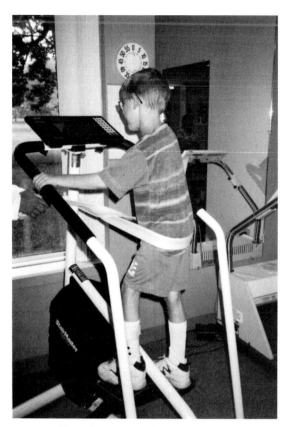

Figure 7.13 ■ Exercise on standard exercise equipment may not only improve endurance, but may also help improve strength. The stair stepper improves control in hip extensors and abductors, knee extensors, and ankle plantar flexors. The strap at the hips provides a cue to maintain hip extension alignment and to increase weight bearing on the more involved side.

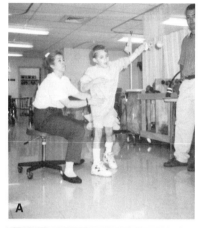

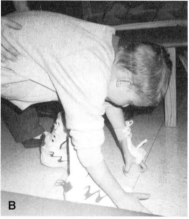

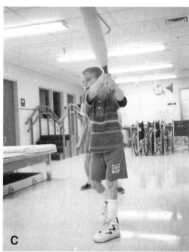

 Prevention

Prevention is the key to decreasing the annual incidence of TBI. Effective prevention involves decreasing the intensity of the impact to the brain, increasing options for direct prevention, and mandating protective laws.

BICYCLE HELMETS

The consistent use of bicycle helmets can decrease the incidence of injury, as unhelmeted riders are eight times more likely to have a brain injury than helmeted bicyclists.[108] Fit of the helmet is important, as poor fit has been associated with an increased risk of TBI in children, especially in boys.[109] Use of helmets can also potentially prevent brain injuries from occurring in sports and recreational activities including baseball, football, horseback riding, rollerblading, skateboarding, hockey, roller skating, skiing, and sledding.[2] Barriers to helmet use include the lack of awareness of recreational risks and the effectiveness of helmets, cost, and negative peer pressure. Increasing the use of helmets may be accomplished by advocating for educational

Figure 7.14 ■ Sports can be incorporated into therapeutic activities to enhance coordination, balance, and motor planning. A game of baseball can incorporate gross motor tasks of **(A)** throwing with the involved arm, **(B)** picking up a ground ball, and **(C)** batting.

programs, discount coupons, helmet subsidies, role modeling by parents, and mandatory legislative change.

PLAYGROUND EQUIPMENT

Prevention can also be aimed at preventing falls from playground equipment onto unprotected surfaces. The severity of the injuries can be remarkably decreased if the height of equipment does not exceed 5 feet and materials such as sand, pea gravel, or wood chips are used under the playground equipment.[2] Surface materials must be continually maintained if they are to be effective.

BABY WALKERS

Infant walker use in children between 6 and 18 months of age is very common in the United States, and parent surveys report that 30% to 40% of children using walkers experience some form of injury while in an infant walker.[110] It is important for parents to understand that infant walkers do not promote early walking skills. In addition, the physical therapist needs to offer some alternative, such as the use of safety gates or a playpen, which will allow the baby to move safely and freely within the home.

TRAFFIC BEHAVIOR

The inability of a child under 11 years of age to assess distances and speeds, combined with his or her normal impulsiveness, results in unsafe traffic behavior.[111] Even after training programs, the majority of young children still exhibit risky behavior and parents should be cautious of children crossing traffic alone. More effective community approaches should focus primarily on decreasing the traffic speed, enforcing laws governing pedestrian–motor vehicle interaction, and separating the pedestrian from the traffic[2] (see Case Study).

CAR RESTRAINTS

The use of occupant seat belt restraints is clearly an effective strategy for preventing injury if a crash occurs. The placement of the child in the back seat of the car and the correct use of car seats can prevent up to 90% of serious and fatal injuries to children under 5 years of age.[2] Unfortunately, misuse of child seats is still a common problem. In older children and adolescents, the use of lap and shoulder belts can prevent approximately 45% of serious and fatal injuries.[2]

CASE STUDY

Justin: Patient Client Management Applied to Preferred Practice Pattern 5C

Element of Patient/Client Management	Application for a Child with Acquired TBI
Examination	*Examples of history:* Age of child, past medical history, prior functional status, medications
	Examples of systems review: Blood pressure fluctuations, abrasion or other problem with skin integrity, inability to make needs known
	Examples of tests and measures: Postural observation, FIM, WeeFIM, PEDI, range of motion, muscle strength testing, gait analysis
Evaluation	*Synthesis* of observed impairments with *interpretation* from functional examination tools commonly used, such as the FIM and PEDI
Diagnosis	Physical therapy diagnosis based *impairments* and *functional limitations*
Prognosis and plan of care	*80%* of the patients in the preferred practice pattern will achieve the anticipated goals and expected outcomes within *six to 90 visits per episode of care*
Intervention	*Examples of coordination, communication, and documentation:* Case management, patient/client family meetings, outcome data
	Examples of topics for patient/client-related instruction: Current condition, plan of care, fitness program, risk factors, transitions across settings
	Examples of procedural interventions: Balance training, flexibility exercises, postural stabilization, neuromotor development training, gait training, device and equipment use, biofeedback, passive range of motion
Outcome	Use the *anticipated goals* and *expected outcomes* to assist with monitoring progress and documentation

---

Justin is an 8-year-old boy who experienced a traumatic brain injury secondary to a pedestrian-motor vehicle accident. He was unconscious at the scene of the accident and was life-flighted to the nearest pediatric trauma center. On arrival to the emergency room, he had a GCS of 2 and his pupils were fixed and dilated. Justin was in a coma. Diagnostic studies revealed diffuse right intracranial hemorrhage, a right pneumothorax, fracture of the left orbit, and multiple contusions. An ICP monitor, chest tubes, and placement of a tracheostomy tube were required for acute management.

Justin lives at home with his parents and a 6-year-old sister in a two-story home with five steps to enter. His bedroom and bathroom are on the second floor. His past medical history is unremarkable. Justin is a second-grade student at Jones Elementary.

The brain injury rehabilitation team was consulted 3 days after admission, and Justin was determined to be at a Rancho Los Amigos Scale level II. The brain injury team implemented a coma stimulation program. Caution was taken implementing the program due to his multiple injuries, monitors, and tube placements. In addition, the physical therapist initiated an inhibitory casting program to manage his left ankle plantar flexion posturing, which was measured at 45 degrees. A resting splint was made to maintain the right ankle in a neutral position. Based on the physical therapist's screening, systems review, and examination, Justin's medical diagnosis fits in the physical therapist preferred practice pattern 5C.[3]

Justin slowly emerged from the coma over a period of 2 weeks. Subsequent treatment focused on increasing tolerance to upright on the tilt table, facilitation of head control and sitting balance, and contracture management. During the next 2 weeks Justin's medical condition stabilized and he progressed to a Rancho Los Amigos Scale level V. Due to the severity of his brain injury and the presence of multiple impairments, the acute care team anticipated that Justin would require additional care in an acute rehabilitation setting and an outpatient setting, and additional services at his school setting. His episodes of care would most likely be on the higher end of the range anticipated for preferred practice pattern 5C.

As Justin awoke, his tracheostomy was removed and he was transferred to a pediatric rehabilitation center. The WeeFIM and the PEDI were used to examine his status upon admission and to determine his projected goals for improvement during his stay. Inhibitory casting was continued for the left ankle plantar flexion contracture, which was now measured at 20 degrees. Justin was given a high-back wheelchair for mobility with a custom-fit modular seating system for postural control. In addition to the previous intervention strategies, Justin also began to work on transfers from supine to sit and from the wheelchair to a mat with moderate assistance. He also engaged in standing activities and gait training. Decreased motor control and hemiplegia on the left were more evident as he increased his activity level. Justin moved in synergistic patterns for both the upper and lower extremity. Strength on the right side of the body was fair. Balance and coordination in upright were poor and he required maximal assistance for standing activities.

As rehabilitation progressed, Justin's condition improved and he began to follow commands consistently and showed some recall of newly learned tasks. His parents participated regularly in family conferences and family education and were instructed how to assist Justin during tasks of functional mobility as well as how to perform prescribed exercises. At the time of discharge from rehabilitation, Justin was able to propel himself in a regular wheelchair using the right extremities. He was able to transfer from the wheelchair to the mat with supervision and was able to walk short household distances with a forearm crutch on the right. He was still limited in his mobility by the left-sided spasticity. Justin had been evaluated for orthotics and was to receive a left dynamic AFO. Neuropsychological testing was completed prior to discharge and revealed deficiencies in short-term memory, attention span and focus, judgment, and agility to learn new material.

By four months after the injury, Justin was transitioning back into his school. His school program was modified for a half-day of inclusion in his regular classroom and a half-day of specialized classroom services. Justin would continue to receive physical therapy through the school setting. He was independent in his transfers and was ambulating with the left forearm crutch and the dynamic AFO more consistently. Justin used the wheelchair only for community mobility.

REFERENCES

1. Harrison CL, Dijkers M. Traumatic brain injury registries in the United States: an overview. Brain Inj 1992;6:203–212.
2. Rivara FP. Epidemiology and prevention of pediatric traumatic brain injury. Pediatr Ann 1994;1:12–17.
3. Guide to physical therapist practice. 2nd edition. Phys Ther 2001;81(1):1–768.
4. Centers for Disease Control and Prevention. Traumatic brain injury–Colorado, Missouri, Oklahoma and Utah, 1990–1993. Morb Mortal Wkly Rep 1997;46:8–11.
5. Varon J, Marik PE. The management of head trauma in children. Crit Care Shock 2002;5:133–143.
6. Guerrero JL, Thurman DJ, Sniezek JE. Emergency department visits associated with traumatic brain injury: United States, 1995–1996. Brain Inj 2000;14:181–186.
7. Kraus JF. Epidemiology of head injury. In: Cooper PR, Golfinos JG, eds. Head Injury. 4th Ed. New York: McGraw-Hill Companies, Inc., 2000:1–25.
8. Rivara FP. Child pedestrian injuries in the United States. Am J Dis Child 1990;144:692–696.
9. Tepas JJ, Ramenofsky ML, Barlow B, et al. Mortality in head injury: the pediatric perspective. J Pediatr Surg 1990;58:236–240.
10. Division of Injury Control, Center for Environmental Health and Injury Control, Centers for Disease Control. Childhood injuries in the United States. Am J Dis Child 1990;144:627–646.
11. Mazzola CA, Adelson PD. Critical care management of head trauma in children. Crit Care Med 2002;30(11 Suppl.):S393–S401.
12. Gedeit R. Head injury. Pediatr Rev 2001;22:118–124.
13. Adelson PD, Kochanek PM. Head injury in children. J Child Neurol 1998;13:2–15.
14. Bijur P, Golding J, Haslum M, et al. Behavioral predictors of injury in school-age children. Am J Dis Child 1988;142:1307–1312.
15. Davidson LL, Hughes SJ, O'Connor PA. Preschool behavior problems and subsequent risk of injury. 1988;82:644–651.
16. Goldstein F, Levin H. Epidemiology of pediatric closed head injury: incidence, clinical characteristics and risk factors. J Learn Disabil 1987;20:518–525.
17. Ponsford J, Willmott C, Rothwell A, et al. Cognitive and behavioral outcome following mild traumatic head injury in children. J Head Trauma Rehabil 1999;14(4):360–372.
18. Kraus JF, Rock A, Hemyari P. Brain injuries among infants, children, adolescents and young adults. Am J Dis Child 1990;144:684–691.
19. Williams RA. Injuries in infants and small children resulting from witnessed and corroborated free falls. J Trauma 1991;31:1350–1352.
20. Chadwick DL, Chin S, Salerno C, et al. Deaths from falls in children: how far is fatal? J Trauma 1991;31:1353–1355.
21. Zimmerman RA, Bilaniuk LT. Pediatric head trauma. Pediatr Neuroradiol 1994;4:349–366.
22. Centers for Disease Control and Prevention. Factors potentially associated with reductions in alcohol related traffic fatalities, United States, 1990–1991. Morb Mortal Wkly Rep 1992;41:213–215.
23. Rivara FP, Gurney JG, Ries RK, et al. A descriptive study of trauma, alcohol and alcoholism in young adults. J Adolesc Health 1992;13:663–667.

24. Wintemute GJ, Sloan JH. Head injury by firearm: epidemiology, clinical course, and options for prevention. J Head Trauma Rehabil 1991;6:38–47.

25. Rivara FP. Epidemiology of violent deaths in children and adolescents in the United States. Pediatrician 1983–1988;12:3–10.

26. Duhaime AC, Alairo AJ, Lewander J, et al. Head injury in very young children: mechanisms, injury types, and ophthalmologic findings in 100 hospitalized patients younger than 2 years of age. Pediatrics 1992;90:179–185.

27. Bonadio WA, Smith DS, Hillman S. Clinical indicators of intracranial lesion on computed tomographic scan in children with parietal skull fracture. Am J Dis Child 1989;143:194–196.

28. Hahn YS, McLone DG. Risk factors in the outcome of children with minor head injury. Pediatr Neurosurg 1993;19:134–142.

29. Kaufman BA, Dacey RG. Acute care management of closed head injury in childhood. Pediatr Ann 1994;23:18–28.

30. Pang D. Pathophysiologic correlates of neurobehavioral syndromes following closed head injury. In: Ylviasaker M, ed. Head Injury Rehabilitation. Austin, TX: Pro-Ed, 1985:3–70.

31. Griffith ER, Rosenthal M, Bond MR, et al., eds. Rehabilitation of the Child and Adult with Traumatic Brain Injury. 2nd Ed. Philadelphia: FA Davis, 1990.

32. Marion DW. Pathophysiology and initial neurosurgical care: future directions. In: Horn LJ, Zasler ND, eds. Medical Rehabilitation of Traumatic Brain Injury. Philadelphia: Hanley & Belfus, Inc., 1996:29–52.

33. Masters SJ. Evaluation of head trauma: efficacy of skull films. AJR Am J Roentgenol 1980;135:539–547.

34. Phillips WE. Brain tumors, traumatic head injuries, and near-drowning. In: Campbell SK, ed. Physical Therapy for Children. Philadelphia: WB Saunders Company, 1994:549–570.

35. Graham DI, Gennarelli TA. Pathology of brain damage after head injury. In: Cooper PR, Golfinos JG, eds. Head Injury. 4th Ed. New York: McGraw-Hill Companies, Inc., 2000:132–153.

36. Mysiw JW, Fugate LP, Clinchot DM. Assessment, early rehabilitation intervention, and ter-tiary prevention. In: Horn LJ, Zasler ND, eds. Medical Rehabilitation of Traumatic Brain Injury. Philadelphia: Hanley & Belfus, Inc., 1996:53–76.

37. Robertson CS, Contant CF, Narayan RK, et al. Cerebral blood flow, AVD02, and neurologic outcome in head-injured patients. J Neurotrauma 1992;9:S349–S358.

38. Konotos HA. Oxygen radicals in central nervous system damage. Chem Biol Int 1989;72:229–255.

39. Fullerton Long D. Diagnosis and management of intracranial complications in TBI rehabilitation. In: Horn LJ, Zasler ND, eds. Medical Rehabilitation of Traumatic Brain Injury. Philadelphia: Hanley & Belfus, Inc., 1996:333–362.

40. Hahn YS, Fuchs S, Flannery AM, et al. Factors influencing posttraumatic seizures in children. Neurosurgery 1988;22:864–867.

41. Weiner HL, Weinberg JS. Head injury in the pediatric age group. In: Cooper PR, Golfinos JG, eds. Head Injury. 4th Ed. New York: McGraw-Hill Companies, Inc., 2000:419–456.

42. Yablon SA. Posttraumatic seizures. In: Horn LJ, Zasler ND, eds. Medical Rehabilitation of Traumatic Brain Injury. Philadelphia: Hanley & Belfus, Inc., 1996:363–393.

43. Blendonohy PM, Philip PA. Precocious puberty in children after traumatic brain injury. Brain Inj 1991;5:63–68.

44. Bijur PE, Haslum M, Golding J. Cognitive and behavioral sequelae of mild head injury in children. Pediatrics 1990;86:337–344.

45. Ruijs MB, Keyser A, Gabreels FJM. Assessment of posttraumatic amnesia in young children. Dev Med Child Neurol 1992;34:885–892.

46. Kriel RL, Krach LE, Sheehan M. Pediatric closed head injury: outcomes following prolonged unconsciousness. Arch Phys Med Rehabil 1988;69:678–681.

47. Jaffe KM, Fay GC, Polissar NL, et al. Severity of pediatric traumatic brain injury and neurobehavioral recovery at 1 year—a cohort study. Arch Phys Med Rehabil 1993;74:587–595.

48. Teasdale G, Jennett B. Assessment of coma and impaired consciousness: a practical scale. Lancet 1974;2:81–84.

49. Hahn YS, Chyung C, Barthel MJ, et al. Head injuries in children under 36 months of age. Neurosurgery 1988;4:34–39.

50. Reilly PL, Simpson DA, Sprod R, et al. Assessing the conscious level in infants and young children: a pediatric version of the Glasgow Coma Scale. Childs Nerv Syst 1988;4:30–33.

51. Simpson DA, Cockington RA, Hanieh A, et al. Head injuries in infants and young children: the value of the Pediatric Coma Scale. Review of the literature and report on a study. Childs Nerv Syst 1991;7:183–190.

52. MacPherson V, Sullivan SJ, Lambert J. Prediction of motor status 3 and 6 months post severe traumatic brain injury: a preliminary study. Brain Inj 1992;6:489–498.

53. Wilson B, Vizor A, Bryant T. Predicting severity of cognitive impairment after severe head injury. Brain Inj 1991;5:189–197.

54. Fletcher J, Ewing-Cobbs L, Miner M. Behavioral changes after closed head injury in children. J Consult Clin Psychol 1990;58:93–98.

55. Lieh-Lai MW, Theodorou AA, Sarnaik AP, et al. Limitations of the Glasgow Coma Scale in predicting outcome in children with traumatic brain injury. J Pediatr 1992;120:195–199.

56. Gagnon I, Forget R, Sullivan SJ, et al. Motor performance following a mild traumatic brain injury in children: an exploratory study. Brain Inj 1998;12(10):843–853.

57. Ewing-Cobbs L, Levin HS, Fletcher JM, et al. The Children's Orientation and Amnesia Test: relationship to severity of acute head injury and to recovery of memory. Neurosurgery 1990;27:683–691.

58. Cockrell J. Pediatric brain injury rehabilitation. In: Horn LJ, Zasler ND, eds. Medical Rehabilitation of Traumatic Brain Injury. Philadelphia: Hanley & Belfus, Inc., 1996:171–196.

59. Russell WR. The Traumatic Amnesias. Oxford: Oxford University Press, 1971.

60. Hagen C, Makmus D, Durham P, et al. Levels of cognitive functioning. In: Rehabilitation of the Head-Injured Adult: Comprehensive Physical Management. Downey, CA: Professional Staff of Rancho Los Amigos Hospital, 1979:87–90.

61. Johnston MV, Hall K, Carnevale G, et al. Functional assessment and outcome evaluation in traumatic brain injury rehabilitation. In: Horn LJ, Zasler ND, eds. Medical Rehabilitation of Traumatic Brain Injury. Philadelphia: Hanley & Belfus, Inc., 1996:197–226.

62. Bowers MC, Edwards P. Outcome one to three years after severe traumatic brain injury. Br J Acc Surg 1991;22:315–320.

63. Staff from Denver Child's Hospital. Notes from Pediatric Rehab: Traumatic Brain Injury. Denver, CO, 1989.

64. Finger S. Brain damage, development, and behavior: Early findings. Dev Neuropsychol 1991;7:261–274.

65. Rivara FP. Epidemiology and prevention of pediatric traumatic brain injury. Pediatr Ann 1994;23:12–17.

66. Vargha-Khadem F, O'Gorman AM, Watters GV. Aphasia and handedness in relation to hemispheric side, age at injury and severity of cerebral lesion during childhood. Brain 1985;108:677–696.

67. Thomen IV. Late outcome of severe blunt head trauma. A 10–15 year second follow-up. J Neurol Neurosurg Psychiatry 1984;46:870–875.

68. Gagnon I, Swaine B, Friedman D, et al. Children show decreased dynamic balance after mild traumatic brain injury. Arch Phys Med Rehabil 2004;85:444–452.

69. Aitken ME, Jaffe KM, DiScala C, et al. Functional outcome in children with multiple trauma without significant head injury. Arch Phys Med. Rehab 1999;80(8):889–895.

70. Kuhtz-Buschbeck JP, Hoppe B, Dreesmann M, et al. Sensori-motor recovery in children after traumatic brain injury: analyses of gait, gross motor and fine motor skills. Dev Med Child Neurol 2003;45:821–828.

71. Jaffe KM, Brink JD, Hays RM, et al. Specific problems associated with pediatric head injury. In: Griffith ER, ed. Rehabilitation of the Adult and Child with Traumatic Brain Injury. 2nd Ed. Philadelphia: FA Davis Company, 1990: 539–556.

72. Haley SM, Dumas HM, Rabin JP, et al. Early recovery of walking in children and youths after traumatic brain injury. Dev Med Child Neurol 2003;45:671–675.

73. Taylor HG, Yeates KO, Wade SL, et al. Influences on first-year recovery from traumatic brain injury in children. Neuropsychology 1999;13(1):76–89.

74. Berger MS, Pitts LH, Lovely M, et al. Outcome of severe head injury in children and adolescents. J Neurosurg 1985;62: 194–199.

75. Rivara JB. Family functioning following pediatric traumatic brain injury. Pediatr Ann 1994;23:38–43.

76. Koch L, Merz MA, Lynch RT. Screening for mild traumatic brain injury: a guide for rehabilitation counselors. J Rehabil 1995;61:50–56.

77. Levin HS, Eisenberg HM. Neuropsychological impairment after closed head injury in children and adolescents. Childs Brain 1979;5:281–292.

78. Coffey RJ. Pediatric neurological emergencies. In: Pierog JE, Pierog LJ, eds. Pediatric Critical Illness and Injury: Assessment and Care. Rockville, MD: Aspen Systems Corporation, 1984: 95–106.

79. Sakai CS, Mateer C. Otological and audiological sequelae of closed head injury. Semin Hear 1984;5:157–173.

80. Griffith JT, Dodge PR. Transient blindness following head injury in children. N Engl J Med 1968;278:648–651.

81. Harwood-Nash DC. Abuse to the pediatric central nervous system. Am J Neuroradiol 1992;13:369–375.

82. Buys YM, Levin AV, Enzenauer RW, et al. Retinal findings after head trauma in infants and young children. Ophthalmology 1992;99:1718–1723.

83. Hurvitz EA, Mandac BR, Davidoff G, et al. Risk factors for heterotopic ossification in children and adolescents with severe traumatic brain injury. Arch Phys Med Rehabil 1992;73: 459–462.

84. Djergaian RS. Management of musculoskeletal complications. In: Horn LJ, Zasler ND, eds. Medical Rehabilitation of Traumatic Brain Injury. Philadelphia: Hanley & Belfus, Inc., 1996:459–477.

85. Sobus KML, Alexander MA, Harcke HT. Undetected musculoskeletal trauma in children with traumatic brain injury or spinal cord injury. Arch Phys Med Rehabil 1993;74:902–904.

86. Johns JS, Cifu DX, Keyser-Marcus L, et al. Impact of clinically significant heterotopic ossification on functional outcome after brain injury. J Head Trauma Rehabil 1999;14(3):269–276.

87. Molnar GE, Perrin JC. Head injury. In: Molnar GE, ed. Pediatric Rehabilitation. 2nd Ed. Baltimore: Williams & Wilkins, 1992:254–292.

88. Blasier D, Letts M. The orthopedic manifestations of head injury in children. Orthop Rev 1989;18:350–358.

89. Braun SL, Granger CV. A practical approach to functional assessment in pediatrics. Occup Ther Pract 1991;2:46–51.

90. Feldman AB, Haley SM, Coryell J. Concurrent and construct validity of the Pediatric Evaluation of Disability Inventory. Phys Ther 1990;70:602–610.

91. Kothari DH, Haley SM, Gill-Body KM, et al. Measuring functional change in children with acquired brain injury (ABI): comparison of generic and ABI-specific scales using the Pediatric Evaluation of Disability Inventory (PEDI). Phys Ther 2003;83(9): 776–785.

92. Bruininks RH. Bruininks-Oseretsky Test of Motor Proficiency: Examiners' Manual. Circle Pines, MI: American Guidance Services, 1978.

93. Haley SM, Cioffi MI, Lewin JE, et al. Motor dysfunction in children and adolescents after traumatic brain injury. J Head Trauma Rehabil 1990;5:77–90.

94. Fletcher JM, Miner ME, Ewing-Cobb L. Age and recovery from head injury in children: developmental issues. In: Levin HS, Greyman J, Eisenberg HM, eds. Neurobehavioral Recovery from Head Injury. New York: Oxford University Press, 1987.

95. Hall KM, Cope DN. The benefit of rehabilitation in traumatic brain injury: a literature review. J Head Trauma Rehabil 1995;10:1–13.

96. Conine TA, Sullivan T, Mackie T, et al. Effects of serial casting for the prevention of equinus in patients with acute head injury. Arch Phys Med Rehabil 1990;71:310–312.

97. National Head Injury Foundation. Directory of head injury, rehabilitation services. Southborough, MA, 1990.

98. Giles GM. The status of brain injury rehabilitation. Am J Occup Ther 1994;48:199–205.

99. Sosnowski C, Ustik M. Early intervention: coma stimulation in the intensive care unit. J Neurosci Nurs 1994;26:336–341.

100. Seif-Naraghi AH, Herman RM. A novel method for locomotion training. J Head Trauma Rehabil 1999;14:146–167.

101. Bronkjorst AJ, Lamb GA. An orthosis to aide in reduction of lower limb spasticity. Orthot Prosthet 1987;41:23–28.

102. Hinderer KA, Harris SR, Purdy AH, et al. Effects of "tone-reducing" vs. standard plaster-casts on gait improvement of children with cerebral palsy. Dev Med Child Neurol 1988; 30:370–377.

103. Sankey RJ, Anderson DM, Young JA. Characteristics of ankle-foot orthoses for management of the spastic lower limb. Dev Med Child Neurol 1989;31:466–470.

104. Karman N, Maryles J, Baker RW, et al. Constraint-induced movement therapy for hemiplegic children with acquired brain injuries. J Head Trauma Rehabil 2003;18:259–267.

105. Gordon WA, Sliwinski M, Echo J, et al. The benefits of exercise in individuals with traumatic brain injury: a retrospective study. J Head Trauma Rehabil 1998;13:58–67.

106. Telzrow CF. Management of academic and educational problems in head injury. J Learn Disabil 1987;20:536–545.

107. Dickerson-Mayes S, Pelco LE, Campbell CJ. Relationships among pre- and post-injury intelligence with severe closed-head injuries. Brain Inj 1989;3:301–313.

108. Thompson RS, Rivara FP, Thompson DC. A case-control study of the effectiveness of bicycle safety helmets. N Engl J Med 1989;320:1361–1367.

109. Rivara FP, Astley SJ, Clarren SK, et al. Fit of bicycle safety helmets and risk of head injuries in children. injury prevention. J Int Soc Child Adolesc Inj Prevent 1999;5:194–197.

110. Board of Trustees, AMA. Use of infant walkers. Am J Dis Child 1991;145:933–934.

111. Rivara FP. Child pedestrian injuries in the United States. Current status of the problem, potential interventions and future research needs. Am J Dis Child 1990;144:692–696.

Traumatic and Atraumatic Spinal Cord Injury in Pediatrics

Heather Atkinson and Elena M. Spearing

A s with all pediatric conditions requiring care from a physical therapist, working with a child poses special challenges. Treatment of a child with traumatic or atraumatic spinal cord injury not only demands attention to their current age-specific needs, but also requires special consideration of their physical, cognitive, and emotional development. Spinal cord injury is a lifelong disability, and physical therapists have the responsibility to anticipate the variety of changes a child will encounter as he or she grows and develops over his or her lifetime. A catastrophic illness or injury such as a spinal cord injury has profound effects on both the child and his or her family. A physical therapist has the unique opportunity to be not only a teacher, a guide, and an advocate, but also a coach who empowers his or her clients to live life to its fullest potential.

The National Spinal Cord Injury Association (NSCIA) defines pediatric spinal cord injury as an acute traumatic lesion of the spinal cord and nerve roots in children from newborn through 15 years of age.[1] According to the NSCIA, there are an estimated 11,000 new cases of SCI per year, with 10% affecting children ages 1 to 15. In the United States, there are currently 250,000 to 400,000 people living with spinal cord injury. The average age of injury is 33 and the most frequent age of injury is 19.

Eighty-two percent of those affected are men and 18% are women. This is most likely related to greater male participation in higher risk-taking behaviors.[2]

General mechanisms of traumatic spinal injury for adults include flexion/extension, axial loading, burst, and compression fractures. A child's spine, however, does not fully mature until between the ages of 8 and 10 years and therefore can lend itself to a different mechanism of injury. These immature features can predispose a child under 11 years old to an upper cervical spine injury at the level of C-3 or above.[3] Ligamentous laxity, disproportionately large head size, and relatively horizontal facet joints can create a fulcrum for a sagittal force and allow a large amount of translatory movement. A child over 11 years of age has a greater tendency toward injury to the lower cervical spine (C-3 and below) as opposed to the adult population.[3] Thoracolumbar injuries in young children are also unique due to anatomic differences from adults. Specifically, the ring apophysis in the growing pediatric spine can slip or separate into the spinal canal from an axial traumatic force and mimic the symptoms of a herniated intervertebral disk.[3] Finally, the ligamentous laxity in the pediatric spinal column can allow the vertebra to stretch and recoil during a force to the spine or head; however, this action also causes the relatively inflexible spinal cord inside to stretch as well. This stretching can cause distraction or ischemia to delicate neuropathways and cause an invisible spinal cord injury that is not picked up on radiographic assessment as there is no obvious fracture or dislocation. This phenomenon is known as spinal cord injury without radiographic abnormality (SCIWORA) and can present as a complete or incomplete injury. SCIWORA is a prevalent manifestation and has been reported in 19% to 34% of all children who experience spinal cord injury.[4] All children who have experienced a trauma should have both head injury and SCIWORA ruled out, due to the increased potential for neurologic devastation. SCIWORA can also have a delayed onset, so all medical staff including the physical therapist should carefully monitor the child's clinical presentation.

Additional causes of traumatic spinal cord injury include motor vehicle accident, violence, falls, and sports. The causes of spinal cord injury that are unique to pediatrics include birth trauma, child abuse, and motor vehicle lap belt injuries.[3] Motor vehicle restraints are designed to dissipate force over bony areas of the body to prevent injury during a crash. Small children are often improperly positioned in a car with the lap belt riding higher than the pelvis, causing a fulcrum of force in the thoracic or lumbar spine and severe pressure on the abdomen. Children with this type of injury often have a burn mark across the abdomen and may have significant visceral injury as well.[3,5]

Atraumatic spinal cord injury includes all other spinal cord dysfunction such as myelopathies, cancer, and stroke. Clinically, atraumatic spinal cord injury often presents similarly to either a complete or incomplete spinal cord injury. Myelopathies include both compressive and inflammatory disorders. Compressive myelopathies are often caused by an underlying structural abnormality (stenosis, spondylolisthesis) combined with some antecedent trigger such as a fall or car accident with resultant compression on the spinal cord. Chiari malformations and protruding discs also have the potential to cause compression on the spinal cord. Inflammatory myelopathies include an entire spectrum of neuroinflammatory disorders including acute transverse myelitis (ATM), Guillain-Barré syndrome (GBS), multiple sclerosis (MS), acute disseminated encephalomyelitis (ADEM), and neuromyelitis optica (NMO).[6]

Acute transverse myelitis affects both children and adults and has the potential to be significantly disabling.[7] The cause of transverse myelitis is not clearly defined, although more information is becoming available about its neuropathology and possible treatments. An underlying systemic inflammation or autoimmune disorder can trigger the development of any inflammatory myelopathy including transverse myelitis.[6,8] In addition, infection is also considered in these disorders and may initiate the cascade of events resulting in spinal cord dysfunction. There is some documentation relating the onset of transverse myelitis with vaccination, although the benefits of vaccination still far outweigh the risks.[6,8] There is also a high incidence of

an antecedent infection (respiratory, gastrointestinal, systemic) prior to the development of transverse myelitis. It is thought that this antecedent infection initiates a cascade of cellular and immune-mediated events that ultimately result in attack of the spinal cord. A specific protein byproduct in this cellular reaction (interleukin-6) has a unique affinity for the spinal cord and has been demonstrated to kill spinal cord cells. Additionally, the spinal cord itself responds differently from other internal organs in how it responds to autoimmune dysfunction.[6,8] Although it is still unknown why a specific transverse segment of the spinal cord is targeted, increased knowledge about the immunopathogenesis of transverse myelitis is leading to better treatment options. These options will be discussed later in this chapter.

Atraumatic spinal cord injury can also be caused by cancer. This may be a primary tumor with focal dysfunction or it could be in the form of metastases with more diffuse dysfunction. Nonetheless, the physical effects can include sensory and motor abnormalities as well as spasticity and bowel and bladder dysfunction.[9]

Another form of atraumatic spinal cord injury is stroke. This can be caused by arterial or venous ischemia, watershed infarct, arteriovenous malformation (AVM), or a dural arteriovenous fistula. Onset can be either sudden or gradual, depending on the type of bleed. The overall course of recovery may vary as well.[10]

Although traumatic and atraumatic injuries can present similarly, understanding the exact nature of the injury can assist the clinician in formulating a hypothesis that will guide the examination, evaluation, diagnosis, prognosis, intervention, and ultimately outcome that the child achieves.

 Examination

HISTORY

The physical therapist begins with a thorough history taken from all available resources. This may include any or all of the following.

HISTORY OF PRESENT ILLNESS

- Mechanism and date of injury
- Any loss of consciousness at the time of injury or potential brain injury
- Any acute medical treatment received (spinal stabilization, steroids, etc.)
- Description of onset and progression of symptoms if atraumatic
- Any medical tests, labs, procedures, or films relating to the injury
- Any complications or comorbidities apparent during hospital course
- Medications for current or any other condition

MEDICAL HISTORY

- All other pertinent medical information including hospitalizations or procedures
- Birth history if applicable to mechanism or onset of injury

DEVELOPMENTAL HISTORY

- Developmental history, including prior level of function
- Any previously owned adaptive equipment

SOCIAL HISTORY

- Cultural beliefs and behaviors
- Primary caregivers, family, and resources
- Learning style of client and caregivers
- Current living situation including living environment, community characteristics, and projected discharge destination
- Social interactions, activities, and support systems
- Current and prior school situation (services received, individualized education plans)
- Leisure activities/sports/dreams for the future

SYSTEMS REVIEW

Guided by the history and initial information, the physical therapist proceeds to examine the patient system by system.

CARDIOVASCULAR/PULMONARY

Vital signs such as blood pressure, heart rate, and respiratory rate are taken before, during, and after activity. Evaluating tolerance for the upright position can sometimes be a slow process as patients with spinal cord injury are at risk for orthostatic hypotension. Compression stockings and abdominal binders are helpful to aid in vascular support. Patients with a lesion above T-6 are also at risk for autonomic dysreflexia (Display 8.1).

Patients with neuromuscular weakness also have decreased respiratory efficiency. Quality of cough, breathing pattern, and chest and diaphragmatic excursion measurements should be taken. Access to medical tests such as vital capacity and forced expiratory volume are also helpful. For patients on ventilators, parameter settings should be noted. Collaboration with medical, nursing, and respiratory staff can help in assessing respiratory potential. These measurements may need to be repeated, especially if the child is weaning ventilatory support. In some practice settings, physical therapists have an active role in airway clearance interventions. Therefore, a complete examination of the pulmonary system is necessary.

INTEGUMENTARY

The skin of a child with a spinal cord injury must be fully assessed. This includes color, integrity, bruising, and the presence of any scar formation. Neurovascular signs such as pulses, skin temperature, and edema should also be assessed regularly. Decubitus ulcers can be a chronic problem for children with spinal cord injury, and vigilant pressure relief and proper skin care are the only way to prevent this problem. Education regarding position changes and pressure relief should begin during the initial examination (Displays 8.2 through 8.4).

MUSCULOSKELETAL SYSTEM

Range of motion (ROM), tone, strength, symmetry, and posture are assessed. In the acute phase, tone may initially be flaccid and ROM full, but special precautions are required to prevent loss of flexibility. Spasticity can begin quickly and interfere with the child's flexibility goals. ROM assessment should be performed with overall diagnosis and prognosis in mind. For example, shortening of

---

» DISPLAY 8.1

Autonomic Dysreflexia

Autonomic dysreflexia is the body's response to lack of sympathetic input during noxious stimuli. The noxious stimulus may include kinked catheter tubing, constipation, muscle spasm, ingrown toenail, or even range-of-motion exercises. Symptoms vary but most often include elevated blood pressure, diaphoresis, headache, and bradycardia and require immediate attention. Treatment requires removal of the noxious stimulus, positioning to decrease blood pressure, and pharmacologic intervention if needed. If left untreated, autonomic dysreflexia may progress to a life-threatening situation.

» DISPLAY 8.2

Nutrition

It is important for any person with a new spinal cord injury to have a full nutritional workup in order to ensure that caloric intake is meeting new energy demands and that there is a healthy balance between intake and output. Patients with spinal cord injury are at risk for lowered immunity and decreased nutritional status.[51] Unfortunately, both of these issues can delay wound healing so it is important for the physical therapist to discuss nutritional status with the child's physician and nutritionist if there is any disruption in skin integrity. The physical therapist may also refer a child with a spinal cord injury to a nutritionist at any point along the continuum of care in order to promote a healthy and balanced diet that is individualized for that child's unique needs.

DISPLAY 8.3

Latex Allergy

Patients with significantly increased exposure to latex products, such as children with myelomeningocele or spinal cord injury, can develop an allergy to latex. In order to decrease their exposure to latex, products that are latex-free should be used whenever possible. Due to the need for catheterization supplies and gloves, over the course of a lifetime, many institutions now advocate a "latex-free" environment in which health care workers and other caregivers utilize latex alternatives to provide care. Many products commonly found in both the home and hospital environment contain latex and have the potential to cause a reaction in the client. Care must be taken to ensure that the client does not encounter latex if he or she already has an allergy to it or to prevent one from occurring. Products that contain latex include Thera-Band, Ace wraps, catheters, many toys, balloons, and even Band-Aids. Many companies offer a latex-free substitute for therapeutic modalities.

certain structures (long finger flexors, low back extensors) may be desirable in some situations. Similarly, over-lengthening of certain muscle groups such as the hamstrings and shoulder internal rotators may be desirable depending on the expected functional outcomes.

Spasticity assessment is performed by using the modified Ashworth scale while noting any clonus or spasms (Displays 8.4 and 8.5). Spasticity may vary throughout the day or with different activities and may even be useful in some functional situations. For example, someone with significant lower extremity weakness may rely on his or her spasticity for stability in weight bearing for transfers or ambulation. Some patients can even learn to trigger a spasm in order to help their lower extremity move in a certain way. Conversely, excessive spasticity can lead to problems with ROM, positioning, or comfort. For incomplete spinal cord

DISPLAY 8.4

Advantageous Muscle Imbalances

Allowing shortening of the long finger flexors can allow a tenodesis grasp for someone who is able to extend his or her wrist but is unable to actively grasp. It can also allow someone who cannot extend his or her wrist to use his or her hand as a hook. Tightening of low back extensors can improve sitting stability and assist in moving the lower part of the body in someone with paraplegia. Conversely, excessive shoulder extension and external rotation can combine to substitute for absent triceps, and a straight leg raise of 120 degrees is imperative to allow floor-to-wheelchair transfers.

DISPLAY 8.5

Modified Ashworth Scale[52]

0 = No increase in tone

1 = Slight increase in muscle tone, manifested by a catch and release or by minimal resistance at the end range of motion (ROM)

1+ = Slight increase in muscle tone, manifested by a catch, followed by minimal resistance throughout the remainder (less than half) of the ROM

2 = More marked increase in muscle tone through most of the ROM, but the affected part is easily moved

3 = Considerable increase in muscle tone, passive movement is difficult

4 = Affected part is rigid

injuries and those experiencing neurologic recovery, spasticity can mask underlying neuromuscular recovery; however, it may be necessary for functional activities. A thorough knowledge of the child's spasticity and movement patterns will assist the therapist in understanding the child's process of recovery. It will also allow the therapist to make valuable contributions to the medical team. Medical management often requires a balance between decreasing and increasing spasticity based on the child's goals and functional needs. Therapists should have a thorough understanding of the medical management of spasticity in order to provide educated recommendations to the physician.

For strength assessment in the pediatric population, performing manual muscle testing can provide valuable information if the child is able to fully participate in the examination. Games such as "Simon Says" can be useful in helping the child understand the task. For the very young or those with cognitive impairments, strength testing can be performed with observation, noting whether the child has the ability to move against gravity or against any resistance (i.e., reaching for a toy in different planes of movement or lifting/kicking against something with force). In the case of spinal cord injury, the therapist should note both gross and individual muscle strength and prevent substitution by the patient. It is important for the physical therapist to assess motor abilities of all spinal levels as this information will have significant impact for the physical therapy diagnosis and prognosis. Strength assessment should be performed on a regular basis in the early phases of recovery as the period of spinal shock can produce different results.

Sensory examination includes a thorough screen of all sensory spinal tracts and further individualized testing when warranted. Light touch, temperature, pinprick, and proprioception are important indicators of spinal function. The clinician can further pinpoint where the breakdown occurs using a dermatomal chart indicating spinal level.

The presence or absence of any sensory or motor function in the lowest sacral segment is an indication of prognosis, and should not be overlooked in the examination process. Often this information is obtained by the examining physician; however, in some practice settings a physical therapist may also perform this assessment.

Position, posture, and alignment must be assessed in children with spinal cord injury. Children with muscular weakness and imbalances are at risk for developing spinal deformities and scoliosis. Proper positioning is a crucial component to maintaining proper alignment. Radiographic films of the bones and joints can assist the therapist in determining the child's skeletal alignment (Display 8.6).

NEUROMUSCULAR SYSTEM

In the neuromuscular system, the physical therapist examines all functional movements. Movements can be isolated or synergistic during functional activity. Functional movements are related to available ROM, tone, and strength. While the therapist may strive for assisting the client to achieve the most "normal" movement pattern, it may be more important to the client to be able to perform the activity in any way possible. Neuromuscular assessment also includes gross coordinated movements including functional mobility, transfers, locomotion, balance, and coordination. In the acute stages of a new spinal cord injury, functional movement may be limited to bed mobility and sitting balance on the edge of the bed. When the injury is no longer acute or during re-examination, the client may be able to withstand more rigorous examination. For those with spinal cord injury, this portion of the examination also includes wheelchair mobility and skills.

In these cases, the wheelchair is considered as an extension of the person's body.

The physical therapist also examines the client's communication, affect, cognition, language, and learning style. This includes the client's level of consciousness; orientation to person, place, and time; ability to make his or her needs known; expected emotional and behavioral responses; and learning preferences (for both the child and the caregiver). If the child has sustained either a mild or more severe traumatic brain injury as a result of the accident, the physical therapist should also consider examination techniques outlined in Chapter 7 (Display 8.7). A knowledge of normal cognitive development will assist the therapist in determining what may be a new cognitive deficit versus a deficit that was present prior to the onset of the spinal cord injury.

TESTS AND MEASURES

The physical therapist has a wide variety of tests and measures to further characterize and quantify the information gathered during the examination. These include, but are not limited to:

- Aerobic capacity and endurance
- Anthropometric characteristics
- Assistive and adaptive devices
- Arousal, attention, and cognition
- Circulation
- Cranial and peripheral nerve integrity
- Environmental, home, and work (job/school/play) barriers
- Ergonomics and body mechanics
- Gait, locomotion, and balance
- Integumentary integrity
- Joint integrity and mobility
- Motor function (motor control and motor learning)
- Muscle performance (including strength, power, and endurance)
- Neuromotor development and sensory integration
- Orthotic, protective, and supportive devices

» DISPLAY 8.6

Heterotopic Ossification

Patients with upper motor neuron lesions such as spinal cord injury are at risk for the development of heterotopic ossification (HO). Primary areas affected are large joints such as the hip, shoulder, knee, and elbow. Patients are most at risk during the first 1 to 4 months after injury. There is no acute treatment for the pediatric population since medications that are used for the prevention of HO in adults have not been approved for use with the pediatric population. HO can be surgically excised but only after the abnormal bone formation is completely mature, usually 1 to 2 years after onset. Current best practice advocates the use of gentle range of motion (ROM) to affected joints and avoiding immobilization or aggressive ROM.[52,53] The entire team should be vigilant in screening for the development of heterotopic ossification since it can be a major setback for the child.

» DISPLAY 8.7

Traumatic Brain Injury

Because of the high velocity and trauma often associated with spinal cord injury, there is an increased risk of associated traumatic brain injury, which may be as high as 24% to 59%.[54,55] Consequently, cognition should always be screened and neuropsychological testing may be indicated with any person who has sustained a spinal cord injury in order to rule out any mild deficits.

- Pain
- Posture
- Range of motion (including muscle length)
- Reflex integrity
- Self-care and home management (including activities of daily living [ADLs] and instrumental ADLs [IADLs])
- Sensory integrity
- Ventilation and respiration
- Work (job/school/play), community, and leisure integration or reintegration (including IADLs)

 ## Evaluation, Diagnosis, and Prognosis

During the evaluation process, the physical therapist synthesizes the information that was discovered during the history, systems review, and tests and measures. He or she then formulates a physical therapy diagnosis and prognosis. In the case of spinal cord injury, the type and severity of the injury is central to establishing a prognosis and a plan of care.

Standards for neurologic and functional classification of spinal cord injury were identified by the American Spinal Injury Association (ASIA) in 1982.[11] This multidisciplinary group of experts established common terminology and a standard classification system for the medical field. It was last revised in 2006. Using the information from the examination and the guidelines set forth by the ASIA, the clinician can assess the client's myotomes and dermatomes, allowing the therapist to determine a sensory and a motor diagnostic level for both the right and left sides of the body. Furthermore, the ASIA classification states whether the injury is complete or incomplete. The clinician can then assign an ASIA level of impairment (Display 8.8) for classification. Some spinal cord lesions present as a clinical syndrome, as described in Display 8.9, and this terminology can also be used universally when dis-

cussing the client's presentation with other health care professionals. Although the ASIA has not yet published a specific worksheet for children and youth, current study supports the notion that several modifications may be applicable.[12] ASIA testing is widely inappropriate for children under 4 due to their inability to understand directions of the examination, and children under 8 may have unreliable pinprick examinations due to anxiety.[18] Further study and suggestions for the pediatric client are warranted in order to describe a truer classification of spinal injury.[18]

Physical therapy diagnoses for this population may include the following: decreased strength, decreased ROM, decreased endurance, decreased airway clearance and respiratory efficiency, decreased functional mobility, and decreased independence in the home, school, or community due to spinal cord injury.

After establishing a physical therapy diagnosis, the clinician can prognosticate the optimal level of function the child may achieve. The amount and intensity of physical therapy services required to achieve that level of function can be discussed as well as future episodes of care that may be needed over the course of the child's lifetime. Formulating a physical therapy prognosis incorporates information from the examination and should be based on evidence from current scientific literature. The physical therapist is also guided by the medical prognosis in developing goals that the child may be able to achieve. Prognoses for someone with a complete injury and someone with an incomplete injury can be very different based on neurologic potential for recovery. Studies suggest that some individuals with spinal cord injury may skip to the next level on the ASIA Impairment Scale during the period of neurologic recovery.[13–15] Ongoing reassessment of the patient using the ASIA Impairment Scale is

---

> ## DISPLAY 8.9

ASIA Clinical Syndromes[18]

Central cord syndrome: Presents with greater weakness in the upper extremities than the lower extremities and presents with sacral sparing

Brown-Sequard syndrome: Presents with ipsilateral proprioceptive and motor loss and contralateral loss of pinprick and temperature

Anterior cord syndrome: Presents with variable loss of motor function and sensation to pinprick and temperature and has sparing of proprioception

Conus medullaris syndrome: May present with areflexic bladder, bowel, and lower extremities or may show preserved bulbocavernosus and micturition reflexes

Cauda equina syndrome: Presents with areflexic bladder, bowel, and lower extremities

---

> ## DISPLAY 8.8

ASIA Impairment Scale[18]

A = Complete. No sensory or motor function is preserved in sacral segments S-4 to S-5.

B = Incomplete. Sensory but not motor function is preserved below the neurologic level and extends through the sacral segments S-4 to S-5.

C = Incomplete. Motor function is preserved below the neurologic level, and the majority of key muscles below the neurologic level have a muscle grade <3.

D = Incomplete. Motor function is preserved below the neurologic level, and the majority of key muscles below the neurologic level have a muscle grade ≥3.

critical not only to understand the patient's current status and potential ability, but also to monitor for possible change. The most significant recovery is expected in the first year after injury, but some patients show improvement for up to 5 years.[21]

Although the principles of examination, evaluation, and diagnosis are similar to those of clients with traumatic injuries, atraumatic spinal cord injuries can be more unpredictable in their outcomes. Transverse myelitis can have varying functional outcomes. Approximately 30% of those afflicted have full recovery, 30% have partial recovery, and another 30% have little to no recovery.[16] There are some medical factors that help prognosticate recovery including speed of onset, amount of paralysis, and speed of recovery in the first month, but these are never certain, as the Case Study at the end of this chapter will illustrate. Published research also demonstrates that a high level of interleukin-6 in the cerebrospinal fluid correlates with a poor functional outcome.[8,17] The potential for a large amount of neurologic recovery can alter the entire focus of physical therapy from goals of learning to compensate with the remaining intact musculature to a goal for recovering lost function. Atraumatic spinal cord injury caused by a tumor may present with similar clinical symptoms to a traumatic spinal cord injury, but cancer treatment such as radiation and chemotherapy can have profound effects on the child's functioning, physical therapy treatment, and the family as a whole. This can greatly impact the child's prognosis.

When considering the child's prognosis, the clinician should keep in mind both the child's potential for neurologic recovery and the functional outcomes that can be realistically achieved. Although no standard functional outcome measure for pediatric clients with traumatic or atraumatic spinal cord injury has been documented, the clinician can identify anticipated functional outcomes based on both the adult spinal cord injury literature and myelodysplasia literature. A discussion of general functional expectations by level of involvement is discussed in Table 8.1.[18]

Understanding the child's prognosis for functional outcomes leads the clinician to develop a plan of care that includes specific interventions and the frequency, intensity, and duration of those interventions. It also incorporates anticipated goals, expected outcomes, and discharge plans. When working in an interdisciplinary model, the plan of care may involve other health care professionals in both establishing interdisciplinary goals and providing the intervention to achieve them. For example, a child working on transfers in the hospital should have the opportunity to practice these transfers in a variety of environments and situations that incorporate the family, nurses, and other therapists and to help simulate the situations the child will encounter after discharge.

Standardized outcome measures performed prior to and after physical therapy intervention are useful in meas-uring the progress the child has made over the course of an episode of care. Some outcome measures include the WeeFIM (Functional Independence Measure), Pediatric Evaluation of Disability Inventory (PEDI), and Gross Motor Function Measure (GMFM).[19] Creativity may sometimes be useful in modifying existing outcome measures for a patient with paralysis. For example, the 9-minute walk/run can be modified into a 9-minute "wheelchair run" to measure endurance. The physical therapist should be familiar with all available outcome measures in order to choose the most appropriate one for the client. Standardized outcome measures can help the therapist pinpoint weaknesses as well as focus and modify the plan of care.

Intervention

MEDICAL INTERVENTION

SURGERY

MUSCLE TRANSFERS Recent advances in surgical techniques have allowed for the transfer of muscle function from one group to another. If there is sufficient remaining muscle strength in two or more muscle groups that work together to perform a movement, one of the muscles can be transferred biomechanically to perform another movement. There is little or no adverse effect on the original motion. Most commonly elbow extension is achieved by transferring the posterior deltoid to the triceps. Similarly, wrist extension is achieved by transferring the brachioradialis to the extensor carpi radialis. Active grasp is achieved by transferring the brachioradialis and using it as a thumb flexor.[20]

Processes such as tenodesis, arthrodesis, tendon lengthenings, rerouting, releases, and tendon transfers have the capacity to restore function to persons with tetraplegia. There is an abundance of literature on these procedures in the adult population. Although there are fewer studies performed on children, the results are similar.[26]

SPASTICITY

Spasticity is the clinical manifestation that accompanies upper motor neuron disease. A muscle displays an increased resistance to passive motion that results from the hyperactivity of the spinal and brainstem reflexes. In spinal cord injury, acutely, there is usually flaccidity, and then flexor spasticity presents and then finally extensor spasticity. Options for this population are similar to those with central nervous system dysfunction. Oral baclofen, intrathecal baclofen, botulinum toxin, and neurologic and orthopedic surgery are options when spasticity interferes with daily function.

The medical management of spasticity with movement can be conservative by removing the noxious stimuli,

> **TABLE 8.1**
>
> **Functional Expectations by Level of Involvement**

Level of Injury	Mobility	Transfers	Activities of Daily Living
C-1–C-4	• Sipping or blowing to independently control a power wheelchair, power tilt mechanism and environmental controls	• Dependent for all transfers	• Dependent for dressing, bathing, and bowel and bladder management
C-5: Addition of biceps and deltoids	• Can propel a manual wheelchair with hand rims for short distances on level surfaces • Power wheelchair for longer distances	• Able to assist with transfers and bed mobility	• Able to assist with feeding, grooming with adaptive equipment and setup • Dependent for dressing and bathing
C-6: Addition of pectorals	• Able to independently use manual wheelchair with projections on the hand rims	• Independent with self-care with equipment • Independent with upper extremity dressing, assists with lower extremity • Independent with bowel program, needs assistance with bladder program • Can drive with a specially adapted van	• Assists with sliding board transfers
C-7–T-1: Addition of triceps	• Able to independently propel a manual wheelchair on level surfaces	• Independent with adaptive equipment • Can drive a car with hand controls	• Independent transfers with or without sliding board
T-4–T-6: Addition of upper abdominal	• Can ambulate with RGOs for short distances with a walker	• Independent for grooming, bowel and bladder, dressing and bathing	• Independent transfers with or without sliding board
T-9–T-12: Addition of lower abdominals	• Household ambulation with RGOs or HKAFOs and assistive device	• Independent for grooming, bowel and bladder, dressing and bathing	• Independent transfers with or without sliding board
L-2–L-4: Addition of gracilis, iliopsoas, and quadratus lumborum	• Functional ambulation with KAFOs with crutches	• Independent for grooming, bowel and bladder, dressing and bathing	• Independent transfers with or without sliding board
L-4–L-5: Addition of hamstrings, quadriceps, and anterior tibialis	• Able to ambulate with AFOs with or without assistive device	• Independent for grooming, bowel and bladder, dressing and bathing	• Independent transfers with or without sliding board

AFO, ankle–foot orthosis; HKAFO, hip–knee–ankle–foot orthosis; KAFO, knee–ankle–foot orthosis; RGO, reciprocating gait orthosis.

stretching, positioning, orthotics, biofeedback, and electric stimulation. These all have short-term effects. When that is not enough, there are other agents that have been shown to reduce muscle spasticity.[21] Pharmacologically, baclofen acts as a γ-aminobutyric acid (GABA) analog at the site of the spinal cord. A common side effect, however, is that baclofen can cause drowsiness, fatigue, and weakness.[22,27] Baclofen administered intrathecally acts directly on the spinal cord with less risk of drowsiness and weakness than oral baclofen. There is risk of infection with the pump insertion.[27] Dantrolene sodium acts on the muscle to

inhibit the release of calcium from the sarcoplasmic reticulum. This medication carries the same effects of drowsiness and fatigue and can damage liver function. Clonidine via the oral route or patch acts centrally as an α agonist. Clonidine can lead to hypotension; however, side effects are limited to dry mouth and drowsiness. Diazepam (Valium) acts on the limbic system. Adverse reactions can include drowsiness and fatigue, and use can lead to drug dependency.[27]

Chemical nerve blocks work at the motor point. Lidocaine is a short-acting agent. Phenol can last up to

6 months. Botulinum toxin is so specific that it goes straight to the muscle.[27]

PAIN

The adult literature has shown that patients with spinal cord injury experience many different complaints of pain.[23,27,28] Studies of chronic pain reported by children are few but do report the same results. They report that pain associated with pediatric-onset spinal cord injury is common. Reports of nociceptive pain were greater than neuropathic pain.[30] Data suggest that although it is common, chronic pain in childhood SCI has a significantly smaller impact on daily activities than that reported in the literature for adult-onset SCI.[24]

Studies have looked at multiple interventions for pain, including medications, physical therapy, psychotherapy, and spinal cord stimulators. There is consistency in the reports of pain in patients with spinal cord injury; the reports of pain continue through the postacute stage, with 60% of patients with a spinal cord injury reporting pain at 6 and 12 months postinjury.[27] The International Association for the Study of Pain has proposed a scheme for characterizing spinal cord injury. It classifies pain into two types: neuropathic and nociceptive. Nociceptive pain is musculoskeletal and visceral. Neuropathic pain is classified as above the level, at the level, or below the level of injury. Nociceptive pain is characterized by dull, aching, movement-related pain that is eased by rest and responds to opioids. Neuropathic pain is usually described as sharp, shooting, burning, and electrical with abnormal sensory responsiveness (hyperesthesia or hyperalgesia). Antidepressants and anticonvulsants are usually used for SCI; however, neither is particularly effective for SCI pain. Recent reports have shown promise for opioids and α-adrenergic antagonists, as well as baclofen, a GABA-b agonist, when there is spasticity interfering with function.[27]

Sodium channel blockers such as lidocaine and tetracaine hydrochloride have shown decreases in allodynia (pain from a stimulus that is not usually painful). Opioids have been demonstrated to help neuropathic pain as well as nociceptive pain. Intrathecal clonidine in combination with morphine had an analgesic effect in patients with spinal cord injury.[27]

SURGICAL PROCEDURES Surgical procedures such as cordectomy, cordotomy, and myelotomy are most effective for spontaneous lancinating or shooting pain. They are not effective for burning or aching pain. Complications associated with these procedures include contralateral pain, bowel and bladder dysfunction, loss of sexual function, and development of spasms.[27]

SPINAL CORD STIMULATORS Spinal cord stimulators were first used in the 1970s to manage severe pain such as reflex sympathetic dystrophy (RSD). Spinal cord stimulators inhibit spinal transmission of pain through electrical stimulation via the gate control theory. One to two leads are placed in the epidural space of the spinal cord, and a small electric current is sent through the electrodes. A receiver or battery pack is placed under the skin in the abdomen.[25] Results have been mixed; some subjects have reported decreased pain. It has been shown to be most effective in patients with incomplete pain or postcordotomy pain,[27] and less effective in patients with complete injury. Complications may include infections, allergic reaction, electrode migration, cerebrospinal fluid (CSF) leak, and bleeding. Deep brain stimulation was also used in the 1970s and 1980s; however, it has not been used recently because the Food and Drug Administration (FDA) has not approved it for any pain indications.[27]

THERAPEUTIC AND FUNCTIONAL INTERVENTIONS

When working with a child or adolescent with a spinal cord injury, physical therapy interventions in pediatrics are similar to the interventions that would be used with adults with spinal cord injury, but the approach may be different.

The physical therapist provides interventions that consist of a variety of procedures and techniques that are individualized for each client. These will produce changes in the client's overall function and help him or her make progress toward his or her goals. The therapist should always be assessing the patient's response to the interventions and modifying them as needed. There are some differences, however, that should be considered when working with children with spinal cord injuries, which will be highlighted here. Interventions will be discussed as generalizations, though some specifics to the type and level of spinal cord injury will also be mentioned.

THERAPEUTIC EXERCISE

Therapeutic exercise should include range of motion for specific areas of limitations. Special attention should be given to the areas where tone is abnormal. Hamstrings, heel cords, and adductors often develop contractures early. In some cases, however, contractures are necessary to improve function. As mentioned previously, examples of this include maintaining a shortening of the long finger flexors to achieve finger flexion when the wrist is extended (Fig. 8.1). Some children can use this active tenodesis for a functional grip. There are other situations where excessive ROM is necessary. For example, having increased hamstring flexibility will allow a patient with a spinal cord injury to be able to perform lower extremity dressing independently.

The implementation of therapeutic exercise in children is similar to that with other populations, with a few exceptions. Some muscle groups may not be able to be strengthened or improved due to complete denervation. In contrast,

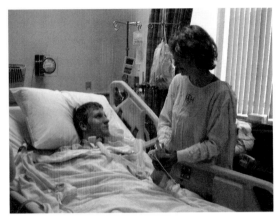

Figure 8.1 ■ *Physical therapy begins in the intensive care unit with positioning, passive and active range of motion, and family education.*

some muscle groups may require greater than normal strength to compensate for other muscle groups that are no longer functioning. When considering pediatric clients, age-appropriate interventions will likely provide greater success. For example, it is unlikely that a 4-year-old will perform biceps curls with a free weight as instructed; however, he or she may engage in pulling against resistance in a tug-of-war activity. Therapeutic exercises can often be incorporated into play, but it is imperative to remain focused on the goals being worked toward. In other situations, a child may perform traditional sets of strengthening exercises but may need to be rewarded with a fun and equally therapeutic play activity such as shooting basketballs with wrist cuff weights. Other therapeutic interventions to provide include:

- Aerobic and endurance conditioning or reconditioning
- Balance, coordination, and agility training
- Body mechanics and postural stabilization
- Flexibility exercises
- Gait and locomotion training
- Relaxation
- Strength, power, and endurance training for head, neck, limb, pelvic-floor, trunk, and ventilatory muscles

Therapeutic exercises as described above can be performed in a land or aquatic environment. Aquatic therapy can be very useful as the buoyancy of the water can assist in neuromuscular re-education in clients with neurologic disorders who have several muscle groups with ⅗ or less strength.[26] An aquatic environment can also be very fun for children, and they often perform more work while having more fun.

FUNCTIONAL TRAINING IN SELF-CARE AND HOME MANAGEMENT (INCLUDING ACTIVITIES OF DAILY LIVING AND INSTRUMENTAL ACTIVITIES OF DAILY LIVING)

Devices and adaptive equipment for the pediatric population with spinal cord injury include wheelchairs, standers, braces, and ADL devices. The physical therapist may provide the following types of interventions:

- ADL training
- Devices and equipment use training
- Functional training programs
- IADL training
- Injury prevention or reduction

For an adult, IADLs include caring for dependents, home maintenance, household chores, shopping, and yard work. For children, IADLs include participation in school and play activities. Play is an integral part of a child's life and is necessary for development and maturation. Training a child how to utilize new movement patterns in playing an age-appropriate game or sport is very important in a child's life. Other IADLs may include performing basic household chores depending on family desire and eventually prevocational and vocational training. ADL or IADL training might include collaboration with an occupational therapist.

DRIVING

Adaptations for driving make it possible for some people with spinal cord injury to operate a vehicle. Adolescents who are candidates for driving should be referred to rehab centers for driving assessment and training (Fig. 8.2).

MOBILITY

WHEELCHAIRS A wheelchair may be the primary means of locomotion for a child with a spinal cord injury. Children as young as 18 to 24 months can independently propel a wheelchair.[27] Evaluation for the appropriate wheelchair should take place as part of a team assessment. There are many options to allow children to function independently in a wheelchair. Reclining-back wheelchairs can be used to accommodate braces when sitting at

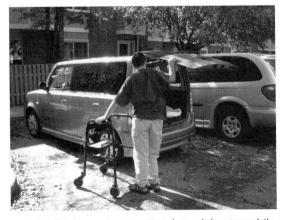

Figure 8.2 ■ *Adolescents can attend special automobile driving classes for people with disabilities and learn what modifications they may need to safely drive a vehicle.*

a right angle is difficult. Seating principles such as distribution of weight, propulsion, and environmental controls should be considered with children with spinal cord injury (Fig. 8.3).

BRACES AND AMBULATION

Reciprocating Gait Orthoses Versus Hip–Knee–Ankle–Foot Orthoses The reciprocating gait orthosis (RGO) is a bracing system that is composed of a bilateral hip, knee, and ankle orthosis with the right and left side connected by a cable. More recently, a version has been designed to be cableless (isocentric RGO [IRGO]).[28] The cableless connection allows one side of the orthosis to flex when the other extends. The user biomechanically extends one side by weight shifting onto one side while extending his or her trunk. This unweighting mechanism allows the opposite side to flex. Repeating this action on the contralateral side simulates the gait pattern. Some IRGO models allow hip abduction to occur for the purpose of self-catheterization. Physical therapy and rehabilitation training for RGOs involves assessment for appropriateness.[35]

There are many things to consider when recommending RGOs. In order to use RGOs, patients should have lower limb weakness with the inability to control the knees and hips. Additionally, children need to have sufficient upper extremity strength for weight bearing and advancing an assistive device. Patients must be free of lower extremity contractures and be able to sit comfortably with hips and knees flexed to at least 90 degrees. Children should also be cognitively able to follow directions and be motivated to do activities that will allow them to use the RGO system. Prior to the RGO fitting, special attention should be paid to upper extremity strengthening and stabilization activities, especially in the upright position. With the RGOs, weight shifting is key to adequate advancement of the lower extremities. This weight shift consists of a diagonal weight shift, pushdown through upper extremities, and unweighting of the contralateral side while extending the trunk. No active hip flexion is required to use RGOs. Training for RGO use begins in the parallel bars. Mirrors can help provide visual feedback for this motion. Hands-on facilitation of the weight shifting by the physical therapist can provide mechanical and tactile feedback to help the child learn the movement. The therapist should be aware of any substitutions, particularly lateral trunk movement and the urge to pull the limbs through using the abdominals. This is usually very typical for those patients who have learned a swing-through pattern prior to using RGOs or for those who have sustained spinal cord pathology after they were independently ambulating. In addition to ambulation, other functional skills such as donning and doffing the braces, coming to and from standing to sitting, and negotiating all levels and uneven surfaces, elevations, and inclines must be learned.

Learning to ambulate with RGOs requires intensive rehabilitation. Therapy should be daily until independent ambulation is achieved. At that time, the child should be given the opportunity to practice the ambulation skills within the context of his or her everyday activities. It is important to establish realistic goals with the patient, family, therapists, orthotist, physician, and other members of the health care team (Figs. 8.4 and 8.5; Display 8.10).

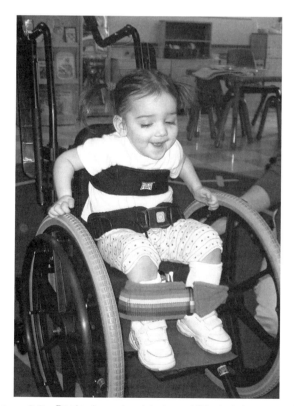

Figure 8.3 ■ *Beginning wheelchair mobility training as early as possible allows the child to experience a sense of freedom and explore his or her environment for learning opportunities.*

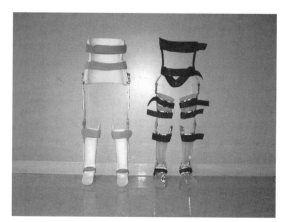

Figure 8.4 ■ Braces. **(A)** Reciprocating gait orthoses. **(B)** Hip–knee–ankle–foot orthoses.

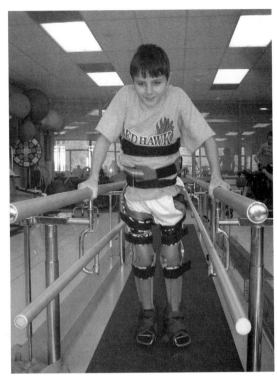

Figure 8.5 ■ Ambulation training requires excellent upper body strength and endurance and begins in the parallel bars until the child is ready to progress to an assistive device.

There is evidence to support the decision making when determining the appropriate brace system. When ambulation is compared between RGOs and hip–knee–ankle–foot orthoses (HKAFOs), it was found that for thoracic-level injury, the oxygen cost for ambulating with the HKAFOs was higher than for the RGOs. There was no significant difference in oxygen cost with a high lumbar–level injury. Additionally, velocity of ambulation was faster for RGOs than HKAFOs for thoracic-level patients.[29] Again, there was no difference in the high lumbar–level patients. In this study seven out of eight patients preferred RGOs to HKAFOs.[37]

PARTIAL WEIGHT-BEARING SYSTEMS Locomotor training with a treadmill and body weight support systems have been shown to be efficacious for retraining gait in some persons with SCI.[30] Body weight support systems are designed to allow suspension of a client in order to vary the amount of vertical weight bearing according to a client's ability to maintain a standing position. When used over an appropriate treadmill, the combination of unweighting the body and varying the speed of the treadmill allows specificity of gait training.

FUNCTIONAL ELECTRIC STIMULATION

For those children and adolescents with SCI resulting in C-4 tetraplegia, active functional upper extremity move-ment is limited to shoulder shrug. Assistive technology such as joysticks and head arrays assist these patients with communication and mobility. Options for self-care are limited for those with this level of injury. There are some devices that use robotics, but these are expensive and cumbersome. Some patients who have retained shoulder retraction may be able to use mobile arm supports; however, these have shown little promise for those with cervical injury due to decreased control of the glenohumeral joint.[31] Functional electrical stimulation (FES) uses surface electrode stimulation to produce functional movement. Grasping, wrist flexion, extension, and elbow extension have been used with voice activation systems.[38] Intramuscular stimulation systems have also been used to achieve flexion and extension with sip and puff control activators.[38] The literature also describes a system of using FES and stimulating hand grasp and release, elbow movement, and arm abduction by using proportionally controlled movement of the contralateral shoulder with glenohumeral joint stability achieved by a suspended sling.[38] Researchers at Shriners Hospital have shown that the combination of FES and surgical reconstruction provided active palmar and lateral grasp and release in a laboratory setting. The study also showed that FES systems increased pinch force, improved the manipulation of objects, and typically increased the independence in six standard ADLs as compared to pre-FES hand function. Subjects also reported preferring the FES system for most of the ADLs tested.[32]

Patterns of home use for electric stimulation have described a persistent but sporadic pattern of FES use that was influenced by the patient's perception of standing as a separate but occasional activity performed for an increased sense of fitness and well-being.[33] Studies have shown that the FES system generally provides equal or greater independence in seven mobility activities as compared with long leg braces, provided faster sit-to-stand times, and was preferred over lower leg braces in a majority of cases.[42]

 Coordination, Communication, and Documentation

Coordination, communication, and documentation are very important when working with a child with a spinal cord injury. Practice Pattern 5H in the *Guide to Physical Therapy Practice* outlines specific important components to remember when working with children with a spinal cord injury. Specifically, the child's school setting and special education requirements should be emphasized when planning for discharge.

The physical therapist plays an integral part in the health care team and may assist in coordinating care between

>> **DISPLAY 8.10**

To Walk or Not to Walk, and Family-Centered Care

One of the first questions a child or caregiver will ask when first faced with a spinal cord injury is, "Will I/he/she ever walk again?" Although many physical therapists will defer to the physician on this difficult topic, the therapist inevitably will discuss walking at some point with the client and should be well prepared to answer the question before it is asked. For some clients with spinal cord injury, walking *is* a possibility. This "walking" may require long leg bracing, implantable electric stimulation, and/or assistive devices; however, it may not be the type of walking the child is expecting. The physical therapist should always be honest in what current best practice can achieve and the child and family can then make an informed decision about whether walking is a goal they want to pursue. Walking as exercise even with bracing and assistive devices has benefits that are not only physical but emotional.[56] Walking can also improve quality of life for children as they can be on an eye-to-eye level with their peers. Many studies have been performed looking at energy expenditure with ambulation and wheelchair use in the myelodysplasia population, but little research has been done on the pediatric spinal cord injury population. Generally, as a child grows and becomes larger, it becomes increasingly difficult to keep up with peers while ambulating. Often the child ends up choosing a wheelchair as his or her primary means of mobility. The most important concept is that the child is choosing that means of mobility for him- or herself.

During the process of rehabilitation, it is the physical therapist's responsibility to help the client deal with his or her body in its current condition, and to help the child achieve the highest level of independence possible. Striving for independence also requires reintegration back into the community and bridging the client with others in the community. One of the most valuable things a therapist can give his or her client is to put him or her in a situation that challenges him or her to think and solve problems. The therapist can show the patient all the things that he or she can do—the way he or she is now—and provide support as the patient goes through the emotions of losing the way he or she used to be.

A therapist can also provide hope for the future. For a child with an incomplete or atraumatic injury, the period of recovery can last up to 5 years. Being realistic while allowing some hope can help focus and motivate the patient and sustain him or her through this difficult period. The child should come to understand that even though something isn't probable doesn't always mean it isn't possible. A child with a complete injury should learn all of the skills necessary as though he or she is going to be a primary wheelchair user. The opportunity for ambulation with an assistive device should be provided if the patient and family desire and if there is potential. To walk or not to walk is not an easy question. It requires careful consideration of the child's diagnosis and prognosis, the known functional potentials based on the literature, and input from the child and family. Being realistic while hopeful and working with the child and family on establishing goals together is the essence of family-centered care.

disciplines or between care settings. One of the goals of family-centered care is to ensure a smooth transition for patients and families across professionals and institutions. Communication is critical to coordinating a child's care and the physical therapist often participates in case conferences, patient care rounds, and family meetings when in an interdisciplinary setting. The therapist may need to make referrals to other sources and communicate with other providers if practicing in an ambulatory or school setting. The physical therapist must manage admission and discharge planning and coordinate this with other professionals when necessary. Discharge planning also includes the need to communicate a patient's care and needs among equipment suppliers and community resources. Discharge planning also requires the therapist and the team to use available funding wisely, and to assist the family in procuring charitable funds if needed. Planning for re-entry into the school and the community requires ongoing open communication and coordination of care (Fig. 8.6). Documentation should follow the American Physical Therapy Association's Guidelines for Physical Therapy Documentation as described in the *Guide to Physical Therapist Practice*. It is imperative for the profession as a whole to have a consistent and reliable means of documenting patient status, changes in function, changes in

interventions, elements of patient/client management, and outcomes of intervention.

EDUCATION

Caregiver instruction is as important when working with children as the patient education itself. Caregivers must be independent with all aspects of the home program recommendations so as to be able to facilitate their child's independence.

The primary focus for all physical therapy intervention should be patient and family education. Incorporating the family goals, the therapist establishes the plan of care and seeks to educate the child and family according to their learning style to help them make progress toward their goals, with the ultimate goal being discharge and reintegration into the community. Education begins in the earliest stages of rehabilitation and includes basic education about the client's diagnosis, the role of physical therapy, the prognosis, the plan of care, and what is needed for the family to help the child achieve his or her goals. Tasks such as performing ROM, bed and wheelchair positioning, pressure relief maneuvers, and donning/ doffing splints and equipment begin in the acute phases of treatment. Often the family members are thankful to

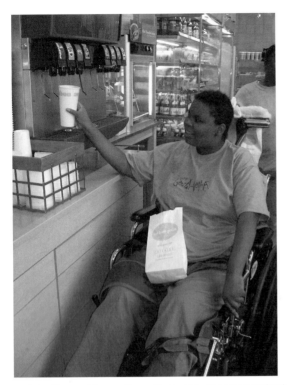

Figure 8.6 ■ Therapists can focus their plan of care to assist their clients in returning to activities enjoyed prior to their injury.

be able to start doing something for their child. It is important for the client and his or her family to receive education about skin integrity, autonomic dysreflexia, and stretching multiple times over the course of the admission since these are issues that the child will face over his or her lifetime. As the child advances through the phases of rehabilitation, he or she and his or her family change from being less active participants to becoming more active participants. Families must learn and demonstrate all aspects of patient care, and the child needs to learn how to teach others how to care for him or her. Caregivers of children with a spinal cord injury often need support to prevent "burnout" in these types of cases. The physical therapist may be the health care professional referring the caregiver to a support group or mental health professional. Some children perform better in physical therapy when family members are present, but other children may not. In cases when caregivers are asked to step out of a session to enable the child to become a more active participant, the therapist will follow up with a brief education session and explain what the child was able to do and what they can practice together that night. Children often demonstrate increased motivation for their personal exercise programs if there is some sort of reward associated with it. Parents and pediatric psychologists can be extremely useful in helping to determine a plan to increase desirable behaviors and active participation by the child to help support his or her physical therapy goals.

DISCHARGE PLANNING

Education of the child, the parent, and the child's teacher is critical prior to discharge planning. School visits by the team may be helpful. Medical issues must be stressed with the school including neurogenic bladder, bowel and skin integrity, autonomic dysreflexia, orthostatic hypotension, and thermoregulation.

SCHOOL RE-ENTRY

All children are entitled to a free and appropriate education.[34] Related services include transportation, developmental, corrective, and other supportive services to assist the child with a disability to benefit from special education. Children with spinal cord injury and mobility impairments may need extra time between classes or the use of a peer buddy system to help them manage their school challenges. Community resources include counseling, respite care, financial support, legal rights, and advocacy. There are also national, state, and local government agencies, some of which include the National Spinal Cord Injury Association, the National Parent Network on Disabilities, and the Family Resource Center on Disabilities.

Illness Prevention and Wellness

FITNESS

It is important for the child with a spinal cord injury to remain active (Fig. 8.7). Lack of activity can lead to a child becoming overweight, and children with a spinal cord injury are at increased risk for becoming overweight.[35] Aerobic and endurance conditioning should be performed to improve cardiorespiratory status. Patients with lower extremity paralysis can perform upper extremity activity with ergometers, arm bikes, and seated yoga and dance. There are also various wheelchair sports like track and field, basketball, tennis, etc.

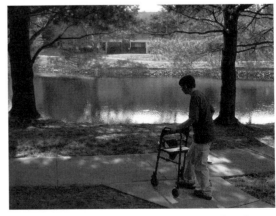

Figure 8.7 ■ Teens with a spinal cord injury often have to problem solve how to access things that they enjoy.

CIRCULATION

Although deep vein thrombosis and pulmonary embolism are rare in children, in order to prevent circulatory problems, children with spinal cord injury are often placed on prophylactic blood anti-coagulation agents. Precautions against injury should be maintained as these children may be at risk for increased bruising.

DYSREFLEXIA/HYPERREFLEXIA

For patients with a spinal cord injury above T-6, interventions to prevent and monitor for autonomic dysreflexia are extremely important. It is important to teach patients who are at risk for autonomic dysreflexia to identify its signs and symptoms as well as educate others about its treatment.

Studies show that there is a similar prevalence of dysreflexia in children with pediatric-onset SCI compared with adult-onset SCI. Dysreflexia is diagnosed less commonly in infants and preschool-aged children, and these two populations may present with more subtle signs and symptoms.[36]

GROWTH ABNORMALITIES

HIP SUBLUXATION

There is a high incidence of hip subluxation/dislocation in children with SCI.[37] The rate is significantly higher among children with onset of injury before 10 years of age.

SCOLIOSIS

The incidence of progressive paralytic scoliosis subsequent to acquired SCI has been reported to range from 46% to 98% in patients injured before their adolescent growth spurt.[38] Other studies have revealed that more severe scoliosis is related to a younger age at onset of paralysis. Age at injury has been shown to be a critical factor influencing development of paralytic scoliosis. Some studies have shown that early bracing in patients whose curve is less than 20 degrees may decrease or prevent surgery. Patients whose curve ranges from 20 to 40 degrees should undergo a trial of bracing with the goal to delay surgery. In patients with large curves greater than 41 degrees, the use of bracing is ineffective and may actually lead to skin breakdown and hindrance of ADLs.[45]

RENAL DISEASE

Good bowel and bladder management is important for prevention of renal disease.[39] Urogenic hygiene education is very important as well. There are many traditional options for handling bowel and bladder incontinence. There is reflex voiding and pressure voiding, where voids are timed and facilitated manually by increasing exter-nal pressure on the bladder. Catheterization is another means of emptying the bladder. There are indwelling catheters, but these are not without problems. External condom-type catheters and pads are also options.

Nurses, physicians, and occupational therapists work together to afford children and young adults the most independence possible. Readiness for this includes having the cognitive abilities necessary. A child must also have the fine motor skills to be able to independently use the equipment for self-catheterization. The typical age a child begins to understand is around 2 to 3 years old. Total independence is expected by 5 years old whether or not the child has spinal cord injury.

There are also surgical procedures like FES and urologic diversion surgeries. The overall goal for these is to avoid infection and to use antibiotics sparingly due to the development of resistant organisms.

The goal for bowel continence is to control constipation, be convenient, and allow independence. Diets rich in fiber with adequate fluid and exercise are the best way to achieve these goals. Training the bowels is done by habitual voids (every other day). Digital stimulation and the use of suppositories and enemas can assist with the process. For bowel and bladder incontinence, it is important that orthoses do not interfere with the ability to self-catheterize. Some brace options allow for abduction to eliminate the need for donning and doffing the braces for catheterization.

SKIN INTEGRITY

The importance of skin inspection and pressure relief is increased in those with decreased sensation. Children can be taught to do independent pressure relief, which may include wheelchair tilts, sitting push-ups off the seat, or unweighting each side in the wheelchair.

BONE DENSITY

Due to decreased weight bearing, patients with a spinal cord injury are at risk for osteoporosis, especially thoracic- and lumbar-level–injured patients. Patients who have spinal cord neoplasm may also suffer from osteopenia due to their chemotherapy regimes. Standing programs are the best way to maintain strong bones. Care should also be taken when performing ROM, positioning, and sometimes transfers and ambulation because of the potential for fractures due to osteopenia and osteoporosis.

ANTICIPATORY PLANNING

This intervention involves planning for things that a child or adolescent may encounter in life. Often these are normal things that are encountered by children and adolescents even without a spinal cord injury.

SEX EDUCATION/REPRODUCTION

Teenagers with spinal cord injury often have questions about their fertility, and they must be educated about this. Boys should learn about fertility options. Females should understand that they are still able to conceive and bear a child with the proper medical care and should understand the implications of potential pregnancy. Male fertility significantly decreases after spinal cord injury due to inability to ejaculate and poor sperm quality. There are options for those males who want to father a child, including intravaginal and intrauterine insemination and in vitro fertilization. In a female with a spinal cord injury, fertility is not affected.[40]

HIGHER EDUCATION/JOB TRAINING

When an adolescent begins to think about his or her life goals, there are many things to consider. Attending college in a manual chair may not be the best option for a patient, even if the upper extremities are not involved. There is an increased risk of upper extremity dysfunction and overuse syndromes with clients who have paraplegia in college and the workforce. Additionally, those entering the workforce need to understand their rights under the Americans with Disabilities Act.

 Outcomes

When determining what the appropriate adult outcomes are, one must determine what the important milestones are in the life of an adult. In this Anglo-American culture, these milestones for young adults include moving away from parents, achieving an education or training, obtaining a job, becoming financially independent, establishing significant relationships, and forming a family.[41]

Overall, it is a young adult's goal to keep pace with his or her peers and achieve these outcomes at the same rate. Other indicators are the ability to move around the community and integrate within it. Some argue that the measure of the means is the individual's satisfaction and quality of life.

One study that looked at outcomes of pediatric-onset SCI showed that adults with pediatric spinal cord injury are not equivalent to their peers.[42] When compared with the general population of the same age, those with spinal cord injury have equivalent education levels but demonstrate lower levels of community involvement, employment, income, independent living, and marriage. They also report lower life satisfaction and perceived physical health. Additionally, there are reports that despite similar education, there is difficulty for adults with SCI to obtain jobs. When they do obtain a job they are not paid similarly to their peers.[49] This presents a challenge for health care providers to work toward transitioning their patients to adult roles.

There is also evidence that adults who were injured as children have better outcomes than adults who were injured as adults. The assumption is that those who were injured at a younger age are enabled to develop the career goals and educational preparation that facilitated their entry into the adult workforce. The most highly correlated items to a positive outcome were education, functional independence, and decreased number of medical complications.[43,48]

VOCATIONAL OUTCOMES

A long-term follow-up study of adults who sustained spinal cord injuries as children or adolescents showed there was a high rate of unemployment as compared to the general population. Predictive factors of unemployment included education, community mobility, functional independence, and decreased medical complications. Other variables that were significantly associated with employment included community integration, independent driving, independent living, and higher income and life satisfaction. This provides insight into areas to target during rehab.[44]

PSYCHOLOGICAL OUTCOMES

Patients with spinal cord injury often experience frustration, loss, and depression. This is especially important to remember with children with spinal cord injury because they are in the midst of developing their personality. Adolescent control, anger, fear, and loss of dignity all contribute to psychological implications for the child with a spinal cord injury.[50]

LIFE SATISFACTION OUTCOMES

In a study of long-term outcomes and life satisfaction of adults who had pediatric spinal cord injuries, life satisfaction was associated with education, income satisfaction with employment, and social and recreational opportunities. Life satisfaction was inversely associated with some medical complications. Life satisfaction was not significantly associated with level of injury, age at injury, or duration of injury.[50]

 Future Directions

PREVENTION

There is currently no cure for spinal cord injury, traumatic or atraumatic. Prevention and public awareness are clearly the best means to avoid the lifelong disability associated with spinal cord injury. Many accidents involving spinal cord injury can be avoided with knowledge and education. Along with car seat guidelines for infants and toddlers, the National Highway Traffic Safety Administration

(NHTSA) recommends that children ages 4 to 8 and under 57 inches tall be placed in a booster seat until they can be properly positioned with a passenger seatbelt. The shoulder harness and lap belt together provide the safest protection for passengers and have decreased the incidence of SCI caused by lap belt alone. Other prevention measures include protective gear in sports and the prohibition of certain full-contact maneuvers such as "spearing" that carry more risk for spinal cord injury. Fall prevention for children can include window and stair guards as well as avoidance of wheeled baby walkers and trampolines. Violence prevention has taken on many forms in public education as well as legislation on both the community and federal levels. Education about prevention can be found extensively on the internet and can be focused toward children, teenagers, parents, or teachers. Vehicle safety, water and diving safety, bike safety, playground and sports safety, and gun safety play a large role in avoiding injury (Display 8.11).

RESEARCH

Although there is no cure at the present time, there is hope for the future. Improved knowledge about the neuropathology of transverse myelitis has given physicians clues on what medications to administer during certain points of the cascade of events. While this is not yet curative, it may help the final outcome.

One of the most exciting areas of research is the use of stem cells for spinal cord regeneration in both traumatic and atraumatic injuries. In motoneuron-injured adult rats, stem cells have been shown to not only survive in the mammalian spinal cord, but to also send axons through spinal cord white matter toward muscle targets.[45,46] With the addition of certain factors and developmental cues, Deshpande et al. have shown these axons to not only reach their muscle targets, but also to form neuromuscular junctions and become physiologically active, allowing partial recovery from paralysis in adult rats. This groundbreaking research is the first time scientists have shown that stem cell axons can form neuromuscular junctions and synapses within a living body's overall neural circuitry.[47] Further research will continue to expand upon these principles with the ultimate goal to one day become a successful treatment for humans with paralysis. The complexity of the original nervous system will unlikely be completely recreated, but rather, the new-growth axons will find their way to muscle in a more primitive manner. Therefore, the plasticity and self-regulation of the nervous system will likely prune and select advantageous motor pathways that will allow for function. This selection process requires appropriate external stimulation such as instructed activities and exercise.[48] Physical therapy will play a key role as stem cell studies advance toward human trials and will be instrumental in this revolution of knowledge, treatment, and possibilities.

SUMMARY

This chapter has detailed the examination, intervention, evaluation, prognosis, and care planning for children who have acquired a spinal cord injury. Specific attention was given to functional implications in both evaluation and treatment. It is important to keep in mind that although there are common themes that emerge with all patients, each child and family is unique and individual. Keeping a family-centered approach to treatment will ensure the most optimal outcomes for each and every child.

CASE STUDIES
CASE STUDY 1

MARK

Mark is a 15-year-old boy who developed transverse myelitis of his cervical spine (C-2 to C-5) with full quadriplegia and ventilator dependency within the first 24 hours. Over the course of the first month of hospitalization, Mark made very little recovery and could only demonstrate trace to poor movement in the right wrist and right ankle. He was transferred to an inpatient respiratory rehabilitation unit with the goal of providing family education for a safe discharge home. Prior to his illness he lived alone with his mother in a two-story condominium. His father recently died from cancer and there was no other family nearby to provide support. Mark was an honor student and wanted to become a pilot for the U.S. Air Force. His past medical history was significant for depression.

Examination

Mark initially presented with 0/5 strength throughout except minimal right ankle dorsiflexion and minimal right wrist extension. Sensation was absent from the neck down, and he was dependent for all mobility. He was unable to tolerate sitting out of bed in a chair due to anxiety and discomfort, and was unable to hold up his head. His tone was flaccid from the neck down and range of motion was within normal limits throughout. He was dependent on a ventilator for all breathing, and he was unable to produce a cough.

Evaluation

Mark presented with the following problems: decreased strength, decreased mobility, decreased airway clearance, and respiratory insufficiency. In addition, he had immense needs for caregiver education. His initial goals for physical therapy included tolerating out of bed in a wheelchair for 8 hours to prepare for return to school, power mobility on level surfaces with supervision, and caregiver education regarding all aspects of dependent care.

Physical Therapy Diagnosis

Impaired strength and decreased functional mobility due to transverse myelitis.

Physical Therapy Prognosis

Good potential to achieve above goals with caregiver assistance. Ambulation not likely due to medical prognostic factors of quick speed and severity of onset, slow rate of neurologic recovery, and complicating factors such as ventilator dependency. Mark did have good potential to use a power wheelchair with a head array or sip-and-puff mechanism in the community.

Physical Therapy Interventions and Re-Examination

Interventions were initially aimed at maintaining range of motion and skin integrity through positioning, pressure relief, and family education. Out-of-bed tolerance was increased with the use of a tilt-in-space wheelchair with elevating leg rests, an abdominal binder, and compression stockings to provide vascular support. Strengthening of available muscle groups was performed using traditional therapeutic exercises as well as biofeedback and neuromuscular electric stimulation (NMES).

As the weeks went on, Mark began to experience neurologic recovery, and it was crucial to re-examine and re-evaluate and adjust goals and interventions as necessary. A time line is provided below to illustrate the highlights of his medical and physical therapy course in rehabilitation:

September: Onset of illness, full quadriplegia, and vent dependency in first 24 hours

October: Interventions as above; began standing program using a tilt table, sitting edge of mat with maximal assistance; development of grip on right upper extremity, development of increased tone (modified Ashworth scale 2–3) throughout all extremities

November: Began stand-pivot transfers; developed gross flexion/extension of right leg, minimal right elbow flexion (brachialis) and bilateral elbow extension

December: Began ambulation training in partial weight-bearing walker (knee immobilizer and molded ankle foot orthosis on left lower extremity); developed right biceps strength; started weaning from the ventilator; received power wheelchair for mobility

January: Began walking with platform rolling walker, rolling supine to prone independently; moved left leg for first time (knee flexion/extension, great toe extension); tracheostomy capped during the day and bilevel positive airway pressure (BiPAP) at night

February: Decannulated with no external support and was transferred from the respiratory rehab service to the neuro-rehab service to achieve new goals of increasing independence with transfers and ambulation

March: Started performing bed mobility, sit to stand, and transfer board transfers with supervision only; ambulating with walker and no bracing and supervision only; starting to propel manual wheelchair with minimal assistance; received Botox injections to bilateral adductors and left hamstrings

April: Ambulating with forearm crutches; stood with quad cane for 30 seconds; moved left ankle for first time; discharged from inpatient setting to outpatient therapies

Currently: Primary power wheelchair user in community; uses walker at home and for short distances; Mark is now working toward long-term goal of independent ambulation in the community

Due to Mark's unexpected but definite neurologic recovery, it was crucial to constantly re-examine and reassess his goals and interventions. It was also important to communicate his changes with the family and the team and to advocate for more time in intensive rehab. Finally, it became very important to Mark, his mom, and the team to return Mark to home and school before the end of the school year to get assimilated back into the community and to re-form peer relationships before the summer, when he would have a bigger chance of isolation.

A constant theme during his physical therapy course included the constant re-examination of strength in upper and lower extremities and the neck and trunk. This also required careful assessment and a good working knowledge of Mark's fluctuating spasticity and subsequent communication with the medical team who adjusted his antispasticity medication. Interventions were progressed to work on Mark's current strengths and to challenge his weaknesses. Gait training and orthotic and assistive device assessment was also ever changing and constant, and a variety of bracing options were tried to correct his left knee. Mark was able to flex and extend his left hip and knee, but he felt unstable in late stance. An articulating ankle–foot orthosis (AFO) did not achieve the stability he needed, so he trialed a stance-control knee–ankle–foot orthosis on loan from a local vendor. He had difficulty making the mechanism work properly for him, so he continued on with the current program and continued to use only an articulating AFO on his left ankle. Another constant theme in his physical therapy course was the consideration of the disablement model (Display 8.12).[49] While addressing Mark's impairments and functional limitations was critical in the achievement of his goals, considering the impact of disability and handicap in his life was also very important to him. Physical therapy played a definite role in assisting Mark and his mother to become advocates for themselves, both to his school and to the community.

Currently, 18 months after his initial diagnosis, Mark remains a primary power wheelchair user in the community and uses a walker at home and for short distances. He is now working toward his long-term goal of independent ambulation in the community and is beginning to take independent steps with a quad cane. Socially, he is active in extracurricular activities and is on the honor role at his school. He currently works for an airplane museum where he is able to enjoy his love of aviation. He continues to work hard and is looking forward to attending college for technical engineering.

This case is an example of the vast diversity physical therapists encounter in patient populations. Although all factors indicated a poor outcome, Mark's immense determination and constant hard work helped him to achieve goals no one dreamed possible. Physical therapists have an awesome responsibility to balance being realistic about expected outcomes while also challenging their patients to achieve their fullest potential. Working together as a team with patients and families, amazing and life-changing things can be accomplished.

CASE STUDY 2

KEITH

Keith is an 11-year-old boy who was involved in a motor vehicle accident. He was an unrestrained rear-seat passenger and was ejected from the car when it struck a tree. He had loss of consciousness and was intubated at the scene. In the emergency room he was noted to have no movement in both lower extremities and computed tomography revealed a T-6 fracture with spinal cord infarct. Other injuries included left epidural hematoma, occipital fracture, bilateral pulmonary contusions, and right iliac fracture with retroperitoneal hematoma. During this time he received acute-care physical therapy to address range of motion, positioning, elevating the head of the bed to increase upright tolerance, and caregiver education. Once Keith was extubated and stabilized, he was admitted to an inpatient rehabilitation program. Socially, he lived with his mother and two younger siblings in a two-story house with his bedroom and bathroom on the second floor and two steps to enter. His father was the driver of the vehicle and his parents were in the process of a divorce. He attended the local public school and was extremely involved in athletics.

Examination
Keith presented with 4+/5 strength above the level of T-6 and 0/5 strength and no sensation below that level. He was wearing a thoracic–lumbar–sacral orthosis (TLSO) for fracture stabilization and was not yet cleared for lower extremity weight bearing. His tone was grossly 2 on the modified Ashworth scale throughout his lower extremities with three beats of clonus in each ankle and occasional flexor spasms in his left lower extremity when touched. His passive ROM was within normal limits throughout, with bilateral straight leg raise to 90 degrees. He was able to roll with minimal to moderate assistance using bed rails and transferred wheelchair to a level surface with a transfer board, push-up blocks, and moderate assistance. He required minimal assistance to sit upright and moderate assistance to reach outside his base of support.

Evaluation
Keith presented with decreased strength, decreased endurance, decreased flexibility, decreased bed mobility, decreased transfers, decreased functional mobility, and need for family education. Goals established at that time to be achieved during the inpatient rehabilitation admission included:

1. Roll independently supine to prone without a bed rail
2. Side-lying to sit with minimal assistance for lower extremities only
3. Transfer to level surfaces with a transfer board and contact guard assistance
4. Transfer to uneven surfaces with a transfer board and minimal assistance of one

5. Transfer floor to wheelchair with assistance only for lower extremities
6. Stand in parallel bars with bracing as needed and contact guard for 5 minutes with vital signs stable
7. Ambulate 25 feet with a walker and bracing as needed and contact guard assistance
8. Independent wheelchair mobility on level surfaces for 3000 feet without fatigue
9. Ascend and descend a 2-inch curb in his wheelchair with a spotter
10. Independence with wheelchair push-ups for pressure relief every 30 minutes
11. Patient independent with self-ROM
12. Caregiver independent with passive ROM, knowledge of skin checks, safe guarding for all levels of functional mobility, and all adaptive equipment management

Physical Therapy Diagnosis

Decreased strength and functional mobility due to ASIA A T-5 spinal cord injury.

Physical Therapy Prognosis

Excellent potential to achieve above goals due to current physical status, motivation, and family support. Based on the evidence, Keith has the potential to ambulate household distances with bracing and an assistive device but will most likely be primary wheelchair user in community.

Interventions

INCREASING UPRIGHT TOLERANCE

Utilized compression stockings, abdominal binder to help prevent orthostatic hypotension. Increased time out of bed in wheelchair and on tilt table using knee immobilizers and solid ankle–foot orthoses for stability in the weight-bearing position.

INCREASING STRENGTH

Worked with interdisciplinary team on increasing arm strength throughout the day. Activities included progressive resistive exercises, trunk strengthening, and upper extremity dynamic activities.

INCREASING FLEXIBILITY

Performed range-of-motion and stretching exercises to the lower extremities, which were carried out by family members as a bedside exercise program under the supervision of nursing staff. Keith was eventually taught to perform self-ROM. Special care was taken to allow enough hamstring flexibility to allow future floor-to-chair transfers and to maintain length in hip flexors and heel cords to allow for standing and assistive ambulation.

INCREASING BALANCE

Keith initially worked on improving sitting balance and reaching outside his base of support with his TLSO but later learned to sit without the TLSO when it was discontinued due to fracture stability and healing.

INCREASING ENDURANCE

Worked on increasing periods of aerobic activity including dynamic activities, wheelchair propulsion, and recreational activities, which will be described later.

MAINTAINING SKIN INTEGRITY

Keith was instructed in performing wheelchair push-ups to provided adequate pressure relief. He was also instructed in performing daily skin checks to all insensate areas. He maintained a positioning program in bed and used a gel cushion on his wheelchair.

IMPROVING BED MOBILITY AND TRANSFERS

Keith was instructed in the head hips relationship and was taught how to move his body without creating shear forces along his bottom. He initially used a transfer board to perform transfers but eventually was able to transfer with no equipment and use a transfer board only for car transfers. He was also trained in techniques for floor-to-chair transfers, scooting along the floor, and bumping up and down steps.

AMBULATION

Keith initially began standing in the parallel bars using knee immobilizers, temporary solid ankle orthoses, and his TLSO. He attempted to learn how to hang on his Y ligaments, but this was very difficult with the TLSO. Once the TLSO was no longer necessary for fracture stabilization, Keith was able to align and position himself in a standing position in the parallel bars. He was extremely motivated to walk using any assistive devices or bracing necessary despite the knowledge of its difficulties. He started with a pair of reciprocating gait orthoses (RGOs) and after much practice preferred to swing through rather than utilize the reciprocating mechanism, which he thought was slower and made him feel more fatigued. He was ordered and received a pair of lightweight single upright THKAFOs (trunk-hip-knee-ankle-foot orthosis) and was trained in donning, doffing, and ambulation.

IMPROVING WHEELCHAIR SKILLS

Keith was trained in propulsion, wheelies, ascending and descending curbs and ramps, and wheelchair recoveries. He was also trained in basic wheelchair maintenance.

EQUIPMENT

Keith received multipodus boots to wear in bed, molded ankle–foot orthoses to wear while in his wheelchair, THKAFOs for standing and walking, forearm crutches, a rigid-frame wheelchair, a transfer board, a commode, and bath equipment.

FAMILY EDUCATION

Keith's mother was trained and independent with safe guarding for all levels of functional mobility, all adaptive equipment management, and coaching Keith with his home exercise program. Keith was independent in pressure reliefs, skin checks, his home exercise program, and training others how to safely assist him when needed. With the aid of the interdisciplinary team, Keith and his family were provided with basic knowledge of spinal cord injury in general and living with a disability.

Re-Examination

Keith was re-examined during several points of his admission but most notably when he had a change in medical status.

Once his spinal fractures were adequately healed and he no longer required the use of the TLSO for fracture stabilization, Keith's entire center of gravity changed, and he needed to learn to use his body in a different way. He was also fully re-examined at the time of discharge from the inpatient setting, and he still had several physical therapy needs that were to be taken care of on an outpatient basis.

The Interdisciplinary Team

As is the case with most inpatient rehabilitation settings, Keith had a full team of professionals working closely on his case to achieve his family goal of safe discharge back to home. Although various disciplines have specific roles in caring for a child with a spinal cord injury, the team must communicate and work closely together. There is often overlap between professionals, and all team members should carry over the teaching of others to provide optimal family-centered care. Keith had a rehabilitation doctor overseeing his medical course with consulting medical services as needed such as orthopedics and urology. He also had nurses who primarily focused on skin, education, bowel and bladder program, and carrying over day-to-day skills such as activities of daily living and transfers. Psychosocial support came from a psychologist, child life staff, social worker, and the hospital chaplain. Educational needs were covered by the education coordinator, teacher, and neuropsychologist. He received speech therapy initially to work on increasing speaking volume and intensive occupational therapy to achieve goals of independence in activities of daily living. Physical therapy, occupational therapy, and nursing worked closely together so that Keith had the opportunity to practice new skills in a variety of environments. Together, the team, Keith, and his mother were able to achieve his family goal of successful reintegration back to home, school, and the community.

Discharge Planning

In order to ensure successful reintegration back to home, school, and the community, discharge planning began from the first day of admission. His family learning styles and needs were assessed and barriers to successful reintegration into the world were identified. First, due to Keith's mild traumatic brain injury, he was fully assessed by the hospital education staff and neuropsychologist to identify any new cognitive or learning needs upon return to school. Several meetings were set up with the staff at his school to problem solve and determine an appropriate educational plan and to remove any physical barriers. To prepare Keith to go home, the physical and occupational therapist performed a home evaluation with both Keith and his mother present. Measurements were taken and the basic layout was assessed in order to make appropriate home modification recommendations, but Keith and his mom also had the opportunity to practice transfers and mobility under the direction of the therapists. The therapists were then able to identify any new physical or occupational needs and what still required more practice in the hospital environment prior to discharge home. Child life and psychology were instrumental in working with Keith's

psychosocial issues regarding transition back into the community, but physical therapy played a large role in helping Keith to identify what types of leisure activities he may enjoy. Previously an athlete, Keith was very interested in pursuing adaptive sports including wheelchair basketball. Physical therapy introduced him to the idea of sled hockey, and Keith soon found it to be his favorite activity. The therapist had a loaner roller sled for Keith to try out while still an inpatient and helped him and his mom connect with community resources so that he could join a team upon discharge. Keith was thrilled at the idea of playing sports again, making contacts with peers and adult athletes with spinal cord injuries, and stated that his new goal was to play sled hockey for the U.S. Paralympic team. This illustrates the importance of considering the entire disablement spectrum in order to treat patients holistically. Follow-up services were established and Keith had a series of scheduled appointments with physicians trained to follow the needs of a person with spinal cord injury through the lifespan. Keith and his mom were given the tools needed to be advocates for themselves in both the health care and school systems as well as community resources to provide help along the way.

The Continuum of Care

Keith was recommended to be followed by outpatient physical therapy closer to his home to continue work on progressing wheelchair and ambulation skills to achieve his ultimate long-term goal of becoming as independent as possible. A recent study noted that patients with SCI who achieve a higher level of independence have improved quality of life and smoother transition to adulthood.[50] Keith may present with new pathologies, impairments, functional limitations, or disabilities as he grows and develops throughout his lifetime and may require future episodes of care from a physical therapist. Emphasis should be placed on resolving those new problems and returning the patient to self sufficiency, wellness, and a healthy lifestyle (Fig. 8.8).

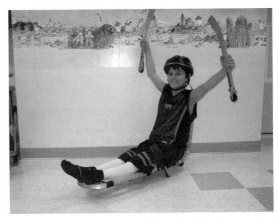

Figure 8.8 ▪ *Adaptive sports such as sled hockey can help fulfill a child's need for peer interaction and participation in the community.*

REFERENCES

1. National Spinal Cord Injury Association. Spinal cord injury statistics. Available at: http://www.spinalcord.org/. Accessed October 9, 2006.
2. National Spinal Cord Injury Statistical Center. Spinal cord injury: facts and figures at a glance. The University of Alabama at Birmingham, June 2006.
3. Segal LS. Spine and pelvis trauma. In: Dormans JP, ed. Pediatric Orthopedics and Sports Medicine: The Requisites in Pediatrics. Mosby. St. Louis: 2004.
4. Buldini B, Amigoni A, Faggin R, et al. Spinal cord injury without radiographic abnormalities. Eur J Pediatr 2006;165(2):108–111.
5. Shepherd M, Hamill J, Segedin E. Paediatric lap-belt injury: a 7 year experience. Emerg Med Australas 2006;18(1):57–63.
6. Kerr DA, Ayetey H. Immunopathogenesis of acute transverse myelitis. Curr Opin Neurol 2002;15(3):339–347.
7. Krishnan C, Kaplin AI, Pardo CA, et al. Demyelinating disorders: update on transverse myelitis. Curr Neurol Neurosci Rep 2006;6(3):236–243.
8. Kerr DA, Calabresi PA. 2004 Pathogenesis of rare neuroimmunologic disorders, Hyatt Regency Inner Harbor, Baltimore, MD, August 19th 2004-August 20th 2004 [Congresses]. J Neuroimmunol 2005;159(1–2):3–11.
9. Pollono D, Tomarchia S, Drut R, et al. Spinal cord compression: a review of 70 pediatric patients. Pediatr Hematol Oncol 2003;20(6):457–466.
10. Meisel HJ, Lasjaunias P, Brock M. Modern management of spinal and spinal cord vascular lesions. Minim Invasive Neurosurg 1995;38(4):138–145.
11. Cruse JM, Lewis RE, Dilioglou S, et al. Review of immune function, healing of pressure ulcers, and nutritional status in patients with spinal cord injury. J spinal Cord Med 2000;23(2)129–135.
12. Bohannon RW, Smith MB. Inter-rater reliability of a modified Ashworth scale of muscle spasticity. Phys Ther 1987;67:206–207.
13. Linan E, O'Dell MW, Pierce JM. Continuous passive motion in the management of heterotopic ossification in a brain injured patient. Am J Phys Med Rehabil 2001;80(8):614–617.
14. Van Kuijk AA, Geurts AC, Van Kuppevelt HJ. Neurogenic heterotopic ossification in spinal cord injury. Spinal Cord 2002;40(7):313–326.
15. Smith JA, Siegel JH, Siddiqi SQ. Spine and spinal cord injury in motor vehicle crashes; a function of change in velocity and energy dissipation on impact with respect to the direction of crash. J Trauma Inj Infect Crit Care 2005;59(1):117–131.
16. Sommer JL, Witkiewicz PM. The therapeutic challenges of dual diagnosis: TBI/SCI. Brain Inj 2004;18(12):1297–1308.
17. Americal Spinal Injury Association. Standard neurological classification of spinal cord injury. Available at: http://www.asia-spinal injury.org. Accessed October 9, 2006.
18. Mulcahey MJ, Betz RR. International Standards for Neurological Classification of SCI: Reliability of Data when Applied to Children and Youth. Conference proceedings, Contemporary Topics in Pediatric Spinal Cord Injury, Shriners Hospital for Children, Philadelphia, October 10–11, 2005.
19. Thaleisnik M, Fishel B, Ronen J, et al. Recovery of neurologic function after spinal cord injury in Israel. Spine 2002;27(16):1733–1735.
20. Marino RD, Ditunno JF Jr, Donovan WH, et al. Neurologic recovery after traumatic spinal cord injury: data from the Model Spinal Cord Injury Systems. Arch Phys Med Rehabil 1999;80(11):1391–1396.
21. Kirshblum S, Millis S, McKinley W, et al. Later neurologic recovery after traumatic spinal cord injury. Arch Phys Med Rehabil 2004;85 (11):1811–1817.
22. Krishnan C, Kaplin AI, Deshpande DM, et al. Transverse myelitis: pathogenesis, diagnosis and treatment. Front Biosci 2004;9:1483–1499.
23. Irani DN, Kerr DA. 14-3-3 protein in the cerebrospinal fluid of patients with acute transverse myelitis. Lancet 2000;355(9207):901.
24. Somers MF. Spinal Cord Injury: Functional Rehabilitation. 2nd Ed. Prentice Hall.
25. Lollar DJ, Simeonssonn RJ, Nanda U. Measures of outcomes for children and youth. Arch Phys Med Rehabil 2000;81(12;Suppl 2):S46–S52.
26. Mulcahey MJ, Betz R, Smith B. A prospective evaluation of upper extremity tendon transfers in children with cervical spinal cord injury. J Pediatr Orthop 1999;19(3):319–328.
27. Burcheil K, Hsu K, Frank P. Pain and spasticity and spinal cord injury. Spine 2001;26(24S):S146–S160.
28. Warms C, Turner J, Marshall H. Treatments for chronic pain associated with spinal cord injuries. Many are tried, few are helpful. Clin J Pain 2002;18(3):154–163.
29. Yap EC, Tow A, Menon EB, et al. Pain during in-patient rehabilitation after traumatic spinal cord injury. Int J Rehabil Res 2003;26(2):137–140.
30. Jan F, Wilson P. A survey of chronic pain in the pediatric spinal cord injury population. J Spinal Cord Med 2004;27(Suppl 1):S50–S53.
31. Forest DM. Spinal cord stimulator therapy. J Perianesth Nurs 2006;11(5):349–352.
32. Kelly M, Darrah J. Aquatic exercise for children with cerebral palsy. Dev Med Child Neurol 2005;47(12).
33. Tefft D, Duerette P, Furumasu J. Cognitive predictors of young children's readiness for power mobility. Dev Med Child Neurol 1999;41:655–670.
34. The Center for Orthotics Design. Isocentric RGO. Retrieved from http://www.centerfororthoticdesign.com. Accessed October 9, 2006.
35. Vogel LC, Lubicky JP. Ambulation in children and adolescents with spinal cord injuries. J Pediatr Orthop 1995;15(4).
36. Katz D, Haideri N, Song K. Comparative study of conventional hip-knee-ankle-foot-orthoses versus reciprocal-gait orthoses for children with high level paraplegia. J Pediatr Orthop 1997;17(3):377–386.
37. Behrman AL, Harkema SJ. Locomotor training after human spinal cord injury: a series of case studies. Phys Ther 2000;80:688–700.
38. Smith B, Mulcahey MJ, Bet R. Development of an upper extremity FES system for individuals with C-4 tetraplegia. Trans Rehabil Eng 1996;4(4).
39. Mulcahey MJ, Betz R, Smith B. Implanted functional electrical stimulation hand system in adolescents with spinal injuries: an evaluation. Arch Phys Med 1997;78.
40. Moynahen M, Mullin C, Chohn J, et al. Home use of a functional electrical stimulation system for standing and mobility in adolescents with spinal cord injury. Arch Phys Med Rehabil 1996;77.
41. Individuals with Disabilities Education Act (IDEA), 20 U.S.C. 1400.
42. Liusuwan A, Widman L, D'Andrea L. Altered body composition affects resting energy expenditure and interpretation of body mass index in children with spinal cord injury. J Spinal Cord Med 2004;27(Suppl. 1).
43. Hickey K, Vogel L, Willis K, et al. Prevalence and etiology of autonomic dysreflexia in children with spinal cord injuries. J Spinal Cord Med 2004;27.
44. McCarthy J, Chavetz R, Betz R. Incidence and degree of hip subluxation/dislocation in children with spinal cord injury. J Spinal Cord Med 2004;27(Suppl 1):S80–S83.
45. Mehta S, Betz R, Mulcahey MJ. Effect of bracing on paralytic scoliosis secondary to spinal cord injury. J Spinal Cord Med 2004;27(Suppl 1):S88–S92.

46. Merenda L, Brown JP. Bladder and bowel management for the child with spinal cord dysfunction. J Spinal Cord Med 2004; 27(Suppl 1):S16–S23.

47. Deforge D, Blackmer J, Garrity C. Fertility following spinal cord injury: a systematic review. Spinal Cord 2005;43(12): 693–793.

48. Anderson CJ, Vogel LC. Employment outcomes of adults who sustain spinal cord injuries as children or adolescents. Arch Phys Med Rehabil 1998;79(12):1496–1503.

49. Vogel LC, Klaas SJ, Anderson CJ. Long-term outcomes and life satisfaction of adults who had pediatric spinal cord injuries. Arch Phys Med Rehabil 1998;79(12):1496–1502.

50. Vogel L, Klaas S, Lupicky J. Long-term outcomes and life satisfaction of adults who had pediatric spinal cord injury. Arch Phys Med Rehabil 1998;79.

51. Anderson CJ, Vogel LC, Betz RR, et al. Overview of adult outcomes in pediatric-onset spinal cord injuries: implications for transition to adulthood. J Spinal Cord Med 2004;27(Suppl 1): S98–S106.

52. Harper JM, Krishnan C, Darman JS, et al. Axonal growth of embryonic stem cell-derived motoneurons in vitro and in motoneuron-injured adult rats. Proc Natl Acad Sci USA 2004; 101(18):7123–7128.

53. Kerr DA, Llado J, Shamblott MJ, et al. Human embryonic germ cell derivatives facilitate motor recovery of rats with diffuse motor neuron injury. J Neurosci 2003;23(12):5131–5140.

54. Deshpande DM, Kim YS, Martinez T, et al. Recovery from Paralysis in adult rats using embryonic stem cells. Ann Neurol 2006;60(1):32–44.

55. Ramer LM, Ramer MS, Steeves JD. Setting the stage for functional repair of spinal cord injuries: a cast of thousands. Spinal Cord 2005;43:134–161.

56. Guccione AA. Physical therapy diagnosis and the relationship between impairments and function. Phys Ther 1991;71(7): 499–503; discussion 503–504.

57. Anderson CJ, Vogel LC, Willis KM, et al. Stability of transition to adulthood among individuals with pediatric-onset spinal cord injuries. J Spinal Cord Med 2006;29(1):46–56.

Neuromuscular Disorders in Childhood: Physical Therapy Intervention

Allan M. Glanzman and Jean M. Flickinger

C hildren with neuromuscular disorders have a lifelong challenge to maintain function. That challenge can be met with the help of a knowledgeable physical therapist. In this chapter, the term *neuromuscular disease* refers to disorders whose primary pathology affects any part of the motor unit from the anterior horn cell out to the muscle itself. Common to all of these disorders is muscle weakness, which may be produced by pathology at any part of the motor unit. When characterizing neuromuscular disorders and their pathology, it is convenient to consider the various anatomic divisions of this motor unit: the anterior horn cell, the peripheral nerve, the neuromuscular junction, and the muscle.

Neuromuscular diseases may be either hereditary or acquired and are variously classified as a myopathy or dystrophy, in which the cause of the muscle weakness is attributable to pathology confined to the muscle itself, or neuropathy, in which the muscle weakness is secondary to an abnormality of either the anterior horn cell or peripheral nerve. Further characterization is based on a particular disorder's characteristic pattern of presentation.

The term *muscular dystrophy* describes a group of muscle diseases that are genetically determined and have a steadily progressive degenerative course. Further classification of the muscular dystrophies is based on their clinical presentation, including the distribution of weakness, mode of inheritance, and pathologic findings. In the past two decades, much has been discovered in the area of molecular science to help us better understand and classify the childhood muscular dystrophies. After the cloning of the gene for Duchenne muscular dystrophy (DMD) in 1987,[1,2] scientists have learned more about the relationship between the different dystrophies and how they relate to the dystrophin–glycoprotein complex (DGC), found within the muscle-cell membrane (Fig. 9.1). The DGC is a group of proteins that links the subsarcolemmal cytoskeleton and extracellular matrix and gives stability to the muscle-cell membrane.[3] When different proteins in the DGC are deficient or made incorrectly, different corresponding muscular dystrophies present themselves. For example, when dystrophin is deficient, the result is Duchenne or Becker muscular dystrophy. When sarcoglycans are deficient, different limb girdle muscular dystrophies present themselves. A deficiency of laminin results in a certain type of congenital muscular dystrophy.

Some of the above dystrophies are categorized by the deficiency of proteins that characterize their disorder. DMD and Becker muscular dystrophy (BMD) are also known as *dystrophinopathies* because dystrophin is deficient in these conditions. Some of the limb girdle muscular dystrophies are also known as *sarcoglycanopathies* because the protein sarcoglycan is deficient in these conditions.

The term *spinal muscular atrophy* refers to neurogenic disorders whose underlying pathology affects the anterior horn cell, as in the spinal muscular atrophies. The term *motor neuropathy* refers to neurogenic disorders

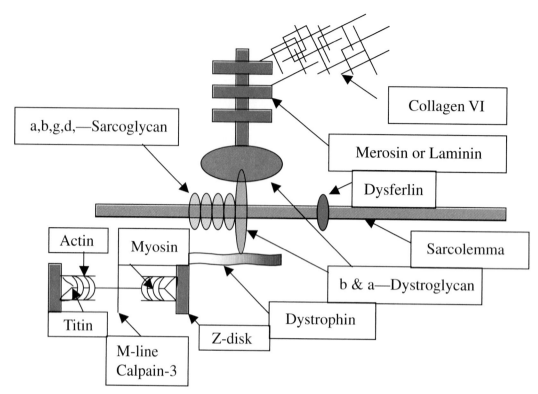

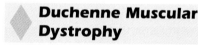

Figure 9.1 ▪ Muscle cell membrane and associated protein complexes implicated in muscle disease.

whose underlying pathology affects the peripheral nerve, as in Charcot-Marie-Tooth disease. Further classification is based on clinical presentation and mode of inheritance.

The neuromuscular disorders vary significantly in their presentation, pathology, and progression but are linked with regard to physical therapy intervention by their common characteristic of muscle weakness leading to loss of function and physical deformity. A physical therapist with an understanding of these disorders can help identify, predict, intervene, and possibly prevent unnecessary complications throughout the course of each disorder. The purpose of this chapter is to provide an overview of select neuromuscular diseases, including clinical presentation, pathology, diagnosis, disease progression, medical treatment, and physical therapy intervention.

Because DMD is one of the most common myopathies and best known of the dystrophies affecting children, much of this chapter is devoted to a discussion of this disorder. Physical therapy interventions and principles that apply to the management of weakness and deformity in patients with DMD are also applicable to other neuromuscular diseases that present with similar symptoms and complications with the exception of strengthening strategies. Knowledge of the various disorders will allow appropriate decisions to be made about the suitability and timing of various physical therapy interventions. Other neuromuscular diseases that are reviewed in this chapter include Becker muscular dystrophy, myotonic dystrophy,

limb girdle muscular dystrophy, congenital myopathy, congenital muscular dystrophy, spinal muscular atrophy, and Charcot-Marie-Tooth disease.

Duchenne Muscular Dystrophy

Duchenne muscular dystrophy, also known as pseudo-hypertrophic muscular dystrophy or progressive muscular dystrophy, is one of the most prevalent and severely disabling of the childhood myopathies, occurring in approximately 1 in 3500 live male births.[2] It is a dystrophinopathy in which the child becomes weaker and usually dies of respiratory insufficiency and/or heart failure due to myocardial involvement in the second or third decade of life.[4] There is an X-linked inheritance pattern to DMD whereby male offspring inherit the disease from their mothers, who are most often asymptomatic. Advances in molecular biology have shown the defect to be a mutation at Xp21 in the gene coding for the protein dystrophin.[1,5]

DIAGNOSIS

The clinical presentation gives the first clues to the diagnosis, which is confirmed by the results of laboratory studies. Laboratory findings include an abnormally high serum creatinine kinase (CK) level, which is 50 to 200 times the nor-

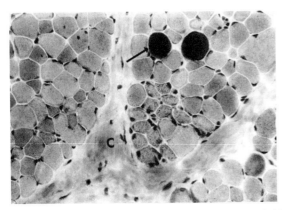

Figure 9.2 ■ Dystrophic changes include a marked variability in fiber size; dark, "opaque" fibers (arrow); and abnormal quantities of fibrous connective tissue (C). (Trichrome, ×300) (From Maloney, Burks, Ringel, eds. Interdisciplinary Rehabilitation of Muscular Dystrophy and Neuromuscular Disorders. Philadelphia: JB Lippincott, 1984:203.)

mal level[6] and usually ranges from 15,000 to 35,000 IU/L (normal <160 IU/L).[7] Electromyogram (EMG) findings show nonspecific myopathic features with normal motor and sensory nerve velocities and no denervation. A muscle biopsy is usually performed to confirm the diagnosis and shows degenerating and regenerating fibers, inflammatory infiltrates, and connective tissue with adipose cells (Fig. 9.2), which can be compared to normal muscle (Fig. 9.3). Immunohistologic staining of the tissue reveals the absence of dystrophin along the muscle cell membranes.[8]

Advances in genetic testing have allowed more specific diagnosis of the type of mutation present in DMD and BMD, providing more information for possible treatments in the future. Approximately 65% of patients with DMD

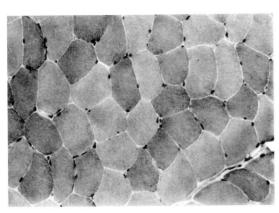

Figure 9.3 ■ Normal adult muscle. Muscle fibers are cut in a plane transverse to their long axis and appear to have round, oval, or slightly irregular profiles. One or more darkly stained nuclei are seen at the edge of most fibers. (Trichrome, ×300) (From Maloney, Burks, Ringel, eds. Interdisciplinary Rehabilitation of Multiple Sclerosis and Neuromuscular Disorders. Philadelphia: JB Lippincott, 1984:202.)

and BMD have gross deletions of the dystrophin gene, which results in either the complete absence of dystrophin in DMD or some levels of truncated protein in BMD.[9] One-third of DMD cases are caused by very small point mutations.[9] There is also a high frequency of new mutations occurring in approximately one-third of the cases of DMD, which may in part be secondary to the very large size of the dystrophin gene.[2] With the availability of genetic analysis, all male family members may be screened for the disorder and all female family members may be screened for their carrier status.

PATHOPHYSIOLOGY

The absence of dystrophin leads to a reduction in all of the dystrophin-associated proteins in the muscle cell membrane and causes a disruption in the linkage between the subsarcolemmal cytoskeleton and the extracellular matrix. The exact cause of muscle cell necrosis is unknown. However, lack of dystrophin is thought to cause sarcolemmal instability and an increased susceptibility to membrane microtears, which may be exacerbated by muscle contractions. This causes increased calcium channel leaks, which raises intracellular calcium levels, leading to muscle cell necrosis.[2,3]

The following describes the clinical features of Duchenne muscular dystrophy. Becker muscular dystrophy also follows a similar pattern of muscle degeneration but at a much slower and variable rate.

CLINICAL PRESENTATION AND PROGRESSION

The onset of the disorder is insidious, usually resulting in symptoms between 2 and 5 years of age; however, symptoms may not be noticed for months or years, and the disease may be misdiagnosed for years.[6]

Earliest symptoms may include a reluctance to walk or run at appropriate ages, falling, difficulty getting up off the floor, toe walking, clumsiness, and an increase in size of several groups of muscles. The gastrocnemius is the most notable muscle that commonly shows this "pseudohypertrophy," but the infraspinatus and deltoid muscles are also commonly enlarged. These pseudohypertrophic muscles have a firm consistency when palpated (Fig. 9.4).

The weakness is steadily progressive with proximal muscles tending to be weaker earlier in the course of the illness and to progress faster (Fig. 9.5). Weakness of the hip and knee extensors often results in an exaggerated lumbar lordosis that is characteristic of the early stages of disease. The lordosis occurs in response to the attempt to align the center of gravity anterior to the fulcrum of the knee joint and posterior to the fulcrum of the hip joint. This realignment gives maximum stability at both joints. The child attempts to broaden the base of support during walking and thus develops a gait that resembles

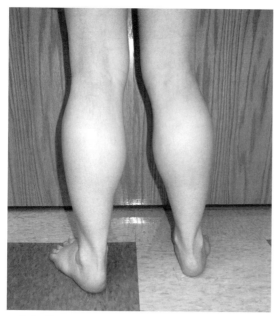

Figure 9.4 ■ Ten-year-old with Duchenne dystrophy. Pseudohypertrophy of the calf.

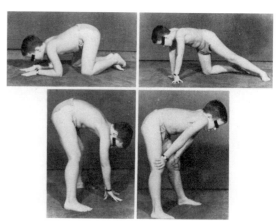

Figure 9.6 ■ Gower's sign. This series of maneuvers is necessary to achieve an upright posture, and it occurs with all types of pelvic and trunk weakness. The child "climbs up the legs" when rising from the floor. (From Lovell WW, Winter RB, eds. Pediatric Orthopaedics. 2nd Ed. Philadelphia: JB Lippincott, 1986:265.)

waddling. The child may develop iliotibial band contractures, which are made worse by this wide-based stance. As the weakness progresses, the child rises from the floor by "climbing up the legs." This maneuver, known as Gower's sign, is indicative of proximal muscle weakness (Fig. 9.6).

As the disease progresses, there is a tendency to develop contractures. These contractures typically result in plantar flexion at the ankle, with inversion of the foot and flexion at both the hips and knees.

This early loss of range of motion (ROM), noted in the hip flexors, iliotibial bands, and heel cords, limits stance and ambulation, in that patients find it difficult to achieve the mechanical alignment necessary to hold themselves in

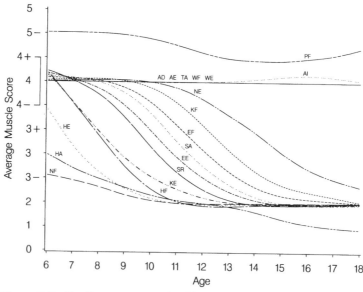

Figure 9.5 ■ The lines represent the 50th percentiles for the strength of individual muscles plotted against age. AD, ankle dorsiflexor; AE, ankle invertor; AI, ankle invertor; EE, elbow extensor; EF, elbow flexor; HA, hip abductor; HE, hip extensor; HF, hip flexor; KE, knee extensor; KF, knee flexor; NE, neck extensor; NF, neck flexor PF, plantar flexor; SA, shoulder abductor; SR, shoulder external rotator; TA, thumb abductor; WE, wrist extensor; WF, wrist flexor. (Courtesy of the Collaborative Investigation of Duchenne Dystrophy [CIDD] Group).

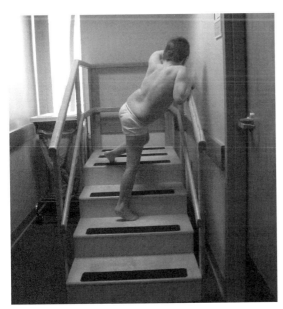

Figure 9.7 ■ Ten-year-old with spinal muscular atrophy type III. Notice the use of the upper extremities to assist climbing the steps. This posture and use of a hand to extend the knee are the two most typical patterns noted with proximal weakness.

an upright posture using their weak musculature. As these children spend more time sitting, an increasing degree of contracture is seen at the hips, knees, and elbows.

Functional activities may be performed more slowly by children with DMD than by normal children, but most of those affected are able to walk, climb stairs (Fig. 9.7), and

stand up from the floor without too much difficulty until 6 or 7 years of age. At this time, a relatively rapid decline in function has been documented, which generally results in a loss of unassisted ambulation at 9 to 10 years of age and loss of ambulation, even in long leg braces, at 12 to 13 years of age.[10] A graphic representation of the ages at which the children have increasing difficulty with various functional activities is presented in Figure 9.8. These functional activities are considered to be "milestones" and represent significant points in disease progression. The arm grades awarded were developed by Brooke and associates[10] (Table 9.1), whereas the leg grades are based on a scale proposed by Vignos et al. (Table 9.2).[11]

As is demonstrated by the range and distribution of percentiles in Figure 9.8, the clinical course of disease progression in individual children is not homogeneous.

The mildest of the X-linked progressive dystrophies has been termed Becker muscular dystrophy. This classification applies to individuals who maintain independent ambulation until after the age of 15 years. The type of mutation on the dystrophin gene causing BMD allows for some dystrophin to be produced. The dystrophin produced is insufficient in quantity and quality, causing muscle breakdown to occur at a slower rate than in DMD. Boys with BMD will usually present with symptoms between 5 and 15 years old, although onset is variable and may not occur until as late as the third or fourth decade.[2] The course of BMD is much less predictable than that of DMD; however, patients with BMD usually live at least until their fourth or fifth decade.[2]

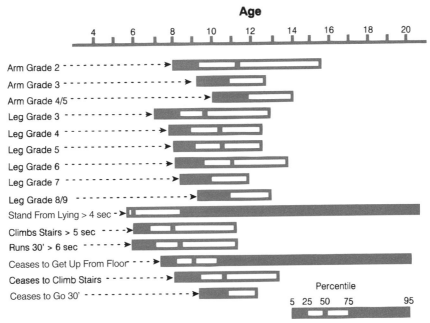

Figure 9.8 ■ Graphic representation of the ages (expressed as percentiles) at which children with Duchenne muscular dystrophy have increasing difficulty with functional tasks. (Courtesy of the Collaborative Investigation of Duchenne Dystrophy [CIDD] Group.)

TABLE 9.1

Functional Grades: Arms and Shoulders

Grades	Functional Ability
1	Standing with arms at the sides, the patient can abduct the arms in a full circle until they touch above the head.
2	The patient can raise the arms above the head only by flexing the elbow (i.e., by shortening the circumference of the movement) or by using accessory muscles.
3	The patient cannot raise hands above the head, but can raise an 8-oz glass of water to the mouth (using both hands if necessary).
4	The patient can raise hands to the mouth, but cannot raise an 8-oz glass of water to the mouth.
5	The patient cannot raise hands to the mouth, but can use the hands to hold a pen or to pick up pennies from a table.
6	The patient cannot raise hands to the mouth and has no useful function of the hands.

Brooke and colleagues have coined the term "outliers"[10] to describe a population of boys who fulfill the diagnostic criteria for DMD but who, when compared to the DMD population's usual pattern of disease progression, fall outside the usual limits. Outliers usually retain the ability to ambulate and climb steps up to age 12 but

TABLE 9.2

Functional Grades: Hips and Legs

Grades	Functional Ability
1	Walks and climbs stairs without assistance
2	Walks and climbs stairs with the aid of a railing
3	Walks and climbs stairs slowly (elapsed time of more than 12 seconds for four standard stairs) with the aid of a railing
4	Walks unassisted and rises from a chair, but cannot climb stairs
5	Walks unassisted but cannot rise from a chair or climb stairs
6	Walks only with assistance or walks independently with long leg braces
7	Walks in long leg braces, but requires assistance for balance
8	Stands in long leg braces, but is unable to walk even with assistance
9	Is in wheelchair
10	Is confined to bed

not beyond age 15.[2] Antigravity neck flexion is also relatively preserved early on in the disease process in these patients[2] as well as in BMD. Investigators are studying genetic heterogeneity with regard to DNA mutations and resulting dystrophin expression in an attempt to explain the varying levels of clinical severity associated with DMD.[12]

SCOLIOSIS

Scoliosis develops as the age of the child with DMD increases; significant curves are generally not noticed until after the age of 11 years.[13] This scoliosis tends to progress as the back muscles become weaker and as the child spends less time standing and more time sitting, resulting in a positional scoliosis, which, over time, becomes fixed.

RESPIRATORY INVOLVEMENT

In addition to the voluntary muscles, DMD affects other organs. As the respiratory musculature atrophies, coughing becomes ineffective and pulmonary infections become more frequent, often leading to the patient's early death. The major cause of respiratory complications in DMD is the progressive weakness of the muscles of respiration. This weakness may or may not be exacerbated by the mechanical disadvantages associated with kyphoscoliosis. The signs and symptoms of respiratory insufficiency include excessive fatigue and daytime sleepiness, headaches on awakening (secondary to increased carbon dioxide levels that may accompany decreased respiratory efficacy while supine), sleep disturbances (nightmares), or feeling the need to strain to "gulp for air."

GASTROINTESTINAL SYSTEM

The muscles of the gastrointestinal tract are also affected, causing constipation and the risk of acute gastric dilation or intestinal pseudo-obstruction, which causes sudden episodes of vomiting, abdominal pain, and distention. If not treated properly, this can lead to death.[3]

CARDIAC ISSUES

Heart muscle is also affected by a deficiency of dystrophin resulting in cardiomyopathy, arrhythmias, and congestive heart failure. In DMD, the posterobasal portion of the left ventricle is affected greater than other parts of the heart. In DMD, heart muscle involvement generally occurs later than skeletal muscle involvement and may not present until the late second decade.[14] In BMD and female carriers of the dystrophin mutation, cardiac involvement can occur later and sometimes may require heart transplantation.[14] Monitoring of these patients should begin in the second decade for DMD and BMD, and in the third or fourth decade for female carriers of the dystrophin mutation.[14]

Motor and sensory neurons are undamaged, and there is no significant change in either the central nervous system (CNS) or in the vascular system. Fortunately, children with DMD seldom lose bowel or bladder control, and other neurologic signs do not appear.

COGNITION

A high rate of intellectual impairment and emotional disturbance has been associated with DMD.[15] Although intelligence may be reduced among children with DMD, this deficit is not progressive and is not related to the severity of disease.[16] IQ scores fall approximately one standard deviation below the mean[15] and affect verbal scores more than performance scores.[2] Although not progressive, this intellectual deficit may hinder the child's development and may make a physical evaluation of the child difficult.

TREATMENT

Although definitive treatment is lacking, proper management, as outlined by Ziter and Allsop, can prolong the maximum functional ability of the child.[17] This program of management begins once the diagnosis is established, and it is initiated concurrently with parental counseling in an attempt to reduce the guilt, hostility, fear, depression, hopelessness, and numerous other emotions commonly experienced by the parents.

The clinician faced with this situation can propose a positive approach based on the following: (1) some of the complications that magnify the functional disability of DMD are predictable and preventable; (2) an active program of physical therapy and the timely application of braces can prolong ambulation and more closely approximate the normal independence of later childhood; and (3) if a specific treatment ever becomes available, those in optimal physical condition are most apt to benefit.[17]

MEDICAL TREATMENT

There is no pharmaceutical treatment that will cure DMD, but several studies[18,19] have confirmed an initial report that glucocorticoid corticosteroids including prednisone, and deflazacort increase strength and improve function from 6 months to up to 2 years in patients with DMD.[20,21] Further investigation has shown that prednisone, despite its many side effects, keeps those affected by DMD "stronger for longer."[22,23] Short-term adverse effects of prednisone include excessive weight gain, cushingoid appearance, behavioral abnormalities, and excessive hair growth.[20] A small study showed that use of deflazacort may result in less weight gain but equivalent strength and functional benefits of prednisone.[24]

Creatine monohydrate, a naturally occurring substance, often used by body builders to increase muscle performance, is sometimes recommended for boys with DMD. When healthy subjects take oral creatine for 1 to 4 weeks, the result is increases in muscle levels of creatine and improvements in maximal exercise performance and recovery from exercise.[25] A study of 30 boys with DMD showed increases in fat-free mass (FFM) and hand-grip strength in the dominant hand after 4 months of creatine supplementation.[26] Studies of the MDX mouse also report benefits of creatine.[27,28]

Myoblast transplant has been proposed as a treatment for DMD with the aim of replacing the missing protein dystrophin.[29] However, at present, this procedure is still being investigated. The use of aminoglycosides, including gentamicin, may have some benefit in the treatment of DMD. Use of gentamicin in the MDX mouse increased dystrophin expression in the cell membrane and provided protection against muscle injury.[30,31] However, two clinical trials of human subjects with DMD found no changes in muscle strength or increased dystrophin in muscle biopsies posttreatment with gentamicin.[31] Further research is needed. Various other strategies for replacing the defective gene and missing protein are under study, but currently none is available for clinical use.[32]

ORTHOPEDIC TREATMENT

Spinal fixation is generally recommended for boys with DMD once their scoliosis begins to progress rapidly and their spinal curve becomes greater than 30 degrees, usually once boys are wheelchair bound.[33] Further indications for surgery include increasing pelvic obliquity, difficulty with bracing, skin breakdown, discomfort and decreased tolerance to sitting, and difficulty using upper extremities secondary to lack of trunk stability requiring propping on arms.[33] The goals of spinal surgery should include providing a stable spine, maximally correcting scoliosis, correcting pelvic obliquity, and providing sagittal-plane alignment for improved comfort and function.[33,34] Spinal stabilization should be segmental, using unit rods and fixating the spine from T2 or T3 at the upper end and attaching into the body of the ilium at the lower end, and should attempt to correct pelvic obliquity and provide a lumbar lordosis.[34] The above surgery allows for immediate postoperative mobilization without an orthosis. Timing of surgery is critical as the risks of surgery become greater as the disease progresses. It is recommended that spinal stabilization occur before the percentage of normal forced vital capacity (FVC) reaches 45 with an absolute cutoff point at less than or equal to 35.[34]

Other orthopedic surgeries include Achilles tendon lengthening, Yount fasciotomies, tibialis posterior transpositions, and percutaneous tenotomies in an attempt to increase joint range of motion for prolongation of ambulation.

Nutrition for the Child with Childhood Myopathy

Rose Ann Manadan, RD, LDN
Clinical Dietitian
Children's Hospital of Philadelphia

Myopathy/neuromuscular disorders in infants and children
- Duchenne muscular dystrophy
- Spinal muscular atrophy
- Myasthenia gravis
- Myotonic dystrophy
- Congenital myopathy

Nutrition-related challenges/issues
- Failure to thrive vs. obesity
- Abnormal swallowing
  Poor coordination
  Delayed swallow
  Nasal regurgitation
  Fatigue on chewing
  Gag reflex
  Delayed peristalsis
  Reduced tongue motility
  Pooling of oral secretions
  Risk of aspiration
  Risk of choking
  High arch palate
  Poor lip closure
- Gastroesophageal reflux (GER)
- Constipation
- Hypotonia/contractions/motor developmental delay
- Adequate hydration
- Reliable and consistent anthropometric measurements due to contractures and scoliosis, which prevent patients from standing and bearing weight
- Increased appetite and weight gain and growth suppression with steroids
- Risk of osteoporosis and osteopenia

Nutrition-related interventions
- Ensuring adequacy of calorie, micronutrients, fluid, and fiber intake
- Increasing calories via concentration of formula and use of additives
- Small frequent feedings
- Assistance with meals
- Occupational, physical, and speech therapy referral to:
  - Retrain sucking and/or chewing mechanism
  - Use adaptive nipples, other feeding equipment
  - Adjust table height, position of arms and body
- Providing nonfood rewards
- Medications for GER, constipation
- Nasogastric or gastrostomy/jejunostomy tube feeding
- Nissen fundoplication procedure

SUGGESTED READINGS

Ekvall S. Pediatric Nutrition in Chronic Diseases and Developmental Disorders. Oxford University Press, Inc., 1993:103–106.

McCrory MA, Wright NC, Kilmer DD. Nutritional aspects of neuromuscular diseases. Rehabilitation of neuromuscular disease. Phys Med Rehabil Clin N Am 1998;9(1):127–143.

Tilton, AH, Miller MD, Khoshoo V. Nutrition and swallowing in pediatric neuromuscular patients. Semin Pediatr Neurol 1998;5(2):106–115.

PULMONARY TREATMENT

A child with DMD will need to be followed by a pulmonologist for regular monitoring of pulmonary status. If the history and pulmonary function test results suggest that the lungs are not being adequately ventilated, the pulmonologist will need to discuss options for assisted ventilation. Nasal positive pressure ventilation may be used at night to assist breathing and to provide a rest for overworked respiratory muscles.[35] An adjustment period is often necessary when this type of ventilation is used, but after a period of time the patient often derives the benefits of improved sleep and increased energy and alertness in the daytime. Ventilatory assistance might be required both day and night for children with advanced respiratory failure. Thanks to modern technology, this is a feasible option.[36] Technology has provided advances so that speech and eating are not severely affected by a tracheostomy, and ventilators are compact, battery-driven devices that can be attached to an appropriately modified wheelchair. The pulmonologist can also recommend various airway clearance techniques and medications to improve pulmonary health.

CARDIAC TREATMENT

Regular cardiac echocardiogram (ECHO) and electrocardiogram (ECG) monitoring by a cardiologist is necessary for boys with DMD and BMD and for female carriers. Cardiac medications for arrhythmias may be necessary. Patients with BMD also may need heart transplantation for dilated cardiomyopathy.

GASTROINTESTINAL/NUTRITION

A gastrointestinal (GI) specialist can help with constipation issues as well as monitor for intestinal pseudo-obstruction. A nutritionist can help prevent weight gain and assist with diet recommendations.

PHYSICAL THERAPY EXAMINATION

The role of the physical therapist in treating DMD and BMD is an important one and requires a solid understanding of the unique features of the disease and a delicate approach to the issues related to treating a progressive and fatal disorder. When discussing examination and treatment of the child with DMD, it is helpful to categorize the disease into three general life stages: the early or ambulatory stage, the transitional phase during loss of ambulation, and the later/wheelchair stage when the child or young adult is wheelchair bound and dependent for most of his functional activities.

Each child with DMD should undergo a physical therapy examination. Such an examination involves the gathering of information that contributes to the development of a plan of care.[37] That care plan will be based largely on the functional significance of the therapist's findings.

HISTORY

A thorough history should be taken during the physical therapy examination process. This should include family history; birth and developmental history; a review of systems including cardiac, pulmonary, gastrointestinal, and musculoskeletal systems; functional mobility; social history; and current durable medical equipment. The primary concerns of the child and family should also be understood prior to examining the child.

FAMILY HISTORY

Understanding the child's family history is important. The child and family may already know someone with the disease and may have a different perspective than someone diagnosed with a new mutation who is unfamiliar with the disease. If the child's mother or sisters are carriers, they will need to understand their risks of cardiomyopathy as well as implications for future family planning.

DEVELOPMENTAL HISTORY

The physical therapist should gather information regarding the child's birth and development. Often, boys with DMD are late walkers, never gain the ability to jump, and lag behind their peers in gross motor skills. Parents often report frequent falling or clumsiness as boys lose their strength. It is common for boys to have a lower IQ and they may have learning disabilities that need to be addressed in school.

REVIEW OF SYSTEMS

PULMONARY

A good pulmonary history is required to determine whether the child has any pulmonary issues that require treatment or referral to a pulmonologist. Does the child have a productive cough? Can the child clear his own secretions? Does the family currently perform percussion and postural drainage or use any devices to aid in airway clearance to maintain pulmonary health? Does the child exhibit any symptoms of respiratory insufficiency or nighttime hypoventilation? If the child demonstrates these symptoms, the child must be referred to a pulmonologist for a possible sleep study. Other systems including cardiac, GI, integumentary, and musculoskeletal systems will also need to be reviewed to determine whether referral to a specialist is necessary.

TESTS AND MEASURES

FUNCTIONAL ABILITY

Systematic and serial recording of standard tasks shows that the child with DMD is in one of two general phases: stable performance or declining performance. During the stable phase, which may continue for several years, the child may demonstrate normal performance of various tasks during the serial evaluations, despite a continuing decline in strength. A discrepancy exists in the age at which the aforementioned tasks have failed, as illustrated in Figure 9.8.

The use of timed testing during examinations in the clinical setting is useful for monitoring patient function. Activities frequently timed include transferring from supine to standing, running a distance of 30 feet, transferring from sitting to standing, and climbing up four steps. Qualitative description along with timing adds useful information in monitoring function and level of fatigue. For example, it is helpful to note during the floor-to-stand transfer whether a Gower's maneuver is present and whether the child requires the use of one or both hands on knees to complete the transfer. When climbing the steps, it is helpful to describe how many rails are required, the pattern or sequence of steps used (reciprocal vs. marking time), and whether use of upper extremities is required to push on knees or to pull up on the rail to ascend steps.

Ziter and associates[38] and Allsop and Ziter[39] have demonstrated that, although functional ability appears to remain at a constant stage in many children with DMD, actual muscle strength continues to decline insidiously. These findings suggest that, although timed functional tests are useful in determining the patient's current status, they have limited value in monitoring the progressive loss of strength in DMD. As a result of these studies, Allsop believes that, when timed trials are used as dependent variables in drug trials, they may overestimate therapeutic efficacy. A patient who appears to be stable in a series of timed trials may actually be experiencing a continual decline in strength, in which case the drug has had no effect on the progression of the myopathy.

Brooke and coworkers[40] and Florence and associates[41] have presented a clinical evaluation protocol for DMD—assessing strength, pulmonary function, and functional tasks in combination—that has been demonstrated to be reliable in documenting disease course in patients with DMD.[42] In addition, the protocol is able to detect not only the therapeutic effect of pharmaceutical intervention, but also the time course and differences in various dose levels of such intervention.[29]

MUSCLE TESTING

Measurement of muscle strength by way of manual muscle testing (MMT) remains a valid approach to assessing the progression of disease in children with DMD.[41] MMT has been shown to be both reliable[32] and sensitive to changes in strength in patients with DMD.[43]

Because muscle weakness is characteristic of all myopathies, MMT must be a routine part of the physical therapy evaluation of the child with myopathy. Serial use of MMT provides data against which the efficacy of management can be monitored. The longitudinal results of MMT

in children with DMD show linearity in the decline of muscle strength. Although some authors describe an apparent stabilization of strength between 5 and 8 years of age, Allsop and Ziter,[39] Ziter and associates,[38] and Brooke et al.[42] have found neither plateaus nor accelerated periods of the disease process. Bracing does not slow down the deterioration, and use of a wheelchair does not increase the rate of decline.

By the time the child reaches 7 years of age, or with serial strength scores recorded for 1 year, it is possible to estimate the rate of progression as either rapid (>10% deterioration per year), average (5% to 10% deterioration per year), or slow (<5% deterioration per year). There is a variation in the rapidity of progression, and MMT, along with performance of functional tasks, helps determine when bracing or wheelchairs will be needed.

Reliability of muscle testing has been documented. It has been demonstrated that, although MMT is a reliable means of assessment in DMD when performed by the same examiner, the interrater reliability of MMT varies among individual muscles and grades.[41,44] It is apparent that one's purpose for performing MMT—whether it is to answer clinical questions or to serve as a research measurement tool—determines the vigor with which one approaches strength testing.

DYNAMOMETRY

Handheld myometry and various fixed tensiometer systems have been used in attempts to better quantify muscle strength in boys with DMD.[45,46] Handheld myometers and grip and pinch dynamometers can be useful in obtaining more objective and specific muscle strength data. Kilmer et al. found handheld dynamometry (HHD) to be reliable in people with neurogenic weakness.[47] Other studies have found that HHD was more reliable in the weaker limbs of subjects with hemiplegia[48] and may be more suitable for use in weaker patients.[47]

RANGE OF MOTION

Standard assessment of joint motion with goniometry should be done periodically. Pandya and associates studied the intratester and intertester reliability of goniometry for children with DMD.[49] They found high intratester values, but intertester values varied. As a result, they have recommended that serial goniometric evaluations be done by the same examiner.[49] Early loss of ambulation is more frequently caused by loss of motion and contracture than by weakness in specific muscle groups. Loss of full ankle dorsiflexion, knee extension, and hip extension, with resultant contractures, occurs commonly in patients with DMD. Measurement of ankle dorsiflexion, knee extension, hip extension, and iliotibial band (ITB) tightness are probably the most important aspects of goniometric testing. Measurement of the popliteal angle is useful in monitoring hamstring flexibility. Special tests including the Thomas test and Ober test[50] can also be useful in monitoring hip flexor and ITB tightness.

PHYSICAL THERAPY INTERVENTION

Physical therapists manage patients and their problems, not diseases. The primary problems encountered by children with DMD include the following:

1. Weakness
2. Decreased active and passive ROM
3. Loss of ambulation
4. Decreased functional ability
5. Decreased pulmonary function
6. Emotional trauma—individual and family
7. Progressive scoliosis
8. Pain

After a physical examination of the patient, the physical therapist can identify current problems and, based on a thorough understanding of the disease process, should be able to predict the next major difficulties to be encountered. Based on the specific areas of concern for each family, it is possible to identify five major goals of management common to all children with DMD:

1. Prevent deformity.
2. Prolong functional capacity.
3. Improve pulmonary function.
4. Facilitate the development and assistance of family support and support of others.
5. Control pain, if necessary.

As the preceding five goals are accomplished, we fulfill our general goal for all individuals with neuromuscular disease, that of helping them be as independent and comfortable as possible within the limits of their disability.

To address the preceding goals, one must think about the specifics of preventing deformity through the prescription of ROM exercises and stretching, splinting, and appropriate positioning. Prolonging functional capacity of ensuring safety while functioning may require the prescription of specific orthotics or adaptive equipment.

Support for the family members may be aided by good rapport with the medical personnel; family education in regard to the disease process and its implications; referral to the Muscular Dystrophy Association (MDA), where they would have access to other families facing similar problems; and the educational, social, financial, and medical care opportunities offered by the MDA. The child and family may be aided by appropriate timing of referral to other associated medical personnel, including orthotist, occupational therapist, nutritionist, adaptive equipment supplier, social service worker, or medical specialists including orthopedic surgeon, pulmonologist, gastrointestinal specialist, or cardiologist.

Pain control may or may not be necessary and is often dependent on how successful stretching and bracing strategies were in the child's earlier years. Appropriate stretching, fit and positioning in wheelchairs, cushions, alternating pressure pads, or specialized mattresses and hospital beds can go a long way in assisting the control of discomfort in these children.

HOME PROGRAM

Because much of the responsibility for daily treatment must be assumed by the family or friends of the patient with DMD, an effective program of care at home is essential. Although sustaining enthusiasm and adherence with the home program may be difficult, the likelihood of success can be improved by giving simple instructions, requesting a limited number of exercises and repetitions each day, and offering extensive feedback and positive reinforcement to people in the support system. By reducing the anxiety associated with nonadherence and outlining both short- and long-term goals for the family, adherence and rapport can be improved. In the case of a single-parent family, we suggest extra support from older siblings, clergy, social groups, neighbors, and schools. The home program is convenient and inexpensive. Outpatient physical therapy once or twice each week at times may be indicated with the primary goal of instructing family members in an appropriate home program, providing safe guidelines for exercise, and monitoring of orthotic or splinting needs. Early intervention physical therapy may be indicated for the younger child if diagnosed early, with a transition to physical therapy in the school setting when the child reaches school age. Periodic re-evaluation, retraining, and motivation sessions for parents are recommended.

PREVENTING DEFORMITY

The tendency for development of plantar flexion contractures is usually the earliest problem. Daily stretching of the Achilles tendons should slow down the development of this deformity. The use of night splints in combination with heel-cord stretching has been shown to play a significant role in preventing the often relentless equinovarus deformity associated with DMD.[51] Use of night splints has been shown to be more effective in preventing deformity of the Achilles tendon than stretching alone.[52] Boys with DMD who used night splints early on (prior to the loss of ambulation) walked independently longer than boys who did not use splints.[53]

No studies are available on which to base a passive stretching prescription, but the regimen often prescribed is between 10 and 15 reps, holding at least 15 seconds, performed at least once, and preferably twice, daily.[54]

As soon as the physical therapist sees any change in length of the hamstring muscles during a periodic evaluation, hamstring stretching is added to the home program.

The ITB, hip flexors, and foot evertors are other structures that must be monitored carefully for loss of ROM, which usually occurs in all these structures as a result of either weakness or static position.

If plantar flexion contractures and the resultant knee, ITB, and hip flexion contractures are allowed to continue unchecked, the child will progress much sooner than necessary to the late ambulation stage and will lose the ability to ambulate at an earlier age than with intervention. At least 2 to 3 hours of standing or walking is recommended daily in addition to stretching to help prevent contracture formation.[54] Therefore, a stander may be considered to aid in the prevention of contractures.

MINIMIZING SPINAL DEFORMITY

As the child's sitting time increases, so does kyphoscoliosis. Previous clinical observations have documented that the convexity will likely be toward the dominant extremity.[55] Because of this relationship, it has been recommended that the child with adequate bilateral manual skills have the wheelchair drive moved from side to side every 6 months in order to prevent the scoliosis from becoming structural. Many boys, however, are resistant to this idea for practical reasons and preferences.

A lateral support and gel or air cushions in wheelchairs have been used in an attempt to provide appropriate pressure relief and spinal positioning while the patient is seated in the wheelchair, but no studies are available to prove their clinical efficacy. Typically spinal orthoses are not used in patients with DMD since they have not been shown to delay development of the spinal curve.

The increasing sophistication of spinal instrumentation within the field of orthopedics has made spinal fixation an option for children with DMD. Previously, the amount of "down time" following surgery precluded these children from choosing this option, both because of the muscle weakness and the risk of respiratory complications. Currently, physical therapy plays an important role in getting these children "up and moving" within days to a week after surgery, depending on their medical status. Initially, referrals for spinal stabilization were attempts to improve or stabilize a patient's respiratory function to alleviate the mechanical disadvantage the kyphoscoliosis placed on the already weak respiratory muscles, as well as to prevent the potentially deleterious effect of this scoliosis on respiratory function. Recent studies have demonstrated no salutary effect of segmental spinal stabilization on respiratory function based on either short- or long-term follow-up, but all studies have documented improved sitting comfort, appearance, and stabilization, or improvement of kyphoscoliosis.[56–58]

ACTIVITY LEVEL/ACTIVE EXERCISE

Normal, age-appropriate activities for a young boy with DMD are encouraged. The family should be instructed to allow the child to self-limit his activities and allow rests when needed. Care should be taken to avoid overusing muscles and causing fatigue. Signs of overuse weakness include feeling weaker 30 minutes postexercise or excessive soreness 24 to 48 hours after exercise.[59] Other signs include severe muscle cramping, heaviness in the extremities, and prolonged shortness of breath.[59] In general, eccentric muscle activities such as walking or running downhill and squats should be avoided if possible as they tend to cause more muscle soreness. Resistive muscle strengthening is not recommended in boys with DMD because of the risk of contraction-induced muscle injury.

STRENGTHENING

Strength training in boys with DMD has been a subject of controversy. Research on strength training and exercise programs in human subjects with DMD has been limited and has had mixed outcomes. There are few well-controlled, randomized studies, and most have had heterogeneous groups of subjects that include different forms of muscular dystrophies with very different pathologies and clinical presentations. Most of the studies looked at short-term strength gains in individual muscles, but few looked at long-term effects and functional benefits after exercise regimens.

In an early study in 1966, Vignos and Watkins found improvements in weight-lifting capacity in subjects with various forms of muscular dystrophy over a 1-year training period. The strength benefits plateaued in the subjects with DMD after approximately 4 months and results were less sustainable than in patients with other dystrophies.[60,61] Little functional benefits were found in the subjects with DMD, although greater strength gains and functional benefits were found in subjects with limb girdle and fascioscapulohumeral forms of muscular dystrophy.[60] In 1979, de Lateur and Giaconi found that isokinetic submaximal strength training minimally improved strength in four boys with DMD without negative side effects.[62] Scott et al. also found absence of deterioration with mild to moderate exercise in the short term.[63] Most of the researchers recommended that exercise programs should be started early on in the course of the disease as individuals with the least amount of muscle impairment benefited the most from training programs.[61,64] There is very little research on exercise in nonambulant patients with DMD.[64]

There is no evidence in humans that increased activity or resistive exercise caused physical deterioration[64]; however, studies of the MDX mouse, a dystrophin-deficient mouse, have indicated damage to muscle cell membranes, which increases during exercise.[65] Eccentric exercise in particular may induce muscle cell damage as was demonstrated in a downhill treadmill running protocol with MDX mice.[66] Connolly et al. showed 40% to 45% fatigue when comparing the first two and last two pulls when measuring repetitive grip strength of MDX mice.[67] Various other MDX mice studies have contributed to the theory of contraction-induced muscle cell damage. Lack of dystrophin increases susceptibility to muscle cell damage. Microtears in the muscle cell membrane increase with muscle contractions and cause an increase in calcium leak channel activity, which in turn causes an increase in intracellular calcium. This increase causes calcium-dependent proteolysis, which eventually leads to cell death.[65,68]

Endurance exercises such as swimming have been found to be beneficial in MDX mice by increasing the resistance to fatigue in muscles by increasing the proportion of type I (slow oxidative) fibers.[69]

Care must be taken in interpreting and transferring data from the MDX mouse model to humans. The muscle sizes and forces experienced by muscle groups vary and the stance of the mouse is quite different from humans. In addition, the natural history of the MDX mouse is different than the course of DMD in humans.[64]

More research is needed in the area of strength training; however, given the current research on mice and humans, general recommendations can be made. Avoidance of maximal resistive strength training and eccentric exercise is recommended in boys with DMD. Submaximal endurance training such as swimming or cycling may be beneficial, especially in the younger child with DMD.

PROLONGING AMBULATION

As patients with DMD become weaker, their gait pattern is altered in an attempt to improve stability during walking. Stride length decreases, and the width of the base of support increases to provide a more stable base. The ITB accommodates to the new, shortened position associated with the wider base of support. Weakness in the gluteus medius becomes more pronounced, and the child assumes the typical waddling gait.

The lordotic curve increases with progressive weakness of the gluteus maximus. As that muscle weakens, the child attempts to increase stability, moving the center of gravity posterior to the fulcrum of the hip joint by pulling the arms back and by exaggerating the lordosis. Stability at the hip joint during standing is now provided passively by structures anterior to the hip joint, primarily the iliofemoral ligament. Even a mild knee flexion contracture or an ankle–foot orthosis (AFO) with its angle set in dorsiflexion would make ambulation difficult or impossible with the child in this position.

Treatment programs combining passive stretching and lower extremity bracing have demonstrated a reduction in the rate of progression of lower extremity contractures and have prolonged ambulation.[70,71] Various surgical interventions—including Achilles tendon lengthening and Yount fasciotomies,[72] tibialis posterior transpositions,[73] and percutaneous tenotomies[74,75]—in combination with vigorous physical therapy and orthotic intervention have been reported to improve and prolong ambulation.[76–78]

A prospective study has demonstrated "that a comprehensive program of single early surgical intervention followed by a definite course of rehabilitation can significantly stabilize and possibly prolong ambulation without resorting to long leg braces."[79]

Whatever the surgical methods, a vigorous postoperative physical therapy program should aim to get the patient up and standing and walking as soon as possible. Active joint stretching will help maintain, and may even increase, ROM at those muscles that have been released. The goal of the postoperative physical therapy program is independent ambulation with a minimum of 3 to 5 hours per day of standing and/or walking. Even when no steps are possible, the child is asked to stand at least 1 hour a day (in a standing table if necessary). Optimal stance is with the back in extension so that the center of gravity falls behind the hip joint.

Before any lengthening surgery is considered, families must thoroughly weigh the benefits and risks involved with surgical intervention. When patients are still ambulatory, an overcorrection of a heel-cord contracture may result in immediate loss of ambulation[54] or may result in ambulation with long leg braces only, which may be cumbersome and not very functional. With the increased use of corticosteroids, many boys are reaping the benefit of prolonged ambulation without the risks of surgical intervention, and many centers do not recommend orthopedic intervention uniformly for all patients with DMD. An alternative to surgical correction for those patients with contractures at the ankle that are limiting ambulation is serial casting. It is vital to ensure that the patient is able to ambulate in the cast, and the casts should be changed either weekly or twice a week to ensure that the period of casting is as short as possible.

WHEELCHAIR USE

When ambulation becomes more difficult, falling becomes more frequent, and the child with DMD is unable to get to the places he needs without undue fatigue, it is time to consider the use of a wheelchair for a primary means of mobility. Because of the rapid decline in function and the fatigue induced by pushing a manual wheelchair, a power wheelchair is generally recommended for a first wheelchair option. Because of the time it takes to order and get insurance approval for a power wheelchair, the therapist will need to estimate when a child will no longer be able to ambulate. According to clinical guidelines developed by Brooke et al.[13] for predicting loss of ambulation, ambulation ceased 2.4 years (range, 1.2 to 4.1 years) after the patient could no longer climb four standard (6-inch) steps in less than 5 seconds and 1.5 years (range, 0.6 to 2.2 years) after more than 12 seconds were needed.[80]

Some boys with DMD and their families initially resist a powered wheelchair and feel a powered scooter is more acceptable socially; however, most scooters do not provide sufficient seating support and can be difficult to transport compared to power wheelchairs. Most school buses are able to transport a wheelchair, but not a scooter. A scooter can be a nice transitional piece of equipment to be used while the child is still ambulatory but requires assistance for longer distances. It is important to consider the timing of this purchase, however, since most insurance companies only reimburse for power mobility every 3 to 5 years. A boy with DMD can quickly decline in function and strength and may require a more supportive wheelchair before funding is available again. It is important to discuss these factors to help patients and their families through the decision-making process.

Initially, a power wheelchair with a conventional joystick and comfortable seat is usually sufficient to meet the needs of the first-time wheelchair user. As scoliosis develops, a lateral support on the convexity of the scoliotic curve is recommended. Bilateral lateral supports are often not used as this may limit the child's ability to shift weight and perform functional tasks in the chair. Patients with DMD often use neck and trunk motions skillfully to compensate for trunk weakness in their daily activities; therefore, a seating device that is too stable may restrict their ability to perform these maneuvers.[81] A proper pressure-relieving seat cushion is also recommended. Potential pressure areas and/or areas of pain or discomfort can vary depending on the type of spinal deformity present.[81] In patients with scoliosis or kyphoscoliosis, patients complained of pain on the lateral thoracic area and ischial area on the convex side of the curve. In patients with extended spines, pain was reported on bilateral posterior aspects of thighs and bilateral ischial areas. In patients with kyphotic spines, pressure was felt on the sacrum.[81] This should be considered when selecting a pressure-relieving seat cushion.

Once a child undergoes a spinal fusion, some adaptations to the wheelchair and seating components are usually indicated as the child will in effect become taller and less able to compensate for antigravity upper extremity movements. The spinal deformity will now be corrected partially and pressure areas may change as a result. Adjustments in the fit and placement of laterals, head rests, and foot rests may need to be made as well as modifications made to the seat cushion. An addition of an adjustable mobile arm support may be indicated to support the upper arm in a position to allow the elbow to move in a gravity-eliminated plane to assist with activities such as eating or brushing teeth as the child will no longer be able to compensate for weakness with trunk flexion.

As the disease progresses, power tilt-in-space capability will be necessary to provide pressure relief and relaxation as neck and trunk musculature weaken. Additional features such as ventilator adaptations will need to be added on as respiratory status declines. As hand strength weakens, a change in the power control may be indicated.

In a recent study by Pellegrini et al., adults with DMD who had lost their ability to drive a power wheelchair without restriction using a conventional joystick were able to regain unrestricted driving once they changed to an alternative control system including mini-joystick, isometric mini-joystick, finger joystick, or pad.[82] In some drivers the position of the control needed to be modified as well as the device, such as using an isometric mini-joystick with the chin or lips. The study also found that restricted ability to drive a power wheelchair correlated significantly with a decrease in key pinch strength.[82]

Power mobility, although often resisted initially, can provide boys with DMD a positive sense of independence and important means of independent mobility. Careful discussion of power mobility options early on in the disease process can help boys with DMD and their families come to accept the positive aspects of power mobility with confidence when the need for such assistance arises.

WEIGHT CONTROL

The need to guard against obesity is especially important now that the use of corticosteroids in patients with DMD has become more prevalent, as weight gain is a significant side effect. Weight management for the ambulatory child is now equally as important as it is for the child who is limited to a wheelchair. Despite good use of transfer techniques and proper body mechanics by others, excessive weight gain can reduce the child's transfers and may restrict both mobility and social activity. Moreover, excessive weight gain in the child with neuromuscular disease may not only reduce mobility, but also have a deleterious effect on self-esteem, posture, and respiratory function.

Edwards has demonstrated that controlled weight reduction in obese children with DMD is a safe and practical way to improve mobility and self-esteem.[83] However, it is probably easier to prevent excessive weight gain in the young, ambulatory child than to initiate severe dietary restriction in an obese, seated adolescent. It has been proposed that this philosophy of weight control be promoted early for children with neuromuscular disease (taking into account the need for fat intake in early development). Normal growth charts make no allowance for the progressive loss of muscle in DMD, so if the child continues to gain weight according to normal standards, accumulation of fat tissue may occur as, at this stage, there is muscle wasting in DMD. Griffiths and Edwards studied the relationships between body composition and breakdown products of muscle.[84] They developed a chart, based on their research, which gives ideal weight guidelines for weight control in boys with DMD.[84] The physical therapist can play a major role in promoting this weight control philosophy with the child and family. When weight control is not effective, use of a hydraulic lift becomes important. One or more family members must be trained in the safe and proper use of such a lift.

FACILITATING SLEEP

Air mattresses or commercial flotation pads often improve sleeping comfort for children with advanced deterioration who have difficulty positioning themselves or changing position at night. These devices also provide relief for family members who might otherwise be up three to five times per night to turn the patient. A hospital bed may be useful in the later stages of disease to assist with positioning and transfers, as well as to elevate the head of the bed in an attempt to ease the respiratory distress that can occur during sleep as the contents of the abdominal cavity push against the diaphragm, increasing the effort required in taking a deep breath.

ACTIVITIES OF DAILY LIVING

The physical therapist should routinely assess the child's ability to perform activities of daily living (ADLs). The patient's ability to feed himself, turn pages in a book, and do necessary personal hygiene tasks must all be assessed periodically. The physical therapist may choose to request an occupational therapy consultation. A home visit is most helpful in assessing adaptive equipment needs.

RESPIRATORY CONSIDERATIONS

The physical therapist's role in the pulmonary care of patients with DMD will vary depending on each individual practice setting. All physical therapists working with boys with DMD, however, should be aware of the importance of maintaining good pulmonary health whether directly or indirectly involved with their care.

As the diaphragm, trunk, and abdominal muscles weaken, tidal volume and the ability of the patient to effectively clear secretions decreases. Spontaneous periodic deep breaths, as occurs with sighs and yawns, which help to reinflate areas of atelectasis zones and spread surfactant, become absent.[85] A good history and periodic pulmonary function testing with the child in both the seated and supine positions are the most effective means of monitoring respiratory insufficiency. In addition, family members should be trained in the techniques of bronchial drainage, chest percussion, and assisted coughing.

Use of inspiratory and expiratory aids has been shown to prolong survival as well as decrease hospitalizations significantly when following an intensive protocol.[86] In this study by Bach et al., the 24 protocol patients with DMD used noninvasive intermittent positive pressure ventilation (IPPV), manually assisted cough, and mechanically assisted cough (using mechanical insufflation–exsufflation). They used these techniques when needed as indicated by an oximeter, to maintain oxyhemoglobin saturation (SaO_2) greater than or equal to 95%. The protocol patients were compared to patients conventionally managed with tracheostomy and IPPV alone.[86]

Another study demonstrated improved pulmonary function after performance of breathing exercises, but this effect was not sustained.[87] Wanke et al. found improvements in respiratory muscle strength in 10 of 15 boys with DMD, and improvements remained at 6 months after inspiratory muscle training had ended. The five subjects that did not show improvements after 1 month of training had less than 25% predicted vital capacity; therefore, the authors concluded that inspiratory muscle training was beneficial in the early stage of DMD.[88] In a study of the long-term effects of respiratory muscle training (RMT) in 21 subjects with DMD and spinal muscular atrophy (SMA) type III, the authors concluded that, despite the rapidly reversible RMT-induced strength benefits, long-lasting improvements in respiratory load perception (RLP) persisted after 12 months.[89]

FACILITATING FAMILY SUPPORT

The physical therapist plays an important role in providing support, motivation, and training of the patient with DMD and his family members. Successful family support depends on the early involvement of the physical therapist and the ability of the therapist to have the family comply with a home program that is monitored and adapted appropriately. Assessment of the social situation of the family should be part of each visit.

The mild to moderate intellectual impairment in these young boys often imposes both educational and emotional handicaps, in addition to the obvious physical changes accompanying DMD. The child learns that the disease will continuously erode the quality and quantity of his existence, and the resultant reliance and dependence on others frequently gives rise to stress within the family. Although not a psychotherapist, the physical therapist must be aware of the emotional factors involved with the illness and must provide strong emotional support, as well as help in reinforcing and attaining goals and preventing conflicts. A healthy emotional environment for the family and the child with DMD is at least as important to the child as the prevention of contractures.

MANAGEMENT OF PAIN

Most of the pain that occurs in these disorders is mechanical in nature and caused by limited ability to move in the bed or wheelchair either because of muscle weakness or joint contracture. If the aforementioned goals are achieved, management of pain should be minimal. Pain occurs at the limits of ROM in all joints, and because contractures reduce the ROM, they also increase the opportunity for the development of pain. If pain becomes a problem, routine methods of treatment and appropriate positioning techniques should help minimize the discomfort.

SUMMARY

A successful treatment program should result in several additional years of independent ambulation, improved self-sufficiency, and the maintenance of the maximal functional independence allowed by the child's level of strength (see the Case Study at the end of the chapter).

 ## Myotonic Dystrophy

Myotonic dystrophy (MTD) is an autosomal dominant disorder whose location is on chromosome 19.[90] In the most typical form of MTD, the symptoms are first noticed during adolescence and are characterized by myotonia, a delay in muscle relaxation time, and muscle weakness. As the weakness progresses, the myotonia often decreases. The individual will present to the clinic with complaints of weakness and stiffness. Stiffness, which is often the major complaint, is characteristic of the myotonia. Patients often have a characteristic physical appearance that includes a long, thin face with temporal and masseter muscle wasting; frontal balding; and weakness and wasting of the sternocleidomastoids. The pattern of weakness in MTD presents first with distal wasting and weakness, manifested by a foot drop and difficulty opening jars. Proximal muscle weakness occurs in the later stage of the disease. The most severe form of MTD is congenital and is associated with generalized muscular hypoplasia, mental retardation, and a high incidence of neonatal mortality. Children with congenital MTD are born to mothers afflicted with the disorder. Because MTD is inherited in an autosomal dominant pattern, an individual with the disease has a 50/50 chance of each offspring having the disease. The severe congenital form of MTD is characterized by maternal transmission only. The latter group is often plagued with mental retardation, speech disturbances, delayed motor milestones, distal weakness, and spinal deformities. With survival to adulthood, these individuals follow the pattern of the classic course of the disease, in which cataracts are common. There is involvement not only of skeletal muscle, but also smooth muscle and cardiac conduction defects are often seen, particularly first-degree heart block. There may be associated infertility, decreased respiratory drive, and numerous endocrine problems. Currently, there is no treatment for the disorder, and the etiology of the genetic defect is unknown. There is no curative pharmacologic treatment, although some medications may be used to ameliorate the symptoms of myotonia. The objectives of current therapeutic intervention are to reduce the distal wasting and weakness and control the spinal deformities.

Death in these individuals is usually caused by heart block or problems secondary to decreased respiratory drive. The respiratory complications may be severe and, once mechanically ventilated, these patients are very difficult to wean. The congenital forms of MTD may be accompanied by severe developmental delays, in which case intervention that employs various motor development approaches may be beneficial.

 ## Limb-Girdle Muscular Dystrophy

Limb-girdle muscular dystrophy (LGMD) is the term used to refer to a group of progressive muscular dystrophies that primarily affect the proximal musculature. The initial presentation can be quite variable, extending from early childhood into adulthood. Unlike Duchenne muscular dystrophy, the underlying pathology of LGMD is quite heterogeneous. There are now 17 different distinct LGMD genes identified (Table 9.3). These have been labeled 1A through G, representing the recessive forms, and 2A through J, representing the dominant forms.[91] With the elucidation of the underlying genetic and biochemical defects that can cause LGMD, it has become apparent that each of these defects is associated with specific phenotypic patterns. It is beyond the scope of this chapter to discuss all of the forms of LGMD; however, we will discuss the ones that present typically in childhood and may present for treatment in pediatric practice.

The sarcoglycanopathies (LGMD C, D, E, and F) represent those forms of LGMD that most closely resemble the progression of DMD. The sarcoglycanopathies are recessively inherited, with a significant number of cases presenting sporadically.[92] These four forms of LGMD are caused by a deficiency of a group of muscle membrane proteins (Fig. 9.1). The sarcoglycan proteins are coded for on four different chromosomes: γ-sarcoglycan at 13q12, α-sarcoglycan at 17q21.1, β-sarcoglycan at 4q12, and δ-sarcoglycan at 5q33. A deletion of any one of these proteins as the primary defect results in problems incorporating the entire complex or portions of the complex in the membrane. In almost half the cases, this results in incomplete incorporation of dystrophin in the membrane.[92] As a result, there is a great degree of phenotypic overlap between these muscular dystrophies.

Findings on medical evaluation include elevated serum CK anywhere from five times to 100 times normal.[93] The EMG examination is marked by myopathic findings similar to those seen in Duchenne's. Muscle biopsy is typically needed to determine the diagnosis and should show a variation in fiber size, degenerating and regenerating fibers, and central nuclei. When stained by immunohistochemical techniques with monoclonal antibodies to the specific sarcoglycan proteins, the specific pathologic basis of the impairment can often be identified. Genetic testing can also be used to finalize the diagnosis.

Patients with sarcoglycanopathies have an increased risk of dilated cardiac myopathy. Politano et al.[93] found a 40% rate of presymptomatic cardiomyopathy in these patients in addition to signs of hypoxic myocardial insults. The

TABLE 9.3		
Limb Girdle Muscular Dystrophy[a]		
Disease Name	**Gene, Inheritance**	**Protein Product**
LGMD 2A Calpainopathy	15q15 Recessive	Calpain-3
LGMD 2B Dysferlinopathy	2p13 Recessive	Dysferlin
LGMD 2C γ-Sarcoglycanopathy	13q12 Recessive	γ-Sarcoglycan
LGMD 2D α-Sarcoglycanopathy	17q21 Recessive	α-Sarcoglycan
LGMD 2E β-Sarcoglycanopathy	4q12 Recessive	β-Sarcoglycan
LGMD 2F δ-Sarcoglycanopathy	5q33–34 Recessive	δ-Sarcoglycan
LGMD 2G Telethoninopathy	17q11–12 Recessive	Telethonin
LGMD 2H	9q33.2 Recessive	TRIM32
LGMD 2I FKRPopathy	19q13.3 Recessive	Fukutin-related protein (FKRP)
LGMD 2J Titinopathy	2q24.3 Recessive	Titin
LGMD 1A Myotilinopathy	5q22–34 Dominant	Myotilin
LGMD 1B Laminopathy	1q11–21 Dominant	Lamin A/C
LGMD 1C Caveolinopathy	3p25 Dominant	Caveolin-3
LGMD 1D	6q23 Dominant	
LGMD 1E	7q Dominant	
LGMD 1F	7q32.1–32.2 Dominant	
LGMD 1G	4p21 Dominant	

[a]From Kirschner J, Bonnemenn CG. The congenital and limb-girdle muscular dystrophies: sharpening the focus, blurring the boundaries. Arch Neurol 2004;61:189–199; and Starling A, Kok F, Passos-Bueno MR, et al. A new form of autosomal dominant limb-girdle muscular dystrophy (LGMD1G) with progressive fingers and toes flexion limitation maps to chromosome 4p21. Eur J Hum Genet 2004;12(12):1033–1040.

patients with dilated cardiomyopathy had primarily γ and δ sarcoglycanopathies and those with hypoxic damage had β, γ, and δ sarcoglycanopathies.

These four proteins, α-, β-, γ-, and δ-sarcoglycan, are closely associated with dystrophin, the defective protein in Duchenne muscular dystrophy. LGMD in general and sarcoglycanopathies in particular can present with a similar albeit somewhat more variable phenotype when compared with DMD. The distribution of muscle weakness is marked by a proximal-to-distal gradient, and in sarcoglycanopathies the adductors of the hip are the most severely and first involved followed by the hamstrings and biceps.

Other muscles of the upper extremity that become involved include the deltoids, pectoralis major, rhomboids, and infraspinatus, and a significant number of patients demonstrate scapular winging emblematic of their proximal weakness. Of the distal muscles the anterior tibialis is the most likely to be weak. Unlike patients with DMD, a compensated Trendelenburg or waddling gait is not typically seen in these patients.[92]

A second form of LGMD, type 2A or calpainopathy, is also recessively inherited and is caused by the absence of calpain-3 that results from a deletion on chromosome 15q15.1–15.3.[94] Calpain-3 is the first enzyme that was identified as the causative defect of a progressive muscular dystrophy. Calpain-3 is part of a larger group of calpain molecules whose exact function is still not entirely clear but may be involved in modulation of cytoskeletal proteins. Calpain-3 can also be reduced in patients with LGMD 2B and 2J because presumably calpain is associated with dysferlin and connectin (titin), the primary protein defects in these forms of LGMD (Fig. 9.1).[95]

Clinical presentation of LGMD 2A includes a typically elevated creatine kinase and muscle biopsy findings with degenerating and regenerating fibers, central nuclei, and a variation in fiber size. The EMG will have typical myopathic features. Patients show no intellectual deficits and cardiac defects have not been reported at increased rates in LGMD 2A.[96] Unlike other muscular dystrophies, there seems to be no direct correlation between the amount of protein identified on biopsy and the severity of clinical presentation,[95] and the age at presentation does not necessarily provide guidance for the timing of ambulation loss.[97] However, patients with in-frame genetic defects on both alleles tend to have a later onset of symptoms and a later diagnosis as compared to those with heterozygous or homozygous null mutations. Ambulation typically continues throughout childhood, with the average child losing ambulation in the late teens or early 20s; however, there can be a significant variability between patients, with some continuing to ambulate into middle age and others losing ambulation in early childhood.[96]

LGMD 2A has a wide variation in the severity of presentation and in the course of the disease. Typically the presentation is in the second decade of life initially with proximal atrophy. This is most commonly expressed as scapular winging. Weakness of the elbow flexors can also be present. The wrist extensors are typically weaker than the flexors and the hip adductors are more affected, while the abductors are preserved long into the disease process. The knee extensors typically remain stronger than the flexors and the ankle evertors are typically weaker than the invertors. Contractures are typically found in the calf muscles along with atrophy of this muscle in most European patients; however, in Brazilian patients hypertrophy can be found in the calf. Finger-flexion and elbow-flexion contractures may also be present early on in the disease process. These muscle imbalances correspond with a typical standing posture of hip abduction, knee hyperextension, and inversion at the ankle that is preserved long into the disease process. Patients with LGMD 2A typically remain able to stand with support far into the disease process because of this pattern of contracture and muscle involvement.[96,97]

The last form of LGMD that will be discussed here is LGMD 2I. LGMD 2I is recessively inherited and caused by a mutation in the fukutin-related protein gene (FKRP). This gene is also the cause of some forms of congenital muscular dystrophy, which we will discuss later. The gene was mapped to chromosome 19q13.3[98] and the encoded protein FKRP is a glycosyltransferase that aids in the glycosylation of α-dystroglycan; as a result, the protein does not form properly.[99] α-Dystroglycan is located in the extracellular space and is associated with the dystrophin complex that spans the membrane. Although the exact function is not known, it is thought to transmit force from the intracellular actin via dystrophin in addition to assisting in stabilizing the muscle membrane during contraction.[100]

Diagnosis is established first by clinical presentation marked by weakness. EMG shows a typical myopathic pattern and serum creatine kinase typically is in the thousands. Muscle biopsy is typically characterized by a variation in fiber size with type 1 predominance, degenerating and regenerating fibers, an increase in central nuclei, and increased connective tissue.[98] Immunohistochemistry in these patients can be variable, with the most common finding being a reduction of laminin α-2; reductions in α-dystroglycan can also be found.[101]

Clinical presentation of patients with LGMD 2I can vary somewhat, with initial onset of symptoms typically in the first two decades of life. A significant number of patients present with a Duchenne-like phenotype. In these patients onset is typically in the preschool years. The pattern of weakness is similar to that of Duchenne with proximal weakness predominating and gastrocnemius/soleus contracture and hypertrophy most pronounced. However, in the more severely involved patients, the shoulder girdle is more involved than the pelvic girdle. In the milder patients, the opposite is true. In the more severe patients respiratory function can become an issue as the disease progresses; however, this appears to progress at a slower rate than Duchenne's. Most patients with LGMD 2I typically maintain fairly good respiratory function throughout the first two decades of life.[102,103] Cardiac defects are also a common characteristic of LGMD 2I. More than half of these patients have cardiac involvement. Male patients with heterozygous mutations are at increased risk for developing dilated cardiac myopathy when compared with female patients or those with homozygous mutations[103] and as a result need to be monitored more closely by their physician.

Clinical care for patients with LGMD revolves around anticipating the development of contractures and conservative management with dynamic or static resting splints to maintain muscle length. Range-of-motion exercises and exercise to optimize muscle endurance such as swimming can be considered but, because this is a dystrophic process, eccentric and strengthening exercise should be avoided.

Congenital Myopathy

Congenital myopathy describes a group of diseases including nemaline myopathy, central core myopathy, and centronuclear (myotubular) myopathy. These as well as the other congenital myopathies typically result from abnormalities of the sarcomeric proteins. These diseases are characterized by weakness and muscle atrophy that typically presents at birth. There are, however, forms that can present later in life. The congenital myopathies represent a group of disorders that are less well characterized when compared to the other disorders we have discussed thus far. The broad diagnostic classifications are based on morphologic characteristics found on muscle biopsy with subtyping based on clinical features. In each broad category there are a number of genetic mutations that can be the predisposing factor; however, there is significant clinical variability that can be seen. Here we will discuss two of the most common congenital myopathies, nemaline myopathy and central core myopathy.

Nemaline myopathy has a wide range in the severity of clinical presentation as well as heterogeneity of genetic causes. There have been five genes identified as possible causes of nemaline myopathy, each related to a different sarcomeric protein (Table 9.4). The inheritance pattern is most often sporadic but can be also dominant or recessive. Pathologically on muscle biopsy there are cytoplasmic inclusions called either rods or nemaline bodies that represent deposits of z-line proteins.[104–106]

Nemaline myopathy has been divided into seven different forms based on severity and other factors by the European Neuromuscular Center. These types include the typical or classic form, the severe form, the intermediate form, the mild form, and the adult-onset form. In addition, there is a severe Amish type with neonatal onset and a category for other forms. The typical form of nemaline myopathy presents at birth or early infancy with respiratory insufficiency being an issue, especially at night. These patients often become ambulatory; however, some will need wheeled mobility. The severe form is characterized by weakness from birth. Often in this type no spontaneous movement is evident. These patients can have arthrogryposis and fractures at birth. Lack of respiratory effort and the resulting respiratory insufficiency and ventilator dependence often lead to death in the first year of life. The intermediate form presents in infancy or at birth. Patients are able to breathe on their own by 1 year and either don't

ambulate at all or progress and develop contractures over time and lose the ability to ambulate by 11 years of age. The mild form presents in childhood, often with a history of normal developmental milestones. This form is often slowly progressive, and in the later stages this form can be clinically indistinguishable from the classic or typical presentation. The adult form tends to be more progressive and can also demonstrate inflammatory changes on biopsy as well as cardiomyopathy.[107–108] The most common form is the classic or typical form representing 43% of cases in one series.[109] The intermediate and severe congenital forms represent 20% and 16%, respectively, with the less severe form with childhood and adult-onset representing the remaining cases.

Central core myopathy is named for the appearance of the presence of histologic cores on muscle biopsy. If the cores appear large, the name *central core myopathy* is used, and if there are multiple small cores, the term *multiminicore myopathy* is used. Despite the use of these two terms, they only represent a pathologic description and may represent different stages in the same disease process. Family members with presumably the same disease process may have both central and multiminicores, and the same patient first with multiminicores may later in the disease process present with central cores.[105] These cores are areas within the muscle that contain no mitochondria, are negative for oxidative enzymes, and contain a collection of proteins that include many of the proteins that have been identified in other muscle diseases as well as many other proteins. The gene identified as responsible for central core disease is found on 19q13; it codes for the ryanodine receptor 1 protein and controls the release of calcium from the sarcoplasmic reticulum.[105,110,111]

Clinically, central core myopathy can be relatively static or mildly progressive over long periods. The pattern of weakness typically includes facial weakness, neck flexor weakness, and proximal weakness with the legs being more involved than the arms.[112] There is a spectrum of patients with central core myopathy and more severe forms have been noted. The other clinical feature of patients with ryanodine receptor 1 mutations is the susceptibility to malignant hyperthermia, which is a severe reaction to anesthesia.

TABLE 9.4	

Gene Locus and Protein Product for Nemaline Myopathy[a]

Gene Locus	Protein
1q21–23	α-Tropomyosin
2q21.2–22	Nebulin
1q42.1	Sarcomeric actin
9p13.4	β-Tropomyosin
19q13.4	Troponin T1

[a]From Goebel HH. Congenital myopathies at their molecular dawning. Muscle Nerve 2003;27:527–48

Congenital Muscular Dystrophy

Congenital muscular dystrophy (CMD) can be divided into those CMDs with central nervous system involvement and those without central nervous system involvement. Fukuyama congenital muscular dystrophy, Walker-Warburg syndrome, and muscle–eye–brain disease all demonstrate muscle, brain, and eye abnormalities. The typical brain abnormalities include a cobblestone lissencephaly with cerebral and cerebellar cortical dysplasia secondary to a neuronal migration abnormality. Eye and vision abnormalities span a wide range of possible abnormalities and vary from one disease to the other but may include myopia and retinal detachment.[113] The muscle abnormalities are based on abnormal glycosylation of dystroglycan resulting from the absence of various enzymes that facilitate the process of glycosylation, which is the addition of glycosyl groups to a protein to form a glycoprotein. As a result of the common pathophysiology, there is significant overlap in the clinical presentation of these diseases and the pathologic findings encountered during the diagnostic workup. All present congenitally in the typical case. Walker-Warburg syndrome is the most severe of the congenital muscular dystrophies and children typically die by 3 years of age. Muscle–eye–brain disease has a variable clinical picture and presents in infancy. The more mildly involved patients may ambulate for a period of time during childhood; however, their functional abilities are limited by spasticity and ataxia resulting from the brain abnormalities as well as the muscle weakness. Most patients with Fukuyama CMD will achieve standing and some can take steps in early childhood. Typically in the second decade respiratory failure becomes a problem beginning with nocturnal hypoventilation. This can progress, limiting the life expectancy of these patients to the third decade of life. Cardiomyopathy is also a feature commonly seen in these patients, and they should be periodically followed by cardiology.

Merosin, also known as laminin, negative CMD is the most common CMD representing half of all cases of CMD. The absence of merosin in the muscle (Fig. 9.1) results from an abnormality of the LAMA2 gene found on chromosome 6q2. Merosin-negative CMD also shows central nervous system involvement in the form of abnormalities of the periventricular and subcortical white matter. The clinical course of this disorder is characterized by severe weakness in early infancy and the development of contractures, particularly at the ankle and eventually at the knee and elbow. The severe weakness can improve over time and most patients will sit by 2 or 3 years of age and upwards of 25% will stand or walk with bracing. Muscle strength can be stable over time; however, nocturnal hypoventilation may be a problem for many of these patients and one-third may have cardiac abnormalities.[114,115]

Ullrich CMD results from the abnormalities of collagen VI resulting from mutations of COL6A1, A2, or A3. COL6A2 is located on chromosome 21q22.3 and COL5A3 is located on chromosome 2q37.[116] Collagen VI is found in the extracellular matrix (Fig. 9.1) and presumably acts to transmit force from the muscle to the bone and tendon. Ullrich CMD is typically recessively inherited; however, dominant negative inheritance has recently been shown to represent a significant minority of these patients' inheritance pattern.[117] A dominant negative exists where the affected allele negatively impacts the nonaffected allele. The milder form of collagen VI abnor-

mality, Bethlem myopathy, is dominantly inherited. On muscle biopsy, findings can range from mild myopathic findings to dystrophic in the more severe patients; however, it is rare to see necrotic and regenerating fibers. Classically, findings include variation in fiber size and infiltration of the muscle by fatty and fibrotic tissue. Patients with Ullrich CMD typically have weakness at birth in all but the mildest cases. There is an increased risk of congenital hip dislocation as well as torticollis and arthrogryposis; the latter two typically improve with stretching. Gross motor skills are typically delayed; however, there are improvements seen in motor skills in the first few years of life and patients typically gain the ability to sit independently and stand with bracing. A significant number of patients also gain the ability to ambulate independently. Contractures of the hips, knees, and elbows are typical and are combined with hyperlaxity of the distal joints as well as the shoulders and hips. Respiratory insufficiency can be a problem for the more severely effected patients as they age.[116]

Physical therapy intervention in CMD and congenital myopathy needs to take into account the natural history of the specific disorder, and realistic goals need to be planned based on the natural history of the disease. A focus on the maintenance of flexibility with stretching and appropriate bracing or serial casting as needed is important. Bracing may be needed for standing or ambulation, and for those who are not ambulatory, standers and wheelchairs as well as bathroom adaptations may provide practical assistance. In those patients with sufficient cognitive skills, power mobility should be considered. Even in those patients who have some household ambulation, power mobility may be necessary for community mobility or for longer distances at school.

Spinal Muscular Atrophy

Spinal muscular atrophy is a disorder that is manifested by a loss of anterior horn cells. This results in a phenotypic spectrum of disease states that have been divided into three types of SMA based on a functional classification system.

Three categories of SMA occur in childhood:

1. SMA type I (Werdnig-Hoffman disease)
2. SMA type II
3. SMA type III (Kugelberg-Welander disease)

The classification of a child with SMA into one of the above types of SMA is solely based on the child's functional abilities. The children who are so weak that they never learn to sit are diagnosed with SMA type I. Those children who learn to sit but never learn to walk without an assistive device have type II SMA. The children that walk independently are diagnosed with SMA type III.

GENETICS

SMA is inherited as an autosomal recessive disorder. The underlying genetic defect is located on chromosome 5q13 where the survival motor neuron (SMN) gene is located and the SMN protein is coded for.[117,118] In this region of the gene there are two homologous genes, SMN1 and SMN2, that code for the SMN protein. Typically there is one copy of SMN1 and multiple copies of SMN2. SMN1 produces most of the protein that the body uses, and when that portion of the gene is deleted, the SMN2 gene must be relied on to produce the SMN protein. Most of the SMN protein that SMN2 produces is not functional. The amount of SMN produced in patients with SMA depends on how many copies of SMN2 the patient has. The number of SMN2 copies also correlates with how severe the phenotypic presentation of the disease is.

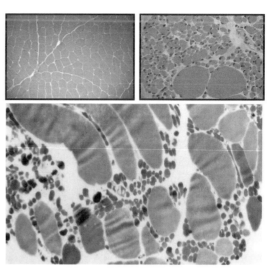

Figure 9.9 ■ Neuropathic changes associated with spinal muscular atrophy. Note the hypertrophic changes and grouped atrophy.

PATHOPHYSIOLOGY

SMN plays a role in the function of all cells, mediating the assembly of a set of proteins that associate with RNA. The α motor neuron appears to be the only cell significantly impacted by the diminished levels of SMN. Patients with SMA as a result have a portion of their α motor neurons undergo apoptosis.

As a result of the loss of motor neurons, EMG results will be characterized by diminished compound motor unit action potentials (CMAPs) that are often of short duration; the diminished CMAPs will track the course of the disease. Positive sharp waves and fibrillations are also found and typically conduction velocities and sensory studies are normal.[120] The number of motor units are also diminished in children with SMA. The number of remaining motor units can be estimated by EMG using motor unit number estimation (MUNE). MUNE reflects the number of lower motor neurons that innervate a given muscle. In addition to CMAPs, MUNE can be used to monitor the progress of the underlying pathologic process affecting the motor neuron.[121]

Typically the histopathology found on muscle biopsy is characterized by groups of small atrophic fibers interspersed with groups of large hypertrophic fibers (Fig. 9.9). This type of grouped atrophy is characteristic of a neurogenic process. The groups of atrophic fibers are the result of lack of innervation to that motor unit. All three types of SMA have underlying pathology that affects the anterior horn cell; as a result they share some common clinical features. All children with SMA will demonstrate some degree of weakness, albeit to varying degrees, depending on the type of the disease. Patients with SMA will typically have absent deep tendon reflexes; however, this is not completely uniform. About half of patients will have fasciculations that can be seen in the tongue as spontaneous small muscle contractions[122]; these can be seen on muscle ultra-

sound at times even if they are not visible in the tongue. Since only the lower motor neuron is affected, sensation is typically intact as is cognitive function in patients with SMA. Since this is a lower motor neuron disease, no upper motor neuron signs should be noted.

SPINAL MUSCULAR ATROPHY TYPE I (WERDNIG-HOFFMAN DISEASE)

SMA type I is almost always noted within the first 3 months of life; however, the diagnosis may not be made for a number of months. The mother often complains of decreased fetal movement during her pregnancy. At birth, the affected child is hypotonic, and may have difficulty feeding. Muscle wasting is often severe, and spontaneous movements are infrequent and of small amplitude. On examination the infant with SMA type I will present with a head lag in the pull-to-sit position and will drape over the examiner's hand when a landau test is performed. The infant will be dominated by gravity and in supine the legs will be abducted and flexed and the arms will move primarily with the elbows on the surface, and if they can be brought to midline this will be with difficulty. In the most severely affected infants axial strength will be so diminished that in supine the head will not be able to be maintained in midline. Prone skills will be similarly limited and infants with SMA type I will not be able to prop and typically cannot turn their heads from side to side in prone. In vertical some infants will demonstrate tenuous head control, while most will not be able to maintain their heads erect.

Infants with SMA type I typically have significant oral motor weakness that makes feeding progressively more difficult. These infants have difficulty taking in sufficient calories to gain weight and thrive. Medical options for supplemental feeding in these patients include nasogastric feeding or the surgical placement of a gastrostomy tube.

Patients with SMA type I also have limited respiratory function and develop an abnormal pattern of breathing, with the diaphragmatic muscles playing the primary role in ventilation. In these infants inspiration is diaphragmatically initiated, and as negative pressure develops in the thoracic cavity, the intercostals and other thoracic muscles that typically stabilize the ribcage fail and the ribcage collapses with each breath. Typically the belly also rises as the diaphragm lowers. In the weakest infants the chest and the abdomen will be directly out of phase. In the infants who are a bit stronger the chest will stabilize or expand briefly with the abdomen prior to collapsing, which is in contrast with the normal condition of almost simultaneous abdominal and thoracic expansion. Pulmonary infections are common in infants with SMA type I, and pulmonary management is an important facet of care for these patients. Both the inability to take a deep breath and the lack of an effective cough can cause serious respiratory complications, including atelectasis and pneumonia. Percussion and postural drainage should be recommended for use when the infant has upper respiratory infections to move the secretions from the small airways. These infants may also be treated with a mechanical insufflator–exsufflator that delivers a positive pressure insufflation followed by an expulsive exsufflation that simulates a cough as an additional means of airway clearance[123] and as a way of maintaining flexibility of the lung and ribcage. Most children with infantile SMA do not survive beyond 3 years of age without the assistance of mechanical ventilation. For those that do choose to have tracheostomies the life span can be extended significantly beyond this.[8,124]

Children with SMA type I have such severe weakness that it is difficult for them to take part in play activities. Switch toys are appropriate to allow the child access to play for those children that survive past 8 months when cause and effect begins to develop. In addition, younger infants may benefit from a sling-and-spring setup that can be made from Thera-Band tubing and Velfoam cuffs and attached to their infant carrier to aid them in antigravity shoulder movement and allow access to their toys. The approach to physical therapy for these children must be aimed at quality of life for both the child and family.

SPINAL MUSCULAR ATROPHY TYPE II

Type II SMA also affects infants but is more benign than SMA type I. Initial presentation is typically later in the first year of life when the child is not pulling to stand. These children are characterized by weakness and wasting of the extremities and trunk musculature. Fasciculations are common on examination of the tongue in these patients. There is also often a fine tremor when the child attempts to use the limbs. This is not a true intention tremor, but has been referred to as a mini-polymyoclonus.[8]

In children with SMA type II there is a delay in the acquisition of motor skills that is somewhat variable between children. Approximately one-third of children with SMA type II will sit by the normal time of 6 months and 90% will be able to sit by their first birthday.[125] Some children may continue to gain skills throughout their preschool years, but there is typically a peak after which a slow decline in skills ensues, the rapidity of which depends largely on the underlying disease severity. Of the children who become independent sitters, 75% will remain independent sitters until 7 years and half will remain sitting at 14 years of age.[126] Motor skills that employ a long lever arm are most difficult for these patients and as a result prone and quadruped skills are most delayed because it is difficult to maintain head control in these positions. Transitions to and from sit will also be difficult because of the weight of the head during the transition. Despite a slow overall decline in function as these children grow up, there are often long periods of relative functional stability. Despite what one would anticipate based on the decline in function, there is not a loss in strength over time in children with SMA.[127] However, these data represent a group of patients over the age of 4 years, since younger children cannot be reliably tested.

The pattern of weakness seen in the extremities is most notable for the relative strength in the distal muscles as compared to the proximal muscles. On average, strength in patients with type II and III SMA falls between 20% and 40% of predicted based on age. Quadriceps strength tends to be the most diminished, averaging 5% of normal. However, in patients with SMA who ambulate, the variation in quadriceps strength can be threefold as compared to patients who do not ambulate.[128,129]

Contracture is also an issue in the management of patients with SMA type II. Limitations of the knee extensors and ankle plantar flexors are frequently the most significant contractures in the lower extremity, and contractures of the elbow flexors and wrist flexors are the most significant in the arm. For the hands, resting hand splints are appropriate for night use and for the legs knee–ankle–foot orthotics (KAFO) as discussed in the next section will aid in maintaining range of motion. In addition, a daily stretching program will help maintain the patients' flexibility.

By definition, these children do not ambulate independently; however, some of these children may learn to walk with bracing or an assistive device,[130] although often the ambulation is not functional. Nonetheless, it is important to encourage standing in patients with type II SMA. Standing will act to maintain joint mobility, maintain bone stock, prevent problems associated with long-term wheelchair sitting, and attempt to keep the patient's back as straight as possible for as long as possible. These patients often require KAFOs for standing, and as they become weaker the addition of a pelvic band may be necessary. The proximal portion of the KAFO may be shaped for ischial weight bearing for comfort and improved control of the proximal femur (Fig. 9.10). During the school-age years when the child becomes too heavy to lift into standing, a transition to a more traditional stander becomes appropriate and bracing may be necessary only to stabilize the foot and ankle. Some children will become too contracted to maintain a standing program. For those children who can continue in a standing program, there are a number of options, some that will accommodate flexion contractures and others that assist in the transfer, alleviating some of the burden on the parent.

Feeding and swallowing difficulties are seldom a problem early in the course of the disease, but many children do not gain weight well and some require supplemental feeding as they get older to maintain optimal body weight.

These children often survive into adulthood but are vulnerable to pulmonary infection and may require mechanical ventilation either at night secondary to nocturnal hypoventilation or full time. The use of a mechanical insufflator–exsufflator in this population is also helpful in airway clearance, as are percussion and postural drainage, since these patients also lack the muscle strength to produce a strong cough.[123]

Children with SMA type II are predisposed to kyphoscoliosis, similar to that which affects other children with neuromuscular weakness. Spinal bracing has been characterized as not preventing progression of the spinal curve,[131] and when spinal bracing is worn, pulmonary function is limited as compared to pulmonary function without bracing.[132] However, as a practical matter for patients who have pain as well as scoliosis, a soft spinal orthosis can provide support for the trunk and allow improved tolerance in sitting for those patients that choose not to have a fusion. Typically scoliosis in this population and in patients with type III SMA has been treated with segmental spinal fusion. This prevents the inevitable progression of the curve, which can be more rapid once the patient is in a wheelchair full time.[133] However, there is a down side to spinal fusion. Fusion can also be associated with some loss of functional skill. When the flexibility of the spine is taken away, some tasks can become more difficult, especially in the weaker patients. Ambulatory patients are also at risk of functional decline following a fusion.[134] Despite this, typically the benefits of preventing the inevitable progression of the scoliosis and the associated pulmonary decline outweigh the risks associated with the surgery, and patients typically report improved comfort and sitting balance following surgery.[135]

SPINAL MUSCULAR ATROPHY TYPE III (KUGELBERG-WELANDER DISEASE)

SMA type III is characterized by symptoms of progressive weakness, wasting, and fasciculations. Age of presentation can vary from the toddler years into adulthood, the latter

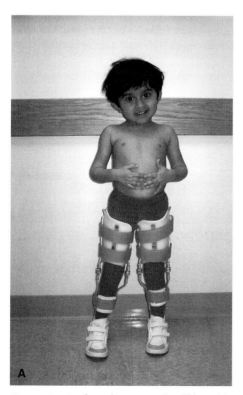
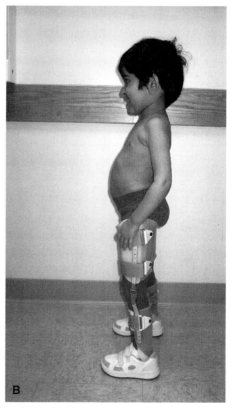

Figure 9.10 ■ Anterior–posterior **(A)** and lateral view **(B)** of 3-year-old with type II spinal muscular atrophy wearing ischial weight-bearing knee–ankle–foot orthoses.

of which some would classify as type IV. Proximal muscles are usually involved first, and because of the age of presentation, this disease may be confused with the muscular dystrophies. Deep tendon reflexes are decreased, but contractures are unusual, and progressive spinal deformities are uncommon as long as the child remains ambulatory. Diagnosis is established on the basis of the clinical picture and the results of diagnostic laboratory studies, including an electromyogram and muscle biopsy, which show denervation as in the other forms of SMA. In addition, genetic testing will show a deletion of the SMN gene on the fifth chromosome.

Prognosis in patients with SMA type III can be aided by a good developmental history. Patients who have symptoms that begin prior to 2 years of age have a relatively poorer prognosis when compared with patients who have symptoms that begin after the age of 2. Russman et al. followed 159 patients with SMA and found that in patients with SMA type III, if symptoms begin after 2 years of age, on average patients continued to ambulate until 44 years of age. In those who began to have symptoms prior to 2 years of age, ambulation was maintained until an average of 12 years of age.[126]

Treatment from a physical therapy standpoint is focused primarily on the maintenance of function and flexibility. Patients need to be braced appropriately while they are still ambulating and for standing after they stop ambulating. Once patients become more difficult to handle in braces for standing, standers, which aid patients to standing from a sitting position, like the Grand stand can be helpful to maintain flexibility and bone stock through a standing program.

Charcot-Marie-Tooth Disease

Charcot-Marie-Tooth (CMT) disease, also known as hereditary motor and sensory neuropathy (HMSN), is a slowly progressive neuropathy that affects peripheral nerves and causes sensory loss, weakness, and muscle wasting primarily in the distal musculature of the feet, lower legs, hands, and forearms. It is the most frequently inherited peripheral neuropathy affecting 1 in 2500 persons.[136] There are many different types and subtypes of CMT depending on the specific gene defect, inheritance pattern, age of onset, and whether the primary defect is in the myelin or axon of the nerve. CMT1, a demyelinating form, is the most common form of CMT and is characterized by an autosomal dominance inheritance pattern and onset of symptoms in childhood or adolescence.[137,138] In the most common subtype, CMT1a, a defect of the gene PMP22 or peripheral myelin protein 22 on chromosome 17 is present.[139] CMT2 shares the inheritance pattern and time of onset of CMT1; however, it primarily affects the axon of the nerve.[137] CMT1 and CMT2 share the same clinical features as noted above. CMT3, also known as Dejerine-Sottas (DS)

disease, is an autosomal dominant congenital hypomyelinating neuropathy with onset in infancy and more severe weakness.[59,138] CMT4 also presents in infancy but is autosomal recessive. There are other forms of CMT including an X-linked form (CMTX) and a mild congenital form.

CMT is diagnosed by physical examination, genetic testing, EMG, and nerve conduction velocity (NCV) tests. Symptoms of weakness usually begin in the feet and ankles with a foot drop and later in the hands and forearms. Many people with CMT develop contractures in the feet causing cavovarus deformity involving the forefoot, hindfoot, midfoot, and toes (Fig. 9.11).[139] Contractures in the long finger flexors may also develop. Decreased sensation to heat, touch, and pain is also present distally.

A physical therapy program can benefit individuals with CMT by improving strength, range of motion, and functional activities. Orthotic assessment and prescription can greatly improve the gait and functional mobility of a person with CMT by preventing contracture formation and providing a more stable base for ambulation. Custom braces may also improve aerobic performance and decrease energy expenditure, as was demonstrated in a single subject with CMT.[140] Stretching, night splints, and serial casting also can improve range of motion, but if a fixed deformity develops, orthopedic surgery to correct the deformity may be necessary to produce a plantigrade foot.[54]

A resistance training program of 3 days per week for 12 weeks was found to improve strength and ADLs in a study of 20 subjects with CMT (18 with CMT1A and two with CMT2).[136] These subjects were also randomized to either a placebo or creatine monohydrate group. The authors concluded that creatine added no benefit.[25] Another study by Lindeman et al. found increases in

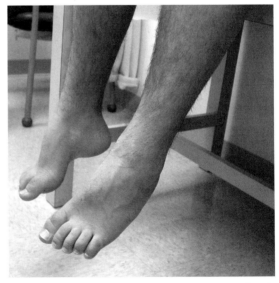

Figure 9.11 ■ Sixteen-year-old with Charcot-Marie-Tooth disease. Notice the high arch and hammertoes on both feet as well as the varus position of the ankle.

strength and function after a moderate to moderately high-resistance home-based strengthening program in subjects with CMT but not in the subjects with myotonic dystrophy.[141,142]

SUMMARY

The disorders discussed in this chapter are all characterized by weakness and wasting of the skeletal musculature, progressive deformity, and increasing disability. The physical therapist plays an important role in the management of these disorders. The therapist's role centers around the maintenance of function, both through the management of what is often a progressive process and the provision of assistive technology. This may be as simple as recommending bath equipment to make transfers more manageable or as involved as prescribing power mobility to compensate for the loss of ambulation. The therapist is also in a position to provide teaching surrounding the natural history of the disease process and the necessary emotional support for the affected child and family. These additional roles may be as important as the actual physical assistance that physical therapists traditionally provide.

CASE STUDY

A.M. is a 10-year-old Caucasian boy with a diagnosis of Duchenne muscular dystrophy. He was diagnosed at 4 years of age when it was noted that he was slow getting up off the floor after story time at preschool and appeared unable to keep up with his school mates. He has been followed periodically by physical therapy since that time for family education in range-of-motion and active stretching exercises and for monitoring the status of his muscle strength, function, and joint contractures.

At 4 years of age, the family had been instructed in stretching of the heel cords to be performed on a daily basis and A.M. had been fitted with night splints to maintain a neutral position at his ankles during sleep. (He was encouraged to wear his "moon boots" throughout the night, but if it was only 2 to 3 hours at neutral before he took them off, this shorter period was considered beneficial.) A.M. was started on prednisone by his neurologist and became somewhat stronger and was able to run better. These functional gains, however, came with a price. A.M. initially gained some weight, but since his parents knew to watch for this, his weight gain was not as great as it could have been. In addition, A.M. was somewhat more active and inattentive in school. Despite the side effects, his parents chose to keep him on the medication because they felt the benefits outweighed the side effects. At 5 to 6 years of age, the stretching of hip flexors and iliotibial bands had been added to the

daily stretching regimen because he had developed mild flexion and abduction contractures.

At this time, A.M. comes to physical therapy with the chief complaint of an increased number of falls (approximately four per day), increased difficulty rising from a chair and ascending and descending stairs, and no longer being able to get off the floor without the use of "furniture" along with his Gower's maneuver.

Strength in the upper extremities (UE) graded in the "good" range, with the lower extremities (LE) grading "fair" to "poor," in the proximal muscle groups. Measurements of joint contractures revealed hip flexors that measured –10 degrees bilaterally, iliotibial bands at 0 degrees bilaterally, knees at neutral, and –10 degrees at the right ankle and –8 degrees on the left. In the UE, ROM was within normal limits bilaterally and functionally still independent.

Stretching exercises were reviewed and emphasized with the family. Contracture releases were also discussed with the family as an option and a future referral to the orthopedic surgeon was discussed. A.M. and his family were instructed to return to physical therapy in conjunction with being fitted by the orthotist with the long leg braces should they opt for surgery. The need for a wheelchair, only to be used for long-distance transport and on uneven terrain, was addressed, and since it had been discussed at previous visits they were ready to order this and chose a power wheelchair. They had a "buggy" that they used for long distances, but it was clear that this didn't provide the independence that A.M. wanted, especially outdoors with his friends.

Contact was made with the treating physical therapist in the school district for his or her suggestions or comments regarding power mobility, and issues related to home and school accessibility was discussed with the family and therapist, both in terms of transport and access. A.M. became a full-time wheelchair user at 12, and despite the lateral support on his chair, he developed scoliosis, which required fusion when it reached 40 degrees. Following the fusion, A.M. had trouble feeding himself and was ordered a mobile arm support and also began to use the tilt feature on his most recent power chair not only for pressure relief, but also to clear the door while entering his adapted van since he grew 3 inches following the surgery.

As A.M. got older the focus of therapy shifted to maintaining hand function, and resting hand splints and range of motion for the long finger flexors and elbow flexors were taught. At 22, A.M. was having increasing difficulty driving his chair. He was unable to drive in reverse and could no longer reposition his arm when he went over bumps. In addition, through further discussion it became apparent that he had been having trouble accessing his computer and had not discussed this at previous clinic visits. A.M. was ordered a mini-joystick to drive his wheelchair and a mouse emulator so he could access the computer with his wheelchair control. In addition, he was referred for evaluation for an on-screen keyboard word prediction software and a dictation program.

REFERENCES

1. Koenig N, Hoffman EP, Bertelson CJ, et al. Complete cloning of the Duchenne muscular dystrophy (DMD) cDNA and preliminary genomic organization of the DMD gene in normal and affected individuals. Cell 1987;50:509–517.

2. Tsao CY, Mendell JR. The childhood muscular dystrophies: making order out of chaos. Semin Neurol. 1999;19:9–23.

3. Mendell JR, Sahenk Z, Prior TW. The childhood muscular dystrophies: diseases sharing a common pathogenesis of membrane instability. J Child Neurol 1995;10:150–159.

4. Melancini P, Vianello A, Villanova C, et al. Cardiac and respiratory involvement in advanced stage Duchenne muscular dystrophy. Neuromusc Disord 1996;6:367–376.

5. Hoffman EP, Brown RH, Kunkel LM. Dystrophin: the protein product of the Duchenne muscular dystrophy locus. Cell 1987;51:919.

6. Crisp DE, Ziter FA, Bray PF. Diagnostic delay in Duchenne muscular dystrophy. JAMA 1982;247:478–480.

7. Behrman RG, Kleigman R, Jenson HB. Nelson Textbook of Pediatrics. 16th Ed. WB Saunders, 2000.

8. Brooke MH. Clinicians' View of Neuromuscular Disease. 2nd Ed. Baltimore: Williams & Wilkins, 1986:117–159.

9. Blake DJ, Weir A, Newey SE, et al. Function and genetics of dystrophin and dystrophin-related proteins in muscle. Physiol Rev 2002;82:291–329.

10. Brooke MH, Fenichel G, Griggs R, et al. Clinical investigations in Duchenne dystrophy. Part 2. Determination of the "power" of therapeutic trials based on the natural history. Muscle Nerve 1983;6:91–103.

11. Vignos PJ, Spencer GE, Archibald KC. Management of progressive muscular dystrophy of childhood. JAMA 1963;184:89–96.

12. Koenig M, Biggs AH, Moyer M, et al. The molecular basis for Duchenne vs Becker muscular dystrophy: correlation of severity with type of deletion. Am J Hum Genet 1989;45:498.

13. Brooke MH, Fenichel G, Griggs R, et al. Duchenne muscular dystrophy: patterns of clinical progression and effects of supportive therapy. Neurology 1989;39:475–481.

14. McNally EM, Towbin JA. Cardiomyopathy in Muscular Dystrophy Workshop 28–30 September 2003, Tucson, Arizona. Neuromusc Disord 2004;20:1–7.

15. Leibowitz D, Dubowitz V. Intellect and behavior in Duchenne muscular dystrophy. Dev Med Child Neurol 1981;23:577–590.

16. Prosser JE. Intelligence and the gene for Duchenne muscular dystrophy. Arch Dis Child 1969;44:221–230.

17. Ziter FA, Allsop K. The diagnosis and management of childhood muscular dystrophy. Clin Pediatr 1976;15(6):540–548.

18. Brooke MH, Fenichel G, Griggs R, et al. Clinical investigation of Duchenne muscular dystrophy. Interesting results in a trial of prednisone. Arch Neurol 1987;44:812–817.

19. Mendell JR. Randomized, double-blind six-month trial of prednisone in Duchenne's muscular dystrophy. N Engl J Med 1989;320:1592–1597.

20. Manzur AY, Kuntzer T, Pike M, et al. Glucocorticoid corticosteroids for Duchenne muscular dystrophy. Cochrane Database Syst Rev 2004;2.

21. Drachman DB, Tokya RV, Meyer E. Prednisone in Duchenne muscular dystrophy. Lancet 1974;2:1409–1412.

22. DeSilva S, Drachman D, Mellits D, et al. Prednisone treatment in Duchenne muscular dystrophy. Long-term benefit. Arch Neurol 1987;44:818–822.

23. Fenichel G, Florence J, Pestronk A, et al. Long-term benefit from prednisone therapy in Duchenne muscular dystrophy. Neurology 1991;41:1874–1877.

24. Bonifati MD, Ruzza G, Bonometto P, et al. A multicenter, double-blind, randomized trial of deflazacort versus prednisone in Duchenne muscular dystrophy. Muscle Nerve 2000; 23:1344–1347.

25. Chetlin RD, Gutmann L, Tarnopolsky MA, et al. Resistance training exercise and creatine in patients with Charcot-Marie-Tooth Disease. Muscle Nerve 2004;30:69–76.

26. Tarnopolsky MA, Mahoney DJ, Vajsar J, et al. Creatine monohydrate enhances strength and body composition in Duchenne muscular dystrophy. Neurology 2004;62:1771–1777.

27. Passaquin AC, Renard M, Kay L, et al. Creatine supplementation reduces skeletal muscle degeneration and enhances mitochondrial function in mdx mice. Neuromusc Disord 2002;12: 174–182.

28. Pulito SM, Passaquin AC, Leijendekker WJ, et al. Creatine supplementation improves intracellular Ca2+ handling and survival in mdx skeletal muscle cells. FEBS Lett 1998;439:357–362.

29. Mendell J, Kissel J, Amato A, et al. Myoblast transfer in the treatment of Duchenne muscular dystrophy. N Engl J Med 1995;333(13):832–838.

30. Barton-Davis ER, Cordier L, Shoturma DI, et al. Aminoglycoside antibiotics restore dystrophin function to skeletal muscles of mdx mice. J Clin Invest 1999;104:375–381.

31. Howard MT, Anderson CB, Fass U, et al. Readthrough of dystrophin stop codon mutations induced by aminoglycosides. Ann Neurol 2004;55:422–426.

32. Wolff J, Malone R, Williams P, et al. Direct gene transfer into mouse muscle in vivo. Science 1990;247:1465.

33. Bentley G, Haddad F, Bull TM, et al. The treatment of scoliosis in muscular dystrophy using modified Luque and Harrington-Luque instrumentation. J Bone Joint Surg Br 2001;83-B1:22–28.

34. Miller F, Moseley CF, Koreska J. Spinal fusion in Duchenne muscular dystrophy. Dev Med Child Neurol 1992;34:775–786.

35. Leger P, Jennequin J, Gerard M, et al. Home positive pressure ventilation via nasal mask for patients with neuromuscular weakness or restrictive lung or chest-wall disease. Respir Care 1989;34:73–79.

36. Bach J, O'Brien J, Krotenberg R, et al. Management of end-stage respiratory failure in Duchenne muscular dystrophy. Muscle Nerve 1987;10:177–182.

37. Florence J, Brooke M, Carroll J. Evaluation of the child with muscular weakness. Orthoped Clin North Am 1978;9(2): 421–422.

38. Ziter FA, Allsop KG, Tyler FH. Assessment of muscle strength in Duchenne muscular dystrophy. Neurology 1977;27:981–984.

39. Allsop KG, Ziter FA. Loss of strength and functional decline in Duchenne dystrophy. Arch Neurol 1981;38:406–411.

40. Brooke MH, Griggs R, Mendell J, et al. Clinical trial in Duchenne dystrophy. The design of the protocol. Muscle Nerve 1981;4:186–197.

41. Florence JM, Pandya S, King W, et al. Clinical trials in Duchenne dystrophy. Standardization and reliability of evaluation procedures. 1984 Phys Ther 64:41–45.

42. Brooke MH, Fenichel G, Griggs R, et al. Clinical investigations in Duchenne dystrophy. Part 2. Determination of the "power" of therapeutic trials based on the natural history. Muscle Nerve 1983;6:91–103.

43. Griggs R, Moxley R, Mendell J, et al. Prednisone in Duchenne dystrophy. A randomized, controlled trial defining the time course and dose response. Arch Neurol 1991;48:383–388.

44. Florence J, Pandya S, King W, et al. Intrarater reliability of manual muscle test (Medical Research Council Scale) grades in Duchenne muscular dystrophy. Phys Ther 1992;72:115–126.

45. Stuberg W, Metcalf W. Reliability of quantitative muscle testing in healthy children and in chil-dren with Duchenne muscular dystrophy using hand held dynamometers. Phys Ther 1988;68(6):977–982.

46. Brussock C, Haley S, Munsat T, et al. Measurement of isometric force in children with and without Duchenne muscular dystrophy. Phys Ther 1992;72(2):105–114.

47. Kilmer DD, McCrory MA, Wright NC, et al. Hand-held dynamometry reliability in persons with neuropathic weakness. Arch Phys Med Rehabil 1997;78:1364–1368.

48. Riddle DL, Finucane SD, Rothstein JM, et al. Intrasession and intersession reliability of hand-held dynamometry measurements taken on brain-damaged patients. Phys Ther 1989;69:182–189.

49. Pandya S, Florence JM, King W, et al. Reliability of goniometric measurements in patients with Duchenne muscular dystrophy. Phys Ther 1985;65:1339–1342.

50. Magee DJ. Orthopedic Physical Assessment. 2nd Ed. Philadelphia: WB Saunders, 1992.

51. Brooke MH, Fenichel G, Griggs R, et al. Duchenne muscular dystrophy: patterns of clinical progression and effects of supportive therapy. Neurology 1989;39:475–481.

52. Hyde SA, Floytruuup I, Glent S, et al. A randomized comparative study of two methods for controlling Tendo Achilles contracture in Duchenne muscular dystrophy. Neuromusc Disord 2000;10:257–263.

53. Scott OM, Hyde SA, Goddard C, et al. Prevention of deformity in Duchenne muscular dystrophy. Physiotherapy 1981; 67:177–180.

54. McDonald CM. Limb contractures in progressive neuromuscular disease and the role of stretching, orthotics, and surgery. Phys Med Rehabil Clin N Am 1998;9:187–209.

55. Johnson E, Yarnell S. Hand dominance and scoliosis in Duchenne muscular dystrophy. Arch Phys Med Rehabil 1976; 57:462–464.

56. Miller F, Moseley C, Koreska J, et al. Pulmonary function and scoliosis in Duchenne dystrophy. J Pediatr Orthop 1988;8: 133–137.

57. Miller R, Chalmers A, Dao H, et al. The effect of spine fusion on respiratory function in Duchenne muscular dystrophy. Neurology 1991;41:37–40.

58. Shapiro F, Sethna N, Colan S, et al. Spinal fusion in Duchenne muscular dystrophy: a multidisciplinary approach. Muscle Nerve 1992;15:604–614.

59. Carter GT. Rehabilitation management in neuromuscular disease. J Neurol Rehabil 1997;11:69–80.

60. Vignos P, Watkins M. The effect of exercise in muscular dystrophy. JAMA 1966;197:121–126.

61. Ansved T. Muscle training in muscular dystrophies. Acta Physiol Scand 2001;171:359–366.

62. de Lateur B, Giaconi R. Effect on maximal strength of submaximal exercise in Duchenne muscular dystrophy. Am J Phys Med 1979;58:26–36.

63. Scott, OM, Hyse SA, Goddard C, et al. Effect of exercise in Duchenne muscular dystrophy. Physiotherapy 1981;67(6): 174–176.

64. Eagle M. Report on the muscular dystrophy campaign workshop: exercise in neuromuscular diseases Newcastle, 2002. Neuromusc Disord 2002;12:975–983.

65. McCarter GC, Steinhardt RA. Increased activity of calcium leak channels caused by proteolysis near sarcolemmal ruptures. J. Membrane Biol 2000;176:169–174.

66. Brussee V, Tardif F, Tremblay J. Muscle fibers of mdx mice are more vulnerable to exercise than those of normal mice. Neuromusc Disord. 1997;7:487–492.

67. Connolly AM, Keeling RM, Mehta S, et al. Three mouse models of muscular dystrophy: the natural history of strength and fatigue in dystrophin-, dystrophin/utrophin-, and laminin α2-deficient mice. Neuromusc Disord 2001;11:703–712.

68. Alderton JM, Steinhardt RA. How calcium influx through calcium leak channels is responsible for the elevated levels of calcium-dependent proteolysis in dystrophic myotubes. Trends Cardiovasc Med 2000;10:268–272.

69. Hayes A, Lynch GS, Williams DA. The effects of endurance exercise on dystrophic mdx mice I. contractile and histochem-ical properties of intact muscles. Proc R Soc Lond Biol Sci 1993;253:19–25.

70. Harris SE, Cherry DB. Childhood progressive muscular dystrophy and the role of physical therapy. Phys Ther 1974;54: 4–12.

71. Scott OM, Hyde SA, Goddard C, et al. Prevention of deformity in Duchenne muscular dystrophy. A prospective study of passive stretching and splintage. Physiotherapy 1981;67:177–180.

72. Archibald DC, Vignos PJ Jr. A study of contractures in muscular dystrophy. Arch Phys Med Rehabil 1959;40:150–157.

73. Spencer GE. Orthopaedic care of progressive muscular dystrophy. J Bone Joint Surg Am 1967;49:1201–1204.

74. Roy L, Gibson DA. Pseudohypertrophic muscular dystrophy and its surgical management: review of 30 patients. Can J Surg 1970;13:13–20.

75. Siegel IM. Management of musculoskeletal complications in neuromuscular disease. Enhancing mobility and the role of bracing and surgery. In: Fowler WM Jr, ed. Advances in the Rehabilitation of Neuromuscular Diseases: State of the Art Reviews. Vol. 4. Philadelphia: Hanley & Belfus, 1988: 553–575.

76. Ziter FA, Allsop KG. The value of orthoses for patients with Duchenne muscular dystrophy. Phys Ther 1979;59:1361–1365.

77. Heckmatt JZ, Dubowitz V, Hyde SA, et al. Prolongation of walking in Duchenne muscular dystrophy with lightweight orthoses. Review of 57 cases. Dev Med Child Neurol 1985;27: 149–154.

78. Vignos PJ. Management of musculoskeletal complications in neuromuscular disease: limb contractures and the role of stretching, braces and surgery. In: Fowler WM Jr, ed. Advances in the Rehabilitation of Neuromuscular Diseases: State of the Art Reviews. Vol. 4. Philadelphia: Hanley & Belfus, 1988:509–536.

79. Bach JR. Orthopedic surgery and rehabilitation for the prolongation of brace-free ambulation of patients with Duchenne muscular dystrophy. Am J Phys Med Rehabil 1991;20:323–331.

80. Bach JR, Campagnolo DI, Hoeman S. Life satisfaction of individuals with Duchenne muscular dystrophy using long-term mechanical ventilatory support. Am J Phys Rehabil 1991; 70:129–135.

81. Liu M, Kiyoshi M, Kozo H, et al. Practical problems and management of seating through the clinical stages of Duchenne's muscular dystrophy. Arch Phys Med Rehabil 2003;84:818–824.

82. Pellegrini N, Guillon B, Prigent H, et al. Optimization of power wheelchair control for patients with severe Duchenne muscular dystrophy. Neuromusc Disord 2004;14:297–300.

83. Edwards RHT. Weight reduction in boys with muscular dystrophy. Dev Med Child Neurol 1984;26:384–390.

84. Griffiths R, Edwards R. A new chart for weight control in Duchenne muscular dystrophy. Arch Dis Child 1988;63: 1256–1258.

85. Perez A, Mulot R, Vardon G, et al. Thoracoabdominal pattern of breathing in neuromuscular disorders. Chest 1996;110: 454–461.

86. Bach JR, Ishikawa Y, Kim H. Prevention of pulmonary morbidity for patients with Duchenne muscular dystrophy. Chest 1997;112(4):1024–1028.

87. Adams M, Chandler L. Effects of physical therapy program on vital capacity of patients with muscular dystrophy. Phys Ther 1974;54:494–494.

88. Wanke T, Toifl K, Merkle M, et al. Inspiratory muscle training in patients with Duchenne muscular dystrophy. Chest 1994; 105:475–482.

89. Gozal D, Thiriet P. Respiratory muscle training in neuromuscular disease: long-term effects on strength and load perception. Med Sci Sports Exerc 1999;31(11):1522–1527.

90. Griggs R, Mendell J, Miller R. Evaluation and Treatment of Myopathies. Philadelphia: FA Davis, 1995:114–128.

91. Kirschner J, Bonnemenn CG. The congenital and limb-girdle muscular dystrophies: sharpening the focus, blurring the boundaries. Arch Neurol 2004;61:189–199.

92. Khadikar SV, Singh RK, Katrak SM. Sarcoglycanopathies: a report of 25 cases. Neurol India 2002;50:27–32.

93. Politano L, Nigro V, Passamano L, et al. Evaluation of cardiac and respiratory involvement in sarcoglycanopathies. Neuromusc Disord. 2001;11:178–185.

94. Richard I, Roudaut C, Saenz A, et al. Calpainopathy-a survey of mutations and polymorphisms. Am J Hum Genet 1999; 64:1524–1540.

95. Chrebakova T, Hermanova M, Kroupova I, et al. Mutations in Czech LGMD2A patients revealed by analysis of calpain3 mRNA and their phenotypic outcome. Neuromusc Disord 2004;14:659–665.

96. Zatz M, de Paula F, Starling A, et al. The 10 autosomal recessive limb-girdle muscular dystrophies. Neuromusc Disord 2003;13:532–544.

97. Pollitt C, Anderson LVB, Pogue R, et al. The phenotype of calpainopathy: diagnosis based on a multidisciplinary approach. Neuromusc Disord 2001;11:287–296.

98. Driss A, Amouri R, Hamida B, et al. A new locus for autosomal-recessive limb-girdle muscular dystrophy in a large consanguineous Tunisian family maps to chromosome 19q3.3. Neuromusc Disord 2000;10:240–246.

99. Brockington M, Blake DJ, Prandini P, et al. Mutations in the fukutin-related protein gene (FKRP) cause a form of congenital muscular dystrophy with secondary laminin α-2 deficiency and abnormal glycosylation of α-dystroglycan. Am J Hum Genet 2001;69:1198–1209.

100. Haliloglu G, Tapaloglu H, Glycosylation defects in muscular dystrophies. Curr Opin Neurol 2004;17:521–527.

101. Poppe M, Cree L, Bourke J, et al. The phenotype of limb-girdle muscular dystrophy type 2I. Neurology 2003;60:1246–1251.

102. Mercuri E, Brockington M, Straub V, et al. Phenotypic spectrum associated with mutations in the fukutin-related protein gene. Ann Neurol 2003;53:537–542.

103. Poppe M, Bourke J, Eagle M, et al. Cardiac and respiratory failure in limb-girdle muscular dystrophy 2I. Ann Neurol 2004;56:738–741.

104. Clarkson E, Costa CF, Machesky LM. Congenital myopathies: diseases of the actin cytoskeleton. J Pathol 2004;204:407–417.

105. Goebel HH. Congenital myopathies at their molecular dawning. Muscle Nerve 2003;27:527–48.

106. Bönnemmann CG, Laing NG. Myopathies resulting from mutations in sarcomeric proteins. Curr Opin Neurol 2004;17:1–9.

107. Sanoudoud, Beggs AH. Clinical and genetic heterogeneity in nemaline myopathy-a disease of skeletal muscle thin filaments. Trends Mol Med 2001;7:362–368.

108. Wallgren-Pattersson C, Laing NG. Report of the 70th ENMC International Workshop: Nemaline Myopathy 11–13 June 1999, Naarden, the Netherlands. Neuromusc Disord 2000;10: 299–306.

109. Ryan MM, Schnell C, Strickland CD, et al. Nemaline myopathy: a clinical study of 143 cases. Ann Neurol 2001;50:312–320.

110. Zhang Y, Chen HS, Khanna VK, et al. A mutation in the human ryanodine receptor gene associated with central core disease. Nat Genet 1993;5(1):46–50.

111. Quane KA, Healy JM, Keating KE, et al. Mutations in the ryanodine receptor gene in central core disease and malignant hyperthermia. Nat Genet 1993;5(1):51–55.

112. Quinlivan RM, Muller CR, Davis M, et al. Central core disease: clinical, pathological, and genetic features. Arch Dis Child 2003;88:1051–1055.

113. Muntoni F, Voit T. The congenital muscular dystrophies in 2004: a century of exciting progress. Neuromusc Disord 2004; 14:635–649.

114. Voit T. Congenital muscular dystrophies: 1997 update. Brain Dev 1998;20:65–74.

115. Jones JK, Morgan G, Johnston H, et al. The expanding phenotype of laminin 2 chain (merosin) abnormalities; case series and review. J Med Genet 2001;38:649–657.

116. Demir E, Ferreiro A, Sabatelli P, et al. Collagen VI status and clinical severity in Ullrich congenital muscular dystrophy: phenotype analysis of 11 families linked to the COL6 Loci. Neuropediatrics 2004;35:103–112.

117. Baker NL, Morgelin M, Peat R, et al. Dominant collagen VI mutations are a common cause of Ullrich congenital muscular dystrophy. Hum Mol Genet. 2005;14:279–293.

118. Guillian T, Brzustowicz L, Castilla L, et al. Genetic hemogeneity between acute and chronic forms of spinal muscular atrophy. Nature 1990;345:823–825.

119. Brzustowicz L, Lehner T, Castilla L, et al. Genetic mapping of chronic childhood-onset spinal muscular atrophy to chromosome 5q 11.2–13.3. Nature 1990;344:540–541.

120. Dumitro D. Electrodiagnostic Medicine. Philadelphia: Hanley and Belfus, 1995.

121. Lomen-Hoerth C, Slawnych MP. Statistical motor unit number estimation: from theory to practice. Muscle Nerve 2003; 28(3):263–272.

122. Iannaccone ST, Brown RH, Samaha FJ, et al., DCN/SMA Group. Prospective study of spinal muscular atrophy before age 6 years. Pediatr Neurol 1993;9:187–193.

123. Miske LJ, Hickey EM, Kolb SM, et al. Use of the mechanical in-exsufflator in pediatric patients with neuromuscular disease and impaired cough. Chest 2004;125:1406–1412.

124. Wang TG, Bach JR, Avilla C, et al. Survival of individuals with spinal muscular atrophy on ventilatory support. Am J Phys Med Rehabil 1994;73:207–211.

125. Rudnik-Schoneborn S, Hausmanowa-Petrusewicz I, Brokowska J, et al. The predictive value of achieved motor milestones assessed in 441 patients with infantile spinal muscular atrophy types II and III. Eur Neurol 2000;45:174–181.

126. Russman BS, Bucher CR, Shite M, et al., DCN/SMA Group. Function changes in spinal muscular atrophy II and III. Neurology 1996;47:973–976.

127. Iannaccone AT, Russman BS, Browne GH, et al., DCN/Spinal Muscular Atrophy Group. Prospective analysis of strength in spinal muscular atrophy. J Child Neurol 2000;15:97–101.

128. Merlini L, Bertini E, Minetti C, et al. Motor function-muscle strength relationship in spinal muscle atrophy. Muscle Nerve 2004;12:561–6.

129. Koch BM, Simenson RL. Upper extremity strength and function in children with spinal muscular atrophy type II. Arch Phys Med Rehabil 1992;73:241–245.

130. Granata C, Cornelio F, Bonfiglioli S, et al. Promotion of ambulation of patients with spinal muscular atrophy by early fitting of knee-ankle-foot orthoses. Dev Med Child Neurol 1987;29(2): 221–224.

131. Shapiro F, Specht L. Current concepts review. The diagnosis and orthopaedic treatment of childhood spinal muscular atrophy, peripheral neuropathy, Friedreich ataxia, and artrogryposis. J Bone Joint Surg Am 1993;75A:1699–1714.

132. Tangsrud SE, Lodrup Carlsen KC, Lund-Petersen KC, et al. Lung function measurements in young children with spinal muscle atrophy; a cross sectional survey on the effect of position and bracing. Arch Dis Child 2001;84:521–524.

133. Rodillo E, Marini ML, Heckmatt JZ, et al. Scoliosis in spinal muscular atrophy: review of 63 cases. J Child Neurol 1989; 4:118–123.

134. Furumasu J, Swank SM, Brown JC, et al. functional activities in spinal muscular atrophy patients after spinal fusion. Spine 1989;14:771–775.

135. Phillips DP, Roye DP, Farcy JPC, et al. Surgical treatment of scoliosis in a spinal muscular atrophy population. Spine 1990; 15:942–945.

136. Chetlin RD, Gutmann L, Tarnopolsky M, et al. Resistance training effectiveness in patients with Charcot-Marie-Tooth Disease: recommendations for exercise prescription. Arch Phys Med Rehabil 2004;85:1217–1223.

137. Shy ME, Blake J, Krajewski K, et al. Reliability and validity of the CMT neuropathy score as a measure of disability. Neurology 2005;64:1209–1214.

138. Muscular Dystrophy Association. Charcot-Marie-Tooth Disease and Dejerine-Sottas Disease. Available at: www.mdausa.org. Accessed May 1, 2005.

139. Azmaipairashvili Z, Riddle EC, Scavina M, et al. Correction of cavovarus foot deformity in Charcot-Marie-Tooth Disease. J Pediatr Orthop 2005;25:360–365.

140. Bean J, Walsh A, Frontera W. Brace modification improves aerobic performance in Charcot-Marie-Tooth Disease: a single subject design. Am J Phys Med Rehabil 2001;80:578–582.

141. Lindeman E, Leffers P, Spaans F, et al. Strength training in patients with myotonic dystrophy and hereditary motor and sensory neuropathy: a randomized clinical trial. Arch Phys Med Rehabil 1995;76(7):612–620.

142. Kilmer DD. The role of exercise in neuromuscular disease. Phys Med Rehabil Clin N Am 1998;9(1):115–125.

143. Starling A, Kok F, Passos-Bueno MR, et al. A new form of autosomal dominant limb-girdle muscular dystrophy (LGMD1G) with progressive fingers and toes flexion limitation maps to chromosome 4p21. Eur J Hum Genet 2004;12(12):1033–1040.

Mental Retardation: Focus on Down Syndrome

Dolores B. Bertoti and Dale E. Smith

he physical therapist plays a challenging and important, multifaceted role in the management of children with mental retardation. This challenge is inherent within the clinical presentation of a child with mental retardation who exhibits simultaneous and interactive impairments in the neuromotor, musculoskeletal, developmental, cognitive, and affective domains. The physical therapist not only must be able to accurately assess the child, but also must innovatively develop, implement, modify, and share with parents and other providers of service an accurate plan of care. In this chapter, an approach is offered to assist the entry-level physical therapist with examination, intervention, and management of the child with mental retardation. The strategy presented is from a functional perspective, delineating the interactive effects of common impairments associated with mental retardation and the role of the physical therapist in managing these impairments to promote maximum best function of the child within his or her environment. Physical therapy management for the child with Down syndrome is outlined as a model strategy.

Historical Review

The history of society and its treatment of people with mental retardation have had an intriguing, interesting, and still-unfolding interactional relationship. As societal trends followed a path of increased education and understanding, the quality of these interactions oscillated along a pathway from severe humiliation, to tolerance and protection, to understanding and acceptance, and now evolving to a pathway of full inclusion. In the earliest of recorded interactions between the two groups, people with mental retardation were ignored, received little or no care, or were even left to die.[1] Spartan society believed in survival of only the fittest, and many people, including the physically and mentally handicapped, were left to perish.

Conversely, during the Middle Ages and in ancient Rome, it was not uncommon for wealthy people to help a "fool" or "court jester" in return for the amusement these people provided for the household and its guests.[1] Artistic work of the Middle Ages shows people serving as clowns and jesters who depict the physical characteristics of what we now identify as Down syndrome.[2] In the later Middle Ages, particularly in Europe, superstitious beliefs led to the execution of many people who were considered to be "witches and warlocks." People with mental retardation were undoubtedly included in these groups.[1] This idea that people with mental retardation were social menaces persisted throughout the 19th century, with the eventual trend away from execution but still toward punishment, imprisonment, and isolation.[3]

In the early 20th century, there was a publicly perceived need to shelter and protect people with mental retardation from the misunderstanding, abuses, and wrath of society. As a result, people with mental deficiency were isolated in asylums, shelters, and farm communities. These communities, however, rapidly became overcrowded. The goal of this public effort was clearly housing, not the provision of services.

Interest in providing services to assist people with mental retardation had a difficult beginning. In the early 1800s, Jean Marc Itard, a French physician, became intrigued with a mentally retarded youngster whom the physician had captured in the forests of Aveyron in France. Acting on his then-revolutionary premise that intellectual performance could be affected by environmental stimulation, Itard succeeded in teaching this "wild boy of Aveyron." Although Itard's work helped the boy improve over a 5-year period, the gains were not sufficient for acceptance of the boy into Parisian society at that time. Society frowned on the child, and Itard believed he had failed.[4]

Johann Jacob Guggenbuhl, in 1840, established a center in Switzerland for a then-innovative approach involving group teaching for children with mental retardation. His work received worldwide acclaim as a major reform. This reform influenced the work in Europe and in the United States of Edouard Sequin, who was a world leader in the development of educational and residential services for people with mental retardation. In 1876, Seguin was made president of the newly formed Association of Medical Officers of the American Institutions for Idiotic and Feeble-Minded Persons. This association later (1876) became the American Association of Mental Deficiency (AAMD), currently called the American Association on Mental Retardation.[5]

In the United States, the social organization accompanying the Industrial Revolution reinforced this concept of group care of children, as well as stimulating a sense of social responsibility.[1] Throughout the 1800s, small gains fluctuated with a sense of frustration and futility, and

there was a large-scale movement to house the "incurables" in large, overcrowded facilities in isolated areas.[2]

During the midpart of the century, an interesting development began, referred to as "special education." The notoriety of famous people like Samuel Gridley Howe and Horace Mann who publicized the educational experiences of Laura Bridgman, a child who was blind and came to be educated at a school for the blind, then housed at the Perkins Institute in Massachusetts, furthered the efforts. Howe's description of the processes used at the Institute with Bridgman was further distributed in reports written by Charles Dickens. Dickens' articles were widely read, aided by his popularity at that time, and helped give fuel to the special education movement.[6] Special education first promoted for use with individuals with severe disabilities, including those with mental retardation, were "generally provided in large institutions designed as much to protect persons with disabilities from the public as to protect the public from them. As the enterprise gained permanence and legitimacy, the population expanded. With more children encompassed, special segregated classes in the public schools became a feature by about 1910."[7]

By the end of World War II, emphasis for care of people with mental retardation evolved to include "programming." This shift to a plan of activity was mainly the result of efforts by the National Association for Retarded Citizens (NARC) and other parent or professional advocacy groups.[2] A growing awareness of the negative effects of residential segregation and the limitations of existing programs led to a critical reappraisal of existing kinds of care available for people with mental retardation. Influenced by the Civil Rights Movement, the 1960s represented a time of expansion in program legislation and funds allocation for all people with disabilities. Discrimination against and segregation of people with mental retardation were finally recognized as negative and undesirable.[2]

In the early 1970s, American visitors to Scandinavian countries encountered the concept of "normalization," which was defined as the principle of educating persons with handicaps to the maximum extent feasible within the "normal" environment of the nonhandicapped.[8] This process obviously required major development and use of community support systems. This era became known as the era of "deinstitutionalization." As an example, in 1972 the Association for Retarded Citizens won a landmark decision against the Commonwealth of Pennsylvania that provided access to public education for children with mental retardation. In this decision, it was stated that "it is the Commonwealth's obligation to place each mentally retarded child in a free, public program of education and training appropriate to the child's capacity. . . . Placement in a regular school class is preferable to placement in a special public school class and placement in a special public school is preferable to placement in any other type of program of education and training." Eight similar landmark cases were happening in states across the country. This deinstitutionalization movement continued into the 1980s and public interest was further stirred by a series of investigations and publications of the conditions of several institutions, one in particular being broadcast by a television station in New York City that was part of the ABC network. These televised broadcasts "exposed abuse, neglect, and lack of programming at Willowbrook, a state institution for persons with mental retardation on Staten Island."[9] This occurrence spurred the interest of Jacob Javits, then a state senator from New York, to propose legislation to regulate practices in institutions.[8] Since that time, many changes have occurred as a result of public interest and educators. Most of the nation's institutions serving the population with mental retardation have closed, and other types of educational facilities and housing have been developed. Living arrangements in the community have now become the norm for the long-term care and support of people with mental retardation.

The most current approach to programming in the field of mental retardation is a functional, integrated model. Society as a whole and, therefore, the countless legislatures and service providers of today's society view mental retardation along a changing paradigm, with a more functional definition and a focus on the interaction between the person, the environment, and the intensities and patterns of needed supports. The term readers will hear most frequently since the 1990s is *support,* including needed level of support for maximum function of the individual with mental retardation in the environment.[9]

 Definition

Mental retardation is a disability characterized by significant limitations in both intellectual functioning and adaptive behavior expressed in conceptual, social, and practical adaptive skills. In order to be classified as mental retardation, the onset of this disability occurs before age 18. According to the DSM-IV-TR, 4th edition, the essential feature of mental retardation is significantly subaverage general intellectual functioning, accompanied by significant limitations in adaptive functioning in at least two of the following applicable adaptive skill areas: communication, self-care, home living, social/interpersonal skills, use of community resources, self-direction, health and safety, functional academic skills, leisure, and work.[10]

This present definition reflects a continued emphasis on the adaptive behavior dimensions that differs from earlier definitions. The current definition further narrows adaptive behaviors to the major areas of conceptual thinking, social development, and adaptive behavior. These major areas were identified through statistical analysis utilized in conducting research on a variety of factors that affect behavioral performance.[11] Thus, mental retardation is generally regarded as a condition existing in an individual that is described by the specific performance of the individual not

due to a specific trait, although it is influenced by certain characteristics or capabilities of the individual. Rather, mental retardation describes a performance *state* in which functioning is impaired. This distinction is central to understanding how the present definition broadens the concept of mental retardation and how it shifts the emphasis from measurement of traits to understanding the individual's actual functioning in everyday living. For any individual with mental retardation, the description of its current state of functional behavior requires knowledge of the individual's capabilities as well as an understanding of the behavior within the structure and expectation of the individual's personal and social environment.

 Incidence

About 3% of the population of the United States is assumed to have mental retardation, but only 1% to 1.5% are actually diagnosed with this condition.[10] In 80% of the cases, the cause of the mental retardation is unknown. Mental retardation is four times more prevalent among men than women. Seventy-five percent of all people with mental retardation have a mild form, 20% a moderate form, and 5% a severe or profound form.[10] One of the most prevalent forms of mental retardation is Down syndrome, with an incidence of 1 in 800 to 1000 live births.[12,13]

 Diagnosis

A diagnosis of mental retardation is based on the criteria embodied within the definition reflecting intellectual functioning level and adaptive skill level.

ASSESSMENT OF INTELLECTUAL FUNCTIONING

The determination that a child's intellectual functioning is significantly below average is arrived at through the administration of a standardized intelligence test, usually administered by a psychologist. Fulfillment of this criterion for diagnosis of mental retardation is made on the basis of an IQ of 70 or 75 or below.[5,10] The instruments most commonly used for the assessment of intellectual functioning in children are the Stanford-Binet Intelligence Scale, 5th edition[14]; one of the Wechsler Scales, such as Wechsler Intelligence Scale for Children-IV[15] or Wechsler Preschool and Primary Scale of Intelligence III[16]; and the Kaufman Assessment Battery for Children.[17]

ASSESSMENT OF ADAPTIVE SKILL LEVEL

Impairments in adaptive functioning, rather than low IQ, are usually the presenting symptoms in individuals with mental retardation.[10] Adaptive skills are those skills considered to be central to successful life functioning and are frequently related to the need for supports for persons with mental retardation. The adaptive areas in which limitations are specifically exhibited are in any one of the following areas: communication, self-care, home living, social skills, community use, self-direction, health and safety, functional academics, leisure, and work. In order to fulfill the diagnostic criteria for mental retardation, deficits in two or more areas of adaptive functioning must be present, thus showing a generalized limitation in adaptive skill level.[5,10] In order to address the level of adaptive behaviors, the practitioner must perform a functional examination of the child's behavior across all environmental settings. To do this, several scales are available to measure adaptive functioning, such as the Vineland Adaptive Behavior Scales[18] and the American Association on Mental Retardation Adaptive Behavior Scale.[19] Table 10.1 describes the general adaptive behavior characteristics of children and adults with different levels of mental retardation.[20]

 Classification

In keeping with contemporary views of disablement,[21–23] the key elements in the definition of mental retardation are *capabilities*, *environment*, and *function*. The previously used terms of mildly, moderately, severely, or profoundly mentally retarded are no longer widely used. This classification language was in use until 1992 and was closely correlated with IQ scores.[24] Current classification carries with it an application of the new diagnostic criteria directly correlated to need for support. Needed supports will vary along a number of dimensions. First, support may be necessary in some areas of adaptive skills but not in others; second, support requirements may be time limited or ongoing; and third, the intensities of the supports required, the types of support resources, and the support functions will be specific to the individual and the life cycle. It is important to note that the need for supports may vary across environments as well as across the life span. There are basically four intensities of support: intermittent, limited, extensive, and pervasive. Support services may come to the child with mental retardation from four sources: the individual child (e.g., ability to make choices), other people (e.g., parent, teacher), technology (e.g., assistive devices), or habilitation services (e.g., physical therapy, occupational therapy, speech therapy).[5]

EDUCATIONAL CLASSIFICATION

The original but more familiar educational classification system, first defined by Scheerenberger in 1964, is rarely used as a sole classification system.[24] Terms such as educable, trainable, and dependent are considered to be out of date but may still be seen in some educational placement descriptions. Current special education practices are shaped by both the definition of mental retardation and the need for supports. Contemporary educational placement terms follow a more functional approach, highlighting the need for support and thereby being descriptive of the child's needs for educational success.

TABLE 10.1

Adaptive Behavior Characteristics of Persons with Mental Retardation

| IQ | Age of the Person with Mental Retardation | | |
	Preschool	School-aged	Adult
50–55 to 70	Often appears unimpaired; develops functional social and communication skill	Academic skills of sixth grade are possible; special education support is needed for secondary school	Can learn social and vocational skills
35–40 to 50–55	Impaired social skills; can communicate; may need supervision	Can develop up to fourth-grade academic skills with special training/ modification	Unskilled or semiskilled vocation
20–25 to 35–40	Severely impaired communication; impaired motor skills	May learn to communicate; basic personal health habits; limited academic skills	Needs complete support and supervision for any self-support activity
<20–25	Requires full support; dependent for care; limited sensorimotor development	Some motor development; continues to be dependent for care; limited success with training	Limited motor ability and communication; continued dependency for care

Updated by author from original reference: Sloan W, Birch JW. A rationale for degrees of retardation. Am J Ment Defic. 1955;60:262.

This descriptive terminology for educational support includes:

- Academic support or gifted support
- Learning support
- Life skills support
- Emotional support
- Sensory and communication support
- Visually impaired support
- Speech and language support
- Physical support
- Multiple disabilities support[25]

Physical therapy in the educational setting is detailed in Chapter 19 of this text.

MEDICAL CLASSIFICATION

Medical classification, according to the DSM-IV-TR,[10] uses a classification based on the degree of severity of intellectual impairment as detailed in the following Box.

DSM-IV-TR Diagnoses and Codes	
317	Mild Mental Retardation
	IQ level 50–55 to approximately 70
318.0	Moderate Mental Retardation
	IQ level 35–40 to 50–55
318.1	Severe Mental Retardation
	IQ level 20–25 to 35–40
318.2	Profound Mental Retardation
	IQ level below 20 or 25
319	Mental Retardation, Severity unspecified
	Untestable by standard tests

Etiology and Pathophysiology

Over 350 etiologies for mental retardation have been identified.[26,27] These can be broadly categorized into prenatal, perinatal, and postnatal causes. Etiologic causes with examples are depicted in Display 10.1. Movement disorders are associated with some etiologies more than others. Many children also present with a variety of associated disorders such as visual, hearing, or additional medical problems. In approximately 30% to 40% of individuals seen in educational or clinical settings, no clear etiology can be determined despite extensive evaluation efforts.[10]

Primary Impairments

NEUROMOTOR IMPAIRMENTS

Many types of mental retardation have associated neuro-muscular, musculoskeletal, and cardiopulmonary impairments. Display 10.2 details the most common mental retardation conditions and their associated neuromotor impairments.[28–43] Most neuromuscular impairments are present as a result of primary pathology in the central nervous system (CNS). Secondary impairments then include deficits typically of concern to the physical therapist such as deficits in motor control, coordination, postural control, force production, flexibility, and balance.[44] Physical therapy examination and intervention for these impairments for children with mental retardation are similar to those procedures used in any pediatric setting. Display 10.2 can guide the pediatric physical therapist in anticipating typical management concerns associated with common mental retardation disorders. The mental retardation itself, viewed as an additional or confounding coimpairment, requires some adaptation in evaluation and intervention because of the specific cognitive limitations presented by the child.

LEARNING IMPAIRMENT

Learning is impaired in children with mental retardation. Children with mental retardation demonstrate an impaired ability to utilize advanced cognitive processes, manage simultaneous or multiple demands, and successfully organize complex information, with subsequent effects on task performance as well as task mastery.[45] Physical therapists must be able to adapt examination and intervention approaches to accommodate the coimpairment of deficient intellectual functioning. Clearly, the range of cognitive deficit and ability found in children with mental retardation is indicative of variant levels of performance, functioning, and potential.[46] It is the task and the challenge of the therapist to assist the child to maximize his or her potential for optimum functioning across environments.

Physical Therapy Examination and Intervention Principles

KEY ELEMENTS OF EXAMINATION

Meaningful examination always maintains a focus on the child's functioning as the key issue. A successful and effective physical therapy examination of the child with mental retardation depends largely on the therapist's approach to the child. Four important elements should facilitate the process of examination.

First, throughout the examination, the therapist must analyze not only what the child can do, but also the *processes underlying the observed skills and behaviors.*[47] Thus, the therapist must determine not only what tasks the child can do, but also why the child can do those specific tasks and not others. Movements must be broken down into components, and basic mental, physiologic,

>> **DISPLAY 10.1**

Etiologic Classification of Mental Retardation

Prenatal Onset	Examples
1. Chromosomal disorder	Down, Turner, or Klinefelter syndrome
2. Syndrome disorders	Neurofibromatosis, myotonic muscular dystrophy, Prader-Willi, tuberous sclerosis
3. Inborn errors of metabolism	Phenylketonuria, carbohydrate disorders, mucopolysaccharide disorders (e.g., Hurler type), nucleic acid disorders (e.g., Lesch-Nyhan syndrome)
4. Developmental disorders of brain formation	Neural tube closure defects (e.g., anencephaly), hydrocephalus, porencephaly, microcephaly
5. Environmental influences	Intrauterine malnutrition, drugs, toxins, alcohol, narcotics, maternal diseases
Perinatal Causes	
6. Intrauterine disorders	Placental insufficiency, maternal sepsis, abnormal labor or delivery
7. Neonatal disorders	Intracranial hemorrhage, periventricular leukomalacia, seizures, infections, respiratory disorders, head trauma, metabolic disorders
Postnatal Causes	
8. Head injuries	Intracranial hemorrhage, contusion, concussion
9. Infections	Encephalitis, meningitis, viral infections
10. Demyelinating disorders	Postinfectious and postimmunization disorders
11. Degenerative disorders	Syndromic disorders (e.g., Rett syndrome), poliodystrophies (e.g., Friedreich ataxia), basal ganglia disorders, leukodystrophies
12. Seizure disorders	Infantile spasms, myoclonic epilepsy
13. Toxic–metabolic disorders	Reye syndrome, lead intoxication, metabolic disorders (e.g., hypoglycemia)
14. Malnutrition	Protein-calorie, prolonged IV alimentation
15. Environmental deprivation	Psychosocial disadvantage, child abuse/neglect

From American Association on Mental Retardation (AAMR). 1719 Kalorama Road, NW, Washington, DC, 20009-2683; and International Classification of Diseases (ICD). Ann Arbor, MI: World Health Organization; 1992.

and physical processes must be analyzed in relation to those tasks.

Second, evaluative procedures used for children, particularly children with mental retardation, often differ from the more rigid clinical procedures used for adults. As in all of pediatrics, much information can be gathered by interacting with the child through observation and during play. Standard evaluative tests and procedures may be used as rapport is established, depending on the functional level of the child. Owing to the attention deficits and associated problems of the child with mental retardation, the evaluation should be done serially, and should be ongoing. Consistent with the functional approach to curriculum planning, the physical therapist should perform an evaluation with as many *functional aspects,* using age-appropriate materials, as is reasonable.

The third important element necessary for appropriate examination is related to the basic orientation of the therapist. As with other areas of physical therapy, but more importantly with the child with multiple disabilities, the therapist must be able to identify not only the disability, but also the child's abilities, however minimal.

The skilled therapist will identify even the smallest of abilities and effectively communicate the importance of those abilities to the child, parents, and other professionals working with the child. A major focus of intervention involves attempts to increase those abilities. This "positive" orientation and approach will have a beneficial effect on the child's self-image and on those people working with the child.[48] If our actions suggest a true concern and expectation for progress, however limited that progress may be, the effect of this attitude should encourage the child, the teachers, and the family to strive toward goals that have been identified.[48]

The fourth important element in evaluation is that the therapist must always concurrently assess sensory processes and attention. Children experience their world through sensory (afferent) pathways and the feedback received from sensory input and attempts at interaction with the world. They assimilate the information; they take action; and they consequently modify subsequent actions. The therapist must understand by what means—or even whether—the child is perceiving the world, including you, the evaluator, before continuing with the evaluation.

>> DISPLAY 10.2

Neuromuscular, Musculoskeletal, and Cardiopulmonary Impairments Associated with Selected Conditions of Mental Retardation

Condition	Neuromuscular	Musculoskeletal	Cardiopulmonary
Cri-du-chat syndrome[28]	Hypotonia in early childhood, sometimes later hypertonia	Minor upper extremity anomalies, scoliosis	Congenital heart disease common
Cytomegalovirus[29] (prenatal infection)	Hypertonia, seizures, microcephaly	Secondary to neuromuscular problems	Mitral stenosis, pulmonary valvular stenosis, atrial septal defect
de Lange syndrome[30,31]	Spasticity, seizures, intention tremor, microcephaly	Decreased bone age, small stature, small hands and feet, short digits, proximal thumb placement, clinodactyly fifth digit, other hand and finger defects, limited elbow extension	Neonatal respiratory problems, cardiac malformations, recurrent upper respiratory tract infections
Down syndrome[32,33]	Hypotonia, low muscle force production, slow postural reactions, slow reaction time, motor delays increasing with age	Joint hyperflexibility, ligamentous laxity, foot deformities, scoliosis, atlanto-hypertension axial instability (20%)	Congenital heart disease (40%), lung hypoplasia, with pulmonary
Fetal alcohol syndrome[31,34]	Fine motor dysfunction, visual–motor deficits, weak grasp, ptosis	Joint anomalies with abnormal position or function, maxillary hypoplasia	Heart murmur—often disappears after first year
Fragile X syndrome[35,36]	Hypotonia, poor coordination and motor planning, seizures	Hyperextensible finger joints, prominent jaw, scoliosis	Mitral valve prolapse
Hurler's syndrome[27,31]	Hydrocephalus	Joint contractures, claw-like deformities of hands, short fingers, thoracolumbar kyphosis, shallow acetabular and glenoid fossae, irregularly shaped bones	Cardiac deformities such as cardiac enlargement due to right ventricular hypertension, death frequently due to cardiac failure
Lesch-Nyhan syndrome[37]	Hypotonia followed by spasticity, chorea, and athetosis/dystonia; compulsive self-injurious behavior	Secondary to neuromuscular problems	
Prader-Willi syndrome[38,39]	Severe hypotonia and feeding problems in infancy, excessive eating and obesity in childhood, poor fine and gross motor coordination	Short stature, small hands and feet	May be associated with cor pulmonale (most common cause of death)
Rett syndrome[40–43]	Hypotonia in infancy, then gradually increasing hypertonia and lack of acquired skills; ataxia, apraxia, choreoathetosis and/or dystonia, progression from hyperkinesia to bradykinesia with age, slow reaction time, stereotypic hand movements (clapping, wringing, clenching) drooling, involuntary rhythmic tongue movement/deviation, seizures	Scoliosis, kyphosis, joint contractures, hip subluxation or dislocation, equinovarus deformities	Immature respiratory patterns, breathing irregularities, such as hyperventilation, apnea
Williams syndrome[31,34] (elfin facies)	Mild neurologic dysfunction, poor motor coordination	Hallux valgus	Variable congenital heart disease

Adapted with permission from McEwen I. Mental retardation. In: Campbell SK, ed. Physical Therapy for Children. Philadelphia: WB Saunders, 1994.

SENSORY EXAMINATION AND INTERVENTION

The therapist must determine the basic responsiveness of the child before deciding on an appropriate interaction strategy for the rest of the evaluation or intervention. Kinnealy distinguished two broad categories of behaviors typical of children with mental retardation on the basis of their reactions to various sensory stimuli or environmental input.[49] She described one group as having difficulty monitoring the intensity of sensory input and, therefore, difficulty in modulating the response. The other group was described as having reduced perception of the incoming stimuli. This group required more intense input for arousal or elicitation of a response. This initial difference in perception of sensory stimulus is a critical point of departure that the therapist must ascertain during the first attempt at interaction with the child.

VISUAL When assessing the child's visual sense, the therapist should note the ability of the child to orient to, focus on, and track a visual stimulus. Getman and associates have suggested that horizontal tracking is easier than vertical tracking, and that diagonal tracking is the most difficult.[50] Notable responses include difficulty in tracking across the midline and resting eye movements (nystagmus). The term *cortical blindness* describes an inability to interpret visual information owing to severe brain damage or occipital lobe atrophy.

During intervention and integration into classroom activities, visual stimulation activities can be used to provide practice in both focusing and tracking. Children who have poor head control may have an inadequate base of support for eye movements. Intervention aimed at improving postural mechanisms may improve visual skill.[47] Adaptive aids to ensure proper body positioning should be used as needed. Vestibular input may also improve visual focusing and processing because vestibular reflexes, in combination with optic and tonic neck reflexes, maintain a stable image on the retina while the head and body are in motion.[47] The vestibulo-oculomotor pathways contribute to skilled movements of the eyes that can be used for educational skills, including reading and writing.[51]

AUDITORY

The child's response to auditory stimuli may range from an absence of response, to simple orientation to and movement toward the stimulus, to a startle response.[47] Although it is difficult to assess hearing loss in a child with mental retardation or multiple handicaps, referral for a complete audiologic evaluation is indicated whenever there is a possibility of a hearing loss. Audiologic testing can be used to identify a hearing loss, to differentiate between conductive and sensorineural loss, and to quantify the degree of loss. Tympanometry (an objective measure of eardrum function) helps identify a conductive loss when behavioral testing is unreliable. Testing for brainstem-evoked response traces the passage of an auditory stimulus from the ear to the brainstem. Central or cortical deafness describes a lack of interpretation of auditory information due to brain damage.

Vestibular stimulation is a component of intervention aimed at enhancing auditory integration. Although the vestibulocochlear nerve (cranial nerve VIII) has been described as comprising two separate entities (vestibular and auditory), it developed phylogenetically as a unit, and its portions appear to be related functionally.[47] There is clear clinical evidence that difficulties in hearing interfere with equilibrium responses. Vestibular input may not only improve equilibrium reactions, but also sometimes enhance auditory attention and integration.[52]

TACTILE

The tactile system is the largest sensory system, and it plays a major role in both physical and emotional behavior.[53,54] The tactile system develops earliest in utero, and the ability to process tactile input is important for neural organization. The sensation of touch is, in fact, the "oldest and most primitive expressive channel" and is a primary system for making contact with the external environment.[54,55] When threatened, there is a predominant response of increased alertness and increased affect. When not challenged, however, the person is free to explore and manipulate the environment.[56,57]

Many children with brain damage show a disordered tactile system. With neurologic impairment, many children show an aversive response to some types of tactile stimulation. This aversion to tactile stimuli, called *tactile defensiveness,* is often manifested by such behavior as hyperactivity or distractibility.[56] Children who show tactile defensiveness may display avoidance reactions around the hands, feet, and face. This behavior has obvious implications for the manner in which a child explores the environment, appreciates tactile sensation, and thus learns. Tactile defensiveness in the oral area may cause the child to reject textured or flavored food in preference to smoother, blander foods.

Although no data are available to support the idea, some professionals suggest that tactile defensiveness is part of a generalized "set" of the nervous system by which the child interprets stimuli as "danger."[56] Tactile functions were among the first means by which the child received information about his or her environment in order to adapt appropriately. The result of developmental disorders is often behavior that appears to be less sophisticated and less discriminatory than normal. Tactile defensiveness or overresponsiveness may be seen in this context as poorly developed mechanisms for the interpretation of information. Clinically, the child may appear anxious, emotionally labile, or threatened and unable to cope. Compensatory behavior may be characterized by withdrawal, irritability, or distractibility.[56]

Ayres has suggested various intervention approaches designed to facilitate increased organization of the tactile system and increased integration of this subsystem into effective environmental interaction. The proprioceptive system serves a cooperative role in this functional scheme.[56,57]

The physical therapist can easily incorporate appropriate activities into intervention to address both the tactile and proprioceptive systems. Heavy touch and pressure or weight bearing are excellent activities for decreasing tactile hypersensitivity and promoting proximal joint stability. Light touch or stimuli that tickle or irritate the child should be avoided in favor of activities that offer deep pressure.

The response of the child with mental retardation to tactile input must be observed and monitored during assessment and intervention. The therapist must note whether the child responds to the stimulus (i.e., the touch of the therapist's hand), and if a response is noted, the therapist must identify the type of response. If the input is noxious, does the child respond with a grimace, or does the child move actively to avoid the stimulus? One might surmise that the child who actively removes or withdraws from the noxious stimulus is not only aware of the stimulus, but also has some proprioceptive sense by which to locate and remove the stimulus. Conversely, the therapist must be aware of the child who is so totally unaware of sensory input that the therapist is unable to penetrate and reach the child by any means. Clearly, knowing the level of awareness of the child will direct the therapist through subsequent stages of the evaluation and intervention process.[46]

VESTIBULAR SYSTEM

Along with the tactile system, the vestibular system is one of the earliest developing sensory systems in the human being. The tracts within the vestibular system are fully myelinated by 20 weeks of gestation.[56] Information from the vestibular system tells us our position exactly in relation to gravity, whether or not we are moving, and our speed and direction of movement.[53] Semicircular canals within the inner ear are the vestibular receptors that provide dynamic information regarding angular acceleration around the body's axis. The utricles are receptors that provide static information concerning the position of the body in relation to gravity.[58] The vestibular system is so sensitive that changes in position and movement have a powerful effect on the brain, and this effect changes with even the most subtle adjustments of movement or posture.[56]

Vestibular sensations are produced mainly within the vestibular nuclei and the cerebellum.[56] Stimuli are sent caudally in the spinal cord and into the brainstem, where they serve a powerful integrative function. Some stimuli are also sent rostrally from the brainstem to the cerebral hemispheres.[53]

The vestibular system has a strong effect on muscle tone and movement. This influence is mediated through the lateral and medial vestibular nuclei and affects efferent transmission down the spinal cord. Vestibular influence usually exerts a facilitatory effect on the γ motoneuron to the muscle spindle and may influence the α motoneurons supplying skeletal muscle. By activating the γ efferent to the muscle spindle, the afferent flow from the spindle is maintained and regulated for assistance with motor function. This basic role in muscle function and mobility gives the vestibular system an important role in the development and maintenance of body scheme that depends on interpretation of movement.[56] Impulses ascending to higher brainstem and cortical levels synapse with tactile, proprioceptive, visual, and auditory impulses to provide both perception of space and orientation of the body within that space.[53] Vestibular input seldom enters conscious thought or awareness except when the stimulus is so intense that one is rendered dizzy.

Vestibular function can be assessed clinically by noting the presence of and duration of nystagmus after vestibular stimulation, such as spinning. Nystagmus is a slow movement of the eyes in one direction, followed by a rapid movement in the opposite direction.[47,59] It is important to know whether the child overreacts to or is threatened by movement, or has difficulty in attending to and assimilating movement experiences.

The physical therapist may choose to include various movement or vestibular activities in a child's program with the hope of achieving several goals. With a knowledge of the child's response to vestibular stimulation, activities can be chosen to improve balance, simulate experience of movement, activate muscle contraction (specifically, antigravity extensors), promote awareness and eye contact, and increase spatial awareness and perception. Examples of equipment used in these movement activities include swings, barrels, and scooter boards.

SELF-STIMULATION

Self-stimulation in some children with mental retardation is an area of concern. This type of behavior can take many forms, including self-abuse. Examples of self-stimulation include constant mouthing of objects or the hand, spinning, head banging, hand or arm flapping, teeth grinding, rocking, and self-biting. Evaluation of the sensory status of the child may identify the reason for self-stimulation. The child may be performing self-stimulation to fulfill a basic sensory need, or he or she may be overstimulated and may be reacting out of frustration or an inability to cope with sensory overload.[47]

In educational programs, the tendency is to discourage self-stimulation, especially when the stimulation is abusive or socially unacceptable. An appropriate sensory input must be substituted or the child may substitute another form of self-stimulation. A child who cannot cope with the sensory stimuli in the environment and is being overstimulated needs to have sensory input graded to tolerance.[47] As in all other areas of evaluation and intervention, the therapist must look beyond the behavior to the processes that are initiating it. Underlying sensory abnormalities or deficiencies must be recognized and intervened with before a change in behavior can be expected.[60]

The manner in which the child provides self-stimulation can suggest strategies that may be effective in improving or eliminating the behavior. Slow, rhythmic rocking may be the distractible child's method of calming himself or herself, whereas violent, irregular rocking may be the hypotonic child's method of providing sensory input that will increase muscle activation and alertness. The type of behavior must also be considered in light of the developmental age of the child. Constant mouthing of objects and hands is socially unacceptable for a school-aged child. If, however, that child is functioning at a developmental and functional level less than chronologic age would dictate, oral exploration is a primary component of the learning process.[47] Rather than restricting such oral exploration and stimulation, the child must be provided means of oral stimulation, such as tooth brushing, and foods of various textures, in order to help facilitate progression to the next developmental and functional level.

To summarize, the physical therapist assessing the child with mental retardation must have various skills and must approach the evaluation with a flexible but organized strategy. Examination must include not only developmental testing, functional assessment, goniometrics, posture, and strength, but also a complete evaluation of the sensory systems. Because the main goal of intervention is to enhance basic developmental processes and to improve function,

there must be a thorough examination of all sensory and motor components of development. It is challenging and rewarding to evaluate such a complex group of skill areas and still have a concise picture of the whole child.

 ## Key Elements of Physical Therapy Intervention

GENERAL PRINCIPLES

Intervention with and management of the child with mental retardation must be directed toward the development of the child's full potential in all areas of learning: motor, cognitive, and affective. The child's ability to respond appropriately and effectively in terms of movement, intellectual function, and attitudes and feelings serves as the major long-range goal of intervention. This concept of intervention applies to the total function of the child. A deficit in one type of behavior may influence all other types. The child who needs motor stability may also benefit from psychological stability. Influences used to change the former may also have an effect on the latter and vice versa.[48]

There are several important elements to remember when designing effective intervention programs for children with mental retardation. The therapist must recognize the importance of choosing activities that accommodate the mental age of the child but that are also as age appropriate as possible. Display 10.3 offers several examples of how developmentally appropriate activities can be translated into functional but age-appropriate activities.

Activities in the intervention program should be interesting, fun, and meaningful. Because children with mental retardation often have a poor attention span, therapeutic activities should be chosen that most effectively and effi-

---

> > > **DISPLAY 10.3**

Examples of Functional Activities that Incorporate Developmental Skills

Examination Item	Underlying Skill	Examples of Alternative Materials/Activities
Walks on balance beam	Balance	Walking on bleachers, walking between rows of chairs
Holds toy for 5–10 sec	Can hold an object for 5–10 sec	Cup, spoon, book, hairbrush, coin, pencil, and ball
Stacks three wooden blocks	Perceptual–motor coordination of stacking	Glasses, bowls, dishes, trays, cassette tapes, CDs, books
Strings three 1-inch beads	Perceptual–motor coordination of inserting and pushing/pulling through	Lace shoe
Places peg in pegboard	Eye–hand (or hand–hand) coordination of placing an object in another object	Straw in milk carton, sock in shoe, toast in toaster, coin in vending machine slot, key in lock, pencil in sharpener
Picks up raisin with pincer grasp	Uses pincer grasp to pick up small items	Food, table game pieces, coins, pages of book, vocational items (nails, hooks)
Anticipates being picked up	Anticipates routine event	Being fed, bathed, tickled, greeted, and put to bed

Updated and revised from Downing J, Bailey B. Presented at the TASH Annual Conference, Washington, DC, December 9, 1988.

ciently meet the identified goal. Rather than asking a child to do a standard exercise regimen for strengthening, the necessary therapeutic activities can be translated into a functional task or social game. This approach not only sustains interest, cooperation, and enthusiasm, but also emphasizes carryover into activities of daily living. It may also promote achievement of goals in other areas, such as social, emotional, self-help, and cognitive skills. The therapist must be imaginative and should integrate many different approaches in order to develop an effective intervention approach for a particular child in a particular situation.

Repetition and consistency are crucial aspects of any program in which learning is expected to occur. Because repetition is important for learning any task, the therapist must design several activities that teach the same component task but do so in different ways. For example, if the goal is to improve extension of the trunk, the therapist may use activities such as a basketball drop or scooterboard games. These activities are varied but enjoyable methods of attaining the same goal. This approach to program planning not only ensures the necessary repetition of activities, but also offers the dimensions of interest and fun for a child with limited comprehension or attention.

One of the most important yet most difficult skills for the therapist to master is the ability to delineate priorities for intervention and to establish effective and appropriate long-term plans. When the therapist is faced with the challenge of a child with numerous deficits in many areas of development, it is easy for the therapist to become overwhelmed. When developing intervention plans, it is important to consider the child as a whole person. All pieces of the examination puzzle should merge to provide the therapist with a composite picture of how the child is or is not functioning within the child's world. The priorities for programming should become clear by looking at the child's overall development in this functional sense.

LEARNING CHARACTERISTICS

DIFFERENCES IN THE CHILD WITH MENTAL RETARDATION

An overview of cognitive development is necessary in order to understand the cognitive limitation of the child with mental retardation and to design effective intervention programs to overcome those cognitive limitations.

PIAGET'S THEORY OF INTELLECTUAL DEVELOPMENT

Jean Piaget, in order to explain normal and abnormal intellectual development, divided the developmental process into four stages: the sensorimotor period (0 to 18 months); the preoperational stage (2 to 7 years); the stage of concrete operations (7 to 12 years); and the period of formal operations (12 years and older).[61] The delineations offered by

Piaget's stages provide a basis for understanding the sequence of normal development and the limitations that are typical at each stage of cognitive development. Utilizing the Piagetian theory of development can be useful in understanding the various degrees of cognitive impairment seen in mental retardation.

Children learn mainly through exploration of the senses and through movement during the sensorimotor stage, which Piaget explained as an equilibration process. The unknown is presented as a confrontation with the unexplained and less understood and the child learns by his or her attempts to manipulate the environment with strategies with which to create new understandings, called accommodations. The ability to coordinate sensorimotor activity to reach certain goals is apparent in immature forms of intelligence displayed by children with behaviors reflective of seriously impaired cognitive abilities. Children thought to be functioning at this early stage explore their environment through much experimentation, which may even be repeated over and over. Accommodations to manage the environment are not routinely understood; therefore, learning cannot be generalized to new situations during this period. In fact, most learnings are discoveries made by trial and error. A child who is severely impaired may never progress beyond this stage of intellectual development.[61]

The preoperational stage is characterized by the development of language and the beginnings of abstract thought. Children at this stage can use symbols to represent objects that are not present, and may be able to classify and group objects, although not proficiently. A child with an IQ between 35 and 55 may not develop beyond this stage.[61]

During the concrete operations stage, the ability to order, classify, and relate experience to an organized whole begins to develop.[62] The child can solve some mathematical problems and can read well. The child can generalize learning to new situations and can begin to recognize another person's point of view. There is still a limited ability to deal with hypothetical problems. Persons with mild cognitive impairments often remain at this level of development.[61] Piaget's final stage—formal operations—normally begins at 12 years of age and continues throughout life. The abilities to reason and hypothesize are characteristic of this stage. The child with mental retardation seldom reaches this level of cognitive development.

INTERVENTION TO LIMIT COGNITIVE IMPAIRMENT

CONCRETE CONCEPTS COMPARED WITH ABSTRACT CONCEPTS

Children with mental retardation are less able to grasp abstract concepts than concrete concepts.[63] When working with children with mental retardation, the therapist must present concepts using meaningful, concrete directions.

Activities are best understood when demonstrated, done passively first, or translated into familiar activities pertaining to daily life. Using step-by-step examples and pictures to represent activities would be useful to building understanding of the expectations. The child learns from the telling, the retelling, the demonstrating, the practicing, and ultimately the actual performing in the "real" environment. Therapists need to understand the performance level in order to plan and direct the intervention plan.

MEMORY

The literature regarding the person with mental retardation's ability to remember shows that that ability is related to the type of retention task involved.[62] Use of short-term memory is consistently difficult for the child with mental retardation.[64–66] Smith indicates that a high level of distractibility by external, irrelevant stimuli is associated with these short-term memory deficits. However, overcoming this short-term memory problem can be dealt with by repetitions to enhance the use of long-term memory, an area that tends to be a relative strength for children with mental retardation. With this knowledge in mind, some of the following strategies can be used during physical therapy intervention:

1. Remove irrelevant, distracting material from the activity area. Do not work with the child in distracting surroundings, even if room dividers or curtains must be used to separate a small space from a larger, busy area.
2. Present each component of the task clearly and separately.
3. Begin with simple tasks and then progress to more difficult tasks.
4. Explain your expectations of the child at each stage of the intervention.
5. Try to support the tasks with visual aids, or model the task repeatedly.
6. Give immediate and consistent positive reinforcement.
7. Repeat directions as often as necessary.
8. Check the accuracy of performance frequently.
9. Keep the child informed of progress, and give the child an opportunity to demonstrate or practice the new skill independently.

Most researchers agree that practice, review, and overlearning help the child with mental retardation with long-term retention of skills. The therapist can promote learning and retention with much repetition of both the directions and the steps needed to complete the intended skill. It is important to provide ample opportunity to practice and use the newly learned material. Physical therapists inform parents and teachers of a child's progress and should encourage practice of the newly learned task at home or in the classroom. Learning cannot occur or be retained when the physical therapy intervention is an isolated segment of the child's day. Here again, the use of pictures and examples to extend the learning could be developed for the child to use in the home or community. Extended practice and communication with other team members are both vital. The current inclusion model of service delivery facilitates carryover of learning.

TRANSFER OF LEARNING

Transfer of learning is regarded as the ability to apply newly learned material to new situations having components that are similar to those of the material that was newly learned.[65] The Piagetian term for this process is assimilation. The learning challenge has been understood and the child has invented new strategies that are found to be useful in performing within the environment. The literature on transfer of learning suggests that two factors, in particular, be considered when formulating a plan for intervention.

Meaningfulness is an important element in transfer of learning for the child with cognitive impairment. A meaningful task is both easier to learn at the outset and easier to transfer to a second setting than one that has no meaning for the learner. This concept strongly supports the use of functional activities during physical therapy as opposed to meaningless "splinter skills."

Moreover, learning can be transferred best when both the initial task and the transfer task are similar. If, for example, the therapist is working on the ability to push rather than to pull on crutches, all of the therapy tasks, such as pushing in a prone position, sitting push-ups, and other tasks, can be transferred more readily to the task of pushing on crutches. *Consistency* also helps the child see the connection between therapy tools and their function.

Knowledge of basic learning concepts and an understanding of cognitive development are crucial for the physical therapist working with a child who is intellectually impaired. One can comprehend the utility of the Piagetian theories to the understanding of good therapy practices; learning is supported through the challenge stage while the child is learning to apply the strategy. The process is enhanced through repetitions and the use of visual aids, with demonstrations of the usefulness of the habilitation skill, all of which support the accommodation and the understanding, and thus fosters generalization of the skill. Physical therapy is a learning situation, and some modifications in approach will be necessary to accommodate the differences in performance seen in the child with mental retardation.

INTERVENTION TO LIMIT PHYSICAL IMPAIRMENTS AND FUNCTIONAL LIMITATIONS

Pediatric physical therapists traditionally have focused their efforts on interventions designed to limit musculoskeletal, neuromuscular, and cardiopulmonary impairments; reduce functional limitations; and prevent secondary impairment.[44] Early identification of these musculoskeletal, neuromuscular, and cardiopulmonary problems and anticipation of their recognition as associated within specific diagnoses give the therapist an insight into appropriate lifespan management of the child with mental retardation. A glance again at Display 10.2 gives the therapist familiarity with some of the specific musculoskeletal, neuromuscular, or cardiopulmonary risks associated with common types of mental retardation. Within this chapter, a focus on physical therapy management for the child with Down syndrome will offer the entry-level therapist a strategy for applying this management model to any child with any type of mental retardation diagnosis. The child's needs as they change throughout the lifespan will determine the level of support intervention required by physical therapy. Although this text is a pediatric physical therapy resource, this author will discuss lifespan management issues relevant to the client with developmental disabilities as he or she moves into and through adulthood. Again, those issues will be discussed using Down syndrome as the management model, consistent with the intent of this chapter.

THE IMPORTANCE OF FOCUSED INTERVENTION

Interventions designed by the therapist should be directed by the results of the multifaceted assessment and guided too by the findings of the functional assessment. Together these assessments will provide the therapist and the intervention team the data by which their evaluation should be directed in order to design focused interventions that address not only skills, but also their application in the various environments interfaced by the child. After the design of the intervention plan, multiple task analyses will guide the specific intervention strategies.

To ensure the desired learning, the therapist is encouraged to design discrete tasks that reflect the child's participation within the current environments and to set goals that increase the participation levels. This will address the child's need for meaningful, purposeful, and concrete activities to more naturally provide the motivation to learn.

Children with cognitive impairment learn better through multimodal teaching. Therapists are encouraged to use these techniques while teaching new tasks and practicing those previously introduced. In order to do this, the authors encourage the use of the "Practitioner's P's" methodology: *Plan, Present, Picture, Practice, Perform.* First, it is important to *Plan* the procedures for learning in specific discrete steps. Next, the therapist needs to *Present* tasks in ways that are understood by the child, being aware of any communication needs uncovered during the examination stages. Following the presentation of the tasks to be learned during the session, the *Picture* of the task to be performed should be presented as well. This

can be done through the use of pictures taken of the specific skill performance or through the use of available commercially produced stick-figure diagrams. Another form would be the therapist modeling the task in step-by-step fashion. The fourth step is to have the patient *Practice* the task. In this portion of the session the therapist guides the child through the steps of the task using the hand-over-hand methodology. The fifth and final "P" is for the child to *Perform* the task. Using these five P's, the therapist will be encouraged to use the multimodal methods more routinely.

The Team Concept and Collaboration

When working with the child with mental retardation, physical therapists must view themselves and their intervention goals as part of a total management plan. Use of a transdisciplinary team of professionals is the standard approach for children with special needs. The current inclusion model offers a strong support for the team concept. Comprehensive delivery of services for the child with mental retardation is beyond the scope of any one professional discipline. One of the main values of a transdisciplinary approach is the pooling of knowledge so that a composite and relevant course of action can be made. Because the child with mental retardation will have delays in many areas of development, the skills of many professionals can be used. No single professional has the necessary scope of expertise nor the resources to effectively provide care and education throughout the life of the child with mental retardation.[67,68]

To be effective, each professional on the team must understand the periodic shift of authority and emphasis at different times and different stages of development. Input from the physical therapist will sometimes be of paramount importance, whereas at other times, the priorities will lie in other areas of care. During these latter periods, the physical therapist may play a consultative or advisory role. Success of the team in its primary purpose of helping the child achieve his or her maximum potential will depend on each professional considering the whole child while offering the needed expertise to alleviate specific problems.[48] Communication among team members and respect for one another's unique knowledge and skills are keys to making the team process truly collaborative and therefore effective.

Effective use of all team members will ensure that consistency and reinforcement are present throughout the child's total program. For example, if certain sounds are being taught in speech therapy, the learning of these sounds can be reinforced by using them during physical therapy sessions. The physical therapist and special education teacher must work as partners in caring for the child. The therapist is uniquely qualified to assist the teacher in understanding the impact of impaired sensorimotor function on the achievement of cognitive milestones. For example, consider the child with severely impaired movement control, average head control, and preferred movement patterns dominated by strong tonic neck reflex patterns. In such a case, knowledge of the basics of normal movement control development could be invaluable to the teacher when working on a cognitive skill with the child, such as performing a simple cause-and-effect activity (e.g., manipulating a "busy box"). A simple suggestion from the therapist that the child be side-lying rather than supine could enable the child to reach for and manipulate the "busy box." Such a cooperative approach both facilitates the child's accomplishment of the educational goal and reduces the frustration of the teacher. The physical therapist must communicate and work with all members of the team, including the nurse, occupational therapist, psychologist, physician, teacher, physical education teacher, speech therapist, and parent (Fig. 10.1). The present-day model of inclusion certainly facilitates this collaborative team concept.

Whenever they work with children, physical therapists must recognize the importance of the family as part of the therapeutic team. Program carryover into the home is important for maximum effectiveness. The parents must learn how to work effectively with the child and must be able to help achieve the goals of the program (Fig. 10.2). This concept is true not only for physical therapy, but also for all areas of intervention and education. When asking family members to participate in a home program of care, physical therapists must be able to assess the abilities of the parents and siblings. The therapist must recognize problems or conditions in the home that may limit the successful participation of the parents.[68] Referral to appropriate agencies may help parents alleviate or resolve those problems or conditions. Several books that discuss the special needs of families of children with mental retardation may

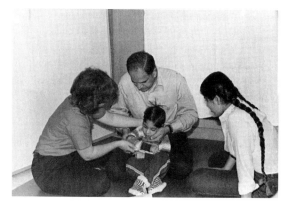

Figure 10.2 ▪ A physical therapist teaches proper handling techniques and proper positioning skills.

be useful for physical therapists.[69–72] The long-term nature of problems associated with mental retardation and management of those problems usually require a major commitment from the family.

A Management Model for Physical Therapists for the Child with Down Syndrome

DEFINITION

Down syndrome is a chromosomal disorder resulting in 47 chromosomes instead of 46.[73–75] Commonly called trisomy 21, Down syndrome results from faulty cell division affecting the 21st pair of chromosomes, either owing to a nondisjunction (95%), translocation (3% to 4%), or, least commonly, a mosaic presentation (1%).[76]

HISTORY AND INCIDENCE

Down syndrome is the most common cause of mental retardation and is a diagnosis frequently encountered by pediatric physical therapists. Approximately 4000 infants with Down syndrome are born annually in the United States with an incidence of 1 in 800 to 1000 live births.[9,13,77]

Evidence of an awareness of Down syndrome dates back to early times, with the earliest anthropologic record stemming from excavations in the 7th century of a Saxon skull that had many of the structural changes associated with Down syndrome.[76] Artwork throughout the Middle Ages contains depictions of children with the now-recognized facial characteristics of Down syndrome. Despite these early historical conjectures, there are no published documented reports of Down syndrome until the 19th century. This is understandable from a historical perspective because of the prevalence of infectious diseases and malnutrition that overshadowed research into genetic problems. Also, until beyond the mid-19th century, only half of the mothers survived beyond their 35th birthday (and

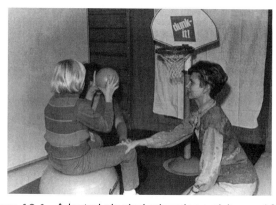

Figure 10.1 ▪ Adapted physical education activity used for therapeutic endeavors in a recreational mode. It is important for the adapted physical education teacher to have a thorough understanding of the sensory and motor skills being developed.

it is well known that there is an increased incidence of Down syndrome in mothers of advanced maternal age), and many children who indeed were born with Down syndrome probably died in early infancy.[76]

In 1846, Edouard Sequin described a patient with features suggestive of Down syndrome. In 1866, John Langdon Down published a paper describing the characteristics of the then-recognizable syndrome, which has since borne his name.[76] It was not until the mid-1950s that progress in methodologies to visualize chromosomes allowed more accurate studies of human chromosomes, leading to Lejeune's discovery that an alteration in the 21st chromosomal pair is the characteristic hallmark of Down syndrome.[78]

Pathophysiology and Associated Impairments of the the Child with Down Syndrome

Down syndrome results in neuromotor, musculoskeletal, and cardiopulmonary pathologies, which all require management by pediatric physical therapists. As with any etiology of mental retardation, an awareness of the pathologies and impairments indigenous to that specific etiology will offer the practicing therapist a model for lifespan management for the child.

NEUROPATHOLOGY

The primary neuropathology causing CNS disorder in children with Down syndrome is owing to several well-documented brain abnormalities. Overall brain weight in individuals with Down syndrome is 76% of normal, with the combined weight of the cerebellum and brainstem being even smaller: 66% of normal. There is also microcephaly, and the brain is abnormally rounded and short with a decreased anterior–posterior (AP) diameter, specifically called microbrachycephaly.[79–80] The number of secondary sulci is reduced, resulting in a simplicity of convoluted patterns in the brains of children with Down syndrome.[81] Several cytologic distinctions of the brain in Down syndrome include a paucity of small neurons, a migrational defect involving small neurons, and decreased synaptogenesis owing to altered synaptic morphology.[81] There are also structural abnormalities in the dendritic spines in the pyramidal tracts of the motor cortex that possibly underlie the motor incoordination so often seen in children with Down syndrome.[82] Research also shows evidence of a lack of myelination as well as a delay in the completion of myelination between 2 months and 6 years of age, which may explain the overall developmental delay typically seen in children with Down syndrome.[83] Some studies claim that up to 8% of children with Down syndrome also have some form of seizure disorder.[84]

SENSORY DEFICITS

Visual and hearing deficits, as well as speech impairments, are common in children with Down syndrome and have a direct impact on physical therapy examination and intervention. Visual deficits include congenital as well as adult-onset cataracts, myopia (50%), farsightedness (20%), strabismus, and nystagmus.[84] Other ocular findings of less clinical significance include the presence of Brushfield spots in the iris and the classic presence of epicanthal folds.

Many children with Down syndrome (60% to 80%) are found to have a mild to moderate hearing loss.[84] Otitis media is a frequently occurring medical problem that may contribute to intermittent or persisting hearing loss in children with Down syndrome.[73]

CARDIOPULMONARY PATHOLOGIES

Forty percent of children with Down syndrome are born with congenital heart defects, most commonly, atrioventricular canal defects and ventriculoseptal defects.[73] Although usually repaired in infancy, heart defects not corrected by age 3 are highly associated with greater delays in motor skill development.[85]

MUSCULOSKELETAL DIFFERENCES

Children with Down syndrome demonstrate many musculoskeletal differences that are of concern to the physical therapist. Linear growth deficits are observed, including a decrease in normal velocity of growth in stature, with the greatest deficiency between 6 and 24 months of age,[86–88] leg length reduction,[89] and a 10% to 30% reduction in metacarpal and phalangeal length. Muscle variations may also be present including an absent palmaris longus and supernumerary forearm flexors. There is also a lack of differentiation of distinct muscles bellies for the zygomaticus major and minor and the levator labii superior,[90] which may account for the typical facial appearance of the child with Down syndrome.

The most significant musculoskeletal differences, however, are owing in large part to the hypotonia and ligamentous laxity characteristic of this disorder. Ligamentous laxity is thought to be owing to a collagen deficit and commonly results in pes planus, patellar instability, scoliosis (52%), and atlantoaxial instability.[86,91,92] Atlantoaxial subluxation with risk for atlantoaxial dislocation is caused by laxity of odontoid ligament, whereby there may be excessive motion of C1 on C2 (12% to 20% incidence).[93–96] Hip subluxation is also commonly seen in children with Down syndrome.

Generalized hypotonia, found in all muscle groups of extremities, neck, and trunk, is a hallmark feature in children with Down syndrome. It is a major contributing factor to developmental motor delay.[97,98] Grip strength, isometric strength, and ankle strength have all been found to be deficient in studies on school-age children with Down syndrome.[99,100]

ADDITIONAL PHYSICAL CHARACTERISTICS

The back of the head is slightly flattened (brachycephaly), and the fontanels are frequently larger than normal and take longer to close. There may be areas of hair loss, and the skin is often dry and mottled in infancy and rough in the older child. The face of the child with Down syndrome has a somewhat flat contour, primarily because of the underdeveloped facial bones and facial muscles and a small nose. Usually, the nasal bridge is depressed and the nasal openings may be narrow. The eyes are characterized by narrow, slightly slanted eyelids, with the corners marked by epicanthal folds. The mouth of the child with Down syndrome is small, the palate narrow, and the tongue may take on a furrowed shape in later childhood. Dentition is often delayed and may be spotty. The abdomen may be slightly protuberant secondary to hypotonia and the chest may take on an abnormal shape secondary to congenital heart defect. More than 90% of children with Down syndrome develop an umbilical hernia. Hands and feet tend to be small, and the fifth finger is curved inward. In about 50% of children with Down syndrome, a single crease is observed across the palm on one or both hands (simian crease). The toes are usually short, and in the majority of children with Down syndrome, there is a wide space between the first and second toes, with a crease running between them on the sole of the foot.

Physical Therapy Examination and Intervention for the Child with Down Syndrome

Physical therapy examination of the child with Down syndrome should be holistic, viewing the child from multiple perspectives. The therapist must be aware of coexisting medical problems and especially alert to those typically associated with Down syndrome such as cardiac status, atlantoaxial stability, hearing and visual status, and the presence of seizure disorders. Speech difficulties may be present and therapists may be additionally challenged to effectively communicate during examination and subsequent intervention. The therapist must also integrate the child's cognitive capabilities into the evaluation process, including discussion of formal intelligence tests with appropriate team members and parent interviews, as well as conducting a brief cognitive assessment as part of a comprehensive developmental test battery.

Evaluation includes any or all of the following measures as appropriate for the age and setting within which the child is evaluated: comprehensive developmental testing, component testing of gross and fine motor skills including qualitative observational examination of movement, musculoskeletal examination, assessment of automatic reactions and postural responses, and, ultimately,

a functional examination. These pediatric evaluation procedures are discussed elsewhere in this text. Evaluation of the child with any type of mental retardation disorder, including Down syndrome, additionally encompasses examination of the musculoskeletal, neuromotor, and cardiopulmonary impairments associated with the specific diagnosis (see Display 10.2) and knowledge of the coexistence of the cognitive deficit associated with mental retardation and how that affects physical therapy examination and intervention.

LEARNING DIFFERENCES

Generally, children with mental retardation have been found to:

1. be capable of learning,
2. benefit from frequent repetitions in order to learn,
3. have difficulty generalizing skills,
4. need to have more frequent practice sessions in order to maintain learned skills,
5. need extended time in order to respond, and
6. have a more limited repertoire of responses.[101,102]

The levels of cognitive impairment seen in children with Down syndrome vary, from profoundly to mildly impaired, with a mild to moderate impairment being most common. As with any child with coexistent visual or hearing deficits, therapists must adapt interaction, examination, and teaching to accommodate these coimpairments. Children with mental retardation typically demonstrate attentional difficulties and difficulties with information processing. Research also shows myriad specific cognitive problems encountered in children with Down syndrome, including difficulties in sequential verbal processing, social–cognitive skills, auditory memory, and motor planning.[103–107] Children with Down syndrome appear to have significant impairments in verbal–motor interactions, with learning least proficient when the mode of response or reception calls for auditory or vocal skill.[108] It is important, therefore, for therapists to utilize frequent visual demonstration, practice and rehearsal, and perhaps multimodal sensory avenues in order to best interact with the child with Down syndrome. Oftentimes, the child may benefit from hand-over-hand demonstrations to aid in pattern development. The child with Down syndrome is more likely to remember the rules and patterns of a new activity if he or she is presented with input over many modalities—visual and kinesthetic as well as verbal.[109]

ASSOCIATED MOTOR DEFICITS

The ligamentous laxity and generalized muscular hypotonia associated with Down syndrome contribute the most to the motor delays and secondary musculoskeletal impairments that are of utmost concern to pediatric physical therapists. The degree to which muscular hypotonia is present will vary, but most investigators agree that it is the most frequently observed characteristic in children with Down syndrome.[75,110–113] Hypotonia is distributed to all major muscle groups including neck, trunk, and all four extremities.[114]

DEVELOPMENTAL DELAY

Clinically, muscular hypotonia has been well established to be highly correlated with developmental delay, including delay in attainment of gross motor and fine motor milestones,[85,115] as well as with delay in other areas of development such as speech acquisition and cognitive development.[98,116–118] Studies also have shown the persistence of reflexive movement patterns beyond the time when they should be integrated into more sophisticated movement patterns.[98] Consistent with delayed integration of reflex or immature movement patterns, a slower rate of development of postural reactions has been noted in children with Down syndrome.[119] Additional studies by Harris and Rast and Shumway-Cook also demonstrated difficulties in postural control, antigravity control, deficits in postural response synergies when balance perturbations were introduced, and, consequently, the development of compensatory movement strategies as children with Down syndrome attempted to learn to move and stabilize themselves.[119–121] These investigators attribute the movement deficiencies seen in children with Down syndrome primarily to disturbances in postural control and balance.

Not only is developmental delay to be anticipated when evaluating children with Down syndrome, but there is also some evidence to suggest that the underlying muscular hypotonia, ligamentous laxity, and postural difficulties contribute to some of the movement differences frequently observed in children with Down syndrome. Examples include "W" sitting, where the child will characteristically spread his or her legs to a full 180-degree split while in prone and then advance to a sitting posture by pushing up with his or her hands into sitting.[122] Gait acquisition is delayed and is immature, characterized by a persistent wide base and out-toeing.[122,123] It has been suggested that these differences in movement qualities are caused by muscular hypotonia, ligamentous laxity, and a resultant lack of trunk rotation. Hypotonia has also been shown to contribute to slower reaction time and depressed kinesthetic feedback.[124] Children who have motor impairments are at subsequent risk for secondary impairments because of their restricted ability to explore the environment, especially cognition, communication, and psychosocial development.[125–127]

PHYSICAL THERAPY EVALUATION AND INTERVENTION IMPLICATIONS

1. Evaluation should include administration of a comprehensive or component test to measure and track the developmental delay.

2. Qualitative examination of movement will alert the therapist to movement differences and possible emergent compensatory strategies.

3. Intervention must include an understanding from a functional, dynamic systems perspective and of the control parameters most likely to cause a responsiveness shift when attempting to influence developing motor strategies.[128]

4. General goal: Anticipate gross and fine motor delay and provide interventions to minimize it.
   - Utilize positioning and handling activities throughout early infancy and childhood to promote antigravity control and weight bearing.
   - Facilitate antigravity extension in prone and weight shifting within and as transition from prone.
   - In supine and supported sitting, encourage midline orientation, antigravity bimanual activities including eye–hand coordination, and activities to promote anterior neck and trunk antigravity muscle strength.
   - Emphasize trunk extension and extremity loading, which tend to increase axial muscle strength.[129]
   - Encourage emergence of righting and postural reactions through use of rotation within and during movement.
   - Allow for dynamic rather than static exploration of movement.
   - Introduce developmental milestones when chronologically appropriate, including supported sitting and standing, when trunk control and alignment are able to be established.
   - Anticipate delay in postural control responses and provide functional opportunities to enhance development in areas of cognition, language, and socialization.
   - Teach parents and other team members activities and position choices that will enhance the child's overall development.

MUSCULOSKELETAL PROBLEMS

In addition to generalized muscular hypotonia, ligamentous laxity is a hallmark musculoskeletal characteristic of Down syndrome and commonly results in pes planus, patellar instability, scoliosis (52%), and atlantoaxial instability.[86,91,92] The previously noted atlantoaxial relationship is identified by sagittal plane radiographs of the cervical spine in three different positions: flexion, neutral, and extension.[130–132] A joint interval of 6 to 10 mm is considered symptomatic. A joint interval of more than 4.5 mm carries precautions with it. Early signs of atlantoaxial dislocation include gait changes, urinary retention, reluctance to move neck, and increased deep tendon reflexes (DTRs).[96] In cases of dislocation with symptomatic atlantoaxial instability, posterior arthrodesis or fusion of C1 and C2 is recommended.[130] In addition to atlantoaxial instability, thoracolumbar scoliosis is also an associated vertebral column musculoskeletal impairment frequently seen in children and adolescents with Down syndrome, usually defined as of a mild to moderate degree.[92]

In the lower extremities, hip instability, patellar instability, and foot deformity are the most common musculoskeletal concerns for the physical therapist managing the child with Down syndrome. Hip subluxation is secondary to developmental acetabular dysplasia and long, tapered ischia that result in decreased acetabular and iliac angles as well as laxity of ligamentous support.[91] Pes planus and metatarsus primus varus are the major foot deformities seen in children with Down syndrome.[92]

PHYSICAL THERAPY EVALUATION AND INTERVENTION IMPLICATIONS

1. Ligamentous laxity makes any joint less resistant to any trauma, malalignment, or uneven forces. Alignment and support are crucial. At the atlantoaxial joint, this laxity makes the joint less resistant especially to superimposed flexion, where the joint interval is already widened.
2. Therapists should avoid exaggerated neck flexion, extension, rotation, and positions or movements that may cause twisting or undue forces. With caution, joint approximation or compression of the cervical spine should be performed gently with all children with Down syndrome and is contraindicated in children with identified atlantoaxial instability. Therapists should also use caution when placing a child in the inverted position or in other positions that increase risk of a fall onto the head.[96]
3. In the infant and child under the age of 2 years, a radiograph will not reliably detect atlantoaxial instability. Extreme caution must be taken and any activity that may result in cervical spine injury may be contraindicated.
4. Physical therapists must closely monitor children with Down syndrome for changes in neurologic status and be vigilant in assessing risk of atlantoaxial instability. Parent education should include issues of atlantoaxial instability, symptoms of neurologic compromise, periods and activities that may carry increased risk, and activities to avoid if instability is identified.[96]
5. The Committee on Sports Medicine of the American Academy of Pediatrics recommends an initial set of cervical spine radiographs at 2 years of age and follow-up radiographs in grade school, at adolescence, and in adulthood.[130]
6. Contact sports and physical activities that may result in cervical spine injury may be contraindicated.[133] The following activities are considered to be restricted for children with even asymptomatic atlantoaxial intervals of greater than 4.5 mm: gymnastics (somersaults), diving, high jump, soccer, butterfly stroke in swimming, exercises that place pressure on the head and neck, high-risk activities that involve possible trauma to the head and neck, and participation in pentathalons.[130,134]
7. Screening for scoliosis should be a routine part of lifespan management of the child with Down syndrome,

especially during periods of increased risk such as growth spurts, puberty, and throughout adolescence. Parents should be taught to perform routine screening for scoliosis. Activities and exercises should promote symmetry and alignment.
8. Musculoskeletal examination also should include biomechanical examination of the lower extremity and orthotic management, if indicated, for pes planus. In the infant, examination of hip stability is a routine part of a physical therapy evaluation and referral is indicated for orthopedic examination if hip instability if suspect. Supported standing in a stander should not be instituted unless hip stability and proper alignment has been established.
9. General goal: Maintain alignment and encourage normal movement forces in order to promote optimal biomechanical forces for best musculoskeletal development and prevention of anticipated malalignments and instabilities.
   - Use of aligned compression or weight-bearing forces in order to stimulate longitudinal bone growth as well as thickness and density of the bone and shaft
   - Aligned, supported weight bearing in order to promote joint stability and formation
   - Facilitation of normal cocontraction, force production, and increased muscle tone

In summary, the impact of all of these associated motor deficits in Down syndrome on physical therapy can be viewed as how they affect the child's development and overall functioning. Most of these movement problems have their basis in CNS pathology or primary musculoskeletal differences, which then often lead to secondary impairments in flexibility, stability, force production, coordination, postural control, balance, endurance, and overall efficiency. The specific intervention used will depend on the identified problems and on the consequences that can be predicted and perhaps prevented.

Neuromuscular Impairments	Functional Implications
Hypotonia, low force production	Motor delay, poor contraction
	Movement paucity
Slow automatic postural reactions	Balance limitations
	Slow reaction time
Joint hypermobility	Decreased speed
	Instability, movement anxiety
Atlantoaxial Instability, scoliosis, foot deformities	May preclude access to activities or limit participation level in activity

CARDIOPULMONARY FITNESS

General physical fitness is often below desired levels in children with mental retardation, and specifically, in children with Down syndrome.[135] Children with Down syndrome are at risk for restrictive pulmonary disease with concomitant decreased lung volumes and a weak cough, because of generalized trunk and extremity weakness.[136–138] Reduced cough effectiveness may contribute to a high incidence of respiratory infections.[139] Decreased lung volumes including vital capacity and total lung capacity may contribute to a deficiency of the pulmonary system to oxygenate the mixed venous blood or remove the carbon dioxide from the same blood.[140] If there is a reduction in the maximum amount of oxygen available for transport, the energy available for activities is lowered, and consequently a poorer level of physical fitness is achieved.

PHYSICAL THERAPY EVALUATION AND INTERVENTION IMPLICATIONS

The implications for lifespan management of the child with Down syndrome are obvious.

1. Greater emphasis on physical fitness may increase cardiopulmonary endurance and muscular strength. Programming should begin with children of primary age in order to prevent a slowing of activity and the subsequent onset of obesity and long-term atherosclerotic risk profiles.[135] Knowledge of improvement reported from training programs for children with Down syndrome supports the ability of these children to respond to early intervention.[141,142]
2. Physical therapists have an excellent opportunity to impact the health of children with Down syndrome through direct intervention or in consultation with special educators or physical/recreational educators.
3. General goal: Encourage commitment to wellness by promoting cardiopulmonary endurance, overall physical fitness, and parent/caregiver/client education.

The Person with Mental Retardation Moving into and Through Adulthood: Key Management Issues

Mental retardation and Down syndrome both fall under the broad descriptive definition as types of developmental disabilities. The Developmental Disabilities Assistance and Bill of Rights Amendment of 1987 defines a "developmental disability" as a severe and chronic disability that manifests before age 22, is attributable to a mental and/or physical impairment, results in substantial functional limitations in three or more major life activities, and reflects a need for a combination and sequence of special, individualized services that are of extended duration or lifelong.[143,144] With increased sensitivity to lifespan issues and the recent availability of both retrospective reviews and good clinical case reports, the literature is now available

documenting typical lifespan management concerns. Concurrently, the current practice of physical therapy focuses attention on wellness and preventative management. It is imperative that the practitioners of today integrate a proactive, wellness-focused preventative bias into a client's management plan. Since persons with mental retardation, including Down syndrome, typically begin intervention in childhood, the pediatric physical therapist is most likely to be the clinician who will have contact with that client into and through adulthood. This section will highlight some of the most typical challenges facing persons with mental retardation and/or Down syndrome as they move into and through the adult years.

People with mental retardation and other developmental disabilities including Down syndrome are enjoying a lengthened life expectancy and will experience the same age-related changes that occur in the general population.[145,146] The aging process does, however, start earlier in persons with mental retardation, perhaps as early as age 35, and generally at around age 55.[146–149] The onset and the impact of the age-related changes are influenced by the severity of the person's existing disabilities and are likely to have a more significant effect if the person has multiple coimpairments.[145]

A review of the literature reveals several features of the aging process that are pertinent for integration into a lifespan physical therapy management approach. Therapists should be alert to the following anticipated issues: early menopause with the related secondary effects, such as increased risk for osteoporosis; thyroid dysfunction; obesity; diabetes mellitus; late onset of seizure disorder; increased visual or hearing impairment; cardiac disease; depression; dementia; and Alzheimer's disease.[150–154] Physical therapy evaluation and intervention should include proactive preventative management for the possible early onset of any number of these disorders. Evaluation methods may require that standardized tests be modified for use with the cognitively impaired individual.[155]

As emphasized throughout this chapter, a main focus of examination and intervention is always on the preservation of safe, independent function or caregiver assistance, as required. Therapists need to use a holistic and multidimensional approach to meet these wide-ranging needs of adults with developmental disabilities.[156]

SUMMARY

In the management of the child with mental retardation, the physical therapist is challenged to use various skills. The many complex and persistent difficulties encountered by children with mental retardation often require innovative methods of physical therapy evaluation and intervention. It is easy to understand that physical therapists may feel overwhelmed by the complexity of this population.

This chapter has attempted to give therapists a "user-friendly" strategy for physical therapy management, including evaluation and intervention, for *any* child with a diagnosis of mental retardation. Therapists are reminded to view the mental retardation itself as only a partial description of that child's learning impairment, which may vary in severity from having anywhere from a mild to a profound influence on that child's functional learning capabilities. This may be further confounded by other concomitant sensory deficits, including visual, hearing, or sensory organizational problems. Physical therapy evaluation and intervention must incorporate not only the basic principles of pediatric physical therapy, but also an understanding of the principles of teaching and learning as they relate to the child with mental retardation.

Additionally, although there are at least 350 known etiologies for mental retardation, the therapist can easily investigate any of those specific etiologies and acquaint himself or herself with any commonly associated neuromuscular, musculoskeletal, or cardiopulmonary impairments. This investigative approach will sharpen the therapist's examination skills and alert him or her to the presence of likely coimpairments or associated medical problems. An understanding of the primary pathology and associated motor deficits readily assists the therapist in establishing goals and priorities. Effective lifespan physical therapy management of the child can then encompass the anticipation of secondary deformities and risks for that child, which can then be shared with parents and other team members. This chapter illustrated the application of this investigative strategy to the physical therapy management of a child with Down syndrome. This same investigative strategy can be utilized for any mental retardation diagnosis encountered in pediatric physical therapy practice.

Communication of the changing needs of children with mental retardation to parents and other professionals requires not only technical expertise on the part of the therapist, but also the ability to be a sensitive listener and creative teacher. Through an effective transdisciplinary and collaborative approach to the child and his or her family, one can strive to help the child with mental retardation to function at his or her best in society.

CASE STUDY

Ashir

This case study will summarize physical therapy management for this child who presented with multiple disabilities, followed from initial referral at 2 months of age until death at age 8. This case study will illustrate how the role and level of service changes and fluctuates in response to a child's changing needs during the course of his or her lifespan.

Ashir was born at 36 weeks' gestation via a spontaneous vaginal delivery to a 38-year-old college professor. Pregnancy was uneventful with the exception of the mother retrospectively reporting a paucity of fetal movement. Neonatal course was characterized by poor suck, difficulty feeding, marked irritability, and failure to thrive. Developmental delay characterized by poor visual regard and following poor head control and persistent feeding difficulties precipitated a referral for early intervention services by the pediatrician when Ashir was 2 months old. The family was also very concerned and described Ashir as unresponsive, irritable, and difficult to manage.

Evaluation consisted of a physical therapy examination of multiple systems and the administration of a developmental test battery. The physical therapist was a member of a transdisciplinary evaluation team. Ashir presented with limited voluntary motor control with most movements characterized by primitive or tonic reflex patterns and strong extension muscular hypertonus with signs of spasticity. Deep tendon reflexes were scored at 5 with a few beats of unsustained clonus elicited at both the ankles and the biceps. Posture was typically asymmetric with head and trunk laterally flexed to the left and all movements jerky and rigid in quality. Respiration was shallow and suck and swallow not rhythmic. When positioned with his head in the midline, he would quiet to a voice but did not demonstrate visual regard or the ability to track a visual stimulus. Function was significantly impaired in multiple domains. Ashir was a handsome child who was observed to smile when quieted and comforted.

Physical therapy during infancy focused on educating the family, facilitating caregiving, making appropriate referrals for diagnosis, baseline assessment and social agency support, and promoting the development of sensorimotor skills. During infancy, the main physical therapy goals were established as follows:

1. Handling and care. Ashir's family learned positioning, carrying, feeding, bathing, and dressing techniques to promote skeletal alignment and symmetry, to minimize secondary impairments such as contractures and spinal deformity, to promote respiratory hygiene, and to facilitate the emergence of functional and purposeful movement. Basic principles employed were to teach methods that used a variety of movements and postures to promote sensory variety, including positions that would promote full lengthening of spastic or hypoextensible muscles, and using positions that promoted functional voluntary movement.
2. Facilitation of optimal sensorimotor development. Therapy focused on the development of well-aligned postural stability along with smooth mobility to allow for the emergence of motor skills such as reaching, rolling, sitting, floor mobility, and transitional movements. Movements that included trunk rotation, dissociation, weight bearing, weight shifting, and selected isolated movements were incorporated into everyday activity. Activities or specialized equipment was introduced to allow for the attainment of functional skills because the severity of the impairments was preventing the natural emergence of those skills. For

example, adapted equipment was used to support and encourage upright sitting, which then allowed Ashir to begin to visually explore the world and begin developing upper extremity skills. Toys were modified to allow for these skills to emerge with support.

3. Family-centered care. Since infancy is a crucial time to establish a trusting relationship with parents, maintain hope, and empower parents to be informed, effective advocates for their child, the family was actively involved as collaborative members of the team.

During the preschool years, Ashir continued to present with multiple disabilities and a significant need for support within all areas of function. A main goal of intervention was to maximize function while simultaneously minimizing secondary impairment or further disabilities. The focus expanded to include intervention for the support of self-care activities such as dressing, toileting, and feeding as well as play, communication, and social interaction. Functional examinations included evaluation of the ability to bear weight and assist with transfers, and the need for assistive devices/adaptive equipment. Intervention and education centered on reducing impairments and preventing secondary impairments within a functional context. Optimal postural alignment and movements that are conducive to musculoskeletal development, neurophysiologic control, and function through exercise, positioning, and equipment were the main aims of most interventions.

During the preschool years, the main physical therapy goals were established as follows:

1. Increase functional strength. For children with significant impairment, muscle strength is evaluated within a functional context. Ashir continued to present with limited voluntary motor control, weakness, and symptoms of spasticity. Functional strengthening through movement activity will result in a clinical reduction in the influence of spasticity on motor control. Movement activities focused on assisted functional skills integrated into activities of daily living and exploration of the environment.

2. Management of spasticity. Spasticity is best viewed as a symptom of disordered motor control. The diminishment of spasticity through pharmaceutical, neurosurgical, or orthopedic intervention may be appropriate at this age. For Ashir, medication was prescribed to alleviate the spasticity but more invasive options were discarded because of high risk and questionable life quality value.

3. Preservation of range of motion. Active and passive stretching activities were taught to all family members and caregivers, including school professionals. Prolonged stretching using splints was employed for nighttime use.

4. Skeletal alignment and weight bearing. Alignment of the body is important and should be promoted in a variety of positions with and without adaptive equipment. The benefits of standing include mineralization and increasing bone density, as well as promoting normal skeletal modeling and joint formation. Personal experience has shown that children with severe postural control problems may require

several shorter periods per day because they cannot tolerate sessions longer than 20 minutes at a time. Ashir enjoyed the use of a stander for several 20-minute sessions per day, offering him the opportunity to be upright.

5. Mobility and the attainment of functional skills. The persistence of obligatory primitive reflexes at 12 to 24 months of age suggests limited motor control and is highly predictive of nonlocomotion.[157] Physical therapy focused on decreasing the effect of functional limitations during these preschool years. Optimal treatment frequency is unknown, but periods of increased frequency have shown improvements in the attainment of specific intervention goals when these skills were incorporated into daily functional activities. Physical therapy was delivered in a transdisciplinary inclusion model within the preschool setting.

6. Family involvement. Family-centered management suggests that the therapist and family communicate openly and listen carefully to each other so that the child's and family's unique needs can be most effectively met. Siblings, grandparents, and daycare providers were all included as appropriate (see Fig. 10.2).

School age is typically a time when the extent of the functional limitations and differences becomes poignantly clear. Therapists must be supportive of children and their families while facilitating communication and role definition with school service providers. For Ashir, the goals and intervention concerns were an extension of those listed in the preschool period, with continued emphasis on maximizing some level of functional performance and prevention of secondary impairment. Growth spurts were monitored carefully so that secondary impairments such as limitations in range of motion did not contribute to decreased function. Physical therapy within the school system offers unique opportunities and challenges for therapists. For an in-depth discussion of issues pertinent to school-based therapy, refer to Chapter 19.

Ashir died at the age of 8 after pneumonia. His family members were devoted to his care and were able to move through this final process knowing that they had offered Ashir a short but meaningful life of supportive care.

ACKNOWLEDGMENTS

I wish to gratefully acknowledge the children and parents from whom I have learned so much. I congratulate all of them for their courage, spirit, and unconditional love.

REFERENCES

1. Nichtern S. Helping the Retarded Child. Grosset and Dunlap, 1974.
2. Sebelist RM. Mental retardation. In: Hopkins HL, Smith HD, eds. Willard and Spackman's Occupational Therapy. 9th Ed. Philadelphia: JB Lippincott, 1996.
3. National Institute on Mental Retardation: Orientation Manual on Mental Retardation. Ontario, Canada: York University, 1981.
4. Itard J. The Wild Boy of Aveyron. Englewood Cliffs, NJ: Prentice-Hall, 1962.
5. American Association on Mental Retardation (AAMR). 1719 Kalorama Road, NW, Washington, DC, 20009-2683.

6. Sorrells AM, Rieth HJ, Sindelar PT. Critical Issues in Special Education: Access, Diversity, and Accountability. Boston: Pearson Education, Inc., 2004.

7. Winzer MA. A tale often told: the early progression of special education. Remedial Special Educ 1998;19(4):212–219.

8. *PARC v. Commonwealth of Pennsylvania*, 1972. In: Heward WL, ed. Exceptional Children. Upper Saddle River, NJ: Merrill Prentice Hall, 2003.

9. National Association of Protection and Advocacy Systems. Early history. Online webpage. Available at: http://www.napas.org/I-5/early-history_home.htm. Accessed September 11, 2004.

10. Diagnostic and Statistical Manual of Mental Disorders. 4th Ed, Text Revision. Washington, DC: American Psychiatric Association, 2000.

11. Taylor LT, Richards SB, Brady MP. Mental Retardation. Boston: Pearson Education, 2005:44–45.

12. Berkow R. Mental illness and developmental disabilities. In: Ginsberg L, ed. Social Work Almanac. 2nd Ed. Washington, DC: National Association of Social Workers Press, 1992.

13. National Dissemination Center for Children with Disabilities (NICHCY). Online webpage. Available at http://www.nichcy.org/pubs/factshe/fs4txt.htm. Accessed September 26, 2004.

14. Roid GH. Stanford-Binet Intelligence Scale. 5th Ed. Chicago: Riverside, 2003.

15. Wechsler D. Wechsler Intelligence Scale for Children-IV. San Antonio, TX: Psychological Corporation, 2003.

16. Wechsler D. Wechsler Preschool and Primary Scale of Intelligence III. San Antonio, TX: Psychological Corporation, 2002.

17. Kaufman AS, Kaufman NL. Kaufman Assessment Battery for Children. Circle Pines, MN: American Guidance Service, 2003.

18. Sparrow SS. Vineland Adaptive Behavior Scales. Circle Pines, MN: American Guidance Service, 1984.

19. Adams GL. Comprehensive Test of Adaptive Behavior. Columbus, OH: Merrill, 1984.

20. Sloan W, Birch JW. A rationale for degrees of retardation. Am J Ment Defic 1955;60:262.

21. Nagi SZ. Disability and Rehabilitation. Columbus, OH: Ohio State University Press, 1969.

22. World Health Organization. International Classification of Functioning, Disability, and Health. Geneva, Switzerland: World Health Organization, 2001.

23. National Institutes of Health. Draft V: Report and Plan for Rehabilitation Research. Bethesda, MD: National Institutes of Health, National Center for Rehabilitation and Research, 1992.

24. Bertoti DB. Physical therapy for the mentally retarded child. In: Tecklin JS, ed. Pediatric Physical Therapy. Philadelphia: JB Lippincott, 1993.

25. Chinn PC, Drew CJ, Logan DR. Mental Retardation: A Life Cycle Approach. St. Louis: CV Mosby, 1979.

26. International Classification of Diseases (ICD). Ann Arbor, MI: World Health Organization, 1992.

27. Carter CH. Handbook of Mental Retardation Syndromes. Springfield, IL: Charles C Thomas, 1970.

28. Nyhan WL, Sakati NO. Genetic and Malformation Syndromes in Clinical Medicine. Chicago: Year Book Medical Publishers, 1976.

29. Bergsma D. Birth Defects: Atlas and Compendium. Baltimore: Williams & Wilkins, 1973.

30. Berg JM. The de Lange Syndrome. New York: Pergamon Press, 1970.

31. Jones KL, Smith DW, eds. Recognizable Patterns of Malformation. Smith's recognizable Patterns of Human Malformation. 5th Ed. Philadelphia: WB Saunders, 1996. p. 88–89.

32. Harris SR, Shea AM. Down syndrome. In: Campbell SK. Pediatric Neurologic Physical Therapy. 2nd Ed. New York: Churchill Livingstone, 1991.

33. Shumway-Cook A, Woollacott MH. Dynamics of postural control in the child with Down syndrome. Phys Ther 1985;65: 1315–1322.

34. Bloom AS, et al. Developmental characteristics of recognizable patterns of human malformation. In: Berg JM, ed. Science and Service in Mental Retardation: Proceedings of the Seventh Congress of the International Association for the Scientific Study of Mental Deficiency (LASSMD). New York: Methuen, 1985.

35. Kastner T, Nathanson R, Keenan J, et al. A statewide public and professional educational program on fragile X syndrome. Ment Retard 1992;30:355–361.

36. Rinck C. Fragile X syndrome. Dialogue Drugs Behav Dev Disabil (University of Missouri) 1992;4(3):1–4.

37. Anderson LT, Ernst M. Self-injury in Lesch-Nyhan disease. J Autism Dev Dis 1994;24:67–81.

38. Aughton DJ, Cassidy SB. Physical features of Prader-Willi syndrome in neonates. Am J Dis Child 1990;144:1251–1254.

39. Dykens EM, Cassidy SB. Prader-Willi syndrome: genetic, behavioral and treatment issues. Child Adolesc Psychiatric Clin North Am 1996;5:913–927.

40. Borrelli J, Rany E, Guidera KJ, et al. Orthopaedic manifestations of Rett syndrome. J Pediatr Orthop 1991;11:204–208.

41. Holm VA, King HA. Scoliosis in the Rett syndrome. Brain Dev 1990;12:151–153.

42. Nomura Y, Segawa Y. Characteristics of motor disturbance in Rett syndrome. Brain Dev 1990;12:27–30.

43. Brady DK, Crowe TK, Stewart KB, et al. Rett syndrome: a literature review and survey of patients and therapists. Phys Occup Ther Pediatr 1989;9(3):35–55.

44. McEwen I. Mental retardation. In: Campbell SK, ed. Physical Therapy for Children. 2nd Ed. Philadelphia: WB Saunders, 2000.

45. Detterman DK, Mayer JD, Canuso DR, et al. Assessment of basic cognitive abilities in relation to cognitive deficits. Am J Ment Retard 1992;97:251–286.

46. Horvat M, Croce R. Physical rehabilitation of individuals with mental retardation: physical fitness and information processing. Crit Rev Phys Rehabil Med 1995;7(3):233–252.

47. Montgomery PC. Assessment and treatment of the child with mental retardation. Phys Ther 1981;61:1265–1272.

48. Pearson PH, Williams CE, eds. Physical Therapy Services in the Developmental Disabilities. Springfield, IL: Charles C Thomas, 1972.

49. Kinnealy M. Aversive and nonaversive responses to sensory stimuli in mentally retarded children. Am J Occup Ther 1973; 27:464–472.

50. Getman GN, Kone ER, et al. Developing Learning Readiness. St. Louis: McGraw-Hill, 1966.

51. DeQuiros JB. Diagnosis of vestibular disorders in the learning disabled. J Learn Disabil 1976;9:50–58.

52. Moore J. Cranial nerves and their importance in current rehabilitation techniques. In: Henderson A, Coryell J, eds. The Body Senses and Perceptual Deficit. Boston: Boston University, 1973:102–120.

53. Ayres AJ. Sensory Integration and the Child. Los Angeles: Western Psychological Services, 1979:34–35.

54. Collier G. Emotional Expression. Hillsdale, NJ: Lawrence Erlbaum Associates, 1985.

55. Royeen CB, Lane SJ. Tactile processing and sensory defensiveness. In Fisher AG, Murray EA, Bundy AC, eds. Sensory Integration: Theory and Practice. Philadelphia: FA Davis Company, 1991.

56. Ayres AJ. Sensory Integration and Learning Disorders. Los Angeles: Western Psychological Services, 1972.

57. Ayres AJ. Tactile functions: their relation to hyperactive and perceptive motor behavior. Am J Occup Ther 1964;18:6–11.

58. Clark RG, Gilman S, Wilhaus-Newman S. Essentials of Clinical Neuroanatomy and Neurophysiology. 9th Ed. Philadelphia: FA Davis, 1996.

59. Westcott SL, Lowes LP, Richardson PK. Evaluation of postural stability in children: current theories and assessment tools. Phys Ther 1997;77:629–645.

60. Lemke H. Self-abusive behavior. Am J Occup Ther 1974;28:94–98.

61. Batshaw NL, Perret YM. Children with Handicaps: A Medical Primer. 2nd Ed. Baltimore: Paul H. Brookes, 1986.

62. Hardy RD, Cull JB. Mental Retardation and Physical Disability. Springfield, IL: Charles C Thomas, 1974.

63. Weiner H. Comparative Psychology of Mental Development. New York: International University Press, 1948.

64. Bird EKR, Chapman RS. Sequential recall in individuals with Down syndrome. J Speech Hearing Res 1994;37:1369–1381.

65. Smith R. Clinical Teaching: Methods of Instruction for the Retarded. New York: McGraw-Hill, 1968.

66. Hale CA, Borkowski JG. Attention, memory, and cognition. In: Matson JL, Mulick JA, eds. Handbook of Mental Retardation. New York: Pergamon Press, 1991.

67. Scheerenberger RC. Mental retardation: definition, classification, and prevalence. Ment Retard Abstr 1964;1:432–441.

68. Connolly BH, Anderson RM. Severely handicapped children in the public schools—a new frontier for the physical therapist. Phys Ther 1978;58:433–438.

69. Odel SJ, Greer JG, Anderson RM. The family of the severely retarded individual. In: Anderson RM, Greer JG, eds. Educating the Severely and Profoundly Retarded. Baltimore: University Park Press, 1976:251–261.

70. Barsch RH. The Parent of the Handicapped Child. Springfield, IL: Charles C Thomas, 1968.

71. Roos P. Parents and families of the mentally retarded. In: Kauffman JM, Payne JS, eds. Mental Retardation: An Introduction and Personal Perspectives. Columbus, OH: Charles E. Merrill, 1975.

72. Farber B. Family Organization and Crisis: Maintenance of Integration in Families with a Severely Retarded Child. Lafayette, IN: Child Development Publication, Society Research Child Development, 1960.

73. Coleman M. Down's syndrome. Pediatr Ann 1978; 7:90.

74. Kirman BH. Genetic errors: chromosome anomalies. In: Kirman BH, Bicknell J, eds. Mental Handicap. Edinburgh: Churchill Livingstone, 1975.

75. Harris SR, Shea AM. Down syndrome. In: Campbell SK, ed. Pediatric Neurologic Physical Therapy. 2nd Ed. New York: Churchill Livingstone, 1991.

76. Pueschel SM. Cause of Down syndrome. In: Pueschel SM. A Parent's Guide to Down Syndrome: Toward a Brighter Future. Baltimore: Paul H Brookes Publishing Co., 1990.

77. Huether C. Demographic projections for Down syndrome. In: Pueschel SM, Tingey C, Rynders CE, et al., eds. New Perspectives on Down Syndrome. Baltimore: Paul H Brookes Publishing Co., 1987.

78. Lejeune J, Gauthier M, Turpin R. Les chromosomes humain en culture de tissus. CR Acad Sci (D) 1959;248:602.

79. Roche AF. The cranium in mongolism. Acta Neurol 1966; 42:62.

80. Penrose LS, Smith GF. Down's Anomaly. London: Churchill Livingstone, 1966.

81. Becker LE, Petit TL, Scott BS, et al. Neurobiology of Down's syndrome. Prog Neurobiol 1983;21:199.

82. Marin-Padilla M. Pyramidal cell abnormalities in the motor cortex of a child with Down's syndrome. J Comp Neurol 1976; 67:63.

83. Schmidt-Sidor B, Wisniewski KF, et al. Postnatal delay of myelin formation in brains from Down's syndrome. Clin Neuropathol 1989;6(2):55.

84. Pueschel SM. Medical concerns. In: Pueschel SM, ed. A Parent's Guide to Down syndrome: Toward a Brighter Future. Baltimore: Paul H Brookes Publishing Co., 1990.

85. Zausmer EF, Shea A. Motor development. In: Pueschel SM, ed. The Young Child with Down Syndrome. New York: Human Sciences Press Inc., 1984.

86. Shea AM. Growth and development in Down syndrome in infancy and early childhood: implications for the physical therapist. In: Touch Topics in Pediatrics, Lesson 5. Alexandria, VA: American Physical Therapy Association, 1990.

87. Castells S, Beaulieu I, Torrado C, et al. Hypothalamic versus pituitary dysfunction in Down's syndrome as a cause of growth retardation. J Intellect Disabil Res 1996;40:509–517.

88. Cronk CE, Crocker AC, Pueschel SM, et al. Growth charts for children with Down syndrome; 1 month to 18 years of age. Pediatrics 1988;81:102–110.

89. Rarick GG, Seefeldt V. Observations from longitudinal data on growth and stature and sitting height of children with Down syndrome. J Ment Defic Res 1974;18:63–78.

90. Bersu ET. Anatomical analysis of the developmental effects of aneuploidy in man: the Down syndrome. Am J Med Genet 1980;5:399.

91. Dummer GM. Strength and flexibility in Down's syndrome. In: American Association for Health, Physical Education and Recreation: Research Consortium Papers: Movement Studies, vol. 1, book 3. Washington, DC: American Association for Health, Physical Education and Recreation, 1978.

92. Lynne D, Sigman B, Diamond LS, et al. Orthopedic disorders in patients with Down's syndrome. Orthop Clin North Am 1981;12:57.

93. Giblin PE, Michele LJ. The management of atlanto-axial subluxation with neurological involvement in Down's syndrome: a report of two cases and review of the literature. Clin Orthop 1979;140:66.

94. Gray WD, Whaley WJ, et al. Atlantoaxial dislocation and Down syndrome. Can Med Assoc J 1980;123:35.

95. Brenneman S, Stanger M, Bertoti DB. Age-related considerations: pediatric. In: Saunders RM, ed. Saunders Manual of Physical Therapy Practice. Philadelphia: WB Saunders, 1995.

96. Gajdosik CG, Ostertag S. Cervical instability and Down syndrome: review of the literature and implications for physical therapists. Pediatric Phys Ther 1996;8:1:31–36.

97. Carr J. Mental and motor development in young Mongol children. J Ment Defic Res 1970;14:205.

98. Cowie VA. A Study of the Early Development of Mongols. Oxford: Pergamon Press, 1970.

99. Morris AF, Vaughan SE, Vaccaro P. Measurements of neuromuscular tone and strength in Down syndrome children. J Ment Defic Res 1982;26:41–47.

100. Mezzomo JM, MacNeill-Shea SH, et al. Relationship of ankle strength and hypermobility to squatting skills of children with Down syndrome. Phys Ther 1985;65:1658–1666.

101. Brown L, et al. A strategy for developing chronological age appropriate and functional curricular content for severely handicapped adolescents and young adults. J Spec Educ 1979;12:81–90.

102. Orelove FP, Sobsey D. Designing transdisciplinary services. In: Orelove, Sobsey D, eds. Educating Children with Multiple Disabilities: A Transdisciplinary Approach. Baltimore: Paul H Brooks, 1991.

103. Horvat M, Croce R. Physical rehabilitation of individuals with mental retardation: physical fitness and information processing. Crit Rev Phys Rehabil Med 1995;7(3):233–252.

104. Hartley XY. Lateralization of speech stimuli in young Down's syndrome children. Cortex 1981;17:241.

105. Marcel MM, Armstrong V. Auditory and visual sequential memory of Down syndrome and nonretarded children. Am J Ment Defic 1982;87:86.

106. Edwards JM, Elliott D, Lee TD. Contextual interference effects during skill acquisition and transfer in Down's syndrome adolescents. Adapt Phys Act Quart 1986;3:250.

107. Elliott D, Weeks DJ. A functional systems approach to movement pathology. Adapt Phys Act Quart 1993;10:312.

108. Griffiths MI. Development of children with Down's syndrome. Physiotherapy 1976;62:11–15.

109. Hagen C. A approach to the treatment of mild to moderately severe apraxia. Top Land Dis 1987;34:8.

110. Cummins H, Talley C, Platou RV. Palmar dermatoglyphics in mongolism. Pediatrics 1950;5:241.

111. Levinson A, Friedman A, Stamps F. Variability of mongolism. Pediatrics 1955;16:43.

112. McIntire MS, Dutch SJ. Mongolism and generalized hypotonia. Am J Ment Defic 1964;68:669.

113. Wagner HR. Mongolism in orientals. Am J Dis Child 1962; 103:706.

114. McIntire MS, Menolascino FJ, Wiley JH. Mongolism—some clinical aspects. Am J Ment Defic 1965;69:794.

115. Harris SR. Relationship of mental and motor development in Down's syndrome infants. Phys Occup Ther Pediatr 1981;1:13.

116. Canning CD, Pueschel SM. Developmental expectations: an overview. In: Pueschel SM, ed. A Parent's Guide to Down Syndrome: Toward a Brighter Future. Baltimore: Paul H Brookes Publishing Co., 1990.

117. LaVeck B, LaVeck GD. Sex differences in development among young children with Down syndrome. J Pediatr 1977;91:767.

118. Cicchetti D, Sroufe LA. The relationship between affective and cognitive development in Down's syndrome infants. Child Dev 1976;47:920.

119. Haley SM. Postural reactions in children with Down syndrome. Phys Ther 1986;66(1):17–31.

120. Rast MM, Harris SR. Motor control in infants with Down syndrome. Dev Med Child Neurol 1985;27:682–685.

121. Shumway-Cook A, Woollacott M. Dynamics of postural control in the child with Down syndrome. Phys Ther 1985;65: 1315–1322.

122. Lydic JS, Steele C. Assessment of the quality of sitting and gait patterns in children with Down's syndrome. Phys Ther 1979;59(12):1489–1494.

123. Parker AW, Bronks R. Gait of children with Down syndrome. Arch Phys Med Rehabil 1980;61:345–351.

124. O'Connor N, Hermelin B. Speech and Thought in Severe Subnormality. London: Oxford Press, 1963.

125. Hays RM. Childhood motor impairments: clinical overview and scope of the problem. In: Jaffe KM, ed. Childhood Powered Mobility. Washington, DC: RESNA, 1987:1–10.

126. Affoltier FD. Perception, Interaction and Language: Interaction of Daily Living: The Root of Development. New York: Springer-Verlag, 1991.

127. Kermoian R, Campos JJ, et al. Locomotor experience: a facilitator of spatial cognitive development. Child Dev 1988;59: 908–917.

128. Ulrich BD, Ulrich DA, Collier DH, et al. Developmental shifts in the ability of infants with Down syndrome to produce treadmill steps. Phys Ther 1995;75:20–29.

129. Long TM, Cintas HL. Handbook of Pediatric Physical Therapy. Baltimore: Williams & Wilkins, 1995.

130. American Academy of Pediatrics, Committee on Sports Medicine. Atlantoaxial instability in Down syndrome. Pediatrics 1984;74:152–154.

131. Pueschel SM, Scola FH. Atlantoaxial instability in individuals with Down syndrome: epidemiologic, radiographic, and clinical studies. Pediatrics 1987; 80:555–560.

132. Singer SJ, Rubin IL, Strauss KJ. Atlantoaxial distance in patients with Down syndrome: standardization of measurement. Radiology 1987;164:871–872.

133. Micheli LJ, Giblin PE, et al. The management of atlanto-axial subluxation with neurological involvement in Down syndrome. Clin Orthop 1979;140:66.

134. Cooke RE. Atlantoaxial instability in individuals with Down syndrome. Adap Phys Act Q 1984;1:194–196.

135. Dichter CG, Darbee JC, Effgen SK, et al. Assessment of pulmonary function and physical fitness in children with Down syndrome. Pediatr Phys Ther 1993;5(1):3–8.

136. Polacek JJ, Wang PY, Eichstaedt CB. A Study of Physical and Health Related Fitness Levels of Mild, Moderate, and Down Syndrome Students in Illinois. Normal, IL: Illinois State University Press, 1985.

137. DeCesare J. Physical therapy for the child with respiratory dysfunction. In: Irwin S, Tecklin JS, eds. Cardiopulmonary Physical Therapy. 3rd Ed. St. Louis: Mosby–Yearbook, 1995.

138. Connolly BH, Michael BT. Performance of retarded children, with and without Down syndrome, on the Bruinicks Oseretsky Test of Motor Proficiency. Phys Ther 1986;66:344–348.

139. Harris SR, Tada WL. Genetic disorders in children. In: Umphred DA. Neurological Rehabilitation. Princeton, NJ: CV Mosby, 1985.

140. Ruppel G. Manual of Pulmonary Function Testing. 3rd Ed. St. Louis: CV Mosby, 1982.

141. Skrobak-Kaczynski J, Vavik T. Physical fitness and trainability of young male patients with Down syndrome. In: Berg K, Eriksson BO, eds. Children and Exercise IX. Baltimore: University Park Press, 1980.

142. Weber R, French R. The Influence of Strength Training on Down Syndrome Adolescents: A Comparative Investigation. Texas Women's University.

143. Herge E, Campbell J E. The role of the occupational and physical therapist in the rehabilitation of the older adult with mental retardation. Top Geriatr Rehabil 2004;13(4):12–22.

144. Amadio AN, Lakin KC, Menke JM. 1990 Chartbook Services for People with Developmental Disabilities. Minneapolis: Center for Residential and Community Services, 1990.

145. Nochajski SM. The impact of age-related changes on the functioning of older adults with developmental disabilities. Phys Occupat Ther Geriatr 2000;18:5–21.

146. Lubin RA, Kiley M. Epidemiology of aging in developmental disabilities. In: Janicki MP, Wisniewski HM, eds. Aging and Developmental Disabilities: Issues and Approaches. Baltimore: Paul H. Brookes Publishing Co., 1985:95–113.

147. Connolly BH. General effects of aging on persons with developmental disabilities. Top Geriatr Rehabil 1998;13(3):1–18.

148. Campbell JE, Herge E. Challenges to aging in place: the elder adult with MR/DD. Phys Occupat Ther Geriatr 2000;18: 75–90.

149. Seltzer MM, Seltzer GB. The elderly mentally retarded: a group in need of service. J Gerontol Social Work 1985;8:99–119.

150. Gill CJ, Brown AA. Overview of health issues of older women with intellectual disabilities. Phys Occupat Ther Geriatr 2000; 18:23–36.

151. Rapp C. Improved lifespan for persons with Down syndrome: implications for the medical profession. Exceptional Parent 2004;34:70–71.

152. Finesilver C. Down syndrome. RN 2002;65:43–49.

153. Platt LS. Medical and orthopaedic conditions in special Olympics athletes. J Athlet Train 2001;36:74–80.

154. Post SG. Down syndrome and Alzheimer disease: defining a new ethical horizon in dual diagnosis. Alzheimer Care Quart 2002;3:215–224.

155. Bruckner J, Herge E. Assessing the risk of falls in elders with mental retardation and developmental disabilities. Top Geriatr Rehabil 2003;19:206–211.

156. Hotaling G. Rehabilitation of adults with developmental disabilities: an occupational therapy perspective. Top Geriatr Rehabil 1998;13:73–83.

157. Montgomery PA. Predicting potential for ambulation in children with cerebral palsy. Pediatr Phys Ther 1998;10:148–155.

11

Adaptive Equipment and Environmental Aids for Children with Disabilities

Emilie J. Aubert

P hysical therapists have many products at their disposal to help children with disabilities with positioning, achieving mobility, and performing activities of daily living. New products are being developed every year in an attempt to satisfy the needs of children with disabilities. Products and materials are available in both standard, commercially produced forms and custom-fabricated forms to meet individualized specifications for each child.

The great variety of products and materials available and the constantly changing and expanding market present a challenge to the therapist who tries to give parents useful suggestions regarding equipment. How can students, recent graduates, or physical therapists inexperienced in treating children acquaint themselves with these products, in order to feel confident in guiding families who need adaptive equipment for their children? What conditions should be evaluated before making decisions regarding adaptive equipment? What is the true role of adaptive equipment for children with physical disabilities, and are there particular dangers or contraindications with adaptive equipment? These questions are addressed in this chapter, the main

goal of which is to provide the student and the therapist who is inexperienced in pediatrics with a theoretical construct to facilitate decision making about adaptive equipment, regardless of familiarity with any particular piece of equipment. Common types of equipment such as prone standers, side-lyers, and wheelchairs are discussed, along with approaches to practical clinical decision making. There are few, if any, clear, scientific, objective guidelines on which to base a decision about adaptive equipment. The selection of adaptive equipment for children is still an art, rather than a science. As physical therapists, the goal is to try to meet the needs of children with disabilities by using a critical approach to document successes and failures, in the hope of eventually transforming this art into more of a science.

◆ Role of Adaptive Equipment

Adaptive equipment is becoming increasingly necessary as an adjunct to direct treatment. No child can realistically receive the constant handling needed throughout the day to prevent abnormal movement patterns and postures or support more independent function. Although the physical therapist may teach families, daycare providers, and teachers about methods of handling the child to encourage optimal development, the child must be allowed time to move, explore, and relax without constant help. The increased cost of direct care and the increasing number of children needing therapeutic intervention suggest a need for alternatives to direct patient handling.

One alternative is the judicious use of adaptive equipment to allow correct positioning during a child's free, independent time. Adaptive equipment can also provide reinforcement for and use of positions, movements, and skills introduced to the child during treatment sessions. Similarly, abnormal or undesirable positions or movements can often be prevented by use of correct equipment.

Adaptive equipment can facilitate functional skills that the child might otherwise be unable to accomplish. These uses of adaptive equipment not only promote motor and sensory development, but also concurrently improve cognitive, perceptual, emotional, and social development.

Adaptive equipment, in addition to having direct therapeutic benefits, can play an important role in caregiving and parenting by assisting in the daily management of the child at home. Some indispensable items include bathtub seats, hydraulic lifts, and adapted high chairs. Adaptive items that facilitate safe and effective transportation may include many types of car seats, strollers, and wheelchairs.

Although adaptive equipment should be prescribed with the goal of achieving maximum benefits with the least restriction, this ideal approach may occasionally need to be compromised. For example, some families may be unwilling to adjust the routines of all family members to meet the needs of only one member. Also, ideal goals may not be possible because of architectural barriers that prohibit the use of certain adaptive devices. When barriers (behavioral, architectural, or financial) exist, the therapist must analyze the short-term needs of the family and the long-term goals for the child before making a decision or recommendation. Decisions to use adaptive equipment should be made jointly by the physical therapist and the family. Also, the child's input should be considered if he or she is able to participate in such decision making. Whenever adaptive equipment is recommended, its use must be monitored to ensure that therapeutic goals and family needs are being met.

◆ **Precautions When Using Adaptive Equipment**

Can adaptive equipment be dangerous? This is a difficult question to answer, especially because most equipment has a design that is inherently free of dangers. Problems may arise from the way in which equipment is used by various caregivers. Although a particular piece of equipment may

have been prescribed, fitted, and properly explained, its overuse or misuse may cause difficulties.

MISUSE

Adaptive equipment is often static, and in spite of the benefits of a particular device, it may not provide a rich environment for exploration or for learning new movements and transitions from one position to another. Gross motor development in normal children requires learning through doing, moving, and feeling. Sensory, vestibular, and tactile input are all required to produce varied and effective motor output. Static positioning, which occurs when some adaptive equipment is used excessively, can retard motor development by modifying sensory input and limiting spontaneous movement activity.

A carefully developed plan for therapeutic use of a piece of adaptive equipment must take into consideration not only the potential benefits, but also the potential deleterious effects. Normal motor development relies on coordination of both agonist and antagonist muscle groups to complete a pattern of movement. Adaptive equipment tends to fix a child into one pattern, albeit therapeutic, while denying the opportunity to experience the competing or antagonist pattern. For example, a side-lyer provides an opportunity for the child to play while placed in a neutral, midline orientation. Although a neutral, midline orientation may be an appropriate goal, it is important to note that an asymmetric orientation is not inherently bad or undesirable. An asymmetric orientation is a normal precursor to weight shifting, lateral flexion, and lateral rotation. Also, although the pathologic pattern or orientation may compete strongly with the pattern facilitated by the equipment, the therapist is responsible for teaching normal or balanced movement patterns and positions.

The person who places the child in a position must be aware of the benefits of various positions and must avoid constant and unchanging positioning habits. Inappropriate use of equipment that places the child in static postures can also lead to other complications, such as joint contractures or skin breakdown, either of which may eventually require surgical repair. Anyone who has responsibility for the child must understand the therapeutic goals and must monitor equipment use to maximize the benefits and minimize the deleterious effects.

POOR PLANNING

A child's age and developmental level are first considerations when planning for equipment needs. However, poor planning for growth and change can lead to equipment that fails to meet the child's needs for the short and/or long term. With the increasing difficulty experienced in receiving third-party payment for expensive equipment for the child with a physical disability, the therapist must anticipate and plan carefully for the child's physical growth, developmental changes, and acquisition of new skills. The inexperienced therapist may overlook the changing needs of the child. A child who requires positioning in sitting during the early years may be given an expensive chair that will provide positioning in sitting and optimal use of the upper extremities for fine motor skills. However, in spite of the initial advantages of the chair, it may be inappropriate for future mobility and socialization needs. Predicting the child's needs in the areas of growth and development, education, and recreational alternatives (e.g., wheelchair sports) is a monumental task, but one in which physical therapists must often participate at the request of insurers and local and state funding agencies.

Therapists must learn how various agencies and providers prefer to reconcile future needs and reimbursement patterns with the child's current needs. Some providers prefer to pay initially for less expensive devices that must be replaced more frequently, even though a costlier device might be more cost effective in the long term. Other providers prefer an initial, larger expenditure for a device that will last for 3 to 5 years. These considerations must be contemplated carefully. The consequences of miscalculations in these decisions may be a child poorly accommodated in an ill-fitting device that does not meet his or her current needs or that will meet his or her needs for only a short period of time. In such instances, the therapist must then explore difficult alternatives, such as borrowing or adapting old equipment, until the patient is eligible for new equipment. The growth potential of various pieces of equipment is discussed later in this chapter. Clearly, in addition to a child's current age and developmental level, growth and developmental change are critical aspects to consider when selecting adaptive equipment.

EQUIPMENT USE COMPARED TO FACILITATION OF FUNCTION

The use of equipment in place of facilitating the development of nonassisted skills is a concern when recommending adaptive equipment. As already discussed, positioning devices may not allow for balanced development because of their static nature. Unfortunately, some therapists and parents have the idea that, because there are so many equipment options, equipment is equivalent to therapy. The child is thus plugged into many types of equipment (e.g., progressing from high chair to car seat to side-lyer to stander). The equipment then becomes a substitute for handling or positioning of the child by the parent or physical therapist. This occurrence can be a detriment to parent–child relationships as well as a barrier to continued skill acquisition by the child. Equipment is not a substitute for treatment. Equipment may restrict the learning of active postural transitions and movement for exploration, two major aspects of normal motor development. In some cases, a child who uses no adaptive equipment may fare better through verbal instructions, feedback, and handling than the child who is extensively equipped. This suggestion does not advocate denial of needed equipment in order to maximize therapeutic input; rather, it recognizes that, just as appropriate equipment can be useful for satisfying the overall needs of a child, overuse or misuse of equipment can be detrimental.

SAFETY ISSUES

Ensuring the safe and correct use of the equipment is a top priority. Caregivers, and the child him- or herself when age appropriate, must be taught the correct methods of donning, doffing, and using equipment. Strategies such as color coding and numbering straps, to make sure they are fastened to the proper endpoint in the proper sequence, help avoid mistakes in donning the device. This is particularly helpful when caregivers include a number of people in addition to the parents, such as grandparents, babysitters, daycare staff, teachers, and teachers' aides.

Another safety issue relates specifically to mobility equipment. Equipment that gives a nonlocomotive child the ability to locomote requires attention to the environment in which the equipment is used as well as attention to the child's cognitive and judgment abilities. If the equipment makes it possible for the child to maneuver in an area of the home in which he or she could not maneuver previously, is the area adequately childproofed? Or in the case of a motorized wheelchair instead of a manual wheelchair, does the child exhibit sufficient judgment to use the motorized chair safely, regarding both his or her own safety and the safety of others?

PSYCHOSOCIAL ISSUES

Although carefully selected and fitted adaptive equipment can open many otherwise closed doors and increase a child's independence, the use of equipment can be psychosocially disadvantageous. Equipment, especially extensive equipment, often has a way of drawing attention to a child's disabilities and therefore his or her differences. Children tend to be honest, sometimes brutally so. Adaptive equipment, or anything else that separates a child from peers, can be emotionally and socially challenging for the child with a disability.

In addition to socially and psychologically separating a child from others, adaptive equipment can actually physically separate a child. A child who is strapped into plastic, vinyl, wood, and metal often seems to be the recipient of fewer hugs and physical affection. This may be simply because of the physical barriers caused by the equipment, but it may also be the result of adults and children who feel intimidated by the equipment and are fearful of disturbing something if they get too close to the child.

Determining a Child's Equipment Needs

The therapist who provides routine continuing care for a child with a disability is often not the same therapist responsible for purchasing adaptive equipment. Sometimes, because of the size or nature of the facility at which the child receives routine treatment, a referral to a larger, better equipped institution may be appropriate to determine equipment needs. Whether the child is referred to a children's hospital, to a wheelchair clinic in a major medical center, or directly to the vendor's establishment, the provision of appropriate apparatus depends mainly on detailed and accurate information about both the child and the child's environment. If possible, the primary therapist should be present during the evaluation for equipment to give an accurate assessment of the child's needs. In lieu of the physical therapist's presence, a detailed report with an assessment of the child's needs and recommendations for equipment should be included in the referral.

An initial assessment, assessing the child in relation to a specific piece of apparatus, is required whether a therapist is serving in a direct care or a consulting role. Because of time restrictions, the assessment may concentrate on one specific type of equipment or functional need (e.g., sitting), and additional assessments may be required for other equipment needs. Once a piece of equipment has been received, the therapist must examine the child to ensure that the apparatus suits the child, that it meets the identified goals, and that those people who will be using the equipment understand its correct use.

INITIAL EVALUATION

The parameters to be considered when evaluating a child's need for adaptive equipment are similar to those of most other evaluations. The goal of such an evaluation, however, is to clarify and direct the therapist to the most appropriate equipment options available. The following specific items should be considered in the evaluation.

RANGE OF MOTION

Range of motion (ROM) is important in selecting most equipment because accommodation of the patient in most apparatuses will depend on adequate ROM and joint mobility. The device being considered will dictate the motions that are necessary for success.

Critical ranges of motion that need to be addressed when using various adaptive devices include adequate head and neck rotation to bring head to midline, trunk rotation to achieve trunk symmetry, a minimum of 90 degrees hip and knee flexion for functional sitting, and plantigrade feet (neutral dorsiflexion/plantarflexion) for standing and use of footrests or the floor when sitting. Contractures of the knees, if present, should not exceed 20 degrees if lower extremity orthoses will cover the knee joint (knee–ankle–foot orthosis [KAFO] or hip–knee–ankle–foot orthosis [HKAFO]).

MUSCLE TONE, CONTROL, AND STRENGTH

Muscle tone, control, and strength deserve careful consideration when selecting equipment. The degree of strength or motor control needed for functional use of the device must be determined. For example, use of a manually controlled wheelchair requires strength and coordination of the upper extremities. If the child does not have adequate upper extremity function, or if the child is functioning asymmetrically, a manually controlled wheelchair is an inappropriate choice. A motorized device that does not require the strength needed for a manually controlled chair may be more useful for the child. A motorized chair also has options for control that do not require any upper extremity function. A specific, detailed assessment by an experienced technician can help the therapist identify alternative methods to attain optimal management of the equipment. In the example of a motorized device, strength is only one determinant of success. One must also evaluate cognitive, visuomotor, perceptual, and social functions as well as the child's judgment.

Motor control and muscle tone are particularly important factors in equipment decisions for children with sensorimotor impairments, such as children with a diagnosis of cerebral palsy. Positioning devices, such as standers, sidelyers, and seats, often have a modifying effect on muscle tone in these children. The child's orientation to gravity may have significant bearing on muscle tone when the child tries to assume an upright position. In addition to active muscle control and strength, the therapist must assess patterns of movement with regard to spasticity, athetosis, flexor predominance, or extensor predominance.

Does the child exhibit uncontrolled, extraneous, and involuntary movements (dyskinesias); hypotonus; or hypertonus? Are movement patterns of mild, moderate, or severe magnitude? Does the patient have cortical control, manifested by a voluntary ability to initiate a pattern of movement? Does the child's body exhibit attempts to compensate, whether volitional or not, for uncomfortable positioning and/or movement? For example, a child positioned in a prone stander with too much forward tilt from the vertical position may show increased extensor tone in an attempt to achieve a more upright position against the force of gravity. Increased scapular retraction and hyperextension of the neck in the child with hypertonia may occur secondary to positioning the child in supine or reclined sitting. These patterns will interfere with optimal upper extremity function. Sometimes the child with extensor hypertonus will attempt to counteract the body's pull into extreme extension when sitting by protracting the shoulder girdle, posteriorly tilting the pelvis, and holding the head forward. Any position the child exhibits must be assessed for the contributing causes, including compensation.

REFLEXES

A change of position with respect to gravity will also influence a child whose motor patterns are dominated by reflexes. The prone or supine position may increase or decrease the tonic labyrinthine reflex. Side-lying may facilitate the asymmetric tonic lumbar reflex. Because inadvertent facilitation of primitive reactions may create a block in the normal developmental pattern, each piece of equipment should be evaluated for its effect on reflexes. For example, some devices for mobility, such as tricycles and bicycles, may aggravate a persistent asymmetric tonic neck reflex. As the child pushes the pedal with the right foot, the head is turned toward the right side to enhance the effectiveness of the push. The child reverses this pattern when pushing with the left foot. Only in unusual circumstances would a therapist choose to use a technique that encourages using obligatory reflexes. The use of devices to restrict or inhibit primitive reflexes is more common, thus providing an opportunity for the development of more normal and symmetric patterns of movement.

SENSATION

Children with myelomeningocele, or other pathologies with compromised sensation to touch, offer tremendous challenges to the therapist attempting to develop a program involving the use of adaptive equipment. Priorities for the child with myelomeningocele include providing safe, pressure-tolerant seating and upright positioning. The therapist must have a thorough knowledge of the patient's sensation in order to achieve these goals. The patient and family should be consulted with regard to sensation, as they usually have a keen awareness of the sensory loss, as well as potential danger zones. This situation is especially true for the older child. Particular attention must be paid to bony prominences, including the ischial tuberosities, greater trochanters, sacrum, femoral and tibial condyles, tibial tuberosities, fibular heads, and malleoli, as well as the skin over the spinal lesion, in a child with myelomeningocele. These bony prominences also must be monitored in a child with intact sensation but limited ability to reposition him- or herself because of poor motor control, weakness, or severe spasticity.

PERCEPTION, COGNITION, AND SOCIAL/EMOTIONAL FACTORS

Most physical therapists are not trained specifically to assess perception, cognition, or social/emotional development; as a result, these areas are often ignored. This is a serious omission with the pediatric patient, whose prognosis for function with adaptive equipment often depends more on perception, cognitive function, and social/emotional skills than on physical abilities. Motivation, intelligence, and normal perception often overcome even severe physical impairments. The opposite is also true. Limitations in perception, cognition, or social/emotional skills may result in function that is lower than would be predicted by physical findings alone. In order to develop realistic goals for a child, the physical therapist must know the whole child and must integrate information obtained from the teacher, social worker, occupational therapist, and psychologist into the therapeutic plan.

FUNCTION

Assessing functional skills requires integration of all available information, in an attempt to determine why a child behaves in a certain manner. The physical therapist must discover what functions the child is able to perform and how, what functions he or she is unable to perform and why, and why the child does not do more. For example, some children tend to bunny hop rather than creep. It is important to know if this tendency to bunny hop is secondary to a strong symmetric tonic neck reflex, muscle weakness in the extensors of the hip and/or knee, or both. Determining appropriate physical therapy interventions and recommendations is based on this type of analysis and understanding.

A similar thought process should be used when deciding whether or not the child needs equipment. For example, if a 2-year-old child is not rolling or exploring the environment, is a device aimed at the goal of improving mobility an appropriate acquisition? The therapist must first assess why the child does not move and explore. Does the child have a cognitive disability that limits his or her natural curiosity to explore his or her environment? Is the child afraid of moving because of visual or hearing impairments? Does the child exhibit a strong asymmetric tonic neck reflex or hypertonia that poses physical limitations? Has the child been placed in devices at home that limit the opportunity to develop independent mobility? Once a determination has been made as to why a child has decreased mobility, realistic recommendations for equipment can be offered. Only when working with a child who is severely limited in his or her mobility, without reasonable short- or long-term expectations of gaining device-unaided mobility, would it be appropriate to opt immediately for adaptive equipment for remediation of the problem(s).

The child with profound cognitive deficits may not use equipment that is provided because he or she lacks the motivation to explore his or her environment. In order for the child with visual or hearing impairments to learn to manipulate his or her environment, methods for exploration of that environment need to be improved by first addressing the specific sensory impairments. If a child lacks experience in exploring the environment due to lack of opportunity, the therapist must offer as much freedom of movement and equipment-free mobility as is possible. Although equipment may eventually play a role in each of these situations, adaptive equipment should not be the first type of treatment used. Adaptive equipment should supplement and complement function with the least amount of restriction of the child.

The child who is physically limited may show great improvement in cognitive ability, social interaction, and independence when mobility is improved. When adaptive equipment or devices are used judiciously, the improvement in mobility should occur without increases in abnormal reflexes or patterns of movement in children with sensorimotor impairments.

Evaluation of ROM, muscle tone, motor control, strength, reflexes, perception, cognition, and social/emotional status is an integral component of the assessment of the child. Only when these parameters are considered, and it is understood why a child has particular motor behaviors, can the child be treated effectively, including recommending appropriate adaptive equipment.

Once the goals for the device and the type of device being considered are identified, the therapist should evaluate the family and school environments. Goals for the child must be compatible with the goals of the caregivers at home and school. Because adaptive equipment is often used in several settings, there may be many conflicts and problems to solve while trying to achieve the short- and long-term goals for the child. Problems with adaptive aids may arise for the child who is institutionalized or in a school placement. For example, the opportunity to teach the correct use of equipment to members of a changing or rotating staff is a major consideration. Minimizing the number of easily lost parts is important. Also, in institutional care, in particular, ease of equipment maintenance must be considered.

ASSESSMENT OF THE FAMILY AND HOME

Useful information can be obtained by asking the family members about their expectations for the apparatus being considered. This opportunity for family members to express their opinions promotes a dialogue between family and therapist, allowing the therapist to determine whether the family goals are realistic or whether compromises are necessary. Objective data about the family and home include the following categories and questions:

1. *Physical layout of the dwelling*
   - Is the dwelling a house or apartment?
   - How many steps are found in the home?
   - Is there easy access to the home from the outdoors (i.e., no stairs, availability of an elevator, etc.)?
   - How large are the rooms?
   - Are the structure and size of the home adequate for equipment to be used in the home, particularly mobility equipment?

- Is there space for equipment use and storage?
- How wide are the doorways and hallways?
- Are the floors carpeted?
- Are bathrooms, tubs, and toilets accessible?

2. *Community factors.* The therapist should determine whether the family lives in an urban, suburban, or rural community in order to assess the availability of and options for transportation and socialization within the community. The availability of privately owned vehicles and/or public transportation is important when the therapist is considering the type of mobility equipment to be purchased. Issues such as the weight of mobility equipment, its versatility on various surfaces, and its ease of transport are important considerations.

3. *Socioeconomic factors.* The cost of equipment may have a serious impact on the final decision regarding apparatus for the child with a disability. When making a decision about buying adaptive equipment, the therapist, often in conjunction with a social worker, must examine insurance coverage, other third-party payment systems, funding agencies within the community, and potential rental options. Before equipment is ever ordered, it is essential that the availability and source of funding is determined. Size of the family, daily routine, and the time available to spend with the child with special needs, as well as potential options for others to help the family, must be considered. Compliance with the suggested use of adaptive equipment may ultimately be the main issue to be considered in the decision to obtain the equipment. If there is little realistic expectation that the child will benefit from having the equipment or that the equipment will be used by the family, there may be little justification for its purchase.

4. *Other cultural factors.* In addition to socioeconomic factors, other cultural factors must be considered and respected. Increasingly, physical therapists and other health care professionals find themselves working with patients and clients with cultures different from their own. It is imperative that physical therapists become not only culturally sensitive, but also culturally competent. Some cultural issues that need to be addressed when obtaining equipment for children include the following:
   - Who makes the decisions in the family?
   - Are there cultural sensitivities regarding receiving financial aid to purchase equipment?
   - Does the equipment being considered violate any religious beliefs that the family may have?
   - If there are language barriers, do the family and child understand the need for the equipment as well as the process for acquiring the equipment?
   - Will language differences possibly interfere with teaching the family and child the proper use of the equipment, and can these problems be overcome?
   - Is the type of home structure amenable to the safe and easy use of the equipment being considered?

- Are there cultural beliefs that preclude the use of certain equipment? For example, in some cultures an infant is never placed on the floor. Therefore, a positioning device used on the floor may be unacceptable to the family. Another example is that technology such as electricity or computers is not used in some cultures. These beliefs may eliminate the use of power wheelchairs, home suctioning equipment, and some communications aids.

All of these questions obviously apply to obtaining equipment for any child. However, they are worth special mention in regard to a child whose culture differs considerably from the dominant culture of the community. It is the therapist's responsibility to learn enough about a child's culture to effectively and competently provide interventions, including recommendations of adaptive equipment.

SCHOOL ASSESSMENT

When assessing a child's need for equipment, the physical therapist must consider the school setting in which the child may spend a large portion of the day. It is important to determine whether the child is enrolled in a special school for children with disabilities or mainstreamed into a regular school and/or classroom. In a special school, teachers and staff are usually very open to suggestions and are well equipped to handle any devices being considered. It is often these teachers who initiate the purchase or procurement of the equipment, and they are eager to learn and work with the child.

When the child is mainstreamed into a regular school, teachers and other staff may be reluctant to accept adaptive equipment because of their limited experience with special apparatuses. This reluctance of the staff may be related not only to the health and developmental needs of the child, but also to concerns about the time, space, liability for, and acceptability of these devices in a classroom of children, most of whom do not have disabilities. A thoughtful compromise is often necessary in order to meet the physical, educational, emotional, and social needs of the child with a disability. Examples of equipment that might be recommended for use in the classroom include the following:

1. Special chairs, seating devices, or adaptations to the regular desk chair
2. Wheelchair lapboards
3. Wheelchair or desk easels
4. Standing frames, tables, and prone standers
5. Wedges for seating in chairs
6. Wedges or bolsters for positioning on the floor

The physical therapist can be a valuable resource person for teachers and other staff by making suggestions and helping procure equipment that can enhance a child's educational experience. Often, a piece of adaptive equipment can make the difference between a child feeling fully included in, rather than excluded from, classroom work and activities.

 ## Equipment Selection

When the evaluation of the child is completed and goals are established, the types of equipment available, or alternatively, the practicality of making equipment, are determined.

PURCHASING EQUIPMENT

Many companies make devices and equipment that are identical in concept. Criteria that must be considered in choosing a specific device include the following:

1. *Dimensions of the apparatus.* The device should not only be adequate when purchased, but should also, if feasible, allow for some future growth. Some pieces of equipment have a built-in system for extending or enlarging the device. The therapist must determine which company makes the particular size best suited for a given child.
2. *Availability of optional adaptations.* Are there parts that help improve the fit and specificity of the device? Are these options cost effective, easily adjusted, and durable?
3. *Reputation of the manufacturer.* Is the product covered by a guarantee? Has the company previously provided support when problems with equipment have arisen? Is service readily available, and is equipment for trial use available? Will a company representative instruct the staff in optimal use of the device?
4. *Promptness of delivery.* Is the product kept in stock by most local vendors or medical supply houses? Is there a backlog of orders that will delay the equipment's delivery? Is the product custom made?
5. *Cost.* Is the price reasonable for the anticipated use of the product, or will less expensive alternatives provide the same benefits?
6. *Aesthetics.* Is the device cosmetically acceptable to the child and family, or might it be rejected on this basis?
7. *Weight, size, and manageability.* Is the device easy to use, and can it be stored? Can it be transported if necessary? Does it fold or disassemble in some way that makes storage and/or transport easier?

Brochures or catalogs available from the manufacturer or vendor will provide much of this information. Local vendors who may have extensive experience with the equipment can help in answering many questions. Physical therapists in local hospitals or in the community can recommend vendors or specific salespeople. The therapist should not feel obligated to order from any vendor or person in particular. Although one salesperson might be knowledgeable about wheelchairs, another person may have more experience with positioning devices or self-help equipment.

Anyone procuring or fabricating equipment on a regular basis should keep records on the various devices, manufacturers, and vendors used. Records should indicate ease of fit, wear of the device (how well it holds up over time), acceptance or criticism from patients and families, and the efficiency of customer service, including the elapsed time from placement of an order to delivery of equipment. Records may be kept on computer or in card catalog form (or some similar system), and may be a useful resource for future recommendations and orders. In addition, the file may provide the basis for quantitative data regarding benefits and deficits of various adaptive devices. Perhaps the compilation of these data can serve to help the profession evolve from an art to a science.

RENTING OR BORROWING EQUIPMENT

Some types of equipment for short-term use can be rented. However, if particular customized features are needed in a device, the likelihood of finding the precise, appropriate apparatus is decreased. Often, concessions can be made regarding some equipment options, if renting the equipment proves to be highly cost effective. Compromising correct fit and safety for the sake of cost effectiveness should not be an option.

Some communities have what is commonly referred to as an equipment closet. These closets, usually run by not-for-profit organizations or agencies, are repositories for used equipment in good repair that parents no longer need for their children. This equipment is then available for other children and parents to borrow for the period of time such equipment is needed, often until the child outgrows the size of the equipment. Also, in today's Internet-connected world, it is not unusual for parents to make contact with other parents who have adaptive equipment that is no longer being used. These parents are often willing to sell or give away functional used equipment, or make a trade for another piece of equipment. However, the same exceptions and cautions mentioned regarding renting equipment also apply to borrowing equipment from closets or other individuals.

MAKING EQUIPMENT

The decision to make equipment is based on many variables that must be considered carefully.

PERSONNEL

Will physical therapists be building the equipment themselves, or will they be serving as consultants to other builders? Other people who might build equipment for children include commercial woodworkers, woodworking hobbyists, volunteer organizations with appropriately skilled members, and the child's parents. If the therapist builds the apparatus, how will his or her schedule allow for this time expenditure? Will patients be canceled or will special time be allotted? Will overtime hours be needed? If the physical therapist is a consultant, how will this time be allocated and at what expense? If other people are building the equipment, will they be compensated, and if so, by whom? Will parents pay directly, or will insurance companies pay the cost? Will the facility offering the services assume the cost? Will permission be given to build the equipment only after approval by third-party payers of the needed funding, or will the facility assume the cost in the hope that funds will be forthcoming? Who will bear the cost if funds are unavailable?

SPACE

Is adequate space available for building the apparatus on the premises? If space is available, will the safety and comfort of patients be compromised by this building site? Building is noisy, dirty, and potentially dangerous because of the tools and materials used. Ventilation must be provided if fumes from toxic paint or varnish are expected.

COST

A decision must be made initially about the cost effectiveness of making equipment. Items that must be accounted for include tools, space needs, building materials, time for planning and designing, time for measuring and building, and time away from patient care. In making a decision, the advantages of customized equipment must be weighed against the expense of designing, planning, and building the apparatus. Will adapting a commercially available device be the best compromise?

FAILURES

Can and will the facility absorb the loss in revenue that may occur if equipment is fitted incorrectly or is inappropriate when completed? This issue of equipment failure must be considered, because even the most experienced equipment technician will make mistakes.

TIMING AND SETTING

An advantage of noncommercial devices is evident when equipment is needed immediately. Therapist-fabricated equipment is usually available in days or weeks rather than the months often required for bureaucracies to approve, fund, order, and receive the equipment. Building the equipment might also be an attractive alternative when the device is required only for one specific setting, such as the classroom, but not for transport or home use.

LIABILITY

Who assumes liability for the correct and safe use and performance of equipment made by a therapist, hobbyist, or volunteer? This is an important consideration in today's society wherein manufacturers are liable for the safe use of their products. If a child is injured or otherwise harmed using noncommercial equipment, the person who made the equipment may be legally and financially responsible. This is a dangerous position for a physical therapist. The liability issue alone may be sufficient reason for a physical therapist not to fabricate equipment.

SUMMARY

In spite of the potential drawbacks, many therapists still choose to fabricate equipment themselves or have a parent do so. This may be particularly useful for the young child who is growing rapidly or for the child whose need is only temporary. In each of these situations, a simply made piece of equipment could satisfy the short-term needs of the patient. The child could use the fabricated equipment until he or she outgrows it, at which time another piece could be made, or if growth has slowed, a commercially available piece could be substituted. One of the main reasons for building equipment is that commercially available equipment often does not satisfy the needs of a child with unique problems. Recently, however, manufacturers have shown an increased interest in children with physical impairments, which has resulted in a wider variety of and improvements in devices.

SELECTION OF MATERIALS

Adaptive equipment can be built using various materials, each of which has unique qualities, advantages, and disadvantages. Personal preference often plays a major role in the decision to use a particular type of material. Although each material has its specific properties, most can be adapted to various uses. Some materials are lighter in weight, some are easier to use, some are easier to wash and keep clean, and some are more durable. Because none of the products is perfect, the therapist should have knowledge of several different materials. The therapist can try to match the material's advantages to the specific needs of the child. Wood, triwall, and Adaptafoam are materials used commonly by pediatric therapists.

WOOD

Wood is inexpensive, durable, and available, but requires a moderate measure of skill. Large work areas are required because fabrication using wood can produce a lot of sawdust and often requires many different hand and power tools, some of which are expensive. Many therapists prefer to have professional carpenters construct adaptive devices from wood because of the level of skill required. Parents, however, are often familiar with woodworking, and a therapist may enlist the help of such a parent, providing plans and specifications for the equipment needed. Fabrication by family members can be a rewarding and satisfying means of helping in the care of their child. Wooden equip-

ment is often heavy, but it is also durable. Strength and durability are particularly important qualities when equipment is to be used by a larger child. Wooden devices often need padding for comfort and either painting, varnishing, or sealing for protection against liquids. Wood is often used for making inserts for seats, side-lyers, prone standers, and various ingenious mobility toys.

TRIWALL

Triwall consists of triple-thickness corrugated cardboard that is lightweight, firm, and inexpensive. Triwall is fast and easy to use, although its use requires an electric saw, glue gun, and hand tools, such as a hammer, screwdriver, and utility knife. Although it is not waterproof, triwall can be treated with acrylic latex paint or fabric for sealing and preservation. Triwall is less durable than wood, which makes it most appropriate for temporary or trial pieces of equipment, or for children who are growing rapidly (Fig. 11.1). Like wood, triwall is a firm, solid medium and may require padding for comfort. Many therapists consider triwall useful for making customized chairs that must be measured precisely for the child. A bolster-type chair available commercially and a similar chair made from triwall are shown in Figures 11.2 and 11.3. Although selection of a design and measuring the child and the triwall are time-consuming chores, actual building with triwall is a fast process. Working with this material is noisy, messy, and potentially dangerous because of the tools. A separate workplace is recommended. As with wood, family members and volunteers

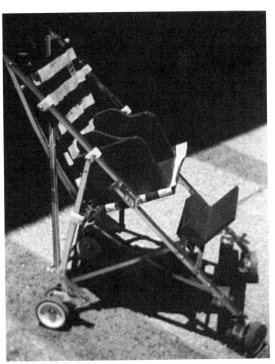

Figure 11.1 ■ Umbrella-type stroller with a triwall insert and foot support.

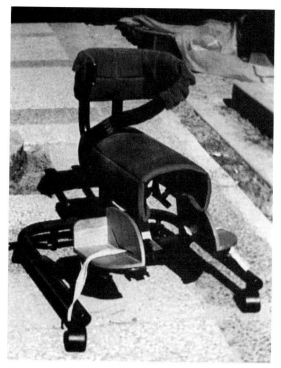

Figure 11.2 ■ Commercially made bolster chair.

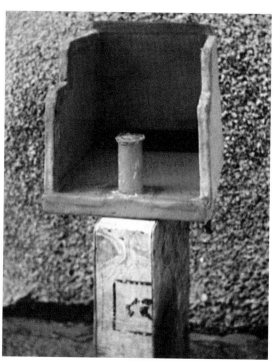

Figure 11.4 ■ Triwall seat insert.

can be recruited to make apparatuses from triwall. Special training is usually necessary, and many parents are reluctant to try because of fear of mistakes and failure. Some judicious support and praise for the family member can help overcome reluctance, and the parent may become an essential part of the team that is making the adaptive equipment

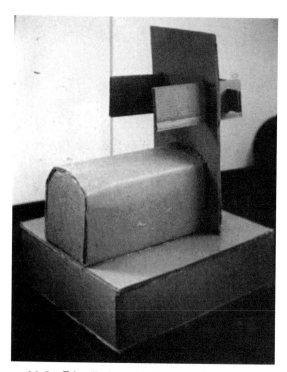

Figure 11.3 ■ Triwall alternative to the commercially made bolster chair shown in Figure 11.2.

for the child. A seating insert made from triwall is shown in Figure 11.4.

ADAPTAFOAM

Adaptafoam is another commonly used medium for pediatric equipment because it is a dense, nonporous, nontoxic foam that is both fast and easy to use, but is more expensive than wood or triwall. The need for tools is minimal (e.g., heat gun, electric knife, and utility knife). Although a work area is useful, Adaptafoam is less messy than wood or triwall and poses less risk because of the limited use of tools. A special coating, Adaptavinyl, is the only paint that can be used, and its safe application requires excellent ventilation. However, because Adaptafoam is nonporous, it can be left unpainted and cleaned with soap and water when it becomes soiled. Covers can be made for the apparatus if the family prefers. Adaptafoam is available in several dimensions and different densities. With some experience, a physical therapist can determine the best use of the various types of Adaptafoam. Adaptafoam is easy to use because it bonds to itself when heated for a short time. Glue and nails are unnecessary. However, this self-bonding property loses some attractiveness when Adaptafoam is used with other materials, such as wood, to which Adaptafoam will not bond. Adaptafoam is commonly used to make pronelyers, seats, inserts, small standers, and various components, including headrests and utensil handles for other apparatuses. Adaptafoam, unlike triwall, is easy to adjust for growth by inserting an additional piece of material when necessary. Like wood and triwall, Adaptafoam provides a firm surface and may need to be padded or covered to improve comfort.

 ## Commonly Used Equipment for Positioning

Having discussed general uses for equipment as adjuncts to treatment, it has been noted that benefits can accrue with proper equipment and frequent changes in position. Among those benefits are inhibition of pathologic tone and movement, reduction of abnormal reflexes, reduction of asymmetries, improved circulation, improved bone health, improved upper extremity functioning, prevention of soft tissue contractures, and prevention of decubiti. Some of the issues involved in providing children with equipment to support various activities as well as the sitting, standing, and side-lying positions will now be addressed.

SITTING

GENERAL CONSIDERATIONS

The sitting position is optimal for upper extremity function and, therefore, is important for the child and adult. Maintained sitting posture is a goal achieved by most typical infants before 1 year of age, and sitting is required for many functions throughout life. By watching children in preschool and kindergarten, it is apparent that a goal of many teachers is sitting for a reasonable amount of time for group activities. Children in the early school years younger than 7 years of age also require frequent changes in position. They prefer to play and work in the prone position, standing by a table, and in other positions that allow for easy transitional movements and change. Sitting, as a position for optimal function, occurs only after the children learn to sit for prolonged periods of time. Sitting is defined as ". . . a position in which the weight of the trunk is transferred to the support area mainly by the ischial tuberosities and surrounding tissues."[1] Proper alignment in sitting is thought to enhance overall functioning by providing an adequate and secure base of support, inhibiting abnormal tone, providing a stable base from which the upper extremities can function, and improving perception of the environment. There are also significant social benefits to being upright in sitting and mobile.

Although there is a large body of literature devoted to seating for the pediatric age group, most of the literature reports clinical experience and empirical data rather than controlled scientific studies. The result of this lack of scientific documentation is poor standardization when evaluating and providing adaptive seating devices. Conflicts regarding the value of various positioning options could be more easily and completely resolved if a scientific basis existed for each option. Because the literature on pediatric seating is limited, the adult literature has been examined

and applied to the pediatric age group. Several factors should be considered when evaluating a chair.

The first factor is the intended purpose of the chair. Chairs can be function specific. A lounge chair is uncomfortable when a person is eating a meal, yet a straight-backed chair with little padding is undesirable for relaxation. Similarly, a physical therapist must consider function when designing chairs for children with special needs. Many therapists believe that a custom-built chair is always preferable, but whether one is buying or making a chair, the following parameters, established for adults, should be considered.

SEAT

HEIGHT The height of the chair seat should allow the feet to be placed flat on the floor or a foot rest. Height should be such that with feet flat, hips are flexed to at least 90 degrees. Slightly more hip flexion is even more desirable to prevent some children from going into extensor posturing. Comfortable placement of the feet should prevent excessive pressure from the front edge of the seat on the popliteal fossae.[1,2]

DEPTH The seat should be shallow enough to provide for flexion of the knee without pressure in the popliteal area and without slouching. Slouching occurs when the child goes into a posterior pelvic tilt in order to allow the knees to flex over the edge of a seat that is too deep. This slouching causes sacral sitting, with the child transferring his or her weight to the chair seat through the sacrum rather than the ischial tuberosities. In addition, normal sitting posture requires an anterior pelvic tilt, whereas this abnormal posture caused by too much seat depth enhances a posterior tilt of the pelvis. The seat should be deep enough to allow maximal distribution of weight.[2] If the seat is too shallow, weight is borne over a smaller area of the body, thereby increasing pressure per square inch on the posterior thighs. Increased pressure over a smaller area of contact means increased risk of skin breakdown. Also, a seat that is too shallow decreases the hip flexion to less than 90 degrees. This increased extension at the hips may cause the child to slide out of a chair. In a child who has extensor hypertonus, increased extension of the hips also may trigger increased extensor tone throughout the body. A good rule of thumb for determining seat depth for children is to have one finger width between the edge of the seat and the popliteal space. Keep in mind that as the child grows, the length of the femur will increase, and the space between the edge of the seat and the popliteal fossae will naturally increase.

PADDING Padding helps to distribute pressure beyond the 6-mm^2 surface of each ischial tuberosity that normally bears most of the weight in sitting. This allows for increased sitting tolerance.[3,4] However, surfaces that are too soft increase the difficulty with which postural changes are made during sitting, and this lack of postural change can lead to back strain and potential skin breakdown. Akerblom judged movement while sitting to be the most important requirement of a comfortable chair.[3] He designed a chair that allowed for various conditions (i.e., the trunk away from the back support, sitting with lumbar support, or reclining back with both lumbar and thoracic support). These options reduce muscle strain and increase tolerance.[3]

BACKREST

Consideration must be given to trunk musculature and spinal ligaments when sitting in order to avoid back discomfort. The anterior and posterior longitudinal ligaments of the trunk provide their best support with the back in neutral position. Increasing the normal lordosis may stretch the anterior longitudinal ligament, whereas exaggerated kyphosis will stretch the posterior longitudinal ligament and may cause posterior protrusion of degenerating intervertebral discs. These changes produce low back pain and may cause difficulty in achieving adequate thoracic and lumbar extension needed to rise from sitting. The chair backrest should accommodate adequate movement while in the chair, to help offset muscular fatigue and for pressure relief. However, the backrest also should provide adequate support of the trunk to prevent muscular fatigue. Support for the weight of the trunk reduces the muscular work of sitting. The height of the backrest must be appropriate for the individual child. The child who needs extensive head, neck, and trunk support needs a tall backrest that extends above the head. Such a child may also benefit from a reclining backrest, which can provide periodic relief of muscles to combat fatigue. The height of the backrest need not extend above the shoulder in many clients. Freedom to change position and improved mobility are available when limiting the height of the backrest to this level.[5] In fact, for patients with excellent trunk stability and balance, the top of a wheelchair backrest often is just below the inferior angles of the scapulae. This shorter backrest allows great mobility of the upper trunk, use of the upper extremities, and general freedom of movement while in a wheelchair. These shorter backrests are usually seen on wheelchairs used by very active young people and wheelchair athletes. Finally, support for the lumbar curve and allowance for the posteriorly protruding sacrum and buttocks are also recommended for good seating.

ARMRESTS

Armrests should be positioned to bear approximately 50% of the weight of the patient's arms. Armrests are also used to move from a sitting to a standing position and vice versa, to do wheelchair transfers, and to do sitting push-ups for regular and frequent pressure relief for the buttocks. Armrests that are too low or too high decrease the mechanical advantage of the flexed elbow when the individual performs sitting push-ups and transfers.

ANGLE OF THE BACK OF THE SEAT

The angle formed between the seat and backrest of a chair is most comfortable between 95 and 110 degrees. However, this angle may cause the person to slide forward, particularly a problem in persons with increased extensor tone in the hips and back musculature. Using a wedged cushion, with the greatest height in the front, may help counteract this problem. Bergan suggests that chair seats provide sensory feedback and a spatial orientation for the child so that he or she is sitting with a slight inclination backward.[6] The word *dump* in wheelchair seating refers to the number of inches closer to the ground the back of the wheelchair seat is, compared to the front of the wheelchair seat, thereby providing a slightly backward spatial orientation as described by Bergan. Dump can be accomplished or enhanced in a chair by using a wedged cushion as described above, or the dump can be built into the chair by decreasing, to less than 90 degrees, the angle between the seat and the backrest. Wheelchair dump for adults is usually 1 inch. For children, a 2-inch dump is more appropriate.

Another way of increasing dump in a wheelchair is to tilt the seat and backrest unit of the chair slightly backward, in relationship to the wheelbase and floor, so that gravity pushes the child back into the chair to avoid the problem of sliding forward. In this case, particular attention must be paid to avoiding pressure in the popliteal spaces.[1] Lumbar supports are also recommended when a chair is reclined slightly.

Orthopedic and biomechanical needs of a child must be considered when planning seating for all children. For children with cerebral palsy or other neuromuscular disorders, the effects of various seating or wheelchair components on muscle tone, reflexes, and function must also be considered. Most therapists use an empirical or trial-and-error approach to determine good positioning for a particular child. However, most physical therapists agree that a stable pelvis serves as the keystone for seating, especially with children with neurodevelopmental disorders. Once the pelvis is aligned properly, the trunk, head, and lower extremities will have a more stable base. This often means that fewer assistive devices and wheelchair options are necessary for optimal function in the child with cerebral palsy.

The specific approaches to, options for, and adaptations of seating, particularly wheelchair seating, are too numerous to review here and are constantly evolving. However, the objectives of providing seated weight bearing on the ischial tuberosities, as occurs with adults, and maintaining a slight lumbar lordosis are reasonable expectations for the child as well. Hip flexion of at least 90 degrees (slightly more being even better) during seating is advocated by many physical therapists, especially when seating the child with cerebral palsy. The 90-degree angle at the hips and knees will aid stabilization by providing solid weight bearing on ischial tuberosities and feet. Furthermore, this position corrects sensory input and decreases the likelihood of posterior pelvic tilt that may result in increased dorsal kyphosis, scapular protraction, and hyperextension of the neck.

One of the problems associated with wheelchair seating of the child with a neurodevelopmental disorder such as cerebral palsy is an increase in extensor tone thought to accompany the sling effect of most wheelchair seats and backrests. A firm seat and backrest can reduce this sling effect.

In addition to altering the hip angle, the chair itself may be tilted, anteriorly or posteriorly, relative to the floor, until the desired results of positioning are achieved. The issues of concern when making these adjustments continue to be pelvic alignment for stability while in a sitting position and the effects on tone of the various angles of the hip and of the seat itself. Nwaobi and colleagues, using electromyograms, found that orientation of the body and head in relation to gravity plays a significant role in controlling extensor activity in children with extensor hypertonus.[7] Perception and hand function will also be altered as differing angles and positions are used. Therefore, an individualized approach, examining the effects of each change in position, will be necessary in determining optimal seating arrangements for children.

Once it appears that the various angles of hips, seat, and chair have been established and pelvic stability has been achieved in the child with cerebral palsy, the therapist must consider the trunk, head and neck, and the lower extremities of the child. Ninety degrees of knee flexion and good weight bearing on the feet should be encouraged to enhance stability. Too much weight bearing on the plantar surface can result in a primitive extensor thrust pattern in children with neuromotor impairments that will significantly reduce stability. Alignment of the trunk should encourage maximal symmetry, yet provide for movement and active postural adjustment. A headrest or supports should be used only if needed to improve positioning or to protect the child during mobility. The ultimate goal of the sitting position should be to align the child without restricting the movements and postural adjustments available to the child. Reassessment of the seating device is necessary when the patient's postural tone improves and new skills are acquired.

CONSIDERATION OF THE SPECIFIC DISABILITY

The criteria and limits described for seating are applicable to all types of seating systems and for all disabilities. The emphasis changes with the disability, but the concepts are constant. Appropriate seating for the child with cerebral palsy, for instance, must take into consideration the effects on tone and abnormal reflexes. Padding and pressure relief warrant increased attention in the child with myelodysplasia. Height of armrests is of particular concern for the child with a myopathy such as muscular dystrophy. The limitations of the seating devices and concerns regarding their use will be reasonably constant across disability groups.

These limitations and precautions include limitation of joint motion secondary to static positioning; poor skin tolerance as a result of prolonged use of the seating devices and a limited ability to change position; decreased sensation to touch characteristic of certain pathologies; and reduced independent functional mobility resulting from overuse of seating devices.

WHEELCHAIRS

Providing a wheelchair for a patient requires an understanding and application of all the criteria previously discussed about proper alignment and positioning in sitting. It is also beneficial to know about the options available in purchasing a wheelchair and the compromises involved when selecting certain options over others.

Before continuing, it is worth stating that the wheelchair industry is in constant flux. This is why a well-informed and capable vendor or manufacturer's representative is critical to the rehabilitation team. The representative can provide information about changes and innovations in durable medical equipment (DME), as well as about the comparative adaptability, durability, cost, and features of wheelchairs and other equipment supplied by competing manufacturers.

It may be easiest to discuss options by looking at a typical order form for a pediatric chair (see Display 11.1). These forms are traditionally completed by the vendor, patient, patient's family, and physical therapist working together to meet the patient's needs.

The first consideration is wheelchair design. For independent mobility, two basic options exist: a rigid frame and a cross-braced (X-frame) folding wheelchair. Most people are familiar with a cross-braced folding wheelchair and opt for this type as it is easiest to transport in cars and store in the home. The rigid-frame chair does not fold, but the wheels are removable and the back drops down, leaving a small box-type structure. The rigid-frame chair offers increased stability and ease of rolling, and it is always the chair of choice for sports and recreation. In many instances, once the child adjusts to it, families find the rigid chair to be as manageable as the folding chair. The disadvantage of the rigid-frame wheelchair is its limited growth adjustability resulting in it sometimes being overlooked for the pediatric population. If properly fitted, however, in many instances it can provide years of use.*

In children who are not independently mobile due to cognitive function, upper extremity involvement, asymmetry, or other problems, a manual wheelchair may not be the best option. The vendor should be consulted regarding alternatives, which are beyond the scope of this chapter. For older and cognitively able individuals who have very

---

*Modified rigid wheelchairs have now been devised that combine rigidity but allow for some growth. Additional information can be obtained from an informed vendor.

►► DISPLAY 11.1

A Sample Order Form for a Pediatric Wheelchair

Effective July 5, 1993

ORDER FORM

Date: _____ P.O.#: _____
Buyer: _____ Customer#: _____

Bill To:
Name _____
Mailing Address _____
City _____ State _____ Zip _____
Phone (___) _____

☐ **Drop Ship/Ship To:**
Name _____
Street Address _____
City _____ State _____ Zip _____
Phone (___) _____ Marked For _____

QUICKIE 2   ☐ *Adult*   ☐ *Kids*

COLOR
☐ *Blue* ☐ *Black* ☐ *Red* ☐ *Midnight Purple* ☐ *Silver*
☐ *Sky White* ☐ *Teal* ☐ *Hot Pink* ☐ *Ultra Yellow* ☐ *Lavender*
☐ *Blue Sapphire* ☐ Blk Diamond ☐ Candy Red

FRAME DIMENSIONS
Frame Width   ☐ *11″** ☐ *12″* ☐ *13″* ☐ *14″* ☐ *15″*   (Seat Width: 1/2″ Narrower)
☐ *16″* ☐ *17″* ☐ *18″* ☐ *19″* ☐ *20″*   (*11″ Wide by Upholstery)

Sling Depth   ☐ 10″ ☐ 11″ ☐ *12″* ☐ 13″
☐ 14″ ☐ 15″ ☐ *16″* ☐ 17″[1] ☐ 18″[1]

Cushion   ☐ *2″* ☐ *3″* ☐ *4″*
☐ Solid Seat[3] ☐ Omit Cushion ☐ Omit Seat Sling

BACKREST   (Push Handles Std.)   ☐ *Low* (8 1/2″–12″)[17]   ☐ *Med* (12″–15 1/2″)[17]   ☐ *Tall* (15 1/2″–19″)[17]
Backrest Options   ☐ 8° Bend (Med & Tall)[17]   ☐ Omit Push Handles[17]   ☐ Depth Adjustable[18,11]
☐ Omit Depth Adj Solid Back & Hardware   ☐ Omit Depth Adj Solid Back Include Hardware
☐ Swing-Away Adj Stroller Handles (Avail w/ Depth Adj Back Only)   ☐ Solid Back[3,17]
☐ Backrest Cushion[17]   ☐ Adj Upholstery (Avail w/ 14″–20″ Frame Widths and Med or Tall Back Heights)[17]
☐ Omit Back Upholstery[17]   ☐ Omit Back Post & Upholstery[17]

FRAME SPECIFICATIONS
Frame Length   ☐ Kids ☐ *Reg* ☐ Long ☐ Hemi[5] ☐ Long Hemi (17″–18″ Deep)[5]

Hanger Type   ☐ *60°* ☐ *70°* ☐ *90°* ☐ *70° V*[19] ☐ Hemi (60°) ☐ Omit Hangers
☐ Articulating-Adult (15″–20″ Widths)[2]
☐ Articulating-Kids (11″–16″ Widths; Std w/ 2″ footrest Ext Tubes and Adj Flip-Up Footplates)[2]
☐ Impact Guards—Plastic   ☐ Impact Guards—Neoprene

Footplates   ☐ *Composite*[9]   ☐ Plastic Cover ☐ Reverse ☐ High Mount[6]
☐ Foam[4]   ☐ Angle Adj[9] ☐ Angle Adj High Mount[9] ☐ Omit Footplate
☐ 90° Adj Flip-Up[4,8] ☐ 90°/90° Footboard[4,7] ☐ Extended[9]
☐ Heel Loops   ☐ Omit Leg Strap

Footrest Ext Tubes[20] ☐ *Short* (14″–16 1/2″; N/A w/Articulating Legrest) ☐ *Med* (16 1/2″–19″) ☐ *Long* (19″–21 1/2″)
☐ Omit Ext Tubes

CASTERS   ☐ *8″ Pneumatic* ☐ 8″ Polyurethane ☐ 5″ Low-Profile Polyurethane
☐ 6″ Pneumatic ☐ 6″ Polyurethane ☐ Aluminum Caster Rim

Caster Options   ☐ 3/4″ Longer Fork Stem Bolt ☐ 1 1/2″ Longer Fork Stem Bolt
☐ Caster Pin Locks ☐ Omit Caster Wheels ☐ Quick-Release Caster Stems[21]

ARMRESTS   ☐ *Padded Swing-Away*[17]   ☐ Omit Armrests
☐ Adult—Height Adjustable w/Std Pad (10″)   ☐ Adult—Height Adjustable w/Full-Length Pad (14″)
☐ Kids—Height Adjustable w/Std Pad (10″)   ☐ Kids—Height Adjustable w/Full-Length Pad (14″)

Stroller Handles   ☐ Stroller Handles (Reg)[10,17] ☐ Stroller Handles (Tall)[10,17]

AXLE PLATE   ☐ *Std* ☐ Amputee[11] ☐ Quad Release Axle Nuts
☐ One-Arm Drive (Attach One-Arm Drive Supplemental Order Form)

REAR WHEELS
Rim   ☐ Mag[12] ☐ *Spoke* ☐ Omit Rear Wheels/Axles

Size   ☐ 20″ ☐ 22″ ☐ *24″* ☐ 26″ (3/4″ Stem Bolt Std w/26″ Wheels)

Tire   ☐ *Pneumatic* ☐ Full-Profile Polyurethane[12] ☐ Airless Insert[12]
☐ Low-Profile Polyurethane[13] ☐ Kevlar[13] ☐ High-Pressure Clincher (24″, 26″ Only)[18]

Handrim   ☐ *Aluminum* ☐ Plastic Coated ☐ Long Tabs ☐ Omit Handrims

Projections ☐ Vertical[14]   20″/22″ _____   24″/26″ _____
☐ Oblique   ☐ 6   ☐ 8   ☐ 10   ☐ 12

WHEEL LOCKS   ☐ *High-Push* ☐ Low ☐ Omit
☐ High-Pull ☐ Do Not Mount

Wheel Lock Options   ☐ 6″ Ext Handles ☐ 9″ Ext Handles
☐ Grade Aids (N/A w/ Polyurethane High-Pressure Clincher Tires or Kids Length Frames)

ACCESSORIES
☐ Anti-Tip Tubes
☐ Armrest Pouch (Hgt Adj)
☐ Caddy
☐ Crutch Holder
☐ Front-End Stabilizer
☐ Leg Strap
☐ Leg Strap-Double
☐ Spoke Guards
☐ Transfer Board
☐ Tool Kit

Backpack & Seat Pouch
(Specify Color)
☐ Adult _____
☐ Kids _____
☐ Seat Pouch _____

Clothing
(Specify Color and Size)
☐ Long Sleeve Shirt _____
☐ Sweatshirt _____
☐ Golf Shirt _____
☐ T-Shirt _____
☐ Jacket _____
☐ Barrel Bag _____
☐ Hat _____
☐ Eyeglass Holders _____

Lifting Straps
☐ Q2 Low[10,17]
☐ Q2 Medium[10,17]
☐ Q2 Tall[10,17]

Positioning Bolts
☐ Long Velcro® Style (67″)
☐ Short Velcro® Style (57″)
☐ Long Buckle (64″)
☐ Short Buckle (54″)

Side Guards
☐ Fabric Kids
☐ Fabric Regular
☐ Plastic Kids[15]
☐ Plastic Reg[15]

Touch-Up Paint
☐ Color: _____

Wheelchair Tray Table
☐ Extra Small 10″–12″
☐ Small 13″–14″
☐ Medium 15″–17″
☐ Large 18″–20″

Special Instructions _____
_____
_____
_____
_____
_____

Items in Bold Italic Print are Standard
1. Available only on long frame.
2. N/A w/high-push wheel locks.
3. 8° bend not available: 11″–15″ wide, 10″–15″ deep only.
4. Not available with heel loops: single leg strap standard.
5. Hemi hangers only.
6. Only available on 60° hangers and hemi hangers.
7. Available only with 11″–16″ frame widths.
8. Available only with 11″–16″ frame widths and 90° hangers.
9. Available on 14″–20″ widths.
10. Omit push handles.
11. Not available with swing-away armrest; height adj. available at swing-away price.
12. Not available on 26″ wheels.
13. Only available on 24″ wheels.
14. Not available with low-profile polyurethane tires.
15. Not available with height adjustable armrests.
16. Not available with mag wheels.
17. Not available with depth adjustable back.
18. Standard with 20″ solid back height and stroller handles.
19. Available with 16″–20″ frame widths and composite footplates only.
20. Not available with 90° hangers or articulating legrest-kids.
21. Not available with caster pin locks; not available with 3/4″, or 1 1/2″ lock stem bolt.

Specifications Subject to Change without Notice

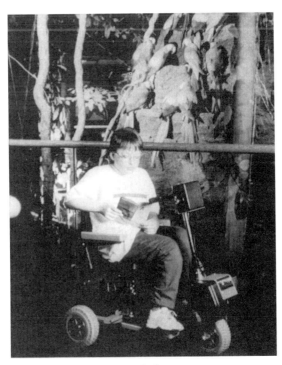

Figure 11.5 ■ The three-wheeled scooter.

limited upper extremity use, asymmetry of the upper extremities, significant hypertonus, and/or profound weakness, a motorized device may be considered. The three-wheeled scooter has become increasingly popular and available and is often a wonderful alternative to power wheelchairs. The scooter (Fig. 11.5) is much less expensive than a standard motorized wheelchair (approximately $1800 to $2300 compared to $14,000),† can be disassembled into components that are lighter and easier to move from home to car, and is relatively simple to learn to operate and maintain. Any seating system, from a simple standard molded plastic seat to the most elaborate custom-made system, can be adapted to the scooter. To be noted, however, is that the patient must have bilateral hand use and some degree of reach in order to hold the scooter's handlebars, push the accelerator, and steer. Also, the individual needs at least fair sitting balance.

Traditional power wheelchairs are extremely heavy, do not disassemble easily into component parts, and generally require a van for transport and ramps or a stair-free entrance to the home. Additionally, they are usually quite sophisticated electronically, which may mean frequent fine-tuning and adjusting. However, they usually accommodate environmental control systems, can allow for changes in position (e.g., reclining), and can be operated using a variety of switches or other types of controls. Traditional motorized wheelchairs require more of a trial-and-error approach to perfect fit and to train the patient, and maintenance may

be more involved. The scooter may be preferred for a marginal ambulator who requires a device for long distances, whereas the traditional motorized wheelchair is usually reserved for the individual who requires a more extensive mobility system for full-time use. Specialists should be consulted if a traditional power wheelchair system is being considered, and one should never be ordered casually by an inexperienced clinician.

Once a wheelchair style has been selected, either manual or power, the size, fit, and options must be determined. The physical therapist should bear in mind the following criteria, as well as the principles of good seating discussed earlier in this chapter:

1. Seat width should allow for growth and should be able to accommodate outerwear for cold winter climates. Most vendors consider 1 inch on each side to be appropriate. Too much room makes it very difficult to propel the wheelchair effectively, especially when armrests are used. In most pediatric models, chairs can be ordered in 1-inch increments to custom-fit any child. In an X-frame wheelchair, growth in width is accommodated by replacing the cross braces and upholstery of the wheelchair. (No growth adjustment is available in a rigid frame wheelchair.) In the pediatric population, almost all patients are provided with a solid seat, used with a cushion, to avoid the slinging effect of upholstery. Cushions are available made of dense foam, or gel, as well as air filled. Cushions are used not only to protect skin from breakdown, particularly over bony prominences, but also to change the patient's placement and alignment within the chair. Increasing the cushion height lowers the functional height of the wheelchair backrest and armrests, lowers the foot plates relative to the patient, and changes the patient's effective arm length and access to the wheels. This technique is often used to extend the use of a chair for several months for a patient who is growing tall but who has not outgrown the width of the chair. It is important, when measuring a chair, to remember to account for changes relating to cushion use (Fig. 11.6).

2. Seat depth should permit comfortable knee flexion without popliteal pressure. In the pediatric population, a solid seat back with hardware placed between the uprights often allows for several inches of growth. The insert is placed forward of the uprights and is moved back as the child grows. However, the most energy-efficient alignment of a patient for manual propulsion places the greater trochanter over the axis of the back wheels and only 40% of the combined weight of the wheelchair and occupant on the front casters. It is, therefore, unwise to use cushions behind the child to temporarily decrease the seat depth or use inserts to accommodate an excessive increase in seat depth. Axle plate adjustments are available, but the extent of modification depends on many factors, including the frame

---

†Prices vary dramatically based on the seating and positioning options required and the need for additional electronic options.

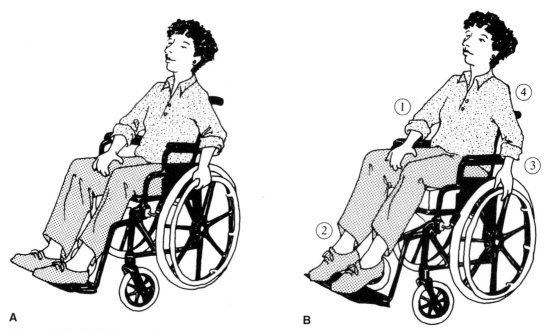

A   **B**

Figure 11.6 ∎ **(A)** *Patient is accommodated without cushion.* **(B)** *Use of a cushion will change: (1) position of arm on armrest; (2) relative leg length; (3) relative arm length in relation to the wheel; and (4) the amount of back support (decreased).*

size of the chair. A sling wheelchair backrest can, if it does not compromise good positioning or alignment, improve mobility, increase sitting tolerance, and decrease the weight of the wheelchair by eliminating heavy inserts and hardware. Other recommendations for wheelchair seat depth were discussed previously in this chapter under general seating principles.

3. The preferred backrest height for maximum independent propulsion of a manual wheelchair is below the scapulae, for optimum freedom of movement as discussed previously, but many patients require additional support. A serious dilemma arises when using a head support for bus transport to school. Automobile safety standards require headrests, and a patient is often safer using a headrest for transportation only (i.e., the patient who has fair head control when in a static position but who experiences fatigue or becomes compromised with excessive movement). It is difficult to mount a headrest on a sling-type backrest; thus, selection of even a removable headrest often implies changing to a solid backrest. In certain instances, this combination may be contraindicated for independence and energy-efficient mobility. This problem remains unresolved unless the patient can transfer into a federally approved car seat when in the bus, thus negating the need for a headrest mounted on the wheelchair itself.

4. Selection and placement of foot plates and leg rests are dictated by patient size and the wheelchair caster wheel size. Although many therapists believe that 90-degree knee flexion is optimal for weight bearing through a flat foot, this position may not be feasible. Vendors are the best resource for determining which options are available considering the frame size, the wheel size, and the patient. Multiple-angle foot plates allow for the braced and nonbraced foot. Removable leg rests are desirable in most cases if leg rests are used, and elevating leg rests should only be requested if absolutely necessary, since they add weight to the chair. Also, elevating the legs when sitting in a wheelchair for prolonged periods should not be done unless medically advised. Elevation of the leg rests shifts the body weight posteriorly, increasing the amount of weight borne directly on the ischial tuberosities, thereby increasing the risk of skin breakdown.

5. Wheel size is critical in achieving the most energy-efficient propulsion. Ideally, the elbow should be extended 120 degrees when the handrim is grasped at the highest point.[8] Pneumatic tires give a smoother ride (adding some shock absorbency) but require considerable maintenance for consistent and proper inflation pressure. For small children, the low weight of the child may not justify the need for pneumatic tires considering the extra maintenance required, but in older, heavier children, riding on rough terrain is clearly better on pneumatic tires.

6. Caster size is the ultimate compromise. In the small-framed chair, adjustability of the rear axle is lost if the caster is too big, as the clearance between the two wheels is minimal. Small tires add maneuverability but get stuck in cracks, ditches, and the like. The author recommends the smallest tire that will still allow wheelchair management on the terrain that is navigated most often.

The options range from 5- to 8-inch-diameter caster wheels.

7. Armrest height should be comfortable, should allow the patient to take some weight off the shoulders, and should allow easy access to the wheels. Essentially, the type of armrest should be dictated by ease of management. Many experienced wheelchair users prefer to be without armrests; however, bus drivers, parents, and other caregivers often rely on them for added support when transferring the chair into and out of vehicles.

8. Brakes should be placed for easiest management and can be operated either by pushing or pulling, depending on the patient's preference and abilities. Many companies also offer high- or low-mount options for brakes.

9. A seat belt is essential on a child's wheelchair. The seat belt should not come around the child from the middle of the backrest of the wheelchair. Rather, the belt should originate at the angle of the seat and backrest on both sides, closing over the child low on the pelvis.

10. Antitippers are also a must on a child's wheelchair, especially the young child and the novice wheelchair user.

11. Lapboards or trays are particularly helpful for children, especially the school-age child. The lapboard, if used, must be carefully fitted to the chair so as not to increase the overall width of the chair. Lapboards that are made of clear Lucite or a similar material are preferable to opaque lapboards. The see-through lapboard helps facilitate positive body image by allowing the child to see his or her own lower extremities and lower trunk. Likewise, the ability of others to see the whole child through the lapboard tends to have a positive impact on the child's interactions with others.

Children with special needs such as a deformity that must be accommodated in the wheelchair will benefit from a wheelchair that is customized to the child's shape by a foam product. The child sits on or back against a container filled with foam. The foam takes approximately 2 minutes to solidify. The foam forms around the deformity. Once hardened, the foam is padded as necessary and covered (Fig. 11.7).

Once a wheelchair prescription is complete, the therapist should feel satisfied that the decisions made are the best for a given child. Any misgivings should be discussed with more experienced therapists, another vendor, or a manufacturer's representative. Therapists should always remember that they are ordering expensive equipment and, more importantly, that the equipment selected will affect the quality of the child's life for the next 3 to 5 years.

SPECIAL SEATS

A variety of special chairs are available commercially or can be constructed for specific seating problems. Chairs that incorporate the basic principles of seating as discussed in this chapter can have many adaptations to facilitate a desired posture.

The corner chair (Fig. 11.8) is a chair that has lateral supports for the upper trunk. These supports position the child in shoulder girdle protraction, a strategy that tends to decrease extensor spasticity in children with tone problems such as cerebral palsy.

Bolster chairs are chairs with a bolster-type seat (see Figs. 11.2 and 11.3). These chairs also aid in inhibiting excessive extensor tone by flexing and abducting the hips.

STANDING

PRONE STANDERS

Prone standers are used frequently for children who require, but cannot achieve, the position of hands-free upright standing or its approximation. The child is placed in a prone position on the device. The trunk, buttocks, and lower extremities are all supported. The angle of the board is then increased toward a vertical position, depending on the child's tolerance and the therapist's goals. When the board is at its maximal angle, usually slightly less than 90 degrees to the floor, weight bearing is optimal through the lower extremities and feet. A knee-standing position can also be used. A prone stander is shown in Figure 11.9. The patient benefits from the physiologic changes associated with weight bearing, the freedom to use hands while upright, and the social and perceptual opportunities afforded by an upright position. As the angle of the prone stander decreases to less than upright, the benefits of lower extremity weight bearing will decrease because weight is borne more completely by the trunk.

Several other aspects of the use of the prone stander should be considered. Upper extremity function may range from almost total weight bearing in the child whose prone stander is less than 45 degrees above horizontal to completely free use of the upper extremities in the child who is in an upright position.

When the prone stander is less than 45 degrees above the horizontal, activities involving not only bilateral weight bearing in the upper extremities, but also weight shifting, unilateral weight bearing, and reaching can be performed. Extensor muscle function of the neck and back will also vary significantly with different angles. As the patient approaches the upright position, the muscular effort for head righting will decrease. The physical therapist can either facilitate or inhibit muscle activity in different muscle groups by varying the angle of the prone stander.

The therapist must assess the quality of movement shown by the child in the prone stander. The function of the head, neck, scapulae, and upper extremities should be included in this assessment, as should trunk alignment and positioning of the lower extremities. Hyperextension of the neck, exaggerated retraction of the scapulae with the upper extremities in the high-guard position, and poor symmetry and midline position of the trunk secondary to muscle imbalance are all common postural problems of the child placed

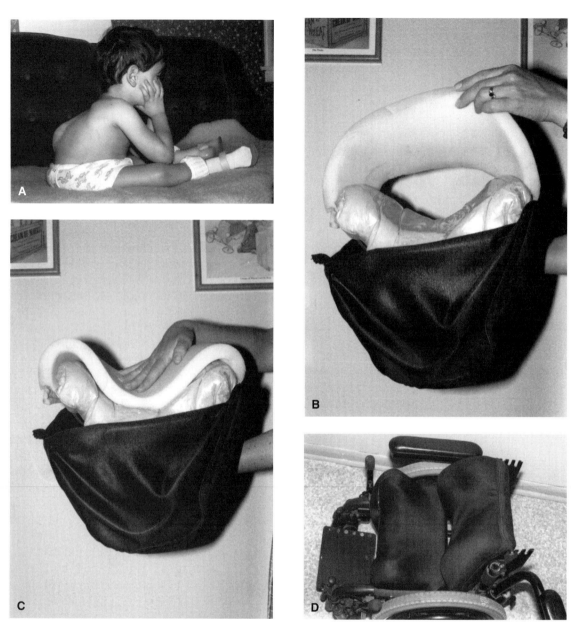

Figure 11.7 ■ **(A)** Child with myelomeningocele with gibbus on back may require a custom-fitted wheelchair back. **(B)** (1) Solidified foam that conforms to child's back during fitting; (2) soft foam for added protection from pressure; (3) wheelchair back upholstery. **(C)** (1) Solidified foam; (2) soft foam; (3) wheelchair back upholstery. **(D)** Finished wheelchair with custom conformed back.

in a prone stander. The therapist also must consider weight-bearing alignment. Proper weight bearing for normal standing requires dynamic pressure through the heels, with the center of gravity passing slightly posterior to the ankle joint; this position is not feasible in a prone stander. Therefore, the use of the prone stander must be evaluated carefully. The prone stander is useful if the physiologic benefits of weight bearing are the major goal or if it is being used to accommodate hands-free standing. If the prone stander is considered for preambulation skills and conditioning, its use may be inappropriate and counterproductive.

When the prone stander is introduced into the child's program, the entire treatment regimen should be re-

evaluated. Although the child may appear to adapt well to use of the prone stander for 1 hour each day, overuse of the prone stander may cause undesirable changes. Increased extensor tone is an example of a change sometimes seen with prolonged use of a prone stander. The increased tone may affect the previously adequate positioning for sitting and may decrease function at home and school. This negative effect might require adjustments in the amount of time spent in the prone stander, or it may require a different approach to positioning in the stander.

One of the most important benefits of using a prone stander is to allow the child to interact with peers in play or school situations. Being able to work at a table or play

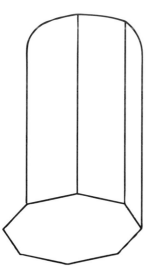

Figure 11.8 ■ Corner chair. The angled sides aid in protraction of the shoulder girdle, inhibiting extensor hypertonia.

at an elevated sandbox with peers has important social and emotional benefits.

SUPINE STANDERS

A supine stander is an alternative to the prone stander and may better meet the needs of some children whose goal is to achieve an upright position. Similar to a standard tilt table, a supine stander allows weight bearing through the trunk and lower extremities, with the degree of weight bearing proportional to the angle of the supporting surface. The child is secured around the trunk, hips, and knees, with these areas as close to neutral alignment as possible. With those criteria achieved, the supine stander is angled toward a 90-degree upright position. Unlike the prone stander, the supine stander does not provide for weight

bearing for the upper extremities, and lower extremity weight bearing occurs through the heels rather than the forefeet. This makes the supine stander a better option if a goal is good weight-bearing alignment for ambulation. The supine stander also affords the child the numerous physiologic benefits of upright weight bearing provided by the prone stander and allows the child to perceive and interact with the environment from an upright posture. Variations of the supine stander are shown in Figures 11.10 and 11.11.

As with all adaptive devices, use of the supine stander must include a careful assessment of the child for compensations, some of which may be pathologic. Commonly noted deviations that occur with a child in a supine stander include thoracic kyphosis with forward protrusion of the head, hyperextension of the cervical spine, and asymmetry secondary to imbalanced muscle control. If tolerance for an upright position is limited and the child is reclined, increased evidence of asymmetric tonic neck reflex and the Moro reflex may be seen. These abnormal reflexes may occur in a supine or semi-reclined position for any patient with poorly integrated reflex activity. The patient will fix into gravity (progravity). Because normal development requires the acquisition of antigravity control, the increased reflex activity in a supine position may be counterproductive. Upper extremity function for the child in a supine stander usually requires a special table or easel, thus restricting the child's participation in group activities. The supine stander, although used less commonly than the prone stander, has become increasingly popular. As with other pieces of adaptive equipment, periodic evaluation is necessary to determine the long-term benefits and hazards associated with the supine stander.

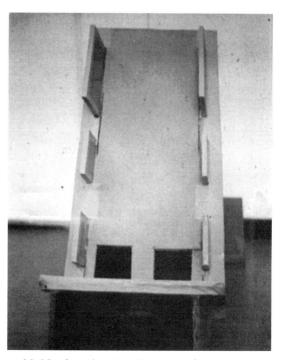

Figure 11.10 ■ A supine stander made of triwall.

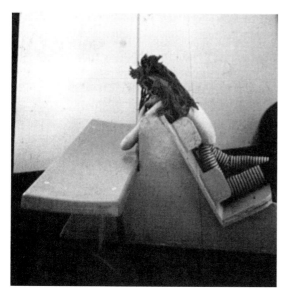

Figure 11.9 ■ A triwall prone stander covered with enamel paint is used for kneeling.

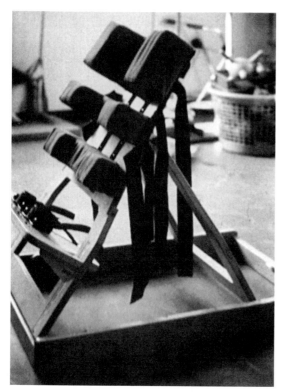

Figure 11.11 ■ *Supine stander made of wood. It is padded for comfort and was designed and built entirely by parents.*

SIDE-LYING

SIDE-LYERS

Side-lyers are particularly useful for young children or large children of low developmental function who require an alternative to sitting, lying in bed, or lying on the floor. Side-lyers can be elaborately constructed or be very simple devices with pillows, straps, and other commonly available items. A typical fabricated side-lyer is shown in Figure 11.12. When using a side-lyer, the objective is to place the child in a side-lying position according to the following criteria:

1. The trunk should be as symmetric as possible.
2. The head should be supported, in neutral alignment with the trunk.

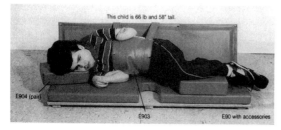

Figure 11.12 ■ *A commercially available side-lyer.*

3. Weight-bearing limbs (upper and lower) should be slightly flexed.
4. Non–weight-bearing limbs should be free to move.

This position encourages play in the midline, dissociation between the limbs, and neutral head and trunk alignment. It is also a position that is relatively neutral regarding most abnormal reflex activity. Straps are commonly used to support the trunk, the pelvis, and, occasionally, the weight-bearing leg. Pillows or pommels usually support the upper leg in a neutral position for hip abduction/adduction and for internal/external rotation. The device should accommodate the child on either side unless circumstances prevent the child from lying on both sides. Frequent reassessment is required to ensure that no compensations occur either when using or after being removed from the side-lyer. Areas of potential problems include hyperextension of the neck from pushing against the head support and flexion and retraction of the shoulder on the non–weight-bearing side. When using a side-lyer, the therapist must be careful when aligning the child with chronic hyperextension of the neck or a tracheostomy. Positioning in either of these cases must not cause an airway obstruction or compromise the child's ventilation.

Although the side-lyer allows for easy manipulation of toys and objects because one hand is fixed in good alignment, the position is not optimal for perceptual development because the child must play with objects in a horizontal plane when the environmental backdrop is vertical. That is, toys are rotated 90 degrees with respect to the visual field. This ironic occurrence is not a contraindication to using a side-lyer unless the child has obvious or suspected difficulties with perception or cognition. Most children compensate easily for the problem, especially when sides are alternated, and enjoy these changes of position.

OVERALL CONSIDERATIONS

Although not a complete list of positioning devices, examples have been provided to illustrate the issues to be considered in choosing and using equipment and the negative consequences that may occur. Negative consequences can be minimized by periodic reassessment of the child and by education of the family and staff. When people who work with the child are aware of the potential negative effects of the equipment, they are more likely to anticipate and recognize early signs of those effects.

Because all physical therapists who work with children and adaptive equipment will be required to suggest the frequency and duration of use, it seems appropriate to discuss the issue of endurance. Unfortunately, a uniform answer rarely exists. Endurance depends on variables that change daily. Rather than suggesting specific times for use, the therapist may choose to let the warning signs of fatigue guide the usage. Those warning signs include difficulty maintaining the desired posture, increased asymmetry, complaints of discomfort, and verbal requests to be moved. The therapist can recommend that the device be used until any one of those signs is apparent or a maximum time limit has been reached. Depending on the child and the type of equipment, 20 to 30 minutes is a recommended maximum for a child who can make few, if any, postural adjustments. For a child able to make postural adjustments while in the equipment, varying the distribution of weight bearing, for example, 1 hour at a time is probably a maximum. It may be worthwhile to encourage attempts to increase endurance gradually over the course of several weeks or months, with the realization that minor variations in tolerance will occur daily. Because daily variations in activity level are normal for everyone, we should acknowledge these variations in the child with physical disabilities.

Prolonged positioning in any one posture is contraindicated. In addition to fatigue, negative effects of prolonged positioning include pressure ulcers, joint stiffness, and decreased passive and active range caused by hypertonus.

Mobility Equipment

In addition to providing assistance with positioning, adaptive equipment can supplement a child's existing manner of independent locomotion or offer mobility to children who otherwise have no form of locomotion. Some devices, such as a scooter board or a sit-and-propel device, are appropriate only within the home or classroom, whereas other devices such as wheelchairs (already discussed in this chapter) make it possible for the child to be mobile within the community.

SCOOTER BOARDS

A scooter board is a flat, padded board with casters (Fig. 11.13). Prone on the board, a child propels himself or herself using hands on the floor. Scooter boards are especially helpful for the toddler or young child who has no prone locomotion and is therefore limited in floor play and exploration. Sometimes a scooter board is incorporated into a prone stander, such that the child can be mobile on the floor and then elevated in the stander without changing equipment.

PREWHEELCHAIR DEVICES

These devices allow children 18 months to 5 years of age to play at peer level. A child long-sits on this device and propels himself or herself by moving the large wheels with the upper extremities, similar to propelling a manual wheelchair. Several commercial designs are available or one could be constructed (Fig. 11.14).

TRICYCLES

Tricycles are a fun and functional way for some small children to locomote. Specially adapted tricycles are available commercially, or a standard tricycle can be modified. Modifications may include vertically turned handgrips (to inhibit flexor hypertonia of the trunk and facilitate antigravity trunk extension in children with tone disorders), abduction pommels, back supports, and foot straps. Foot straps are usually applied at the angle of the foot and lower leg, rather than across the toes, thereby preventing a stimulus to the ball of the foot, which could cause uncontrolled plantar flexion and generally increase abnormal extensor tone in the lower extremities and trunk of some children. Tricycles, although sometimes awkward to transport, are appropriate for use within the community and can be an important adjunct to a child's independence.

OTHER MOBILITY AIDS

A variety of other aids to mobility may be used, depending on the child's impairments and degree of involvement. Mobility aids commonly used with adults can be used with children and include the following:

1. Lofstrand, platform, or axillary crutches
2. Canes (J-cane, T-cane, quad-cane)

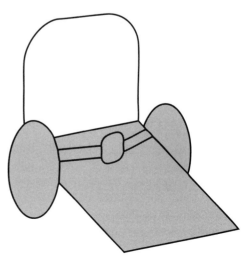

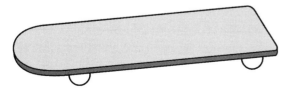

Figure 11.13 ■ The scooter board is a wheeled mobility device that allows the child to locomote on the floor with his or her peers.

Figure 11.14 ■ The prewheelchair device allows the child to be mobile on the floor and teaches the use of the upper extremities for propelling the wheelchair.

3. Walkers (wheeled, reverse-wheeled, platform, walkers with up-turned handgrips)
4. General lower extremity orthoses (supramalleolar orthosis [SMO], ankle–foot orthosis [AFO], KAFO, HKAFO)
5. Specialized orthotic devices (parapodiums, Orlau swivel orthosis, reciprocating gait orthosis)

Equipment for Infants and Toddlers

In examining the needs of the infant and toddler and the availability of devices for these younger children, one must keep in mind that children in this age group are often undiagnosed, or they may show a developmental delay that may or may not result in a long-term disability. Children who require long periods of hospitalization for cardiac, pulmonary, gastrointestinal, and other disorders are also included in this group, as are children who are developing typically but whose parents request information about various types of apparatus to enhance motor development.

HOSPITALIZED CHILDREN

Normal motor development is an integrated process that requires sensory input and freedom to respond to that input through general motor output, exploration, and play. Normal patterns of movement develop when agonist and antagonist muscles learn balanced and synergistic cooperation. Because equipment may disrupt or interfere with this process by limiting or restricting sensory input as well as movement, its use in infants and toddlers is almost always discouraged.

Movement in hospitalized children is often restricted by monitors, telemetry devices, and therapeutic medical equipment. It would be counterproductive to the child's motor development to add to these necessary devices other types of apparatus. The objective for the hospitalized child is often to provide optimal freedom of movement within the limits imposed by medical interventions and equipment. Physical therapy for these hospitalized children should encourage increased activity, if safe, and should facilitate movement patterns that, because of the external limitations, are difficult for the child to initiate. As the child's medical status improves, or when the child returns home, equipment use should still be limited, except when indicated to promote physical control or safety.

In the United States, car seats for the transport of infants and young children are required in all 50 states. Some states now require by law the use of approved car seats for children until the age of 8 years. A few car seats for individuals with disabilities are now available commercially. Check with equipment vendors regarding seats that could meet specific needs. Also, simple modifications, such as adding an abduction pommel or a small seat wedge to a standard car seat, can be made, as long as the integrity of the seat and safety are not compromised by the adaptation.

Standard strollers and high chairs can be used with many infants and toddlers. However, they should be used sparingly with the child who has sensorimotor impairments, just as other adaptive seating options are used. The goal for using seating equipment for feeding is for the child to be in a stable position that allows for optimal oral motor function, head righting and control, and freedom of movement of the upper extremities.

Concepts of seating and positioning already discussed in this chapter should be applied to the use of strollers and high chairs. For example, the toddler who is able to sit in a high chair should have adequate hip flexion (90 degrees) and enough support to facilitate trunk symmetry and midline use of the hands. Umbrella strollers are not suitable for many infants and toddlers because they encourage adduction and internal rotation of the hips and posterior tilt of the pelvis, all of which are not components of good postural alignment for sitting.

Physical therapy interventions for the infant and toddler should concentrate on encouraging the normal development of controlled motor patterns, and assistive devices should not predominate. The therapist working with the young child should make recommendations to the parents about facilitating movement and avoiding static positioning when the child is left alone to play.

As these children grow older, some may no longer have a disability, but others will develop additional manifestations, and a diagnosis may become more evident. Children in the latter group are likely to have continued treatment and equipment needs, and should be evaluated as previously outlined when appropriate.

Ventilator-dependent children represent a small but growing population with major equipment needs. With increasing frequency, the physical therapist will be called on to assist in the discharge planning and management of ventilator-dependent children. Technologic advances have prolonged life expectancy for many children with chronic illnesses, including those with myelomeningocele with symptomatic Arnold-Chiari malformation. Portable ventilators and third-party funding have aided in transforming these once chronically hospitalized children into active members of the community. These children often return home, attend their local schools, and participate in recreational and social activities. Such participation requires a transport system for essential life-support equipment, which includes a portable ventilator and battery, electric cascade humidifier (if the patient will be in one setting for many hours), oxygen source, airway suction unit with catheters and hoses, a bag of supplies, and other items. An innovative approach must be taken with this population in order to address their developmental, orthopedic, and respiratory needs. It is essential to find a vendor who is interested in working with the family and who is able to tailor the specific apparatus to the child's unique requirements. A great deal

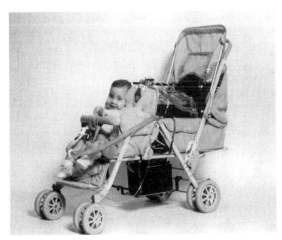

Figure 11.15 ■ A commercially available double stroller.

of trial-and-error effort often is extended in an attempt to resolve the problems presented by the weight of the ventilators, unusual balance points, difficult maneuverability, and the child's need to be in close proximity to these devices.

The two systems shown in Figures 11.15 and 11.16 were designed to meet the specific needs of both child and family. Figure 11.15 shows a commercially available double stroller that has been reinforced to house the ventilator in the rear seat with the battery suspended between the seats. The child can recline or sit upright and has use of an age-appropriate and cost-effective device that is both aesthetically pleasing and manageable. Figure 11.16 shows an Alvena frame adapted for a Snug Seat with the battery on the front foot plate and the ventilator positioned behind the seat. The patient is positioned high enough to allow easy access to the equipment stored underneath and to accommodate the comfort of caregivers who may perform suctioning and other procedures. The Snug Seat tilts 45 degrees in space and allows for easy adjustments for postural changes or growth. As the child grows and independent mobility becomes a concern, manual or motorized wheelchairs can be adapted for the child's use.[‡]

INFANTS AND TODDLERS WITH NORMAL NEUROMOTOR DEVELOPMENT

Let us consider the equipment used frequently for babies and toddlers without special needs, including infant swings, jumpers, and baby walkers. It has become common practice for families to purchase these devices for their children, in spite of little knowledge about their advantages or disadvantages.

Swings are probably the most benign device of the three mentioned. There is little evidence to indicate that swings

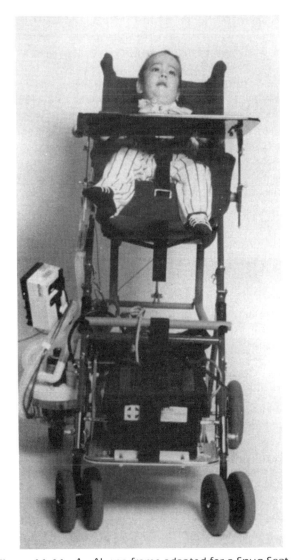

Figure 11.16 ■ An Alvena frame adapted for a Snug Seat.

are unsafe during the first year of life, as long as they are used with supervision. Swings do provide vestibular stimulation through linear movement. Vestibular stimulation is important to development of normal balance and postural responses, especially during the first 2 years of life. The regular rhythm of the swinging action can also be calming to an infant. Although swings are pleasant for the child and family, they should be used sparingly so as not to limit the child's opportunities to move about and explore his or her environment.

Jumpers are devices that are suspended from doorways by large cables, springs, and clamps. The jumper enables the child to bounce up and down by extending the lower extremities and pushing against the floor. Although the child may enjoy the vestibular stimulation provided during such an activity, caution must be exercised. The child must be supervised constantly to ensure that he or she does not fall, bang against the doorframe, or become entrapped in the cables or springs when reaching out for a toy. Even

[‡]A very special thank you to the DME Shoppe and Joe Thieme (Naperville, IL) for creating these units and many more similar devices.

restricted use of the jumper may lead to the development of patterns of exaggerated extensor activity with components of strong internal rotation of the hips and plantar flexion of the ankles. As a result, some children develop a tendency to toe-walk. Also, the high impact loading on the child's young bones and joints may be injurious. In addition to these potential hazards, the jumper, like other devices, impedes development of normal motor skills by eliminating the opportunity to make transitions from one pattern to another and by restricting free movement and the learning of new sequences of movement. For reasons of safety, as well as the potential for the development of abnormal movement patterns, physical therapists generally discourage the use of these jumpers by all children.

Unlike swings and jumpers, walkers have been implicated in injuries severe enough to be fatal. In 1993 more than 23,000 walker-related injuries, mostly to children between the ages of 5 and 15 months, were seen in hospital emergency rooms.[8,9] The number of injuries is most likely significantly higher when one considers those injuries that are never reported or are treated in clinics or at home. A study by Shields and Smith revealed 197,200 baby-walker–related injuries among children under 15 months of age in the United States.[10] During the period of 1989 through 1993, 11 walker-related deaths occurred.[8,9] Most injuries have been the result of the walker tipping over, falls down stairs, walker collapse because of poor structural design, and finger entrapment. Injuries have included abrasions, lacerations, fractures, burns, poisonings, severe head trauma, and death.[8]

In 1994, a stationary-type device, similar to the original walker but an activity center without wheels, was developed. Since that time, the number of walker-related injuries and deaths has decreased dramatically, but the use of second-hand walkers manufactured prior to that time continues, with resultant injuries.[10] Walkers have been often used by parents because of the mistaken impression that walking skills are helped by these devices. Not only are baby walkers potentially dangerous, but also they do not facilitate the development of normal walking and, in fact, may actually impede motor development. Ridenour studied the effects of frequent and regular use of a baby walker on bipedal locomotion in human infants. She found that walkers modified the mechanics of infant locomotion in several ways. Infants who used walkers were able to commit numerous mechanical errors while still succeeding in bipedal locomotion.[11] The patterns of locomotion with an infant walker are neither normal nor advantageous. Children who use these walkers are in poor weight-bearing alignment, holding their trunk and lower extremities in flexion. There is also frequent asymmetry as the child leans, and toe-walking is common. Additionally, a 1986 study by Crouchman found prone locomotion to be delayed in many normal babies who spent excessive time in infant walkers.[12]

These observations suggest that walkers may have a significant adverse effect on motor development, even though the adverse effects may be of short duration once walker use is discontinued.[11-13] Although further study is needed to confirm findings relative to infant walker use and the development of motor skills, particularly ambulation, most physical therapists discourage the use of walkers by infants with apparent normal neuromotor development and strongly discourage their use in infants with documented or suspected neurologic deficits.

Activities of Daily Living

Although not strongly emphasized in this chapter, activities of daily living (ADLs) should be mentioned briefly. ADLs are not major concerns for infants or toddlers with impairments, but they grow increasingly important as these children grow older and become more capable of caring for themselves. Because families can usually manage the ADL needs of a young child, the issue of ADLs as a therapeutic goal may be overlooked or not considered as the child grows older.

Equipment for ADLs, particularly for toileting and bathing, should be assessed according to guidelines similar to those used for other pieces of apparatus described in this chapter. Toilets may be modified by adding abduction pommels, vertical handgrips (to keep the child symmetric and decrease flexor hypertonia), corner-style backrests, and foot rests. Essential to good positioning on the toilet is for the child's hips and knees to be flexed to 90 degrees with feet flat on the floor, foot rests, or a stool. This position helps limit extensor spasticity in those children affected by hypertonia and also helps all children relax their abdominal muscles and feel secure. If the child feels secure, confident, and relaxed, toileting may proceed more rapidly and easily.

When choosing a bathtub seat, ease of management in the tub and safety of the child are the major objectives. Although many bathtub seats exist, seats that are completely satisfactory for both use and safety are difficult to find for all children, but they are particularly difficult to find when the child becomes older and heavier. Vendors should provide sample bathtub seats for both inspection and mock usage trials. The family must decide which tub seat provides the safest and most suitable solution depending on the particular environmental barriers of the home and the physical needs of the child.

Communication Aids

Although most of this chapter has focused on adaptive equipment relative to positioning, mobility, and ADL needs (i.e., the physical needs of the child), it is important that we give brief consideration to another category of adaptive equipment used with pediatric clients. Augmentative communication strategies frequently involve equipment.

As physical therapists, we must be familiar generally with communication devices for two reasons. First, out interaction with children in the therapeutic environment necessarily requires our ability to communicate with them. This brief synopsis is intended to broadly familiarize the reader with various types of communication devices that may be encountered.

A second reason for physical therapists to have an understanding of augmentative communication is that many of these strategies require controlled movement as a means of communicating. Knowing about these systems can help the physical therapist address movement issues that can facilitate the child's successful use of a communication strategy. In fact, the physical therapist at times may work closely with a speech and language pathologist in developing appropriate motor control for a communication system. Augmentative communication strategies are classified as gestural, gestural assisted, or neuro-assisted.[14]

GESTURAL STRATEGIES

Gestural strategies are unaided strategies, requiring no instrumentation and therefore no adaptive equipment. Movement, generally of the face and upper extremities, is used to transmit messages visually. Smiling, nodding, shaking of the head, and other head and eye movements and hand gestures are typically used gestural communication strategies.

Additionally, several gestural communication systems may be used. These include American Sign Language (Ameslan), American Indian Hand Talk (Amer-Ind), manual shorthand, left-hand manual alphabet (a left-hand variation of the American Manual Alphabet used in Ameslan), eye-blink encoding, and gestural Morse code.[14]

GESTURAL-ASSISTED STRATEGIES

These aided communication strategies require adaptive equipment in the form of a communication board or display that is activated by gesture or movement. Users of this type of strategy use gestures to point to components on the display to transmit their messages.[14]

Gestures may be direct movement of the head, upper extremity, or eyes. If head movements are used, a headpointer is required. Indirect use of movement occurs when the display is controlled by an electronic switching device activated by muscle contractions and includes the use of microcomputers. Movements used to activate switches include finger, head, foot, and eyebrow movements. Switches may be controlled by joysticks, pushbuttons (such as keyboards), pads, squeeze bulbs, and blowing or sucking on the end of a tube (sip and puff switches). Gestural-assisted communication aids may simply be visual symbol sets such as photographs, drawings, the alphabet, and printed words on the display. This classification of communication strategies also includes several

specific systems of symbols such as Picsyms, Sigsymbols, Blissymbolics, and Rebuses.[14]

Gestural-assisted communication devices are available commercially. However, they are generally most effective for function when they are customized for a specific child.

NEURO-ASSISTED STRATEGIES

These aided communication strategies also use a display, but unlike the gestural-assisted strategies that rely on gestural manipulation of a switching mechanism, the display is activated by bioelectrical signals from the body such as muscle action potentials. This type of device is most needed in the child who has motor impairments so severe that he or she is unable to control body movements adequately for gesturing. The same displays are used as in the gestural-assisted systems, but the switches are controlled by surface electrodes on the brain (electroencephalogram) or a selected muscle (electromyogram).[14]

SUMMARY

The purchase, building, and use of adaptive equipment are complex and time-consuming aspects of pediatric physical therapy. These processes are further complicated by the lack of scientific documentation to help with the appropriate and objective choice of equipment. The available options are so numerous that even the most experienced physical therapist is unlikely to feel that all equipment has been considered before making a choice. The safest and most realistic approach to the selection of adaptive devices for children lies in a theoretic construct based on careful evaluation of the child. The goals and status of the child must be known before therapeutic needs can be met with various types of equipment. When this information is known, the therapist can develop a therapeutic program that includes safe and effective use of equipment without unwanted negative effects. When the child's needs and goals are considered, the specific details of the numerous devices available become less intimidating and confusing. Frequent re-evaluation by the therapist will ensure that the child receives continuing benefits from adaptive equipment. Input from teachers, aides, parents, and the child will provide valuable feedback regarding the child's use of the equipment. The scheme suggested in this chapter provides the therapist with the opportunity to document the needs of the child, to select or make the equipment, to evaluate the effects of the equipment, and to reassess the child's status periodically.

REFERENCES

1. Marks A. On making chairs more comfortable—how to fit the seat to the sitter. Fine Woodworking 1981;31:11.
2. Keegan J. Alterations in the lumbar curve related to posture and sitting. J Bone Joint Surg 1973;35A:7.
3. Akerblom B. Chairs and Sitting. Presented at the Symposium on Human Factors in Equipment Design, Sweden, 1954.

4. Knutsson B, Lindh K, Telhag H. Sitting: an electromyographic and mechanical study. Acta Orthop Scand 1966;37:415–426.
5. Keegan J. Evaluation and improvement of seats. Industr Med Surg 1962;31:137–148.
6. Bergan A. Positioning the Client with Central Nervous System Deficits: The Wheelchair and Other Adapted Equipment. 2nd Ed. New York: Valhalla Press, 1985.
7. Nwaobi O, Brubaker C, Cusick B, et al. Electromyographic investigation of extensor activity in cerebral palsy children in different seating positions. Dev Med Child Neurol 1983;25: 175–183.
8. Brubaker C. Ergonomic considerations. J Rehabil R D [Clin Suppl] 1990;27:37–48.
9. Consumer Product Safety Commission. Baby walkers: advance notice of proposed rulemaking. Fed Reg 1994;59:39306–39311.
10. Shields BJ, Smith GA. Success in the prevention of infant walker-related injuries: an analysis of national data, 1990–2001. Pediatrics 2006;117:452–459.
11. Ridenour M. Infant walkers: developmental tool or inherent danger? Percept Mot Skills 1982;55:1201–1202.
12. Crouchman M. The effects of babywalkers on early locomotor development. Dev Med Child Neurol 1986;28:757–761.
13. Kauffman I, Ridenour M. Influence of an infant walker on onset and quality of walking pattern of locomotion: An electromyographic investigation. Percept Mot Skills 1977;45:1323–1329.
14. Silverman F. Communication for the Speechless. 3rd Ed. Needham Heights, MA: Allyn & Bacon, 1995.

BIBLIOGRAPHY

Bull M, Stroup K, Stout J, et al. Establishing special needs car seat loan program. Pediatrics 1990;85:540–547.
Hulme JB, Shaver J, Acher S, et al. Effects of adaptive seating devices on the eating and drinking of children with multiple handicaps. Am J Occup Ther 1987;41:81–89.
Mazur MD, Shurtleff D. Orthopedic management of high-level spina bifida—early walking compared with early use of a wheelchair. J Bone Joint Surg 1989;71A:56–61.
Stout J, Bull M, Stroup K. Safe transportation for children with disabilities. Am J Occup Ther 1989;43:31–36.
Trefler E, ed. Seating for Children with Cerebral Palsy—A Resource Manual. Memphis, TN: University of Tennessee, 1984.
Zacharkow D. Posture: Sitting, Standing, Chair Design and Exercise. Springfield, IL: Charles C Thomas, 1988.

PART

III

Musculoskeletal Disorders

Orthopedic Management

Meg Stanger

he term *orthopedics* in pediatric physical therapy is often used to refer to a specific group of pediatric diagnoses. Within the profession of physical therapy, orthopedics refers to a subspecialty of practice. Many of the medical professions have a tendency to compartmentalize their profession and the patients they see by body systems, such as children with orthopedic disabilities or children with neurologic disabilities. This practice lends itself to specialization or the development of clinical expertise in a well-defined area. However, this practice also may fragment the care of patients and even the thinking of the professionals involved.

The various systems of the body are intertwined and normal or atypical influences on one system almost always have an impact on other body systems. This is especially true of a young child whose musculoskeletal system is immature and susceptible to external and internal influences. The action of muscles working within a normal neurologic system is necessary for the development of joints and the shape and contour of a child's bones. When the neurologic or muscular systems are altered or impaired, many times secondary skeletal impairments develop.

This chapter discusses the growth and development of a child's musculoskeletal system and pediatric musculoskeletal assessment, introduces a classification system based on morphogenesis, and provides an overview of pediatric orthopedic diagnoses commonly encountered by pediatric physical therapists. This chapter contains the term *orthopedic* in the title and focuses on specific orthopedic diagnoses. However, the effects of normal and atypical forces on an immature musculoskeletal system and the secondary impairments that may develop, as well as the discussion of the components of a pediatric musculoskeletal assessment, can be applied to many children seen in pediatric physical therapy. For example, most children with a primary diagnosis of neurologic origin present with impairments of their musculoskeletal system that may impact their overall function.

Musculoskeletal Development

The formation of the musculoskeletal system occurs during the embryonic period (second to eighth weeks postconception). The limb buds arise from mesenchymal cells and appear during the fourth week, with the upper limb developing 2 days ahead of the lower limb. Mesenchymal cells begin to differentiate into cartilage within 4 to 5 days of the formation of the limb bud. The formation of a cartilaginous skeleton occurs rapidly and is completed during the first fetal month (3 months from conception). The cartilaginous template then begins to be replaced by bone with the appearance of primary ossification centers in the diaphysis of the long bones. Secondary ossification centers appear near the end of fetal development and remain until puberty, when skeletal growth is complete.[1,2]

Joint formation begins as the cartilaginous template is being formed. An area of flattened undifferentiated cells forms between two areas of cartilage. The flattened area transforms into three layers, and the peripheral layers maintain contact with the cartilage and eventually become the joint capsule. The middle layer cavitates and forms the joint cavity. The original cartilage at the interface of the joint capsule remains and becomes the articular cartilage.[1,2]

The extremities are susceptible to major morphologic abnormalities during the embryonic period when the limb buds are developing. For example, exposure of the embryo to pharmacologic agents while the limb buds are forming may result in congenital limb deficiencies. During the fetal period, structures increase in size and cartilage begins to be replaced by bone formation; however, minimal bone remodeling occurs. During this time, the fetus is more susceptible to minor morphologic abnormalities that are the result of position constraints and abnormal mechanical forces.[2] For example, torticollis or clubfeet may result from position constraints late in the pregnancy. Postnatally, much bone remodeling occurs at a rapid rate of 50% annually in the infant and toddler and gradually slows to the adult rate of 5% annually.

Bone grows in length through the continuation of the process of endochondral ossification begun during the fetal period. Endochondral ossification is often referred to as epiphyseal growth because longitudinal growth occurs at the epiphyseal plate. Increases in the diameter of bone or bone thickness occur through appositional growth or the laying down of new bone on top of old bone. These two types of bone growth respond differently to mechanical loading and the forces associated with weight bearing and muscle pull. Appositional bone growth is stimulated by increased compressive forces. Increased weight bearing results in increased thickness and density of the shaft of the tibia.[3,4] However, decreased weight bearing, as seen with immobilization, results in atrophy of the bone.[3]

The response of epiphyseal growth to mechanical forces is dependent on the direction, magnitude, and timing of the force. Intermittent compressive forces applied parallel to the direction of growth cause longitudinal bone growth; however, constant compressive forces of excessive or high magnitude retard bone growth.[5] A compressive force may be applied unevenly across the epiphyseal plate, resulting in slowing of growth on one side only. The uneven growth produces an angulation of the epiphyseal plate and changes the direction of growth.[3] Mechanical loads or forces that are applied perpendicular to the longitudinal growth of the bone result in a change of direction or deflection of bone growth. New growth is deflected and results in displacement of the epiphysis if the load is maintained. A torsional stress to the epiphyseal plate deflects columns of cartilage around the circumference of the epiphyseal plate in either a clockwise or counterclockwise direction. New bone then grows away from the epiphyseal plate in a spiral pattern resulting in a torsional deformity.

In summary, the growth and development of the musculoskeletal system is dependent on the normal interplay of multiple factors including hormones, nutrition, and mechanical forces.[5,6] The immature musculoskeletal system is vulnerable to abnormal mechanical forces and pressures; alterations in the timing, direction, or magnitude of forces may have a deleterious effect on the growing and developing musculoskeletal system. Congenital deformities and secondary musculoskeletal impairments that are seen in children with neurologic diagnoses are examples of the vulnerability of the immature musculoskeletal system to abnormal extrinsic forces. However, the immaturity of a child's musculoskeletal system can also be an advantage and is often used as the rationale for many treatment interventions that will be discussed throughout this chapter.

◆ Musculoskeletal Assessment

A thorough musculoskeletal assessment should be included as part of a comprehensive evaluation of a child seen by a physical therapist. Depending on the history or diagnosis, certain aspects of the musculoskeletal assessment should be performed and other aspects may be omitted. However, for those children with a diagnosis that includes multiple joint or system involvement, a complete musculoskeletal assessment should be performed. The assessment may begin as a postural screen with a more in-depth assessment dependent on the findings of the initial screen. The assessment should be completed in a timely and organized manner. The order of the assessment outlined in the following sections may need to be altered depending on the comfort and interaction of the child.

HISTORY

A thorough history should be obtained from the parents and the child if the child is able to convey the information to the examiner. The history should obtain information regarding onset or a history of the presenting complaint, if pain is present, what aggravates or alleviates the pain, and any changes in posture or activity noted. Useful information can often be obtained by asking the parents to report to you a typical day for their child. While talking with the parents, the physical therapist should be observing the child's posture, play, spontaneous movements, and activities with relevance to the child's posture, noted asymmetries and difficulty with age-appropriate skills.

POSTURAL SCREEN

During the postural screen, the therapist assesses skeletal alignment in a variety of positions, depending on the age of the child. Skeletal alignment should include spinal and lower extremity alignment and limb length. Spinal alignment is viewed from both a sagittal plane and posterior view. The therapist looks for a normal kyphosis and lordosis of the spine relative to the age of the child. From the posterior view, the physical therapist visually assesses symmetry of shoulder, scapulae, and pelvic height. Any asymmetries in rib position, such as a rib hump, would indicate a rotational deformity of the spine.

Lower extremity alignment should also be screened from a sagittal view as well as an anterior and posterior view. The therapist looks at symmetry of pelvic height; rotational variations of the lower extremities, such as the knees or feet pointing in or out; and a valgus or varus position of the knees or feet. From a sagittal view, the physical therapist assesses pelvic position and alignment of the hip, knee, and ankle.

Limb length should be assessed in both a weight-bearing and non–weight-bearing position using the accepted bony landmarks of the anterior superior iliac spine and the medial malleolus. The postural screen will direct the physical therapist to where to focus the next portion of a more in-depth musculoskeletal assessment.

RANGE OF MOTION

Although the goniometric techniques used to measure active or passive joint range of motion (ROM) in children and adults are similar, several factors must be kept in mind when assessing range of motion in children. Age-related differences exist in ROM values between adults and infants and young children. For example, a full-term newborn will exhibit flexion contractures of the hips and knees secondary to intrauterine positioning.

Before any goniometric measurement is taken, attention must be given so that the child is relaxed and remains calm. Movements should be slow so as to limit anxiety and to avoid eliciting a stretch reflex in children with increased muscle tone. Slow movements should also be used if pain is present or suspected and for those children who may have more brittle bones or recent fractures.

Reliability studies of the use of goniometry in children are present in the literature and should guide physical therapists in their use of goniometric measures to document ROM. Haley et al. demonstrated acceptable levels of interrater and intrarater reliability ($r = 0.77$ to 0.89) of spinal mobility in normal young children.[7] Several researchers have investigated the reliability of goniometric measurement of children with Duchenne's muscular dystrophy and children with cerebral palsy. High intrarater reliability was present in those studies, but interrater reliability was shown to be variable throughout the studies.[8–10] When measuring ROM in children, the most reliable results are obtained when the same therapist assesses changes in ROM over time.

Muscle length tests should also be included in the overall joint motion assessment. Specific tests and their procedures do not differ from standard procedures used with the adult population; however, several tests may be used more frequently in pediatrics. Hip flexor muscle length is assessed using the Thomas test or the prone hip extension test. Hamstring length is usually assessed in adults using the straight leg raise test; however, the passive knee extension (PKE) test is commonly used with pediatrics (Fig. 12.1). The PKE test can be used in the presence of a knee flexion contracture; therefore, it is useful for children who present with involvement of multiple joints.[11] The PKE test is also easier to perform and more reliable with smaller limbs than the lower extremities of large adults.[12]

STRENGTH

An accurate assessment of strength requires careful consideration in the pediatric population but yields important information regarding deficits and changes over time. A variety of methods to assess strength are available, and their use may depend on the age and ability of the child. For infants and children younger than the age of 3 or 4 years, assessment of strength is most often accomplished through observation of movement and function. A child must be able to follow the directions of the testing procedure to ensure accurate results using either manual muscle testing (MMT) or dynamometry.[13] Strength may also be reliably assessed using isokinetic machines if the child is tall enough to reach the componentry.[14]

MMT has the same inherent weaknesses with the pediatric population as with adults. The grades of "good" and "normal" are very subjective and do not account for any changes that may occur in a child over time secondary to maturation. Several authors have determined that MMT may not identify strength deficits until they are greater than 50%.[15,16] Handheld dynamometry has been found to be a reliable and sensitive method of assessing strength in various populations of children.[17–19] Gajdosik[20] determined that handheld dynamometry could be used reliably with typical developing children between the ages of 2 to 5 years as long as they could follow the directions and understand

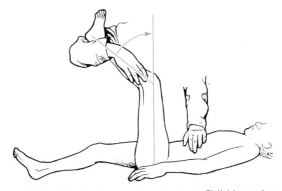

Figure 12.1 ▪ Passive knee extension test. Child is supine, hip is flexed to 90 degrees, and the knee is slowly extended until resistance is felt. The angle between the anterior aspect of the lower leg and a vertical line corresponding to the thigh is recorded as a measure of hamstring contracture.

the command to push as well as agree to participate in the process. Children in the 2-year age range were more likely than the 3- and 4-year-olds to refuse to participate in the testing sessions.

LOWER EXTREMITY ALIGNMENT (ROTATIONAL AND ANGULAR)

Normal skeletal development includes rotational or torsional and alignment changes of bones and joints. These normal developmental processes may be altered secondary to abnormal muscle pull or weight-bearing forces. Consequently, impairments that impact function often result from the combination of abnormal forces on a developing skeletal system. The bones remain susceptible to deforming forces until growth is complete; therefore, the impairments may increase in severity over time.

Staheli et al. have developed a rotational profile to assess lower extremity alignment and assist in determining which component of the lower extremity contributes to the rotational variation. The rotational profile consists of six measurements: (1) foot–progression angle; (2) medial rotation of the hip; (3) lateral rotation of the hip; (4) thigh–foot angle; (5) angle of the transmalleolar axis; and (6) configuration of the foot. Normal values have been established for the first five measurements and can be used to determine whether the variation falls within the wide range of normal or if intervention is indicated.[21]

ROTATIONAL PROFILE

FOOT–PROGRESSION ANGLE The foot–progression angle (FPA) is defined as the angle between the longitudinal axis of the foot and the line of progression of the child's gait. The FPA provides an overall summation of the child's rotation during gait but does not identify the contributing factors. A positive sign denotes out-toeing and a negative sign denotes in-toeing. The FPA can be objectively measured using a variety of footprint measures, including ink or chalk on the feet or more expensive commercially available methods. Many times in the clinic, the FPA is assessed subjectively to give the clinician an overall view of the child's rotation during gait. The procedures listed in the following sections assist the clinician with identifying the contributing factors to the overall rotational profile of the child (Fig. 12.2A).

HIP ROTATION Medial and lateral hip rotation in prone are assessed to determine femoral torsion. The child is in prone with hips extended and knees flexed to 90 degrees, and medial and lateral hip rotation measurements are then taken goniometrically. Soft tissue limitations may influence the final measure of hip rotation as well as the degree of femoral torsion. Normal medial hip rotation is less than 60 to 65 degrees (Fig. 12.2B,C).

The literature also describes a second test of femoral torsion referred to as Ryder's test. The child sits with knees flexed to 90 degrees over the edge of a table. The greater trochanter is palpated while rotating the leg. When the greater trochanter is palpated most laterally, the angle of medial hip rotation is measured goniometrically; the femoral neck should be parallel to the examining table and the measure of medial hip rotation should correspond to the degree of femoral anteversion.[10,22]

THIGH–FOOT ANGLE The child is in the prone position with the hips extended, the knee flexed to 90 degrees, and the foot in a natural resting position; do not attempt to align the foot. The angle formed from the bisection of the axis of the thigh and the axis of the foot is measured. This thigh–foot angle (TFA) is used to determine rotational variation of the tibia and the hindfoot. If the foot is in an out-toeing position, the value is positive; if the foot is in an in-toeing position, the value is negative (Fig. 12.2D).

TRANSMALLEOLAR AXIS The child is positioned in prone, as previously described. A line perpendicular to the axis between the lateral and medial malleoli is drawn. The angle formed from between the perpendicular line and the axis of the thigh is measured. This angle assesses the contribution of the distal tibia to the rotational profile (Fig. 12.2E).

The contribution of the foot must also be included when assessing rotational variations. Assessing the alignment of the hindfoot and forefoot will determine whether a pronated or supinated position of the foot or metatarsus adductus is contributing to the FPA.

ANGULAR ALIGNMENT

If the initial postural screening revealed suspected lower extremity alignment deviations, such as a varus or valgus posture, an objective angular measurement should be performed. Expected values for genu varus and valgus will differ depending on the age of the child. Genu varum is measured with the child in supine with legs extended and the patella facing upward and the medial malleoli touching. The distance between the femoral condyles is measured. Genu valgus is measured in the same position but with the knees touching. The distance between the malleoli is measured.[23] The contribution of angular variations must be delineated from rotational variations.

Additional areas that may be included in the musculoskeletal assessment include assessment of muscle tone, sensation testing, and developmental skill level. An assessment of muscle tone may reveal hypertonicity or hypotonicity of specific muscle groups and an imbalance of muscle forces around specific joints. These unbalanced muscle forces may produce impairments over time that cause pain or interfere with the child's functional abilities.

Sensation testing is performed with children just as with adults and incorporates the same rationale for inclu-

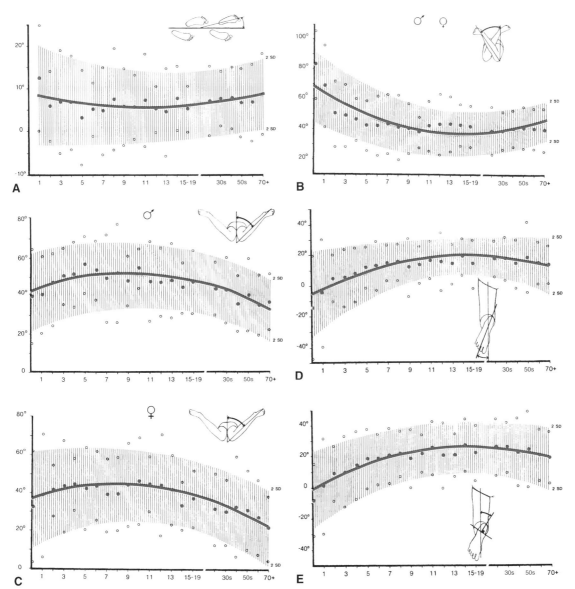

Figure 12.2 ■ The five measurements in Staheli's rotational profile plotted as the mean values plus or minus two standard deviations (SDs) for each of the age groups. The dark line indicates the mean values as they change with age, and the shaded areas indicate the normal ranges. **(A)** Foot–progression angle. **(B)** Lateral rotation of the hip in males and females. **(C)** Medial rotation of the hip in females and males (separate). **(D)** Thigh–foot angle. **(E)** Angle of the transmalleolar axis.

sion of testing. Sensory testing is indicated when nerve involvement is suspected, such as with fractures or after an amputation or application of an external fixator.

Assessment of a child's developmental level is indicated if the orthopedic condition is suspected of delaying or interfering with development. For the ambulatory child, this includes an assessment of gait. Gait assessment is similar to assessing an adult and can be performed through systematic clinical observation or with more objective measures, ranging from video analysis to an instrumented gait laboratory. The age of the child must be considered when assessing gait and knowledge of the characteristics of early walking must be incorporated into the assessment (see Chapter 5).

Classification of Errors of Morphologic Development

The terminology adopted by the World Health Organization's (WHO) International Classification of Functioning, Disability, and Health (ICF)[24] will be utilized in this chapter when discussing various diagnoses and their impact on the functional ability of the child. The ICF model also includes environmental and personal factors that will differ from one child to another and are not related to the child's diagnosis or health condition but may impact his or her activity or participation levels.

To illustrate the ICF model, a child with osteogenesis imperfecta (OI) will be used as an example. For a child with OI, the pathophysiology is the abnormality in the connective tissue at the cellular level. One of the impairments that results is fragile bones susceptible to deforming forces and fracture. The child may sustain multiple lower extremity fractures resulting in misalignment, short stature, weakness, and a slow labored gait. The slow labored gait is an activity limitation that may lead to an inability of the child to keep up with his or her peers during play or at school. Participation restrictions may include not permitting the child to attend a daycare of peers or to play outside at recess owing to a fear of increased risk of fractures. Environmental factors such as a teacher's fears or a crowded recess area have contributed to the child's ability to participate.

Spranger's classification of morphogenesis will also be used to introduce and discuss a multitude of diagnoses that fall under the category of pediatric orthopedics. This classification system provides a framework from which to understand the pathophysiology resulting in a particular diagnosis, the impairments that may develop as the child grows, the impact of the impairments on the child's activities and participation levels, and how physical therapy may have an impact. With an understanding of the pathophysiology, the reader will be able to identify impairments that may be present or may develop and the impact of physical therapy on preventing or limiting the impairments, with the ultimate goal of minimizing the activity limitations and participation restrictions for the child.

Spranger's classification of disorders of morphogenesis consists of four divisions: malformations, disruptions, deformations, and dysplasias.[25] Malformations are morphologic defects of an organ or body part from an intrinsically abnormal developmental process. Because the abnormality is intrinsic from the moment of conception, the organ or body part never had the potential to develop normally. Examples of malformations include longitudinal limb deficiencies, cleft lip and palate, and septal defects of the heart.

Disruptions are morphologic defects of an organ or body part resulting from the extrinsic breakdown of an originally normal developmental process. Normal development is interrupted at the cellular level by an external factor such as a teratogen, trauma, or infection. Transverse limb deficiencies commonly seen with the use of thalidomide are an example of a disruption.

Deformations are abnormalities in form, shape, or position of a body part caused by mechanical forces. The deforming forces may be extrinsic to the fetus, such as intrauterine constraint, or intrinsic to the fetus, such as fetal hypomobility resulting from a neuromuscular defect. Examples of deformations include torticollis and metatarsus adductus. Deformations can be delineated into prenatal and postnatal deformities versus pathologic processes. Examples of postnatal deformities include tibial varum and rotational variations. Pathologic processes are

usually deformities as the result of an insult to the epiphyseal plate or other area of the bone. These processes include the diagnoses of Legg-Calvé-Perthes disease, slipped capital femoral epiphysis, and limb length discrepancies resulting from insults or abnormal forces to the growth plate. Deformations can often be ameliorated with the application of forces in the opposite direction of the deforming mechanism. The application of forces must be timed correctly with expected maturation of the musculoskeletal system to allow for normal growth and remodeling to occur.

The final division in Spranger's classification is dysplasia. Dysplasias result from an abnormal organization of cells into tissues, which leads to abnormal tissue differentiation. OI is an example of a dysplasia. Dysplasias usually involve whole systems of the body with multiple impairments present that will lead to activity limitations and possibly participation restrictions.

Congenital Limb Deficiencies

Using the International Society for Prosthetics and Orthotics (ISPO) classification system, congenital limb deficiencies are described as either longitudinal or transverse (Fig. 12.3A,B).[26] Longitudinal limb deficiencies are described as reduction or absence of an element or elements within the long axis of the limb. There may be normal skeletal elements distal to the affected bone or bones.[26] A longitudinal limb deficiency is an example of a malformation in which a morphologic defect of an organ or larger region of the body occurs when normal organogenesis is interrupted. Any combination of skeletal limb involvement is possible, but certain distinct entities are more commonly seen than others. For this chapter, congenital longitudinal deficiency of the radius will be used as an example of upper extremity involvement and proximal femoral focal deficiency (PFFD) as an example of a lower extremity longitudinal limb deficiency. Both are examples of congenital malformations and are more frequent in their incidence; they are also examples of children with limb deficiencies typically seen by therapists.

Longitudinal deficiency of the radius, often commonly referred to as radial clubhand, occurs in 1 per 100,000 live births, with bilateral involvement present in 50% of the children. Radial deficiencies can be defined as the failure of formation of parts of deficiencies on the radial side of the upper extremity, including the radius, carpals, metacarpals, and phalanges of the first ray and thenar musculature.[27,28] Heikel classified radial deficiencies into four types, ranging in severity from type I (consisting of delayed appearance of the distal radial physis) to type IV (involving complete absence of the radius).[29] Type IV is the most common presentation and is present in 50% of children with a radial deficiency.[23] Clinically, children with type IV radial deficiency present with a shortened forearm of no greater than

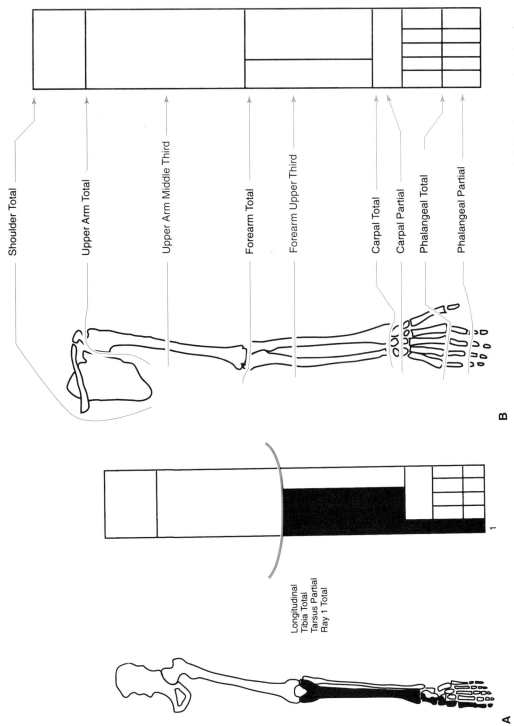

Shoulder Total

Upper Arm Total

Upper Arm Middle Third

Forearm Total

Forearm Upper Third

Carpal Total

Carpal Partial

Phalangeal Total

Phalangeal Partial

B

Longitudinal
Tibia Total
Tarsus Partial
Ray 1 Total

A

Figure 12.3 ■ **(A)** Example of a longitudinal deficiency of the lower extremity. **(B)** Example of transverse deficiencies at various levels of the upper extremity.

50% of the length of the contralateral forearm, an elbow extension contracture, and radial deviation of the hand with an absent or deficient thumb.

The incidence of PFFD is 1 per 50,000 live births and is bilateral in 15% of children with PFFD.[30] Aitken first described and classified four classes of severity of PFFD with class A exhibiting the least involvement and class D being the most severe (Fig. 12.4).[31] PFFD includes absence or hypoplasia of the proximal femur with varying degrees of involvement of the acetabulum, femoral head, patella, tibia, fibula, cruciate ligaments, and the foot. Clinically, infants with PFFD present with an abnormally short thigh held in hip flexion, abduction, and external rotation (Fig. 12.5). Hip and knee flexion contractures are often present along with anteroposterior instability of the knee and a significant leg length difference, with the foot of the involved leg often at the height of the opposite knee.

In transverse limb deficiencies, the limb develops normally to a particular level beyond which no skeletal elements exist.[26] Transverse limb deficiencies are an example of a disruption using Spranger's classification of morphogenesis and resemble in appearance a residual limb after surgical amputation. Most transverse deficiencies are unilateral, with a frequently seen scenario being a transverse forearm deficiency (Fig. 12.6).[27] This type of transverse deficiency occurs more frequently in females and exhibits a 2:1 left-sided predominance.[32]

NONSURGICAL AND SURGICAL MANAGEMENT OF CONGENITAL LIMB DEFICIENCIES

Children with longitudinal limb deficiencies often require multiple surgical procedures to obtain maximal function

TYPE		FEMORAL HEAD	ACETABULUM	FEMORAL SEGMENT	RELATIONSHIP AMONG COMPONENTS OF FEMUR AND ACETABULUM AT SKELETAL MATURITY
A	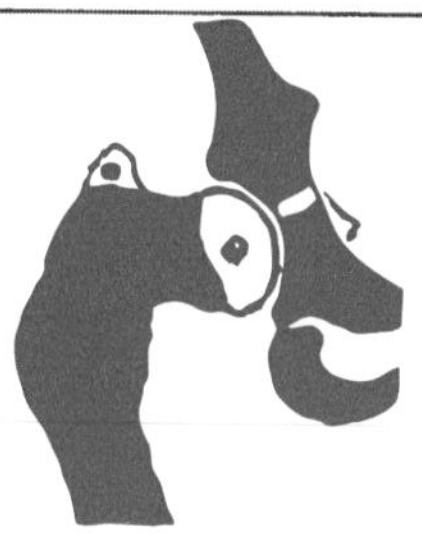	Present	Normal	Short	Bony connection between components of femur Femoral head in acetabulum Subtrochanteric varus angulation, often with pseudarthrosis
B	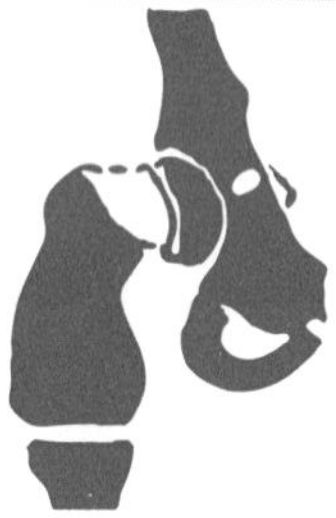	Present	Adequate or moderately dysplastic	Short, usually proximal bony tuft	No osseous connection between head and shaft Femoral head in acetabulum
C	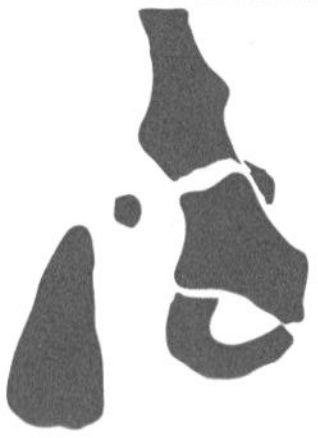	Absent or represented by ossicle	Severely dysplastic	Short, usually proximally tapered	May be osseous connection between shaft and proximal ossicle No articular relation between femur and acetabulum
D	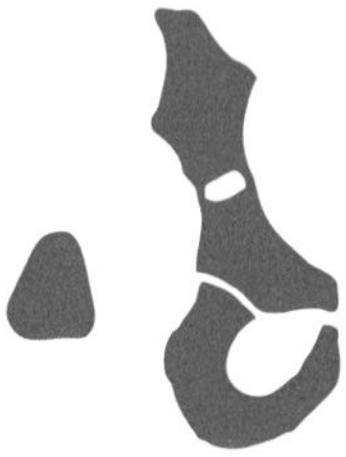	Absent	Absent Obturator foramen enlarged Pelvis squared in bilateral cases	Short, deformed	(none)

Figure 12.4 ■ Aitken classification of proximal femoral focal deficiency.

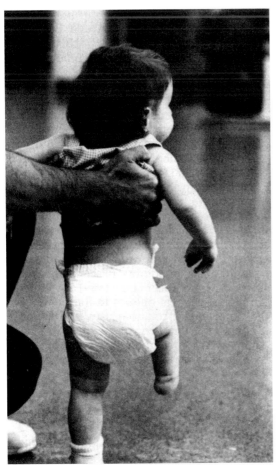

Figure 12.5 ■ Child with unilateral proximal femoral focal deficiency who underwent a Boyd amputation of his right foot. Note popliteal crease near the diaper line indicating where his knee is located.

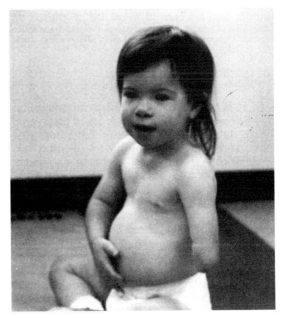

Figure 12.6 ■ Child with congenital transverse below-elbow limb deficiency.

of the involved limb. Surgical procedures may include tendon transfers, realignment or repositioning of the hand and/or fingers, and osteotomies for the upper extremity and most commonly include a combination of amputation, fusion, limb lengthening, and osteotomies for lower extremity limb deficiencies. Surgical correction is rarely required for children with transverse limb deficiencies.

UPPER EXTREMITY: LONGITUDINAL RADIAL DEFICIENCY

Shortly after birth, the child's hand should be serially splinted or casted to stretch the shortened soft tissues and realign the hand as centrally as possible over the distal forearm. At the same time, therapy goals should also focus on increasing elbow ROM, especially elbow flexion. Stretching of the soft tissues is necessary before any surgical procedures. Between 6 months and 1 year of age, centralization of the hand by an orthopedic surgeon is often performed. The goal of centralization is a stable wrist centered on the distal ulna while maintaining functional wrist motion.[33]

Postoperatively, the child's hand is splinted in the newly aligned position on the distal ulna. Compliance with wearing of the splint is crucial for long-term success of the surgical centralization. The splint should be worn throughout the day and night during the healing phase. After the initial healing phase is complete, a splint should be worn at night until skeletal maturity is achieved. By skeletal maturity, the ulna has undergone epiphyseal adaptation to accommodate the centralized carpus to ensure stability of the wrist position and use of a night splint is no longer necessary.[33]

Centralization of the hand is contraindicated in older children or adolescents who have adapted to their hand position, when severe deformity of the hand is also present that would limit hand function and when elbow flexion is less than 90 degrees. Adequate elbow flexion is needed prior to surgery so that when the hand is realigned, the child is still able to bring his or her hand to the mouth.

LOWER EXTREMITY: PROXIMAL FEMORAL FOCAL DEFICIENCY

Surgical intervention for children with PFFD is varied, must be individualized, and can include any combination of amputation, reconstruction, fusion, or limb-lengthening procedures. Surgery addresses the issues of the unstable hip joint and the inequality of limb lengths, the two issues that interfere with the child's overall functional abilities. Many children require multiple surgical procedures; thought must be given early to develop a long-term surgical plan for family education and to condense surgeries into one procedure when possible. Surgery is generally not recommended for children with bilateral PFFD, because their limb length is equal or near equal and they are able to ambulate with or without extension prostheses.[23,34,35]

Surgical options can be divided into those that involve amputation and reconstruction for eventual prosthetic fitting and those that involve limb-lengthening techniques. Three typical surgical scenarios are discussed in the following sections. Prior to surgical intervention, physical therapy should be initiated in early infancy to improve ROM at the involved hip, promote developmental activities (including symmetry of skills and weight bearing at the age-appropriate times), and assist with the development of age-appropriate balance skills.

FOOT AMPUTATION AND PROXIMAL RECONSTRUCTION After this combination of surgical procedures, the child's limb resembles and functions as an above-knee amputation. The foot is amputated at an early age, often before 8 months of age, so that the child may be fitted with a prosthesis. Proximal reconstruction, including forming a connection between the femoral head and the proximal femur and fusion of the knee, is usually performed when the child is between 2 and 6 years of age. Reconstruction of the proximal femur is only recommended if sufficient bone density is present and if gains in stability will be achieved. Fusion of the knee allows the limb to function as a single lever arm. This combination of surgical procedures is indicated for those children with the more severe manifestations of PFFD, including a very short femur and involvement of the femoral head and neck.

ROTATIONPLASTY Rotationplasty, or the turn-about procedure, is a surgical technique that allows the child to function similarly to a child with a below-knee amputation. In children with PFFD the rotationplasty procedure is often performed as an amputation through the knee joint, and the limb is rotated 180 degrees and then reattached with a knee fusion. The neurovascular supply is left intact, and the lower leg muscles are reattached to corresponding muscles of the thigh. The child's ankle then functions as a knee joint, with ankle plantar flexion acting as knee extension and ankle dorsiflexion acting as knee flexion (Fig. 12.7).[23,36] Indications for a rotationplasty procedure include (1) a normal ankle joint; (2) unilateral involvement; (3) a predicted limb length that would place the ankle of the involved limb at the knee of the uninvolved limb at skeletal maturity; and (4) a stable hip.[23]

Postoperatively, the child's leg and pelvis are typically placed in a hip spica cast until healing is complete. After cast removal, physical therapy must emphasize ROM of the ankle. Maximum plantar flexion range is needed to promote knee extension in the prosthesis. Sitting and other activities involving knee flexion will require close to 20 degrees of ankle dorsiflexion. Strengthening of these muscle groups is also important; ankle plantar flexion and dorsiflexion strength provides stability in stance and powers the prosthesis during gait.

LIMB LENGTHENING Limb lengthening may be indicated when more than 60% of predicted femoral length is pres-

ent[34,37] or the discrepancy in femoral length is predicted to be less than 15 cm. Limb-lengthening procedures include unilateral frames such as the Wagner or circular frames, also called the Ilizarov. Limb-lengthening procedures for children with PFFD are often performed when the child is between 8 and 10 years of age. Contraindications include bilateral PFFD, an unstable hip such as with Aitken type C or D, and poor carryover of care at home.[37,38] An in-depth description of limb-lengthening procedures is provided later in this chapter under Limb Length Discrepancies.

PROSTHETIC TRAINING

Physical therapy intervention should begin before the fitting of the initial prosthesis. During infancy, physical therapy may be initiated on a weekly basis or a consultative basis, depending on the needs of the child and the family. Infants with a longitudinal limb deficiency have contractures or ROM limitations that must be addressed before surgery or prosthetic fitting. The infant with a radial deficiency requires stretching of the soft tissues, including passive exercises and splinting before surgery. The infant with PFFD requires ROM exercises to increase hip extension and adduction motions before surgery or prosthetic fitting. Infants with transverse limb deficiencies rarely exhibit contractures.

Infants with congenital limb deficiencies should also be monitored for their developmental skills. Symmetry of skills is emphasized as well as weight-bearing skills through both the upper and lower extremities. Early weight-bearing skills promote proximal joint stability that may be needed later to use a prosthesis. Children with an upper extremity transverse limb deficiency are usually fitted with a prosthesis by 6 months of age when they begin simple two-handed activities. Children with lower extremity limb deficiencies are generally fitted with a prosthesis between 8 and 10 months, when they begin weight-bearing skills.

When an infant or child first receives a prosthesis, the fit, alignment, and overall function are assessed. The child and family must be shown the proper donning and doffing techniques, instructed in a wearing schedule, and shown how to check the skin for redness or possible breakdown. The initial goal is for the infant or toddler to accept wearing the prosthesis and gradually increase the wearing time throughout the day. The prosthesis is usually removed for naps and should be removed when going to sleep for the night.

UPPER EXTREMITY PROSTHETIC TRAINING

An infant's first prosthesis has a terminal device that is soft and cosmetically appealing but nonfunctional (Fig. 12.8). A more functional terminal device is added when the child begins to engage in bimanual play. Functional terminal devices are either voluntary opening or voluntary closing. Voluntary-opening terminal devices open as the child

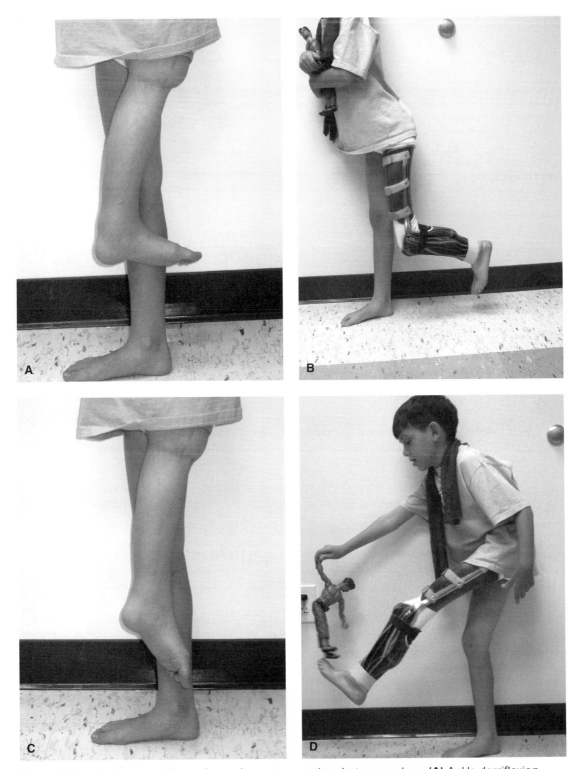

Figure 12.7 ■ *An 11-year-old boy who underwent a rotationplasty procedure.* **(A)** *Ankle dorsiflexion.* **(B)** *Ankle dorsiflexion produces prosthetic knee flexion.* **(C)** *Ankle plantar flexion.* **(D)** *Ankle plantar flexion produces prosthetic knee extension.*

reaches forward with the arm, whereas voluntary-closing devices mimic reaching and grasping and close as the child reaches forward to grasp an object.

The initial goals for an infant or young toddler are to wear the prosthesis, become adjusted to the weight of the prosthesis, and begin to use the prosthesis for propping in prone or sitting and bimanual skills. By the age of 15 to 18 months of age, training on the use of an active terminal device should begin (Fig. 12.9). The child is taught to open the terminal device, grasp an object, and then release

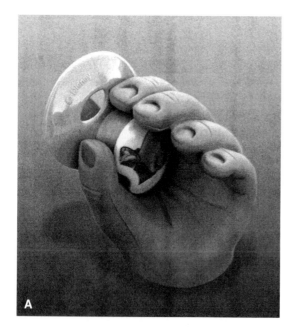

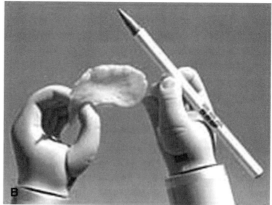

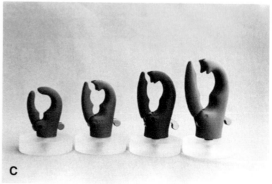

Figure 12.8 ▪ Terminal device options: **(A)** Passive Infant Alpha Hand (TRS, Boulder, CO). **(B)** L'il E-Z Hand promotes grasping when thumb is moved (TRS, Boulder, CO). **(C)** ADEPT voluntary closing hand (TRS, Boulder, CO).

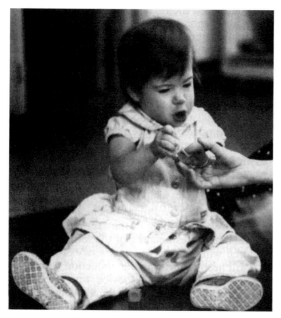

Figure 12.9 ▪ Child is wearing a right below-elbow prosthesis with an ADEPT voluntary closing hook. Therapist assisting child to operate the terminal device.

the object.[39] This order of skill acquisition mimics the normal developmental sequence. The therapist must be familiar with the type of terminal device and how it operates before instructing the child. If the child has an above-elbow prosthesis, the elbow is locked when the child is initially learning to control the terminal device so that the child only learns one movement at a time. The child with an above-elbow limb deficiency activates the terminal device through scapular movements and a cable connected to the terminal device.

Some clinicians and parents may opt to have a young toddler fitted with an externally powered myoelectric device. Initially the child is fitted with a myoelectric hand that opens when one electrode is activated through forearm muscle contraction. By 3 to 4 years of age the child's myoelectric hand can be converted to two electrodes so that both opening and closing of the hand are controlled by the child.[40]

As the child progresses, the use of the terminal device should include manipulation of small objects and using the prosthesis as the helper hand to hold paper for writing or coloring, holding the handlebars of a tricycle, feeding, and dressing. Expectations need to be reasonable, because the child will use the uninvolved hand as the dominant hand. By school age, the child should be independent with self-care activities including dressing, toileting, and eating. Activities should always focus on independence with age-appropriate skills. By the time the child is in high school, he or she may want to participate in various activities, including sports, driving, and social events. Various terminal device options are available to promote participation in numerous sports and to facilitate driving and control of the steering wheel, and cosmetic terminal devices are available for social times when cosmesis may be more important than function. The child, teenager, and young adult should always be a part of the discussion for therapy goals and prosthetic options.

LOWER EXTREMITY PROSTHETIC TRAINING

An infant or toddler younger than 2 years of age may be fitted with a prosthesis without a knee joint. The goals for initial prosthetic training are toleration of the prosthesis and to begin standing weight-bearing activities. The prosthesis will interfere with the child's method of floor mobility and will require an adjustment period by the child. Initial standing activities should include transitions in and out of standing at a support, weight-shift activities in preparation for gait and balance reactions, and protective skills. Gait training may be initiated with an assistive device; the assistive device is often discarded voluntarily by the child when it is no longer necessary. During the early preschool years, a prosthesis with a knee should be introduced to the child. Various prosthetic knee options are available that provide additional stability during the early years.

Recently, several clinics have begun using articulated prosthetic knees for toddlers in their initial prosthesis. The prosthetic knee allows more typical movements seen in toddlers such as crawling, squatting, and kneeling and promotes a more normal gait pattern (Fig. 12.10).[41,42] Previously, it was difficult to fit an articulating knee in the small shank of a toddler's prosthesis, but advances in prosthetic design have enabled prosthetists to overcome this challenge.

Growth is an issue with children and lower extremity prostheses. Young infants and toddlers can outgrow their prosthesis every 6 months. For this reason, many prosthetists will fit a child with a prosthesis that accommodates some growth, stage the introduction of components, and utilize components that can be replaced as the child grows. For toddlers, spacers can be added to increase the length of the prosthesis and prolong the fit and use of the prosthesis. However, children will typically need to have their prosthesis replaced every 9 to 12 months because of growth and durability issues.

The range of prosthetic options available to children who are school age and younger has greatly expanded but lacks the variety that is available for adolescents and adults. Some older children may require a second prosthesis or additional distal components for specific activities such as sports or water activities.

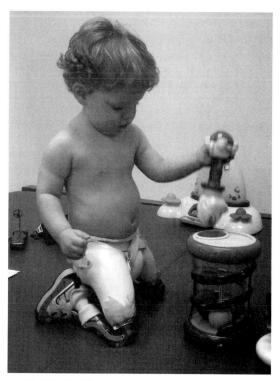

Figure 12.10 ■ *Toddler wearing bilateral transfemoral prosthesis with knee joint to promote age-appropriate ambulation skills and play activities on the floor.*

 Prenatal Deformations

A deformation is an abnormal form, shape, or position of a part of the body caused by mechanical forces. Deformations are normal responses of the tissue to abnormal mechanical forces that may be extrinsic or intrinsic to the fetus. Intrauterine constraint is an example of an extrinsic force, whereas fetal hypomobility secondary to a nervous system impairment such as myelomeningocele is an example of an intrinsic force. If the deforming force is removed, normal development or maturation of the body part would be expected to occur.

This chapter discusses congenital muscular torticollis (CMT) as an example of an extrinsic deformation and clubfeet as an example of either an extrinsic or intrinsic deformation. Both of these diagnoses may also have other causative factors; abnormal mechanical forces are only one of the possible contributing factors. Developmental dysplasia of the hip is an example of a deformation that probably begins prenatally, continues to progress if the deforming forces are not altered, and may not be recognized until much later in postnatal life. Lastly, this section discusses arthrogryposis as an example of an intrinsic deformation that begins very early in fetal development and consequently results in significant deformations at birth and throughout later life.

CONGENITAL MUSCULAR TORTICOLLIS

An infant with congenital muscular torticollis (CMT) presents with unilateral shortening of the sternocleidomastoid muscle, with subsequent limited cervical ROM. The infant's head is laterally flexed toward the shortened muscle, with the chin rotated to the opposite side. An infant with shortening of the right sternocleidomastoid muscle exhibits a posture of right lateral neck flexion with rotation of the head toward the left (Fig. 12.11). Facial asymmetry and plagiocephaly (flattening of the skull) are also often noted.

CMT is usually noted in the first 2 to 3 weeks after birth, with a reported incidence of 0.4% to 1.9%.[43] The etiology of CMT is not clearly understood at this time. Intrauterine malposition and birth trauma have been hypothesized as causative factors. Infants with CMT have a higher incidence of breech presentations[44,45] and associated congenital musculoskeletal diagnoses, such as hip dysplasia and foot deformities.[44,46]

A palpable mass or fibrotic tumor is often observed or is palpable within the belly of the sternocleidomastoid muscle and appears within the first few weeks after birth and then gradually disappears. The exact cause of the fibrotic tumor within the sternocleidomastoid muscle is not known. Researchers have hypothesized that occlusion of blood vessels with resultant anoxic injury to the sternocleidomastoid

muscle may produce the fibrotic changes observed within the muscle. The occlusion could result from intrauterine malposition or trauma at birth.[47] Several authors propose that fibrosis of the sternocleidomastoid muscle is present in all children with CMT and ranges on a continuum of no palpable mass to a firm palpable mass.[44,46] Consequently, CMT is often classified into three categories: (1) sternocleidomastoid tumor (SMT), when a definitive mass or tumor is palpable within the SCM muscle; (2) muscular torticollis (MT), when contracture of the SCM muscle is present but no palpable mass is present; and (3) positional torticollis (POST), when both contracture of the SCM muscle and a palpable mass are absent.[48,49]

The "Back to Sleep" program initiated by the American Academy of Pediatrics in 1992 to reduce the incidence of sudden infant death syndrome (SIDS) recommended sleeping in supine for infants.[50] Since the inception of this program, the incidence of plagiocephaly and positional torticollis has increased dramatically.[51–53] The torticollis associated with positional plagiocephaly develops as a secondary impairment from the plagiocephaly. This is the direct opposite of what is seen with CMT, where the plagiocephaly develops secondary to the persistent asymmetric positioning of the head. Ultimately, the treatment for positional torticollis would follow an approach very similar to that for CMT.

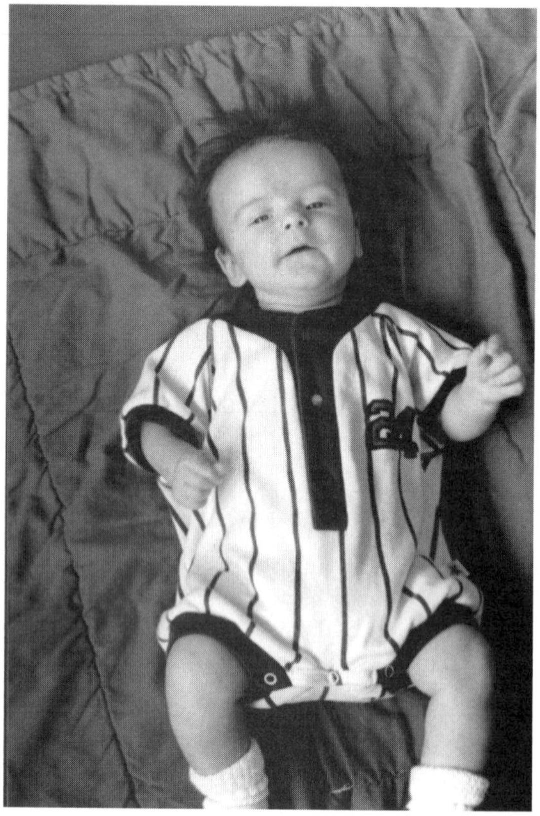

CONSERVATIVE MANAGEMENT

Conservative management of CMT is generally recommended during the first 12 months. Conservative management includes prolonged passive stretching of the sternocleidomastoid muscle through positioning and handling, active cervical ROM with subsequent strengthening exercises, and symmetric developmental activities to correct the infant's head position. Several studies have demonstrated the success of conservative management during the first year. Morrison and MacEwen achieved good to excellent results in 84% of patients diagnosed before 1 year of age.[45] Binder et al. reported complete resolution in 70% of children treated before 1 year of age regardless of the severity or the presence of a fibrotic mass. Of the 15 children who underwent surgery, seven had severe CMT and had been referred for treatment after 12 months of age.[44] Persistent facial asymmetry, intermittent head tilt with fatigue or illness, and functional asymmetry resembling hemiplegia but with a normal neurologic examination have been observed in children with full resolution, indicating the complexity of this disorder as well as possible long-lasting implications.[44] Emory's study of 101 infants with CMT further supports the use of conservative management in children younger than 1 year of age, with full recovery reported for 99% of the infants. Further delineation was made for duration of treatment in which infants with a fibrotic mass required 6.9 months of treatment compared with 4.7 months for children without a

Figure 12.11 ■ Infant with a resolving congenital muscular torticollis. Note the facial asymmetry in the region of his mandible.

mass to achieve full resolution.[46] Taylor and Norton obtained good to excellent outcomes in 22 out of 23 infants with CMT after an average of 3.8 treatment sessions. Their treatment sessions also included prolonged passive stretching of the SCM through positioning and strengthening activities for the weaker muscles.[54] None of these studies included a control group to assist with determining the extent of time and maturation on the resolution of the CMT.

Conservative management consisted of specific physical therapy intervention in both Binder's and Emory's studies. Physical therapy intervention included passive stretching of the sternocleidomastoid and upper trapezius muscles on the involved side, active rotation of the head toward the involved side, and handling and positioning during feeding and sleeping to promote active rotation or stretch of the sternocleidomastoid muscle. At 3 to 4 months of age, lateral neck flexion to strengthen the lengthened sternocleidomastoid muscle on the uninvolved side was initiated through developmental activities such as head righting and rolling. Several authors recommend limiting the passive stretching to prolonged stretches through positioning to avoid the pain associated with passive ROM and the possibility of producing micro-trauma of the soft tissues, resulting in further fibrosis.[49,54] A treatment strategy algorithm based on age and cervical ROM was developed by Van Vlimmeren and colleagues based on the evidence currently available in the literature.[49]

ORTHOTIC DEVICES

An orthotic device may be beneficial for infants and young children with torticollis that is not responding to conservative treatment. The goal for use of an orthotic device is to help maintain cervical ROM or limit the ability to tilt toward the involved side. The TOT collar (tubular orthosis for torticollis) is a soft tubular collar with struts of varying lengths that are positioned to elongate targeted muscles and limit motion in the opposite direction (Fig. 12.12). The TOT collar is recommended for infants at least 4 months old who have a consistent head tilt of 5 degrees or greater for more than 80% of the day and perform all movements with a head tilt. Appropriate candidates for use of the TOT collar must also exhibit a minimum of 10 degrees of lateral neck flexion toward the noninvolved side or demonstrate the ability to laterally flex the head away from the involved side.[55] Orthotic devices should only be used when the child is awake and supervised.

Plagiocephaly resulting from positioning should be treated in early infancy with a cranial orthosis aimed to correct the cranial–facial asymmetry. There are many devices available commercially and through local vendors, but the dynamic orthotic cranioplasty (DOC) band was the first cranial device approved by the Food and Drug Administration (FDA) (Fig. 12.13). The DOC band is a cranial band that applies pressure to the anterior and posterior

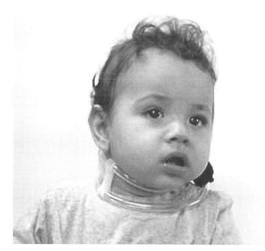

Figure 12.12 ■ Infant with left-sided congenital muscular torticollis wearing a TOT (tubular orthosis for torticollis) collar. (Photo courtesy of Symmetric Designs Ltd.)

prominences of the cranium but allows growth in the flattened areas. Other authors report the successful use of custom-molded helmets to facilitate symmetry of the cranium.[56–58] A DOC band or molding helmet is generally recommended between 3 and 4 months and not for children older than 12 months of age. The band or helmet is initially worn 23 to 24 hours per day and only while sleeping once symmetry is achieved.

It is difficult to draw conclusions for the use of helmets or DOC bands to correct plagiocephaly as the population is not always defined and the time periods for treatment vary greatly. The studies often do not differentiate between plagiocephaly resulting from CMT or positional plagiocephaly, and therefore the length of the time for helmet

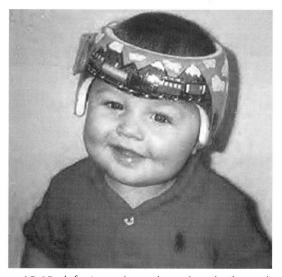

Figure 12.13 ■ Infant wearing a dynamic orthotic cranioplasty (DOC) band to correct plagiocephaly. (Photo courtesy of Cranial Technologies, Inc.)

versus no helmet intervention is very varied. The outcome scores vary greatly, ranging from a cosmetic score assigned by the parents to anthropometric measurements.

SURGICAL MANAGEMENT

Surgical treatment is indicated for infants with CMT that does not respond after 6 months of conservative treatment, who present with a residual head tilt, and who exhibit deficits of passive rotation and lateral flexion of the neck greater than 15 degrees.[48] The need for surgical intervention can also be predicted based on the classification of CMT. Cheng and colleagues followed 821 infants with CMT classified as SMT, MT and postural torticollis (PT). Surgery was needed for 8% of the infants in the SMT group, 3% in the MT, and none in the PT group.

Surgical intervention usually involves release of the muscle distally at one or both of the heads, depending on the severity; excision of a portion of the muscle may also be indicated.[23] Postoperatively, physical therapy is indicated for achieving and maintaining cervical ROM and for strengthening of musculature to maintain newly achieved alignment of the head.

CMT, if left untreated, either by conservative management or surgical intervention, may lead to increased facial and cranial asymmetries secondary to abnormal growth of soft tissues, including the sternocleidomastoid muscle and surrounding fascia and vessels. The development of a cervical scoliosis with compensatory thoracic curvature as well as ocular and vestibular impairments have been reported in cases of unresolved CMT.[23,47]

CONGENITAL METATARSUS ADDUCTUS AND CLUBFOOT DEFORMITY

Metatarsus adductus is characterized by adduction of the forefoot in relation to the midfoot and hindfoot. The lateral border of the foot is convex with the curve beginning at the base of the fifth metatarsal.[59] Metatarsus adductus is an example of a deformation caused by intrauterine positioning and is associated with other positional deformations, such as congenital muscular torticollis and dysplasia of the hip.[60]

Metatarsus adductus is classified as mild with clinical correction of the forefoot to neutral and beyond, moderate with correction of the forefoot to midline, or severe when the forefoot is rigid and any correction toward midline is not possible.[61] Severe metatarsus adductus may also be referred to as metatarsus varus and may include medial subluxation of the tarsometatarsal joint.[23]

Mild metatarsus adductus resolves spontaneously without treatment by 4 to 6 months of age.[62,63] Infants with moderate or severe metatarsus adductus should be treated with serial casting until a flexible forefoot with proper alignment is achieved.[62] The height of the serial cast may need to extend above the knee to control any tibial rotation.

Clubfoot, or congenital talipes equinovarus, is a complex deformity involving ankle plantar flexion, hindfoot varus, and forefoot adduction. The incidence is 1 per 1000 live births, but the etiology is unclear.[59] Intrauterine positioning may be a causative factor in milder forms or when a primary neuromuscular impairment, such as myelomeningocele or arthrogryposis, is present. In the latter cases, decreased or absent fetal movement secondary to the primary neuromuscular impairment could lead to prolonged abnormal fetal positioning and the resultant clubfoot deformity at birth.

In the severe forms of congenital talipes equinovarus, pathologic deformities in the anatomy and alignment of the bony and cartilaginous structures of the foot are present. The muscles are also hypoplastic, giving an overall smaller appearance to both the foot and lower leg on the involved side. The etiology may be a defect in the mesenchymal cells forming the template for the cartilaginous model of the hindfoot structures, indicating a dysplasia rather than a deformation.[23,64] More recently, researchers have begun to suspect a genetic link to idiopathic clubfoot.[65,66]

The goal of treatment for congenital clubfoot is to restore alignment and correct the deformity as much as possible and to provide a mobile foot for normal function and weight bearing. Initial treatment is begun shortly after birth and consists of splinting or casting. The cast must address the forefoot adduction, hindfoot varus, and ankle plantar flexion deformities but differing opinions exist as to which deformity should be addressed first.[23,62,67] Ideally, the cast extends above the knee to limit any rotary compensation from the tibia. Casting should continue until the foot is plantigrade and adequate alignment is documented by radiograph, improvement in foot position has ceased, or progress is very slow. Approximately one-third of infants with clubfoot deformity can be successfully managed with serial casting alone.[63] However, if dislocation of the talocalcaneonavicular joint is present, surgical reduction is warranted.[23]

Surgical correction is usually performed before 6 months of age to limit the extent of secondary deformities from developing. The surgical procedure is dependent on the age of the child and the severity of the deformity but typically includes releases of the tight structures to promote realignment of the foot and ankle. Postoperatively, the infant or child may wear a night splint to maintain correction.

DEVELOPMENTAL DYSPLASIA OF THE HIP

Developmental dysplasia of the hip (DDH) is a term used to cover a broad spectrum of hip anomalies in infants and young children that result from abnormal growth and development of the joint. The etiology of DDH most likely includes multiple factors, such as malposition and mechanical factors in utero, hormone-induced ligamentous laxity, genetics, and cultural or environmental factors. Malposition and mechanical factors include breech presentation in which the fetus hip lies against the mother's sacrum and a small intrauterine space. Cultures that swaddle their infants or use cradle boards that maintain the infant's hips in extension have higher incidences of DDH.[2] The incidence of DDH is very variable and is dependent on environmental factors, age of diagnosis, and inclusion criteria for the diagnosis of DDH.[23] However, the incidence of DDH increases in infants with other congenital deformations, such as torticollis or metatarsus adductus.[60,68]

During early fetal development, the acetabulum is very deep and the femoral head is spherical. Consequently, the femoral head is well covered by the acetabulum and the hip is a stable joint. With fetal growth and development, the acetabulum increases in diameter and becomes shallower, providing less coverage for the femoral head. The shallow acetabulum, less rounded femoral head, and increased femoral anteversion values present normally in infants at birth result in a very unstable hip. In the immediate postnatal period, depth of the acetabulum increases relative to diameter, producing a more stable ball-and-socket joint. The increased movement available to the newborn creates modeling forces that deepen the acetabulum as growth occurs. The most significant acetabular growth occurs during the first 18 months and minimal acetabular growth occurs after 3 years of age.[2]

Any interference with the normal growth and development of the hip joint may result in DDH. Interference can include abnormal forces resulting from positioning and confined space in utero, positioning that restricts normal kicking movements postnatally, and abnormal or absent muscle pull in utero and postnatally. The timing of these factors impacts the severity of the joint changes. DDH, which results from malpositioning late in the last trimester, shows less anatomic changes and responds quickly to intervention compared with an infant whose hip development was affected early in fetal life. DDH in a newborn can be classified as subluxatable, dislocatable, subluxed, or dislocated (see Table 12.1).

TABLE 12.1

Classification of Newborn Infant's Hips

Classification	Criteria
Normal	No instability of hip joint
Subluxatable	Femoral head within the acetabulum but can be partially displaced out from under the acetabulum
Dislocatable	Femoral head within the acetabulum but can be fully dislocated using the Barlow maneuver
Subluxed	Femoral head rests partially out of the acetabulum but can be reduced
Dislocated	Femoral head is completely out of the acetabulum

ASSESSMENT

Newborn screening for DDH includes the Ortolani test and the Barlow maneuvers (Fig. 12.14A,B). Both of these tests are more reliable when the infant is calm and not crying and before 2 months of age. A crying infant tenses the soft tissues surrounding the hip joint and prevents the examiner from observing any joint laxity or instability. As the infant grows, the unstable hip either remains in the acetabulum through normal development or remains outside the acetabulum and is prevented from relocating. Therefore, the Ortolani and Barlow maneuvers are much less reliable for infants older than 2 to 3 months of age.[23,62] Additional signs that may be noted in the newborn period include asymmetry of thigh or gluteal folds, limitation of hip abduction ROM or asymmetric hip abduction ROM, and apparent unequal femoral lengths, referred to as Galeazzi's sign. These signs become strong indicators of DDH in the older infant when the Ortolani or Barlow maneuvers are no longer reliable. In older children who are ambulatory, DDH is usually diagnosed by an abnormal gait pattern. Children with unilateral DDH exhibit a positive Trendelenburg sign, and children with bilateral DDH walk with a waddle.[23,62]

When DDH is suspected from your assessment, the infant is referred for an ultrasound or radiography dependent on his or her age. Ultrasound is used for young infants when ossification of the femoral head is minimal and would not be detected on radiography. Any time an infant is referred for physical therapy, regardless of diagnosis, hip stability should be assessed. If risk factors are present, such as breech presentation or other congenital deformities, and your assessment is normal, the infant may still benefit from a referral for an ultrasound to confirm that DDH is not present.

MANAGEMENT

The aim of treatment is to return the femoral head to its normal relationship within the acetabulum and to maintain this relationship until the abnormal changes reverse.[68] The earlier the treatment is initiated, the less abnormal changes are present in the structures of the hip joint and the less time is needed for the structures to return to their normal relationship. Treatment regimens will vary slightly between facilities and preference of the physician, but the same general concepts are followed in the management of infants and children with DDH.

NEWBORN TO 6 MONTHS
The goal of treatment is to maintain the femoral head within the acetabulum. An orthosis, typically the Pavlik harness, is used to maintain the infant's hips in a flexed and abducted position.

The Pavlik harness consists of a shoulder harness with two anterior and two posterior straps, stirrups for the legs, and booties to secure the feet (Fig. 12.15). In the Pavlik harness the infant's hips are flexed 90 to 100 degrees,

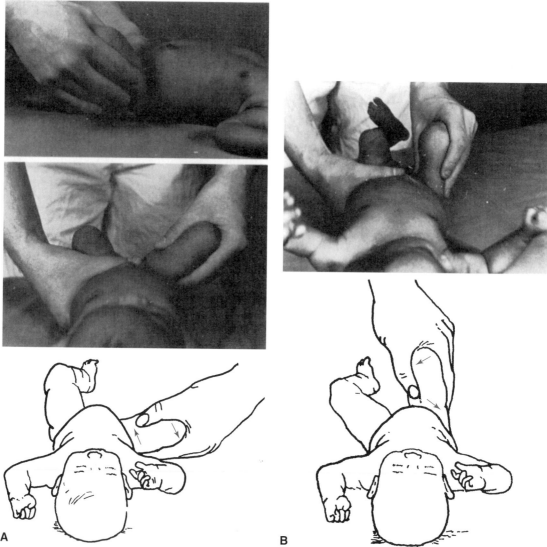

Figure 12.14 ■ **(A)** The Ortolani maneuver. From a flexed and adduced position, the hip is abducted; the examiner feels a clunk as the femoral head moves into the socket. The examiner's other hand stabilizes the infant's pelvis. **(B)** The Barlow test. The examiner holds the infant's hip in flexion and slight abduction. The infant's hip is adduced while applying pressure in a posterior direction. Dislocation of the femoral head with pressure indicates an unstable hip.

which locates the femoral head in the acetabulum. With the infant in supine, the hips are allowed to fall into abduction; they are not forced into abduction. The abducted position stretches the hip adductor muscles and allows the femoral head to slide over the posterior rim into the acetabulum. The anterior and posterior straps permit active hip flexion and abduction but limit hip extension and adduction. Therefore, the Pavlik harness has a dynamic component that promotes active movement and modeling of the hip joint.

The Pavlik harness is worn 24 hours a day until the hip is stable; full-time use of the harness is continued after stability is achieved, and then a period of weaning out of the harness is instituted. The child's progress must be closely monitored to detect complications or decide alternative treatments if hip stability is not developing.

Complications that can develop with the use of the Pavlik harness include avascular necrosis of the femoral head, femoral nerve palsy, and inferior dislocation.[23,69] These complications can be avoided through regular monitoring of the child's hips, parent or caregiver education, and proper fit of the harness. At many centers, the physical therapist works with the orthopedist and instructs the family in proper donning and doffing of the Pavlik harness. In an outpatient facility, an infant you are treating for another impairment may be wearing a Pavlik harness. It is imperative that the physical therapist be knowledgeable in the fitting of the Pavlik harness and recognize signs of ill-fit when he or she is working with these infants.

6 TO 12 MONTHS After 6 months of age, it may become more difficult to relocate the femoral head in the acetabu-

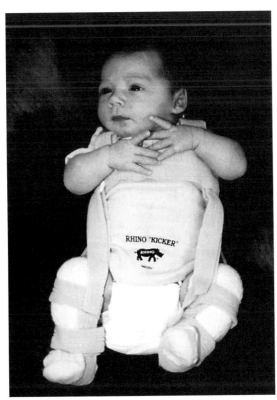

Figure 12.15 ■ The Pavlik harness maintains the infant's hips in flexion and allows active movement of the hips into abduction. (Photo courtesy of RhinPediatric Orthopedic Design, Inc.)

lum. Traction for a period of time may be attempted to relocate the hip and then institute wearing of the Pavlik harness. If the child is ambulatory, an abduction orthosis may be more practical than a Pavlik harness. Closed reduction under anesthesia may be required with the application of a hip spica cast to maintain the hip in the located position.[23]

AFTER 12 MONTHS Rarely will the child's hip be able to be relocated without surgical intervention. Conservative methods, such as home traction followed by closed reduction, may be attempted before a surgical procedure. Surgical correction may include release of tight soft tissue structures or osteotomy of the proximal femur to allow the femoral head to move into the acetabulum. Older children may require removal of a portion of the femoral shaft to reduce the forces on the femoral head when it is relocated in the acetabulum, femoral osteotomy, or acetabular osteotomy to aid in relocating the femoral head.[23,62]

ARTHROGRYPOSIS MULTIPLEX CONGENITA

Arthrogryposis multiplex congenita (AMC), also referred to as multiple congenital contracture (MCC), is a nonprogressive disorder characterized by multiple joint contractures and muscle weakness or imbalance. The reported incidence of AMC varies from 1 in 3000 to 1 in 4000 live births.[70,71] The disorder is related to a paucity of movement early in fetal development, leading to multiple contractures at birth. The exact etiology is unknown but is probably multifactorial. AMC is associated with multiple neurogenic or myopathic disorders that exhibit a defect in the motor unit including the anterior horn cells, roots, peripheral nerve, motor end plates, or muscle, resulting in weakness and decreased fetal movement early in development. Fetal immobility results in multiple joint contractures, fibrosis of muscles, and fibrosis of the periarticular structures.[71,72]

There is much variability among infants with AMC; however, common clinical features are generally present. These features include (1) featureless extremities that are often cylindric in shape with absent skin creases; (2) rigid joints with significant contractures; (3) dislocation of joints, especially the hips; (4) atrophy and even absence of muscle groups; and (5) intact sensation, although deep tendon reflexes (DTRs) may be diminished or absent.[71] The infant's contractures are usually symmetric and typically include shoulder internal rotation, elbow flexion or extension, wrist flexion with ulnar deviation, hip flexion with either internal rotation or a frog-legged posture, knee flexion or extension, and equinovarus deformities of the feet (Fig. 12.16).[23]

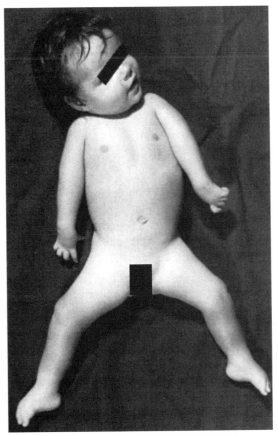

Figure 12.16 ■ Arthrogryposis multiplex congenita in an infant. The shoulders are internally rotated and adducted, and the elbows and wrists are extended. The hips are flexed, externally rotated, and abducted, and the feet demonstrate talipes equinocavus.

MANAGEMENT

Intervention requires multiple disciplines working toward the same goal and timeline. The goal of intervention is to achieve the maximum functional level for each child. Treatment techniques include passive stretching through positioning, casting and splinting, strengthening activities, developmental skills, surgical procedures, and the use of adapted or rehabilitation equipment. The family is crucial in planning the long-term goals for the child and assisting with the carryover of activities.

INFANCY Positioning and passive stretching exercises should begin shortly after birth. Serial casting begins in the first few months for foot deformities, knee flexion contractures, and wrist flexion contractures. Caution must be used to stretch only to the end range and maintain the stretch with a cast or splint. Forceful aggressive stretching of a rigid joint can result in damage to the joint capsule and surrounding soft tissues.[23] Any gains in ROM must be maintained with a splint or positioning device, or the contracture will recur.

Usually between 6 and 12 months of age, residual contractures at the feet and knees are surgically corrected.[62] Surgical correction involves release of the tight joint capsule and soft tissues. Surgical correction is maintained by splinting, strengthening exercises, and active functional movement. For example, a child who had a bilateral release of posterior structures of the ankle to correct an equinovarus deformity should have a splint fabricated to maintain the ROM as well as begin a standing program with the use of a standing device or ambulation aid.

The goals of intervention for the child's upper extremities must be well planned. For optimum function and independence with self-care skills, the child should have the ability to flex and extend the elbows. If this is not possible, treatment should aim to ensure that one elbow is able to flex for feeding activities and that the other elbow is able to extend for reaching and toileting activities.

During this age range, the child should develop some mobility skills. Rolling is often difficult secondary to the lower extremity contractures. Some children may learn to scoot on the floor on their belly or their back initially. Most children can learn to sit but have difficulty achieving the sitting position independently. From sitting, floor mobility should be encouraged. Creeping on hands and knees is often difficult, and children often learn to scoot on their bottom. Pulling to stand may be limited by contractures of the lower extremity. Surgical techniques should be timed to prepare the child to stand when the child is developmentally ready. Preambulation activities should begin before 1 year of age.

12 MONTHS THROUGH PRESCHOOL The goal of treatment during this age range is to develop the maximum level of independence with mobility and self-care skills. Ambulation is possible for many children with AMC and

should be considered a viable goal until proven otherwise. Upper extremity skills focus on feeding and dressing activities. Maintenance of acquired ROM is crucial, as are continued gains in ROM. Strengthening exercises through age-appropriate activities, as well as specific mobility training, are incorporated into the program.

SCHOOL AGE The school-age time period often highlights the functional impairments that may exist for a child with AMC. The child's ambulation speed may be slow compared with his or her peers, and fine motor difficulty may interfere with writing speed and clarity. Adaptive and rehabilitation equipment may be necessary to assist the child with functioning independently in the school setting and maintaining social interaction with his or her peers.

Postnatal Deformations

Deformations can also occur postnatally secondary to the immaturity of the musculoskeletal system of a growing and developing child. The effect of growth on the musculoskeletal system can be used to correct prenatal deformities, such as seen in the treatment rationale for congenital muscular torticollis or metatarsus adductus. However, the effect of growth can also produce additional deformities postnatally if a force is abnormal or unopposed.

ROTATIONAL DEFORMITIES

The variation of a child's rotational profile that occurs with normal growth and development produces many questions for parents and subsequent visits to an orthopedist or a physical therapist. The child with a rotational variation presents with either an in-toed or out-toed gait. Clarification on what is a true normal rotational variation, when the rotation becomes a deformity, and appropriate assessment and intervention are necessary to answer parents' questions, recognize true problems, and possibly impact those problems. The causative factors of the in-toeing or out-toeing must be evaluated and the rotational components measured using Staheli's rotational profile outlined earlier in the chapter. Staheli's rotational profile includes foot–progression angle as an overall measure, hip rotation ROM to assess femoral torsion, TFA to assess tibial torsion and the hindfoot, angle of the TMA to assess the distal tibia, and the configuration of the foot. The measurements can then be compared with the normative values to determine whether the child falls within the range of normal for his or her age and which component or components of the lower extremity are contributing to the in-toed or out-toed gait pattern (see Fig. 12.2).

FPA shows the greatest variability in infancy before leveling off to a mean of 10 degrees with a range of −3 to 20 degrees in childhood. Hip rotation ROM is divided into medial and lateral rotation of the hip and is a clinical measure to assess femoral torsion. The sum of medial and lateral hip rotation is approximately 100 degrees and slightly more in infants.[73] Lateral rotation of the hip is greater than medial rotation in infants secondary to tightness of soft tissues from intrauterine positioning. Femoral anteversion is present in infancy but is not as noticeable because of the infant's position of lateral rotation. Femoral anteversion is usually noticeable in young children but continues to decrease from infancy throughout childhood. Persistent femoral anteversion may be classified as a rotational deformity when the following values exist: mild if medial rotation is 70 to 80 degrees and lateral rotation is 10 to 20 degrees, moderate if medial rotation is 80 to 90 degrees and lateral rotation is 0 to 10 degrees, and severe if medial rotation is greater than 90 degrees and no lateral rotation is present.[73] The TFA increases from a negative angle in infancy to a positive angle throughout childhood. The angle of the TMA also increases from infancy through childhood. The tibia is medially rotated in infancy secondary to intrauterine positioning. Derotation of the tibia toward the normal lateral tibial torsion values in adulthood occurs normally through growth and development.

Infants and young children exhibit greater femoral anteversion and medial tibial torsion that gradually decrease through normal growth and development. An in-toeing gait is most common during the second year after the child begins to walk. If the measured values fall outside the two standard deviation values for normal, a rotational deformity exists. Intervention is necessary only if that rotational deformity is cosmetically unappealing for the child or adolescent or if the deformity interferes with function.[73]

Previously, treatment has included exercise, bracing, shoe modifications, and orthopedic correction. Studies have shown that shoe modifications are ineffective in correcting in-toeing problems.[23,74] Various orthotic devices, such as the Denis Browne bar or twister cables, have not been shown to be effective and may actually cause secondary deformities at the knee.[63] Orthopedic surgery consisting of a femoral or tibial osteotomy may be indicated for children who exhibit deformities greater than three standard deviations from the normal values and when the deformity interferes with function or is cosmetically an issue for the child.

◆ Dysplasias

A dysplasia is an abnormal organization of cells into tissue that leads to abnormal tissue differentiation.[6,25] Children born with a dysplasia exhibit widespread involvement because the abnormal tissue differentiation is present wherever the tissue is present.

OSTEOGENESIS IMPERFECTA

OI is a congenital disorder of collagen synthesis that affects all connective tissue in the body and occurs with an inci-

dence of from 1 in 20,000 to 1 in 30,000.[75] The musculoskeletal involvement is diffuse and includes osteoporosis with excessive fractures, bowing of long bones, spinal deformities, muscle weakness, and ligamentous laxity.[75–77] In addition to the musculoskeletal involvement, other clinical features of children with OI may include blue sclera, dentinogenesis imperfecta, hearing loss, growth deficiency, cardiopulmonary abnormalities, easy bruising, excessive sweating, and loose or dislocated joints[75] (Fig. 12.17).

The clinical presentation of children with OI varies greatly and may be of genetic origin or a spontaneous mutation. Silence developed a classification system based on genetic, clinical, and radiographic findings that broadly divides OI into four groups, type I through type IV[78] (Table 12.2). Children classified as OI Silence type I to VI have a very heterogeneous clinical presentation as well as a wide range functional abilities. Many reports in the literature will break down the Silence types into subgroups labeled OI IIB or OI VIA. Several authors have further delineated the Silence classification to include additional OI types V, VI, and VII.[79–82] The specific characteristics for OI types I to VII are outlined in Table 12.2.

Binder et al.[77] developed a classification system based on body size and limb proportions and their expected functional outcomes (Table 12.3). Consequently, physical therapy interventions can then be aimed at potential musculoskeletal deformities that presently interfere with the child's expected functional abilities or at preventing those deformities from developing.

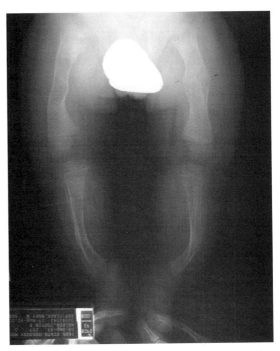

Figure 12.17 ■ Radiograph of 13-month-old child with type III osteogenesis imperfecta. Note the poor bone density, previous fracture sites, bowing of the bones, and the length of the femurs in relation to the tibias.

TABLE 12.2

Classification of Osteogenesis Imperfecta (OI)

Type*	Severity	Inheritance	Characteristics	Mobility Status
I	Mildest form of OI	Autosomal dominant	Blue sclera, dentinogenesis imperfecta, fewer bone fractures and progressive deformity, mild short stature or normal height	Ambulatory—may use an orthotic device
II	Lethal in perinatal period	Autosomal dominant	Severe bone fragility with multiple rib and long bone fractures at birth. Bones are "crumpled"; ribs may be beaded	Not applicable
III	Severe form	Autosomal dominant or recessive	Blue or normal sclera, dentinogenesis imperfecta, variable bone fragility but often severe, progressive skeletal deformity, scoliosis, very short stature	Variable; may be ambulatory with assistive device and orthotic devices, may use wheelchair for all or partial mobility
IV	Moderate	Autosomal dominant	Gray or normal sclera, dentinogenesis imperfecta, moderate fragility of bones, scoliosis, moderate short stature	Often independent at home and community with or without assistive device
V	Moderate	Autosomal dominant pattern	Normal sclera and teeth, abnormalities of forearm including frequent dislocation of radial head, calcification of interosseous membrane, moderate to severe bone fragility, mild to moderate short stature	Ambulatory
VI	Moderate	Autosomal dominant	Normal sclera and teeth, often see vertebral compression fractures, more fractures than seen in type IV but at birth, scoliosis, moderately short stature	May be ambulatory or use wheelchair
VII	Moderate	Autosomal recessive	Blue sclera, normal teeth, moderate bone fragility with fractures at birth, very short humeri and femurs with coax vara, mild short stature	May be ambulatory or use wheelchair

*Types I to IV are based on Sillence classification system. Types V, VI, and VII are newer types that have been added to the classification of OI by Rauch and Glorieux.

MANAGEMENT

PHARMACOLOGIC Several pharmacologic and vitamin supplements have been studied in an attempt to decrease the fragility of the bones of children with OI. These agents have included calcitonin, fluoride, hormones, and vitamins C and D. All of these interventions have been shown to be ineffective in preventing fractures.[75]

More recently, drugs from the bisphosphonate family such as pamidronate and alendronate have been administered to children and adults with OI to improve their bone density. Bisphosphonates act to inhibit osteoclast activity and have been used in postmenopausal women to decrease osteoporosis. Bisphosphonates can be administered orally or intravenously at cyclic periods. Oral administration of bisphosphonates has been shown to be effective in reducing the fracture rate and improving bone density, improving the functional status of some subjects, and improving subjective well-being in children with OI types I, III, and IV.[83–85] Due to the position restrictions after administration of oral bisphosphonates, cyclic IV administration has been utilized and has found to be effective in improving bone density, especially vertebral body; decreasing back pain; improving sense of well-being; and improving function.[86–88] Unanswered questions at this time regarding use of bisphosphonates include how long the child should receive the medications, whether the results are reversed if the medication is stopped, and which patients should receive the medications.

ORTHOPEDIC Fractures are managed with a soft splint or fiberglass cast for immobilization. The period of immobilization is kept short to minimize the bone demineralization that normally occurs with inactivity. Frequent fractures can lead to further demineralization, refractures, and bony deformity, specifically bowing of the long bones. Muscle pull on long bones can also cause significant anterior bowing of the long bones of the lower extremity.[75] Osteotomy and intramedullary rod fixation may be used to correct bowing deformities to facilitate use of orthotic devices and standing programs as well as to provide support to the bones to decrease the fracture rate.

TABLE 12.3

Functional Classification for Osteogenesis Imperfecta and Focus of Rehabilitation

Type	Physical Characteristics	Functional Expectations	Focus of Rehabilitation Interventions
A	Most severely involved group Large head relative to body, very short stature, bowing of long bones with joint contractures and weakness May have severe scoliosis and/or vertebral compression fractures	Dependent for ADLs except for feeding May use manual wheelchair; more likely to use power wheelchair	Positioning, including molded seating systems, therapeutic water activities Soft tissue mobilization to increase shoulder and MCP joint ROM and soft tissue mobilization techniques to alleviate back pain
B	Severe short stature, high incidence of femoral bowing, scoliosis, hip flexion contractures Strength generally at least 3/5	Stand and/or ambulate with assistive devices and braces Partial independence with ADLs Contractures of hips and shoulders and limited forearm supination interfere with function	Posture and active ROM exercises aimed at limiting contractures Strengthening with emphasis on abdominals, hip extensors and abductors, and quadriceps Endurance through swimming and biking, developmental activities through normal sequence Many children will not crawl but scoot in sitting
C	Less growth deficiency, poor LE alignment including hip abduction and external rotation contractures Joint laxity with LE valgus and pronation of the feet Strength of 3/5 or greater, poor endurance	Community ambulation with or without orthotic devices Independent with ADLs	Strengthening exercises with weights *proximal* on limb Conditioning exercise to improve endurance and long-distance ambulation May use orthotic devices for alignment but all orthotic devices should be articulated

ADLs, activities of daily living; LE, lower extremity; MCP, metacarpophalangeal; ROM, range of motion.
From Binder H, Conway A, Gerber LH. Rehabilitation approaches to children with osteogenesis imperfecta: a ten-year experience. Arch Phys Med Rehabil 1993;74:386–390.

REHABILITATION Several practitioners from the Children's Hospital Medical Center, Washington, DC, and the National Institutes of Health have developed and revised a rehabilitation protocol for children with OI.[75-77,89] Much of this information is now published in a book with clear explanations of exercises from early infancy through gaining independence for adolescents.[90] Due to the wide variability among children with OI, the protocol is meant to serve as a guideline and must be individualized for each child and family. The goals for the child with severe OI are to (1) prevent deformities of the head, spine, and extremities; (2) avert cardiorespiratory compromise by avoiding constant positioning in supine; and (3) maximize the child's ability to move actively.[76] These goals are based on the theory that muscle strengthening and weight-bearing programs for upper and lower extremities promote active earlier use of the extremities and may lead to increased bone mineralization and less severe musculoskeletal deformities.[76,89]

Instruction in handling of an infant with OI is crucial for all parents and caregivers. The infant should be held with the head and trunk fully supported. For infants with severe OI, caregivers may be more comfortable holding the child on a pillow. Careful positioning of an infant with OI should begin in the first few days after birth with instruction from a knowledgeable physical therapist. Positioning aims to align the infant's head, trunk, and extremities and to protect the infant from hitting hard surfaces with activity. Emphasis is on midline orientation of the head and position changes to prevent the development of a laterally tilted head and misshapen skull. Active movement is encouraged as beginning strengthening exercises.

Strengthening activities progress from active movement to playing with lightweight toys and rattles. Active movement can be further encouraged in water either at bath time or in a swim program with the parent present. Standard active-assistive and resistive exercises can be incorporated as the child becomes a little older. Emphasis is also placed on the development of head control and head righting in a variety of positions because children with OI often have a very large head. Developmental activities such as prone skills and rolling are encouraged. Independent sitting is encouraged when developmentally appropriate, as is some type of floor mobility. Those children who do not have the ability to develop independent sitting skills should be fitted for a custom-molded seat to promote head and trunk alignment and afford the child the opportunity to play in an upright position. Throughout the developmental progression, increasing or maintaining ROM and strength, especially of the pelvic girdle, is incorporated into activities.

Children should be fitted with orthoses when they have developed independent sitting skills and balance and are beginning to pull to stand. Those children who cannot sit independently but have developed head control should be fitted for a standing frame. The orthoses recommended in the protocol are containment or clamshell hip–knee–ankle–foot orthoses (HKAFOs).[76,90] Clamshell orthoses are similar to standard HKAFOs except that a contoured anterior shell is present to support the thigh and lower leg. Gait training begins with an assistive device and may or may not progress to independent ambulation without an assistive device. With ambulation and upright positioning, attention must be directed to the pelvic girdle. Hip flexion contractures often develop, and children with OI typically require ongoing strengthening of their hip extensors and abductors.[90]

Children who may not develop independent functional ambulation should be fitted with a manual or power wheelchair as appropriate. Positioning remains key with any seating system and attention is given to head and trunk alignment.

In a 10-year follow-up report, Binder and colleagues emphasized the need for rehabilitation to focus on the child's functional needs.[77] These key rehabilitation strategies are outlined in Table 12.3. Binder et al. reported progress with functional skills in all groups of children with OI, ranging from improved head control to community ambulation. Progress appears related to severity of the disease but should be expected for all children with OI if the goals address functional needs. Those factors that impair independence include joint contractures and muscle weakness for those children with severe forms of OI and endurance capabilities for those children with less severe forms of OI.

 Traumatic Injuries

AMPUTATION

The cause of traumatic amputations in the pediatric population varies according to age and geographic location. Accidents involving farm machinery and power tools are the leading causes of traumatic amputations in pediatrics, followed closely by vehicular accidents, gunshot wounds, and railroad accidents.[91,92] Lawn mowers and household accidents account for most amputations in the 1- to 4-year-old population, whereas vehicular accidents, gunshot wounds, and power tools and machinery are common causes of traumatic amputations in the older child. As a comparison, acquired amputations from both trauma and disease account for 40% of childhood amputations, whereas congenital limb deficiencies account for 60% of childhood

amputations. The highest incidence for traumatic amputations is in the 12- to 16-year-old age range.[91]

MANAGEMENT

The general management principles utilized with adults with amputations can be applied to children with amputations, with a few exceptions. The immature musculoskeletal system of the child offers advantages and disadvantages when managing traumatic amputations. Children tolerate surgical procedures that include skin grafts or closure of the wound under tension because they present with an adequate blood supply as compared with an adult with peripheral vascular disease. The use of skin grafts may allow preservation of limb length rather than amputation at a higher level without use of a skin graft.

Preservation of limb length is crucial not only for use of a prosthesis, but also to ensure continued growth of the limb. Amputation results in loss of physes and therefore limits the amount of possible growth from the affected limb. The physes at the shoulder and wrist account for the majority of growth in the upper extremity, whereas the physes around the knee contribute to the majority of growth in the lower extremity.[91]

Amputation through the midshaft of a long bone may result in terminal overgrowth. Terminal overgrowth is a painful, spike-like prominence of appositional bone growth on the transected end of the residual limb. The result is significant pain that interferes with weight bearing and use of a prosthesis. Terminal overgrowth occurs most frequently in the humerus, followed by the fibula, tibia, and femur.[91] When a child or adolescent complains of pain at the distal end of his or her residual limb, immediate consideration should be given to terminal overgrowth. On palpation, the body prominence may be felt and will elicit increased pain. The child should be referred to his or her orthopedist; the use of the prosthesis may need to be temporarily stopped to avoid further pain and the development of skin breakdown. Surgical correction for terminal overgrowth includes revision of the residual limb and, at times, capping of the distal end with an allograft for frequent recurrences.

PROSTHETIC TRAINING

Most children are fitted with an immediate-fit prosthesis in the operating room to control edema and begin early gait training. For those children who sustained significant trauma to the surrounding tissue or if a skin graft was necessary, an immediate-fit prosthesis is not used. Without an immediate-fit prosthesis, attention must be given to wrapping of the residual limb to control edema and help shape the distal end. Immediately postoperatively, education must begin for positioning to prevent contractures, especially hip and knee flexion and hip abduction contractures.

Gait training begins postoperatively, and weight-bearing status is dependent on the physician. Initial gait training may be begun with a walker but should progress to crutches for most children over 6 years of age. Crutches will allow the development of a reciprocal gait pattern easier than most walkers. Many children will progress to ambulation without an assistive device depending on the level of their amputation.

Many prosthetic options are now available for the pediatric population ranging from passive terminal devices to myoelectrics for upper extremity amputations, to energy-storing feet and modular component systems for the lower extremity. An in-depth review of prosthetics is beyond the scope of this introductory discussion of pediatric amputations. Refer to the earlier section in this chapter on congenital limb deficiencies for general guidelines regarding prosthetic training for various ages.

Pathologic Processes

Pathologic processes are a broad category of conditions that are abnormal and may impact the developing and growing musculoskeletal system of a child. These processes are varied in their origin and may include vascular, infectious, metabolic, mechanical, traumatic, or structural.

LEGG-CALVÉ-PERTHES DISEASE

Legg-Calvé-Perthes disease is a self-limiting disease of the hip initiated by avascular necrosis of the femoral head. The precise cause of the avascular necrosis that disrupts blood flow to the capital femoral epiphysis is not known. Trauma, transient synovitis, infection, congenital or developmental vascular irregularities, and thrombotic vascular insults have all been theorized as producing the avascular necrosis of the femoral head.[94] The disease typically occurs between 3 and 13 years of age, with boys affected three to five times more frequently than girls. Legg-Calvé-Perthes disease is most commonly seen in boys between 5 and 7 years of age. Bilateral presentation is seen in 10% to 20% of children with the disease.[23,95]

Legg-Calvé-Perthes disease progresses through four clearly defined stages: (1) condensation; (2) fragmentation; (3) reossification; and (4) remodeling. During the initial phase a portion or all of the femoral head becomes necrotic and bone growth ceases. The necrotic bone is resorbed and fragmented; at this time revascularization of the femoral head is initiated. During this second stage, the femoral head often becomes deformed and the acetabulum becomes flattened in response to the deformity of the femoral head. With revascularization, the femoral head begins to reossify. As the femoral head grows, remodeling of both the femoral head and the acetabulum occur.[94,96] The stage of the disease at the time of diagnosis, sex of the child, and age at onset impact the final outcome and congruency of the hip joint.

There are several classification systems aimed at assisting with predicting outcomes of children with Legg-Calvé-Perthes disease. Catterall's classification is divided into four categories and is based on the severity of femoral head involvement.[96] This classification has been widely used but has been shown to have poor interobserver reliability.[97] Herring et al. developed a classification system that is based on the involvement of the lateral aspect of the femoral head. They found this lateral pillar classification to demonstrate good to excellent reliability among users.[97]

Clinically, children with Legg-Calvé-Perthes disease present with a limp and pain referred to the groin, thigh, or knee.[23,95] If the condition is undetected, hip ROM limitations may develop with restrictions in hip internal rotation and abduction, a hip flexion contracture may be present, and a Trendelenburg-type gait may be observed. Muscle spasm of the hip adductors and iliopsoas may also be noted.[94,95] Children who may present to a physical therapist with the preceding symptoms and unknown etiology should be referred to a pediatric orthopedist.

MANAGEMENT

The goals of treatment are to relieve the symptoms of pain and muscle spasm, contain the femoral head in the acetabulum while bone remodeling occurs, and restore ROM. Treatment for relief of pain includes anti-inflammatory medications, traction, and partial weight bearing with the use of crutches. Containment of the femoral head may be achieved through the use of traction, orthotic devices such as a Petrie cast or Scottish-Rite orthosis, or surgical procedures such as a femoral or innominate osteotomy (Figs. 12.18 and 12.19).

If an orthotic device has been used as the method of femoral head containment, it may need to be used for a prolonged period of time, up to 1 to 2 years. While wearing the orthosis and after healing, physical therapy is often

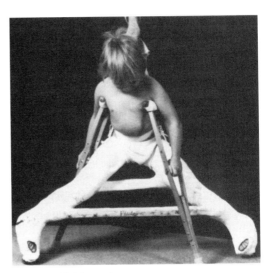

Figure 12.18 ■ Petrie cast.

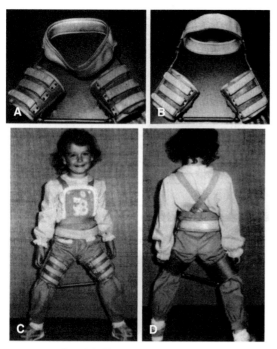

Figure 12.19 ■ Scottish-Rite orthosis. The abduction bar contains a swivel joint that allows reciprocal motion of the legs.

warranted to address ROM limitations and strength deficits. After removal of the orthotic device, children may continue to walk with a Trendelenburg-type gait because of weakness of their hip extensors and hip abductors. Physical therapy after surgical intervention focuses on gait training and restoration of hip ROM and strength.

A recent prospective multicenter study compared five different treatment options: no treatment, brace treatment, ROM exercise, femoral osteotomy, and innominate osteotomy.[98] The investigators found that the revised lateral pillar classification developed by Herring and colleagues and the age of onset were the strongest predictors of outcomes. Children who are under 8 years of age at the time of onset and have minimal involvement of the lateral aspect of their femoral head have very favorable outcomes regardless of the type of treatment received. Children who have complete collapse of the lateral aspect of their femoral head have poor outcomes that are linked to the type of treatment received. However, children who are over the age of 8 years at the time of onset and have moderate involvement of the lateral aspect of the femoral head have improved outcomes with either surgical intervention compared to the nonsurgical interventions.

SLIPPED CAPITAL FEMORAL EPIPHYSIS

Slipped capital femoral epiphysis (SCFE) occurs when the femoral head slips, or is displaced, from its normal alignment with the femoral neck. Excessive stresses on the growth plate are thought to contribute to the displacement of the femoral head. Stresses may include mechani-

cal problems such as excessive weight, torsional forces secondary to trauma, or weakness of the growth plate secondary to sudden growth. The incidence of SCFE varies according to age, sex, and race. The incidence is higher in males and the African-American population, and is often associated with the onset of puberty.[99,100] Bilateral occurrence is present in 22% of young adolescents.

SCFE is classified by both duration of symptoms and radiographic findings. Acute SCFE is defined as a sudden onset of painful symptoms of less than 3 weeks' duration, whereas chronic SCFE is characterized by a gradual onset of symptoms for greater than 3 weeks. The third type is acute-on-chronic SCFE with a history of mild pain for greater than 3 weeks and a recent sudden exacerbation of symptoms.[99] Classification according to the severity of the displacement of the femoral head is defined as follows: grade I, displacement of the femoral head up to one-third of the width of the femoral neck; grade II, greater than one-third but less than one-half displacement; and grade III, displacement greater than one-half (Fig. 12.20).[23]

Clinical presentation of young adolescents with SCFE includes pain in the groin, medial thigh, or knee; limping; external rotation of the leg; and limited hip ROM, especially flexion, abduction, and internal rotation.[63] External rotation is noted with attempts to flex the affected hip. With an acute onset, pain is often severe and the adolescent is unable to bear weight on the affected lower extremity. History may include a traumatic or gradual onset. If an undiagnosed young adolescent presents to physical therapy with the preceding symptoms, he or she should be immediately referred to a pediatric orthopedist for further workup.

MANAGEMENT

The goals of treatment include stabilization of the growth plate to prevent further displacement and prevention of complications, including avascular necrosis, chondrolysis, and early osteoarthritis.[23,101] Stabilization is achieved through surgical pin fixation. Nonsurgical treatment, including bedrest, traction, and casting, have not been successful with long-term outcomes of limited hip ROM, pain, and surgical procedures necessitated by early osteoarthritis. Physical therapy includes gait training with an assistive device postsurgically; weight-bearing status is usually non–weight bearing during the acute recovery period.

TIBIA VARA (BLOUNT'S DISEASE)

Tibia vara, or Blount's disease, is a growth disorder of the medial aspect of the proximal tibia, including the epiphysis, epiphyseal plate, and metaphysis.[23] Tibia vara is classified as three types, depending on the age of onset: (1) infantile, less than 3 years of age; (2) juvenile, between 4 and 10 years of age; and (3) adolescent, 11 years of age or older.[102] Diagnostic radiographic changes include sharp varus angulation in the metaphysis, beaking of the medial tibial meta-

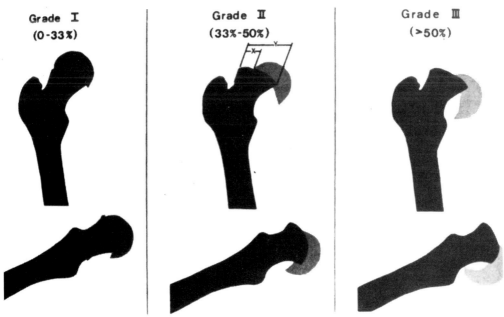

Figure 12.20 ■ Classification of the three grades of slipped capital femoral epiphysis.

physis, wedging of the medial epiphysis, widening of the growth plate, and the presence of cartilage islands in or near the metaphyseal beak (Fig. 12.21).[103] This growth disturbance is thought to be the result of asymmetric excessive compressive and shear forces across the proximal tibial growth plate.[23,104]

Clinically, the child with tibia vara presents with a bowlegged stance. Infantile tibia vara must be distinguished from normal physiologic genu varum and medial tibial torsion. Physiologic genu varum gradually decreases until a genu valgus alignment is present between 2.5 and 3 years of age. Toddlers with tibia vara are often obese, are often early walkers, and may exhibit a lateral thrust of the knee during stance.[23,105] Tibia vara increases in severity, whereas physiologic genu varum decreases as the child grows and develops. Other diagnoses that must be ruled out include various skeletal dysplasias, rickets or vitamin D deficiency, or a fracture that involved the growth plate of the proximal medial tibia. Juvenile or adolescent tibia vara may result from infection or trauma that disrupted growth of the proximal medial tibia.

MANAGEMENT

Treatment is dependent on the age of the child and the stage of the disease. Langenskiöld differentiated tibia vara into six stages with guidelines for prognosis and intervention.[106] Stage I occurs between 18 months and 3 years of age, and is characterized by beaking of the medial metaphysis and delay in growth of the medial epiphysis of the tibia. The stages progress in severity until stage VI. Stage VI is seen between 10 and 13 years of age and is characterized by fusion of the medial aspect of the epiphyseal plate while growth continues laterally.[23,103,106]

Treatment options include orthotic devices or surgical procedures. Orthotic intervention is recommended for children under 2 to 3 years of age with radiographic findings consistent with stage I or II. An HKAFO is recommended to be worn 23 hours a day.[103,105] Valgus correction of the orthosis is increased every 2 months. Physical therapy intervention may include family instruction in donning and doffing the orthosis, development of a wearing schedule, and instruction in skin inspection while the orthosis is used. Gait training with or without an assistive device may also be warranted.

After the age of 4 years, surgical options produce better outcomes than orthotic devices.[103] Tibial osteotomy is indicated for children under 5 years of age and for those toddlers who present with more advanced stages of tibia vara. After age 5 years, additional surgical procedures other than a tibial osteotomy are often indicated. The disease has often progressed to the more advanced stages and surgical options, such as a lateral epiphysiodesis or removal of a medial bony bridge, may be necessary.[105]

LIMB LENGTH DISCREPANCY

A limb length discrepancy may be caused by shortening or overgrowth of one or more bones of the leg. Inequality of leg lengths may result from congenital conditions such as limb deficiencies or hemihypertrophy, infections or fractures that injure the physis, neuromuscular disorders, tumors, or trauma that results in overgrowth and disease processes. Injuries to the physes are often asymmetric and result in angular deformities in addition to the shortening of the affected limb. Leg length differences range from 1 to 10 cm or greater.

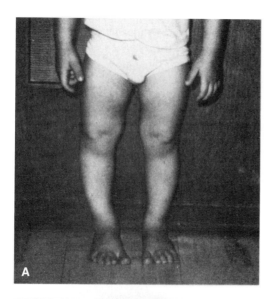

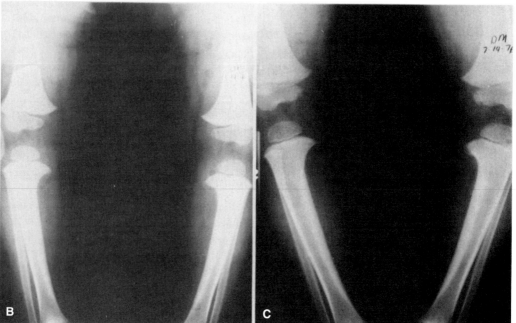

Figure 12.21 ■ **(A)** A 2-year-old child with varus on weight bearing. **(B)** A radiograph of the same child at 2 years of age showing early Blount's disease. **(C)** Same child at 2 years of age and progression of the Blount's disease; note the varus angulation and beaking of the medial tibial metaphysis.

Measurements must be taken when a leg length difference is suspected. Clinical measurements can be taken by placing blocks of known height under the shorter leg or by measuring from the medial malleolus to the anterior superior iliac spine. The pelvis must be level prior to recording of measurements. More precise measurements are needed to predict the leg length discrepancy that will be present at maturity, evaluate treatment options, and predict the timing of surgical intervention if necessary. To assist with prediction of future growth and treatment options, the orthopedist uses radiographic methods to obtain accurate measurements and determine bone age, and uses growth charts to predict future skeletal growth of the child.

Intervention is generally not indicated for leg length differences of less than 2 cm.[23] A lift inside the shoe may be used for differences of 1 to 2 cm. Significant leg length discrepancies are a cosmetic as well as functional issue. Gait is less efficient and awkward, and postural compensations of the pelvis and spine often develop. Postural compensations may not lead to a structural deformity, but they may cause discomfort in adulthood.

MANAGEMENT

Treatment is dependent on the age of the child and growth remaining, severity of the leg length difference, and preference of the family and child. Surgical treatment options involve either shortening of the longer limb or lengthening of the shorter limb. Limb shortening is commonly achieved through epiphysiodesis. The predetermined physes are surgically destroyed by the physician to arrest growth in the longer leg. Epiphysiodesis is indicated for leg length discrepancies of 2 to 5 cm.[23,63] Most physicians opt for lengthening the shorter limb when the discrepancy is greater than 5 cm.

If the adolescent has reached skeletal maturity and epiphysiodesis is not an option, shortening of the longer limb can be accomplished through osteotomy. A portion of the bone is removed to equalize leg lengths; 5 to 6 cm is the maximum for removal in the femur and 2 to 4 cm is the maximum for the tibia. The disadvantages of shortening by osteotomy are the reduction in overall height of the individual, body proportions may be cosmetically unappealing, the amount of equalization is limited, and the uninvolved leg has undergone surgery.

Limb-lengthening techniques are directed at the involved leg and allow for equalization of greater discrepancies. Limb lengthening may be indicated for discrepancies greater than 5 cm.[23] Limb-lengthening techniques involve either metaphyseal or diaphyseal distraction and are based on the principles of fixation of the fragments to allow vascular ingrowth; the distraction rate correlates to the osteogenic activity and goals of minimal disruption of intramedullary vessels and the periosteum.[23,63] The Wagner and Ilizarov methods are two lengthening techniques used in pediatrics.

The Wagner technique utilizes the principle of diaphyseal lengthening. An osteotomy is performed followed by rapid distraction of the bone that is stabilized through an external device. When the desired length is achieved, the external device is removed and internal fixation and bone grafting are performed to support the gap in the bone. When the gap is filled through new bone growth, the internal fixation is removed. The Wagner method is relatively quick, depending on the length to be achieved and the number of external pins is minimal. However, the entire process involves three operative procedures and cannot be used to correct angular or rotational deformities.

The Ilizarov method utilizes metaphyseal lengthening and involves a corticotomy rather than an osteotomy. Circular rings are placed above and below the level of the corticotomy and are attached to the bone through multiple pins existing in the skin. The rings are connected by telescoping rods with a dial (Fig. 12.22). The dial is turned to provide a slow distraction force that keeps pace with the body's ability to lay down new bone. Postoperatively, the distraction rate is 1 mm/day performed in increments of 0.25 mm four times a day.[63] After the desired length is achieved, the external fixator device is kept in place until bone consolidation is complete. The pins are then removed without the need for an additional operative procedure. The Ilizarov method is used to correct angular and

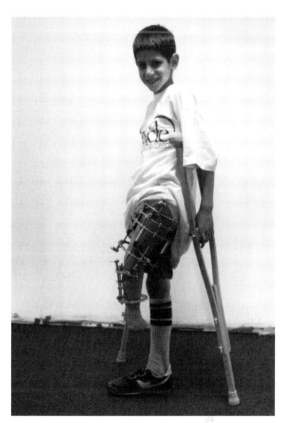

Figure 12.22 ■ A 9-year-old boy with a diagnosis of proximal femoral focal deficiency who is presently undergoing an Ilizarov lengthening. The lengthening will provide a longer level arm when wearing his prosthesis and bring the height of his knees closer together.

rotational components of limb leg discrepancies. The disadvantages of the Ilizarov method are the multiple pin sites, bulkiness of the apparatus, and the length of time required to achieve the desired length.

Limb-lengthening procedures bring their own set of problems to the child, family, and professionals involved in the care of the child. Families must be able to make multiple appointments over a period of time, perform daily pin care, and carry out exercise programs. Problems that may be encountered during the course of a lengthening procedure include infection at the pin sites, joint stiffness, subluxation or dislocation (especially of the proximal tibia), nonunion, and fractures. The rate of distraction with the Ilizarov method is meant to keep pace with bone growth and therefore minimize the complications of nonunion and fracture. With both techniques, ROM limitations occur secondary to shortening of the soft tissues and the rate of soft tissue growth compared with that of bone.

PHYSICAL THERAPY

Immediately after surgery, the physical therapist is involved for gait-training activities and promoting early weight bearing for most children who have undergone the

Ilizarov procedure. Instruction in pin care must also begin immediately postoperatively. Joint ROM limitations occur but should be minimized. Ankle dorsiflexion ROM is often difficult to maintain. Preventive splinting should be implemented early on to maintain the ankle in a planti-grade position. Knee flexion and extension ROM can also become limited. Again, splinting can be implemented to maintain a prolonged stretch on the soft tissues. Muscle weakness is also usually present as the muscles lengthen to accommodate the new limb length. Strengthening exercises should begin early on and continue throughout the duration of the lengthening procedure.

SCOLIOSIS (IDIOPATHIC)

Scoliosis is a lateral curvature of the spine. Idiopathic denotes that the scoliosis is of unknown origin and is the most common form of scoliosis. Idiopathic scoliosis can be further delineated by age of onset: infantile occurs in children from birth to 3 years of age, juvenile occurs between the ages of 3 and 10 years, and adolescent develops after 10 years of age.[23] This section will focus on adolescent idiopathic scoliosis. The prevalence of idiopathic scoliosis in North America is 2% to 3% for curves 10 degrees or less and decreases to 0.2% to 0.3% for curves of 20 degrees or greater.[23,107]

Scoliosis is defined as either structural or nonstructural. Structural curves are fixed and do not correct with lateral trunk bending or traction. Structural curves have a rotary component that is visible when the trunk is flexed forward. Nonstructural curves correct on lateral trunk bending and often have as their etiology a pelvic obliquity, limb length discrepancy, or medical factors such as a tumor or muscle spasm. Structural scoliosis is further identified by the location and direction of the apex of the curve. For example, a curve with the apex in the thoracic region and convexity toward the right would be labeled as a right thoracic curve. Most curves have a primary curve and a compensatory curve. The compensatory curve is the body's attempt to keep the head and trunk aligned vertically. In the preceding example of the right thoracic curve, there may be smaller compensatory curves in the cervical or lumbar regions with their convexity toward the left (Fig. 12.23).

Multiple structural changes occur with scoliosis, and their severity is related to the severity of the curve.[23] Changes occur in the growing spine in response to compression and distraction forces that are altered in the presence of a curvature. The vertebrae become wedge shaped, higher on the convex side, and compressed on the concave side, and muscles on the concave side become shortened. The vertebral body rotates toward the convex side so that the spinous process is rotated toward the concave side. Because the ribs are attached to the thoracic vertebrae, they also rotate. The rotation of the ribs produces a rib hump posteriorly, which is noted on the forward-bend test (Fig. 12.24).

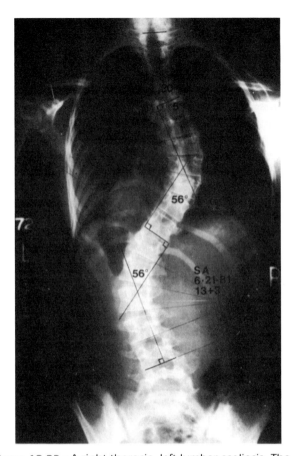

Figure 12.23 ■ A right thoracic, left lumbar scoliosis. The degree of curvature is measured using the Cobb method. The end vertebrae, or the vertebrae that tilts toward the concavity the most, are identified. Lines are drawn extending the end plate of the top and bottom vertebrae for each curve. Perpendicular lines to the end plate lines are then drawn. The degree of curvature is defined as the angle of the intersection of the end plate and perpendicular lines.

SCREENING

Screenings for scoliosis occur in many schools and target the early adolescent population between 10 and 15 years of age.[108] The goal of school screenings is early detection to limit progression of the curvature. A screening should include anterior and posterior views of the trunk with the shirt removed and a forward-bend test (Fig. 12.24). On the anterior and posterior views, the examiner is looking for asymmetries in shoulder, nipple, scapular, or pelvic heights; asymmetric folds of the trunk; and curvature of the spine. The adolescent is then asked to bend over, keeping the knees extended and allowing the arms to dangle toward the floor. During the forward-bend test, the examiner is looking for asymmetries in the contour of the back indicating a rotary component to the curvature.

When a scoliosis is detected, the adolescent should be referred to an orthopedist. Accurate measurement of the curve is performed through a variety of methods. A common method of measurement is a radiograph and the

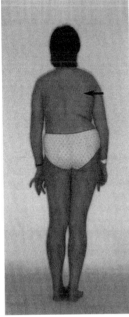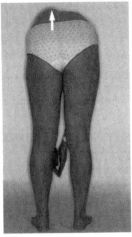

Figure 12.24 ■ Forward-bend test. Rib hump is visible on bending forward.

Cobb measure. To limit radiographic exposure, other measurement methods include Moire topography and the integrated shape investigation system (ISIS).[109] Moire topography is a photogrammetric technique that visually depicts shadow patterns that assess asymmetries. ISIS utilizes computer images in the transverse, frontal, and sagittal planes to develop contours of the adolescent's trunk. The goal of measurement is to determine a baseline and monitor progression of the curve.

MANAGEMENT OF SCOLIOSIS

Treatment intervention is based on the sex, age, and skeletal maturity of the adolescent and the severity of the curvature.[23,110] Young adolescents who are prepuberty are almost certain to exhibit progression of their curvature. Females with a bone age of 15.5 years and males with a bone age of 17.5 years generally do not require treatment. Curves less than 25 degrees can be observed on a regular basis to monitor progression of the curve. Curves between 25 and 40 degrees should be treated with nonsurgical methods. Adolescents with curves greater than 40 degrees are candidates for surgical intervention.

NONOPERATIVE MANAGEMENT The goal of nonoperative intervention is to maintain the curvature, not to correct the curvature. Nonoperative intervention methods have included exercise, electrical stimulation, and orthoses. Exercise or physical therapy has not been proven beneficial in reducing or altering the progression of a curvature. Exercise is indicated to maintain strength of muscles when an orthotic device is used. Electrical stimulation was attempted as a means of strengthening the paraspinal

muscles on the convex side of the curve but has been shown to be ineffective.[111]

Orthotic devices have been used in the treatment of scoliosis for many years. Most orthotic devices operate on the principle of three-point pressure against the apex of the curve and may also incorporate a traction component. The Milwaukee brace was one of the first orthotic devices developed for scoliosis. The orthosis consists of a collar that supports the chin and occiput and a pelvic component connected by metal uprights. Lateral pads are present in the pelvic component to provide pressure against the lumbar component of the curve and a thoracic pad is attached to a metal upright to provide pressure against the thoracic component of the curve.

Many orthoses presently incorporate a lower profile system that eliminates the chin and occiput component of the Milwaukee brace and are often referred to as a thoracic–lumbar–sacral orthosis (TLSO) (Fig. 12.25). The pelvic stabilization and lateral pressure pads are present in a TLSO. Adolescents are generally instructed to wear the orthosis between 18 and 23 hours a day until skeletal maturity or unless the curve continues to progress and surgery is indicated.

Instruction in donning and doffing the orthosis, developing a wearing schedule, skin care, and an exercise program to maintain ROM and strength while wearing the orthosis are provided by a physical therapist. Exercise should

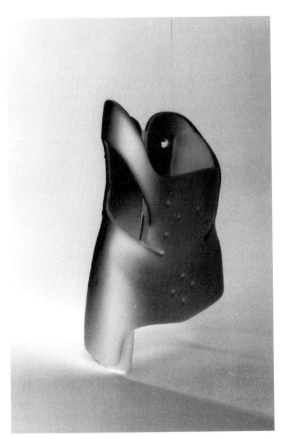

Figure 12.25 ■ Boston brace (thoracic–lumbar–sacral orthosis).

be focused on maintaining flexibility and muscle strength. Hip flexion contractures can develop with use of the orthosis; routine stretching of the hip flexors should be instituted when orthosis wearing is initiated. Muscle strength must be maintained while wearing the orthosis so that the trunk muscles are strong when the use of the orthosis is discontinued. Exercise should include strengthening for abdominals, gluteal muscles, and paraspinal musculature.

OPERATIVE MANAGEMENT Surgical intervention is warranted if the curve is greater than 40 degrees, the curve is progressing with conservative management, or there is decompensation of the spine or thoracic cavity.[23] The goal of surgery is to obtain as much correction as possible and to stabilize the spine and maintain the correction over time.

There are many types of instrumentation available, but the main principles of instrumentation are distraction and compression of the curve appropriately, correction or minimization of the rotary component, and stabilization of the spine to maintain the correction. Harrington rods, both a compression and a distraction rod, were the standard instrumentation for many years. Alterations have been made to the Harrington rods, and many other types of instrumentation have been introduced. Much of the instrumentation aims to maintain the normal lordotic and kyphotic curves of the spine, control the rotary component of the curve, and provide additional stability to the spine.

PHYSICAL THERAPY Ideally physical therapy has been involved preoperatively with ROM and trunk-strengthening exercises. Instruction in deep breathing and coughing exercises should be initiated preoperatively and adhered to immediately postoperatively. Depending on the instrumentation used, the adolescent is encouraged to begin early mobilization, including transfers and gait training. Time frames for ambulation depend on the instrumentation, surgeon's preference, and whether or not a supportive orthosis is needed.

SUMMARY

The growth and development of a child's musculoskeletal system were discussed in this chapter. The immature musculoskeletal system of a child is susceptible to abnormal forces and stresses. Physical therapists must be alert to those forces and the consequences they may have on an immature musculoskeletal system. Many orthopedic diagnoses were discussed in this chapter as examples of the effect of abnormal forces on the developing child and how those forces can at times be beneficial in treatment. However, the principles that were discussed and the assessment procedures that were outlined can be applied to any child seen by a physical therapist, not just those children with a diagnosis of orthopedic origin. Identifying potentially deforming forces and developing treatment protocol based on your findings is the challenging but very rewarding aspect of pediatric physical therapy.

REFERENCES

1. Crelin ES. Development of the musculoskeletal system. Clin Symp 1981;33:2–36.
2. Walker JM. Musculoskeletal development: a review. Phys Ther 1991;71:878–889.
3. Arkin AM, Katz JF. The effects of pressure on epiphyseal growth. J Bone Joint Surg Am 1956;38:1056–1076.
4. Storey E. Growth and remodeling of bone and bones. Dent Clin North Am 1975;19:443–454.
5. LeVeau BF, Bernhardt DB. Developmental biomechanics: effect of forces on the growth, development and maintenance of the human body. Phys Ther 1984;64:1874–1882.
6. Dunne KB, Clarren SK. The origin of prenatal and postnatal deformities. Pediatr Clin North Am 1986;33:1277–1297.
7. Haley SM, Tada WL, Carmichael EM. Spinal mobility in young children: a normative study. Phys Ther 1986;66:1697–1703.
8. Florence JM, Pandya S, King WM, et al. Clinical trials in Duchenne dystrophy: standardization and reliability of evaluation procedures. Phys Ther 1984;64:41–45.
9. Pandya S, Florence JM, King WM, et al. Reliability of goniometric measurements in patients with Duchenne muscular dystrophy. Phys Ther 1985;65:1339–1342.
10. Stuberg WA, Metcalf WK. Reliability of quantitative muscle testing in healthy children and in children with Duchenne muscular dystrophy using a hand-held dynamometer. Phys Ther 1988;68:977–982.
11. Bleck EE. Orthopedic Management in Cerebral Palsy. Philadelphia: JB Lippincott, 1987.
12. Donovan BM, Munson SH, Richtel A. Correlational analysis between goniometric values obtained from straight leg raise testing and a passive knee extension test for measurement of hamstring length. Unpublished Masters Thesis, Philadelphia College of Pharmacy & Science, February 1998.
13. Kendall FP, McCreary EK. Muscles: Testing and Function. Baltimore: Williams & Wilkins, 1993.
14. Merlini L, Dell'Accio D, Granata C. Reliability of dynamic strength knee muscle testing in children. J Sports Phys Ther 1995;22:73–76.
15. Beasley WC. Quantitative muscle testing: principles and applications to research and clinical services. Arch Phys Med Rehabil 1961;42:398–425.
16. Bohannon RW. Manual muscle test scores and dynamometer test scores of knee extension strength. Arch Phys Med Rehabil 1986;67:390–392.
17. Effgen SK, Brown DA. Long-term stability of hand-held dynamometric measurements in children who have myelomeningocele. Phys Ther 1992;72:458–465.
18. Hinderer K, Gutierrez T. Myometry measurements of children using isometric and eccentric methods of muscle testing (Abstract). Phys Ther 1988;68:817.
19. Stuberg WA, Koehler A, Wichita M, et al. Comparison of femoral torsion assessment using goniometry and computerized tomography. Pediatr Phys 1989;1:115–118.
20. Gajdosik CG. Ability of very young children to produce reliable isometric force measurements. Pediatr Phys Ther 2005;17(4):251–257.
21. Staheli LT, Corbett M, Wyss C, et al. Lower-extremity rotational problems in children. J Bone Joint Surg 1985;67A:39–47.
22. Cusick BD, Stuberg WA. Assessment of lower-extremity alignment in the transverse plane: implications for management of children with neuromotor dysfunction. Phys Ther 1992;72:3–15.
23. Tachdjian MO. Pediatric Orthopedics. 2nd Ed. Philadelphia: WB Saunders Co., 1990.

24. World Health Organization. International Classification of Functioning, Disability, and Health. Geneva, Switzerland: World Health Organization, 2001.

25. Spranger J, Benirschke JG, Hall W, et al. Errors of morphogenesis: concepts and terms. J Pediatr 1982;100:160–165.

26. Day HJB. The ISO/ISPO classification of congenital limb deficiency. Prosth Orthot Int 1991;15:67–69.

27. Wright PE, Jobe MT. Congenital anomalies of the hand. In: Canlae ST, Beaty JH, eds. Operative Pediatric Orthopedics. Philadelphia: Mosby–Year Book, 1991:253–330.

28. Swanson AB, Barsky AJ, Entin MA. Classification of limb malformations on the basis of embryological failures. Surg Clin North Am 1968;48:1169–1179.

29. Heikel HVA. Aplasia and hypoplasia of the radius. Acta Orthop Scand (Suppl) 1959;39:1.

30. Morrissy RT, Giavedoni BJ, Coulter-O'Berry C. The limb-deficient child. In: Lovell, WW, Winter, RB, eds. Pediatric Orthopedics. 5th Ed. Philadelphia: Lippincott Williams & Wilkins, 2001:1217–1272.

31. Aitken GT. Proximal femoral focal deficiency: definition, classification and management. In: Proximal Femoral Focal Deficiency: A Congenital Anomaly. Washington, DC: National Academy of Sciences, 1969:1–22.

32. Shurr DG, Cook TM. Prosthetics and Orthotics. East Norwalk, CT: Appleton & Lange, 1990:183–193.

33. Bayne LG, Klug MS. Long-term review of the surgical treatment of radial deficiencies. J Hand Surg Am 1987;12:169–179.

34. Herzenberg JE. Congenital limb deficiency and limb length discrepancy. In: Canale ST, Beaty JH, eds. Operative Pediatric Orthopedics. Philadelphia: Mosby–Year Book, 1991:187–252.

35. Kruger LM. Lower-limb deficiencies: surgical management. In: Bowker JH, Michael JW, eds. Atlas of Limb Prosthetics: Surgical, Prosthetic, and Rehabilitation Principles. Philadelphia: Mosby–Year Book, 1981:795–834.

36. Krajbich JL. Rotationplasty in the management of proximal femoral focal deficiency. In: Herring JA, Birch JG, eds. The Child with a Limb Deficiency. Rosemont, IL: American Academy of Orthopedic Surgeons, 1998:87.

37. Gillespie R. Principles of amputation surgery in children with longitudinal limb deficiencies of the femur. Clin Orthop Rel Res 1990;256:29–38.

38. DeVito D. Lengthening and Shortening Solutions of Lower Extremity Deficiencies. Presentation and handout at APTA Combined Sections Meeting, 1996.

39. Gover AM, McIvor J. Upper limb deficiencies in infants and young children. Infants Young Child 1992;5:58–72.

40. Cummings DR. Pediatric prosthetics, current trends and future possibilities. Phys Med Rehabil Clin N Am 2003;11:653–679.

41. Wilk B, Karol L, Halliday S, et al. Transition to an articulating knee prosthesis in pediatric amputees. J Prosthet Orthot 1999;11:69–74.

42. Coulter-O'Berry C. Physical therapy considerations in pediatric acquired and congenital lower limb amputees. In: Smith DG, Michael JW, Bowker JH, eds. Atlas of Amputations & Limb Deficiencies: Surgical, Prosthetic and Rehabilitation Principles. 3rd Ed. Rosemont, IL: American Academy of Orthopedic Surgeons, 2004:831.

43. Suzuki S, Yamamura T, Fujita A. Aetiological relationship between congenital torticollis and obstetrical paralysis. Int Orthop 1984;8:175–181.

44. Binder H, Eng GD, Gaiser JF, et al. Congenital muscular torticollis: results of conservative management with long-term follow-up in 85 cases. Arch Phys Med Rehabil 1987;68:222–225.

45. Morrison DL, MacEwen GD. Congenital muscular torticollis: observations regarding clinical findings, associated conditions, and results of treatment. J Pediatr Orthop 1982;2:500–505.

46. Emery C. The determinants of treatment duration for congenital muscular torticollis. Phys Ther 1994;74:921–929.

47. Bredenkamp JK, Hoover LA, Berke GS, et al. Congenital muscular torticollis. Arch Otolaryngol Head Neck Surg 1990;116:212–216.

48. Cheng JCY, Wong MWN, Tang SP, et al. Clinical determinants of the outcome of manual stretching in the treatment of congenital muscular torticollis in infants. J Bone Joint Surg 2001;83A(5):679–687.

49. Van Vlimmeren LA, Helders PJM, Van Adrichem LNA, et al. Torticollis and plagiocephaly in infancy: therapeutic strategies. Pediatr Rehabil 2006;9(1):40–46.

50. American Academy of Pediatrics. Changing concepts of sudden infant death syndrome: implications for infant sleeping environment and sleep position. Pediatrics 2000;105:650–656.

51. Kane AA, Mitchell LE, Craven KP, et al. Observations on a recent increase in plagiocephaly without synostosis. Pediatrics 1996;97:877–885.

52. Persing J, James H, Swanson J, et al. Prevention and management of positional skull deformities in infants. Pediatrics 2003;112:199–202.

53. De Chalain TM, Park S. Torticollis associated with positional plagiocephaly: a growing epidemic. J Craniofac Surg 2005;16(3):411–418.

54. Taylor JL, Norton ES. Developmental muscular torticollis: outcomes in young children treated by physical therapy. Pediatr Phys Ther 1997;9(4):173–178.

55. Jacques C, Karmel-Ross K. The use of splinting in conservative and post-operative treatment of congenital muscular torticollis. Phys Occup Ther Pediatr 1997;17:81–90.

56. Pollack IF, Losken HW, Fasick P. Diagnosis and management of posterior plagiocephaly. Pediatrics 1997;99:180–185.

57. Vles JSH, Colla C, Weber JW, et al. Helmet versus nonhelmet treatment in nonsynostotic positional posterior plagiocephaly. J Craniofac Surg 2000;11(6):572–574.

58. Loveday BPT, de Chalain TB. Active counterpositioning or orthotic device to treat positional plagiocephaly? J Craniofac Surg 2001;12:308–313.

59. Hensinger RN, Jones ET. Developmental orthopedics: the lower limb. Dev Med Child Neurol 1982;24:95–116.

60. Dunn PM. Congenital postural deformities. Br Med Bull 1976;32:71–76.

61. Bleck EE. Metatarsus adductus: classification and relationship to outcomes of treatment. J Pediatr Orthop 1983;3:2–9.

62. Beaty JH. Congenital anomalies of the lower and upper extremities. In: Canale ST, Beaty JH, eds. Operative Pediatric Orthopedics. Philadelphia: Mosby–Year Book, 1991:73–186.

63. Staheli LT. Fundamentals of Pediatric Orthopedics. Philadelphia: Lippincott-Raven, 1992.

64. Irani RN, Sherman MS. The pathological anatomy of idiopathic clubfoot. Clin Orthop Rel Res 1972;84:14–20.

65. Dietz F. The genetics of idiopathic clubfoot. Clin Orthop Rel Res 2002;401:39–48.

66. Lochmiller C, Johnston D, Scott A, et al. Genetic epidemiology study of idiopathic talipes quinovarus. Am J Med Genet 1998;79:90–96.

67. Lovell WW, Hancock CI. Treatment of congenital talipes equinovarus. Clin Orthop Rel Res 1970;70:79.

68. Hensinger RN. Congenital dislocation of the hip, treatment in infancy to walking age. Orthop Clin North Am 1987;18:597–616.

69. Mubarak MD, Garfin S, Vance R, et al. Pitfalls in the use of the Pavlik harness for treatment of congenital dysplasia, subluxation, and dislocation of the hip. J Bone Joint Surg Am 1981;63:1239–1247.

70. Darin N, Kimber E, Kroksmark A, et al. Multiple congenital contractures: birth prevalence, etiology, and outcome. J Pediatri 2002;140:61–67.

71. Thompson GH, Bilenker RM. Comprehensive management of arthrogryposis multiplex congenita. Clin Orthop Rel Res 1985; 194:6–14.

72. Banker BQ. Neuropathic aspects of arthrogryposis multiplex congenita. Clin Orthop Rel Res 1985;194:30–43.

73. Staheli LT. Torsional deformity. Pediatr Clin North Am 1977; 24:799–811.

74. Knittel G, Staheli LT. The effectiveness of shoe modifications for intoeing. Orthop Clin North Am 1976;7:1019–1024.

75. Marini JC. Osteogenesis imperfecta: comprehensive management. Adv Pediatr 1988;35:391–426.

76. Binder H, Hawks L, Graybill G, et al. Osteogenesis imperfecta: rehabilitation approach with infants and young children. Adv Pediatr 1984;65:537–541.

77. Binder H, Conway A, Gerber LH. Rehabilitation approaches to children with osteogenesis imperfecta: a ten-year experience. Arch Phys Med Rehabil 1993;74:386–390.

78. Sillence D. Osteogenesis imperfecta: an expanding panorama of variants. Clin Orthop Rel Res 1981;159:11–25.

79. Glorieux FH, Rauch F, Pltkin H, et al. Type V osteogenesis imperfecta: a new form of brittle bone disease. J Bone Miner Res 2000;15(9):1650–1658.

80. Glorieux FH, Ward LM, Rauch R, et al. Osteogenesis imperfecta type VI: a form of brittle bone disease with a mineralization effect. J Bone Miner Res 2002;17(1):30–38.

81. Ward LM, Rauch F, Travers R, et al. Osteogenesis imperfecta type VII: an autosomal recessive form of brittle bone disease. Bone 2002;31(1):12–18.

82. Rauch F, Glorieux FH. Osteogenesis imperfecta. Lancet 2004; 363:1377–1385.

83. Sakkers R, Kok D, Englebert RH, et al. Skeletal effects and functional outcome with olpadronate in children with osteogenesis imperfecta: a 2-year randomized, placebo-controlled study. Lancet 2004;363:1427–1431.

84. Cho TJ, Choi IH, Chung CY, et al. Efficacy of oral alendronate in children with osteogenesis imperfecta. J Pediatr Orthop 2005;25(5):607–612.

85. Seikaly MG, Kopanati S, Salhab N, et al. Impact of alendronate on quality of life in children with osteogenesis imperfecta. J Pediatr Orthop 2005;25(6):786–791.

86. Glorieux FH, Bishop NJ, Plotkin H, et al. Cyclic administration of pamidronate in children with severe osteogenesis imperfecta. N Engl J Med 1998;339:947–952.

87. Plotkin H, Rauch FH, Bishop NJ, et al. Pamidronate treatment of severe osteogenesis imperfecta in children under 3 years of age. J Clin Endocrinol Metab 2000;85:1846–1850.

88. Astrom E, Soderhall S. Beneficial effect of long term intravenous bisphosphonate treatment of osteogenesis imperfecta. Arch Dis Child 2002;86:356–364.

89. Gerber LH, Binder H, Weintrob J, et al. Rehabilitation of children and infants with osteogenesis imperfecta. Clin Orthop Rel Res 1990;251:254–262.

90. Cintas HL, Gerber LH. Children with Osteogenesis Imperfecta: Strategies to Enhance Performance. Gaithersburg, MD: Osteogenesis Imperfecta Foundation, Inc., 2005.

91. Tooms RE. Acquired amputations in children. In: Bowker JH, Michael JW, eds. Atlas of Limb Prosthetics: Surgical, Prosthetic and Rehabilitation Principles. St. Louis: Mosby, 1992:735–741.

92. Trautwein LC, Smith DG, Rivara FP. Pediatric amputation injuries: etiology, cost and outcome. J Trauma Inj Infect Crit Care 1996;41:831–838.

93. Herring JA, ed. Growth and development. In: Tachdjian's Pediatric Orthopedics. 3rd Ed. Philadelphia: WB Saunders, 2002:3–21.

94. Canale TS. Osteochondroses. In: Canale TS, Beaty JH, eds. Operative Pediatric Orthopedics. Philadelphia: Mosby–Year Book, 1991:743–775.

95. Wenger DR, Ward WT, Herring JA. Current concepts review: Legg-Calvé-Perthes disease. J Bone Joint Surg Am 1991;73: 778–788.

96. Catterall A. The natural history of Perthes disease. J Bone Joint Surg Br 1971;53:37–53.

97. Herring JA, Kim HT, Browne R. Legg-Calve-Perthes disease. Part I: classification of radiographs with use of the modified lateral pillar and Stulberg classifications. J Bone Joint Surg 2004; 86A(10):2103–2120.

98. Herring JA, Kim HT, Browne R. Legg-Calve-Perthes disease. Part II: prospective multicenter study of the effect of treatment on outcome. J Bone Joint Surg 2004;86A(10):2121–2134.

99. Aaronson DD, Loder RT. Treatment of the unstable (acute) slipped capital femoral epiphysis. Clin Orthop Rel Res 1996;322: 99–110.

100. Loder RT. The demographics of slipped capital femoral epiphysis: an international multicenter study. Clin Orthop Rel Res 1996;322:8–27.

101. Ordenberg G, Hansson IL, Sandstrom S. Slipped capital femoral epiphysis in southern Sweden: long-term result with closed reduction and hip plaster spica. Clin Orthop Rel Res 1987;220: 148–154.

102. Thompson GH, Carter JR. Late-onset tibia vara (Blount's disease). Clin Orthop Rel Res 1990;255:24–35.

103. Schoenecker PL, Meade WC, Pierron RL, et al. Blount's disease: a retrospective review and recommendations for treatment. J Pediatr Orthop 1985;5:181–186.

104. Carter JR, Leeson MC, Thompson GH, et al. Late-onset tibia vara: a histopathologic analysis, a comparative evaluation with infantile tibia vara and slipped capital femoral epiphysis. J Pediatr Orthop 1988;8:187.

105. Johnston CE. Infantile tibia vara. Clin Orthop Rel Res 1990; 255:13–23.

106. Langenskiöld A. Tibia vara: osteochondrosis deformans tibiae: a survey of 23 cases. Acta Chir Scand 1952;103:1–8.

107. Rogala EJ, Drummond DS, Gurr J. Scoliosis: incidence and natural history, a prospective epidemiological study. J Bone Joint Surg Am 1978;60:173–177.

108. Lonstein JE. Natural history and school screening for scoliosis. Orthop Clin North Am 1988;19:227–237.

109. Cassella MC, Hall JE. Current treatment approaches in the nonoperative and operative management of adolescent idiopathic scoliosis. Phys Ther 1991;71:897–909.

110. Hall JE. Nonoperative and Operative Management of Adolescent Idiopathic Scoliosis. Presented at APTA Combined Sections Meeting, February 1998.

111. Sullivan JA, Davidson R, Renshaw TS. Further evaluation of the scolitron treatment of idiopathic adolescent scoliosis. Spine. 1986;11:903–906.

Traumatic Disorders and Sports Injuries

Joe Molony and Donna Merckel

t is a natural part of growth and development for children to explore movement and challenge their bodies to acquire new motor skills. Some children are zealous in their achievement of these skills and climb the highest trees, swing quickly on the swings and monkey bars, and are thrilled by the speed of a fast bike or scooter. Others are tentative and cautious as they test the waters in exploration. In either case, accidents and falls are inevitable, causing traumatic childhood injuries.

As the rise in sports participation climbs to 30 million children, so has the incidence of sports-related injuries. Sports injuries include both traumatic and overuse conditions, accounting for about 25% of all childhood reported injuries.[1] As health care providers, it is our responsibility to unite with parents, coaches, and other health care disciplines to minimize and prevent injuries. Injuries are the most frequent reason for sports attrition.[2] Physical activity, whether it is playing in the backyard or on a sports field, is important in establishing a lifetime of good fitness practices. The risks of injury should not overshadow the positive psychological, social, and moral developments that can be achieved through sports activities.[2]

In treating childhood injuries, health care workers need to be cognizant that children are not just "little" adults. Besides suffering from different injuries due to their immature musculoskeletal system, children and adolescents have different psychosocial needs and pressures that can escalate a minor injury into a traumatic event. In our society today, the large financial rewards achieved by college and professional athletes often create large pressures on the young athlete to become a star. It takes a multidisciplinary team to provide optimal and appropriate care for the young athlete.

This chapter will provide basic knowledge in recognition and treatment of common pediatric (child and adolescent) traumatic and sports injuries. Omitted from the chapter are emergency care of these injuries, dermatology, nutrition, and first aid for skin abrasions, blisters, and wounds. Specializing in sports physical therapy requires the knowledge base of these content areas to provide comprehensive care for the young athlete.

 Tissue Response to Injury

OVERVIEW OF INFLAMMATION AND REPAIR

Inherent in the concept of traumatic disorders and sports injuries is the fact that healing must occur. Understanding the healing process of the various bodily tissues and how those processes differ between the mature and immature body is a cornerstone of effective treatment planning and clinical decision making. It is important to note that the inflammatory response does not always correlate with the severity of injury, and as such, an overexuberant response can occur. Early efforts to control inflammation can go very far in maximizing the rate and efficacy of recovery. Table 13.1 summarizes the inflammation and repair process as well as the goals of treatment for each phase. There is no significant tensile strength in this early phase of repair, yet, in order for a quality repair to be made, tension through

the injured tissue should be initiated to promote collagen deposition that parallels the tensile forces.[3,4]

ACUTE INFLAMMATORY PHASE

During the acute inflammatory phase of healing, the goals of intervention are to minimize atrophy, the loss of conditioning, the loss of range of motion (ROM), the loss of proprioception, and the development of edema, and to facilitate the development of a healthy repair. In some cases strict immobilization is necessary for proper tissue healing and may result in muscle atrophy. With the injured structure protected, it is important to maintain the athlete's conditioning level. Cross-training exercises can consist of nonimpact activities such as a stationary bike, aquatics, and circuit training. Typically, isometrics are performed in this stage and perhaps isotonics if the injury is minor or if they can be performed in a pain-free range. An example would be performing isotonics in a pain-free range for a grade 1 ankle sprain. In this example, strengthening can proceed without placing the injured structures at risk for disruption or adverse irritation. For a low grade 2 sprain, isometrics would be the most likely starting point once they could be performed with little to no pain. Isometrics most likely can be performed before isotonics and therefore allow earlier initiation of muscle activity. Note that generally speaking, when an injury occurs the impact is regional, not local. For instance, the hip abductors may become weak in the presence of an ankle sprain. This weakness can unfortunately then be augmented by diminished weight bearing.

Regarding flexibility and ROM during this stage, the primary goals are to protect the injured tissue structure

TABLE 13.1

Summary of Inflammation and Repair Process

Phase	Name	Time Frame	Activity	Treatment Goals
Phase 1	Acute vascular inflammatory phase	From onset of injury to 48–72 hr	Cell death Hematoma Clotting	Pain control Decrease edema Protect injured structures Minimize range-of-motion loss and atrophy
Phase 2	Repair and regeneration phase	Beginning 48–72 hr after injury and lasting up to 8 wk	Deposition of repair tissue (bone or type II collagen) Decreased tensile strength Removal of damaged tissue	Promote healthy repair via tissue loading
Phase 3	Remodeling and maturation phase	Beginning several weeks after injury and lasting up to or beyond 1 yr	Remodeling of bone Type I collagen deposition May be up to 30% weaker than original tissue	Promote full-strength repair

and promote quality healing. In the case of minor soft tissue injuries, gentle tension can be placed through the injured structure. These forces need to be sufficient to promote appropriate remodeling without damaging the tissue. The amount of appropriate tension can be gauged by the patient's response. Pain should be minimal and short lived after icing. The patient should not have significantly greater difficulty with function of the involved body part after stretching, and there should be no significant edema or effusion resulting from the activity. Joint pain should not be produced unless ROM is an issue and additional range needs to be obtained. In this case, the pain is related to the forces on the injured structures that are being stressed to prevent or reverse adherence. More significant injuries will need to be immobilized during this stage to allow for adequate healing. Examples would be a knee collateral ligament tear or a partial tendon rupture. In cases of significant injury, early motion may not be tolerated nor warranted.

REPAIR/REGENERATION PHASE

During the repair/regeneration phase the aggressiveness of exercise can be augmented. Again, if the injury is at the joint level, care must be taken not to enhance the inflammatory response for intra-articular injuries. If ROM is an issue, pain at the joint or muscle level is acceptable if tissue elongation is desired. Unfortunately, in this case pain will be necessary during this stage in order for quality recovery to occur. This will be the case with ROM and flexibility but generally not with strengthening. During strengthening for an intra-articular injury, there is rarely a reason to exercise in pain. If the injury is in the contractile element or tendon, pain may be a part of exercise at this stage. Placing forces through the injured structure facilitates proper collagen alignment along the vectors of force. If some level of discomfort is being obtained, then the injured tissue is receiving appropriate stress to stimulate this response. Too little stress will only promote a haphazard matrix of scar; too much stress will cause the structure to fail. Ensuring that the patient has only mild discomfort, which dissipates rapidly after icing, is the best way to ensure appropriate stress to the injured structure.

Generally speaking, concentric and eccentric exercises as well as tonic/isometric exercises, where appropriate, are utilized in this phase for all types of injuries. The key is to match the muscular contraction with the demands that will be placed upon those muscles in the athletes' daily lives and recreational endeavors, as mentioned previously.

REMODELING AND MATURATION PHASE

During the remodeling and maturation phase, high-intensity exercises of all modes are performed. At this point in the healing process, the injured structure is largely healed and can progressively tolerate normal loads. Exercise progression is gradual, systematic, and based upon the individual's response. Some discomfort may occur, but should be relieved by the next day. In the end the patient needs to demonstrate the ability to function in the situations that he or she may be subjected to in his or her daily life or recreation/sporting endeavors prior to discharge. The treating therapist needs to not only recreate these scenarios, but also verify that the patient is prepared for the duration of the activity as well.

As with all aspects of sports rehabilitation, reassessment needs to occur every visit. Children and adolescents heal more rapidly than adults, and as such their rate of progression in rehabilitation is more rapid, mandating this constant reassessment and adjustment/augmentation of the rehabilitation program.

BONE HEALING

During phase 1 bone needs to be immobilized to allow for healing. During phase 2 a bone callus forms within 2 weeks of the fracture through endochondral bone healing. This type of healing occurs during nonrigid immobilization (such as casting). At this time the callus does not have the strength of normal bone. At the beginning of phase 3, 4 to 8 weeks following the initial injury in a young individual, significant stresses can begin to be tolerated. The status of the healing and resultant ability to tolerate forces should be determined by radiography.

Remodeling occurs in the middle of the repair phase and lasts up to several years, long after clinical healing. During the remodeling phase the callus converts to woven bone. Through this process woven bone is replaced with lamellar bone. Of note is that in the presence of internal fixation, direct bone healing occurs, allowing deposition of woven bone without callus formation.[3]

SYNOVIUM

Normally only a few milliliters of synovial fluid exist in a joint. Reactive synovitis (resulting from an insult to a joint or surrounding tissues) will cause an outpouring of synovial fluid, which will create an effused joint. Note that effusion can also be caused by bleeding, as in the case of an anterior cruciate ligament (ACL) rupture. Therefore, in the presence of an effusion reactive synovitis versus bleeding is the differential diagnosis.

◆ Examination

A thorough history is extremely important for a pediatric athlete. It provides critical information for accurate diagnosis and treatment of the injury and can facilitate an athlete's safe and timely return to sport. Often pediatric patients are not accurate historians and additional input from a parent, coach, or medical staff covering the event may be necessary. Remember to ask if the child has hit his or her head during the fall or accident. See Displays 13.1 and 13.2 for a comprehensive list of information gathered during a subjective evaluation.

All recent changes should be noted. Knowing the athlete's playing position, level of player (recreational to elite), years of participation, and primary sport will not only help with assessment of the injury, but also provide needed information for rehabilitation for return to play. Nutritional information and other medical information, such as whether the patient has asthma, are important to know as they may have an impact on rehabilitation. A referral to a sports nutritionist or primary care provider may be necessary to help the athlete have a healthy return to sport and prevent future injuries. Discussion of the patient's goals and important upcoming events assists in structuring the rehabilitation process and provides a medium for appropriate goal setting for the practitioner and the athlete.

PHYSICAL ASSESSMENT

This section will provide additional objective evaluations that are specific to an athletic injury. Traditional evaluation procedures like ROM, strength, flexibility, edema, and discoloration are always necessary. It is important to evaluate the noninjured side of the body for a normal point of reference for these evaluation procedures. In addition to clearing the joint above and below the area of pain, a screen of the entire extremity, including the axial skeleton, is warranted to eliminate the possibility of referred pain or secondary injuries. Although the athlete appears to have suffered a sports injury, other pathologic reasons for pain need to be ruled out or considered. Proper evaluation attire is important for accurate assessment: shorts and a T-shirt with shoes off for a lower extremity injury and sports bra for girls with T-shirt off for an upper extremity injury. Palpation of bone landmarks, ligaments, and joint lines can help localize pain. It is often helpful to ask the patient to "point with one finger" to the spot that is most tender. Injury-specific special tests, which are used to evaluate adult sports injuries, are also implemented in the

pediatric population, such as the Speed's test for the shoulder or the anterior drawer test of the ankle and knee. Evaluation of hands and feet for blisters, calluses, and other signs of altered mechanics and/or overuse is important for equipment modification and recommendations.

Generalized ligament laxity should be assessed. The Beighton-Horan ligament laxity scale is one assessment tool[5] (Display 13.3). This test provides information about the hypermobility of the athlete's joint throughout various parts of his or her body: 0 of 9 is normal; 9 of 9 is highly lax. Biomechanical evaluation of the entire kinetic chain identifies sources of the pain, musculoskeletal malalignments, abnormal joint motion, muscle atrophy, and muscular weakness. The athlete should be evaluated both statically and dynamically. Note the differences in body positions at rest and then while moving. Functional tests provide information regarding balance, alignment, body awareness, strength, control, and core stability. Refer to Display 13.4 for lower extremity functional tests and Figure 13.1 for single-leg squatting correct and incorrect forms.

While the athlete is performing the functional test, the clinician is evaluating the quality of movement, not just the ability to perform the task. During single-leg squatting activities, the pelvis should remain parallel to the floor and the trunk vertical, not laterally flexed to one side or the other. The knee should remain in neutral alignment

---

Sports Nutrition Guidelines for the Young Athlete

Kimberly Cover, RD, LDN
Clinical Nutritionist
Sports Nutritionist
Attended Training in Child/Adol Wt Mgt
Eating Disorder Specialist
Children's Hospital of Philadelphia

Fielding nutrition questions for clients can be a daunting experience even for the health-food enthusiast. The practitioner working with young athletes should prioritize optimal growth and development at all times. Key nutrients for this age group include fluid, protein, carbohydrates (CHO), calcium and iron. Estimated needs will vary according to body weight, stage of development, condition of the athlete, age, sport, and the position played. Protein and CHO needs vary widely during adolescence. The following table delineates a wide range of nutritional requirements for a diverse, young athletic population.

Age of athlete in years		Fluid (oz/day)	Protein (gm/day)	CHO (gm/day)	Calcium (mg/day)	Iron (mg/day)
	4–8	40–45	14–52	130–210	800	10
Male	9–13	50–76	21–97	130–520	1300	8
	14–18	50–107	34–138	130–740	1300	11
Female	9–13	50–78	20–100	130–540	1300	8
	14–18	50–93	34–120	130–640	1300	15

Fluid: Basic fluid needs should be met each day. On top of this, fluid breaks should be mandatory as children are less efficient at dissipating heat. Extreme care should be taken with exercise on hot and humid days. Extra fluid may be needed on these days with an emphasis on water, milk, 100% fruit juice and or a commercial sports drink for practice and games.

Protein: Most Americans and athletes consume more protein than they need. Care should be taken with the adolescent athlete who chooses a vegetarian eating style, as this can develop into a disordered eating pattern that could progress to an eating disorder. High-protein foods include dairy products, meat, fish, poultry, eggs, legumes, nuts, and vegetarian soy meat analogues.

CHO: A key function of the CHO is to provide primary energy to exercising muscles and to spare protein from being used as an energy source. This allows muscle accretion and tissue repair to be prioritized. High CHO foods include milk, yogurt, whole grain breads/pasta/cereal, rice, fruit, legumes, and vegetables.

Calcium: Calcium is a core element and needs to be offered at all meals and at least one or two snacks per day. Adolescence represents a period of peak bone mass development. Adequate calcium is crucial to maximize bone density, especially in an athlete who presents with the female athlete triad. High-calcium foods include: dairy products, deep green vegetables, and certain legumes. There is a plethora of calcium-fortified foods available; look for foods with at least 20–30% calcium. Examples include tofu, orange juice, cereal/energy bars, and some brands of breads and margarines.

Iron: Because of an increase in blood volume and rapid growth during adolescence, iron-rich foods should be emphasized. These include meat, poultry, fish, sunflower seeds, apricots, raisins, and deep green vegetables such as spinach and broccoli.

REFERENCES

1. Dietary Reference Intakes: Recommended Intakes for Individuals, Vitamins, Minerals and Macronutrients. National Academies of Sciences. 2001.
2. Pediatric Manual of Clinical Dietetics, 2nd Edition. Nutrition for the Child Athlete. American Dietetic Association. 2003, pp. 113–122.
3. Sports Nutrition: A Guide for the Professional Working with Active People, 3rd Edition. CA Rosenbloom. American Dietetic Association. 2000.

over the second toe. The foot also should be in a neutral position. Note supination or pronation and calcaneal varus or valgus. The same process occurs for all functional tasks of the lower body. It is also important to note the athlete's gait for abnormalities as he or she walks into the clinic without the pressure of being evaluated.

In assessing the athlete performing push-ups, evaluate the position of wrists and elbows. Do the scapulae wing or contour the thoracic wall? Can the athlete maintain the spine in a neutral position or is a sway back or pike position noted? Refer to Display 13.5 for upper extremity functional tests. Core strength should be evaluated for all injuries. Sport-specific activities, which aggravate the pain, should also be assessed. For instance, have a pitcher

throw or a runner run. Video analysis of the athlete during the evaluation is another helpful tool. Having the athlete bring in videotapes of his or her performance is another way of analyzing his or her form and techniques. Equipment and footwear are evaluated for proper size, excessive wear, and appropriateness for the sport (i.e., a basketball player should not be playing in running shoes).

The thorough evaluation of an athlete is comprehensive, time consuming, and necessary. Only after all the subjective and objective information is gathered can the injured tissue structure and the cause/predisposing factors be accurately identified. Examples of cause/predisposing factors include biomechanical malalignment, muscular weakness, loss of motion, and improper athletic technique. At times the cause/predisposing factors and injured tissue are the same, but often they are different. The cause/predisposing factors for a shoulder injury may be a weak hip, causing altered throwing mechanics. For full recovery and prevention of future injuries, the identification and treatment of the cause/predisposing factors, not just the injured tissue, is paramount.

◆ Rehabilitation Principles

In order to effectively treat patients with traumatic and sports injuries, a solid understanding of basic strength and conditioning principles is requisite and a thorough understanding optimal. This section will review the general concepts of strengthening, range of motion, and conditioning.

STRENGTHENING

Strength training is not contraindicated in children and adolescents.[6,7] Considering the activities that a normal child performs recreationally and in sports, strength training is a safe activity when performed under the supervision of a trained adult. Strength gains of roughly 30% to 40% have been evidenced in children and gains of up to 74% have been reported.[8]

Strengthening essentially falls into three categories: hypertrophy, endurance, and strength. Hypertrophy is the process of increasing muscle size, as in the case of body building. The parameters for obtaining hypertrophy

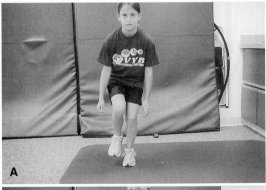

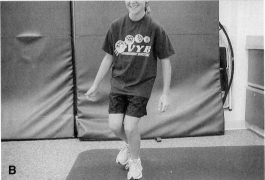

Figure 13.1 ■ Correct **(A)** and incorrect **(B)** forms of single-leg squats.

are strength training of moderate intensity (50% to 75% of one maximum repetition, or RM) and moderate to very high volume (three to six sets of 10 to 20 reps) with a short rest between sets.[8]

Endurance training is achieved through submaximal contractions (low intensity) over a large number of repetitions (12 or more reps over two to three sets) with little recovery between sets.[9] It can be noted that the difference between hypertrophy training and muscular endurance does not vary greatly; the key components that differentiate the two are that endurance training consists of lower intensity exertion and shorter rest than hypertrophy training.

Strength training prepares muscle for maximal exertion.[9] Many studies have been unable to support an exact set and rep scheme to promote maximal increases in strength.[9] Generally, the protocol consists of high-resistance near-maximal contractions for a small number of repetitions (three sets of 10 reps after a warm-up) where there is fatigue by the 10th repetition followed by a full recovery period between sets.[9]

Plyometrics are a form of resistance training in which quick, powerful movements are performed using a pre-stretch or countermovement that involves the stretch shortening cycle. The stretch shortening cycle stores energy in the series elastic component of muscles to promote a maximal contraction in a short period of time. The most crucial phase of plyometrics is the amortization phase, which occurs between the eccentric and concentric contractions. Optimally, the shorter the amortization phase is, the better. This prevents dissipation of accumulated forces and provides for a contraction force beyond that of an isolated contraction.[9] Plyometrics can be used in the upper or lower body. For example, in the lower body plyometrics are often jumps, and in the upper body ballistic medicine ball tosses are common. Care must be taken not to create an overuse injury to the lower extremities when performing plyometrics. Typical repetition volumes are 80- to 100-foot contacts for most rehabilitation applications.[9] Recovery following plyometric training is longer between sets and workouts due to the high-intensity nature of this type of exercise. Plyometrics are typically used later in rehabilitation in the return-to-sports preparation phase.

Core strengthening is another component of rehabilitation that deserves attention. Core strength is the ability to use the trunk and pelvis muscles in a coordinated pattern to provide proximal stability for dynamic mobility. The core is a box with abdominal muscles anteriorly, paraspinal and gluteal muscles posteriorly, the diaphragm at the roof, and hip girdle musculature at the bottom. The core serves as the center of the functional kinetic chain. It is the command center for the transmission of force and power. The core is also an essential component of balance. Conceptually, a few parameters should be followed regarding core strengthening during rehabilitation. First, transverse abdominus should be facilitated through drawing in of the abdomen during all activities. Eccentrics during rotation should be incorporated to facilitate external obliques. Given that the core musculature consists largely of tonic muscles, isometric and eccentric modes should be employed. Hip flexor stretching helps to allow for appropriate contraction of lower abdominal musculature by allowing the pelvis to obtain optimal alignment, rather than maintaining an anteriorly tilted position that elongates the anterior core muscles and places them at mechanical disadvantage. The core should be integrated into all activities. It cannot be assumed that firing of the core musculature will be automatic during functional activities simply as a result of performing core-specific exercises.

CONDITIONING

Regarding conditioning, it should be noted that there are three ways in which the body produces energy to fuel muscular activity. For immediate fuel needs the body utilizes the phosphagen system, which is one of two anaerobic energy systems. The phosphagen system is needed for short bursts of energy as found in sports such as football, basketball, and volleyball. This system is also needed for endurance athletes who may use a sudden burst of speed, such as a distance runner who exerts him- or herself maximally at the end of a race for a finishing kick.[9] In order to train the phosphagen system, high-intensity activities should be performed with significant rest to provide for full recovery between bouts. The duration of activity is generally under 10 seconds, and several minutes of recovery are utilized to prevent lactic acid accumulation, which will impair performance during the subsequent bout.[9]

The second system is anaerobic glycolysis. This is needed for moderate-intensity efforts, which exist across many sports, such as ice hockey, boxing, downhill skiing, and wrestling. To activate this system moderate-intensity activities are performed with shorter rest periods that do not allow for full recovery and elimination of lactic acid. In essence, a goal of training for this system is to enable the body to more effectively buffer acids in the muscles.

Activities that will activate these two anaerobic systems typically consist of agility, sprints, shuttles, plyometrics, and high-intensity strength training. The parameters used for these will determine which energy system is primarily utilized, though training of both systems individually and together is paramount as most athletes will need to utilize both of these systems in their sports.[9]

The third system for energy production is the aerobic system. The primary stimulus for developing aerobic capacity is short rest; that is, high-intensity activities can develop aerobic power if the rest between bouts is short.[9] Therefore the notion that continuous exercise is the only way to develop aerobic capacity is incorrect. Aerobic training is important not only for aerobic sports, but also as a preseason base for largely anaerobic sports. Care must be taken to match the training to the sport as typical aerobic training, such as long-distance running, can be detrimental to power sports. Instead, aerobic power for those athletes should be developed via alternative methods such as interval training with short rest periods. This allows lactate to be maintained and obligates adaptation. Athletes who are initiating a rehabilitation program will benefit from aerobic training, but the methods used need to be specific to the upcoming sport.

DEVELOPING A REHABILITATION PROGRAM FOR THE YOUNG ATHLETE

When making decisions regarding strengthening parameters for rehabilitation, intensity selection should be based on multiple factors including the athlete's prior level of conditioning, current level of conditioning (i.e., how much rest/deconditioning has occurred), type of injury, extent of injury, extent of repair based on phases of healing, pain levels, concomitant injury or potential for iatrogenic injury (i.e., patellofemoral pain syndrome can easily be developed when rehabilitating an injury in the lower leg), and type of injury. "No pain—no gain" is rarely operative in sports and traumatic orthopedic rehabilitation, with the exception of joint stiffness, where contracted soft tissues must be stretched. The goal of strength training in rehabilitation is to facilitate rapid strength gains and/or prevent atrophy without enhancing inflammation. Patients should be closely monitored and instructed to report any discomfort. Often in the pediatric and adolescent population patients may be reluctant to offer spontaneously that they are having discomfort either because they are embarrassed to admit it or they have discomfort at another site than their injury and do not think it is relevant (e.g., a patient with an ankle sprain performing single-leg squats and having patellofemoral pain).

QUALITY OF MOVEMENT

One of the cornerstones of sound rehabilitation for traumatic and sports injuries is the development of strength and neuromuscular control. In order for this to be effective, quality of movement must be emphasized. This is best accomplished by closely supervising and giving feedback to the patient during exercises. Care must be taken to choose appropriate exercises such that the patient has the capacity to perform them successfully; otherwise, the process will lead to frustration and lost confidence. Attention to detail must be emphasized to facilitate the desired neuromuscular recruitment pattern. For example, a patient performing scapular retraction to strengthen middle trapezius needs to have the shoulders depressed and the humerus elevated in abduction adequately to avoid compensatory firing of the rhomboids and upper trapezius muscles. It is easy to allow this compensation if close attention is not being paid to the exercise. Another helpful technique is to simply ask the patient where there is a feeling of fatigue as a result of the exercise. It may be best not to tell the individual ahead of time where to expect to feel the activity. Patients often will be reluctant to express that they don't feel it where the therapist indicated they would, most likely to avoid embarrassing the therapist by suggesting that the therapist was wrong. By keeping the question open ended, the patient may be more likely to be truthful about the report of fatigue.

RETURN TO SPORT/ACTIVITY

In designing a rehabilitation program and making decisions about return to activities, it is important to consider the patient's desires, demands of the sport, issues relating to scholarships, championship competitions, and worst-case scenarios of participation. Active children and athletes often want to return to activities as rapidly as possible and think that they will be safe. It is not uncommon to hear that they "will be careful." What has to be considered is the worst-case scenario of that participation and what impact it would have on their injury. For example, if a child with a knee injury wants to ride a scooter, the decision needs to be based on what could happen if the child fell, not whether or not propelling him- or herself on the scooter would be detrimental. Regarding the decision to return to play for an athlete, the amount of risk that will be acceptable should be determined by the athlete and his or her family. Clearly there are risks that the sports physical therapist cannot ethically support, but as healing progresses and function improves there is a gray zone where risks approach normal. These decisions can be some of the most challenging for the sports therapist. They are best made in conjunction with the sports medicine team.

Two athletes with the same diagnosis and at the same point of recovery may follow two different paths regarding return to their sport. In one case may be the athlete who values full recovery and the best chance at having no long-term sequelae and is willing to sacrifice his or her season to obtain full recovery. On the other end of the spectrum, and what is seen frequently in sports medicine, is the athlete who wants to return to his or her sport as soon as possible out of a strong desire to participate, because of potential scholarship issues, or perhaps because this is the last season of active participation prior to graduation. In this latter scenario the risks of return to sport will need to be clearly identified to the patient and his or her family and the decision to return well documented. In this process realize that risk is inherent not only in sports, but also in all aspects of life. For a summary of Exercise Guidelines, refer to Addendum A at the end of the chapter.

 Injuries to Bone

FRACTURES

Fractures occur often in childhood due to falls or collisions with other youngsters or objects and are the result of direct or indirect forces placed on the bone. Both complete and incomplete fractures occur in children. Due to increased blood supply and a thick periosteum, immature bone quickly heals more rapidly than mature (adult) bone.[1,3,9] Complete fractures present as transverse, oblique, or spiral in form.[3] Fractures are described by their location. Diaphyseal fractures are located in the central shaft of long bones. Metaphyseal fractures are located at the expanding end of bone adjacent to the physis. Physeal fractures are at the epiphyseal growth plate, and epiphyseal fractures involve the epiphysis, which is the portion of the bone closest to the joint space. Physeal fractures heal generally twice as rapidly as diaphyseal fractures[2,4] (see Fig. 13.2). There are three common incomplete fractures present in children: greenstick, torus/buckle, and plastic bowing. A greenstick fracture is identified by a fracture on the tension side of the bone with the compression side remaining intact. Often plastic bowing is observed with a greenstick fracture. For an upper extremity greenstick fracture, a child is casted in a long or short arm cast for 4 weeks.[1] A torus fracture, referred to frequently as a buckle fracture, is often the result of a fall on an outstretched hand, referred to as a FOOSH.[1] This fracture occurs at the diaphyseal–metaphyseal junction when the stronger diaphyseal cortex compresses the metaphysis. If the fracture is nondisplaced, 3 weeks in a short arm cast is the course of treatment. Plastic bowing refers to a bone that is deformed into a bowed shape due to overt pressures placed upon it. Even when these pressures are removed, the bone cannot rebound back to its original form. Sometimes surgery is necessary to reverse the deformity.[10]

PHYSEAL FRACTURES

Physeal fractures or growth plate injuries are common in children and account for 15% to 20% of all fractures in children.[4] Although children heal quickly and most often without sequelae, caution is taken in monitoring growth plate disturbances. A complete closure of the growth plate or formation of a physeal bridge over a localized area of the growth plate can impair bone growth. This occurs with significance in about 10% of physeal injuries.[4] The most commonly used classification system for growth plate fractures is Salter-Harris type I through V. Figure 13.3 and Display 13.6 provide a diagram representation of the Salter-Harris classification.[1,3,4] Range's type VI and Ogden's types VII, VIII, and IX describe fractures that do not directly involve the physis but during the repair process may develop physeal bridges that impact growth.

Types I and II have favorable outcomes without growth arrest. Types III IV often require surgical fixation and continuous monitoring for growth arrest. Type V is often difficult to identify and may go unnoticed until growth arrest is taking place.

AVULSION FRACTURES

Avulsion fractures occur in children and adolescents as a result of tendon and ligament attachments to immature bone.[1,3] A strong muscle contraction or maximum stretch of a muscle, which creates a high force across the attachment site, causes the osseous structure to break away from the bone. This injury can occur in many different areas of the body. Common sites as well as treatment are discussed under each specific body section below.

STRESS FRACTURES

Stress fractures occur when repetitive microtrauma to the bone accumulates faster than the body's ability to repair itself.[3] Both normal and abnormal bone are affected.[10,11] Stress fractures can occur in most of the bones of the body. Symptoms are diffuse in the beginning with a dull ache during activity, which is relieved by rest. As the cyclic process continues of repeated stress and inadequate time to repair, the athlete's symptoms increase in intensity and duration until pain becomes constant at rest. Pain now becomes localized and increases with palpation. Swelling may or may

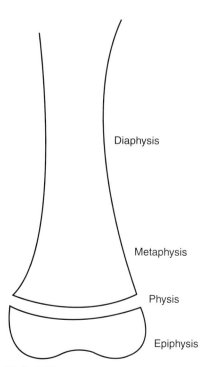

Diaphysis

Metaphysis

Physis

Epiphysis

Figure 13.2 ■ Different areas of bone.

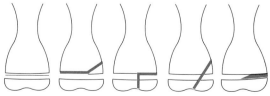

Figure 13.3 ■ Salter-Harris classification. White area between bones is the physis. Thick blue line indicates the fracture. See Display 13.6.

not be present. Common reasons for acquiring a stress fracture include malalignment, overtraining, improper technique, inappropriate footwear, poor nutrition, and inadequate rest. Stress fractures occur in the lower extremity, with the tibia and metatarsal most effected.[12] Stress fractures account for about 10% of all sports-related overuse injuries.[11,13]

General treatment is rest, activity modification, and splinting. Alteration in weight-bearing status may also be needed depending on the severity of the fracture and its location. During the rehabilitation process, maintaining the athlete's conditioning level is important. Cycling and aqua jogging at the same intensity and duration of a practice can be implemented if performed pain free. Strengthening and flexibility exercises are added as healing progresses. A gradual return to sport is allowed with continuous monitoring of pain. Identifying the culprit and correcting it are integral parts of the rehabilitation process. This may involve coordinating care with coaches, athletic trainers, nutritionists, and physicians.

APOPHYSITIS

An apophysis is a cartilaginous structure that is located at the end of long bones.[3] It is an attachment site for the muscle–tendon unit in the immature skeleton. Inflammation is caused by excessive tensile forces at the tendon–cartilage interface that are not large enough to create an avulsion injury. Apophysitis is primarily an overuse injury but can occur acutely. It frequently occurs in preteen girls and teenage boys during periods of rapid growth.[1,13] In the adult population, athletes will experience tendonitis since the musculotendon interface occurs into solid bone. Eponyms are commonly used to describe specific areas of apophysitis. These will be discussed in more detail later.

CARTILAGE INJURY

Osteochondritis dissecans (OCD) occurs in different areas of the body. Typically, only one area is problematic. The knee is most affected, followed by the elbow and the ankle. OCD is described as an osteochondral lesion that occurs as subchondral bone separates from the overlying articular cartilage. It is observed in adolescents from 13 to 17 years of age. The definitive cause is unknown but probable cause appears to be trauma, uneven or excessive pressure, disruption of blood supply to the bone, and genetics. Symptoms include generalized pain that increases with activity, increase in pain with rotation movements, and swelling. Athletes may complain of instability and locking. OCD can be characterized in four stages according to severity (Display 13.7).

Treatment is based on the severity of presentation. Conservative treatment is initiated with activity modification. More severe cases are managed with immobilization and surgery if symptoms persist or decline. Surgery is performed to stimulate blood flow to the area promoting healing and/or to remove loose fragments in the joint space. Cartilage has little capacity for self-repair because it has no direct blood supply, lymphatic circulation, or nerves.[3] Cartilage defects that extend into the underlying cancellous bone will repair to some extent due to the inflammatory response initiated at the bone level. The repair undergoes the same sequence as other tissues with inflammation repair and remodel and the cells differentiate into articular cartilage, but not completely into hyaline cartilage. Instead, they form a fibrocartilaginous matrix, which is not as strong as hyaline cartilage.[3] This repair process is much more effective in the skeletally immature individual due to increased vascularity of the periosteum and metaphysis.

Chondromalacia is a softening of articular cartilage resulting from either macrotrauma or persistent overload, typically shear. It is graded using the Outerbridge classification of I = softening, II = fraying/fibrillation up to ½ inch in diameter, III = fraying/fibrillation over ½ inch in diameter, and IV = exposure of subchondral bone (also referred to as eburnation). Pain is caused by shedding of matrix breakdown byproducts and secondary irritation of the synovium.[3]

Concussion

A concussion is a "transient traumatic disruption of cognitive function."[13] Estimates regarding the likelihood of an athlete in a contact sport experiencing a concussion may be as high as 19% per season.[14] Injuries associated with participation in sports and recreational activities account for 21% of all traumatic brain injuries among children in the United States.[15] Display 13.8 lists the symptoms associated with postconcussion syndrome.[15]

The ImPACT concussion management system (http://www.impacttest.com/) is a computerized testing system that is gaining popularity for concussion management. Optimal results can be obtained if baseline tests are performed prior to sports participation, but the system is able to assess cognitive status without baseline tests by comparing postconcussive results to normative data. Using a system such as ImPACT is a preferred method of assessment in comparison to physical examination and subjective questions.

Management of an athlete with a concussion consists of (1) removal from sports participation; (2) placing rehabilitation on hold (as exertion can increase symptoms); and (3) tracking of cognitive function (note that subdural hematomas can create evolution of symptoms over days). Postconcussive syndrome symptoms can last for up to several weeks, depending on the severity of the concussion. Many guideline systems exist and vary in their recommendations regarding return to sports and recreational activities. In general, the individual must be symptom free for 1 to 4 weeks before returning and may participate in rehabilitation if symptoms are not reproduced. If any symptoms are present, the athlete is not able to participate in sport. Second-impact syndrome describes the occurrence of a second concussion before complete resolution of the preceding concussion.[16] Both mortality and morbidity can be very high for individuals following second-impact syndrome. Ultimately, a physical therapist treating athletes needs to be aware of the signs of concussion and to alert the sports medicine team if there is concern about the possibility of a concussion. Athletes will often hide symptoms to avoid being removed from athletic participation. Unfortunately, the risks of playing with a concussion are significant, which obviates the importance of the physical therapist being able to recognize its presence.

Spine Care

SPINE EXAMINATION

Posture should be the initial aspect of the spinal examination, followed by ROM (flexion, extension, side bending, rotation); strength assessment (core, scapulothoracic/hip, extremities); extremity flexibility (shoulder flexion/horizontal abduction, hip flexion, hamstring length, ankle dorsiflexion); and, if needed, palpation of the appropriate sites. Special tests for the spine include Spurling's (combined extension, lateral flexion and rotation)[17]; straight leg raise; FABER (combined flexion, abduction, and external rotation of the hip); end-range spinal motions with overpressure; segmental mobilization (for the lumbar and thoracic spine); and sacroiliac (SI) joint tests. In addition, most spinal disorders should have radiographs in the skeletally immature population.

SPINAL DISORDERS IN THE YOUNG ATHLETE

Spondylolysis is the most common spine injury seen in the young athlete.[13] Physiologically, spondylolysis represents a fracture of the pars interarticularis of the spine, usually in the lower lumbar spine. The mean age for spondylolysis is 15 to 16 years old. This pattern of injury contrasts to the adult population, in which discogenic injury and pain is the most common cause. Spondylolysis is often seen in dancers, gymnasts, and ice skaters due to repeated hyperextension in these sports. Clinical examination findings include pain with extension on the Spurling test and grossly painful free flexion. On radiography a "scotty dog fracture" is usually seen at the pars interarticularis. Plain films can be negative, and if so, usually a bone scan or single photon emission computed tomography (SPECT) scan can assist with diagnosis.

Spondylolisthesis also occurs in this population, and is marked by anterior migration of one vertebra on another. One differentiating clinical examination finding is that of a "step sign." Radiography can provide evidence of spondylolisthesis and allow grading to be performed.[3] There is controversy regarding sports participation, but the rule of thumb is that grade 3 to 4 (those with 75% to 100% migration of the spinal segment relative to the segment below) should not participate. General treatment strategies for the spine will be discussed shortly, but regarding specific details for spondylolysis and spondylolisthesis, spinal extension should be avoided and principles of neutral positioning should be followed. Additionally, custom brace immobilization for several weeks may be warranted.

>> **DISPLAY 13.8**

Postconcussion Syndrome Symptoms

- Chronic headaches
- Fatigue
- Sleep difficulties
- Personality change (e.g., increased irritability, emotionality)
- Sensitivity to light/noise
- Dizziness when standing quickly
- Deficits in short-term memory, problem solving, and general academic functioning

Apophysitis is another common cause of pain in the spine of the young athlete. Clinically it is marked by mechanical pain that is irritated with repeated motions of the spine and improves with rest. If it occurs at iliac crest, the patients will have pain with contraction of obliques and with palpation over the iliac apophysis. In the spine the apophysis is a ring at the vertebral end-plates. This will not be palpable.

A Schmorl's node occurs when the end-plate of a vertebral body fails under discal pressure.[13] These are more often seen on magnetic resonance imaging (MRI), even when not visible on plain film radiography. The most common age and location for Schmorl's nodes is 14 to 18 years in the mid- to low back. These may or may not be symptomatic, and the etiologic significance for back pain is controversial.

Pain caused with muscular contraction or stretch of a muscle group is consistent with a muscle strain. Symptoms will be local and pain will be superficial. Swelling and discoloration may also be present.

A "burner" is a traction injury of the brachial plexus that usually involves the C-5 and C-6 nerve roots, although it may extend down to T-1. The athlete commonly has deltoid weakness and often biceps and serratus anterior weakness as well. Usually symptoms will extend distally into the hand. The athlete will often shake his or her arm and bend over toward the injured side. Stinging pain is produced, as well as numbness and tingling without neck symptoms. A burner may resolve quickly with return of full strength, sensation, and ROM and reduction of pain, thereby allowing the athlete to return to play. Electromyographic (EMG) findings are not an accurate guideline for return to play, as EMG deficits may be noted long after clinical resolution is obtained. X-ray examination is recommended for recurrent burners or those which exhibit symptoms for longer than 24 hours. Other less common disorders of the spine include Scheuermann's disease (juvenile kyphosis), which consists of anterior wedging of the vertebral bodies as demonstrated on plain films. The patient will be kyphotic.

SPINE TREATMENT

The initial approach to successful treatment of the spine is to remove offending forces (improper movement patterns and postures). Postural correction and cessation of irritating activities can be effective in reducing symptoms. Another general concept of intervention is to stretch tight muscle groups and other tissues. Typically this entails stretching the hip flexors, hamstrings, quadriceps, and ankles for thoracolumbar injuries and stretching the anterior chest wall soft tissue to reduce symptoms of neck injuries. Core strengthening is also an essential component to the treatment of the spine in the youth athlete (refer to Fig. 13.4A through D). In addition to the concepts mentioned earlier in the chapter, trunk extensors should be strengthened in functional positions.

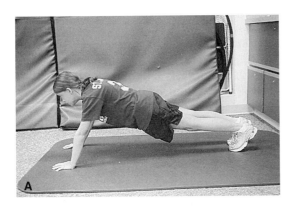
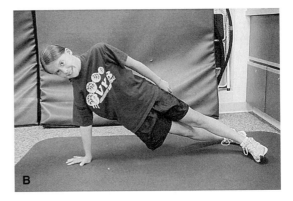
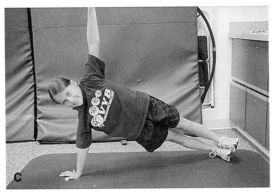
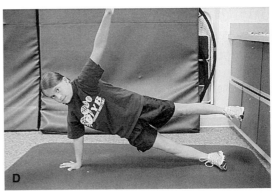

Figure 13.4 ■ Core progression. **(A)** Plank. **(B)** Side plank. **(C)** "T" position. **(D)** Star.

Other principles important to include in the treatment of spinal injuries include combining strength, control, and endurance as well as creating an even distribution spinal mobility. If there is hyper- or hypomobility at one spinal segment, that segment will be overstressed. This is often seen in gymnasts and dancers with excessive spinal extension in the lower lumbar spine. Often treatment will be incomplete and ineffective until extension throughout the rest of the spine is increased to decrease stress on the lower lumbar spine. "Return to play" guidelines for spinal injuries follow the simple rule of avoiding activities that are likely to be painful. The spine is a complex region that usually takes a long time to heal. If this is understood by both the therapist and the athlete, expectations will be appropriate regarding the timeframe for return to sport and frustration will be minimized. Prevention strategies for spinal injuries at present have no clear answer. It is likely that good posture, core strength, flexibility, and proper sports technique all contribute to spinal health.

 ## Shoulder

EXAMINATION

Examination of the athlete's shoulder should begin with a postural assessment. Optimally the head should be upright rather than forward, and shoulders should be neutral in the sagittal plane rather than protracted. There should be normal thoracic spine kyphosis, the inferior angles of the scapulae should be lateral to the superior angles (indicating good serratus anterior muscle tone), and minimal shoulder height differences should be present.

Next, in examining ROM, a key concept is the arc of rotational motion, rather than isolating each motion in comparison to norms. Within 90 degrees of abduction the total arc should approximate 180 degrees. It is common in throwing athletes to have increased external rotation equal to a loss of internal rotation when compared to the nonthrowing shoulder. For example, if an athlete has 60 degrees of internal rotation and 120 degrees of external rotation, the total arc is 180 degrees and demonstrates a normal arc of motion. The contralateral shoulder may have the same arc but distributed as 70 degrees of internal rotation and 110 degrees of external rotation. Despite a mismatching of expected motions in each direction, the presence of an adequate total arc is sufficient for proper participation. The practitioner is therefore cautioned not to look solely at a decrease in internal rotation and assume that the athlete has a tight posterior capsule. In the scenario provided, the humerus is simply retroverted.[18] If, conversely, the total arc of motion is 150 degrees with 110 degrees of external rotation and only 40 degrees of internal rotation, there is concern regarding a tight posterior capsule because the complete arc is clearly below the expected 180 degrees. Assisted ROM should be

viewed from the front and back of the patient, with note of scapular dyskinesia made.

In addition to the special tests listed in Addendum B, which are used to directly identify specific injuries, some other tests are noteworthy. In the throwing athlete, the core, hip, and lower extremity are also important to examine and evaluate. With power being generated from ground reaction forces, all of these components must function appropriately in order to deliver that power to the upper extremity. Issues such as an incompletely healed or rehabilitated ankle injury, hip muscle weakness, or core muscular insufficiency can all be contributory to a shoulder injury.

Also noteworthy are the phases of throwing. Understanding these phases (Display 13.9) can help the physical therapist better identify both the injury and potential causal factors. A key element of the phases of throwing is that high forces are generated at the glenohumeral joint during late cocking, acceleration, and deceleration phases. During late cocking and acceleration, greater forces are generally exerted on the anterior aspect of the shoulder and in the posterior aspect during deceleration.

PROGRAM PLANNING

Interventions for most shoulder disorders in young athletes are similar and should begin with good posture, scapular stabilization, and avoidance of offending activities. Customization should be based on specific examination findings of weakness, ROM deficits, and the status of the injured tissue. One basic tenet of quality shoulder rehabilitation is that rotator cuff strengthening should be performed with the scapula and the body in good alignment and functional positions. Isometrics may be used in early rehabilitation for the rotator cuff if symptoms and stage of healing indicate; otherwise, isotonic exercises at varying speeds should be utilized. Begin exercising with the limb below shoulder level, within pain-free ROM prior to exercising above 90 degrees of shoulder elevation.

Scapulothoracic musculature, particularly posterior muscles such as middle and lower trapezii, is another important focus of quality rehabilitation. The focus should be on stabilization and endurance. It is important that

---

》》 DISPLAY 13.9

Phases of Throwing

- Wind-up
- Early cocking
- Late cocking
- Acceleration
- Deceleration
- Follow-through

these muscles are able to appropriately position the gleno-humeral joint for optimal function throughout all activities.

OTHER CONSIDERATIONS IN SHOULDER REHABILITATION

The role of the core and hip/pelvic musculature in shoulder rehabilitation is also important. As mentioned earlier, these muscles act as the force generators and transmitters of ground reaction forces to the shoulder. The core musculature, as with the posterior scapulothoracic musculature, should be exercised with an emphasis on endurance and stability. The hip musculature, particularly abductors and external rotators, also must be able to stabilize the pelvis as well as guide it appropriately during functional activities.

Another concept worth mentioning is that of the speed of exercises. The humerus is able to rotate on the glenoid at several thousand degrees per second during overhead throwing.[19] Plyometric activities for the upper extremity can grossly simulate these speeds and will help to properly prepare the athlete for return to play.

Altering the position of the extremity during exercises to mimic functional positions and to change the intensity of the resistance in various portions of the range of motion is also helpful. External rotation does not have to be performed at only neutral and 90 degrees of abduction as is often done. Performing external rotation with the resistance parallel to the individuals' body at all times is not realistic either; instead, change the angle of the body relative to the resistance so that maximal resistance is obtained at various points in the range of motion.

Often posterior glenohumeral motion restriction will exist in the injured athlete's shoulder and posterior structures will need to be stretched. This can be accomplished rather effectively by the sleeper stretch (Fig. 13.5).

A frequently used exercise program for the overhead athlete is the Thrower's 10 (Display 13.10). Video content for this program can be found at http://www.asmi.org/SportsMed/throwing/thrower10.html.

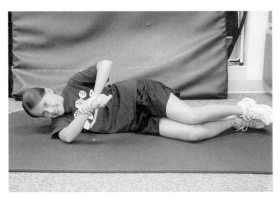

Figure 13.5 ■ Sleeper stretch.

As the throwing athlete regains function, a return-to-throwing program can be initiated. Typically these programs have many phases over many weeks and include warm-up, throwing at progressively longer distances, and significant rest periods between bouts of throwing in a given session.

SPECIFIC PROBLEMS

Generalized shoulder pain resulting from overuse or rapid advancement of training protocols (i.e., significant increase in swimming yardage, volume of throwing) is often caused by tendonitis with secondary impingement in the pediatric and adolescent population. Typical examination findings would be positive special tests, a tight posterior rotator cuff or shoulder capsule, weakness of the posterior scapulothoracic musculature and external rotators, and forward rounded shoulders.

Shoulder multidirectional instability (MDI) is another common problem in this age group. It typically results from generalized ligamentous laxity (testing for this was described earlier in the chapter). Recognition of this disorder and counseling regarding injury risk due to systemic ligamentous laxity will be beneficial to the patient.

One difficulty encountered is when an individual with ligamentous laxity incurs a traumatic dislocation that does not result in a Bankart lesion (tear of the anterior–inferior glenoid labrum) but, rather, simply stretches the capsule. In these cases the course of action is less clear, as reconstruction may not be effective. If surgery is performed, immobilization is necessary to promote adequate healing and provide for long-term stability. During the rehabilitation process, care must be taken not to overstretch the repaired tissue. Avoidance of horizontal glenohumeral extension, such as during a bench-press maneuver, is one of the primary contraindications.

"Little league" shoulder is another entity commonly encountered in the pediatric and adolescent athlete. It is defined as a stress reaction or fracture of the proximal humeral physis.[3] Plain films or bone scans are often used but are sometimes not definitive. Palpatory tenderness over the physis is diagnostic if rotator cuff testing and other tests are negative. Treatment for little league shoulder is primarily rest. Reviewing throwing mechanics, ensuring good balance and core strength/function, scapulothoracic strengthening, a gradual return-to-throwing program, and modification of throwing volume are then added as the injury heals.

Acromioclavicular joint separations and Salter fractures also occur in this population, but are generally not treated surgically despite their appearance. Of note is that the periosteum may remain intact despite that the joint has separated. This periosteal sleeve then fills with bone over time and may appear as a bony abnormality. Rehabilitation proceeds according to tolerance. There may be a permanent elevation of the distal clavicle, but this is only cosmetic and will not affect function.

Clavicle fractures also occur and surprisingly are also not treated surgically in the majority of cases despite their appearance. Treatment generally consists of splinting in a retracted position to allow good alignment during the healing process. A "figure-of-eight brace" is used. As in the case of the acromioclavicular (AC) separation, the individual should be counseled that there will be a cosmetic lump at the clavicle, but this should not be of functional concern. Because after the acute pain subsides the athlete can function rather well while wearing the brace, rehabilitation needs are minor.

Superior labrum anterior-to-posterior (SLAP) lesions occur in adolescents as a result of trauma or overuse. The overuse injury is due to pulling of the biceps tendon on the superior labrum. SLAP lesions can result in laxity of the shoulder since the structural integrity of the shoulder is impaired. The typical subjective complaints of a slap lesion are popping, clicking, and superior shoulder pain. SLAP lesions may mimic rotator cuff tendonitis, and the two can be difficult to differentiate. Neer and Hawkins impingement tests are generally positive, as is the anterior slide test. In the case of a SLAP lesion, performing the O'Brien's test of horizontal abduction with external rotation should be negative—if positive, this indicates a greater likelihood of tendonitis rather than a SLAP lesion.[20]

Initial treatment of SLAP lesions consists of rehabilitation for several weeks. The therapist can determine whether the injury can be treated conservatively. If conservative treatment is not reasonable, then the injury is more likely a SLAP lesion and arthroscopy is indicated. Surgery usually consists of debridement and possibly reattachment of the detached labrum in more advanced cases.

From a rehabilitation perspective, postoperative care must not disrupt the surgical site. Hence, in the early phases the primary focus of intervention is on gentle motion restoration and isometrics with progression into the usual comprehensive rehabilitation activities for a shoulder injury. Much of the protocol will depend on the extent of the injury and surgical technique used, as well as surgeon's preference.

Elbow, Wrist, and Hand Injuries

The elbow, wrist, and hand are frequently injured in the pediatric population. The hand suffers the majority of upper extremity fractures.[13] A FOOSH is the most common mechanism of injury. It transmits forces to the hand not only on impact, but also through the kinetic chain to the axial skeleton with occasional clavicle and cervical injury. A growing child's elbow is at risk of injury with its generalized ligament laxity, bony instability due to open growth centers, and bony plasticity.[13] A large effusion at the elbow commonly signifies dislocation or fracture. Immobilization after closed or open reduction is the primary treatment of traumatic fractures. Open fractures of any size are a surgical emergency. An elbow deformity is treated like a fracture until ruled out. Rehabilitation to restore ROM, strength, and function is often necessary. Unrestricted activities are resumed when bone healing is sufficient, full elbow extension has returned, and the majority of elbow flexion has been achieved. Adequate strength in open- and closed-chain positions must also be present.

TRAUMATIC ELBOW FRACTURES

Supracondylar fracture commonly occurs in children younger than 8 years old due to a fall. This is a serious injury that requires surgical attention of an orthopedist. A large amount of swelling is present and nerve injury occurs in 10% to 15% of all supracondylar fractures, with the anterior interosseus nerve most often implicated.[1] When there is suspected nerve involvement, the therapist should examine flexion of the thumb and distal interphalangeal (DIP) joint of the index finger.[1] Caution is always necessary with this injury to prevent or detect early signs of compartment syndrome in the forearm. This is an emergent condition, which, left unattended, can lead to permanent decrease in limb function or loss of a limb. Signs of compartment syndrome include increasing pain with passive finger extension, pallor, paraesthesias, diminished pulse, and paralysis.[13] Compartment pressure measurement confirms diagnosis. A surgical fasciotomy relieves the pressure, which restores blood flow. Sometimes vascular repair is necessary.[13]

A lateral condyle fracture is classified as a Salter-Harris type IV and is the second most common elbow fracture in children. The fracture line continues from the epiphysis through the physeal plate and across the metaphysis, causing a separation of a triangular portion of bone. Open reduction and internal fixation of the free fragment is required with greater than 2 mm of displacement. This fracture's healing process must be monitored closely for growth arrest or formation of a physeal bridge.

Monteggia fracture dislocations describe a radial head dislocation with concomitant ulnar fracture. This is a rare injury but can have serious sequelae. Failure to diagnose the injury in a timely manner may result in failure or loss of radial head reduction, nerve injury, late stiffness, avascular necrosis of the radial head, and radioulnar synostosis.[1]

Fractures to the forearm are very common and can occur to the proximal, midshaft, and distal portions. Ulnar and radial fractures can occur independently or simultaneously. Colles fractures (radius and tip of ulna fracture with associated epiphyseal plate injury) and Buckle fractures (at the diaphyseal–metaphyseal junction when the stronger diaphyseal cortex compresses the metaphysis) typically occur as a result of a FOOSH. Both injuries require cast immobilization for several weeks.

OVERUSE

The term *little league elbow* is used to describe a set of conditions manifested by repetitive valgus extension overloads at the elbow frequently caused by pitching mechanics. This injury is found in young baseball players who throw too many pitches with inadequate rest. Excessive pitching might not occur during a single game but is often the summation of pitches thrown during practice, while at home, or while playing on multiple teams in the same season. During late cocking and acceleration phases in throwing, tension forces are placed on the medial elbow and compressive forces are received on the lateral elbow. During deceleration, shearing forces occur as the forearm fully pronates and the elbow extends. Side arm throwing increases these forces and should be discouraged. Medial elbow injuries include medial epicondyle apophysitis and medial epicondyle avulsion fractures. Lateral elbow injuries include Panner's disease, which can involve the blood supply to the capitellum and OCD, a fragmentation of bone that can lead to loose bodies within the joint. Symptoms include medial and lateral elbow pain, swelling, and loss of motion. Joint locking may occur if loose bodies have been formed. Treatment is activity modification until painless (about 3 to 4 weeks) and full pain-free ROM, a negative clinical examination, and normal strength are achieved, followed by rehabilitation. Specific interventions include scapular and rotator cuff strengthening to support the elbow, flexor and pronator strengthening and stretching, eccentric biceps strengthening for control during the deceleration phase, and core strengthening of abdominal and hip musculature for assistance during single-leg stance. The Thrower's 10 program (see Display 13.10) addresses the majority of these exercises. A return-to-throwing program is then initiated limiting the number of pitches, speed, and distance. Pitching typically begins off the pitching mound. Evaluation of pitching mechanics and education regarding proper pitching are necessary to prevent reoccurrence (Display 13.11).

> ## DISPLAY 13.11
>
> ### Prevention Guidelines
>
> - Change-up (not before 11 years of age)
> - Curveball (not before 14.5 years of age)
> - Slider (not before 18 years of age)
> - Do not participate in more than one youth baseball league at a time
> - Do not play baseball year round
> - Maximum pitches per game: ages 8–10 = 50; ages 11–14 = 75; ages 15–18 = 90–100
> - Maximum innings per week: ages 14 and under = 6; ages 15 and over = 10

PANNER'S DISEASE AND OSTEOCHONDRITIS DISSECANS

Panner's disease (PD) and OCD are the same disease process occurring during different stages of development, thereby accounting for the different presentations and treatment. In PD, lateral compressive forces at the elbow cause avascular necrosis of the ossific nucleus of the capitellum. PD is seen frequently in baseball players and gymnasts from ages 4 to 10 years old. Rest and avoidance of the offending activity can lead to revascularization and reformation of the ossific nucleus. In most cases, surgery is not indicated and a normal capitellum forms. Full return to sport occurs in the next season.[21] OCD is a separation of the subchondral bone from the overlying cartilage and is seen in the 10- to 17-year-old athletes.[22] When conservative treatment fails, drilling through the articulator surface into the cancellous bone to stimulate healing is performed.[23] The elbow is then casted in extension for 6 weeks with complete reconstitution occurring in 12 to 18 months. Symptoms in both PD and OCD include pain, decreased elbow ROM, and swelling and tenderness over the radiocapitellar joint.[23] Other etiologies are investigated when bilateral OCD is identified in an athlete other than a gymnast who performs symmetric, bilateral upper extremity movements.

OTHER DISORDERS OF THE ELBOW

Medial epicondyle apophysitis is the result of repetitive tensile forces from the medial elbow musculature. Symptoms are similar to those of little league elbow, with palpable tenderness over the medial epicondyle. Treatment is as mentioned above for little league elbow. Activity modification includes avoidance of heavy lifting. Triceps apophysitis occurs with increased extension loads at the ulnar–triceps interface. Continued sports participation could result in an avulsion fracture as seen in the lower extremity.

Occasionally, an acute avulsion fracture of the medial epicondyle occurs during throwing. A pop is often heard or felt at the time of injury with an acute onset of pain over the medial epicondyle. Treatment is immobilization with the elbow at 90 degrees of flexion for 3 weeks if the displacement of the epicondyle is less than 5 mm, and surgical pinning is performed when the displacement is greater than 5 mm.[13] Although not typically seen in children, medial epicondylitis can occur in gymnasts who present with a large carrying angle and elbow recurvatum. Repetitive loads during tumbling cause strain of the flexor pronator muscles of the elbow. Differential symptoms between flexor pronator muscle strain and medial epicondylitis occur during palpation, with a flexor pronator muscle strain exhibiting more distal pain over the flexor pronator muscle belly.

"Forearm splints" are produced with excessive weight-bearing activities of the upper extremity.[3] An aching pain is experienced between the radius and ulna. Cheerleaders and gymnasts are most affected. Treatment is rest, ice, and activity modification. As with all upper extremity injuries, a thorough evaluation is needed to identify the weakest link in the kinetic chain. Chronic posterior elbow contusions as observed in football and hockey players lead to olecranon bursitis. Treatment includes rest and reduction of trauma to the area with the use of elbow pads or activity modification.[3]

EXAMINATION OF THE HAND, WRIST, AND FINGERS

Begin examination of the hand, wrist, and finger injuries with a general inspection. Assess fingernail and nail beds for abnormal structure or circulation. Locate diffuse or localized swelling among all fingers, the hand, and the wrist. Then inspect the palmar surface of the hand for proper arch and muscle symmetry. The normal resting hand position is arched with fingers slightly flexed at each joint. Evaluate the alignment of metacarpals and phalanges by opening the palm and extending the fingers, then slowly flexing the fingers into the palm. A finger fracture is suspected if the fingers cross when flexed into the palm.

TRAUMATIC INJURIES OF THE HAND, WRIST, AND FINGERS

A scaphoid fracture is caused by a fall on an outstretched hand. Pain is elicited in the anatomic snuffbox located between the abductor pollicis longus and brevis tendons. ROM is decreased and an increase in pain is noted with radial deviation. The hand and wrist are immobilized in a thumb spica cast for 6 to 10 weeks. If the fracture is displaced or nonunion occurs after immobilization, then surgery is indicated. It is important to identify these fractures as the scaphoid has a tenuous blood supply, which can cause difficulty in healing.

Hook of the hamate fractures occur during racquet sports like baseball, golf, or hockey when excessive forces from the swing are transmitted to the hamate. The mechanism of injury can be a missed swing or striking

of a solid object. Symptoms may include a sharp pain on the ulnar side of the hand or a dull pain only with sports participation. Point tenderness is elicited on the ulnar side of the hand just distal to the flexion crease of the wrist. Treatment is immobilization for 6 weeks in a short arm cast with the fourth and fifth digits postured in flexion. Fragment excision is performed if complete healing has not occurred after immobilization.

A Bennet's fracture occurs as a fracture dislocation at the base of the thumb's metacarpal. The volar fragment remains connected to the trapezium by the volar ligament.[13] Tension from the abductor pollicis longus creates a proximal subluxation of the metacarpal.

A fracture of the neck of the fifth digit, called a "boxer" fracture, occurs during a punching maneuver when the closed fist hits an unforgiving object. Immobilization for 3 weeks followed by gentle ROM and continued splinting for 2 weeks is the common intervention.

In general, if finger fractures are stable and non-displaced, they are immobilized and splinted to adjacent fingers for additional support and alignment. Unstable or multiple fractures may require surgery. Radiographs are used to determine the severity of the fracture or physeal injury. Physeal fractures of the proximal phalanx are the most common[13] and are caused by angular and rotatory forces. Distal phalanx physeal fractures involve the epiphyseal plate, nail, and surrounding soft tissue. The middle phalanx is most often spared from injury due to the collateral ligament attachment to the periosteum of the metaphysis beyond the growth plate.[13]

"Gymnast wrist" is an overuse injury caused by mechanical overload at the distal radius.[1] During intense upper extremity weight-bearing activities, the distal radius receives 80% of the compressive forces during contact. Symptoms include mild discomfort to significant pain over the distal radius. Early detection is important to prevent physeal injury and wrist deformity. Management of the injury includes activity modification from 4 weeks with no radiographic findings to 3 months with positive radiographs.

Ligamentous and tendon injuries occur while participating in both youth and adult sports. Common injuries include boutonniere deformity, mallet finger, jersey finger, ulnar collateral ligament tear of the thumb, and injury to the triangular fibrocartilage complex (TFCC). Additional information regarding these injuries can be found in most sports medicine textbooks. See supplementary readings at the end of this chapter.

◆ Pelvis, Hip, and Thigh Injuries

Whenever complaints of hip, pelvis, thigh, or knee pain occur, careful examination must be performed to rule out pathologic diseases processes. During hip examination, pain and ROM asymmetries may be noted and are significant findings. Acute and overuse injuries to the immature pelvis are not uncommon in young athletes.

Avulsion fractures can occur in multiple areas of the pelvis, with the most common sites being the anterior superior iliac spine (ASIS) and ischial tuberosity. Sports that require running, jumping, sprinting, and cutting are most responsible for these avulsion injuries. X-ray studies are necessary for accurate diagnosis. Management consists of rest, ice, compression, and elevation (RICE); activity modification; and rehabilitation, unless a greater than 3-cm displacement exists, at which point surgery is required. Refer to Display 13.12 for phases of rehabilitation of an avulsion fracture.[13]

Apophysitis most commonly occurs at six major sites in the hip and pelvis: iliac crest, ASIS, anterior inferior iliac spine (AIIS), ischial physis, and greater and lesser trochanters of the femur. Apophysitis is often observed in runners, ice skaters, football players, soccer players, and dancers. Treatment includes activity modification, ice, nonsteroidal anti-inflammatory drugs (NSAIDs), and rehabilitation with an emphasis on flexibility and core strengthening as well as sport-specific activities. Typically, hip fractures and dislocations, which are best treated surgically, are not seen in adolescent sports but are encountered during motor sport activities and vehicular accidents.

Pelvic stress fractures, although uncommon, are found in runners. Symptoms are pain in the inguinal, perineal or adductor region. Protective weight bearing, rest, and inactivity are recommended. A referral to a nutritionist or primary care physician is needed if disordered eating is suspected.

Acetabular labrum tear is an acute injury with severe anterior hip pain. A popping or snapping sensation is often heard or felt. A positive impingement test for an acetabular labrum tear is elicited with flexion, adduction, and internal rotation of the affected leg. Surgical treatment to excise the torn labrum is performed. A slow progressive rehabilitation program follows surgery.

Snapping hip syndrome commonly affects dancers, ice skaters, and gymnasts who require increased hip flexibility with strength and endurance of the hip muscles in order to perform their activities. Two separate mecha-

nisms of injury or overuse cause snapping hip. External snapping hip is created as the tight or shortened iliotibial band repeatedly moves over the femoral greater trochanter. This mechanism may also cause a concurrent trochanteric bursitis. Internal snapping hip is produced by the tight iliopsoas moving over the iliopectineal eminence of the pelvis. In addition, overuse of the iliopsoas muscle during hip flexion is another cause of internal snapping hip. Symptoms include a palpable or audible snap over the greater trochanter or under the iliopsoas muscle. Often the snap will occur in a particular point during the arc of motion. Pain occurs with activity and the offending movement. As the injury progresses, the snapping and pain increase in intensity and frequency. Positive examination findings include Ober test for iliotibial band tightness and Thomas test for hip flexion contracture. The athlete should be taught that engaging the deep abdominal and pelvic floor muscle while lifting and trying to maintain a forward leg position are necessary activities to reduce pain and preventing recurrence.[23]

Trochanteric bursitis of the femur presents with tenderness on palpation over the greater trochanter and complaints of pain while lying on effective side. Biomechanical examination should be performed including leg length measurement and analysis of the sport-specific activity or movement that causes the snapping. The findings of this examination help the therapist develop a comprehensive and rational treatment program and prevention plan. Treatment guidelines include rest, NSAIDs, flexibility exercise for all hip muscles, strengthening of hip abduction and external rotation muscles, core strengthening, and education in proper sports technique. Stretching of the tensor fascia lata (TFL) and iliotibial band (ITB) is necessary in lateral snapping hip syndrome and trochanteric bursitis.[24] This stretching is effective when performed in multiple positions (standing/sitting/lying). Soft tissue massage of the lateral thigh can be performed while side-lying over a foam roller. Although uncomfortable, this technique can be rather effective in relieving symptoms of lateral snapping hip.

Various fractures of the femur can occur is sports. Skier's hip, a season-ending injury, refers to the intertrochanteric and subtrochanteric fractures that occur during a fall. Surgical fixation is required. Femoral fractures can be life threatening and are treated aggressively on and off the field with immobilization on the field followed by rapid transport to the emergency room.

Overtraining can result in stress fracture of the femoral neck in older adolescents. Femoral neck stress fractures are classified as tension side, compression side, or displaced. Severe pain results in decreased or absent ability to bear weight. The pain is referred to the groin or thigh. A tension-side fracture is located on the superior portion of the femoral neck and requires surgical intervention. A compression-side fracture is located on the inferior side of the femoral neck and is treated with protective weight bearing until pain free at rest.[3]

▶▶▶ DISPLAY 13.12

Phases of Rehabilitation of an Avulsion Fracture

Week 1—rest, protected weight bearing and limb position

Week 1 to 3—protected gait and gentle assisted range of motion (ROM) and passive ROM

Week 3—light resistance

Month 1 to 2—return to sport activity

Month 2 to 3—return to play

In the female athlete, osteopenia and osteoporosis may predispose to femoral fracture. The fulcrum test is used to identify femoral shaft stress fractures. With the athlete in a sitting position, the examiner places an arm under the distal portion of the thigh and applies a gentle press to the lower leg. A positive test elicits pain in the femoral shaft. Eight to 16 weeks of rest is indicated from the initial onset of pain.[3] In general, a painful limp or inability to bear weight requires the use of crutches until definitive diagnosis is provided by a physician.

Athletes experience a high incidence of soft tissue injuries to the thigh area. The majority of theses injuries are treated with RICE and gradual return to sport when pain free. A quadriceps contusion is the result of blunt trauma to the thigh. A large hematoma with pain and swelling is often observed. Besides RICE, the knee is immobilized in knee flexion during the acute period to minimize the hematoma and prevent complications of compartment syndrome and myositis ossificans. The thigh is immobilized for 24 to 48 hours followed by active ROM exercise, a gradual return to activity, and continued application of ice. In about 2 to 3 weeks, the athlete can return to sport with protective padding over the contusion. Myositis ossificans is a condition where abnormal bone forms within the muscle at the site of a large hemorrhage. It is treated nonoperatively with ROM and strengthening exercises. If the bony mass interferes with ROM and/or function, surgical excision is indicated. The operation is performed minimally at 6 months after the initial injury, after the bone has matured. Attempts to excise the bone prior to maturation increase the risk of recurrence.

Compartment syndrome in the thigh is rare, but preventive measures are still implemented due to the seriousness of the injury. Swelling occurs within any or all three fascia compartments of the thigh, which produces a rise in intracompartmental pressures. This pressure increase may result in muscle ischemia, cellular acidosis, and necrosis. Signs include an abnormally high pain rating given the extent of injury, and pain described as deep, constant, and not relieved by rest. An increase in pain is noted with passive knee flexion. Motor impairments and diminished pulses are later findings and associated with permanent damage. Diagnosis is confirmed with compartment pressure testing. If testing is positive, a fasciotomy is performed to relieve the pressure.

Muscle strains occur more in the young athlete as the skeletal system matures. Excessive stretch usually during eccentric contraction is typically the mechanism of injury. Acute, sharp, localized pain is described over the area of injury. Hamstrings, quadriceps, and adductors are frequently strained. Recurrence rates are high if the athlete returns to play too quickly or without adequate rehabilitation. Traditional treatment consists of RICE, gentle stretching, and isometrics. As pain diminishes, isotonic strengthening within full ROM is implemented. Sport-specific activities are practiced when the athlete is pain free

prior to return to sporting competition. There are current questions about the effectiveness of this approach versus a functionally based rehabilitation program.

Groin pain is common among soccer, ice hockey, and tennis players due to the increased recruitment of hip abductor and adductor muscles. Besides adductor and iliopsoas strains, multiple nonmuscular causes of groin pain exist. The causes often include inguinal hernia, prostatitis, orchitis, tumors, and testicular torsion, the latter commonly experienced by distance runners and cyclists. Testicular torsion is a urologic emergency.[3]

Meralgia paresthetica is described as burning and stinging sensations on the lateral aspects of the thigh as the result of lateral femoral cutaneous nerve compression. This injury is experienced by gymnasts with impact on the parallel bars and by backpackers and football players due to pad tightness. Pressure relief through activity and equipment modifications will alleviate symptoms.

For many pelvic, hip, and thigh injuries, compression sleeves, wraps, and shorts can be beneficial when returning to sport. These items are only effective if used and fitted properly. As a group, their function is to hold protective pads in place, provide compression, and decrease ROM.

Knee

EXAMINATION

Examination of the knee invariably begins with an assessment of gait as the patient enters the treatment area. Unaware of being examined, the patient's gait pattern is likely to be genuine. Gross abnormalities such as limping and lack of normal knee ROM are often identified at this time.

During the history, the patient with knee pain should be asked specific questions. Answers about typical sitting positions can offer pertinent information. Questions about features common in the patient with insidious anterior knee pain should focus upon positions including "W" sitting, side sitting, or sitting on feet. Other helpful questions regarding symptoms should include the response to going up and down stairs, prolonged sitting (movie-goers sign), prolonged standing, and walking. The presence of the knee joint giving way, locking, or clicking as well as instability should also be ascertained.

Following the history, tests and measurements should begin. The patient should be dressed in shorts and a T-shirt (tucked in to allow visualization of pelvic activity) or a sports bra for females, and be barefoot. If the patient is able to walk, gait should be examined while bearing in mind the gait demonstrated by the patient upon entering the clinic. Obvious changes from that presenting gait should be noted and instructions to the patient presented. Often pediatric and adolescent patients will have difficulty walking genuinely when they know they are being examined. Using distraction techniques and humor can help in these situations so that the patient focuses on something other than gait. Have the patient walk back and forth a few times, observing from the front, back, and sides. Note what is occurring biomechanically starting from the foot up through the trunk. Some of the most common features of altered gait will be excessive foot pronation with concurrent internal rotation of the leg, genu valgus, pelvic abnormalities such as Trendelenburg pattern, side bending or shifting of the trunk over the involved side, decreased stance time on the involved extremity, and lack of full ROM of one or more leg segments during gait. Having assessed gait, observation of the injured area and examination to rule out or clear the foot, hip, and spine can be pursued as described in assessment.

LIGAMENTOUS INJURIES TO THE KNEE

The most common ligament injuries of the knee involve the medial collateral ligament (MCL) and ACL. Valgus trauma is the typical cause of an MCL injury and the patient will present with medial knee pain. Testing involves palpation of the MCL and valgus stress to the knee in extension and flexion. The typical grading for ligament injuries is I through III. Grade I injuries involve strain of the ligament without associated instability. In the case of the MCL this would present as equal medial gapping of the knee in comparison to the uninjured knee, with the test performed in slight knee flexion. Grade II is a partial disruption of the ligament with mild/moderate joint instability. Grade III is a full disruption of the ligament with significant instability. It should be noted that in the skeletally immature individual, distal femoral physeal damage can mimic an MCL strain/tear. The patient will note medial knee pain and gapping can be present if the physis has been disrupted (Salter-Harris I injury).

Management of MCL tear typically consists of rehabilitation rather than surgical reconstruction. Injuries that occur primarily at the femoral end of the ligament tend to repair themselves with more satisfactory scarring and motion can be rapidly initiated. Conversely, tibial-end injuries of the MCL may need comparatively longer immobilization and may progress more slowly. The need for immobilization will also depend on the severity of the injury, with grade I sprains generally requiring little if any immobilization and grades II and III requiring longer periods of immobilization.

Lateral collateral ligament (LCL) injuries generally occur as a result of varus trauma and the athlete presents with lateral knee pain. Testing will consist of palpation of the LCL, the pain noted with varus stress, and the flexion abduction external rotation (FABER) test, in which the injured ankle is placed on the knee of the uninjured extremity with the patient supine. In the FABER position the LCL should feel like a pencil at the lateral aspect of the knee, coursing parallel to the fibula. Management again consists of rehabilitation techniques except in extreme cases.

ACL injuries receive the most attention of all knee injuries. As with MCL injury, bone injury can occur instead of ligament damage in the skeletally immature patient. Tibial spine avulsion fracture can occur and can be ascertained via plain radiographs. In these cases immobilization in extension may prove effective, although surgical repair may be required. The typical mechanism is often noncontact forceful quadriceps contraction while pivoting on a planted foot. The injury may mimic patellofemoral pain syndrome at first due to giving way and anterior knee pain. However, on close questioning the athlete describes hearing and feeling a pop as the injury occurs. Frequent "giving way" or knee buckling often follows. Swelling is progressive and may be described as a "dripping faucet." Loss of motion can be present and a loss of extension can result from a "cyclops" lesion where the retracted stump at the tibial plateau binds in the intracondylar notch near terminal extension. It is possible that the patient may not have pain. Bone bruising is noted frequently on MRI as a result of the joint subluxation that also occurs. Testing for ACL integrity consists primarily of the Lachman test. The Lachman test is the most sensitive test for ACL rupture.[1] Pivot shift testing is also valuable as well as KT 1000/2000 arthrometry.

Management of ACL disruptions in the young population often includes surgery. If the patient is too young for knee reconstruction because of concerns of growth plate disruption, bracing and activity restriction is frequently employed until skeletal maturity necessary for the reconstruction is reached. Unfortunately, patients are often noncompliant and secondary injuries such as meniscus tears occur during this waiting period. New procedures to reconstruct the action of the ACL with physeal sparing may enable earlier reconstruction and minimize reinjury. Unlike adults, adolescent patients most often have reconstruction of their ACL injury. Adults may have good secondary constraints, may not have lifestyles that provoke instability, and may not require reconstruction to live a normal lifestyle.

Prior to reconstruction, prehabilitation is very important to activate muscles inhibited by the injury and teach the patient to exercise properly before reconstructive surgery. Following reconstruction, the patient can typically advance to weight bearing as tolerated. Closed-chain exercises and proprioceptive training activities can be initiated early. Much of the progression will depend on the type of graft and its fixation, as well as concomitant injuries/repair.

Posterior cruciate ligament (PCL) injuries typically occur as a result of landing on the knee or motor vehicle accidents where the knee makes contact with the dashboard. With this type of trauma, posterior movement of the tibia on the femur occurs forcefully, causing a tear in the PCL. Problems with sprinting are one of the most common presenting signs. Clinical testing consists of the posterior sag sign, in which the tibia of the injured leg sags posteriorly to the noninjured leg, and the posterior drawer test. Because the PCL has demonstrated the remarkable capacity to repair itself, typical management of PCL tears is often nonoperative. Rehabilitation again consists of closed-chain strengthening and progressive return to sports activities.

FRACTURES

As mentioned previously, tibial spine avulsion fractures can occur in place of ACL disruptions in the skeletally immature individual and may mimic ACL disruptions. Radiographs can confirm this diagnosis. These fractures are managed with cylinder casting if the fragments are not greatly displaced or by screw fixation in the presence of significant displacement or lack of reduction with casting.[3]

Sleeve fractures most often occur as a result of forceful quadriceps tension at the inferior pole of the patella in children 8 to 12 years old. This avulsion injury can also occur at the proximal pole of the patella. On examination there is significant pain and tenderness over the site and a palpable gap is possible. Patella alta, an abnormally high-riding patella, is frequently noted as well as a quadriceps muscle extensor lag. Imaging procedures confirm the diagnosis and management consists of immobilization followed by rehabilitation. If the fragment is significantly displaced, surgery to reduce the fragment will be necessary.[4]

Tibial tubercle fractures occur most frequently in skeletally mature males participating in high jumping sports and basketball.[4] Pre-existing Osgood-Schlatter disease is common. The typical presentation is pain over the tibial tubercle and displacement of the tubercle noted on radiography. Management can be conservative with closed reduction and immobilization for mild cases and surgical intervention for more displaced cases. Rehabilitation should proceed according to the procedure and will be similar to that for Osgood-Schlatter disease.

Medial distal femoral epiphysis fractures can, as mentioned earlier, mimic MCL injuries. As in MCL injuries, the mechanism is typically a valgus trauma. In the skeletally immature individual the femoral epiphysis fails due to the insertion of the MCL being inferior to the femoral physis (whereas the tibial portion inserts on the diaphysis [i.e., crosses the physis]). As is often the case in the skeletally immature individual, the tensile strength of ligaments and tendons exceeds the tensile strength of the adjacent apophysis or physis. As a result, the bone tends to fail rather than the tendon or ligament. The presentation will be medial knee pain. Clinical examination shows pain with valgus stress and possible knee laxity. Pain to palpation of the medial femur at the physis rather than along the course of the MCL will also be noted. Management consists of cylinder cast immobilization if the fracture is not significantly displaced.[4] Rehabilitation can proceed following healing with precautions to avoid valgus stress initially. As with all growth plate injuries, the potential for growth arrest and resultant deformity is present and follow-up

with the orthopedic surgeon is necessary. A physeal bar can form and tether growth in one area, causing angular deformity. The sports physical therapist must monitor alignment of the extremity and refer the athlete back to the physician if any abnormalities are noted.

OVERUSE INJURIES

Overuse injuries are surprisingly common in the skeletally immature individual. Anterior knee pain, a global term to describe pain in front of knee, is the most common symptom of overuse injury. Pain here can be caused by Sinding-Larsen-Johannson (SLJ) disease, Osgood-Schlatter disease (OSD), an inflamed synovial plica, patellofemoral pain syndrome (PFPS), infrapatellar tendonitis, prepatellar bursitis, and fat pad irritation, as well as a host of other entities. In the pediatric and adolescent population, the most common overuse sources of anterior knee pain are OSD, SLJ, PFPS, and symptomatic plicae.

APOPHYSITIS

OSD and SLJ disease typically affect boys aged 10 to 15 and girls aged 8 to 13. These disorders represent an apophysitis of the tibial tubercle (OSD) and inferior patellar pole (SLJ). The presentation is anterior knee pain at the tibial tubercle (OSD) or inferior patellar pole (SLJ). Testing includes palpation of the injured area and radiographic studies.

Management for both of these disorders includes rest from offending activities, hamstring and quadriceps stretching, straight leg raises, and closed-chain strengthening when tolerated. Long-term flexibility and strengthening will be needed for prevention of these disorders until growth is finished. The patient should be educated that pain may not disappear completely until growth is complete but that mild discomfort is acceptable and not a contraindication to participation in running and jumping sports. In the case of OSD, a bump may be noted at the tibial tubercle and may persist into adulthood.

PATELLOFEMORAL PAIN SYNDROME

PFPS requires special attention and is often seen in the pediatric and adolescent athlete. It is marked by pain at the patellofemoral joint. When asked to point with one finger to the source of pain, patients will often scribe a line along the medial border of the patella or circle the patella. Debate continues as to the source of pain since cartilage is insensate. Clinical correlates with PFPS appear to be malalignment of the lower extremity, with valgus and medial rotation being most common; maltracking of the patella; improper footwear; tight hamstrings, quadriceps, and iliotibial band; and patellar instability, subluxation, or dislocation.

The presentation generally consists of pain about the patella, movie-goers knee, and pain with kneeling and ascending and descending steps. Pain also appears to worsen with squatting and impact activities. Clinical testing includes pain to palpation of the undersurface of patella (be careful not to mistake this with retinaculum) and a positive patellar grind test. Pain with squatting, which can be relieved with patellar realignment via taping or manual techniques, is also indicative of patellofemoral pain.

The management of patellofemoral pain syndrome can be difficult and slow. Stretching is needed for the hamstrings, quadriceps, tensor facia lata muscle and the associated iliotibial band, and hip flexor muscles. Straight leg raising for facilitation of quadriceps function is helpful but may not be well tolerated in terminal extension. As the condition improves the knee can be extended more. Ankle weights can be used in progression to between 10% and 15% of the individual's body weight. This formula has not been scientifically derived, but our experience shows this is a reasonable/effective guideline.

Management also consists of knee squats with good alignment and no patellofemoral pain, up to 100 degrees of knee flexion. There is some debate about how far to allow the knees to progress over the feet and whether they should be maintained behind the forefoot, but we believe that consideration must be given to the demands of the individual's sport or activity—if those demands place the knee beyond the foot, it may be in the best interest of the patient to address this position prior to discharge. The same can be said of valgus and rotational positions.

Techniques useful in the treatment of patellofemoral pain include squeezing a ball between the knees while squatting or performing knee extension exercises. This technique may reduce pain compared to performing the exercise without the squeeze. Over time the squeeze can be eliminated. Taping can also be used to decrease patellofemoral pain. The technique has been well described and consists of attempting to correct malalignment forces (i.e., attempting to medially glide the patella in the presence of lateral maltracking, attempting to laterally rotate the patella in the presence of rotational malpositioning). Knee extension isometrics at 90 degrees of knee flexion may also be beneficial along with medial gliding of the patella if lateral knee structures are tight. Bands of tight fibers from the iliotibial band can tether the patella into lateral tracking and/or a lateral tilt.

The remainder of the biomechanical chain must be considered in patellofemoral pain syndrome. Pronation of the foot, rotational deformity of the tibia or femur, and weakness of the core or hip abductors and rotators may all play a role in patellofemoral pain. The individual must be educated about certain entities that cannot be changed and which compensations may be appropriate or not. For example, structural external tibial rotation will cause the individual to have an externally rotated foot when the knee is in good alignment. This is acceptable. Forcing the foot to face forward in this case will only serve to inappropriately

internally rotate the leg and promote valgus. Other issues that may influence biomechanics include proper footwear and orthotics (either custom or over the counter). These should be utilized both during sports participation and throughout the day.

One of the most frequent mistakes made in the rehabilitation of patellofemoral pain is the lack of questioning regarding the presence of pain with exercises or the outright acceptance that pain with exercise is to be expected. Pain with exercise or activity only serves to prolong the rehabilitation process by perpetuating the irritation that underlies this diagnosis. Therefore, if the patient continues to perform activities or assume positions that cause discomfort, rehabilitation will be protracted. The therapist *must* routinely ask the patient about activities and pain on a daily basis—the best rehabilitation in the world stands little chance of curing this condition if the patient continues to incite irritation outside of the clinic.

Surgery for patellofemoral pain syndrome is a possibility. If the patient has malalignment and conservative measures prove unsuccessful, a lateral retinacular release or medial reefing can be performed. Other surgeries focus on elevation or medialization of the tibial tubercle to optimize alignment and decrease stress on the patellofemoral joint. Rehabilitation following one of these surgeries is similar to conservative treatment of patellofemoral pain and may vary depending on the surgery. Of note is that a lateral retinacular release is a very aggressive technique and requires significant healing time. Postsurgical effusion can last a long time. Hence, aggressive measures should be taken to prevent and reduce effusion perioperatively during the early phases of healing. Progression to activity will be dictated by the absence of pain. Nonimpact activities are used initially and gradually more aggressive activities are introduced as long as there is no pain during or after the activity.

INTRA-ARTICULAR INJURIES

One condition commonly associated with the younger population is a discoid meniscus, where the meniscus is shaped like a disc rather than its normal semilunar shape. Discoid menisci are present in approximately 1% of all lateral menisci[25] but are rare medially.[4,26] Typical symptomatic progression of discoid menisci include complaints of snapping noises in the preschooler and pain in the elementary aged individual. Effusion, giving way, and locking can also be observed.[1,4] These symptoms typically occur as a result of instability or a tear of the meniscus. On examination one is likely to find tenderness at the joint line and a positive McMurray test. Confirmation of the diagnosis is made with MRI.[1] Treatment of discoid menisci ranges from rehabilitation to surgery, the former for largely asymptomatic presentations (such as snapping only) with nondegenerated and stable menisci, the latter for more symptomatic, degenerated, or unstable menisci.[1,4] Whether used as a conservative or postoperative measure, rehabilitation consists of flexibility and strengthening exercises with activity progression as indicated by symptoms or surgeon preference, depending on surgical procedure.

Meniscal tears typically occur as a result of sports trauma or a discoid meniscus.[28] Typical symptoms include joint line pain, effusion, locking, and possibly giving way with a predisposing mechanism of a twisting injury with a notable pop. Associated ligament injuries are common.[28] Clinical testing consists of McMurray test and joint line palpation. Management for meniscal tears consists of immobilization if the tear is in the red zone, the outer border with better blood supply, and is not large. Surgical repair is commonly recommended if the tear is large and has vascular supply, and partial meniscectomy if the tear is in an avascular zone of the meniscus.[1] Children and adolescents generally have greater vascularity in the meniscus and may be more likely to recover with conservative measures.

OCD of the knee most commonly occurs at the lateral aspect of the medial femoral condyle. It is marked by separation of the cartilage from the subchondral bone. OCD is rare in children under the age of 10 and is seen mostly in males. It is classified into three groups. Juvenile OCD occurs in individuals with an open distal femoral growth plate. Adolescent OCD occurs in individuals with a nearly closed distal femoral growth plate. In adult OCD the distal femoral growth plate is closed. The adult type can be seen in the late teenage years. The onset of OCD can be traumatic or insidious. Juvenile cases tend to heal best, with recovery rates as high as 75%. In adolescent cases about half resolve and the other half follow a more adult progression that includes osteoarthritic development.[4]

Presentation of OCD often consists of vague knee pain and possible swelling and stiffness. Clinical examination is generally nonspecific, depending on the lesion. Plain radiographs and MRI confirm the diagnosis. Management consists of immobilization and rest for several weeks in cases where there is no loose fragment.[4] If this approach is insufficient, or in the case of more involved lesions, surgical intervention is required. Typical approaches consist of debridement and/or drilling to stimulate hemorrhage and inflammation in an effort to yield a fibrocartilaginous repair. Postsurgical rehabilitation will depend on the procedure performed. Generally ROM and open-chain exercises are used in the initial phase of rehabilitation, followed by progressive weight-bearing exercises, activities to improve proprioception, and cross-training. Eventual return to impact activities is expected, but the time frame will depend on the extent of the defect and surgeon preference.

OTHER KNEE PAIN SYNDROMES

A plica is a thin wall of fibrous tissue extending from the synovial capsule of the knee. Plicae can be asymptomatic, but they become symptomatic via irritation and by causing irritation of the medial femoral condyle.[28] The presentation is that of anteromedial knee pain that is very similar to patellofemoral pain. Testing consists of palpation of the plicae, which tend to feel like bands oriented in transverse plane from the patella to the medial collateral ligament. Palpation in an inferior to superior direction, transverse to the orientation of the plicae, can identify them, although location is sometimes difficult. Conservative management of symptomatic plicae is the same as for patellofemoral pain syndrome. Surgical excision may be necessary if conservative measures prove unhelpful.

Iliotibial band friction syndrome (ITBF) can occur at the knee as well as the hip. Precursors to this syndrome often include a tight ITB/TFL or weak hip abductors, which result in functional tightness of the ITB during weight bearing. This syndrome is marked by irritation of the lateral femoral bursa. The typical presentation consists of lateral knee pain with knee flexion and extension. Clinical testing includes palpation of bursae and noble compression test of pressure directly over the bursa while the knee slowly extends. The Ober test for tightness of the ITB is also helpful, as is examination of hip abductor strength. Management of ITBF includes ITB/TFL stretching, either by adduction of the leg or by lying on a foam roller to massage the ITB; strengthening weak hip abductors; frequent icing; avoidance of irritation; core strengthening; and, if indicated, correction of a leg length discrepancy.

Multipartite patella often presents in the bipartite form, mostly in males.[4] Anterior knee pain generally at the superior lateral area of the patella is the typical symptom. Unfortunately, this disorder is often misdiagnosed as a patellar fracture. Management generally consists of rest followed by rehabilitation. In unresponsive cases or cases that are severe, surgical intervention to remove the fragment and reattach the tendon can be performed.

Lower Leg, Ankle, and Foot

The lower leg refers to the area of the body below the knee. The tibia and fibula often encounter both traumatic and overuse injuries. The tibia is the most commonly fractured bone of the leg in children.[1] Direct injury usually results in fractures of both the tibia and the fibula. Standard treatment is closed reduction and cast immobilization if the fracture is stable, closed and with limited trauma to the surrounding tissues and nerves.

Growth plate injuries to the proximal and distal physeal area can occur in the tibia and fibula and are described using the Salter-Harris classification system. Management is based on the type of fracture. Physical therapy after immobilization is based on clinical findings, physical function, and physician preference.

Overuse injuries of the lower leg can present as muscle, bone, or nerve injuries. Identifying the specific site of pain narrows the differential diagnosis. For example, pain directly over bone suggests stress fracture, pain in the muscle suggests strain or chronic compartment syndrome, and medial or posteromedial pain suggests medial tibial stress syndrome. Radiating pain indicates radicular or nerve compression injury. Many athletes and coaches use "shin splints" to describe pain in the middle portion of the leg. The term *shin splints* most often represents medial tibial stress syndrome; however, stress fractures, compartment syndrome, and muscle strains should be considered and ruled out. Medial tibia stress syndrome is an inflammation of the periosteum, a fibrous membrane that covers the bone.[27] Initially, pain occurs with activity and is relieved by rest. A positive examination finds pain on palpation over the posterior medial edge of the distal third of the tibia. Musculoskeletal risk factors are varus hindfoot, forefoot pronation, genu valgum, increased femoral anteversion, and external tibial torsion.[28] Potential training errors that predispose to this problem are inadequate conditioning, inappropriate progression of training, overtraining, a hard training surface, and shoes not designed for the athlete's individual body type or activity. Bone scans may confirm the diagnosis by showing diffuse longitudinal area of uptake, as opposed to a transverse line, indicative of a stress fracture. Management includes identifying the predisposing factors and developing a plan for intervention. Activity modification and cross-training are cornerstones of treatment. Strengthening and stretching the gastrocnemius and soleus muscles is usually indicated. Proper shoes with appropriate cushion and support may be recommended. Generic or custom-molded arch supports are often beneficial.[2] The sports physical therapist must know the latest products available in order to make appropriate recommendations for each athlete. Once the athlete is pain free with walking, a graduated return-to-running program is implemented. Running distance, frequency, and intensity should not be increased more than 10% each week for any one item.

Stress fractures in runners usually occur in the middle and distal third of the tibial shaft, in the proximal tibia for jumpers, and at midshaft for dancers. The dreaded "black line," which appears as a transverse line on radiographs, represents anterior stress fracture.[28] Aggressive care is taken to prevent a complete fracture and to promote healing.[30] Surgery may be indicated, as this is often an area of bony nonunion.[30] Point tenderness located a few centimeters above the ankle joint on the fibula is a positive finding for a fibular stress fracture. Single-leg hopping will reproduce symptoms.

Acute compartment syndrome is an emergent condition that results from trauma to the lower leg. Fasciotomy is performed to relieve the compartment pressure and prevent permanent tissue damage. Exertional or chronic compartment syndrome is not an emergency situation but can be functionally disabling to the athlete in time.[29] The commonly reported "aching" pain and a tightness and squeezing sensation are exacerbated by exercise and relieved with rest.[31] Typically, symptoms disappear shortly after exercise ceases. Paraesthesias may be noted over the dorsal or plantar surface of the foot. Pain results from muscle ischemia that occurs when increases in compartment pressures become too great.[31] The pressure changes are caused by the increase in blood volume to the exercising muscle. The anterior compartment is the most commonly affected; however, any of the four compartments of the leg can become involved. Diagnosis of the syndrome is confirmed with compartment pressure testing. Conservative treatment consists of activity modifications; physical therapy including massage to improve ROM, reduce strength deficits, and enhance muscle endurance; orthotic use; and time. When conservative treatment fails, a surgical fasciotomy of all involved compartments is recommended.[31]

ANKLE INJURIES

Ankle injuries are the most common sport-related injury of all ages. The majority of ankle sprains occur on the lateral aspect with the mechanism of injury being inversion and supination of the foot. Only 3% of ankle sprains occur on the medial side.[28] Refer to Display 13.13 for grading of ligament sprains. During the examination, have the athlete pinpoint the area of maximal tenderness. A careful history can determine the foot position at time of injury (inverted, everted, plantar-flexed, dorsiflexed), which will help identify the structures involved. The anterior drawer test assesses the stability of the anterior talofibular ligament. The talar tilt test assesses the integrity of the calcaneofibular ligament. Both should be performed bilaterally to compare for that athlete the normal findings on the uninjured ankle. In the acute stage, the ankle is often too swollen and painful to perform the tests with accuracy. Differential diagnoses are anterior tibial fibular sprain

---

>> **DISPLAY 13.13**

Ankle Sprain Grading

Grade I—Integrity of ligament intact although some tearing occurs, no pathologic laxity, normal range of motion (ROM), minimal to no ecchymosis/edema, ability to bear full weight

Grade II—Ligamentous damage with tearing of fibers, pathologic laxity, motion loss, some resistance to ligamentous stress testing, moderate ecchymosis/edema, bears weight with discomfort and limp

Grade III—Complete rupture, instability to ligamentous stress testing, significant ecchymosis/edema, inability to bear weight

From Dormans JP. Pediatric Orthopaedics and Sports Medicine the Requisites in Pediatrics. St. Louis: Mosby, 2004; and Schenck RC. Athletic Training and Sports Medicine. 3rd Ed. Rosemont: American Academy of Orthopaedic Surgeons, 1999.

(ATFL), posterior tibial fibular sprain (PTFL), calcaneal fibular sprain (CFL), syndesmosis sprain, distal physeal fracture, peroneal longus subluxation, osteochondral fracture of the talar dome, and Maisonneuve fracture, a combination of a distal syndesmosis tear and a proximal fibular fracture.

Plantar flexion and inversion are most often the mechanisms of injury for a lateral ankle sprain. A lateral ankle sprain presents with pain on palpation of one or more of the following structures: ATFL, PTFL, and CFL. Initial treatment includes protection (splint, brace, Ace bandage, cast), rest (activity modification, altered weight bearing), ice (20 minutes every hour), compression (ace bandage, Tubigrip), elevation (minimizing dependent extremity position) (collectively referred to as PRICE).

Management of grades I and II ankle sprains are similar and progress according to resolution of symptoms. Gentle motion and protective weight bearing (using a brace/splint) are implemented early as the patient tolerates. Edema control is very important in re-establishing ROM and function and reducing pain. A J- or U-shaped pad placed around the lateral malleolus held in place with Tubigrip or an Ace bandage is recommended to reduce edema. Retrograde massage is often useful to decrease edema. Thera-Band and intrinsic foot muscle exercises are started early. As soon as the patient can tolerate weight-bearing activities, upright activities are initiated to improve balance, proprioception, strength, and function. Begin the functional intervention with bilateral weight-bearing activities and progress to single-leg weight bearing when the patient is pain free. Exercises are started on even surfaces, then progress to uneven surfaces like wobble boards, foam rollers, DynaDiscs, and BOSU, to name a few. External perturbations, provided manually or with elastic bands and tubes, further challenge the athlete's body awareness and balance. Return to sport activities begins with light jogging in a straight plane, in a controlled environment, on even surfaces with a brace. Activities are progressed from this point as tolerated. Running, jumping, and direction-change (cutting) maneuvers are all performed in therapy prior to returning to practice. The athlete must be able to complete a full practice without pain prior to competition. Most therapists recommend a brace or ankle taping when the athlete returns to play. There are many different ankle-bracing options for sport participation that are slimmer in design and lighter in weight compared to the brace used following the initial injury. Optimally, it is best to match the brace for the individual and the sport. Again, knowing the available bracing options on the market is important. Controversy exists as to when it is safe to discontinue external ankle support for sport.

Continued questioning regarding the presence of pain is warranted because most young athletes will not volunteer this information independently. Additionally, when a patient reports having pain, the specifics about the pain (where, how much, when, what relieves it) should be investigated. Therapeutic exercises, performed at home or in the clinic, should continue for 1 month after the resolution of symptoms with full return to activity.

Initial management of grade III ankle sprains is variable. Three different methods are most often implemented: surgical repair, immobilization with cast or pneumatic brace, and taping and early motion. After initial treatment, rehabilitation proceeds as noted above but often at a slower pace due to the greater severity of the injury.

Syndesmosis sprain often occurs with a dorsiflexed foot. Pain and tenderness are noted at the anterior aspect of the distal tibiofibular syndesmosis and interosseus membrane. Positive clinical tests are the "squeeze" test and external rotation test of the foot with the ankle in dorsiflexion. The squeeze test is performed by squeezing the lower leg at midshaft from the medial and lateral sides with both hands. This action places tension and gapping at the syndesmosis and reproduces pain if injured. The more proximal that pain can be reproduced on palpation, the more significant is the injury and the longer the athlete is immobilized. Treatment of syndesmosis sprain is usually immobilization for a few weeks. General rehabilitation principles as described above are implemented postimmobilization. If a significant diastasis is discovered, immediate surgery may be necessary to correct the instability. Recovery time is twice as long as a lateral ankle sprain.

During examination of what appears to be ankle sprain, the age of the patient must be considered. In children under 12 with an immature skeletal system, a physeal fracture of the distal fibula is highly probable with a lateral ankle injury. Nondisplaced Salter-Harris type I is the most common fracture of the distal fibular growth plate. Pain on palpation is over the physeal growth plate (Fig. 13.6), which is located about one finger width above the distal portion of the lateral malleolus. Management is 3 weeks with cast immobilization followed by rehabilitation, similar to that for a lateral ankle sprain.

Triplane fractures and Tillaux fractures occur as the athlete approaches skeletal maturity. Both fractures are the result of partially closed growth plates. The growth plate closes centrally first, followed by medial then lateral closure.

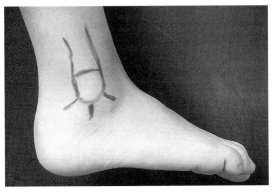

Figure 13.6 ■ Distal fibular physis.

This process leaves the lateral portion vulnerable for injury. A triplane fracture occurs in three planes: coronal, sagittal, and transverse. A Tillaux fracture is a Salter-Harris type III fracture of the unfused anterolateral segment of the distal tibial epiphysis caused by avulsion of the epiphyseal segment by the ATFL when the foot is forcefully externally rotated. Both fractures are managed with a long leg non–weight-bearing cast for 3 to 4 weeks followed by a short leg walking cast for 3 to 4 weeks.

Ankle impingement can be the source of anterior, anterolateral, or posterior pain. Anterior impingement is often seen in football and basketball players and dancers and is often caused by the formation of an osteophyte on the distal tibia.[3] Pain is reproduced with maximum dorsiflexion. As the ankle is dorsiflexed, the osteophyte contacts the talus and causes pain. Anterolateral ankle impingement is often an area of chronic pain, which persists after an ankle sprain. Possible causes are impingement of the tibiofibular ligament, impingement of the synovium, or an osteochondral fracture. Pain is reported in the area between the fibula and the lateral talus (sinus tarsi region) or around the ATFL. Treatment includes rest, NSAIDs, bracing, and possible orthoscopic debridement.

Posterior impingement is described as pain in the posterior ankle when the foot is plantar-flexed and is commonly experienced by ballet dancers. The pain is caused by a bony protrusion such as an os trigonum, a small, round bone behind the ankle joint. The os trigonum is found in about 5% to 15% of normal feet near the posterior talus. When the os trigonum fails to fuse with the talus, it can impinge on the soft tissue during plantar flexion.[3] Management consists of rest, NSAIDs, and surgical excision of the bony ossicle.

Osteochondral fractures of the talar dome can result from an ankle sprain if the talus contacts the medial or lateral malleolus during the excessive motion of the injury. Injury to the bone and overlying cartilage can produce a free-floating painful fragment in the joint space and may limit motion. Osteochondral fractures are difficult to diagnose during the acute stage of an ankle sprain, when much of the surrounding tissue is inflamed. Persistent pain after the sprain with continued edema and intermittent clicking or locking suggests a possible fracture.

FOOT AND HEEL PAIN

Heel pain in the athlete is most often attributed to Sever's disease, Achilles tendonitis, plantar fascitis, and calcaneal stress fracture. Achilles tendonitis and plantar fascitis are observed more frequently in the skeletally mature athlete. Sever's disease is calcaneal apophysitis. It presents as heel pain at the insertion of the Achilles tendon on the posterior calcaneus and sometimes on the distal Achilles tendon. Squeezing the calcaneus by compressing the medial and lateral sides will often reproduce the pain. The typical age of the athlete with Sever's is 9 to 12 years of age.[1]

Athletes who participate in sports requiring repetitive running and jumping are most often affected. Examination findings may include gastrocnemius and soleus muscle tightness, foot pronation, and swelling. Symptoms often appear during a growth spurt, in the beginning of the season, and while training on hard surfaces. The therapist should ask about the training regimen, type of shoe, and whether turf or spiked shoes are necessary. Treatment includes stretching of the involved muscles, gel heel lifts, purchasing a turf shoe or proper sneakers, orthotics, rest, ice, and NSAIDs. Some athletes can continue to participate in sports depending on the severity of symptoms. Recommendations for play or rest vary among clinicians. Activities are always discontinued with antalgic limp, pain at rest, and pain that persists for an extended time after the activity. The condition will usually resolve in a few weeks or months with proper treatment. In persistent cases, casting for immobilization may be an option.

A "pump bump" describes inflammation of the posterior calcaneal bursa with a palpable prominence over the calcaneus. This condition is caused by improper or new footwear and is often observed in ice skaters. A change in footwear improves the problem. Pressure relief pads constructed of foam, felt, or gel may help in the interim.

Plantar fasciitis presents with inferior heel pain along the medial plantar fascia. Pain can be elicited by pressing on the bottom of the heel in a superior direction. The insertion site of the plantar fascia onto the medial tubercle of the calcaneus is often the area of maximum tenderness and is frequently seen in joggers. Pain is often worse in the morning, especially with the first few steps and with increased activity. Rest, ice, and stretching of the plantar fascia multiple times a day relieve symptoms. Proper footwear and arch supports are often beneficial, as is a night splint, to sustain the fascial stretch when the tightness is prolonged. The athlete may continue to cross-train while symptoms are resolving.

Achilles tendonitis is typically reported as pain along the Achilles tendon just proximal to the superior margin of the calcaneus. Ballet dancers, runners, basketball players, and field athletes are susceptible. Foot pronation is believed to be a causative factor by placing increased tension across the Achilles tendon. Examination should include palpation along the entire length of the tendon, starting proximally and continuing inferiorly to the heel pad with the area of maximal tenderness being noted. Swelling, decreased dorsiflexion ROM, and pain with resisted plantar flexion are common findings. Single-leg heel raise and hopping reproduce pain at the Achilles tendon. Intervention begins with rest, ice, NSAIDs, gentle stretching of gastrocnemius and soleus muscles, and changes in footwear. As symptoms improve, light strengthening of the plantar flexor muscles is initiated. Begin strengthening in a non–weight-bearing position and progress to weight bearing with eccentric strengthening performed first on two legs, then on one, and, lastly, concentric contractions on the injured leg.

Balance, proprioception, and entire leg and core strengthening are recommended. Impact activities are added slowly with a graduated return to running.

MIDFOOT

Tarsal coalition is a congenital malformation where two or more of the tarsal bones remain fused. Talocalcaneal and talonavicular articulations are often involved. During the second or third decade of life, symptoms begin to appear as a result of joint immobility. An athlete presents with vague, aching pain over the medial and lateral aspect of the foot and the subtalar joint. Pain increases with activity and foot inversion. Pes planus (flatfoot) and decreased subtalar motion are observed. Treatment is dependent on the symptoms and the athlete. If conservative treatment fails, surgery to restore motion and relieve pain is an option.

An accessory navicular is a bony ossicle that forms on the medial plantar surface of the navicular. Twelve percent of these ossicles are imbedded within the posterior tibialis tendon.[28] Symptoms begin to occur around 12 years of age. Girls are affected three times more often than boys.[3] Pain increases with impact activities and while wearing shoes. A painful bony prominence can be palpated over the medial aspect of the navicular. Management is variable but consists of rest and pain relief by stabilizing the foot. Semi-rigid orthotics, a walking boot, and cast immobilization are all utilized depending on the severity of symptoms and therapist preference. Surgical excision of the accessory bone is successful.

Navicular stress fractures can be complete or partial and are differentially painful to palpation on the dorsum of the navicular. Sports requiring intense running and jumping put athletes at high risk. Radionuclide scanning identifies the presence of a navicular stress injury and computed tomography (CT) scan confirms the diagnosis. Because of the prevalence of nonunion and delayed union fractures, aggressive nonoperative management is implemented. Prolonged immobilization for 6 to 8 weeks with continued re-evaluation of the healing process is the treatment of choice. Rehabilitation after immobilization is a slow, gradual process with pain-free cross-training an important component.

Lis franc fracture dislocation of the tarsometatarsal joint occurs when an athlete lands on a hyperflexed foot as illustrated in football pile-ups and ballet and gymnastic landings. Intense pain and swelling is observed at the tarsal–metatarsal junction. An inability to bear weight is sign of a serious injury. The Lis franc ligament connects the medial cuneiform to the base of the second metatarsal and suffers a sprain. When a sprain occurs without a fracture dislocation, delayed ecchymosis and swelling result. Management of a severe sprain and fracture dislocation requires surgery. Moderate and severe sprains are usually season-ending injuries due to extended recovery time. Mild sprains are treated with rest and non–weight bearing in a cast for 4 to 6 weeks. A full-length custom-molded insert is used for return to play.

FOREFOOT INJURIES

Metatarsal fractures in children are common. A direct blow to the foot is a likely mechanism of injury with the second metatarsal most frequently injured. Stress fractures of the second metatarsal are observed in dancers and runners. Management of a nondisplaced fracture is closed reduction and a short leg walking cast for 4 to 6 weeks. Displaced fractures may require surgery. Significant swelling of the foot may result; therefore, monitoring signs of compartment syndrome is necessary. Avulsion fractures at the base of the fifth metatarsal are the result of increased tension from the peroneus brevis tendon. Pain is elicited with resisted eversion. The mechanism of injury is often forceful inversion. Immobilization in a cast or splint for 2 to 3 weeks is recommended.

A Jones fracture occurs at the proximal diaphysis of the fifth metatarsal. Athletes with skeletal maturity are most affected. This injury can also be caused by an inversion mechanism or by high impact loading.[3,4,30] Due to a decreased blood supply to this area, nonunion fractures are a potential complication. Symptoms are tenderness to palpation over the proximal shaft of the fifth metatarsal, localized swelling, and decreased ability to bear weight. Management is variable depending on the stability of the fracture, the healing process, and the athlete's goal in return to play. Treatment options include acute surgical management, immobilization in either non–weight-bearing or weight-bearing casts, and delayed surgery if nonunion or delayed union presents.[3,4,13,28,32]

Freiberg's disease or infarction is an osteochondrosis of the metatarsal head. Eighty percent occur in the second metatarsal[3] and adolescent females are affected more than males. Its etiology is unknown, but repetitive stress appears to be a factor.[4,32] Localized tenderness and swelling over the implicated metatarsal head is noted with a decreased ROM at the metatarsophalangeal joint. Treatment includes decreased activity, decreased weight bearing, cross-training, metatarsal pads, shoe inserts, and other footwear modifications that reduce stress on the metatarsal head. Intrinsic foot muscle strengthening should be a part of this rehabilitation program as well as for all other foot injuries.

Two sesamoid bones are located on the plantar surface of the first metatarsal head. They can become inflamed with repeated excessive loading of a dorsiflexed first toe. Increases in training schedule, hard surfaces, and flexible footwear can be contributing factors. Football players, field athletes, dancers, and runners are affected. Pain is elicited on direct palpation. Activity modification, changes in footwear, and use of a J-shape pad are recommended.

"Turf toe" is a hyperextension injury to the first metatarsophalangeal joint resulting in damage to the plantar capsule and ligamentous structures. Hard, artificial playing surfaces and footwear with a flexible toe box are causative factors. This is a ligamentous sprain and severity is classified with grades I through III as previously described for sprains. Treatment is implemented accordingly from continued participation to non–weight bearing. Shoe modifications and a stainless steel spring plate insert are recommended for return to play to prevent reinjury.[3]

Skin and toenail injuries to the foot are common in athletes. These injuries are revealed during a foot assessment and may be secondary to the primary treatment. Common problems encountered by the athlete may include ingrown toe nails, onychomycosis (fungal infection of the toenail), subungual hematoma, black toe, athlete's foot, corns, blisters, and calluses.

 ## Female Athlete

In 1972, Title IX of the Education Amendment Act was implemented. This Federal law ensured that female athletic programs and female athletes were given the same opportunities as males. Since that time, the number of female athletic programs and the number of female athletes have increased markedly. As participation numbers rise, care of the female athlete's injuries and special medical considerations are more prevalent.

Prior to puberty, the physical abilities of boys and girls are equal; however, after adolescence, the physiologic differences in the genders lead to inequalities. As girls and boys mature, hormonal changes produce a natural increase in body fat for girls and an increase in lean body mass for boys. With maturation, boys develop larger muscle fibers compared to girls. Eventually, women present with less muscle strength when compared to their male counterparts. After puberty, female athletes have lower maximal oxygen uptake due to physiologic cardiovascular differences.[31] Contributing factors that account for the differences in cardiac output are lower oxygen-carrying capacity of the blood, fewer red blood cells, lower hemoglobin content, smaller hearts, and lower stroke volume. For most endurance events, women cannot perform at the same level as men. Despite the physiologic differences, females have the capacity to achieve similar gains in strength, aerobic capacity, and endurance with equal, adequate, and proper training.

MUSCULOSKELETAL INJURIES IN WOMEN

Anatomic differences often predispose females to certain specific musculoskeletal conditions. Women often have a wider pelvis, anteverted femurs, a larger Q-angle, external tibial torsion, and increased ligament laxity. Women are therefore at higher risk for acquiring shoulder impingement, snapping hip syndrome, ACL rupture, patellofemoral pain syndrome, stress fractures, and metatarsal fractures. Often, the activities in which females participate predispose to higher rates of injury. For example, gymnasts and ice skaters will suffer low back pain from increased lumbar lordosis and ballet dancers will suffer foot injuries from repetitive trauma.

FEMALE ATHLETE TRIAD

The female athlete triad represents the interconnections among three specific medical conditions: disordered eating, osteoporosis, and amenorrhea. Disordered eating includes anorexia nervosa, bulimia nervosa, and eating disorder not otherwise specified (EDNOS). Prevalence of eating disorders among female athletes is estimated at 15% to 62% of all participants.[33] Disordered eating represents a serious medical condition, which affects injury rates, athletic performance, and mortality. If left untreated, 20% of people with anorexia will die secondary to physiologic complications. Display 13.14 includes some general signs of disordered eating.

Over time, the inadequate nutritional habits of an athlete with an eating disorder generate a decline in physiologic function. Fatigue, dizziness, cold intolerance, bradycardia, hair loss, and constipation are a few complications that may be observed. Amenorrhea is classified as primary if the onset of menses has not yet occurred or secondary with the absence of three to six consecutive menstrual cycles. Generally, athletes begin to menstruate later than nonathletes, averaging 13 years of age to 15.5 years of age compared to 12 and 15 years of age, respectively. It is also estimated that the incidence of menstrual dysfunction in athletes can be as high as 60% compared to nonathletes. An athlete with delayed menses and oligomenorrhea (irregular periods) or absent menstrual cycles is at increased risk for premature osteoporosis resulting from a decrease in estrogen, increased bone mineral loss, and decreased bone formation. Sixty to 70% of bone mineral density is acquired before the age of 20 years. Therefore, if an athlete is not laying down strong bone during her younger years, she puts

> ## DISPLAY 13.14
>
> ### General Signs of Disordered Eating
>
> - Food restriction
> - Rigid food patterns (vegetarianism)
> - Inadequate protein
> - Excessive dieting
> - Obsession with size and/or weight
> - Distorted body image
> - Eating alone
> - Vomiting

herself at risk for current and future lower bone mineral densities.[33]

Osteoporosis is diagnosed by dual-energy x-ray absorptiometry (DEXA) scans, which measure bone mineral density. When a DEXA scan measures bone mineral density that falls 2.5 standard deviations below the age norm for an individual, a diagnosis of osteoporosis is made. A smaller decline in bone mineral density of from 1 to 2.5 standard deviations below the norm is called osteopenia. Recurrent or multiple stress fractures for a female athlete require further investigation and identification of the primary cause. Is there an underlying eating disorder and resultant osteoporosis that has caused the stress fractures or are they due to an error in training? Often the answer is multifactorial.

The most effective treatment for an athlete suffering from symptoms of the female athlete triad is a multidisciplinary approach with a primary care physician, a nutritionist, and a psychologist being the most important professionals. Other team members may include orthopedic surgeons, physical therapists, athletic trainers, coaches, and parents. All members must work collaboratively to implement a universal plan to help the athlete achieve wellness and, if possible, return to play. A treatment philosophy should include maximizing performance, improving health and nutrition, improving training, and de-emphasizing weight and body size. Improved health and performance are achieved through increasing muscle mass, balancing nutritional and energy needs, and performing appropriate sport-specific skills. Awareness and prevention of the female athlete triad is the best approach before the cascade of interconnected problems begins. This approach requires education or re-education of the majority of members of society who influence female athletes' goals, perceptions, and performance.

 ### Environmental Conditions

Often athletic events are played in extreme weather conditions of heat, cold, and precipitation. Adjustments in training schedule, equipment, and nutrition are often necessary to maximize safety and performance in these environments. Acclimatization is the process by which an athlete gradually adjusts to changes in environmental conditions of temperature, humidity level, and altitude. Heat acclimatization is necessary for temperatures as low as 60°F and occurs in 4 to 7 days with as little as 90 minutes of exposure.[3]

HEAT-RELATED ILLNESS

Heat-related illnesses occur more rapidly as exposure to unusual conditions continues without intervention. Changes in symptoms can occur quickly and a mild problem can deteriorate rapidly to become a life-threatening situation. Profuse sweating is often an early sign. Heat cramps in the legs, arms, and abdominal area have been associated with dehydration, electrolyte imbalance, and lack of acclimatization. Treatment to reduce muscle cramps includes hydration and rest along with isolated active range of motion with prolonged stretch until symptoms resolve. Some clinicians believe passive range of motion can injure the athlete and the athlete should perform only active range of motion. Heat exhaustion is the body's response to prolonged excessive sweating without replacement of electrolytes or fluids. A vascular imbalance is created with a central decrease in blood volume due to dehydration and an increase in blood being shunted to the periphery to cool the body. The body begins to display signs of shock. See Display 13.15 for signs and symptoms of heat exhaustion and heat stroke.

Treatment of heat exhaustion includes rest in a cooler environment, hydration, removal of heavy or damp clothing and equipment secondary to perspiration, and application of cool towels and water. Heat stroke is a medical emergency caused by a rise in core body temperature due to delayed recognition of or intervention for the above causative factors. The athlete demonstrates symptoms of central nervous system impairments and failures. Anhidrosis occurs when the body's ability to produce sweat becomes impaired due to dehydration. Implementing the emergency medical system is a first priority while cooling the athlete quickly. Move the athlete to a cooler environment, use fans and water, and use ice packs in the axillae and groin. Monitor the physiologic responses and prepare to manage a respiratory or cardiac arrest if necessary. Prevention of heat-related illness requires education of coaches, parents, and athletes (refer to Display 13.16 for heat safety tips).

>> **DISPLAY 13.15**

Signs and Symptoms of Heat Exhaustion and Heat Stroke

Heat exhaustion

- Headache
- Nausea
- Dizziness
- Weakness
- Exhaustion
- Increased thirst
- Cool, moist, pale, ashen skin
- Conscious

Heat stroke

- Irritability, aggressiveness
- Emotionally labile, disoriented
- Glassy stare
- Unsteady gait
- Decreased blood pressure
- Rapid weak pulse
- Hot, dry skin
- Eventual unconsciousness

> **DISPLAY 13.16**

Heat Safety Tips

- Maximize skin exposure.
- Minimize gear and clothing.
- Choose lightweight clothing.
- Wear light colors (white, neutrals, and pastels).
- Change perspired uniforms throughout practice.
- Take rest and rehydration breaks for 10 minutes with every 30 minutes of practice.
- Make fluids available.

> **DISPLAY 13.17**

Signs of Hypothermia

- Shivering
- Clumsiness
- Fumbling
- Stumbling
- Decreased reaction time
- Mental confusion
- Speech difficulties

Monitoring of hydration status can be accomplished by calculating the difference between unclothed weights before and after practice. A pound of weight loss is about equal to a pint of fluid loss. If more than 2% of body weight is lost during practice, the athlete should be withheld from further activity until hydration improves. Using a color chart to monitor hydration level by the color of urine output is also effective. An accurate color chart is located on the back cover of *Performing in Extreme Environments* by Lawrence E. Armstrong, PhD.

LIGHTNING

Although lightning strikes are rare, caution must be observed with approaching storms because lightning can strike from as far as 10 miles away. Athletic fields and outdoor pools are usually in large open areas with minimal cover, thereby exposing both athletes and spectators. A 30-second lightning–thunder count indicates that a storm is within 6 miles of the event. The National Collegiate Athletic Association recommends stopping the event at that time and resuming the event 30 minutes from the last thunderclap.

COLD-RELATED INJURIES

Cold injuries can occur systemically or to localized tissues. Predisposing factors include inadequate insulation from cold and wind, circulatory restriction, poor nutrition, and ingestion of ethanol. The temperature, wind, and amount of time exposed to the elements all impact the severity of the injury. Frostnip and frostbite are localized problems that range from mild without permanent tissue damage to severe that include tissue necrosis. Distal parts of the body are more commonly affected because of diminished blood supply.

Hypothermia occurs when core body temperature falls below 95°F. Mild to moderate hypothermia is experienced when body temperatures are 95°F to 81°F. Severe hypothermia is less than 81°F. Hypothermia can occur with temperatures above freezing. Hypothermia is the body's response to cold, rapidly declining temperatures in a moist environment. Hunger, fatigue, and exertion influence the body's ability to maintain its core body temperature and can be cumulative in a cold environment. Display 13.17 provides common signs of hypothermia.

Intervention for mild cases includes removal of the exposed body part from the elements, removal of wet clothes, and addition of external heat with blankets, hot water bottles, and warm clothes. Warming with steady pressure from an external source such as a warm hand, breath, or another body part can aid rewarming. If the athlete is conscious, warm liquids can be ingested. Tingling and throbbing may occur during rewarming. Redness and tenderness may last for days or weeks depending on the severity. Severe hypothermia and deep frostbite are medical emergencies and activation of the emergency medical system is required.

Prevention of cold-related injuries includes minimizing exposure to the elements by wearing hats, gloves, and breathable rain gear. Wool and other synthetic materials that wick away moisture from the body help a sweating athlete from becoming chilled. Maintaining adequate nutritional status is also important while competing.

 Prevention

Some strategies for prevention of traumatic disorders and sports injuries have already been discussed throughout the chapter. Table 13.2 summarizes these strategies. Responsible decisions and appropriate actions from both adults and athletes are required to minimize sports injuries. Safety rules and safety equipment should be utilized whether the activity takes place at home, at school, in the community, or on the field.

SUMMARY

With good prevention strategies and education of parents, coaches, and health care workers, sports and recreational activities can become safer and more enjoyable to young children and adolescents. As childhood obesity

	TABLE 13.2	
Strategies to Prevent Traumatic Disorders and Sports Injuries		
Extrinsic Factors	**Intrinsic Factors**	**Training Factors**
Appropriate use and fit of equipment	Aerobic and anaerobic fitness	Adequate preseason conditioning
Appropriate type and fit of footwear	Appropriate strength of upper body, lower body, and core, specific for the demands of each sport	Gradual changes in training volume
Adherence to safety rules	Adequate flexibility	Hydration breaks
Adjustment for environmental conditions	Prevention of muscular strength and flexibility imbalances	Limits to training volume: e.g., count pitches and jumps, track amount of miles run
Early problem identification and treatment	Proper rest	Proper form, technique
Communication among multidisciplinary team	Proper nutrition Proper hydration	Maintain good skeletal alignment Proper strength and conditioning program

escalates, emphasis on fun and fitness is paramount. Developing good exercise habits early, through recreational or structured sports, establishes healthier habits in adults. Physiologic and psychological benefits associated with all types of exercise far exceed the risk. The choices are endless for most children, and riding a bike or scooter, gymnastics, dancing, swimming, field sports, running, hop-scotch, rock climbing, mountaineering, and jumping rope are all included.

It is the physical therapist's job to facilitate the prevention, education, and rehabilitation of sports-related injuries through proper recognition and treatment. Collaboration with coaches, athletic trainers, nutritionists, physicians, and parents complete the rehabilitation process. Remember, young children and athletes of all ages have specific needs, which have to be addressed. Knowing the demands of the sport and level of competition is critical in developing the plan of care. Complete rehabilitation with resumption of prior level of fitness is necessary for return to play.

CASE STUDIES
CASE STUDY 1

A 13-year-old female ice skater presents to the clinic with a 2-month history of low back pain, which is increasing. The patient reports an increase in pain whenever she performs skills that require her to grasp her skate behind her head. Her clinical examination findings include decreased shoulder flexion, tight hip flexors, tight hamstrings, and decreased thoracic extension. Posture examination shows forward shoulders, increased lumbar extension, anterior pelvic tilt, bilateral hip anteversion, and genu valgum with mild foot

pronation and tight gastrocnemius. Decreased strength is noted in the following areas: hip abductors, hip extensors, external rotators, quadriceps, and core. During a functional single-leg squat test, the athlete has difficulty keeping her knee over her second toe and falls into genu valgus while performing the squat. Spurling's maneuver is positive. Active spine motion tests show an increase in pain with extension and a decrease in pain noted with flexion or a neutral spine.

Questions

1. Given the examination findings described, what is the most likely diagnosis?
   a. Herniated disc
   b. Scoliosis
   c. Spondylolysis
   d. Muscle sprain/strain
2. Which of the following studies are beneficial in confirming the diagnosis?
   a. Radiography
   b. DEXA scan
   c. Bone scan
   d. a and c
   e. b and c
3. An initial home exercise program would include:
   a. Core strengthening
   b. Repeated spine extensions in prone
   c. Ice
   d. Williams flexion exercises
4. After acute inflammation has decreased, what other structures would be necessary to address in order to prevent recurrence?
   a. Increase lumbar spine extension, increase hamstring flexibility
   b. Increase shoulder flexion, increase thoracic extension

   c. Increase paraspinal strength, increase gastrocnemius strength
   d. Increase rectus abdominus strength, increase hip internal rotator strength
5. Assuming the skater is able to participate in conditioning activities without pain, which of the following would be most appropriate?
   a. Bike
   b. Step aerobics
   c. Slide board
   d. Swimming

CASE STUDY 2

A 10-year-old boy was injured playing soccer. He is hopping into the examination room with help from his parents. He reports that he turned his ankle while playing on an uneven field. He reports having 7 of 10 pain and points to the outside of his ankle. After shoes and socks are removed, the lateral ankle has minimal swelling and no ecchymosis. Palpation findings are negative to the ATFL, CFL, and syndesmosis area. He flinches when his distal fibula is palpated. Radiographs are normal. Mild motion loss in all directions with pain at end-range is noted.

Questions

1. What is the initial treatment of this patient?
   a. Cast immobilization
   b. Stretching of gastrocnemius muscles
   c. T-band exercises
   d. Ice and non–weight bearing
2. What is the most likely diagnosis?
   a. Lateral ankle sprain
   b. Salter-Harris type I fibular fracture
   c. Tarsal coalition
   d. Jones fracture
3. Early on in treatment, initiation of which of the following exercises is important?
   a. Single-leg heal raises
   b. Plyometrics
   c. Knee extension machine
   d. Foot intrinsic muscle exercises
4. What criterion is essential for initial return to sport?
   a. Pain free at rest
   b. Pain free with all sports-related activities
   c. Lower extremity functional tests of 70% involved versus uninvolved side
   d. Isokinetic testing of plantar flexion/dorsiflexion within 10% of uninvolved side

REFERENCES

1. Dormans JP. Pediatric Orthopaedics and Sports Medicine the Requisites in Pediatrics. St. Louis: Mosby, 2004.
2. Patel DR, Greydanus DE, Pratt HD. Youth sports: more than sprains and strains. Contemp Pediatr 2001;18(3):45–72.
3. Schenck RC. Athletic Training and Sports Medicine. 3rd Ed. Rosemont, IL: American Academy of Orthopaedic Surgeons, 1999.
4. DeLee JC, Drez D, Miller MD. Orthopaedic Sports Medicine Principles and Practice. 2nd Ed. Philadelphia: Elsevier, 2003.
5. Jansson A, Saartok T, Werner S, et al. General joint laxity in 1845 Swedish school children of different ages: age- and gender-specific distributions. Acta Paediatr 2004;93(9):1202–1206.
6. Strength Training by Children and Adolescents (RE0048). American Academy of Pediatrics, Committee on Sports Medicine and Fitness. Pediatrics 2001;107(6):1470–1472.
7. Pearson D, Faigenbaum A, Conley M, et al. The national strength and conditioning association's basic guidelines for the resistance training of athletes. Strength Condition J 2000; 22(4):14–27.
8. Baechle TR, Earle RW. Essentials of Strength Training and Conditioning. 2nd Ed. Champaign, IL: National Strength and Conditioning Association, 2000.
9. McKinnis LN. Fundamentals of Orthopedic Radiology. Philadelphia: F. A. Davis Company, 1997.
10. Perron AD, Brady WJ, Keats TA. Principles of stress fracture management-the whys and hows of an increasingly common injury. Stress Fract Manage 2001;110(3):115–124.
11. Miller C, Major N, Toth A. Pelvic stress injuries in the athlete-management and prevention. Sports Med 2003;33(13): 1004–1012.
12. Sullivan AJ, Anderson, SJ. Care of the Young Athlete. Rosemont, IL: American Academy of Orthopaedic Surgeons, 2000.
13. Korpelainen R, Orava S, Karpakka J, et al. Risk factors for recurrent stress fractures in athletes. American J Sports Med 2001; 29(3):304–310.
14. Available at: http://www.impacttest.com/back ground.htm. The Impact™ Team 10/2005 Natl. Ctr Sports Safety. Birmingham, AL 10/2005.
15. Available at: http://www.sportssafety.org.
16. Cantu RC. Second-impact syndrome. Clin Sports Med 1998; 17(1):37–44.
17. Tong HC, Haig AJ, Yamakawa K. The Spurling test and cervical radiculopathy. Spine 2002;27(2):156–159.
18. Crockett HC, Gross LB, Wilk KE, et al. Osseous adaptation and joint range of motion at the glenohumeral joint in professional baseball pitchers. Am J Sports Med 2002;30(1):20–26.
19. Altchek DW, Dines DM. Shoulder injuries in the throwing athlete. J Am Acad Orthop Surg 1995;3:159–165.
20. Tennent TD, Beach WR, Meyers JF. A review of the special tests associated with the shoulder examination. Part II: laxity, Instability and superior labral anterior and posterior (SLAP) lesions. Am J Sports Med 2003;31(2):154–160.
21. Gregg JR, Ganley TJ, Pill SG. Panner's Disease and Osteochondritis Dissecans of the Capitellum-Humeri. Presented at Three B Orthopedics and Sports Medicine Second Annual Philadelphia Sports Medicine Congress, June 15, 2001.
22. Krijnen MR, Lim L, Willems WJ. Arthroscopic treatment of osteochondritis dissecans of the capitellum: report of 5 female athletes. Arthroscopy 2003;19(2):210–214.
23. Micheli LJ, Solomon R. Treatment of recalcitrant iliopsoas tendonitis in athletes and dancers with corticosteroid injection under fluoroscopy. J Dance Med 1997;1(1):7–10.
24. Hip muscle weakness linked to ITBS. Georgia Tech Sports Med Perform Newsletter 2000;9(1):1–2.
25. Solomon DH, Simel DL, Bates DW, et al. The rational clinical examination. Does this patient have a torn meniscus or ligament of the knee? Value of the physical examination. JAMA 2001; 286(13):1610–1620.
26. Morrissy RT, Weinstein SL. Pediatric Orthopaedics. 5th Ed. Vol. 2. Philadelphia: Lippincott Williams and Wilkins, 2001.
27. Kortebein PM, Kaufman KR, Basford JR, et al. Medial tibial stress syndrome. Med Sci Sports Exerc 2000;32(3):S27–S33.

28. Brukner P. Exercise related lower leg pain: bone. Med Sci Sports Exerc 2000;32(3):S15–S26.

29. Blackman PG. A review of chronic exertional compartment syndrome in the lower leg. Med Sci Sports Exerc 2000;32(3): S4–S10.

30. Beaty JH, Kasser JR. Rockwood and Wilkins' Fractures in Children. 5th Ed. Philadelphia: Lippincott Williams and Wilkins, 2001.

31. Ireland ML. Female athlete: are there gender differences? ACSM Team Physician Course, New Orleans, LA, 2002.

32. Beighton P, Grahame R, Bird H. Assessment of hypermobility. In: Hypermobility of joints. 3rd ed. London: Springer Verlag; 1999. p. 9–22.

RECOMMENDED READINGS

Adkins SB, Figler RA. Hip pain in athletes. Am Fam Physician 2000;61(7):2109–2118.

Arendt EA, Griffiths HJ et al; The Use of MR Imaging in the Assessment and Clinical Management of Stress reaction of Bone in High Performance Athletes; Clinics in Sports Med. 16:1997.

Caplinger R. Radial nerve injuries in the throwing athlete. Ann Publ Prof Baseball Athl Trainers Soc 2004;17(1):1–8.

Clifford SN, Fritz, JM. Children and adolescents with low back pain: a descriptive study of examination and outcome measurement. J Orthop Sports Phys Ther 2003;33(9):513–522.

Hosalkar H, Dormans J. Back pain in children requires extensive workup. Biomechanics 2003; June:51–58.

Hutchinson MR. Elbow: functional anatomy. ACSM Team Physician Course; New Orleans, LA, 2002.

Hutchinson MR. Elbow Injuries: Overuse and Traumatic. Chicago: University of Illinois at Chicago.

Kelly AM, Pappas AM. Shoulder and elbow injuries and painful syndromes. Adolesc Med 1998;9(3):569–587.

Khan KM, Brukner PD, Kearney C, et al. Tarsal navicular stress fracture in athletes. Sports Med Injury Clin 1994;65–76.

Korkola M, Amendola A. Exercise induced leg pain: sifting through a broad differential. Physician Sports Med 2001;29(8):35–50.

Lyman S, Fleisig GS, Waterbor JW, et al. Longitudi-nal study of elbow and shoulder pain in youth baseball pitchers. Med Sci Sports Exerc 2001;33(11):1803–1810.

Magee DJ. Orthopedic Physical Assessment. 3rd Ed. Philadelphia: Elsevier, 1997.

Noffal GJ. Isokinetic eccentric–to–concentric strength ratios of the shoulder rotator muscles in throwers and nonthrowers. Am J Sports Med 2003;31(4):537–541.

O'Brien SJ, Pagnani MJ, Fealy S, et al. The active compression test: a new and effective test for diagnosing labral tears and acromioclavicular joint abnormality. Am J Sports Med 1998;26:610–613.

Paterson PD, Waters PM. Pediatric and adolescent sports injuries: shoulder injuries in the childhood athlete. Clin Sports Med 2000;19:4.

Playing it Safe on the Baseball Field: AAOS March 2000. Available at: http://orthoinfo.aaos.org/fact/thr_report.cfm?Thread_ID= 99&topcategory=Sports%20% 2F%20Exercise. Accessed October 15, 2006.

Reid DC. Sports Injury Assessment and Rehabilitation. New York: Churchill Livingstone, 1992.

Standaert CJ. Structural risks raise stakes for athletes with low back pain. Biomechanics 2003;Nov/Dec:53–58.

Tennent TD, Beach WR, Meyers JF. A review of the special tests associated with the shoulder examination. Part I: the rotator cuff tests. Am J Sports Med 2003;31(1):154–160.

Wilk KE, Meister K, Andrews JR. Current concepts in the rehabilitation of the overhead throwing athlete. Am J Sports Med 2002;30(1):15.

Wilson JD, Dougherty CP, Ireland ML, et al. Core stability and its relationship to lower extremity function and injury. J Am Acad Orthop Surg 2005;13(5):316–325.

Woodward TW, Best TM. The painful shoulder: part II. Acute and chronic disorders. Am Fam Physician 2000;61(11):3291–3299.

Young CC, Rutherford DS, Niedfeldt MW. Treatment of plantar fasciitis. Am Fam Physician 2001;63:467–474.

Exercise Instruction Guidelines for the Pediatric and Adolescent Population

General Guidelines

Guidelines for rehabilitation in the clinic include:

- Emphasize proper form. This is essential.
- Exercises should not produce/worsen joint/injury site pain, but will be uncomfortable to the exercising muscles. Pain during rehab is only acceptable when stretching scar tissue, and should resolve by next day.
- Use body weight before free weights (i.e., push-ups before bench press).
- Pain-free cross-training is important to maintain conditioning.
- Vary and advance frequency, intensity, and duration of exercises to address appropriate energy systems and muscle function as well as to ensure progress.
- Continuously reassess status of injury and response to rehabilitation; with young athletes you can typically advance the treatment program each session.
- Prevent iatrogenic complications such as patellofemoral pain and motion loss, etc.
- Work one on one with patients to ensure proper form, particularly as they fatigue. This also allows close monitoring of exercise intensity so that it can be modified as rapidly as possible.
- Practice sport-specific skills and consider having patient bring equipment to treatment.
- Know the limits of the athlete and the diagnosis—exercise intensity and volume will vary from patient to patient.
- With the exception of ice, modalities are rarely indicated, and at times contraindicated in the pediatric/adolescent population.
- Refer to the American Academy of Pediatrics Guidelines.

Guidelines for home exercise programs include:

- Keep exercises simple.
- Minimize number of exercises to maximize compliance (generally fewer than six total).
- Involve the family in the process. Parents know their children and know what is or is not likely to work. They can also play a role in ensuring participation by monitoring or even doing the exercises with their child.

- Discuss the immediate rewards of compliance for motivation such as performance enhancement, rapid return to activities, rapid pain loss, etc.
- Have individual demonstrate exercise independently.
- Provide written handout with pictures and exercise parameters.
- Have patients come in for follow-up to ensure appropriate progress, answer questions, and update program.

Specific Guidelines

Stretching

- Hold for at least 15 seconds (30 seconds is generally the most patients will tolerate well) and perform five to 10 repetitions.
- Perform at least daily (two to three times per day works best).
- It is best to perform after activity to maximize ROM gains.

Strengthening

- Exercise muscles/movements according to function: dynamic/static contractions, eccentric/concentric.
- A burning feeling in the muscle is acceptable but pain should not be produced, for the most part, at the injury site.
- Household items can be useful to aid with exercises (such as soup cans for weights or a sofa cushion to stand on to challenge balance).

Endurance

- Perform 12 or more reps over two or three sets, with little recovery between sets.

Strength

- Perform three sets of 10 reps where there is fatigue by the 10th repetition, followed by a full recovery period between sets.

Hypertrophy

- Perform strength training of moderate intensity (50% to 75% of one maximum repetition, or RM) and moderate to very high volume (three to six sets of 10 to 20 reps), with a short rest between sets.

Conditioning

- Phosphagen: 10 to 30 seconds of activity; train at a 1:3 to 1:5 activity:recovery ratio.
- Glycolysis: 30 to 90 seconds of activity; train at a 1:2 activity:recovery ratio.
- Aerobic: More than 90 seconds of activity; train at a 1:1 activity:recovery ratio.

Rest

- Generally, the more a patient adheres to rest guidelines, the more rapidly he or she will recover.
- Rest should be avoidance of all irritating activities.
- Appropriate rest guidelines during exercise sets maximize exercise effect (more rest between sets for strength development, less rest for endurance development).

Cryotherapy

- Most important is immediate cooling of injury, every hour for 20 minutes for first 12 hours.

- For rehabilitation purposes, the injured tissue needs to effectively be cooled. Equipment that circulates cold fluid (such as Game Ready and Cryocuff with pump) work best to cool without risk of frostbite. Generally 15 minutes of cooling with these devices is sufficient.
- Compress and elevate during cooling to reduce edema and effusion.
- Maintain compression following cooling if edema/effusion are present.
- Athlete should ice at home minimally following exercises or any time injury is irritated (optimally a few times per day).

Return-to-Play Guidelines

- The athlete must pass strength and functional tests and demonstrate adequate stamina/endurance to return to play.
- Athletes may progress back into sport before fully rehabilitated on a case-by-case basis.
- Start with limited practices and limited game time.
- Mild pain at the end of participation is acceptable if it is gone the next day.
- Limping during practice/play is unacceptable.
- Medicating before practice/play is not recommended.

Special Tests

Shoulder

Rotator Cuff	*SLAP*	*Instability*
Empty Can	Speeds	Anterior Apprehension
Full Can	O'Brien's	Relocation
Drop Arm	O'Brien's and ER	Posterior Apprehension
ERLS	Anterior Slide	Load-Shift
IRLS	Crank	Sulcus Sign
Neer Imp.	Biceps Load	
Hawkins Imp.		
Internal Imp.	*Other*	
Lift-Off	Scapular Slide	
	AC Shear	

Elbow

Elbow Valgus	Finkelstein's Maneuver	Phalen's Test
Elbow Varus	Halstead	Tinel's Sign

Hip

Spurling's	PA Mobs	Scour Test; Rectus Femoris
SLR	FABERs	Ober Test
Overpressure	Thomas Test	Prone ER/IR Symmetry

Knee

Lachman's	Posterior Drawer	Plica (30 Degrees/Medial Patella)
Varus	Valgus	Lateral Pivot Shift
Seated ITB Compression Test (30 Degrees)	Patellar Apprehension	Patellar Load/Shear
McMurray	Inhibition Sign	Inverted "J"

Ankle/Foot

Squeeze Test	External Rotation	Anterior Drawer
Thomson's	Five Toe Sign	Talar Tilt

14

Juvenile Idiopathic Arthritis

Susan E. Klepper

Pediatric rheumatology encompasses a wide variety of conditions characterized by acute or chronic inflammation, many of which affect multiple body systems. Because these conditions occur during the growing years, they frequently result in primary and secondary impairments that limit a child's ability to perform necessary and desired activities and participate in home, school, and community situations. Juvenile idiopathic arthritis (JIA) is among the most common of these conditions, although it is not a single disease but a category of disorders that comprise the most common arthritides of childhood. Because the signs and symptoms of these diseases evolve over time, it may take months to years to confirm a specific diagnosis. This can be unsettling for parents and children; however, during this time the rheumatology team carefully monitors the child's condition to manage ongoing problems and support the child's functional abilities.

The purpose of this chapter is to describe the role of the physical therapist in the examination, evaluation, intervention, and overall management of JIA in children and adolescents. Section one describes the criteria for diagnosis and classification, prevalence and incidence, etiology, pathology, and pharmacologic management of the conditions included under the umbrella JIA. Section two provides a framework, based on the *Guide to Physical Therapist Practice* and the World Health Organization's (WHO) International Classification of Functioning, Disability, and Health (ICF) model, for physical therapist examination, evaluation, and goal setting. Standardized assessments and outcome measures developed specifically for children with JIA are discussed. Section three describes interventions to address the most common problems in children with chronic joint disease. Evidence for specific interventions, where available, is presented. Issues related to home, school, and community participation are discussed. A case study illustrates the physical therapist's management of an older child with JIA.

Other pediatric rheumatic conditions that may result in arthritis include connective tissue diseases like scleroderma, juvenile dermatomyositis, systemic lupus erythematosus, and various forms of vasculitis. Rheumatologists also manage noninflammatory disorders in children such as benign hypermobility, localized and diffuse chronic pain syndromes, and heritable disorders of connective tissue. Although this chapter focuses on JIA, the principles that guide physical therapist management for the child with chronic arthritis are applicable to these other diagnoses. The reader will find valuable information about other pediatric rheumatic conditions in Cassidy and Petty's[1] and Melvin and Wright's texts.[2]

Criteria for Diagnosis and Classification of Juvenile Idiopathic Arthritis

Differences in the terminology used to diagnose and classify the heterogeneous group of conditions that result in childhood arthritis often cause confusion among clinicians. Table 14.1 compares the three systems currently reflected in the literature. The American College of Rheumatology (ACR) criteria for juvenile rheumatoid arthritis (JRA) have

> ### TABLE 14.1
>
> **Comparison of Classifications of Childhood Arthritis**

Characteristic	ACR	EULAR	ILAR
Basis of classification	Clinical (onset and course)	Clinical (onset only) and serologic (RF)	Clinical (onset and course) and serologic (RF)
Onset types	Three	Six	Seven
	Systemic juvenile rheumatoid arthritis (SoJRA)	Systemic juvenile chronic arthritis (SoJCA)	Systemic juvenile idiopathic arthritis (SoJIA)
	Polyarticular JRA (PoJRA)	Polyarticular JCA (PoJCA)	Polyarticular RF−
	Pauciarticular JRA (PaJRA)	JRA	Polyarticular RF+
		Pauciarticular JCA (PaJCA)	Oligoarticular JIA (OligoJIA)
		Juvenile psoriatic arthritis (JPsA)	Persistent
			Extended
		Juvenile ankylosing spondylitis (JAS)	Psoriatic arthritis
			Enthesitis-related arthritis (ERA)
			Other arthritis

ACR, American College of Rheumatology; EULAR, European League Against Rheumatism; ILAR, International League of Associates for Rheumatology; RF, rheumatoid factor.

been used primarily in North America, while the European League Against Rheumatism (EULAR) criteria for juvenile chronic arthritis (JCA) are more familiar in the United Kingdom. In 1994, the Pediatric Standing Committee of the International League of Associations for Rheumatology (ILAR) proposed a new classification system for JIA to facilitate research into the etiology, pathogenesis, and treatment of childhood arthritides with no known cause. The committee's goal was to develop a system that achieves as much homogeneity as possible within each disease category and minimizes overlap among categories. In 1999, the WHO endorsed the proposed classification.

The current literature reflects all three terms, although the majority of published data on childhood arthritis is based on either the EULAR or ACR criteria. The ILAR system is gaining international acceptance and a growing number of studies use these diagnostic categories. However, it is important to recognize several factors. The terms JRA, JCA, and JIA are neither synonymous nor interchangeable, the ILAR system does not include all of the childhood arthritides, and the classification system continues to evolve and be refined based on emerging data. This chapter uses the term JIA and the diagnostic categories of the ILAR system. Wherever possible, references to research describing physical therapist examination and intervention clarify the specific disease type included in the population studied.

The term JIA is defined as definite arthritis of unknown etiology beginning before the age of 16 years and lasting for at least 6 weeks. Table 14.2 lists the diagnostic and exclusion criteria for conditions included in the ILAR classification. Each disorder is described by onset type, disease signs and symptoms during the first 6 months after onset, and course type, based on ongoing disease characteristics. The goal of classification is that each disease cate-gory is as homogeneous as possible and mutually exclusive of the other categories.

Systemic onset juvenile idiopathic arthritis (SoJIA), included in all classification systems, occurs in approximately 10% to 11% of children with arthritis using the ACR and EULAR criteria. The disease can begin at any age, with an equal male-to-female ratio. The diagnostic hallmark is a spiking fever of 39°C once or twice a day for at least 2 weeks, accompanied by one or more of the following signs: a migratory, salmon-colored rash on the trunk or limbs; generalized lymphadenopathy; enlargement of the liver or spleen; and serositis. The fever can occur at any time during the day, but is most often found late in the afternoon or evening in combination with the rash. Children are often quite ill while febrile, but feel well during other times. Laboratory findings include negative tests for both the rheumatoid factor (RF) and antinuclear antibodies (ANAs). The presence of or a family history of psoriasis excludes the child from this category. Objective arthritis may be present initially or may not appear for weeks, months, or even years after disease onset, but must be confirmed to make the diagnosis.

Disease course is variable. Systemic symptoms may subside after several months to a few years, although some children experience recurring episodes or persistent systemic disease in conjunction with exacerbations of the arthritis. Some children with systemic disease recover completely after a period of time with arthritis in a few joints, while others follow a progressive course, with persistent arthritis in an increasing number of joints.[3]

Polyarticular onset juvenile idiopathic arthritis (PoJIA), also recognized in each classification system, is defined as arthritis in five or more joints during the first 6 months. Disease onset is usually insidious, with a progressive increase

TABLE 14.2

Classification Criteria for Juvenile Idiopathic Arthritis

Characteristics	Systemic	Polyarticular	Oligoarticular	JPsA	ERA
Diagnostic criteria	Documented typical quotidian fever lasting ≥2 wk plus one of: • Typical rash • Generalized lymphadenopathy • Enlarged liver or spleen • Serositis	Arthritis in four or more joints during first 6 mo of disease	Arthritis in four or fewer joints during first 6 mo of disease	Arthritis and psoriasis or arthritis plus two or more of: • Dactylitis • Nail abnormalities • Family history of psoriasis confirmed by dermatologist in one or more first-degree relatives	Arthritis and enthesitis or arthritis or enthesitis plus two of: • Sacroiliac joint tenderness, inflammatory spinal pain, or both • HLA-B27 • Family history in a first- or second-degree relative of confirmed HLA-B27–associated disease • Acute anterior uveitis
Exclusions	• Psoriasis or family history of psoriasis	• Systemic arthritis	• Systemic arthritis • Psoriasis or family history of psoriasis or HLA-associated disease • Presence of RF • HLA+ male >8 years old	• Systemic arthritis • RF	• Onset of arthritis in a boy age >8 years • Psoriasis or family history of psoriasis confirmed by dermatologist in a first- or second-degree relative

Subtypes	None	• PoJIA RF–: No detectable RF
		• PoJIA RF+:
		  • Five or more joints during first 6 mo of disease
		  • RF detected in two or more laboratory tests 3 mo apart
			• Persistent: total number of joints never greater than four
			• Extended: total number of joints greater than four
				None	None

HLA, human leukocyte antigen; PoJIA RF–, polyarticular rheumatoid factor negative; PoJIA RF+, polyarticular rheumatoid factor positive.

in the number of joints involved. Systemic symptoms, if present, are usually milder and less persistent than in systemic arthritis. Arthritis is symmetric and affects large joints, including the knees, elbows, wrists, and ankles. The cervical spine and temporomandibular joints are frequently involved, as are the small joints of the hands and feet. Figure 14.1 shows the hands of a child with PoJIA.

The ILAR classification identifies two separate categories of polyarthritis, PoJIA RF– disease, characterized by the absence of detectable RF, and PoJIA RF+ disease, diagnosed based on the detection of the RF on two occasions at least 3 months apart. Under the ACR criteria, arthritis in five or more joints during the first 6 months is classified simply as polyarticular onset, although this system also recognizes two subtypes, based on the presence or absence of the RF. In contrast, the EULAR criteria distinguish RF+ polyarthritis, the only disorder classified as JRA, from RF– polyarthritis.

Onset of RF– PoJIA may be at any time before the age of 16 years; about half of this group is younger than 6 years of age at onset, with another peak seen in the preadolescent age group. Arthritis is symmetric, involving both large and

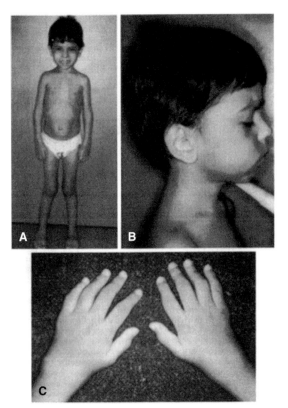

Figure 14.1 ■ **(A)** General appearance, **(B)** Temporomandibular joint, and **(C)** Hands of a child with polyarticular onset juvenile idiopathic arthritis.

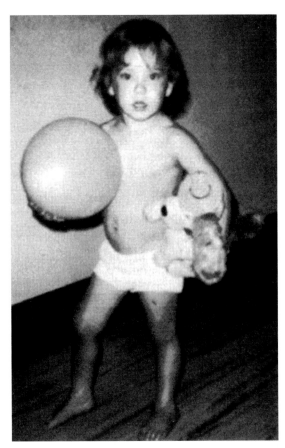

Figure 14.2 ■ A child with asymmetric arthritis resulting in a leg length discrepancy.

small joints, with a tendency for ankylosis of the carpal and tarsal joints. Joint contractures, juxta-articular osteoporosis, muscle atrophy, weakness, and local and generalized growth disturbances are common. Nodules are rarely seen.

One group of children, predominantly female, experiences disease onset in late childhood or adolescence, is RF+, and follows a polyarticular course. About half of these children develop rapid, severe arthritis resembling adult rheumatoid arthritis (RA), with joint erosions seen as early as 6 months after onset. Subcutaneous nodules are often found at the elbow, tibial crests, or fingers. Common symptoms include listlessness, fever, and anorexia. Systemic manifestations, when present, may include a low-grade fever, slight to moderate enlargement of the spleen and liver, and lymphadenopathy. Clinically evident pericarditis or pleuritis is infrequent. About 10% develop chronic uveitis.

Oligoarticular onset juvenile idiopathic arthritis (OligoJIA) is characterized by a low-grade inflammation in four or fewer joints during the first 6 months. This category corresponds to pauciarticular onset in the ACR and EULAR classification systems and represents the largest group of children (about 45% to 60%) with arthritis in all systems. Arthritis is typically asymmetric and affects primarily the lower extremities, with the knees most commonly involved, followed by the ankles and elbows. Figure 14.2 shows a child with asymmetric arthritis resulting in a leg length discrepancy. The hips are rarely involved, and the

small joints of the hands and feet are usually spared, although this is not true in all children. In many children, the disease presents initially as arthritis in one knee, and the physician must be careful to rule out infection or trauma as the cause. Systemic involvement is unusual, but about 20% of children experience uveitis, a chronic anterior nongranulomatous inflammation of the iris and ciliary body that is usually asymptomatic but can lead to functional blindness if left untreated. Frequent eye examinations by an ophthalmologist are necessary.

The ILAR criteria recognize two separate groups of children with OligoJIA disease, persistent and extended. Children who follow a persistent oligoarticular course often go into remission, although they may experience disease flares many years later. Their outcome in terms of joint function is typically very good, although they often remain at risk for eye disease. Approximately 5% to 10% have an extended course after the first 6 months with a progressive increase in the number of joints involved, although these children usually have fewer total joints involved than those with a polyarticular onset disease. Most children with extended OligoJIA follow a pattern similar to those with RF– PoJIA, although a few are RF+ and follow an unremitting course with polyarthritis and joint erosions, similar to that of children with PoJIA RF+.[4]

SPONDYLOARTHROPATHY

The term *spondyloarthropathy* is often used in pediatric rheumatology to describe a group of disorders that includes juvenile ankylosing spondylitis, juvenile psoriatic arthritis, arthritis associated with inflammatory bowel disease (IBD), and reactive forms of arthritis, including Reiter's syndrome (RS). Although these disorders share some characteristics, including the presence of the human leukocyte antigen (HLA) antigen B27, they also have distinct differences. The ACR criteria do not include these disorders as separate categories, although juvenile psoriatic arthritis (JPsA) and juvenile ankylosing spondylitis (JAS) are recognized as subgroups of pauciarticular JRA. In the EULAR classification system, JPsA and JAS are considered separate categories of JCA. The ILAR system avoids the term *spondyloarthropathy*, instead recognizing enthesitis-related arthritis (ERA) and psoriatic arthritis as separate categories. Although arthritis associated with IBD is included under the ERA category, reactive arthritis is excluded because there is usually an identifiable cause.

The term *enthesitis* describes inflammation of the entheses, the attachment sites of tendons, ligaments, or joint capsules to bone. Figure 14.3 shows the most common sites of tenderness associated with enthesitis in the knees, ankles, and feet. The diagnostic criteria for ERA include arthritis and enthesitis, or arthritis or enthesitis with at least two of the following: sacroiliac joint tenderness or inflammatory spinal pain; presence of HLA-B27; family history in at least one first- or second-degree relative of medically confirmed HLA-B27–associated disease; anterior uveitis associated with pain, redness, or photophobia; and onset of arthritis in a boy 8 years or older. Exclusion criteria for ERA are obvious psoriasis in the patient or a family his-tory of psoriasis confirmed by a dermatologist in at least one first- or second-degree relative, the presence of RF on at least two occasions more than 3 months apart, or the presence of systemic symptoms.

This category of JIA includes most children who are eventually diagnosed with JAS, although a specific diagnosis may be delayed until clinical and laboratory signs meet accepted criteria for JAS, including radiologic evidence of inflammation in the sacroiliac joints.

JPsA is defined in a child, younger than 16 years, with arthritis and psoriasis or arthritis and two of the following: dactylitis, nail pitting or onycholysis, and family history of psoriasis in a first-degree relative. Dactylitis represents the combined effects of arthritis and tenosynovitis and is characterized by swelling of one or more digits that extend beyond the joint margins (Fig. 14.4).[5] Children who are RF+ or have signs of another form of JIA are excluded from this category. In many children with JPsA, arthritis precedes the appearance of psoriasis by several years and the disease at onset may appear more similar to asymmetric oligoarthritis than adult psoriatic arthritis. The final category included in the ILAR classification is "other" or "undifferentiated" arthritis. Children included in this category do not meet criteria for any one of the specific diagnoses or exhibit characteristics of more than one condition.

◆ Incidence and Prevalence of Juvenile Idiopathic Arthritis

Reports of the incidence and prevalence of childhood arthritis show wide variations due to differences in the population source, geography, study duration, and criteria used

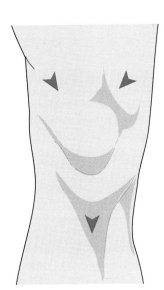
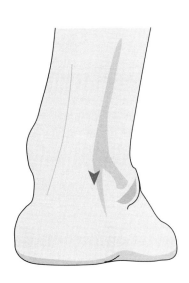
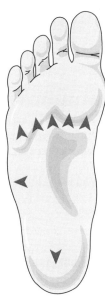

Figure 14.3 ■ The most common sites of tenderness associated with enthesitis in the knees, ankles, and feet.

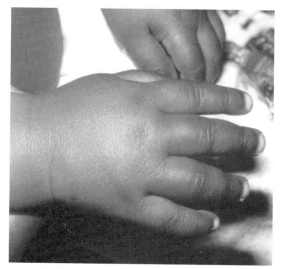

Figure 14.4 ■ Dactylitis represents the combined effects of arthritis and tenosynovitis and is characterized by swelling of one or more digits that extends beyond the joint margins. (Courtesy of Thomas D. Thacher, MD.)

to identify and classify patients. A study by Manners and Bower reported the annual incidence of JIA as 0.008 to 0.226 cases per 1000 children at risk; prevalence rates varied from 0.07 to 4.01 cases per 1000.[6] In an earlier study, Oen and Cheang performed a systematic review of studies published between 1977 and 1995 that examined incidence and prevalence data for childhood arthritis in North America and Europe, using the ACR and EULAR diagnostic criteria.[7] Population-based studies (surveys of general populations in specified geographic areas) reported the highest prevalence rates (132 per 100,000 at risk; 95% confidence interval [CI], 119 to 145), practitioner-based studies (surveys of general practitioners or specified groups of specialty practices) intermediate rates (26 per 100,000; 95% CI, 23 to 29), and clinic-based studies (cases identified in single or multicenter pediatric rheumatology clinics) the lowest rates (12 per 100,000; 95% CI, 10 to 15).

The highest prevalence was reported for pauciarticular (oligoarticular) onset disease, followed by polyarticular onset and then systemic arthritis. All studies indicate that the prevalence and incidence rates for the diseases grouped under the diagnostic category of seronegative spondylo-arthropathy (SSA) were less than for JRA. The weighted average from several studies for SSA was 29 per 100,000 (95% CI, 24 to 35) for practitioner-based studies and 2 per 100,000 (95% CI, 1 to 3) for clinic-based studies. This group presumably included children with JAS, although Burgos-Vargas and Petty estimated the prevalence of JAS to be 12 to 33 per 100,000 in the United States and United Kingdom and 13 to 65 per 100,000 in Mexico.[8] They reported the frequency of JPsA to be 5.2% in a sample of 269, while other studies suggest that 2.3 to 3 per 100,000 children develop JPsA every year, with a prevalence of 10 to 15 per 100,000.[9]

Prevalence data for different racial groups also varies based on geography and the source population, although data from clinic-based studies within North America showed the most homogeneity. Weighted averages from several studies reported prevalence of childhood arthritis as 32 per 100,000 (95% CI, 26 to 38) for Caucasians; 40 per 100,000 (95% CI, 31 to 49) for North American Indian (NAI); and 26 per 100,000 (95% CI, 16 to 36) for "other." One clinic-based study of African-American patients reported a prevalence of 26 per 100,000 at risk in the United States over a 2-year period.[10]

Incidence data for chronic arthritis in childhood, based on the weighted average of values reported by all studies reviewed by Oen and Cheang, showed the following mean values and 95% CI: Caucasians, 2 per 100,000 (CI, 2 to 3); NAI, 9 per 100,000 (CI, 5 to 12); Inuit, Yupik, and Inupiat, 7 per 100,000 (CI, 4 to 10); and "other," 3 per 100,000 (CI, 4 to 5).[7] Using the ACR criteria for JRA, no differences were found in the percentage of patients with systemic onset JRA among racial groups. Among Caucasian patients, the proportion with PaJRA was higher (58%; CI, 56 to 60) than those with PoJRA (27%; CI, 25 to 28). The study by Hochberg et al.[10] reported that the incidence of arthritis among African-American children was 7 per 100,000.

Gender distribution and peak age at onset vary by disease type. Although studies indicate that systemic onset disease occurs with equal frequency in boys and girls, girls outnumber boys in both PaJRA (3:1) and PoJRA (2.8:1). Boys are more highly represented in JAS, with a male-to-female ratio of 7:1. Studies of children with JPsA reported a bias toward girls with a female-to-male ratio ranging from 1.0 to 1.6.

Peak age at onset also varies by disease type. Sullivan et al. in a study of 300 children with JRA reported that peak age at onset was between 1 and 3 years for the total sample and for females who had either PaJRA or PoJRA.[11] In contrast, two separate periods of peak onset were found in boys; one peak onset period at 2 years of age was observed in boys with PoJRA, while another peak onset between the ages of 8 and 10 years appeared to represent those boys later diagnosed with some type of spondylo-arthropathy. For JPsA, one peak onset period appears to occur in the preschool years, mainly in girls, with a second peak during mid- to late childhood. In children diagnosed with JAS, disease onset usually occurs in late childhood or adolescence.

Etiology and Pathogenesis

The exact etiology and pathogenesis of these diseases are not fully understood, although there is general agreement that they represent disorders of the immune system resulting in inflammation in the joints and other body tissues. Research suggests that disease onset occurs in a genetically predisposed host who encounters an external trigger. The trigger may be a viral or bacterial infection. Some parents report that their child sustained some type of physical trauma prior to the onset of symptoms, but it is unclear if the trauma is the cause or simply brings attention to the disease. Different etiologic factors may be responsible for each onset type, or a single pathogen may cause distinct clinical patterns as it interacts with the specific characteristics and vulnerabilities of the child.

The presence of altered immunity, abnormal immunoregulation, and production of proinflammatory cytokines may help explain the onset and persistence of inflammation in childhood arthritis. T-cell abnormalities and the pathology of the inflamed synovium in affected joints suggest that there is a cell-mediated pathogenesis. Humoral abnormalities are evident from the presence of multiple autoanti-bodies, immune complexes, and complement activation. The evidence for genetic predisposition to many of these conditions is increasing but is not completely understood. In one study of over 3000 children with arthritis, there was concordance between siblings with JRA for age at onset, clinical manifestations, and disease course.[12] Although many of the suspected genetic characteristics are within the major histocompatibility complex (MHC) region of chromosome 6, the pathogenesis may involve the interactions of multiple genes. Correlation between HLA specificities and various types of childhood arthritis may have risk and protective effects that are age related for each onset type and some course types.[13]

Nutrition and Juvenile Rheumatoid Arthritis
Megan Johnston Mullin, MS, RD, LDN
Clinical Dietitian
Children's Hospital of Philadelphia

IMPACT ON NUTRITIONAL STATUS
Children suffering from JRA, like any other chronic illness, are at increased risk for developing nutritional inadequacies and growth faltering. There are several factors that may impact on the nutritional status of children with JRA.

Possible Factors Influencing Nutritional Status	Implications	Interventions

Increased caloric expenditure	Especially in children with systemic JRA, due to inflammation and fever	If poor intake or poor weight gain—
		  Increased calories/protein:
		    High calorie additives (oils, butter, etc)
		    Concentrate infant formula
		    Oral supplement/modulars
		  If chewing/swallowing concerns—
		    modify textures
		    Consider multiple vitamin and mineral supplement or supplementation of individual nutrients as needed.
		  Avoid food struggles or battles:
		    Educate parents about: what are the appropriate feeding roles of parent and child, how to provide meals and snacks at consistent times and in a relaxed and loving environment.
		  Consider tube feedings.

Limited motion/ physical activity	Causing an inability to consume adequate calories, muscle wasting, or weight gain	If poor weight gain or poor oral intake, follow guidelines for increasing calorie intake (above).
		If excessive weight gain or risk for obesity:
		  Encourage increase in physical activity.
		  Limit intake of high-calorie/fat foods.
		  Limit juices, sugar-added beverages.
		  Encourage fruits, vegetables, whole grains, lean meats, low-fat dairy products.

(continued)

Nutrition and Juvenile Rheumatoid Arthritis (Continued)

Possible Factors Influencing Nutritional Status	Implications	Interventions
Anorexia	Caused by chronic pain and/or due to medication	Attempt to control pain and minimize side effects of medications. Maximize calorie intake (see above). Other strategies for improving intake: Encourage small, frequent meals. Avoid hot meals that have strong odors. Use colorful foods and foods with appetizing aromas to increase appeal.
Food fads and quackery	Fasting, experimental, or elimination diets may cause nutrient deficiencies	Identify potential nutrient deficiencies. Educate patient and family on rich food sources. Vitamin/mineral supplement as needed.
Drug interactions (Commonly used medications: Salicylates (Aspirin), Tolmetin, Naproxen, Ibuprofen, Methotrexate, Corticosteroid)	Possible gastrointestinal side effects: Decreased absorption of vitamin C and folate, increased or decreased appetite, weight loss of gain, glucose intolerance	Attempt to minimize gastrointestinal side effects of medications. Identify nutrient deficiencies. Educate patient and family on rich food sources. Provide supplementation as needed. Follow guidelines for promoting weight gain or loss (see above). If glucose intolerance: Consistent eating pattern/meal schedule. Limit juices/avoid sugar-added beverages. Plan healthy, balanced meals to avoid excess carbohydrate content.

SUGGESTED READINGS

Behrman RE, Nelson WE, Vaughn VC. Nelson Textbook of Pediatrics 13th Edition. In: Immunology, Allergy, And Related Diseases: Juvenile Rheumatoid Arthritis. WB Saunders Company, 1987; 515-523.

Ekvall SW. Pediatric Nutrition in Chronic Diseases and Developmental Disorders-Prevention, Assessment, and Treatment. In: Lovell D, Henderson C. Juvenile Rheumatoid Arthritis. Oxford University Press, 1993; 263-267.

Lea, Febiger. Modern Nutrition in Health and Disease 8th Edition. In Bollet AJ. Nutrition and Diet in Rheumatic Disease. Volume 2. Waverly Company, 1994; 1362-1372.

Pathology

Figure 14.5 illustrates changes caused by the inflammatory process within and surrounding synovial joints. The cardinal signs of joint inflammation include swelling, end-range stress pain, and stiffness. Changes include villous hypertrophy, hyperplasia of the vascular endothelium, and intra-articular effusion, with swelling and distention of the joint capsule. The joint may also appear enlarged because of bony overgrowth caused by increased blood flow to the inflamed tissues. Distention of the joint capsule from increased synovial fluid, stretching of periarticular tissues, and protective muscle spasm result in pain and stiffness. One commonly measured indicator of disease activity is the presence and duration of morning stiffness, or AM gel, reported by the child.

Synovial cells multiply, forming a massive overgrowth called a pannus, which spreads over the articular cartilage, causing it to soften and weaken. Degradative enzymes are released from the cartilage matrix into the synovial fluid. These enzymes further disrupt the normal cartilage fiber network. Intra-articular adhesions and osteophytes occur later. Articular surfaces become irregular, and joint congruency, alignment, and stability are compromised as erosions occur in articular cartilage and subchondral bone.

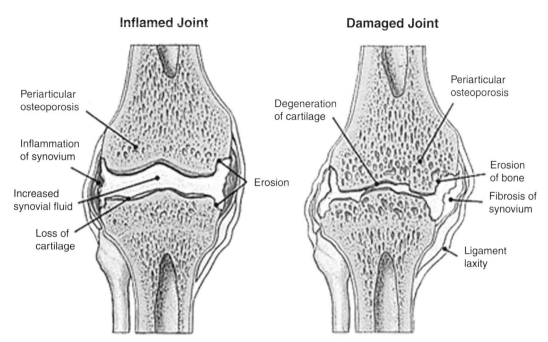

Figure 14.5 ■ Changes caused by the inflammatory process within and surrounding synovial joints.

Fibrosis of periarticular tendons and ligaments results in joint contractures. Subluxation may occur at the wrist and small joints of the hands and feet. Posterior subluxation of the tibia on the femur may occur in the presence of long-standing knee flexion contractures. Muscle imbalance, with a relative weakness of the quadriceps, and impaired mobility of the patella contribute to joint stiffness and instability.

Early radiographic changes include soft tissue swelling, widening of the joint space due to effusions, juxta-articular osteopenia, and periosteal new bone, especially noted in the phalanges, metacarpals, and metatarsals. With persistent disease, radiographs often show joint space narrowing, marginal erosions, and osteophytes due to thinning and loss of articular cartilage. Fibrous or bony ankylosis may occur in joints with severe and persistent inflammation.

Pathologic changes in the apophyseal and sacroiliac joints in JAS include endochondral and capsular ossification. In the early stages of the disease, the surface of the sacroiliac joints shows little change; subchondral inflammation results in granulation tissue with few inflammatory cells and no pannus formation. A balance of erosive synovitis and capsular or ligamentous ossification often occurs in synovial joints, although the ossification process usually dominates in joints of low mobility.

Muscles surrounding joints may atrophy as a result of reflex inhibition from swelling and pain as well as from disuse. Muscle atrophy and weakness is common in children with arthritis, possibly due to protein-energy malnutrition.[14] Soft tissue shortens when the joints are held in flexed positions to accommodate effusions and reduce pain. The result is a loss of joint stability and compliance during loading under motion, increasing the risk for degenerative changes.

Abnormalities in skeletal maturation, with both local and generalized growth disturbances, are common in children with JRA. Increased blood flow to the joint during active disease leads to bony overgrowth, seen most often in the humeral head and radial head of the upper extremities and the femoral head, medial femoral condyle, and proximal tibia in the lower extremities. Active disease may also result in premature epiphyseal closure, as may be seen in the small hands and feet of children with PoJIA. Another example is micrognathia, or undergrowth of the mandible that results from chronic arthritis of the temporomandibular joints (Fig. 14.6).

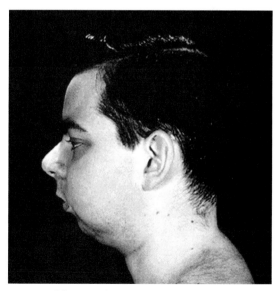

Figure 14.6 ■ Micrognathia, or undergrowth of the mandible, that results from chronic arthritis of the temporomandibular joints.

Juxta-articular osteopenia observed early in JRA may result from the inflammatory process in rheumatoid synovium. The more generalized demineralization seen later appears to be related to continued disease activity, and is associated with an increased risk of fracture in the vertebrae and long bones. Nutritional deficiencies, low body weight, and decreased physical activity result in low bone density and increased risk for fracture in children with long-standing disease.[15] These problems are exaggerated by long-term use of systemic corticosteroids.

Enthesitis, most often found in JAS and JPsA, is characterized by a nonspecific inflammation and localized osteitis whereby granulation tissue replaces the normal bony and cartilaginous attachment of ligament and tendon to bone. During the healing phase of the inflammatory process, bony spurs often form. Calcaneal spurs may develop at the insertion of the plantar fascia into the calcaneus. Enthesitis at the attachment of the outer fibers of the annulus fibrosis to the anterolateral aspects of the rim of the vertebral body may result in syndesmorphyte.[16]

General Goals of Management in Juvenile Idiopathic Arthritis

The overall goals of management in JIA are to (1) quickly control the joint inflammation using the most effective drug therapy with the least adverse effects; (2) preserve joint mobility and integrity and function; (3) promote independence and competence in necessary and desired activities; and (4) provide education and support to the child and family. Many children receive specialized rheumatology care from a multidisciplinary team of health professionals at a tertiary center. The team includes the pediatric rheumatologist, rheumatology nurse, occupational therapist, physical therapist, social worker or psychologist, ophthalmologist, orthopedist, and laboratory and imaging specialists. Occasional consultations with other specialists may be necessary, including podiatrists and orthotists. The day-to-day management of the child's health care needs are typically provided by the family with the guidance of the primary care physician or pediatrician. Children may receive direct physical therapy from a local physical therapist at home, in school as part of their educational program, or in an outpatient clinic.

PHARMACOLOGIC THERAPIES

The purpose of pharmacologic therapy in JIA is to suppress inflammation and decrease or eliminate pain, with the least possible toxicity. The ultimate goal is to prevent or minimize disability. Treatment is guided by a number of parameters, including disease onset and course type, disease severity, and prognostic indicators of outcome. While some children may do well with conservative treatment, others

who are at risk for irreversible joint damage and poor functional outcome may require early and more aggressive treatment. For example, in systemic onset JIA, active systemic disease at 6 months is a strong predictor of a poor functional outcome. Children with polyarticular and extended oligoarticular disease also are at increased risk for joint damage and disability. Other predictors of poor outcome include female gender, presence of rheumatoid factor, subcutaneous nodules, and early arthritis in the small joints of the hands and feet with rapid development of erosions.

The first line of therapy in childhood arthritis includes the nonsteroidal anti-inflammatory drugs (NSAIDs). NSAIDs currently approved for use in children include naproxen, ibuprofen, tolmetin, aspirin, and choline magnesium trisalicylate. Other NSAIDs that may be used in some forms of JIA include indomethacin (Indocin) and diclofenac sodium (Voltaren). NSAIDs reduce fever and inflammation and have an analgesic effect, but do not alter the disease course. Generally, 8 weeks of therapy are necessary to determine the effectiveness of an NSAID; 50% of children show some improvement on the first drug, while another 50% improve on a different NSAID. The most common potential adverse effects include gastrointestinal (GI) upset, liver and kidney toxicity, and pseudoporphyria. Routine monitoring for possible toxicities is necessary for all children.

Disease-modifying antirheumatic drugs (DMARDs) include agents that retard radiologic progression of the disease. Methotrexate (MTX) is the most frequent DMARD prescribed for children with JIA, especially those with an extended polyarticular course. MTX is usually administered in a single oral dose of 10 to 15 mg/m² each week, although higher doses may be used in children with refractory disease. A subcutaneous injection may be useful for children who experience GI upset with the oral dose. Therapeutic effects may not be seen for several weeks to months, but studies indicate that MTX slows progression of the arthritis; 60% to 80% of patients with JRA showed some clinical improvement. Most rheumatology clinics monitor blood counts and liver enzymes every 4 to 8 weeks in children taking MTX. Sufficient data on the immunosuppressive, teratogenic, or oncogenic risks of long-term MTX use in children are not yet available. General precautions include avoiding the use of live vaccines while taking MTX. Patients should also abstain from alcohol, and women of childbearing age should be counseled to avoid pregnancy because of the potential damage to the fetus in the early stages of gestation. Sulfasalazine, another DMARD, has been shown to be more effective than a placebo in suppressing disease activity in some children, primarily those with oligoarticular disease, but the possibility of toxicity is high. Monitoring of blood counts and transaminase levels before initiating treatment and at frequent intervals during treatment is necessary.

Etanercept (ETN) (Enbrel) is a biologic reagent that targets tumor necrosis factor-α (TNF-α), a cytokine responsible for many of the effects of inflammation. In one long-term follow-up study, ETN alone or in combination with MTX was found to be safe and well tolerated in children and adolescents with JIA.[17] Other biologic response modifiers used in inflammatory arthritis include the monoclonal antibodies to TNF-α, infliximab (Remicade), adalimumab (Humira), and anakinra (Kineret). These therapies appear to reduce signs and symptoms of arthritis and delay structural damage in adults with arthritis. Because of concerns about increased susceptibility to infection, children should be brought up to date on their immunizations before receiving ETN. In the presence of infection or exposure to varicella, ETN should be temporarily discontinued.

Systemic glucocorticoids are reserved for children with severe systemic disease. While these drugs have a potent anti-inflammatory effect, they do not alter disease course or duration. Long-term use is associated with serious adverse effects, including Cushing's syndrome, generalized growth deficits, osteoporosis and fracture, diabetes mellitus, obesity, steroid myopathy, and increased susceptibility to infection. Low-dose or alternate-day oral steroids or periodic intravenous pulsed steroid therapy given may be of some benefit to children with severe polyarticular disease who are unresponsive to other treatments.[18] Topical glucocorticoids are often used in the management of acute iritis and chronic uveitis.

Intra-articular steroid injections are increasingly being used to induce disease remission in individual joints when there is insufficient response to a systemic medication. In some children with oligoarticular disease, intra-articular steroid injection may be the first line of therapy. Sherry et al. reported that steroid injections of the lower extremity joints decreased the incidence of leg length discrepancy, a major cause of gait abnormalities in JIA.[19] Another study found decreased pain and improvements in some gait parameters following joint injections in a sample of 18 children with lower extremity polyarthritis. Significant changes included increased hip extensor moment during loading response, increased ankle plantar flexor moment at preswing, increased ankle power during stance phase, and improved knee and ankle range of motion.[20]

There appears to be some disagreement among pediatric rheumatologists as to the number of joints that can be safely injected at one time. Systemic absorption of the steroid from multiple injections performed in a single session may result in a cushingoid appearance; however, this is usually temporary. Other potential adverse effects from injections include steroid leakage and subcutaneous atrophy. These problems can be reduced by scrupulous technique, including aspirating as much synovial fluid as possible from the joint before the injection and using radiographic guidance for difficult joints including the shoulder, hip, and subtalar joint. There is also very little agreement on postinjection protocol, including the necessity or duration of bedrest or weight-bearing precautions following injection and recommendations for specific exercise regimen.

Therapists should consult with the treating physician to determine the preferred postinjection regimen for any given patient.

 Prognosis

The impact of JIA on the child and family is complex, including the burden of physical disease and resulting impairments on the child, as well as the psychological, social, and economic consequences for the family unit. To study outcome in JIA, it is necessary to examine all levels of the ICF framework, including the continued presence of active disease and subsequent impairments, as well as the child's activities and participation in life. Findings from different outcome studies are often contradictory because of differences in the source population and geographic location, specific parameters examined, and length of time after disease onset that patients are followed.

A review of available literature indicates that outcome on all levels is highly dependent on disease type and course, including duration and severity of active arthritis. A study by Oen et al. examined 392 patients diagnosed with JRA by ACR criteria who were at least 8 years old and at least 5 years past disease onset.[21] Mean disease duration by onset type was 4.7 years for PaJRA, 7.0 years for RF–PoJRA, 10.8 years for RF+ PoJRA, and 5.3 years for SoJRA. Of the total sample, 39% met the criteria for disease remission, absence of arthritis while off all medications for 2 or more years. Of those, remission occurred within 5 years after disease onset in 76%, between 5 and 10 years in 15%, and 10 or more years after onset in 9%. Seventeen percent had inactive disease but did not meet criteria for remission, while 41% continued to have active disease. For those children with RF+ PoJRA, the probability of remission after 10 years fell to 10%. Patients who are not in remission by 16 years of age have a high probability of continued active disease into the late 20s or even early 30s. Radiographic evidence of joint erosions in this sample was apparent as early as 2 years after disease onset in children with RF+ PoJRA and SoJRA. Joint space narrowing 5 years after disease onset was most frequent in patients with RF+ PoJRA. Radiographic signs of joint damage correlated with functional disability.

The early course of ERA is often remitting and musculoskeletal complaints are not often recognized as indicators of eventual JAS. Approximately 50% of these children never experience arthritis in more than four joints; however, most children eventually develop peripheral joint disease, with arthritis in the hips, knees, ankles, or feet. The frequency of enthesitis increases during the course of the disease. Long-term follow-up is necessary to monitor for subtle losses in joint motion and tissue extensibility in the thorax and lumbar spine. In one study all patients with ERA had decreased back spinal mobility 5 years after disease onset.[22] In children with JPsA, the outlook is relatively poor compared with other forms of oligoarticular JIA; however, the impact of newer medications, including methotrexate, is not yet known.

Reports of long-term functional outcome in children with arthritis vary. Ruperto and associates, who followed American and Italian patients with oligoarticular disease for 15 years after disease onset, found favorable outcomes on measures of functional status, pain, overall well-being, and quality of life.[23] A recent study conducted in Finland compared health-related quality of life (HRQoL) in adults with a history of childhood arthritis using the RAND 36-item Health Survey. HRQoL was similar in subjects and controls except for the area of physical functioning. Children with extended oligoarticular disease had lower scores in both the physical and mental components than other subgroups of JIA.[24] In contrast to these findings, another study of adults with a history of childhood arthritis reported significantly greater pain, disability, fatigue, and impaired physical function and perception of their health compared to age- and gender-matched controls.[25] Oen et al. found that children with PaJIA had the best functional outcome, while those with RF+ PoJIA developed significant disability. Among those with RF–PoJIA and SoJIA, 40% had no disability, while 33% or more had moderate to severe disability based on their scores on the Childhood Health Assessment Questionnaire.[21] Persistent arthritis and serious damage to the hip joints are significant risk factors for disability in children with RF+ PoJIA and SoJIA. They also found that educational achievements in patients up to secondary levels were comparable to national rates, but fewer females achieved postsecondary education. Additionally, unemployment rates for young adults 20 to 24 years of age were lower than that of the same age group in the general population.

Taken as a whole, these findings suggest the difficulty many children with arthritis have in adapting to the complex demands of adult life. However, over the past 10 years, there has been significant progress in the pharmacologic management of childhood arthritis, as well concerted efforts to identify patients who are at risk of a poor outcome and therefore suitable for early aggressive therapies. Some recent studies indicate improved short-term outcome in children treated with these newer medical therapies. However, long-term studies that follow these patients into adulthood are needed to determine if earlier diagnosis and more affective management improve the overall health status and quality of life in children with arthritis. To this effort, a set of six core response variables (CRVs) and universal definitions of improvement or worsening are now used in most clinical drug trials (Display 14.1).[26] The most commonly used criterion for a positive clinical response is the ACR Pediatric 30, defined as improvement of at least 30% in at least three of the six variables, with no more than one variable worsening by more than 30%. The definition of disease flare is a worsening in any two of the six CRVs by greater than or equal to 40% without concomitant improvement in more than one of the other CRVs by less than or equal to 30%.[27]

DISPLAY 14.1

Core Set of Outcome Measures in Juvenile Idiopathic Arthritis

- Physician global assessment of disease activity on a 10-cm visual analog scale (VAS) anchored by the words "remission" and "very severe" (MD Global)
- Parent or patient global assessment of overall well-being on a 10-cm VAS anchored by the words "very well" and "very poor" (Parent/Patient Global)
- Functional ability
- Number of joints with limited range of motion (JC-ROM)
- Number of joints with active arthritis (NJAA)
- Erythrocyte sedimentation rate (ESR)

◆ Physical Therapy Examination and Evaluation

Display 14.2 shows the components of a comprehensive examination. The physical therapy assessment follows the ICF framework and includes a thorough medical history,

DISPLAY 14.2

Components of the Physical Therapist Examination in Juvenile Idiopathic Arthritis

- Clinical observation
- Medical history
- Examination of the child's ability to participate in typical life settings (home, school, community) through standardized questionnaires or informal interview
- Examination of the child's activities through interview, standardized questionnaires, or performance tests
- Systems review
  - Integumentary system
    - Examine skin for presence of rash, nodules
    - Examine nails for pitting, onycholysis
  - Musculoskeletal system
    - Joint status and integrity
    - Joint range of motion
    - Soft tissue extensibility
    - Muscle bulk
    - Muscle strength and endurance
    - Postural alignment
  - Cardiopulmonary system
    - Resting and exercise heart rate
    - Aerobic capacity or performance on field test
  - Multiple systems
    - Pain
    - Gait pattern and parameters
    - Postural control
- Gross motor skills

an interview to determine the child's ability to perform activities necessary for participation in age-appropriate life situations, and an examination of the body structures and functions to determine specific strengths and impairments. The physical examination includes joint range of motion, soft tissue extensibility, muscle strength and endurance, and aerobic function. In addition, several standardized instruments developed specifically for children with arthritis provide useful information in setting treatment goals and planning intervention. Table 14.3 classifies these measures according to the ICF framework. In general, a top-down approach, beginning with an exploration of the child's activities and participation, allows the therapist to focus the physical examination on those areas that most impact the child's functional abilities and participation in home, school, and community activities. However, because the course of JIA can be erratic and unpredictable, the therapist must also be alert to changes in joint mobility and integrity or loss of muscle bulk and strength that signal a disease flare or damage. Using the ICF framework, the therapist must also consider the age, cognitive and emotional development of the child, and the amount of support and resources available to the family.

EXAMINATION OF ACTIVITIES AND PARTICIPATION

The impact on a child's daily function and ability to successfully participate in age-appropriate activities within home, school, and community environments depends to a great extent on the disease type and course and duration of active arthritis. Children with persistent oligoarthritis usually experience few activity limitations, while those with extended oligoarthritis or polyarthritis may have significant problems. Children with lower extremity arthritis often have difficulty getting up from the floor, walking long distances, climbing stairs, riding a bicycle, or participating in physical education activities or sports. Many children with long-standing disease have subtle motor deficits including impaired balance, coordination, agility, and speed.[28] Chronic arthritis and pain in the upper limbs may cause problems with dressing, bathing, opening jars, cutting food, and handwriting.

The child's personality and drive to be independent, as well as the expectations of parents, other family members, and school and community personnel, also impact the child's functional performance and adaptation to a chronic disease. The fluctuating nature of disease symptoms and functional performance may be confusing and frustrating for the child, parents, and school personnel. School tardiness as a result of morning stiffness and frequent absences due to medical appointments can have a negative effect on the child's education. Children with significant and persistent disease may feel different and somewhat isolated from their peers if their school day is interrupted by the need to rest during the day, the need to visit the nurse for medication, or the inability to participate in the same physical activities. Some studies indicate that many children who report problems in school related to their health condition do not receive the necessary support services recommended by the rheumatology team or required by law.[29,30] Adolescents may have some difficulty making the transition to adult rheumatology care, moving from high school to college or work, and achieving independence. The child and family's ability to successfully adapt to the changing demands of a life with chronic disease often depends on the availability and quality of supportive services within the community.

TABLE 14.3

Standardized Assessment Instruments in Juvenile Idiopathic Arthritis

Level of ICF	Instrument	Outcome Measured	Reference
A, P, I	CHAQ	BADLs and IADLs, pain, overall health status	Singh et al., 1994[33]
A, P, I	JAQQ	BADLs, IADLs, pain, HRQoL	Duffy et al., 1997[36]
A, P, I	PedsQL	BADLs, IADLs, pain, HRQoL	Varni et al., 2002[37]
A, P	JASI	BADLs, IADLs, gross motor activities	Wright et al., 1992[38]
A	JAFAS	BADLs, IADLs	Lovell et al., 1989[39]
I	GROMS	Joint ROM	Epps et al., 2002[44]
I	pEPM-ROM	Joint ROM	Len et al., 1999[45]
I	JC-LOM	Joint ROM loss	Klepper et al., 1992[52]
	JC-Swelling	Joint effusions	
	JC-POM	Joint stress pain	
	JC-Tenderness	Joint tenderness	

ICF, World Health Organization International Classification of Functioning, Disability, and Health; A, activity; P, participation; I, impairment; CHAQ, Childhood Arthritis Health Questionnaire; JAQQ, Juvenile Arthritis Quality of Life Questionnaire; PedsQL, Pediatric Quality of Life Questionnaire; JASI, Juvenile Arthritis Functional Assessment Index; JAFAS, Juvenile Arthritis Functional Assessment Scale; GROMS, Global Range of Motion Scale; pEPM-ROM, Pediatric Escola Paulista de Medicina Range of Motion Scale; JC-LOM, Joint Count Limitation of Motion; JC-POM, Joint Count Pain on Motion; BADLs, basic activities of daily living; IADLs, instrumental activities of daily living; HRQoL, health-related quality of life.

Table 14.3 lists the rheumatology-specific standardized assessments to measure activities, participation, and disability in children with arthritis. Detailed descriptions of these instruments can be found in a special issue of the journal *Arthritis Care & Research*.[31,32] Display 14.3 shows the child-hood Health Assessment Questionnaire (CHAQ), adapted from the Stanford Health Assessment Questionnaire (HAQ) and the most commonly used instrument to examine disability in children with various forms of arthritis.[33] The CHAQ has been translated and validated in multiple languages. The questionnaire is aimed at children age 1 to 19 years old and includes statements about 30 activities organized into eight categories. The respondent (parent for the child or child 9 years or older) scores each statement based on how much difficulty (0 = no difficulty, 1 = some difficulty, 2 = much difficulty, 3 = unable to do) the child has had in performing the task during the previous week. The child or parent scores an item as "not applicable" if the child is too young to perform the task. The highest scored item in each section dictates the score for that category; if the child or parent reports needing an assistive device or assistance from another person to perform any task in that category, the minimum score for the category is 2. The global score for the CHAQ Disability Index (DI) is the unweighted average of the eight category scores; scores range from 0 to 3, with higher scores indicating greater disability. Some studies employ a range of DI scores to categorize levels of disability: 0 = no disability, 0–0.5 = mild, 0.6–1.5 = moderate, and >1.5 = severe.[21] A study by Dempster et al. reported that a minimum decrease of 0.13 in the CHAQ DI correlated significantly with the parent's global assessment of clinical improvement in the child's functional abilities.[34] Conversely, a minimum increase of 0.75 in the DI correlated with parents' assessment of decline in function.

The child, or parent as proxy, also comments on pain intensity during the previous week using a 15-cm visual analog scale (VAS), anchored on the left side with a happy face and the words "no pain" and on the right side with a sad face and the words "worst pain." The Discomfort Index ranges from 0 to 3, with higher scores indicating greater pain. One calculates the score by measuring the distance in centimeters from the left side of the VAS and multiplying by 0.2. A second VAS is completed and scored in a similar way to report overall health status. Higher scores indicate poorer outcome. Both scales can be revised to a 100-mm line using the distance in centimeters from the left end of the line to the respondent's vertical line as the score.

Although the CHAQ remains the most commonly used assessment of functional status in children with arthritis, most recognize that the DI focuses on disability rather than the entire spectrum of the child's functional status. With 0 as the best possible score, the CHAQ DI suffers from a ceiling effect whereby scores are often clustered at the lower end of the scale, making it less sensitive to subtle indicators of disability. It is also very difficult to measure improvement in children whose initial DI is at or close to 0. To address this problem, Lam and colleagues compared the original CHAQ to three revised formats, a 10-cm $VAS_{CHAQ-38}$, a categoric scale ($Cat_{CHAQ-38}$), and a choice scale ($Choice_{CHAQ-38}$).[35] Each of these versions also contained eight additional items asking about the child's ability to perform more physically challenging tasks. For example, one new item asks the child to respond to the statement "I could have played team sports with others in my class" (examples: basketball, baseball, soccer, hockey). In the $VAS_{CHAQ-38}$ the child responds to each item by placing a mark on a 10-cm VAS anchored on the left end by the statement "Much worse than most other kids my age" and on the right side by "Much better than most other kids my age." Results indicated that the $VAS_{CHAQ-38}$ scale was significantly more sensitive than the original or other revised versions in discriminating children with arthritis from healthy controls.

Other self-report or proxy report instruments measuring physical function in children with arthritis include a larger continuum of activities. These include the Juvenile Arthritis Quality of Life Questionnaire (JAQQ),[36] the Pediatric Quality of Life Questionnaire (PedsQL),[37] and the Juvenile Arthritis Functional Assessment Index (JASI).[38] Overall JAQQ and PedsQL scores are measures of health-related quality of life, although individual items measure physical function; each instrument also includes a measure of pain and overall health status. The PedsQL includes both a generic module that can be used for any child and a rheumatology-specific module for children with arthritis or another rheumatic disease. There are also different forms for parents to complete as proxy for young children and for adolescents to complete independently.

The JAQQ includes activities in four categories: gross motor, fine motor, psychosocial, and systemic symptoms. The child responds to each item, using a 7-point scale to indicate how often in the past 2 weeks he or she has had difficulty performing a task. The item is scored 0 if it is not applicable to the child. For each category, the child chooses the five items that he or she views as most problematic or important. Only these items are scored on subsequent tests. The score for each category is the unweighted average of the five highest scoring items, while the total score is the unweighted average of the four category scores. Higher scores indicate lower function and lower quality of life. The JAQQ also includes two pain scales and a categoric scale on which the child indicates if he or she is better, the same, or worse compared to the last clinic visit. The JASI uses a scale similar to that of the JAQQ, but it is unique in that it includes a larger number of gross motor activities than other tests and is completed by the child in the clinic using a computer program. Like the JAQQ, the JASI asks the child to choose the five items that are most important to him or her and considers only those items on subsequent assessments. Unlike other tests, part I of the JASI must be

►► DISPLAY 14.3

Health Assessment Questionnaire*

In this section, we are interested in learning how your child's illness affects his or her ability to function in daily life. Please feel free to add any comments on the back of this page. In the following questions, please check the one response that best describes your child's usual activities (averaged over an entire day) OVER THE PAST WEEK. If your child has difficulty in doing a certain activity or is unable to do it because he or she is too young but NOT because he or she is RESTRICTED BY ARTHRITIS, please mark it as "Not Applicable." ONLY NOTE THOSE DIFFICULTIES OR LIMITATIONS THAT ARE DUE TO ARTHRITIS.

	Without Any Difficulty	With Some Difficulty	With Much Difficulty	Unable To Do	Not Applicable
Dressing and Grooming Is your child able to:					
• Dress, including tying shoelaces and doing buttons?	_____	_____	_____	_____	_____
• Shampoo his or her hair?	_____	_____	_____	_____	_____
• Remove socks?	_____	_____	_____	_____	_____
• Cut fingernails/toenails?	_____	_____	_____	_____	_____
Arising Is your child able to:					
• Stand up from a low chair or floor?	_____	_____	_____	_____	_____
• Get in and out of bed or stand up in crib?	_____	_____	_____	_____	_____
Eating Is your child able to:					
• Cut his or her own meat?	_____	_____	_____	_____	_____
• Lift a cup or glass to mouth?	_____	_____	_____	_____	_____
• Open a new cereal box?	_____	_____	_____	_____	_____
Walking Is your child able to:					
• Walk outdoors on flat ground?	_____	_____	_____	_____	_____
• Climb up five steps?	_____	_____	_____	_____	_____

*Please check any AIDS or DEVICES that your child usually uses for any of the above activities:

_____ Cane	_____ Devices used for dressing (button hook, zipper pull, long-handled shoe horn, etc.)
_____ Walker	_____ Built-up pencil or special utensils
_____ Crutches	_____ Special or built-up chair
_____ Wheelchair	_____ Other (specify: _____)

*Please check any categories for which your child usually needs help from another person BECAUSE OF ARTHRITIS

_____ Dressing and grooming	_____ Eating
_____ Arising	_____ Walking

	Without Any Difficulty	With Some Difficulty	With Much Difficulty	Unable To Do	Not Applicable
Hygiene Is your child able to:					
• Wash and dry entire body?	_____	_____	_____	_____	_____
• Take a tub bath (get in and out of tub)?	_____	_____	_____	_____	_____
• Get on and off the toilet or potty chair?	_____	_____	_____	_____	_____
• Brush teeth?	_____	_____	_____	_____	_____
• Comb/brush hair?	_____	_____	_____	_____	_____
Reach Is your child able to:					
• Reach and get down a heavy object, such as a large game or books, from just above his or her head?	_____	_____	_____	_____	_____

(continued)

>> **DISPLAY 14.3**

Health Assessment Questionnaire* (*Continued*)

	Without Any Difficulty	With Some Difficulty	With Much Difficulty	Unable To Do	Not Applicable
• Bend down to pick up clothing or a piece of paper from the floor?	___	___	___	___	___
• Pull on a sweater over his or her head?	___	___	___	___	___
• Turn neck to look back over shoulder?	___	___	___	___	___

Grip

Is your child able to:

	Without Any Difficulty	With Some Difficulty	With Much Difficulty	Unable To Do	Not Applicable
• Write or scribble with a pen or pencil?	___	___	___	___	___
• Open car doors?	___	___	___	___	___
• Open jars that have been previously opened?	___	___	___	___	___
• Turn faucets on and off?	___	___	___	___	___
• Push open a door when he or she has to turn a doorknob?	___	___	___	___	___

Activities

Is your child able to:

	Without Any Difficulty	With Some Difficulty	With Much Difficulty	Unable To Do	Not Applicable
• Run errands and shop?	___	___	___	___	___
• Get in and out of car or toy car or school bus?	___	___	___	___	___
• Ride bike or tricycle?	___	___	___	___	___
• Do household chores (e.g., wash dishes, take out trash, vacuum, do yardwork, make bed, clean room)?	___	___	___	___	___
• Run and play?	___	___	___	___	___

*Please check any AIDS or DEVICES that your child usually uses for any of the above activities:

___ Raised toilet seat	___ Bathtub bar
___ Bathtub seat	___ Long-handled appliances for reach
___ Jar opener (for jars previously opened)	___ Long-handled appliances in bathroom

*Please check any categories for which your child usually needs help from another person BECAUSE OF ARTHRITIS

___ Hygiene	___ Gripping and opening things
___ Reaching	___ Errands and chores

Pain

We are also interested in learning whether or not your child has been affected by pain because of his or her illness.

• How much pain do you think your child has had because of his or her illness IN THE PAST WEEK? Place a mark on the line below to indicate the severity of the pain.

No Pain   Very Severe Pain

0   100

Health Status

1. Considering all the ways that arthritis affects your child, rate how your child is doing on the following scale by placing a mark on the line.

0   100
Very Well   Very Poorly

2. Is your child stiff in the morning?   _____ Yes   _____ No
   If YES, about how long does the stiffness usually last (in the past week)?   Hours/Minutes _____

*Adapted from Singh G, Athreya B, Fries JF, et al. Measurement of health status in children with juvenile rheumatoid arthritis. Arthritis Rheum 1994;37:1761–1769.

scored using the software, although part II can be scored by hand. The CHAQ and JAQQ are available in the literature or through the test developers for no cost. The PedsQL can be obtained for a trial period through the authors, but must be purchased for ongoing clinical use. The JASI is available from the author for a nominal fee.

The Juvenile Arthritis Functional Assessment Scale (JAFAS)[39] is the only performance measure designed for children with arthritis. The child is observed and timed while performing 10 common daily tasks, including buttoning a shirt or blouse, putting on a shirt over the head, pulling on socks, cutting food with a knife and fork, getting in and out of bed, rising to stand from sitting on the floor, picking up an object from the floor, walking 50 feet, and walking up a flight of steps. The child's time to complete each task is compared to a criterion value based on the performance of a healthy control sample of children. Items are scored as 0 if the time is equal to or less than the criterion, 1 if the time is more than the criterion, and 2 if the child is unable to complete the task. The JAFAS takes about 10 minutes to administer and score and requires minimal training and simple equipment. Directions for administering the test are provided by the authors.[39]

Several other general pediatric assessments may be useful in examining activities and participation in children with arthritis. These include standardized norm-referenced motor tests like the Peabody Developmental Motor Scales–2 and the Bruininks-Oseretsky Test of Motor Proficiency (BOT). Other criterion-referenced assessments based on interviews of parents or teachers that may be useful include the School Function Assessment (SFA)[40] and an informal school checklist (see Appendix 14.1), which can provide valuable information about the child's functional capacity and performance in the home and school settings.

EXAMINATION OF BODY STRUCTURES AND FUNCTIONS

JOINT MOTION AND INTEGRITY

Figure 14.7 shows one format used for recording the findings of the joint examination, including swelling or joint effusion, joint tenderness, stress pain, and limitation of motion. The signs of active joint inflammation include swelling, tenderness, or stress pain. Limited joint motion alone does not indicate active disease, although it may be the result of long-standing disease.[41] Joint effusions are detected by demonstrating fluctuation of synovial fluid from one area of the joint to another. Figure 14.8 illustrates two methods of detecting joint effusions. In examining the fingers and toes, one should place the sensor fingers proximal to the base of the middle phalanx and dorsal to

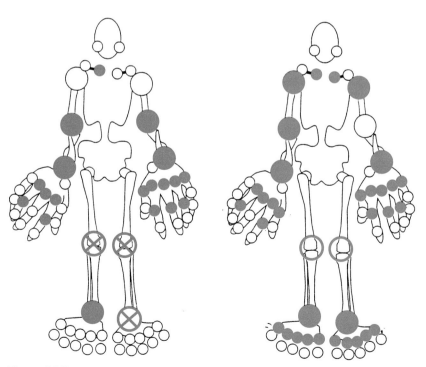

Figure 14.7 ■ Example of the visual format used to record active joint count in a child with polyarticular disease. The left figure shows joints with an effusion (*solid circle*) or soft tissue swelling (*X*). The right figure shows joints with stress pain or tenderness (*solid circle*). (From Wright V, Smith E. Physical therapy management of the child and adolescent with arthritis. In: Walker J, Helewa A, eds. Physical Therapy in Arthritis. Philadelphia: W. B. Saunders; 1996:211–244, with permission.)

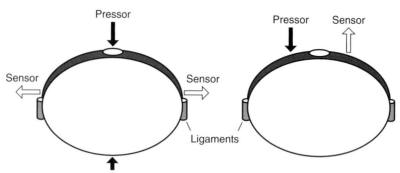

Figure 14.8 ■ Two ways of detecting joint effusions. (From Smythe H, Helewa A. Assessment of joint disease. In: Walker J, Helewa A, eds. *Physical Therapy in Arthritis*. Philadelphia: W. B. Saunders; 1996:129–148, with permission from H. Smythe, MD, FRC[C].)

the collateral ligaments to detect movement of the synovial fluid. Small effusions in the knee joint can be detected by eliciting a bulge sign. This is done by stroking in an upward direction along the medial aspect of the joint to empty the synovial pouch, followed by stroking upward or downward on the lateral side of the joint while using the other hand to detect a bulge of fluid as the pouch refills. The joint is scored as normal if there is not a clear indication of effusion.

Firm pressure applied directly over the joint line may elicit *articular tenderness*. In active disease, tenderness felt by pressure over the joint line should be greater than that elicited by pressure on the bone adjacent to the joint. The amount of pressure applied to detect joint tenderness is about 20% less than that needed to cause pain when squeezing the triceps or lower calf muscles. To assess *stress pain,* the therapist moves the limb to the end of the available range and applies slight overpressure.

An examination of joint motion provides valuable baseline information about joint integrity and function. An initial screening, asking the child to perform a series of movements, directs the therapist's attention to problem areas. In very young children, active motion can be elicited by playing games like "Simon Says." In the presence of limitation of motion (LOM) or pain during active movements, the therapist should use standard goniometry to measure passive range of motion (PROM). Checking accessory joint motions may help determine the cause of impaired joint function. Loss of motion, pain during motion, and bony crepitus may be signs of joint damage in arthritis. Although radiographs may show objective joint damage in long-standing arthritis, magnetic resonance imaging (MRI) studies may be more effective in detecting damage early in the disease course.

The common patterns of joint impairments and subsequent activity restrictions in JIA are shown in Table 14.4. Although there is a bias toward arthritis in the large joints, the small joints of the hands and feet are frequently involved in children with a polyarticular disease course. Arthritis of the hip joint occurs in 30% to 50% of children, primarily in those with a SoJIA and PoJIA.[42] Bekkering et al. found

a significant correlation between loss of motion in the hip joint and higher disability scores on the CHAQ in children with SoJIA.[43] The child with early hip disease often experiences pain in the groin, buttocks, medial thigh, or knee and may have a gluteus medius limp when walking. Hip flexion contractures may result from active inflammation or secondary to knee arthritis or a leg length discrepancy.

The knee is the joint most often involved in OligoJIA, but knee arthritis is common in all disease types. Limited joint mobility, spasm of the hamstrings, and shortening of the tensor fascia latae (TFL) and iliotibial band (ITB) contribute to loss of knee extension and changes in postural alignment and gait. Chronic synovitis often causes overgrowth of the femoral condyle, resulting in a valgus deformity of the knee. Shortening of the TFL and ITB exacerbate this impairment.

Arthritis in the ankle and hindfoot occur in all disease types. Loss of ankle dorsiflexion is common. Subtalar arthritis may result in limited hindfoot motion. Although the literature describes calcaneal eversion and secondary forefoot pronation as the most common deviation, a cavus forefoot and loss of subtalar eversion occurs in some children. The small joints of the feet are often involved in children with a polyarticular disease course. Common problems include hallux valgus, hallux rigidus, hammer toes, and overlapping toes. Metatarsalgia and subluxation of the metatarsophalangeal (MTP) joints cause considerable pain during stance and ambulation.

In the upper limbs, arthritis in the joints of the shoulder girdle complex result in restricted motion or altered biomechanics in shoulder rotation, flexion, and abduction. Elbow flexion contractures are common, occur early in the disease course, and are often accompanied by loss of forearm supination. The severity and pattern of arthritis in the wrists and small joints of the hands depends to some extent on disease type, the child's age, and skeletal maturation. In children with PoJIA with disease onset at a young age, wrist subluxation and undergrowth of the ulna result in ulnar deviation. In children 12 years or older at disease onset, a pattern of radial deviation is more

---

TABLE 14.4 ⟩⟩ ⟩⟩ ⟩⟩ ⟩⟩ ⟩⟩ ⟩ ⟩ ⟩

Common Patterns of Joint and Soft Tissue Impairments in Juvenile Idiopathic Arthritis

Cervical Spine

- Most common in PoJIA and SoJIA
- Loss of extension, rotation
- Loss of normal lordosis
- May develop torticollis if asymmetric
- Chronic inflammation may lead to joint space narrowing with nerve root irritation
- Fusion of zygapophyseal joints—often occurs first in C-2–C-3 but may progress to other levels
- Dysplasia of vertebral bodies
- Instability of C-1–C-2 articulation may occur, but less common than in adult RA

Temporomandibular Joints

- Most common in PoJIA; less common in OligoJIA
- Restriction in opening mouth; pain on chewing
- Greater functional loss if cervical spine extension is limited
- Mandibular asymmetry if unilateral involvement
- Undergrowth of the mandible (micrognathia)
- Malocclusion of the teeth
- May require orthodontic treatment

Shoulder Complex

- Most common in PoJIA
- Limited glenohumeral ABD and MR noted first; limited shoulder flexion
- Shortening of pectorals and scapular abductors
- Overgrowth of humeral head with irregular shape
- Shallow glenoid fossa with increased risk of subluxation
- Functional loss increases if elbow and wrist arthritis is present

Thoracolumbar Spine

- Most common in ERA; sacroiliac arthritis common in JAS
- Motion may be limited by spasm of spinal extensors or short hip flexors
- Scoliosis secondary to long-standing leg length discrepancy
- Kyphosis in association with neck and shoulder arthritis
- Excessive lumbar lordosis secondary to hip flexion contracture
- Long-term systemic steroid therapy contributes to osteoporosis, wedging vertebral bodies, small compression fractures

Hip

- Occurs in PoJIA and SoJIA; primary cause of disability
- Loss of extension, MR, and ABD

- Weakness of gluteus medius and deep hip LR; may cause Trendelenburg gait deviation
- Flexion contracture may be masked by increased lumbar lordosis
- May have marked pain on weight bearing; pain may be referred to groin, buttocks, medial thigh, knee
- Femoral head overgrowth
- Osteoporosis
- Limited weight bearing in young child contributes to poorly developed hip joint with shallow acetabulum and trochanteric growth abnormalities
- Lateral subluxation of femoral head, aggravated by short hip adductors
- Potential for protrusio acetabuli and AVN in persistent severe disease
- Potential for repair of articular cartilage with fibrocartilage during disease remission with improved weight bearing and mobility

Elbow

- Occurs in all types
- Involved early in disease course
- Loss of extension, forearm supination
- Overgrowth of radial head restricts ROM
- Proximal radioulnar joint involved
- Ulnar nerve entrapment possible

Wrist

- Occurs in all types; occurs early in disease course
- Accelerated carpal maturation
- Undergrowth of ulna; ulna may migrate dorsally
- Radial and intercarpal fusion
- Rapid loss of extension; shortening of wrist flexors; volar subluxation
- Wrist rests in flexion and ulnar deviation
- In older onset or RF+ PoJIA, wrist may deviate radially
- Distal radioulnar disease causes loss of forearm pronation and supination
- Flexor tenosynovitis

Hand

- Involvement later in PoJIA and SoJIA than OligoJIA; small joints of hand least commonly affected in JAS
- Premature epiphyseal fusion and growth abnormalities
- MCP and CMC subluxation
- Flexor tenosynovitis
- Loss of MCP flexion, terminal extension
- PIP contractures more common than DIP
- Marked decrease in grip strength
- Boutonniere less common than swan neck deformities

(continued)

> **TABLE 14.4**
>
> **Common Patterns of Joint and Soft Tissue Impairments in Juvenile Idiopathic Arthritis** (Continued)

Knee	Ankle and Foot
• Most common joint involved early in all disease types • Rapid weakness and atrophy of quadriceps, loss of patellar mobility • Flexion contracture; may cause secondary hip flexion contracture • Loss of hip flexion • Overgrowth of distal femur contributes to leg length discrepancy in unilateral disease • Knee valgus aggravated by short hamstrings, TFL, and ITB • Posterior tibial subluxation secondary to prolonged arthritis or aggressive stretching of shortened hamstrings • Risk of femoral fracture associated with osteoporosis	• Occurs in all disease types • Altered growth causes bony changes in the tarsals, with potential for fusion • Growth abnormalities due to early closure of epiphyses • Early loss of ankle inversion, eversion; later loss of D-FL, Pl-FL, especially if standing and walking are limited • Excessive hindfoot valgus or varus • Excessive forefoot pronation or supination • Loss of extension at MTP joints, with subsequent loss of push-off at terminal stance • MTP subluxation • Hallux valgus; hammertoes • Overlapping of IPs • Enthesitis at heel or knee is common in ERA

ABD, abduction; AVN, avascular necrosis; CMC, carpometacarpal; D-FL, dorsiflexion; DIP, distal interphalangeal; ERA, enthesitis-related arthritis; IP, interphalangeal; ITB, iliotibial band; JAS, juvenile ankylosing spondylitis; LR, lateral rotation; MCP, metacar-pophalangeal; MR, medial rotation; MTP, metatarsal phalangeal; OligoJIA, Oligoarticular onset juvenile idiopathic arthritis; PIP, proximal interphalangeal; Pl-FL, plantar flexion; PoJIA, polyarticular onset juvenile idiopathic arthritis; RF+, rheumatoid factor positive; ROM, range of motion; SoJIA, systemic onset juvenile idiopathic arthritis; TFL, tensor fascia latae.
Data in this table is summarized from Cassidy JT, Petty RE, eds. Textbook of Pediatric Rheumatology. 4th Ed. Philadelphia: W. B. Saunders Company, 2001. This listing is not inclusive, nor do all of the characteristics listed occur in every child with arthritis.

common. Persistent arthritis in the joints of the hands and tenosynovitis contribute to pain and loss of motion in the carpometacarpal (CMC), metacarpophalangeal (MCP), and proximal interphalangeal (PIP) joints.

Joint motion can be recorded in standard chart format or on the stick figure used to record joint swelling (Fig. 14.7). Specific goniometric measurements or an ordinal scale—0 = no LOM; 1 = 1% to 25% LOM; 2 = 26% to 50% LOM; 3 = 51% to 75% LOM; 4 = 75% to 100% LOM—may be used. Several standardized scales to measure joint motion in children with arthritis are available, but to date, are used primarily in research. The Global Range of Motion Score (GROMS) includes all joints and provides a single score for global joint motion in children with arthritis.[44] A reduced 10-joint GROMS includes only those joints weighted by experts as essential for function and most often involved in JIA.[44] The Pediatric Escola Paulista de Medicina range of motion (PEPM-ROM) scale also includes 10 joint movements judged to be most often involved and most important for essential functions in children with arthritis. Unlike the GROMS, this scale uses predetermined cut-off points for scoring; scores range from 0 (no limitation) to 3 (severe limitation). The final score for each joint motion is the mean score for the right and left side. The total score for the scale is the sum of each joint movement score divided by 10; the range is 0 to 3. The authors report excellent test-retest and inter-tester agreement for the scale. Although either the PEPM-ROM or the 10-joint GROMS may save time in clinical settings, the full GROMS or traditional recording formats for ROM are more suitable when the child has extensive disease or has arthritis in joints not included in the scale.

MUSCLE STRUCTURE AND FUNCTION

The available research indicates that childhood arthritis results in significant impairments in muscle structure and function. Common patterns include weakness in hip extension and abduction, knee extension, ankle dorsiflexion and plantar flexion, shoulder abduction and flexion, elbow flexion and extension, wrist extension, and hand grip. The coincidence of decreased muscle thickness and strength suggest that this is true weakness rather than simply inhibition of muscle force due to pain or joint swelling.[46] Factors that contribute to muscular impairments include alterations in anabolic hormones, production of inflammatory cytokines and high resting energy use, abnormal protein metabolism, and pain-induced inhibition of motor unit activity.[14,47] Onset of arthritis at a very young age and persistence of active disease may negatively impact muscle development.[48] Deficits are most pronounced near joints with active inflammation, but are also found in distant areas, suggesting a more generalized pattern of weakness.[46,49–51] Muscular impairments often persist years after active disease remits.[50]

Several studies document the effects of reduced strength on physical activity in children with arthritis. Klepper et al. reported that children with polyarticular disease scored significantly below healthy age-, gender-, and size-matched controls on the 1-minute timed sit-up test.[52] Fan et al. found a significant correlation between 50-meter run times and lower limb CHAQ scores in girls with JRA.[53] Takken et al. also found that muscle strength, measured by the Wingate anaerobic test, was significantly related to total CHQ scores in 18 children with arthritis, age 7 to 14 years.[54] Other studies reported weakness in the ankle plantar flexor and dorsiflexor muscle groups that may contribute to altered gait patterns in JIA.[20,51,55] Brostrom et al. used a custom-built isokinetic dynamometer to examine isometric and dynamic muscle torques in the ankle plantar flexors and dorsiflexors in 10 girls with JIA and compared their performance to that of 10 healthy age- and gender-matched controls. Their data showed that ankle plantar flexion and dorsiflexion strength were approximately 40% and 50% less, respectively, in the JIA group than controls.[20] They also found that the ratio of plantar flexor to dorsiflexor strength was similar in children with JIA and controls, suggesting that the disease affects both muscle groups equally.

During the initial and subsequent examinations, the physical therapist should assess muscle bulk, strength, and endurance. Bilateral measures of limb circumference, most often performed on the calf and thigh, help to quantify asymmetries in muscle bulk. To assess strength, the physical therapist has several options. Manual muscle tests (MMTs) are useful to measure isometric strength in older children, but the therapist should be aware of the limitations of MMTs, especially for grades above 3 (fair). Instrumented measurements using either a handheld or isokinetic dynamometer provide more objective and reliable measures of strength in children with arthritis.[56–58] Figure 14.9 shows

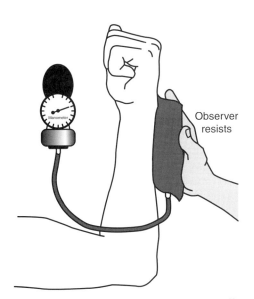

Figure 14.9 ■ Use of modified blood pressure cuff to measure isometric triceps strength. (From Walker J, Helewa A, eds. Physical Therapy in Arthritis. Philadelphia: W. B. Saunders; 1996: 129–148, with permission from H. Smythe, MD, FRC[C].)

a modified blood pressure cuff used as an alternative to the commercial handheld dynamometer.[41] The rolled cuff is placed distally as far as possible on the limb, without crossing a painful joint. The tester applies pressure to the cuff with a flat hand. The patient pushes against the cuff, while the tester increases pressure gradually for 5 seconds. Grip strength can also be measured by having the child squeeze the cuff. The highest pressure sustained by the patient is recorded. With any of these methods, it is important to use consistent procedures and establish reliability among all testers within the clinic.

Testing of dynamic strength provides valuable information about the child's ability to perform necessary and desired activities. Most children with mild to moderate arthritis can tolerate dynamic muscle strength testing. Muscles are usually tested in functional groups; for example, reaching forward in the scapular plane tests the muscle of the shoulder girdle and simulates reaching activities. Special attention is given to the antigravity muscles and those shown in research to be weak in children with arthritis. With very young children, functional strength can be estimated by observing the child perform age-appropriate motor activities like ascending and descending steps to assess strength of the lower extremities. For older children, strength can be assessed using free weights to determine the repetition maximum (RM) for a given muscle group. A 6 to 10 RM (the maximum weight the child can lift through the available ROM, maintaining proper form, for six to 10 repetitions) is a sufficient measure of strength to establish a baseline, determine a training protocol, and evaluate progress.[59] If the child has pain on movement of the limb, the therapist can perform isometric testing at multiple joint angles. This method provides an estimate of dynamic strength and may also reveal specific points within the ROM where the muscle group is weak. Muscle endurance can be measured by asking the child to perform as many repetitions of the movement as possible lifting a specified percentage, usually 60% to 80%, of the six or 10 RM. A warm-up period of light activity should precede all testing. Tests of strength and endurance should be performed on different days to avoid fatigue.

AEROBIC CAPACITY AND PERFORMANCE

A growing body of research documents impairments in aerobic capacity and performance in children with JIA (Display 14.4). In a recent systematic review of the literature, Takken et al. identified five studies that directly measured peak oxygen consumption (VO_{2peak}) during progressive graded exercise in children with JIA.[60] An analysis of pooled data from these studies showed that relative VO_{2peak} was significantly lower in subjects with JIA compared with control subjects or age and gender reference values. In one of these studies, Giannini and Protas also found that children with arthritis (ACR criteria) had a lower peak workload, lower peak exercise heart rate (HR),

Comparison of Physiologic and Performance Variables in Children with and Without Arthritis

Variable	Children with Arthritis Compared with Healthy Children
Peak VO₂	↓
Peak heart rate (HR)	↓
Submaximal HR	↑
Peak workload	↓
Peak anaerobic power	↓
Performance on field tests of aerobic fitness	↓
Muscle strength	↓
Muscle bulk	↓

and shorter exercise time than matched controls.[61] Heart rate during submaximal exercise was also higher in these subjects. Klepper et al.[52] reported that children with polyarticular disease scored significantly lower than matched controls on the 9-Minute Walk-Run Test. Unlike control subjects, most children with JRA were not able to maintain a steady running pace over the 9 minutes. This finding supports the belief that children with arthritis may experience fatigue after short bouts of moderately vigorous physical activity.

The cause of impaired aerobic fitness is most likely multifactorial. Specific physiologic factors related to the disease process may contribute to decreased exercise tolerance and fatigue; these include pain, mild anemia, and poor mechanical efficiency that result from muscle atrophy, weakness, and joint stiffness. These factors may be especially relevant in children who develop arthritis at a very young age and have persistent disease. However, there is also growing evidence that chronic hypoactivity, whether secondary to disease symptoms or lifestyle habits, contributes to low aerobic performance in children with JIA. Several studies failed to find a significant correlation between aerobic fitness and either the number of swollen joints or the severity of disease symptoms.[52,57,61]

These and other studies support the belief that children with arthritis engage in fewer organized sports and less vigorous physical activity than their healthy peers; examined were aerobic fitness (VO₂peak) and physical activity (PA) in 45 children age 4 to 16 years with JIA.[14,54,62] Physical activity was measured over four consecutive days using a Caltrac activity monitor and a parental physical activity rating scale (PAL). Activity counts and VO₂peak values were lower in these subjects than typical values for healthy children, and PA levels and relative VO₂peak were significantly related. PA was also inversely related to the number of swollen joints, suggesting that children with more severe disease were less active.[54] There is also some evidence that children with

arthritis may have deficits in the complex motor skills necessary for participation in sports or perceive themselves as less physically competent than their peers.[28,62]

Aerobic function should be assessed prior to the child's participation in an aerobic conditioning program. Test results can guide intervention and help to monitor the child's response to overall management of the disease. Laboratory assessment of VO₂max should be performed in any child with cardiac or respiratory complications. Assessment of submaximal oxygen consumption can provide an estimate of aerobic fitness in children without systemic symptoms. These tests compare the workload achieved and heart rate response to exercise during a standardized protocol on a treadmill or cycle ergometer.

Alternately, simple, inexpensive field tests, such as a walk-run test, that measure either the time required to travel a specified distance or the distance traveled over a specified time can provide an indication of the child's functional aerobic performance. Results are compared to normative data or health standards, based on age and gender.

PAIN

Despite early studies suggesting that children with arthritis experience less pain than adults with RA, most research using developmentally appropriate measures of pain now concurs that pain is a prominent feature of these disorders and an important predictor of the child's adjustment to the disease. In a recent review of the literature, Anthony and Schanberg discussed the prevalence, demographics, and potential causes of pain in childhood arthritis.[63] Most studies suggest that a high percent of children with arthritis report pain during routine clinic visits. Data on 462 children from the Cincinnati Juvenile Arthritis Databank indicated that 60% of children reported pain at disease onset, 50% reported pain at 1-year follow-up, and 40% reported pain 5 years later.[64] While the majority of children in these and other studies report mild to moderate pain, approximately 25% of the children reported pain intensity in the higher ranges of pain measurement scales.[63]

Acute pain in children with arthritis occurs as a result of the many medical procedures these children endure in routine care, as well as from the inflammatory process. However, the cause of chronic pain in this population is not as clear. Data from daily diaries indicated that some children reported at least mild pain on 70% of the days. Subjects described their pain as "sharp," "aching," "burning," and "uncomfortable." Several groups have studied the factors that might contribute to chronic pain in childhood arthritis. There is some evidence that children with arthritis have a decreased pain threshold and pain tolerance compared with their healthy peers, possibly as a result of increased sensitivity to noxious stimuli due to a change in pain processing that occurs from prolonged activation of both peripheral and central nociceptive systems.[65–67] Yet medical variables, including disease type and severity, do not fully explain the child's report of the distribution and intensity of pain. Several recent studies suggest that psychosocial factors, including parent and family pain histories, fluctuations in mood, stressful events, and the way in which children perceive and cope with their pain, significantly correlate with the child's self-rated pain and physician-rated health status.[63]

Assessment of pain in children with arthritis should be comprehensive and ongoing. Components should include a pain history, self-report for children over the age of 4 years, parent report, and behavioral observations. The Varni/Thompson Pediatric Pain Questionnaire (PPQ) is a self-report and parent (as proxy) report that includes a 10-cm VAS for pain intensity, a list of pain descriptors, and a color body map.[68] The PPQ provides a comprehensive assessment of pain in children, but because of its length, is used primarily in research.

Display 14.5 lists pain assessment instruments useful in the clinic. Self-report measures of pain intensity in young children include the Oucher,[69] Wong-Baker Faces Pain Rating Scale, and the Poker Chip Tool.[70,71] The child can also report pain distribution and intensity on a body map using different colors to represent levels of pain intensity (Fig. 14.10). Children 5 years of age and older can report acute and chronic pain intensity on a numeric scale, a word graphic rating scale, or a visual analog scale.[72] In very young children, the therapist should be alert for validated pain behaviors in JIA, including bracing, guarding, rubbing, rigidity, and flexing.[73]

GROWTH AND POSTURAL ALIGNMENT

Measures of height, weight, body composition, and posture are important components of the initial and ongoing physical therapy assessments to monitor the effects of the disease on growth and skeletal alignment. Postural align-

Pain: | Red | Yellow | Green | Blue |

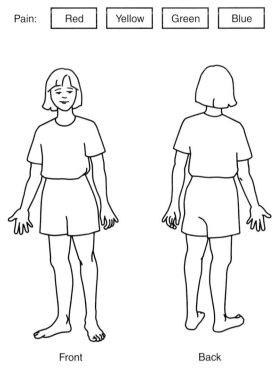

Front   Back

Figure 14.10 ■ *Example of a body outline figure and rating scale used to assess pain intensity and location in children.*

ment is examined in sitting and standing from the front, back, and side. Potential problems include a forward head posture, kyphosis, excessive lumbar lordosis, hip and knee flexion contractures, genu valgus, hindfoot varus or valgus, and other ankle and foot deformities described previously.

The assessment should include screening for scoliosis and restrictions in spinal mobility. Torticollis may occur in children with asymmetric cervical spine arthritis. Differences in leg length may cause pelvic obliquity and the appearance of a scoliosis in standing. Leg length should be examined in supine, measuring from the anterior superior iliac spine (ASIS) to the medial malleolus. The length of the femur and tibia should be measured separately if the child has a hip or knee flexion contracture. When differences are found, recheck spinal alignment after placing small lifts of known thickness under the shorter leg to level the pelvis. Mobility of the lumbar spine should be examined in children with ERA, and particularly in those with JAS. Figure 14.11

>> **DISPLAY 14.5**

Pediatric Pain Assessment Instruments Useful in Children with Juvenile Idiopathic Arthritis

Instrument (References)	Description
Oucher Scale[69]	• Ages 3–12 yr • Measures pain intensity • Includes six faces and a scale from 0 to 100, from happy to very sad, scored as 0–5
Faces Rating Scale[70]	• Suitable for children ages 3 yr and older • Scale includes six faces from happy to very sad, scored as 0–5; record number of face child chooses • Child chooses the face that best represents how he or she feels • Measures pain intensity and affect

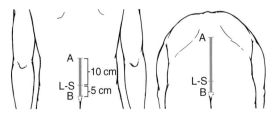

Figure 14.11 ■ *The modified Schober test of lumbar spine mobility. (Modified from Oatis CA.* Kinesiology: The Mechanics and Pathomechanics of Human Movement. *Baltimore: Lippincott Williams & Wilkins, 2004.)*

shows the modified Schober test of lumbar spine mobility. With the child standing with feet together and pointing forward, a line is drawn between the two dimples of Venus to mark the lumbosacral junction. Place a mark on the spine 5 cm below and 10 cm above this line and measure the distance between the two marks. The increase in distance between the marks from baseline to a position of maximum forward flexion is used as an indicator of spinal mobility. Although there are large normal variations at all ages, an increase of less than 6 cm is considered abnormal.

Assessment of sitting posture also is important to determine potential causes of muscle pain and fatigue during functional activities. Habitually sitting in a "slumped" posture characterized by a posterior pelvic tilt, thoracic kyphosis, and forward head position contributes over time to shortening of the anterior chest muscles and overlengthening of scapular stabilizers resulting in limited and/or painful shoulder motion during reaching and other upper limb activities.

GAIT

Several studies document gait deviations in children with JIA.[55,74,75] Early studies found that children with arthritis in the lower extremities have decreased gait velocity, cadence, and shorter step and stride length. Other problems identified included increased anterior pelvic tilt throughout the gait cycle, decreased hip extension at terminal stance, and decreased plantar flexion force at push-off in the patient groups.[55,74] Brostrom et al. examined gait velocity, ground force reactions, and temporal parameters in 15 children with unilateral or bilateral lower limb arthritis JCA, 6 to 14 years old. There was no difference in contact time between the affected and unaffected leg in children with unilateral arthritis, although there was a tendency for this group to have a shorter single support time than similar age controls. Compared with controls, subjects with arthritis had a significantly slower walking velocity, and velocity was negatively correlated with pain, measured on a VAS. Data on ground reaction force indicated lower heel-strike and push-off force in subjects with arthritis.[75] This supports previous reports by Frigo et al. that the ankle joint undergoes less plantar flexion at push-off in children with arthritis and lends support to the clinical observation that children with arthritis often have a "cautious" gait.[74]

Positive changes in some gait parameters, joint angles, and muscle function following intra-articular steroid injections in children with JIA support the belief that pain, stiffness, muscle weakness, and impaired joint mobility contribute to gait deviations.[20] Shortened step length may result from decreased hip extension and ankle plantar flexion at the end of stance. Ankle and foot arthritis and the subsequent joint limitations or deformities contribute to

many of the changes observed in foot pressures and muscle function during stance and decreased push-off.[76]

Although computerized motion analysis is the most valid and reliable method to examine gait parameters, gait assessment in the typical clinical setting involves a simple observational analysis. Ideally, the child should be observed walking with and without shoes, although some children may experience pain walking barefoot. The child's gait pattern should be observed for symmetry, step and stride length, and alignment of the lower limb at heel strike, midstance, terminal stance, and swing. Having the child walk on an instrumented gait mat or pressure-sensitive paper provides objective data. A timed walk can be used to determine gait velocity. The assessment should include walking on level surfaces, inclines, stairs, and curbs, and while running. Use of any assistive devices (orthoses, cane, walker, or wheelchair) for mobility should be noted. A video of the child's gait provides a permanent record and is useful to monitor change.

 ## Evaluation, Diagnosis, Prognosis, and Plan of Care

The therapist synthesizes the examination findings and information from the medical history and interview with the parent and child, analyzes the data, and formulates hypotheses regarding the relationship between disease status, impairments, and activity limitations (Fig. 14.12). The ICF also gives consideration to contextual factors that might impact the prognosis, including the personal attributes of the child, family interactions, and resources available to help the family manage the child's condition. Because of the erratic nature of these disorders, it is not always possible to predict the prognosis early in disease course. Ongoing research to discover predictors of poor outcome in various types of JIA will prove very useful in planning treatment. However, currently the duration and frequency of treatment are often dictated more by the child's health care plan than on evidence-based practice. Exact rehabilitation philosophies and protocols used in JIA vary from clinic to clinic, and there are few studies that provide evidence for the effectiveness of any particular physical therapy techniques or regimen. The therapist must draw from literature in other areas to determine the best interventions to address the child's needs.

 ## Intervention

The general goals of intervention in JIA are to prevent or minimize impairments, maximize the child's functional capacity and performance, and provide education and support to the child and family in their effort to manage the

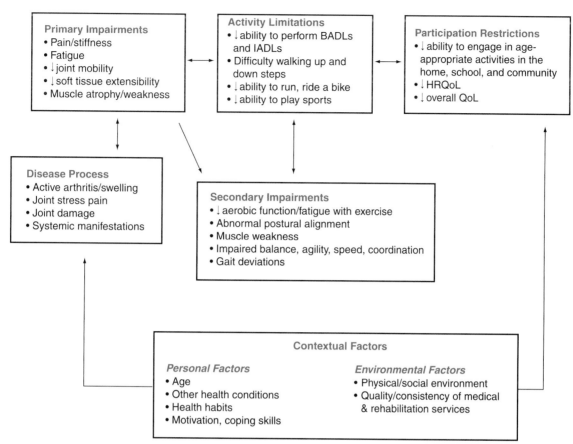

Figure 14.12 ■ The therapist synthesizes the examination findings and information from the medical history and interview with the parent and child, analyzes the data, and formulates hypotheses regarding the relationship between disease status, impairments, and activity limitations. BADLs, basic activities of daily living; HRQoL, health-related quality of life; IADLs, instrumental activities of daily living; QoL, quality of life.

child's condition (Display 14.6). Treatment must be appropriate for the child's cognitive and emotional development to ensure his or her understanding of procedures and active participation in the therapy program. Physical activity and specific exercise must be graded based on disease activity and severity. Although developmentally based play therapy can be very useful to encourage very young children to be active, joints with active disease or limited motion require direct attention.

COORDINATION, COMMUNICATION, AND DOCUMENTATION

Coordination of services and communication among individuals providing care for the child with arthritis can be especially challenging because of the complex nature of these disorders and need to involve multiple disciplines. Most children with JIA receive disease-specific care from a pediatric rheumatology team in a tertiary clinic that is often several hours from the child's home. Therapists working in these centers may perform the initial examination, set treatment goals, and develop an intervention program for the child, but may not provide ongoing care. Children with mild arthritis and no serious physical impairments often

receive a home exercise program (HEP) and suggestions for managing disease symptoms. Children who require direct physical therapy but live far from the rheumatology clinic usually receive services in their home, a local clinic, or school as part of an individualized educational plan (IEP). While coordination of care is typically very good within specialized pediatric rheumatology centers, communication with the local therapists and other health providers is often less than optimal. The treating therapist must make a concerted effort to obtain information from the rheumatology team regarding the child's specific diagnosis, disease status, medications, and precautions. The rheumatology clinic nurse is often in the best position to facilitate communication between the clinic and outside health professionals. Frequent progress reports from the therapist help the rheumatologist monitor the child's response to medical therapies, functional abilities, and adherence to exercise regimens.

PROCEDURAL INTERVENTIONS

PAIN MANAGEMENT AND COMFORT MEASURES

Adequate disease control is the first line of intervention in managing pain associated with inflammation. Many of the

>> **DISPLAY 14.6**

General Goals of Physical Therapist Intervention

Reduce impairments in body structures and functions
- Maintain/improve joint range of motion
- Maintain/improve muscle bulk, strength, and endurance
- Maintain/improve aerobic fitness
  - Reduce fatigue
  - Improve stamina for physical activity
- Reduce postural deviations

Maintain/improve child's ability to perform activities and participate
- Maintain/improve child's mobility in the home, school, and community
- Maintain/improve ability to perform basic and instrumental activities of daily living
- Maintain/improve motor skills to allow child to participate in age-appropriate recreational activities and sports

Provide information and support to the child and family
- Provide information about arthritis and impact on the body systems
- Provide information about the benefits of daily exercise
- Provide information about techniques to manage pain and stiffness
- Consult with school personnel to ensure child's full participation
- Assist child and family to set realistic goals
- Encourage child and family to participate in medical and therapeutic regimen

medications used to treat arthritis also have an analgesic effect. Intra-articular steroid injections are effective in reducing joint inflammation, swelling, and pain that is not well controlled by oral medications. Orthopedic surgery may be necessary for children with joint damage.

Physical modalities to reduce pain include heat, cold, massage, and splinting. Superficial heat applied locally for about 20 minutes increases blood flow to the area, relaxes surrounding muscles and reduces muscle spasm, improves connective tissue extensibility, and facilitates increased joint mobility. Heat can be supplied in the form of warm moist towels or commercial heat wraps. Paraffin wax may help reduce pain and stiffness in the wrist and hands prior to exercise, although young children may refuse to dip their hands into the hot paraffin, preferring to "paint" the wax on their hands. Applied immediately after an injury, rest, ice, compression, and elevation (RICE) reduce inflammation, swelling, and pain.

Balanced rest and exercise are necessary to manage pain and maintain joint mobility and function. Research indicates that children with arthritis report decreased pain following participation in either water- or land-based exercise programs.[77–80] Restful sleep is necessary to help the child manage pain. Simple comfort measures to reduce morning stiffness and pain include using a sleeping bag during the night to maintain body warmth or soaking in a warm bath

upon awakening. Range-of-motion exercises performed before bed or during the morning bath help to relieve morning stiffness and discomfort. Stretch gloves that provide gentle compression and warmth may also relieve stiffness and pain in the wrist and hands. A cervical pillow helps reduce neck pain. One study found that children who received a massage by a parent before bed reported less pain and stress than control subjects.[81]

Cognitive-behavioral techniques, such as progressive muscle relaxation (PMR), meditative breathing, hypnosis, guided imagery, electromyographic (EMG) biofeedback, and modification in pain behaviors, may prove useful in managing the impact of pain on children with JIA. Lavigne et al. found reductions in self-rated pain intensity and expression of pain behaviors in eight children with arthritis who participated in a program of PMR and EMG biofeedback biweekly for 3 months.[82] Parents were counseled in behavior techniques to manage their child's pain behaviors. Walco et al. also found short-term reduction in subjective pain in children with JRA, ages 5 to 15 years of age, after 8 weeks of training to use PMR, meditative breathing, and guided imagery to moderate pain.[83] Effects remained 12 months after completing the program. Distraction and imaginative play are also useful in young children. Children with serious chronic pain may require comprehensive management through a multidisciplinary pain program.

MANAGEMENT OF JOINT IMPAIRMENTS

RANGE-OF-MOTION EXERCISE AND STRETCHING

Techniques to preserve or increase joint mobility and soft tissue extensibility include range-of-motion exercise, positioning, and splinting. All joints with arthritis and adjacent joints should be moved through the available range for three to five repetitions preferably twice a day. Active ROM exercise is optimal, since it preserves muscle function as well as joint mobility. If the child is unable or unwilling to perform active ROM, use active-assisted ROM to encourage the child to move through the full range. PROM should be avoided if there is acute joint inflammation to prevent overstretching and trauma to vulnerable tissues. Games that include functional movement patterns of the limbs and trunk are useful to elicit joint motions in very young children.

Daily positioning in prone for 30 minutes or more makes use of gravity to place a low-load prolonged stretch on shortened or hypoextensible hip and knee flexor muscles. The child can lie prone on a bed or other firm surface with legs extended and feet hanging off the edge. A pillow placed under the abdomen keeps the pelvis level, while a small rolled towel placed under the forehead helps to position the cervical spine to accommodate limited neck rotation. Commercial or custom-made resting splints provide support for inflamed joints, maintain proper joint alignment, and provide a gentle low-load stretch on the soft tissues. Resting splints may be worn while the child sleeps or

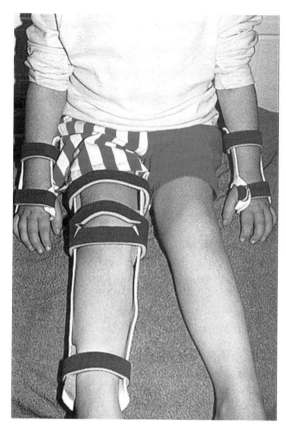

Figure 14.13 ■ *Custom-made resting splints for the hands and knees.*

during the day as needed to provide support, relieve pain, and maintain good joint alignment. Figure 14.13 shows custom-made resting splints for the hands and knees. A posterior "shell" keeps the knee extended and maintains hamstring length during the night; this may reduce stiffness and allow the child to stand and walk more easily upon awakening.

Gentle manual stretching to lengthen shortened soft tissues can begin once the arthritis is under adequate control. Although there is little evidence for the effectiveness of any specific stretching regimen in childhood arthritis, clinical research in adults indicates that holding a static stretch at the end of the available ROM for at least 30 to 60 seconds is necessary to increase muscle extensibility.[84] This stretching method is useful to lengthen tissues prior to placing the limb in a splint. Neuromuscular stretching techniques that make use of autogenic or reciprocal inhibition of the shortened muscle are useful in treating limited joint motion. These include contract-relax, agonist contraction, and a combination of the two techniques. The amount of resistance applied to the active muscle contraction should be varied according to the child's tolerance.

There are several general guidelines for stretching in children with arthritis. Because some joints may respond to medications more quickly than others, ROM and stretching techniques must be graded according to disease status

of individual joints. Stretching should be avoided if there is joint swelling or other indications of active inflammation. It is also important to gain the child's cooperation during stretching, and to minimize pain and reflex muscle spasm. Superficial heat applied locally or through a warm bath prior to stretching facilitates relaxation and tissue extensibility. Aggressive passive stretching is avoided because of the risk for damage to epiphyseal areas at the tendon–bone interface. Aggressive stretching of shortened hamstrings, using a long lever arm contracture, may cause posterior subluxation of the tibia. Stretching should always be combined with active exercise to teach the child to effectively use the previously shortened muscles and the antagonist in their new resting length and to actively use the joint throughout the new range of motion.

Radiologic assessment is necessary to examine available joint space and rule out ankylosis prior to instituting any program to reduce joint contractures. Conservative approaches that provide a static progressive low-load stretch include serial splints or casts and dynamic splints. Custom-made serial splints are convenient because the therapist can mold and easily modify the splint as needed to accommodate the child's ROM. However, because these splints can be easily removed, their effectiveness depends on the child's adherence to the stretching regimen. In contrast, serial casts require a considerable amount of time and skill to apply and cannot be modified, but cannot be removed by the child. Although the exact protocol may vary in different clinics, in the typical regimen, the child wears the cast for 48 to 72 hours, after which it is removed and bivalved. During the next 1 to 2 weeks, the cast is worn for 18 to 24 hours a day, removing it only for exercise sessions. Range-of-motion exercise in a warm pool is especially helpful to encourage use of the joint in its new ROM. If the child still has limited joint mobility, a new cast is applied and the process is repeated until full functional ROM is achieved.

Dynamic splints use springs or rubber bands to provide a constant stretching force to increase soft tissue length. Commercially available dynamic splints can be ordered and fit to specific joints. The tension at the joint can be controlled by the therapist and set to patient tolerance. Commercial orthoses that have a dial-lock joint at the knee allow the therapist to adjust the degree of extension as the child gains motion (Fig. 14.14). Most patients will tolerate a dynamic splint for 1-hour periods during the day. However, this type of splint is not generally used on a joint with acute arthritis.

SURGERY AND POSTOPERATIVE PHYSICAL THERAPY

The apparent success of current medical therapies in controlling inflammation and subsequent joint damage may limit the role of orthopedic surgery in most children with arthritis. However, well-timed selective surgical procedures may be indicated for some children to preserve joint health, relieve disabling pain, or restore function when conservative

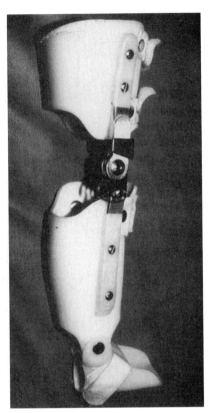

Figure 14.14 ■ Example of a dial-lock knee joint.

measures have failed. The choice of procedure depends on the child's age, disease activity, condition of the involved joint, and functional status. The decision to perform surgery must be made by an interdisciplinary team, based on an analysis of the risks and benefits. The physical therapist is involved in the preoperative assessment and planning, as well as the postoperative rehabilitation.

Soft tissue releases (STRs) are performed to manage joint contractures that do not respond to conservative measures. Reduced intra-articular pressure and increased joint mobility often result in improved joint nutrition and healing of the articular cartilage by fibrocartilage. The most common procedures include adductor and psoas tenotomies to relieve hip flexion contractures, ITB fasciotomy, hamstring lengthening, and posterior capsulotomy to relieve knee flexion contracture. The postoperative period is aimed at preserving the newly acquired muscle length and joint motion through splinting and ROM exercise. Following STR at the hip, the joint is positioned in an abduction and extension splint; following STR for knee flexion contractures, the joint is positioned in extension. However, immobilization is kept to a minimum to avoid further loss of motion, and ROM exercises begin within the first 48 hours unless there are problems with wound healing. Gait training begins as soon as possible. Strengthening exercises can begin when soft tissue inflammation resolves. To maintain ROM following discharge, the child must lie prone for periods during the day and avoid prolonged sit-

ting. The use of splints may be discontinued after about 8 weeks, but the child must continue physical therapy for several months to achieve optimal results.

Supracondylar osteotomy may be performed in conjunction with soft tissue releases for a severe flexion contracture at the knee or when there is a valgus deformity and evidence of joint damage. An arthrotomy is usually done at the same time if there is a poorly formed or overgrown patella that is fixed to the femoral condyle, limiting joint motion.[85] Postoperatively, the leg is immobilized in a cylindric cast, with immediate weight bearing. The cast is removed when there is evidence of adequate bone union.

Synovectomy is not usually performed in children with arthritis, because of problems with postoperative pain and spasm and disappointing long-term results. However, the procedure may be done in combination with STRs to treat hip flexion contractures.[86] It may also be done arthroscopically for acute synovitis of the knee, when effusion and overgrowth of inflamed synovium stimulate the adjacent epiphysis, resulting in lengthening of the limb.[86] Tenosynovectomy may be indicated in a child with severe arthritis in the hand in order to prevent tendon rupture or reduce nerve entrapment from synovial proliferation.

Arthrodesis may be considered when a child has disabling pain on joint motion and there is a high risk for natural joint ankylosis as a result of the disease. Arthrodesis or joint fusion may be beneficial in advanced arthritis of the wrist, interphalangeal joints, and ankle or subtalar joints. Postoperative care includes immobilization in a cast, exercise, and positioning of adjacent joints to maintain mobility. After lower limb surgery, the child is allowed to stand and walk with crutches or walker. Immobilization is maintained until there is radiographic evidence of successful fusion. Temporary epiphysiodesis, or surgical arrest of the growth plate, may be useful in some children with bony overgrowth leading to leg length discrepancy (LLD). In a retrospective study, Skytta et al. studied the long-term efficacy of temporary epiphyseal stapling at the knee in 17 patients.[87] The mean difference between the preoperative LLD (21 mm) and LLD at time of staple removal (4 mm) was −17 mm (5% CI, −10 to −23). Five subjects experienced a reoccurrence of the LLD after staple removal.

Children with irreversible joint damage may be candidates for total joint arthroplasty (TJA). Several factors are considered in the decision to perform TJA in a child with arthritis. These include the child's age, skeletal maturity, physical status, upper limb function, and the potential ability of the child and family to complete the lengthy and intensive postoperative rehabilitation. Ideally, these procedures are delayed until the epiphyses have fused or there is little chance of further growth of the limb, although TJA may be necessary in younger children who have severe joint damage, disabling pain, and loss of function.[88] Custom-designed hip prostheses that are porous are typically used to accommodate the smaller bones in children with JIA and allow for biologic fixation, because cemented prostheses are more susceptible to loosening after several years. Timing of procedures is extremely important in a child who requires multiple joint replacements. In children with severe upper limb arthritis, fusion of a damaged or painful wrist may be necessary first to allow the child to use crutches after hip or knee surgery. When both hips and knees must be replaced, the hip joints are usually done first. When there are severe hip flexion contractures and joint destruction, both hips are replaced at the same time.[89]

Preoperative physical therapy includes a general conditioning exercise program to improve strength, ROM and general stamina, and gait training with crutches or walker. The child also receives instruction in postoperative exercises and precautions to protect the implant during daily activities. The postoperative program for total hip arthroplasty (THA) includes ROM exercise, with precautions to avoid hip flexion past 90 degrees, adduction past neutral, and internal rotation. A foam abduction pillow is used for 6 weeks, alternating with a CPM machine and prone positioning. Submaximal isometric exercises of the hip extensors and abductors and quadriceps may be started early. The child must also practice transfers and activities of daily living (ADLs). Elevated toilet seats and dressing aids help the child maintain hip precautions. Gait training with an assistive device can begin during the first week. Active exercise in shallow water and ambulation in chest-deep water may begin as soon as wound healing is complete. Hip precautions are usually maintained for the first 2 to 3 postoperative months, although this may vary based on the surgeon. Activities that cause high-impact loading on the lower limbs should be avoided.

Total knee arthroplasty (TKA) is usually done using a cemented prosthesis, and may be accompanied by soft tissue releases to resolve a flexion contracture, release of the lateral retinaculum to prevent further valgus deformity, and resurfacing of the underside of the patella. Postoperative therapy begins with ROM exercises on day 2. A CPM machine can be used immediately, with an extension splint worn at other times. Prone positioning is also encouraged to preserve knee extension. The goal is to achieve knee ROM from 0 degrees (full extension) to 100 degrees of flexion. A program to strengthen lower extremity musculature is begun with isometric and straight leg–raising exercises. Aquatic exercise and stationary cycling, using a range limiter on the pedal to control the amount of knee flexion, may also be used. Full weight bearing, using a knee immobilizer, is begun on the second postoperative day. Ambulation without assistive devices is allowed when the child demonstrates at least 90 degrees of knee flexion and adequate lower extremity strength and endurance. Parvizi et al. studied long-term clinical outcome of TKA in 13 children (25 knees) with JIA using the Knee Society Score (KSS). This instrument measures pain and function; each scale has a maximum of 100 points, with higher scores indicating less pain and improved function.[88] The KSS for pain improved from 27.6 (range, 4 to 62) preoperatively

to 88.3 (range, 55 to 100) at the last follow-up period, 10.7 years after surgery. Scores for function improved from 14.8 (range, 0 to 30) preoperatively to 39.2 (range, 10 to 85) at follow-up. The overall arc of knee flexion also improved from a mean of 70 degrees (range, 0 to 115 degrees) to 81 degrees (range, 35 to 120 degrees) at follow-up.

The most common complications reported with TJA include infection, dislocation, and biologic loosening of the components. One long-term follow-up study of 72 patients with THA reported that 30% of the patients required revision surgery after 10 years. Outcome from TJA may be complicated by several factors in children with arthritis, including the smaller bones, extent of osteoporosis, and presence of skeletal malalignment. Also, if the child has significant periarticular changes by the time of TJA, it may be difficult to regain full ROM in the involved and adjacent joints. It may be necessary to perform other procedures at the time of TJA, including STRs, soft tissue transfers, and correction of skeletal deformities, to improve long-term outcomes in children with arthritis. Continued advances in customized prosthetic design and surgical procedures should result in improved safety and longevity of total joint replacements.

EXERCISE TO IMPROVE MUSCLE PERFORMANCE

The term *muscle performance* includes strength, endurance, and power. Impaired muscle performance contributes to joint pain and limited activity in children with JIA. Intervention specifically targets muscles surrounding joints with arthritis, although the exercise prescription must also address other deficits in muscle performance identified during the assessment. Several studies report improved muscle performance with no exacerbation of disease symptoms in children with JIA who completed structured resistance training programs.[49,78,79,90] The mode of exercise and total volume must be graded to the child's age, disease status, condition of individual joints, and current muscle performance. Display 14.7 illustrates the benefits, precautions, and general guidelines of resistance training.

During active disease, the main concern is to maintain muscle strength and endurance to adequately support the joints, prevent deformities, and allow the child to maintain normal daily activities. Isometric exercise is used to prevent atrophy and maintain strength in muscles surrounding inflamed joints when movement is often painful. Resistance can be provided manually or by a stable external object, nonelastic webbing, or heavy elastic bands placed around the limb close to and proximal to the joint. Prolonged maximal isometric contractions of muscle around inflamed joints should be avoided because this may increase the intra-articular pressure and constrict blood flow through the exercising muscles.[91] The child can be taught to regulate the intensity by first contracting the muscle maximally, then letting go slightly and holding that submaximal

>> **DISPLAY 14.7**

Purpose, Recommendations, and Precautions for Isometric and Dynamic Muscle Conditioning Exercises

Isometric	Dynamic
Purpose	
Minimize atrophy	Maintain/increase dynamic strength/endurance
Maintain/increase static strength/endurance	Increase muscle power
Prepare for dynamic and weight-bearing activity	Enhance synovial blood flow
	Promote strength of bone/cartilage
Recommendations	
Perform at functional joint angles; multiple points throughout ROM	Able to perform 8–10 repetitions against gravity before additional resistance
Breathe normally; do not hold breath	Breathe normally; do not hold breath
Intensity: ≤70% one MVC	Use functional movements
Duration: Hold for 6 sec	Progressive resistance regimen
Frequency: 5–10 repetitions daily	Lower weights, 10–15 repetitions for prepubertal child
	Frequency: Two to three times per week, alternate days
	Modify ACSM guidelines as needed for child
Precautions	
Decreased muscle blood flow	May increase biomechanical stress on unstable or malaligned joints
May increase intra-articular pressure	
May increase blood pressure	Avoid deforming forces on hand and wrist

ACSM, American College of Sports Medicine; MVC, maximum voluntary contraction; ROM, range of motion.

Adapted from Minor MA, Westby M. Rest and exercise. In: Robbins L, Burckhardt RN, Hannan MT, eds. Clinical Care in the Rheumatic Diseases. 2nd Ed. Atlanta: American College of Rheumatology, 2001:181, with permission.

contraction for about 6 seconds, exhaling during the contraction, and inhaling during the relaxation phase. EMG biofeedback may help the child isolate the muscle group and learn to regulate the intensity of the contraction. Because strength gains with isometric exercise are specific to the joint angle, isometric contractions should be performed every 15 to 20 degrees throughout the ROM. Five to 10 repetitions daily may be sufficient to maintain muscle strength in individuals with arthritis.[92]

Dynamic exercise can be initiated once the disease is under medical control and the child can move the limb against gravity for eight to 10 repetitions without pain.[92] Training should include both concentric and eccentric muscle contractions and attempt to achieve appropriate balance between agonist and antagonist muscle groups. To increase dynamic strength, external resistance can be provided by the weight of the body part, light free weights, or elastic bands. Oberg et al. reported improved quadriceps strength in children with arthritis following a 3-month program of combined land and water exercise twice a week for 40 minutes.[49] Isokinetic equipment has been used to measure muscle performance in children with JIA and may be useful for training in some children. Fisher et al. examined the effects of individualized resistance training with isokinetic equipment in six children with JRA, age 6 to 14 years, who exercised three times a week for 8 weeks. Subjects showed significant improvement in quadriceps

and hamstring strength and endurance, contraction speed, and performance of timed tasks.[79] Muscle function in control subjects with arthritis who did not exercise declined during the same time period.

As a general rule, young children or older children with musculoskeletal impairments should use lighter weights and perform two to three sets of 10 to 15 repetitions of each exercise to build strength and muscle endurance. Exercise intensity can be based on the amount of weight the child was able to move through the ROM without discomfort for six to 10 repetitions maintaining proper exercise form. Progression is determined by the child's performance at periodic reassessment. If elastic bands are used, lighter bands are used first, progressing to more resistive bands as strength increases, provided there is no joint pain or other signs of active disease. Resistance training twice a week appears to be sufficient for healthy prepubertal children to achieve gains in muscle strength.[93] However, children with arthritis may benefit from shorter exercise sessions three times a week, allowing a day or two between sessions for recovery. Training sessions should begin with a warm-up of light aerobic activity and end with cool-down activity.

The prescription should include diagrams of all exercises to be performed. A useful resource is the Quick-Fit for Kids (SPRI Products, Inc., Buffalo Grove, IL), a complete kit that includes clear, reproducible diagrams and instructions for resistive exercise. Reasonable goals should be established in collaboration with the child and parent. Goals might include increasing strength, reducing fatigue, and improving specific functional abilities, such as climbing stairs. Training in functional movement patterns increases the transfer of strength gains to everyday activities. Nontraditional exercise forms, such as Pilates, yoga, Tai Chi, and modified "kick-boxing," add variety and keep the child motivated. Periodic reassessment of the child's functional abilities, using one of the standardized assessments described earlier, provides information about the impact of training on the child's function.

AEROBIC CONDITIONING EXERCISE

A growing body of research documents the ability of children with JIA to tolerate and benefit from an aerobic training regimen. A review of these studies indicated that children with arthritis who performed moderately vigorous aerobic activity (60% to 85% of HR_{max}) for at least 30 minutes at least twice a week for at least 6 weeks improved their aerobic performance.[94] The exercise regimen in these studies varied, including stationary cycling, water aerobics, and land-based exercise. Most subjects also reported a decrease in disease signs and symptoms following the training program. Children who cannot tolerate a full 30-minute exercise session can begin with more frequent short bouts

of aerobic activity, gradually increasing the duration as their endurance improves. Recommendations for maintaining general health are to accumulate 30 minutes of moderately intense (55% to 70% of HR_{max}) aerobic activity on most days of the week.[92] The child can monitor exercise intensity by counting his or her pulse rate for 6 to 10 seconds, estimating the exercise intensity on a rating of perceived exertion (RPE) scale, or using a portable heart rate monitor.

The mode of exercise depends on the child's age, motor skill, disease status, and individual interests. Nonimpact or reduced-impact aerobic activities, such as swimming, walking, stationary cycling, or low-impact aerobic dance, are encouraged, because they utilize large muscle groups while avoiding excessive loading on the joints. However, whenever possible, weight-bearing exercises should be encouraged to maintain or improve bone density. Activities to improve proprioceptive function, postural control, and coordination can be incorporated into the exercise program. Group exercise sessions or exercising with a friend may be more fun and motivating for the child. Display 14.8 shows an example of a balanced physical conditioning program that includes exercises to improve all components of fitness, including aerobic endurance, muscular strength and endurance, flexibility, and body composition.[95]

Moderation is stressed during any physical conditioning program, because high-intensity exercise or a rapid

---

»» DISPLAY 14.8

Example of a General Physical Conditioning Regimen for Children with Arthritis

Exercise Component	Purpose	Activities	Duration
Warm-up	Increase body temperature Prepare cardiopulmonary system for increased work Increase blood flow to muscles	Gentle movements of upper and lower limbs Low-intensity aerobic activities, e.g., marching, walking, shuttles, "grapevine"	5–10 min
Muscular conditioning	Maintain/improve muscle strength and endurance Improve joint stability Improve proprioception	Submaximal isometric exercise* Dynamic exercises Weight of the body part Light hand/cuff weights Elastic bands Closed kinetic chain activities	12–15 min
Aerobic conditioning	Increase metabolic rate Maintain/improve aerobic fitness and performance Decrease fatigue with exercise Improve gross motor skills	Walking, swimming, biking Aerobic "dance" activities Modified step aerobics Active exercises on therapy ball Other exercise forms (e.g., yoga, Tai Chi, "kick-boxing" can be modified based on child's age, disease activity, and physical ability)	20–30 min; gradually ↑ time
Cool-down and stretching	Gradually lower heart rate Lengthen all muscles used during exercise program Reduce postexercise soreness	Gentle aerobic activities Active stretching	10–12 min

*Isometric exercise is recommended when the child has active arthritis with joint effusion, soft tissue swelling, and pain on motion.

progression in intensity often results in pain or injury and poor adherence. Training in proper exercise form at the beginning of the training program and frequent monitoring are essential to ensure safety and effectiveness of the exercise. Pain reports by the child should be assessed for specific cause. Discomfort from delayed-onset muscle soreness or overstretching may occur early in the program, and should resolve with time. Overuse of a joint, accompanied by swelling, heat, and pain, should be treated with cold, elevation, and rest, and appropriate modification of the program.

The PACE exercise program video, a land-based exercise program designed for adults with arthritis, is available from the Arthritis Foundation (AF). PACE classes are also offered through local YMCA and YWCA centers. The AF recently developed a water exercise program for children with arthritis. This program is not available throughout the country, but may be offered in some centers. Some commercial exercise videos are available for typically developing healthy children and these may be useful for those with JIA. However, the therapist should carefully review the entire video to determine if the activities are appropriate and safe for the child he or she is treating. Therapists can also work with the child to develop their own exercise video and to review commercial exercise videos to determine their safety and usefulness for the child with arthritis. We currently use two exercise videos developed at our center to provide a general conditioning program for children with mild to moderate arthritis.

TRAINING IN FUNCTIONAL ACTIVITIES

SELF-CARE ACTIVITIES A primary goal for the child with arthritis is to achieve independence in age-appropriate basic and instrumental ADLs in all environments. Expectations for independence in a toddler or young child will differ significantly from the skills necessary for older children or adolescents. In younger children, the emphasis may be on acquiring independence in dressing, bathing, feeding, and motor skills within the home and school. Although these skills remain important throughout life, older children become more interested in participating in sports and other social activities. For the adolescent and young adult, independence may revolve around the ability to drive, socialize with friends, and acquire a job.

The role of the therapist is to (1) assess the child's functional abilities using one of the standardized assessments described previously; (2) provide education and direct training in self-care activities, mobility, and motor skills; (3) suggest appropriate assistive devices, environmental modifications, and adaptive equipment, and train the child in their use; and (4) consult with school personnel and suggest adaptations to the child's educational program. A child with minimal joint involvement may only need advice about the most efficient method of performing tasks, whereas a child with more severe limitations may need instruction in the use of adaptive equipment or advice on environmental modifications to promote greater independence. Dressing and hygiene aids that may be useful to the child with arthritis include Velcro closures on clothing and shoes, elastic shoelaces, a dressing stick, a buttonhook, a long-handled shoehorn, and a bath brush. Built-up handles on grooming items, eating utensils, and drawing and writing implements allow the child to be independent in these activities. The child with limited neck extension may need to use a straw to drink from a glass.

Parents and children should receive instruction in the principles of joint protection to reduce pain, muscle fatigue, and potentially deforming mechanical forces on vulnerable joints during activity. The child should be encouraged to use large joints to perform tasks whenever possible, because they tolerate stress better than the small joints. For example, the child should carry large objects on the forearms instead of grasping them with the hands and use a backpack positioned close to the body's center of gravity or a rolling backpack to hold schoolbooks. Diagrams, demonstration, and practice of joint protection techniques may improve adherence.[96] Functional wrist and hand splints may decrease pain with grasping, gripping, or manipulative activities. Splints may also be useful in minimizing deforming mechanical forces during hand use.

Some simple modifications in the home may be necessary to allow a child to be independent. These include replacing traditional doorknobs and faucets with levers, using a raised toilet seat, and installing safety bars in the bathtub or shower and additional handrails in stairways. More substantial modifications may be necessary if the child must use a wheelchair for mobility within the home including widening doorways and adding a ramp or wheelchair lift at the entrance to the house. The child should also have easy and safe access to the tub, toilet, and sink in the bathroom.

FUNCTIONAL MOBILITY Continued weight bearing and walking are vitally important for the child with arthritis to increase bone density, improve muscle strength, and prevent contractures. Standing, cruising, and walking should be encouraged at the expected age. Young children should walk within the home and outside play area and for short distances in the community. Shoes should fit well and provide cushioning and support to the joints of the foot. High heels, platforms, and wedges should be discouraged because they place added stress on the ankles and joints of the feet and may also increase the risk of falling. Sneakers with a flexible sole, good arch support, and deep heel cup are often a good choice for most children. A shoe with a wide, deep toe box may be necessary for children with foot deformities such as hallux valgus, hammer toes, or claw toes. Simple additions to the shoe, such as a thin cushioning liner or a metatarsal pad, can alleviate pressure on the sole of the foot when the child stands and walks.

Custom foot orthoses are sometimes prescribed to reduce pain on weight bearing and improve gait. Careful assessment of the lower quarter, with emphasis on the foot and ankle, should be done to determine the orthotic prescription. The alignment of the lower extremity is noted for rotation, or valgus/varus deformities, and the presence of a normal longitudinal and transverse arch. Range of motion should be assessed at the ankle and subtalar joints, the midtarsals, and the toes. Examination of the sole of the foot helps to identify pressure points from weight bearing or improper alignment. The shoe should also be examined inside and outside for clues to points of pressure or gait deviations. Palpation of the foot can also locate problems such as tenosynovitis or plantar fasciitis.

The choice of an orthosis will vary, based on whether the deformities are fixed or flexible. Flexible deformities may be managed by fabricating the orthosis to hold the joint in correct anatomic alignment. For example, an orthosis with a heel cup molded out of thermoplastic material may help to correct flexible flatfoot. Fixed deformities require accommodative orthoses. For example, a patient with hallux rigidus, with loss of great toe extension, may need a metatarsal bar added to the sole of the shoe to create a mechanical means of rolling over in gait.

Most children with JIA who receive effective medical treatment are able to walk without assistive devices. However, the therapist should remain alert to potential problems that might impact the child's ability or willingness to walk. When changes in gait pattern are observed, or the child refuses to walk, the cause should be determined and addressed immediately. Leg length discrepancy, found most often in children with oligoarticular disease, should be corrected within a quarter-inch to prevent postural compensations, such as knee flexion of the longer limb, pelvic obliquity, or scoliosis. A child with pain or weakness in one leg can use a cane on the opposite side to unload the involved limb. A walker may be necessary for a child who has significant bilateral lower limb impairments. Platform attachments can be added for the child who also has limited upper limb motion, although this is rarely necessary.

Despite these efforts, some children will need to use wheeled mobility to travel long distances to preserve energy and improve function. Powered wheelchairs are generally reserved for children with severe disability. Tricycles or bicycles with training wheels are good alternatives for young children. Older children and adolescents can use a properly fitted lightweight sports wheelchair or powered scooter to move around their school, college campus, or community. The child should be encouraged to get out of the wheelchair often during the day, standing and walking as tolerated to prevent contractures and muscle weakness.

RECREATIONAL ACTIVITIES The child with arthritis should be encouraged to participate in a variety of recreational activities in the school and community. Scull and Athreya provide a useful guide for choosing activities for a child with arthritis.[97] The choice should be based on the child's preferences, age, disease status, physical and emotional

development, and motor skills. Activities suitable for most children with arthritis include music, arts and crafts, drama, and computer activities. Appropriate aerobic activities include cycling, swimming, walking, and low-impact aerobic dance. The height of the bicycle seat should be set so that the knee is at an angle of 10 to 15 degrees of flexion when the child's foot is at the apex of the downstroke.[97] Exercise in a heated pool (88° to 92°F) is recommended throughout the year, especially for children who have difficulty walking and exercising on land. Cooler pool temperatures (82° and 86°F) are more suitable for aerobic exercise.

School-age children should be encouraged to participate in physical education class whenever feasible. The therapist can provide the school with guidelines for adapting the program to meet the child's needs and minimize the potential for injury. Activities such as somersaults and headstands should be avoided to prevent injury to the cervical spine. Children with wrist and hand arthritis should avoid weight bearing on the hands.

Children with mild to moderate arthritis can participate in sports without disease exacerbation.[98] However, activities that cause high-impact loading on inflamed or damaged joints should be avoided. Sports with a high potential for collision, including football, hockey, and boxing, should be discouraged. Figure 14.15 illustrates a flow chart the physical therapist can use to determine if the child's preferred sport or recreational activity is a good "fit" for his or her physical abilities and motor skills. The physical therapist analyzes the activity to determine its collision or contact potential, the demands for aerobic and muscular work, upper and lower body ROM, and neuromuscular skill. If the child lacks the strength, ROM, flexibility, or neuromuscular control to safely play the sport, the therapist can design an exercise program to remediate the deficits and decrease the risk for injury. If the child chooses to play on a sports team, the parents and child should meet with the coach to explain the child's condition and any precautions. The coach must understand that the child's participation on any given day may need to be modified to accommodate disease symptoms and physical status. If there is no preseason conditioning program, the physical therapist can develop an individualized program for the child.

ISSUES RELATED TO SCHOOL PARTICIPATION

Arthritis does not affect cognitive function, but academic problems may occur as a result of frequent absences owing to illness or medical appointments, or decreased attention because of pain, stiffness, and fatigue in school.[99,100] Problems related to school can be assessed by administering the SFA or using a simple school checklist, such as the one shown in Appendix 1. The child indicates problems related to his or her ability to perform necessary tasks in school, the impact of stiffness or pain on various activities,

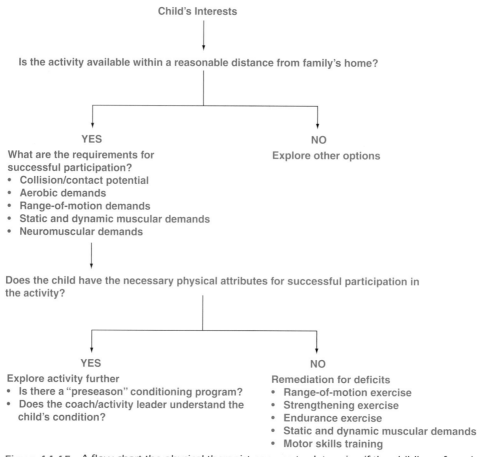

Figure 14.15 ▪ A flow chart the physical therapist can use to determine if the child's preferred sport or recreational activity is a good "fit" for his or her physical abilities and motor skills.

mobility within the school and grounds, and the ability to tolerate the school day.

The therapist can provide information to teachers and other school personnel about specific ways in which arthritis affects the child's school performance, and can suggest possible adaptations to the educational program. Adaptations might include providing a second set of books for home, adapted writing tools or alternatives to writing such as a word processor or tape recorder, or an easel-top desk for a child with cervical spine involvement. Modifications in the schedule may be necessary to allow the child to participate in his or her educational program. These might include time out of the classroom to take medications or rest for brief periods during the day, grouping classes in one area of the building to limit travel time, and allowing the child to stand and move periodically to prevent stiffness from long periods of sitting. Children with lower extremity pain or limitations may need to use the elevators. As mentioned previously, the child should participate in physical education with classmates, even when the program must be modified to accommodate the child's abilities and limitations.

Some schools provide these services and modifications voluntarily, but a formal evaluation by the school and devel-

opment of an IEP may be necessary. Children with arthritis may qualify for related services under the Individuals with Disability Act (IDEA) or under Section 504 of the Vocational Rehabilitation Act. Educational and vocational counseling is often beneficial for adolescents with arthritis to prepare for the transition to postsecondary education or work. Although IDEA requires transition planning for children receiving services to begin at age 16 years, Lovell et al. found that only 8% of children with arthritis received vocational counseling.[29] It is therefore important for parents to advocate for their child in the school system. The manual *Educational Rights for Children with Arthritis* is available from the American Juvenile Arthritis Organization (AJAO) and may be helpful for parents.[101] However, because this manual has not been updated to reflect current changes in IDEA, the reader should refer to Chapter 19 for a thorough discussion of related services in the public schools.

PATIENT AND FAMILY EDUCATION AND SUPPORT

Successful management of the physical problems and prevention of disability in the child with JIA depends to a great extent on adherence to the medical and therapeutic regimen. However, the demands placed on the family can be overwhelming. Active participation in managing the child's health care may be enhanced when the parent and child fully understand the effects of the disease on the body and the benefits of medication, exercise, and other therapeutic procedures. Older children who participate in setting goals and making decisions about their care feel a greater sense of self-efficacy. Physical therapists also play an important role in helping the child and family plan the inevitable transition to adult life and health care.

The therapist should explain to the child and parents how improvements in body structure and function will improve the child's ability to perform necessary and

desired activities and positively affect overall quality of life. Educational materials should be appropriate to the child's level of cognitive development and emotional maturity. Several excellent pamphlets, videos, and books are available for this purpose from the AJAO and the AF. Display 14.9 shows useful resources for children with arthritis, their families, and health professionals who care for them. Home exercise programs should be individualized to target the child's needs and limited to no more than seven simple exercises, requiring 20 to 30 minutes. The book *Raising a Child with Arthritis: A Parent's Guide*, a publication of the AF, provides an illustrated program of ROM and postural exercises.[102] Therapists should demonstrate the exercises to

---

»» DISPLAY 14.9

Resources for Children with Arthritis, Their Families, and Arthritis Health Professionals

Organizations

Arthritis Foundation (AF)

1330 West Peachtree Street

Atlanta, GA 30309

1-800-238-7800

www.arthritis.org

American Juvenile Arthritis Organization (AJAO)

This organization is a council of the AF formed to serve the needs of children with rheumatic disease and their families.

www.arthritis.org or contact local AF chapter

American College of Rheumatology (ACR)

The ACR provides a wealth of educational resources to physicians and other health professionals caring for people with arthritis. Examples include the core curriculum in rheumatology, slide collection, and online case studies. The annual meeting brings together international researchers, educators, and clinicians with the purpose of sharing new and ongoing information related to the care of patients with rheumatic diseases. The three main components of the ACR that would be of interest to physical therapists are the Rehabilitation Section, Pediatric Section, and the Association of Rheumatology Health Professionals.

www.rheumatology.org

Association of Rheumatology Health Professionals (ARHP)

This multidisciplinary organization, a section of the ACR, provides education and resources to all health professionals who care for individuals with rheumatic disease. Educational products and programs include the slide collection, online rehabilitation case studies, phone conferences on current topics and issues in rheumatology practice, position papers on the role of different health professions in rheumatology, and the text *Clinical Care in the Rheumatic Diseases*. ARHP holds its annual meeting in conjunction with the ACR.

www.rheumatology.org

American Academy of Pediatrics (APA)

The Rheumatology Section of the APA works in coordination with the Pediatrics Section of the ACR and presents periodic conferences dedicated to the management of rheumatic diseases in children.

141 North Point Blvd.

Ellagrove Village, IL 60007

1-800-433-9016

www.aap.org

Camps

Several state AF chapters sponsor summer residential camps for children with arthritis or other rheumatic diseases. Contact your local AF chapter for information.

Exercise Programs and Videos

People with Arthritis Can Exercise (PACE) and Aquatic Exercise Program

PACE is an exercise program developed by the AF for adults with arthritis and is suitable for teens and young adults with juvenile idiopathic arthritis. The Aquatic Program is a warm-water exercise program for adults with arthritis or other rheumatic diseases. Local YMCA and YWCA centers often offer one or both programs. The AF also offers the videos of the PACE program for home use. Contact the local AF chapter.

www.arthritis.org

Water Exercise Programs for Children

The National AF, in conjunction with the national office of the YMCA, developed a recreational water exercise program for children with arthritis. This program or others similar in format are offered in some local YMCA and YWCA centers. Contact the local AF chapter or YMCA/YWCA.

(continued)

the child and parent, periodically reassess the child's performance and progress, and make any necessary changes in the program. With young children, it is best to incorporate the exercises into daily activities, such as bathing, dressing, or play. Positive reinforcement with stickers, small prizes, or special outings can be used to encourage a young child to cooperate in the exercise program. Older children and teens might benefit from a contract, listing their personal goals, the necessary medication and exercise regimen, and the reward or incentive for adherence to the therapeutic program.

SUMMARY

This chapter presents information on the heterogeneous disorders that are included under the umbrella term juvenile idiopathic arthritis. These conditions are classified based on signs and symptoms during the first 6 months after disease on-set, although the exact diagnosis may not be clear for some time. The categories include systemic, RF–polyarticular, RF+ polyarticular, oligoarticular—persistent, oligoarticular—extended, enthesitis-related arthritis, psoriatic arthritis, and "other" arthritis. The etiology and pathogenesis of JIA is not completely understood, but research continues to make strides in this area. Most children with JIA do well with early diagnosis and appropriate medical treatment to manage the inflammatory process. However, some children with severe and persistent disease experience significant impairments, including joint pain and swelling, limited ROM, and muscle atrophy and weakness. Secondary impairments in aerobic function and exercise tolerance are common. JIA may also negatively affect the child's ability to perform basic and instrumental ADLs and participate fully in home, school, and community settings. The long-term prognosis depends on the child's age at disease onset, disease type and course, and the quality and consistency of health care services. The goal of management is for the child and family to lead as normal a life as possible. An interdisciplinary team of professionals is necessary to meet the complex needs of the child with JIA. A total program of care should include medical and occasionally surgical management, patient and family education, psychosocial support, and physical and occupational therapy.

CASE STUDY

SARA

Sara is a 13-year old girl with polyarticular JIA of 8 years' duration. After several years of mild disease activity, Sara presents with increased swelling in multiple joints, most notably both knees and the right ankle. She complains of pain and morning stiffness lasting 30 to 60 minutes and neck pain during the day.

Medical History

Sara's arthritis was diagnosed with SoJIA at 5 years of age. Her parents stated that other signs of the disease, including stiffness and irritability upon awakening, "bumps" on her elbows and shins, and altered gait pattern, were evident for at least a year before the diagnosis. At her first visit to the pediatric rheumatologist, she had active disease (obvious swelling or tenderness to palpation, LOM, and pain on motion) in most extremity joints and the cervical spine. Nodules were found on the extensor surface of the ulna and tibial crest bilaterally. She was originally treated with naproxen; however, methotrexate (MTX) given orally once a week was added after 6 months, in which she continued to have active polyarticular disease. Signs of systemic disease were not evident at this time.

Sara's medication regimen remained the same in the intervening years, with the dosage being adjusted based on her weight. She continued to have active disease, and approximately 3 years ago she received seven intra-articular corticosteroid injections (both knees, hips, shoulders, right ankle) to treat the inflammation that was uncontrolled by her systemic medications. Joint swelling and pain decreased dramatically, and Sara was able to walk without pain and participate in most physical activities at school.

Current Complaints

Sara is seen in clinic today to review her medications and home exercise program. Sara takes her MTX each week but often forgets to take the naproxen, missing at least 30% of the prescribed dose each week. She also admits to poor adherence to the HEP, stating that it is boring and takes too long, and she does not see any benefits. According to Sara's mother, she has missed school or been late at least once a week for several months due to disease symptoms. Sara states that she is not able to fulfill her physical education or sports requirement because of her arthritis. At the current time, Sara receives some related services and accommodations to her educational program under an informal agreement with the school system. These include individual "pull-out" physical therapy and occupational therapy sessions once a week, lockers at either end of the school, a second set of books at home, permission to use a laptop computer for class notes, extra time for written exams, and excuse from physical education class when she is unable to participate. Due to her medical problems, Sara is also not bound by the school district's strict attendance policy.

The rheumatologist confirmed that Sara has active arthritis in both of her wrists, knees, and right ankle. Active and passive ROM is limited in the cervical spine, wrists, hips, right knee, and ankle; she has deformities of the toes in both feet. The rheumatologist changed Sara's medication to Enbrel injections once a week and continued the naproxen b.i.d. Intra-articular steroid injections were scheduled for her next visit in 1 week. Sara was referred to physical therapy for an evaluation and review of her HEP and to occupational therapy for revision of her wrist splints and suggestions for adaptive equipment to improve her hand function. An appointment was also made with the child life specialist to help Sara become independent in managing her health care needs.

Physical Therapist Examination
GUIDING QUESTIONS

1. Does Sara currently exhibit activity limitations that negatively impact her participation in home, school, and community settings?
2. Are there impairments in any of the body systems that might negatively impact Sara's ability to perform necessary and desired activities?

ACTIVITY AND PARTICIPATION FINDINGS

To answer the first question, Sara completed the CHAQ and the JAQQ. Her CHAQ DI is 1.50, suggesting moderate disability. Using the 100-mm VAS, Sara scored her pain during the previous week as 60 mm and overall health status as 70 mm. Her total JAQQ score was 5. Using the categoric scale, Sara indicated she was "much worse" than at her last clinic visit. The table below shows the individual category scores and the five highest scoring items in each category.

Category	Score	Item
Gross Motor	5	1. Rising from the floor/getting from standing to sitting on the floor 2. Walking up and down stairs 3. Walking longer than 15 minutes 4. Running 5. Participating in sports
Fine Motor	4	1. Writing 2. Brushing her hair 3. Tying shoe laces 4. Fastening shirt or coat buttons 5. Using eating materials
Psychological	5	1. Interacting poorly with siblings 2. Argued a lot 3. Felt frustrated 4. Felt sad 5. Missed school a lot
Systemic Symptoms	6	1. Poor appetite 2. Stomach pains 3. Difficulty sleeping 4. Joint pain 5. Headaches

Sara's gross motor (GM) skills were examined using three subtests of the BOT GM composite: running speed and agility (RSA), balance (B), and bilateral coordination (BC). The mean and standard deviation (SD) for the normative sample on the BOTMP subtests are 15 and 5, respectively. Sara's scores are shown in the table below.

Gross Motor Subtest	Point Score	Age-Based Standard Score	Compared to Normative Values
Running Speed and Agility	8	7	1.5 SD < mean
Balance	21	6	1.5 SD < mean
Bilateral Coordination	9	5	2 SD < mean

BODY STRUCTURES AND FUNCTION FINDINGS

To answer question two, the physical therapist performed a systems review.

1. Signs of active joint disease
   - Joint effusions, with loss of joint contours, were present in both wrists and knees and the right ankle; swelling was also noted around the Achilles tendon on the right.
   - Complaints of tenderness to palpation and mild withdrawal of the limb were noted at these same joints and at the Achilles tendon on the right.
   - Stress pain was noted at end PROM of the knees, shoulders, wrists, and right ankle.
2. ROM, flexibility, and joint alignment: All joints showed full PROM within normal limits (WNL) with these exceptions:
   - Cervical spine rotation and lateral flexion to either side was limited by 50%.
   - Right shoulder flexion lacked 20 degrees.
   - Elbow extension was limited by 20 degrees (R), 30 degrees (L).
   - Wrist dorsiflexion lacked 25 degrees (0 to 45 degrees) (R), 15 degrees (0 to 55 degrees) (L).
     - Holds right hand in wrist ulnar deviation and MCP and PIP flexion, although alignment can be corrected with passive motion.
   - Pelvis was in anterior tilted position; lumbar spine was positioned in excessive lordosis.
   - Hip extension (modified Thomas test) lacked 10 degrees 0 (R) and (L).
   - There were short TFL (R).
   - Knee extension, measured in supine, lacked 10 degrees (R), 5 degrees (L)
     - Hamstring length test shows −45 degrees (R), −35 degrees (L).
     - Sara's score on the Prudential FitnessGram (PF) Sit & Reach Test was 8 inches, below the health fitness standard (HFS) for her age and gender.

- Feet and ankles
  - Right ankle plantar flexion is 0 to 30 degrees.
  - Right ankle dorsiflexion with the knee flexed is 0 to 5 degrees.
  - Right gastrocnemius: ankle dorsiflexion is limited to neutral with knee extended.
  - Hindfoot eversion is 0 degrees (R) and (L); inversion is WNL.
  - Pes cavus (R) and (L).
3. Muscle strength
   - MMT showed gross strength of lower limb muscle groups to be 4/5; upper limb strength was 3+/5.
   - Plantar flexor muscle endurance was low: Sara was able to perform only eight bilateral heel rises before fatigue.
   - Grip strength measured with a modified blood pressure cuff was 60/20 mm Hg (R) and 80/20 mm Hg (L). According to Smythe and Helewa, a rise of 20 mm Hg from the baseline of 20 mm Hg is equal to approximately 5 lb of force; Sara's grip strength, measured in pounds, was 10 lb (R) and 15 lb (L), considerably below the reported range of values for healthy children (33 to 98 lb [R], 22 to 107 lb [L])[103].
   - Abdominal strength and endurance: Sara's score of 8 on the PF curl-up test was below the age- and gender-based minimum criterion-referenced health fitness standard (HFS) of 18.
   - Upper body strength and endurance: Sara's score of 1 on the modified pull-up test was below the minimum HFS of 4.
4. Aerobic performance/exercise tolerance
   - Sara's score on the PF maximum run walk test (MRWT) was 16 minutes, longer than the HFS of 11.5.
   - Sara rated her worst fatigue during the previous week as 50 on a 100-mm VAS.
5. Body composition
   - Sara's body mass index (BMI) of 23 was within the normal range for her age and gender.
   - Sara's skinfold thickness (sum of calf and triceps) was 30 mm, within the range of the HFS, but at the higher end for her age and gender.
6. Gait pattern: Shoe print analysis with video
   - Decreased velocity: 45 m/min
   - Shortened step length, right versus left leg
   - Majority of weight borne on lateral side of foot throughout stance phase
   - Lack of push-off at terminal stance: decreased active ankle plantar flexion ROM and decreased hip extension

Evaluation and Diagnosis
GUIDING QUESTIONS

1. Which of Sara's current impairments contribute to her activity limitations and participation restrictions?
2. Which impairments must be addressed to prevent or minimize secondary problems?

3. What strengths and resources might help Sara improve her health status and quality of life?

Column one in the table below lists Sara's current activity and participation problems, based on information from the CHAQ and JAQQ. The impairments believed to contribute to each problem are shown in column two.

Participation Restriction	Activity Limitation	Impairment
• Poor school attendance • Unable to participate in physical education and sports	• Walks slowly • Difficulty making transitions between sitting on floor and standing • Difficulty negotiating steps • Difficulty with reach, grasp, and manipulation activities • Difficulty performing physical activity in gym and recreational sports	• Active arthritis • ↓ ROM; ↓ soft tissue extensibility • Muscle weakness • ↓ exercise tolerance • Gait deviations • Pain and fatigue during physical activity • Poor postural control • Poor coordination

- Active arthritis contributes to pain, tenderness, and limited active and passive ROM.
- Limited joint motion and soft tissue shortening contribute to impaired movement patterns and pain during upper and lower limbs activity.
- Poor muscular performance (weakness, poor muscle endurance, poor power) contributes to Sara's difficulty with gross motor activities.
- Both impaired joint mobility and muscle performance contribute to gait deviations.
- Inadequate proprioceptive function may contribute to poor muscular control and postural stability during physical activity.
- Poor adherence to the prescribed medication schedule and HEP and Sara's lack of involvement in her health care contribute to poor disease control and functional outcome.

STRENGTHS AND RESOURCES
Although Sara's adherence to her medical and therapeutic regimen has previously been inadequate, she now appears to be more interested in managing her disease and improving her health status and functional capacity. Her parents are also involved in her health care, and the school appears to be willing to accommodate her needs by making requested modifications to her educational program.

Prognosis
GUIDING QUESTIONS

1. What would improve Sara's active participation in her health care?

2. What is the best plan of care for Sara at this time, with regard to medications and rehabilitation?

Question 1: The rheumatology team believed that some of Sara's current problems were due to inadequate disease control and lack of proper exercise, and they thought adherence might improve if she were involved in setting goals and making decisions regarding her care. Sara stated that she wanted to be like other kids her age and do the same activities. She wanted to participate in physical education and some sports with her family and friends. She is concerned about attending high school next year, transferring between classes in a larger school and keeping up with the work and activities of high school. The child life specialist explained how Sara might achieve these goals if her disease was brought under better control by regular use of medication, and her general physical status was improved through daily exercise.

Question 2: Based on the evidence from the literature, the team believed that Sara's arthritis and functional status would improve following intra-articular injections, a change in her medication to Enbrel, and improved adherence to the nonsteroidal anti-inflammatory drug (NSAID) regimen. Sara agreed to a 3-month contract, listing her functional goals, therapy objectives, and a plan of activities aimed at achieving the goals. An evaluation of her progress was set for the next clinic visit. The contract included following her full medical regimen, performing home ROM and strengthening exercises, and participating in an aerobic training program designed by the physical therapist. She also agreed to wear her night resting splints. Sara and her parents agreed to a 3-month trial of direct physical therapy and occupational therapy twice a week, with the goal of improving ROM and strength. The parents also signed permission for the clinic physical therapist to consult with the school physical education instructor to discuss activities that would be suitable for Sara.

Expected Outcomes (Goals to Be Achieved in 3 Months)

- Improved adherence to medication regimen should result in improved disease control and reduction in pain due to joint inflammation.
  - Goal: Sara will show at least a 75% improvement in adherence to her medication schedule based on a daily log, with entries verified by one parent.
  - Goal: At her 3-month follow-up visit, Sara's self-reported overall health status will show improvement based on a reduced score on the CHAQ VAS.
- Sara's gait pattern will improve following injections of the knees and ankles and supportive physical therapy.
  - Goal: Sara will demonstrate improvements in gait variables, including increased gait velocity and step length.
  - Goal: Sara will demonstrate a more normal weight-bearing pattern during walking, based on footprint analysis.
- Based on the evidence from studies examining the effects of exercise regimen in children with JIA, it is expected that

Sara can achieve (1) improved aerobic fitness if she performs moderate to vigorous aerobic activity at least twice a week for at least 30 minutes, (2) increased muscle strength and endurance if she performs resistance exercise three times a week, and (3) increased independence in self-care and other instrumental activities of daily living.

- Goal: Sara's time to complete the MRWT will meet the minimum HFS for her age and gender.
- Goal: Sara will demonstrate improved scores on the PF curl-up and modified pull-up tests, meeting the minimum HFS for her age and gender.
- Goal: Sara will demonstrate improved ability to perform all self-care and other instrumental ADLs, based on reduced scores on the CHAQ and JAQQ.
- Improved muscle performance and exercise tolerance should result in decreased fatigue following physical activity.
  - Goal: Sara will demonstrate decreased fatigue with physical activity based on self-report using a 100-mm VAS where higher values equal greater fatigue.
- Daily ROM and flexibility exercises should improve joint ROM and soft tissue extensibility, resulting in decreased stiffness and pain.
  - Goal: Sara will demonstrate improved passive joint ROM based on goniometric measurement of the shoulders, hips, knees, and ankles.
- Improved physical status should allow Sara to increase her participation in physical activities with her family and friends.
  - Goal: Sara will demonstrate improved scores on the running speed and agility, balance, and bilateral coordination subtests of the BOTMP.
  - Goal: Sara will actively participate in at least 75% of all physical education activities each week, with or without modifications to the activity.
  - Goal: Sara will participate in at least one recreational physical activity with her family or friends each week for at least 1 hour.

Intervention Plan

Following intra-articular injections to both knees, the right wrist, and the right ankle, Sara was on bedrest and non–weight bearing for 1 day. After 1 week of modified physical activity, she resumed all typical activities.

Coordination, Communication, and Documentation

The rheumatology team worked with Sara and her parents to determine techniques that would improve her adherence to the treatment plan. The nurse provided instruction to Sara and her parents to ensure correct administration of the weekly injections of etanercept and reasons for following the exact prescription for taking the NSAID. The physical therapist provided written and oral instructions, demonstration, and illustrations of the exercises in the HEP. The occupational therapist made new resting wrist splints for Sara and provided assistive devices to improve her ability to perform ADLs. The child life specialist helped Sara establish a sched-

ule for taking her medications and develop a daily diary to keep a written record of her medications, HEP, and use of her splints. Each section of the diary included space for Sara's comments. She was also encouraged to contact the team with any questions about her program or change in symptoms. The team provided, with permission of Sara and her parents, a copy of the physical therapy and occupation therapy evaluations to the school and made a request that therapy services be provided as part of Sara's educational program. The team also requested that the physical education instructor consult with the physical therapist to adjust activities so that Sara could increase her participation.

Patient Education

The clinic physical therapist discussed the findings of the physical examination with Sara and her parents. She discussed the impact of chronic inflammatory arthritis on the joints and muscles, the potential sources of pain and stiffness, and the secondary problems that often occur, including poor exercise tolerance and impaired motor skills. She explained that Sara's current functional problems were likely related to limited joint mobility and soft tissue extensibility, poor muscle performance, movement impairments, and pain. She explained that intervention would be directed toward reducing these impairments. The therapy program would also include specific practice of the activities and motor skills that were difficult for Sara.

Procedural Interventions

- Direct treatment sessions, 30 minutes twice a week
- Instruction in HEP

INTERVENTIONS FOR IMPAIRED JOINT MOBILITY AND MUSCLE FUNCTION

Direct therapy: Initial instruction in maintaining control of the trunk and lumbar spine by engaging abdominal muscles during all activities

1. Active-assisted ROM (AAROM) to shoulder flexion, abduction in scapular plane, medial and lateral rotation, with attention to scapular position, movement, and scapulohumeral rhythm
2. Prone scapular progression exercises; progress to standing scapular exercises against a wall; progress to using light handheld weights when Sara can perform exercises without pain or compensatory movements
3. AAROM and active ROM (AROM) for serratus anterior; progress to resistance exercise
4. Instruction in isometric exercise to improve neck stability
5. Stretching of shortened latissimus dorsi, lateral shoulder rotators and posterior capsule, hip flexors, hamstrings, right gastrocnemius using autogenic and reciprocal inhibition
6. Stretching of right TFL
7. Strength training for hip extensors, deep external rotators, and abductors
   - Begin with AROM to teach correct technique for each muscle group

- Progress to graded resistance exercise using light weights or elastic bands
- Closed kinetic chain (CKC) exercise, including graded squats, lunges, and "step" training to improve strength, endurance, and control of lower extremity musculature

8. Gait training to improve lower extremity weight bearing, weight transfer, and step and stride length

INTERVENTIONS TO ADDRESS IMPAIRED MOTOR SKILLS

1. Once joint mobility, AROM, and strength improve and pain during movement decreases, proprioceptive training and activities to improve postural control, agility, and coordination during movement will be added to the therapy program.
2. Gait training will be included to increase walking velocity, using timed walks.
3. Activity- or sport-specific training will be included to ensure Sara's safe participation in physical therapy activities and her chosen sport, basketball.

HOME EXERCISE PROGRAM

1. AROM exercises concentrating on cervical spine, shoulders, wrists, hips, knees, and ankles using illustrations from the Arthritis Foundation book *Raising a Child with Arthritis*
2. Aerobic training program to include daily physical activity (walking, bike riding, swimming, aerobic dance, etc.); Sara will gradually increase duration to at least 30 minutes a day and intensity to at least 75% of her age-based HR_{max}

RECOMMENDATIONS/REFERRALS

1. Refer to podiatrist for custom insoles to accommodate pes cavus deformity; metatarsal bar to allow better roll-off at terminal stance.
2. Recommend semi-rigid cervical collar when riding in school bus and car.
3. Recommend using easel top for desk to decrease neck strain when reading.

Re-examination

Sara was seen by the physical therapist at her regular rheumatology visit, 3 months after the initial examination. She reported that she now receives physical therapy twice a week at school before classes begin and occupational therapy once a week during school time. Sara's mother reported that Sara now has an IEP that specifies the provision of physical therapy and occupational therapy as well as the previously mentioned accommodations to her educational program. She also now attends all physical education classes each week and is able to participate in approximately 50% of the activities with some modifications. The school physical therapist and the physical education instructor are working together to improve Sara's gross motor skills and adapt difficult activities to allow her to participate with her classmates.

FINDINGS OF RE-EXAMINATION

1. Signs of active joint disease
   - Mild swelling was noted in the right knee.
   - Sara denied tenderness to palpation of any joints.

- Sara complained of stress pain at end of PROM of the right shoulder.
2. ROM, flexibility, and joint alignment
   - Cervical spine lateral flexion and rotation to either side continued to be limited by 50%, although Sara denied pain with any motion.
   - PROM of the right shoulder shows slight improvement: flexion was 0 to 170 degrees; medial rotation was 0 to 40 degrees.
   - Wrist dorsiflexion was 0 to 60 degrees (R), 0 to 65 degrees (L).
   - Passive hip extension limitation was 5 degrees.
   - Passive knee extension was full.
   - Right ankle plantar flexion was improved at 0 to 40 degrees.
   - Right ankle dorsiflexion with knee extended was 0 to 5 degrees.
   - Passive calcaneal eversion was increased to 5 degrees.
3. Standing posture
   - Sara continued to stand with an increased anterior pelvic tilt and lumbar lordosis, although she could correct this upon request by engaging her abdominal muscles.
   - Barefoot, Sara continued to stand with most of her weight over the lateral border of her foot; when wearing her custom-made in-shoe orthoses and sneakers, her weight was borne more evenly over the plantar surface of the foot.
4. Muscle strength and aerobic fitness
   - Sara performed bilateral heel rises 15 times before fatigue, and eight to 10 unilateral heel rises without external support.
   - Grip strength, measured with the modified blood pressure cuff, was 100/20 (20 lb) (R) and 140/20 (30 lb) (L).
   - By report of the school physical education instructor, Sara's scores of 12 on the curl-up test, 5 on the modified pull-up test, and 13 minutes on the MRWT were still below the minimum HFS for her age and gender, but improved since her initial examination.
5. Body composition
   - BMI and skinfold thickness measurements were unchanged at 23 and 30, respectively.
6. Gait variables using footprint analysis, video, and stopwatch
   - Gait velocity increased to 60 m/min.
   - Wearing sneakers and in-shoe orthoses, Sara demonstrated improved heel strike, weight more evenly distributed over the plantar surface of the foot during midstance, improved push-off on the medial side of the forefoot and hip extension at terminal stance, and increased step length.
7. Gross motor skills: Sara's point scores on the BOTMP GM subtests improved
   - Running Speed and Agility improved from 8 to 10.
   - Balance improved from 21 to 24.
   - Bilateral Coordination improved from 9 to 11.

Outcomes

1. A review of Sara's medication and activity diary indicated improved adherence to her medication regimen and HEP program; this conclusion was supported by Sara's parents as well as decreased signs of active arthritis and improved ROM in most joints.
2. Sara's gait pattern and gait velocity improved.
3. Sara's performance on tests of muscle strength showed progress toward the goal of meeting minimum HFS for her age and gender.
4. Activity and participation
   - Sara met her goal of improved performance on the BOTMP GM subtests.
   - Her total CHAQ DI was 1.00, a clinically meaningful improvement over her initial score of 1.50.
   - Her total JAQQ score was 3: GM, 4; FM, 2; Psychological, 3; and Systemic Symptoms, 3.
   - Sara's score of 40 on the 100-mm VAS for pain showed an improvement over her initial pain rating of 60 mm.
   - She rated her overall health status as improved with a score of 30 on the 100-mm VAS from the initial rating of 70 mm; using the ordinal scale on the JAQQ, she rated her condition as "better."
   - She rated her worst fatigue during the previous week as 20 on the 100-mm VAS, an improvement from the initial rating of 50 mm.

Plan

Based on Sara's decreased disease activity and improved physical status, the physical therapist recommended continuing with direct physical therapy in school with an emphasis on increasing aerobic fitness, lower limb and trunk strength and proprioception, and overall flexibility. She also recommended that the physical therapist and physical education instructor work together with Sara on specific training for basketball to allow her to participate in an intramural league at school. Re-evaluation of her program and functional status was scheduled for her next regular rheumatology appointment in 3 months.

REFERENCES

1. Cassidy JT, Petty RE. Textbook of Pediatric Rheumatology. 4th Ed. Philadelphia: W. B. Saunders, 2001.
2. Melvin J, Wright FV, eds. Rheumatologic Reha-bilitation: Pediatric Rheumatic Diseases, vol 3. Bethesda, MD: American Occupational Therapy Association, 2000.
3. Cassidy JT, Levinson JE, Bass JC, et al. A study of classification criteria for a diagnosis of juvenile rheumatoid arthritis. Arthritis Rheum 1986;29:274–281.
4. Sailer M, Cabral D, Petty RE, et al. Rheumatoid factor positive oligoarticular onset juvenile rheumatoid arthritis. J Rheumatol 1997;24:586–588.
5. Southwood TR. Psoriatic arthritis. In: Cassidy JT, Petty RE, eds. Textbook of Pediatric Rheumatology. Philadelphia: E. B. Saunders, 2001.
6. Manners PJ, Bower C. Worldwide prevalence of uvenile arthritis—why does it vary so much? J Rheumatol 2002;29:1520–1530.
7. Oen K, Cheang M. Epidemiology of chronic arthritis in childhood. Semin Arthritis Rheum 1996;26:575–591.
8. Burgos-Vargos R, Petty RE. Juvenile ankylosing spondylitis. Rheum Dis Clin North Am 1992;18:123–142.
9. Southwood TR, Petty RE, Malleson PN, et al. Psoriatic arthritis in children. Arthritis Rheum 1989;32:1007.
10. Hochberg MC, Linet MS, Sills EM. The prevalence and incidence of juvenile rheumatoid arthritis in an urban black population. Am J Public Health 1983;73:1202–1203.
11. Sullivan DB, Cassidy JT, Petty RE. Pathogenic implications of age onset in juvenile rheumatoid arthritis. Arthritis Rheum 1975;18:251–255.
12. Clemans LE, Albert E, Ansell BM. Sibling pairs affected by chronic arthritis of childhood: evidence for a genetic predisposition. J Rheumatol 1985;12:108–113.
13. Murray KJ, Moroldo MB, Donnelly P, et al. Age-specific effects of juvenile rheumatoid arthritis-associated HLA alleles. Arthritis Rheum 1999;42:1843–1853.
14. Henderson C, Lovell D. Assessment of protein-energy malnutrition in children and adolescents with juvenile rheumatoid arthritis. Arthritis Care Res 1989;2(4):108–113.
15. Kotaniemi A, Savolainen A, Kroger H, et al. Weight-bearing physical activity, calcium intake, systemic glucocorticoids, chronic inflammation, and body constitution as determinants of lumbar and femoral bone mineral in juvenile chronic arthritis. Scand J Rheumatol 1999;28:19–26.
16. Petty RE, Cassidy JT. Juvenile ankylosing spondylitis. In: Cassidy JT, Petty RE, eds. Textbook of Pediatric Rheumatology. Philadelphia: W. B. Saunders, 2001.
17. Giannini EH, Lovell DJ, Ilowite NT, et al. Safety outcomes from a phase IV pediatric registry: etanercept therapy in children and adolescents with juvenile rheumatoid arthritis (JRA). Arthritis Rheum 2004;47:S90.
18. Cassidy JT, Petty RE. Juvenile rheumatoid arthritis. In: Cassidy JT, Petty RE, eds. Textbook of Pediatric Rheumatology. Philadelphia: W. B. Saunders, 2001.
19. Sherry DD, Stein LD, Reed AM, et al. Prevention of leg length discrepancy in young children with pauciarticular juvenile rheumatoid arthritis by treatment with intra-articular steroids. Arthritis Rheum 1999;42:2330–2334.
20. Brostrom E, Hagelberg S, Haglund-Akerlind Y. Effect of joint injections in children with juvenile idiopathic arthritis: evaluation of 3-D gait analysis. Acta Paediatr 2004;93:906–910.
21. Oen K, Malleson PN, Cabral DA, et al. Disease course and outcome of juvenile rheumatoid arthritis in a multicenter cohort. J Rheumatol 2002;29:1989–1999.
22. Burgos-Vargas R, Clark J. Axial involvement in the seronegative enthesopathy and arthropathy syndrome and its progression to ankylosing spondylitis. J Rheumatol 1989;16:192.
23. Ruperto N, Ravelli A, Migliavacca D, et al. Responsiveness of clinical measures in children with oligoarticular juvenile chronic arthritis. J Rheumatol 1999;26:1827–1830.
24. Arkela-Kautiainen M, Haapassari J, Kautiainen H, et al. Health-related quality of life of patients with JIA in early childhood. Arthritis Rheum 1996;40:2235–2290.
25. Petersen LS, Mason T, Nelson AM, et al. Psychosocial outcomes and health status of adults who have had juvenile rheumatoid arthritis. Arthritis Rheum 1996;40:2235–2290.
26. Giannini EH, Ruperto EH, Ruperto N, et al. Preliminary definition of improvement in juvenile arthritis. Arthritis Rheum 1997;40:1202–1209.
27. Brunner HI, Lovell DJ, Finck BK, et al. Preliminary definition of disease flare in juvenile rheumatoid arthritis. J Rheumatol 2001;29:1058–1064.
28. Morrison CD, Bundy RC, Fisher AG. The contribution of motor skills and playfulness to the play performance of preschoolers. Am J Occup Ther 1991;45:687–694.
29. Lovell DJ, Athreya B, Emery HM, et al. School attendance and patterns, special needs in pediatric patients with rheumatic disease. Arthritis Care Res 1990;3:196–203.

30. Lineker SC, Badley EM, Dalby DM. Unmet service needs of children with rheumatic diseases and their parents in a metropolitan area. J Rheumatol 1996;23:1054–1058.

31. Klepper SE. Measures of pediatric function. Arthritis Care Res 2003;49:S5–S14.

32. Degotardi P. Pediatric measures of quality of life. Arthritis Care Res 2003;S105–S112.

33. Singh G, Athreya B, Fries J, et al. Measurement of health status in juvenile rheumatoid arthritis. Arthritis Rheum 1994;37:1761–1769.

34. Dempster H, Porepa M, Young N, et al. The clinical meaning of functional outcome scores in children with juvenile arthritis. Arthritis Rheum 2001;44:1768–1774.

35. Lam C, Young N, Marwaha J, et al. Revised versions of the Childhood Health Assessment Questionnaire (CHAQ) are more sensitive and suffer less from a ceiling effect. Arthritis Care Res 2004;51:881–889.

36. Duffy CM, Arsenault HL, Duffy KN, et al. The Juvenile Arthritis Quality of Life Questionnaire–development of a new responsive index for juvenile rheumatoid arthritis and juvenile spondyloarthritides. J Rheumatol 1997;24:738–746.

37. Varni J, Seid M, Smith Knight T, et al. The PedsQL in pediatric rheumatology: reliability, validity, and responsiveness of the Pediatric Quality of Life Inventory generic core scales and rheumatology module. Arthritis Rheum 2002;46:714–725.

38. Wright FV, Longo Kimber JL, Law M, et al. The Juvenile Arthritis Functional Status Index (JASI): a validation study. J Rheumatol 1996;23:1066–1079.

39. Lovell DJ, Howe S, Shear E, et al. Development of a disability measurement tool for juvenile rheumatoid arthritis: the Juvenile Arthritis Functional Assessment Scale. Arthritis Rheum 1989;32:1390–1395.

40. Coster W, Deeney T, Haltiwanger J, et al. School Function Assessment. Boston: Harcourt Brace & Co, 1998.

41. Smythe H, Helewa A. Assessment of joint disease. In: Walker J, Helewa A, eds. Physical Therapy in Arthritis. Philadelphia: W. B. Saunders, 1996.

42. Spencer CH, Berstein BH. Hip disease in juvenile rheumatoid arthritis. Curr Opin Rheumatol 2002;4:536–541.

43. Bekkering WP, ten Cate R, van Suijlekom-Smit LW, et al. The relationship between impairments in joint function and disabilities in independent function in children with systemic juvenile idiopathic arthritis. J Rheumatol 2001;28:199–1105.

44. Epps H, Hurley M, Utley M. Development and evaluation of a single score to assess global range of motion in juvenile rheumatoid arthritis. Arthritis Care Res 2002;47:398–402.

45. Len C, Ferraz M, Goldenberg J, et al. Pediatric Escola Paulista de Medicina range of motion scale: a reduced joint count score for general use in juvenile rheumatoid arthritis. J Rheumatol 1999;26:909–913.

46. Lindehammer H, Backman E. Muscle function in juvenile chronic arthritis. J Rheumatol 1995;22:1159–1165.

47. Knopps K, Wulffraat N, Lodder S, et al. Resting energy expenditure and nutritional status in children with juvenile rheumatoid arthritis. J Rheumatol 1999;26:2039–2043.

48. Vostrejs M, Hollister JR. Muscle atrophy and leg length discrepancies in pauciarticular juvenile rheumatoid arthritis. Am J Dis Child 1988;142:343–345.

49. Oberg T, Karszina B, Gare A, et al. Physical training of children with juvenile chronic arthritis. Scand J Rheumatol 1994;23:92–95.

50. Lindehammer H, Sandstedt P. Measurement of quadriceps muscle strength and bulk in juvenile chronic arthritis: a prospective, longitudinal 2-year survey. J Rheumatol 1998;25:2240–2248.

51. Hendrengren E, Knutson LM, Haglund-Akerlind Y, et al. Lower extremity isometric torque in children with juvenile rheumatoid arthritis. Scand J Rheumatol 2001;30:69–76.

52. Klepper S, Darbee J, Effgen S, et al. Physical fitness levels in children with polyarticular juvenile rheumatoid arthritis. Arthritis Care Res 1992;5:93–100.

53. Fan J, Wessel J, Ellsworth J. The relationship between strength and function in females with juvenile rheumatoid arthritis. J Rheumatol 1998;3:1399–1405.

54. Takken T, van der Net J, Helders P. Relationship between functional ability and physical fitness in juvenile rheumatoid arthritis. Scand J Rheumatol 2003;32:174–178.

55. Lechner DE, McCarthy CF, Holden MK. Gait deviations in patients with juvenile rheumatoid arthritis. Phys Ther 1987;67:1335–1341.

56. Dunn W. Grip strength of children aged 3 to 7 years using a modified sphygmomanometer: comparison of typical children and children with rheumatic disease. Am J Occup Ther 1993;47:421–428.

57. Giannini MJ, Protas EJ. Comparison of peak isometric knee extensor torque in children with and without juvenile arthritis. Arthritis Care Res 1993;6:82–88.

58. Wessel J, Kaup C, Fin J, et al. Isometric strength measurements in children with arthritis: reliability and relation to function. Arthritis Care Res 1999;12:238–246.

59. Kraemer W, Fleck S. Strength Training for Young Athletes. Champaign, IL: Human Kinetics, 1993.

60. Takken T, Hemel A, van der Net JJ, et al. Aerobic fitness in children with juvenile idiopathic arthritis. J Rheumatol 2002;29:2643–2647.

61. Giannini MJ, Protas EJ. Aerobic capacity in juvenile rheumatoid arthritis patients and healthy children. Arthritis Care Res 1992;4:131–135.

62. Hebestreit H, Muller-Scholden J, Huppertz HI. Aerobic fitness and physical activity in patients with HLA-B27 positive juvenile spondyloarthropathy that is inactive or in remission. J Rheumatol 1998;25:1626–1633.

63. Anthony KK, Schanberg LE. Pain in children with arthritis: a review of the current literature. Arthritis Rheum 2003;49:272–279.

64. Lovell DJ, Walco GW. Pain associated with juvenile rheumatoid arthritis. Pediatr Clin N Am 1989;36:1015–1027.

65. Hogeweg JA, Kuis W, Huygen AC, et al. The pain threshold in juvenile chronic arthritis. Br J Rheumatol 1995;4:61–67.

66. Hogeweg JA, Kuis W, Oostendorp RA, et al. General and segmental reduced pain thresholds in juvenile chronic arthritis. Pain 1995;62:11–17.

67. Thatsum M, Zachariae R, Scholer M, et al. Cold pressor pain: comparing responses of juvenile rheumatoid arthritis patients and their parents. Scand J Rheumatol 1997;26:272–279.

68. Varni JW, Thompson KL, Hanson V. The Varni/Thompson pediatric pain questionnaire I: chronic musculoskeletal pain in juvenile rheumatoid arthritis: an empirical model. Pain 1987;28:27–38.

69. Beyer JE, Denyes MJ, Villarruel AM. The creation, validation, and continuing development of the Oucher: a measure of pain intensity in children. J Pediatr Nurs 1992;7:335–346.

70. Wong DL, Baker CM. Pain in children: comparison of assessment scales. Pediatr Nurs 1988;14:9–17.

71. Hester NO, Foster R, Kristensen K. Measurement of pain in children: generalizability and validity of the pain ladder and the poker-chip tool. In: Tyler DC, Kane EJ, eds. Advances in Pain Research and Therapy. New York: Raven Press, 1990.

72. Guidelines for the Management of Pain in Osteoarthritis, Rheumatoid Arthritis, and Juvenile Chronic Arthritis. Glenview, IL: American Pain Society, 2002.

73. Jaworski TM, Bradley LA, Heck LW, et al. Development of an observational method for assessing pain behaviors in children with juvenile rheumatoid arthritis. Arthritis Rheum 1995;38:1142–1151.

74. Frigo C, Bardare M, Corona F, et al. Gait alteration in patients with juvenile idiopathic arthritis: a computerized analysis. J Orthopedic Rheumatol 1996;9:82–90.

75. Brostrom E, Haglund-Akerlind Y, Hagelberg S, et al. Gait in children with juvenile chronic arthritis. Timing and force parameters. Scand J Rheumatol 2002;31:317–323.

76. Spraul G, Koenning G. A descriptive study of foot problems with juvenile rheumatoid arthritis (JRA). Arthritis Care Res 1994;7:144–150.

77. Bacon MC, Nicholson C, Binder H, et al. Juvenile rheumatoid arthritis: aquatic exercise and lower extremity function. Arthritis Care Res 1991;4:102–105.

78. Klepper SE. Effects of an eight-week physical conditioning program on disease signs and symptoms in children with chronic arthritis. Arthritis Care Res 1999;12:52–60.

79. Fisher NM, Venkatraman JT, O'Neil K. The effects of resistance exercises on muscle function in juvenile arthritis. Arthritis Rheum 2001;44(Suppl 9):S276.

80. Takken T, van de Net JJ, Helders PJ. Do juvenile idiopathic arthritis patients benefit from an exercise program? A pilot study. Arthritis Care Res 2001;45:81–85.

81. Field T, Hernandez-Reif M, Seligman S, et al. Juvenile rheumatoid arthritis: benefits of massage therapy. J Pediatr Psychol 1997;22:607–617.

82. Lavigne JV, Ross CK, Barry SL, et al. Evaluation of a psychological treatment package for treating pain in juvenile rheumatoid arthritis. Arthritis Care Res 1992;5:101–110.

83. Walco GA, Varni JW, Ilowite NT. Cognitive-behavioral pain management in children with juvenile rheumatoid arthritis. Pediatrics 1992;89:1075–1079.

84. Bandy WD, Irion JM. The effect of time of static stretch on the flexibility of the hamstring muscles. Phys Ther 1994;74: 845–852.

85. Swann M. The surgery of juvenile chronic arthritis. Clin Orthop Rel Res 1990;259:70–75.

86. McCullough CJ. Surgical management of the hip in juvenile chronic arthritis. Br J Rheumatol 1991;33:178–183.

87. Skytta ET, Savolainen HA, Kautiainen HJ, et al. Long-term results of leg length discrepancies treated with temporary epiphyseal stapling in children with juvenile chronic arthritis. Clin Exper Rheumatol 2003;21:669–671.

88. Parvizi J, Lajam CM, Trousdale RT, et al. Total knee arthroplasty in young patients with juvenile rheumatoid arthritis. J Bone Joint Surg 2003;85:1090–1094.

89. Emery HM, Bayer SL, Sisung CE. Rehabilitation of the child with a rheumatic disease. Pediatr Clin North Am 1995;42: 1263–1285.

90. Feldman BM, Wright FV, Bar-Or O, et al. Rigorous fitness training and testing for children with polyarticular arthritis: a pilot study. Arthritis Rheum 2000;43(Suppl 9):S120.

91. James MJ, Cleland LG, Gaffney RD, et al. Effect of exercise on ^{99m}Tc-StPA clearance from knees with effusions. J Rheumatol 1994;21:501–504.

92. Minor MA, Westby MD. Rest and exercise. In: Robbins L, Burckhardt C, Hannan M, et al, eds. Clinical Care in the Rheumatic Diseases. 2nd Ed. Atlanta: American College of Rheumatology, 2001.

93. Faigenbaum AD, Milliken LA, Laud RL, et al. Comparison of 1 to 2 days per week of strength training in children. Res Q Exercise Sports 2002;73:416–424.

94. Klepper S. Exercise and fitness in children with arthritis; evidence for exercise and physical activity. Arthritis Care Res 2003;49:435–444.

95. Klepper S, Giannini M. Physical conditioning in children with arthritis. Arthritis Care Res 1994;7:226–236.

96. Carmen D, Browne R. Joint protection education for children with arthritis: can handouts replace professional instruction? Arthritis Rheum 1996;39:S1714.

97. Scull S, Athreya B. Childhood arthritis. In: Goldberg B, ed. Sports and Exercise for Children with Chronic Health Conditions. Champaign, IL: Human Kinetics, 1995.

98. Kirchheimer JC, Wanivenhaus A, Engel A. Does sport negatively influence joint scores in patients with juvenile rheumatoid arthritis: an 8-year prospective study. Rheumatol Int 1993;12:239–242.

99. Whitehouse R, Shape J, Sullivan D, et al. Children with juvenile rheumatoid arthritis at school. Clin Pediatr 1989;28: 509–514.

100. Stoff E, Bacon M, White P. The effects of fatigue, distractibility, and absenteeism on school achievement in children with rheumatic disease. Arthritis Care Res 1989;2:54–59.

101. Arthritis Foundation. Educational Rights for Children with Arthritis: A Manual for Parents. American Juvenile Arthritis Organization. Atlanta: Arthritis Foundation, 1989.

102. Arthritis Foundation: Raising a Child with Arthritis. Atlanta: Arthritis Foundation, 1998.

School Activity and Participation Checklist

Children with arthritis or other musculoskeletal disorders may experience difficulty performing some necessary or desired activities in school. These activity limitations may negatively impact the child's participation in school programs. The list below includes many of the typical tasks performed in school. Please check any activity that is difficult for you/your child; please add any other activities that are difficult.

School Attendance

_____ Getting to school on time is difficult for me because
- ☐ I am stiff or hurt in the morning
- ☐ I'm too tired to get ready for school
- ☐ I need help getting dressed

_____ I am often absent, late, or have to leave school early often because
- ☐ I do not feel well
- ☐ I have a doctor's appointment
- ☐ I am tired

Classroom Activities

_____ I have trouble taking off/putting on my coat, hat, gloves, boots, etc.

_____ I have troubled using a pen, pencil, or crayons in school because
- ☐ My arm or hands (fingers or wrist) hurt or ☐ get tired
- ☐ The pen, pencil, crayon is too small to hold

_____ I have trouble writing on the chalkboard

_____ I have trouble raising my hand to ask or answer a question

_____ I get stiff sitting in my chair for a long time

_____ My teacher(s) will not let me stand up or walk around when I'm stiff

_____ I get tired during the day and need to rest

_____ I have trouble finishing my schoolwork on time

_____ I have trouble writing fast when I take a test or class notes

_____ My school doesn't have the things that help me do things at home (splints, easel for writing, chair cushion, other)

Physical Education/Recess

_____ I have trouble opening my gym locker

_____ I have trouble changing clothes for gym

_____ I have trouble taking a shower after gym class

_____ I have trouble walking to the playground as fast as the other kids

_____ I have trouble doing the same things in gym/on the playground as the other kids in my class

_____ My gym teacher is afraid to let me do the same things as the other kids

_____ My gym teacher doesn't understand that I can't do some of the things the other kids do. (List the things you have trouble doing.)

Getting Around School

_____ I have getting around the school (I am often late for the next activity) because
- ☐ My classes are too far apart
- ☐ The cafeteria or gym is too far away

_____ I have trouble standing in lines for a long time, like in the cafeteria or during assemblies

_____ I have trouble carrying my books, lunch tray, or other things while walking in school

_____ I have trouble opening my milk carton, lunch box, or using a knife and fork during lunch

_____ I have trouble opening heavy doors

_____ I have double going up/down stairs

_____ I have trouble using the bathroom at school

_____ I have trouble during fire drills, earthquake drills, and other emergency drills

_____ I often miss field trips because I have trouble walking long distances

Other Problems

_____ My teacher(s) don't understand the problems I have because of my condition

_____ My teacher(s) make a big deal of my condition and it makes me feel different

_____ Other kids make fun of me or say things that make me feel bad

_____ I don't want anyone to know what I have arthritis (other condition)

_____ I have hand splints but don't want to war then in school

_____ I sometimes forget to take my medicine because it is in the nurse's office

Please add any other school-related problems you/your child have because of their arthritis or other health condition

_____

_____

_____

_____

Klepper S, Lopez R, Winn R, 2004

P A R T

IV

Other Medical/ Surgical Disorders

Pediatric Oncology

Victoria Gocha Marchese

ach year more than 11,000 children and adolescents in the United States are diagnosed with cancer.[1] As a result of improvements in diagnostic testing and medical interventions, survival rates of young adults who had cancer in childhood now exceed 75%.[2] It is estimated that 270,000 survivors of childhood cancer are living in the United States, which means that 1 in 570 adults 20 to 34 years of age is a survivor of childhood cancer.[3] Therefore, more young adults than ever before are now living with the short- and long-term effects of the cancer and of the medical interventions used to save their lives. As the numbers of children with cancer and survivors now living with treatment-related effects have increased, so has the need for physical therapists to learn more about early detection, treatment of common types of pediatric cancer, and the short- and long-term side effects from the cancer and the medical interventions. We as physical therapists have a responsibility to understand the full continuum of care for our patients, from the first indication that a diagnosis of cancer is a possibility, to appropriate types of physical therapy interventions, to educating our patients about long-term complications they may experience as they relate to the scope of physical therapy practice primarily in the areas of the musculoskeletal, neuromuscular, integumentary, and cardiopulmonary systems.

Physical therapists are in a unique position to assist patients with cancer and advance the body of research considering our excellent training in the areas that impact patients with cancer so greatly. These areas include pre-vention, education, and intervention, with a focus on range of motion, strength, motor planning, balance and coordination, fatigue, assistive devices, prosthetics and orthotics, functional mobility, activities of daily living, and ultimately improving the patients' quality of life and ability to participate in family and community activities.

Cancer is the uncontrolled growth of cells that are not functioning properly. When these cells overproduce and crowd out normal healthy cells or develop into a solid mass, signs and symptoms of disease begin to appear. Typically the cancer begins to develop at a primary site. If the cancer spreads to other areas of the body, it is said to have *metastasized*. The term *cancer* is often used to refer to various types of cancer. Those that commonly affect adults typically differ from those that affect children. In adults, prostate, breast, lung, colon, and rectal cancer are the most common types of cancer.[4] In children, leukemia, brain tumors, lymphomas, Wilms tumor, neuroblastoma, retinoblastoma, rhabdomyosarcoma, osteosarcoma, and Ewing's sarcoma family of tumors are the most common types.[5]

Common Types of Pediatric Cancer

LEUKEMIA

Leukemia is the most prevalent type of pediatric cancer; it accounts for 31% of all cancer cases in children younger than 15 years of age.[6] The disease takes its name from *leukocyte*, which describes the type of cell (white blood cell), and the Greek word ending *emia,* indicating a condition of the blood. Leukemia, a malignant disorder of the blood and the blood-forming tissues of the bone marrow, is characterized by overproduction of abnormal leukocytes, cells that are essential in helping the body destroy foreign substances such as viruses, bacteria, and fungi. There are several different types of leukemia, and they are typically classified by the type of cell (lymphoid or myeloid) and by whether the leukemia grows quickly (acute) or slowly (chronic).

The most common pediatric leukemia is acute lymphoblastic leukemia (ALL), also known as acute lymphocytic leukemia or acute lymphoid leukemia. ALL accounts for 78% of all childhood leukemia cases in children younger than 15 years of age.[6] It is most common in children 2 and 3 years of age. ALL is considered acute because immature lymphocytes proliferate rapidly, and because the disease is fatal without treatment. However, with appropriate medical intervention, survival rates for children with ALL now exceed 80%.[6]

The second most common pediatric leukemia is acute myeloid leukemia (AML), also referred to as myelocytic, myelogenous, or nonlymphoblastic leukemia; it accounts for approximately 16% of all leukemia cases in children younger than 15 years of age. Furthermore, AML accounts for 36% of leukemia cases in those 15 to 19 years of age.[6] AML is the rapid proliferation of myeloid cells. The survival rate of children with AML is less favorable than that of children with ALL; approximately 41% of children with AML are alive 5 years after diagnosis.[6] Chronic leukemia is less common in children, accounting for less than 2% of the cases of pediatric leukemia.

Genetic factors are assumed to play a role in the cause of acute leukemia. For example, children with Down syndrome, Klinefelter syndrome, and neurofibromatosis are more likely to develop leukemia than are children without these conditions.[7–10] Another possible factor in the development of acute leukemia is exposure to ionizing radiation and certain toxic chemicals.[11]

The signs and symptoms for leukemia are typically caused by an overproduction of a specific cell that crowds out normal healthy cells, causing anemia, thrombocytopenia, and neutropenia and producing the identifiable side effects of leukemia such as fatigue, bruising, bleeding, infection, bone pain, fever, and enlarged lymph nodes and spleen.[11] Medical intervention for children with leukemia includes multiagent chemotherapy, and depending on the specific type of protocol, children with ALL receive multiagent chemotherapy for 2 to 3 years. It is typically only when ALL relapses, that is, when the cancer cells return, that children will receive a stem cell transplant. However, for children with AML, stem cell transplantation is often the first choice of treatment if a donor is available.[12]

CENTRAL NERVOUS SYSTEM TUMORS

Central nervous system (CNS) tumors are the second most commonly diagnosed pediatric cancer, and the most commonly diagnosed solid tumors in children (Table 15.1).[13] CNS tumors account for 16% of childhood malignancies. Most brain tumors occur in children in the first decade of life.[13] The most common types of CNS tumors in children and adolescents are astrocytoma, primitive neuroectodermal tumors (including medulloblastoma), brainstem gliomas, ependymomas, and craniopharyngioma.[14,15] Signs and symptoms of brain tumors in children vary widely according to the size and location of the tumor. They include headaches, seizures, drowsiness, dysphasia (impaired speech), dysphagia (difficulty with swallowing), impaired vision, behavioral changes, sudden vomiting, poor coordination, weakness, impaired balance, and paresthesia.[15–17]

Medical intervention for children with brain tumors depends on the type and location of the tumor and may include surgery, radiation therapy, and chemotherapy.[13] Survival rates for children with CNS tumors vary depending on the type of tumor, size, and location. Children and adolescents with a CNS cancer have a 65% 5-year survival rate.[14]

TABLE 15.1

Common Pediatric Central Nervous System (CNS) Tumors[13–17]

Type of Tumor	Histology	Location	CNS Occurrences (%)	Peak Age of Incidence
Astrocytoma (juvenile pilocytic astrocytoma, anaplastic astrocytoma, glioblastoma multiforme)	Astrocytes (glial cells)	Cerebellum, cerebrum, thalamus, or hypothalamus	52	5
Medulloblastoma	Neuroepithelial	Cerebellum	20	1–10
Primitive neuroectodermal tumor (cerebral, neuroblastoma, cerebral medulloblastoma)	Neuroepithelial	Cerebrum	20	1–10
Brainstem gliomas	Glial cells	Midbrain/pons/medulla	10	5–10
Ependymoma	Ependymal	Fourth ventricle	6	<5

LYMPHOMA

The third most common type of cancer in children is lymphoma, including Hodgkin disease and non-Hodgkin lymphoma (NHL). Lymphoma accounts for 15% of the cases of pediatric cancer.[18] These malignancies arise in the lymphoid tissues and have their own biologic subtypes.[18] Hodgkin disease is more common in older children and adolescents, whereas NHL is more prevalent in younger children.[5] The signs and symptoms of Hodgkin's disease include painless supraclavicular or cervical adenopathy, nonproductive cough, fatigue, anorexia, slight weight loss, and pruritus.[19] NHL is typically classified into four categories[18]:

1. Burkitt and Burkitt-like lymphoma (small noncleaved cell lymphoma)
2. Lymphoblastic lymphoma
3. Diffuse large B-cell lymphoma
4. Anaplastic large cell lymphoma

The clinical signs and symptoms of NHL may include changes in bowel habits; nausea; vomiting; swelling of the abdomen, face, neck, or upper limbs; pain dysphagia; and dyspenia.[20] The survival rate for children and adolescents with Hodgkin disease is 91%; for those with NHL, the rate is 72%.[18] Medical treatment of lymphoma typically includes chemotherapy and radiation therapy.[20]

NEUROBLASTIC TUMORS

The neuroblastic tumors include neuroblastoma, ganglioneuroblastoma, and ganglioneuroma.[21] These tumors develop from primordial neural crest cells and are the most common types of malignancy in infants; 41% of the diagnoses of neuroblastoma are made within the infant's first 3 months of life.[22] Neuroblastoma commonly develops in the adrenal glands, sympathetic nervous system, ganglia of the abdomen, and sympathetic ganglia of the chest or neck.[5,22] The signs and symptoms of neuroblastoma depend largely on the location of the tumor. These include a palpable fixed hard mass in the neck or abdomen area and pain and paralysis if the tumor involves the spinal cord or peripheral nerves.[21] Surgery, chemotherapy, and radiation therapy are used to medically manage cases of neuroblastoma. The survival rate of children with neuroblastoma depends on the child's age, disease stage, and tumor histology.[21] The younger the child is at diagnosis, the greater the chances of survival. Those who are less than 1 year of age at the time of diagnosis have a 5-year survival rate of 83%. The 5-year survival rate of children 1 to 4 years of age at diagnosis of neuroblastoma is approximately 55%, and for children greater than 5 years of age at diagnosis, the 5-year survival rate is 40%.[22]

SARCOMA

The word *sarcoma* means a malignant tumor of mesenchymal cell origin. Sarcoma cells typically mature into skeletal muscle, smooth muscle, fat, fibrous tissue, bone, and cartilage.[23] The medical intervention for sarcoma may include neoadjuvant (preoperative chemotherapy) and adjuvant (after surgery) chemotherapy, surgery, and/or radiation therapy. The primary goal is to improve survival of the patient and to maintain the function of the extremity. Factors used to determine the type of medical intervention include the tumor's size, location, and response to presurgical chemotherapy and containment of the disease to the primary site.[24]

OSTEOSARCOMA

Also called osteogenic sarcoma, osteosarcoma is the most common bone tumor in adolescents.[25] The most common site of occurrence is in the long bones, primarily in the metaphyseal area of the distal femur, proximal tibia, or proximal humerus.[26] Teenagers are at the greatest risk of developing osteosarcoma; this is thought to be due to their rapid growth spurts.[26] The primary symptom of osteosarcoma is pain in the involved site with or without the presence of a palpable mass or a decrease in range of motion.[15,26] Medical intervention for sarcoma includes neoadjuvant chemotherapy, adjuvant chemotherapy, and surgery—limb sparing (salvage), amputation, or rotationplasty (Figs. 15.1 through 15.4). Factors used to determine the form of surgery are the tumor's size, location, and response to presurgical chemotherapy and containment of the disease to the primary site.[24] Survival rates for children with metastatic disease osteosarcoma (30%) are not as favorable as those for children whose disease is localized (75%).[15]

EWING'S SARCOMA

Ewing's sarcoma is the second most common type of bone malignancy in children and adolescents.[27] It is thought that Ewing's sarcoma originates from neural crest cells; however, it is considered to be a tumor primarily of the bone or soft tissue.[27] Common sites for Ewing's sarcoma are the vertebral column, rib, sternum, clavicle, pelvis, sacrum, and coccyx.[25] Approximately 50% of patients who develop Ewing's sarcoma are 10 to 20 years old.[27] Signs

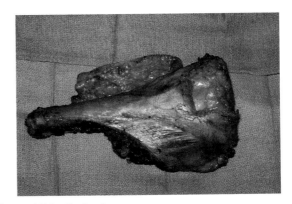

Figure 15.1 ■ Excised osteosarcoma.

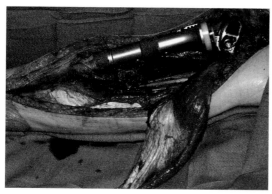

Figure 15.2 ■ Internal prosthesis in place during surgery.

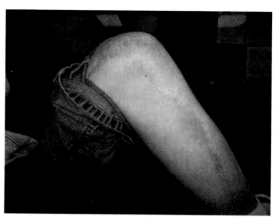

Figure 15.4 ■ Surgically repaired lower extremity approximately 3 months after repair with good wound closure.

and symptoms include pain and/or swelling at the tumor location.[25] Medical intervention for children with Ewing's sarcoma includes surgery, chemotherapy, and radiation therapy. The prognosis for Ewing's sarcoma in children varies widely, depending on the tumor location. The overall 5-year survival rate for children with Ewing's sarcoma is approximately 58%. The rate is lower for patients with Ewing's sarcoma of the pelvis, sacrum, or coccyx.[25]

RHABDOMYOSARCOMA

The most common soft tissue sarcoma in neonates to children 14 years of age, rhabdomyosarcoma is the sixth most common cancer in children and adolescents.[5,28] The most prevalent sites for a rhabdomyosarcoma are the head and neck, then the urinary and reproductive organs, extremities, and trunk.[15,27] Signs and symptoms of rhabdomyosarcoma include the appearance of a mass or a disturbance of normal body function such as a tumor in the nasopharynx that causes an obstruction and discharge.[23] Medical treatment for children with rhabdomyosarcoma includes surgical removal of the tumor, chemotherapy, and radiation therapy.[23] As was the case with the other sarcomas, the survival rate for children with rhabdomyosarcoma depends on the tumor size,

location, and cellular composition; how successful surgical removal was; and whether the tumor is contained to one site. Children younger than 5 years old at diagnosis have a 5-year survival rate of 79% in contrast to those 15 to 19 years of age, who have a 45% survival rate.[28]

RETINOBLASTOMA

Retinoblastoma, a malignancy of the retina that originates from multipotent precursor cells, accounts for only 3% of the cases of cancer in children younger than 15 years of age; however, it accounts for 11% of cancers in infants.[29,30] The disease may be hereditary or nonhereditary; the hereditary form presents primarily in infants.[29,30] The nonhereditary form occurs when the gene develops a new mutation, and is more prevalent in children than in infants.[30] The median age of retinoblastoma is 2 years of age.[29] The child's age at diagnosis strongly predicts whether the child will have unilateral or bilateral eye involvement, with infants more likely to have bilateral eye involvement.[29] The two most common signs and symptoms of retinoblastoma are leukokoria (lack of the normal red reflex of the eye) and strabismus (eyes cross).[30] Medical intervention for children with retinoblastoma is very multifaceted and may include enucleation (removal of the eye), external beam radiotherapy, plaque radiotherapy, laser photocoagulation, cryotherapy, thermotherapy, and systemic chemotherapy.[30] The 5-year survival rate for infants and children with retinoblastoma now exceeds 94%.[15,29]

WILMS TUMOR

Wilms tumor, also called nephroblastoma, is the most common malignancy of the kidney in children.[31] Children younger than 5 years of age are more likely to have Wilms tumor than are older children; it occurs most frequently in the first 2 years of life.[31] The primary signs and symptoms of Wilms tumor are abdominal swelling or mass, fever, anemia, and hypertension.[32] Medical intervention for Wilms

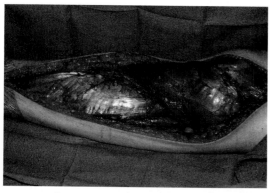

Figure 15.3 ■ Gastrocnemius muscle flap covering the internal prosthesis before closing the surgical wound.

tumor consists of surgical resection, chemotherapy, and radiation therapy.[32] The 5-year survival rate for children with Wilms tumor is 92%.[31]

Disease and Medical Intervention Factors that Influence Physical Therapy Practice

When a patient presents with signs and symptoms of cancer, a physician orders specific diagnostic tests. A complete blood count test is most commonly performed to evaluate the function of the bone marrow. The normal blood values listed in Table 15.2 are only a general range because these values vary slightly according to the child's sex and age.[33] The ranges listed as acceptable for participation in exercise are a guideline only. Because children with cancer often have low blood counts, it is highly recommended that the physical therapist contact the child's physician and discuss these parameters. At the leading children's oncology centers, the physical therapists, with the approval of the physicians, typically continue to provide physical therapy services even when a child has low blood counts. For example, they may encourage gentle active range-of-motion exercises or a light game of toss with a patient who has a platelet count less than 20,000 μg/L or slow walking for a child with a hemoglobin concentration less than 8 g/100/mL rather than no exercise. Therefore, the standard of care must include structured activities with previously agreed upon, by the physical therapist and the physician, parameters guided by the blood count levels.

A bone marrow aspiration or bone marrow biopsy is performed by direct insertion of a needle into the bone, typically the iliac crest bone; the sample is then examined microscopically to detect the presence of cancer cells. A lumbar puncture is performed by insertion of a needle into the lumbar vertebrae area; cerebrospinal fluid is withdrawn to determine whether the cancer involves the cerebrospinal fluid. Physical therapists must understand that a child who has undergone either a bone marrow aspiration or lumbar puncture may experience discomfort with movement or feel sore in these areas for a few days and take this into consideration when performing the physical therapy examination and planning for that session's intervention program. For example, if a patient has difficulty transitioning from a sitting position to standing, it may not be due to lower extremity weakness but instead to discomfort in the hip or low back area and in a few days the problem will resolve.

If a patient presents with pain or swelling in an extremity, radiography, ultrasound, computed tomography (CT), or magnetic resonance imaging (MRI) is performed. Examination of the imaging results is helpful in identifying the tumor's location, but further testing, for example, of a needle biopsy sample, is required to determine the type of tumor on the basis of the cell's morphologic characteristics. This information is important to the physical therapist because the location of the tumor may have an impact on the surrounding tissues such as causing joint contractures or change the patient's lower extremity weight-bearing status, thus limiting ambulation and functional mobility.

Before prescribing a course of medical treatment, the oncologist will determine the tumor's grade and stage by identifying the specific type of cancer on a cellular level, its exact location, and whether the cancer has spread to other areas of the body. The tumor's grade, which indicates its degree of malignancy, is determined on the basis of the microscopic appearance of the tumor cells, the tendency of

TABLE 15.2

Blood Count, Symptoms, and Exercise Guidelines[33]

	Red Blood Cells (Erythrocytes)	Platelets (Thrombocytes)	Hemoglobin	White Blood Cells (Leukocytes)
Function	CO_2 and O_2 transport	Clotting of blood	CO_2 and O_2 transport	Defense against infection
Normal values	Male: 4.7–5.5×10^6/μL Female: 4.1–4.9×10^6/μL	150,000–350,000/μL	10–13 g/100 mL	4500–11,000/mm^3
Name of low value	Anemia	Thrombocytopenia	Anemia	Bacterial, viral, and/or fungal infection
Symptoms of low values	Pallor Fatigue	Bruising Petechiae	Pallor Fatigue	Infection
Exercise guidelines	See Hemoglobin	No exercise: <20,000 Light exercise: 20,000–50,000 Resistive exercise: >50,000	No exercise: <8 Light exercise: 8–10 Resistive exercise: >10	No exercise: <5000 Light exercise: >5000 Resistive exercise: >5000

the tumor to spread, and its growth rate. A system frequently used in the determination of cancer grade is that of the World Health Organization (WHO).[16] The system starts with grade I (a tumor that grows slowly and has a slightly abnormal appearance) and ends with grade IV (a tumor that reproduces most rapidly and has the undifferentiated cells).[17] Staging classifications are used to describe whether the disease is contained to the primary site, and if not, the extent of its spread. Although the exact cause of the cancer is often unknown, genetic and environmental factors have been linked to many of the common pediatric cancers. It is important for the oncologist to understand these genetic factors because they may also affect the type of intervention chosen for the patient. It is also important for the physical therapist to understand the grading and staging systems to tailor the physical therapy intervention program and plan of care around the child's specific needs. For example, if a child has a lower extremity osteosarcoma and the therapist is working on gait training and the patient is becoming short of breath with increased work of breathing, the therapist will want to know if the patient has lung metastases and modify the session accordingly.

Pediatric cancers are typically treated with multiple modalities such as surgery, chemotherapy, radiation therapy, or stem cell transplantation. Medical intervention is based on the type of cancer and the extent of disease. There are different phases of treatment: induction, consolidation, and maintenance. During the induction phase, the patient receives high doses of chemotherapy and possibly other modalities such as radiation therapy, with the goal of achieving remission as quickly as possible (no cancer cells present). To eliminate any remaining cancer cells, patients continue to receive high doses of chemotherapy during the consolidation phase. During the maintenance phase, patients receive lower doses of chemotherapy with the goal of preventing disease relapse.

CHEMOTHERAPY

Chemotherapeutic agents are chemicals used to interfere with rapidly dividing cancer cells, thus resulting in cell death. Multiagent chemotherapy is used to prevent resistance to one drug and allows administration of higher doses. Chemotherapy is the primary intervention for many types of cancers such as leukemia and lymphoma. It is often combined with other treatment modalities such as surgery and radiation therapy. For example, children with osteosarcoma often receive neoadjuvant chemotherapy for approximately 4 months before surgery to help shrink the tumor. They also receive adjuvant chemotherapy to aid in elimination of any cancer cells that have spread into other areas of the body.

Chemotherapeutic agents are administered in a variety of ways, including intravenous, oral, and intramuscular routes. Most do not readily cross the blood–brain barrier;

therefore, to target disease in the central nervous system, these agents are injected directly into the cerebrospinal fluid, typically through a catheter inserted in the lumbar area or in the brain.[34] This mode of administration, which is called intrathecal, is commonly used for administration of methotrexate.

Chemotherapeutic agents cause secondary side effects (Table 15.3).[35–47] Not all agents cause the same side effects, nor do they occur within the same period of time. For example, drugs such as vincristine are known to cause sensory/motor peripheral neuropathy, primarily affecting the hands and feet, within weeks of administration.[35,46,48–51] The earliest and most common clinical sign related to vincristine toxicity is a decreased Achilles tendon reflex, which can occur within a month of chemotherapy. The primary indication of peripheral neuropathy is foot drop, decreased ankle dorsiflexion strength and active range of motion, and neuropathic pain.[41,46,52] However, the order in which the clinical presentation occurs may vary; the physical therapist may observe weakness in a patient's intrinsic muscle of the hands and feet followed by weakness of the anterior tibialis, or the patient may experience neuropathic pain without any signs of muscle weakness. As soon as the dose of the vincristine is decreased or administration of the drug is stopped, the symptoms of neurotoxicity generally decrease; however, some researchers report residual deficits of gross motor skills.[40,49] Drugs such as methotrexate cause problems such as myelosuppression within a week of their administration and long-term neuropsychological problems with memory deficits and visual-spatial and motor coordination impairments.[53–55] Myelosuppression is a process in which bone marrow activity is decreased, resulting in low production of platelets, red blood cells, and white blood cells and a corresponding increase in the risk of bleeding, fatigue, and infection.

RADIATION THERAPY

Radiation therapy uses ionizing radiation to disrupt the structure of the tumor cells' DNA, which limits the cells' ability to further reproduce. Radiation therapy is delivered by an external radiation beam or internal placement of radiation material near the tumor. Radiation therapy is often used alone, or more frequently combined with other treatments such as surgery and chemotherapy.[56,57] Radiation therapy delivered before surgical removal of a tumor can shrink the tumor mass, thus decreasing the amount of damage to the surrounding healthy tissues.[58] It is used after surgery to destroy any cells that may have spread from the primary site.[58] Total body irradiation is also combined with chemotherapy to destroy the child's bone marrow in preparation for receiving a stem cell transplant. Radiation therapy may cause numerous short- and long-term side effects (Table 15.4), which are mainly related to the area and the surrounding tissues that received the radiation.[56–63] Side effects from radiation are

TABLE 15.3

Specific Chemotherapeutic Agents and Common Side Effects Pertinent to Physical Therapy[41-55]

Chemotherapeutic Agents	Common Side Effects		Common Types of Cancer
	Short Term	Long Term	
Vincristine	Hypertension, motor difficulties, central nervous system depression, peripheral neuropathy, alopecia, constipation, anorexia, jaw pain, leg pain, weakness, paresthesia, numbness, myalgia, cramping	Peripheral neuropathy, decreased gross and fine motor skills	Leukemia, Hodgkin disease, neuroblastoma, lymphomas, Wilms tumor, and rhabdomyosarcoma
Cisplatin	Bradycardia, nausea, vomiting, bone marrow suppression, ototoxicity, peripheral neuropathy	Ototoxicity, nephrotoxicity	Osteosarcoma, Hodgkin disease and non-Hodgkin lymphoma, brain tumors
Methotrexate	Malaise, fatigue, dizziness, alopecia, photosensitivity, nausea, vomiting, diarrhea, anorexia, mucositis, glossitis, myelosuppression, arthralgia, osteopenia	Osteoporosis, bone fracture, infertility, renal toxicity, hepatotoxicity, neuropsychological-cognitive deficits	Leukemia, osteosarcoma, non-Hodgkin lymphoma
Dexamethasone	Hypertension, increased susceptibility to infection, myopathy, increased appetite, mental changes	Growth suppression, bone demineralization, osteonecrosis	Leukemia, brain tumors, and other types of malignancy
Ifosfamide	Somnolence, dizziness, polyneuropathy, alopecia, dermatitis, nausea, vomiting, anorexia, diarrhea, constipation, myelosuppression	Cardiotoxicity, nephrotoxicity	Hodgkin disease and non-Hodgkin lymphoma, acute and chronic lymphocytic leukemia, sarcoma
Doxorubicin	Alopecia, nausea, vomiting, mucositis, diarrhea, bone marrow suppression	Cardiotoxicity, myocarditis	Lymphoma, leukemia, soft tissue sarcoma, neuroblastoma, osteosarcoma

TABLE 15.4

Short- and Long-Term Side Effects of Radiation[56-63]

Short Term	Long Term	Implication for Physical Therapists

Skin:
  Redness
  Blistering
  Hair loss
Fibrosis
Fatigue
Cognitive deficits
	Fibrosis
	Pathologic fracture
	Bone-growth abnormalities
	Osteonecrosis/avascular necrosis
	Osteoporosis
	Cardiac complications
	Hypertension
	Thyroid dysfunction
		Pain
		Decreased range of motion
		Decreased strength
		Decreased endurance
		Decreased functional mobility
		Decreased balance
		Decreased neuropsychological function:
		  Motor accuracy, sensory integration,
		  Memory, concentration
		Decreased quality of life and participation
		  in community and family activities

particularly severe in infants and children who are still growing. Their neuropsychological and musculoskeletal systems are affected.

SURGERY

Surgical procedures typically performed for the pediatric patient with cancer include tumor biopsy, central line and shunt placement, and tumor resection, with or without extensive surgical reconstruction.

TUMOR BIOPSY

Typically before any medical intervention takes place, a biopsy of a portion of the tumor or a bone marrow aspiration is obtained. These procedures are performed under general anesthesia, conscious sedation, or local anesthesia. Unfortunately, with some brain tumors, primarily those of the brainstem, a biopsy cannot be performed due to the high risk of damage to surrounding tissue.

CENTRAL LINE AND SHUNT PLACEMENT

Because most children receive intravenous chemotherapy agents over an extended period of time, a surgically placed indwelling catheter that leads directly into a major blood vessel near the heart may be required. These lines are often called a central line, Broviac, or Hickman catheter. The Broviac catheter is an external catheter that leads into a major vessel such as the external or internal jugular. An internal catheter is placed into the same major vessel, but it remains under the skin and is accessed with a needle each time the child needs to receive medication or to have blood drawn. A central line being pulled out accidentally constitutes a medical emergency due to the risk of infection and bleeding. Therefore, special precautions must be taken to keep the area around the catheter clean, dry, and protected from injury.

Surgical placement of a ventriculoperitoneal shunt is often required when a brain tumor results in increased intracranial pressure. It is important for physical therapists to know the following signs and symptoms of increased cranial pressure due to a brain tumor or a shunt malfunction: headaches, vomiting, diplopia, disturbances of consciousness, papilledema, and changes in motor function.[16]

SURGICAL RESECTION

Most solid tumors will require surgical resection. However, some are too large to be resected, or are located where surgical resection would be risky. Examples include brainstem gliomas or neuroblastoma that extends into the spinal cord. However, for malignant tumors, surgical resection is typically the optimal choice. To increase the chance that the tumor does not return or spread to other areas of the body, the surgeon will make every effort to completely resect the tumor with a clean margin of tissue with no cancer cells. Because it is not always known if any cells have spread beyond the primary tumor site, chemotherapy and radiation therapy may also be given to the patient.

OTHER SURGICAL PROCEDURES

For patients with an upper or lower extremity bone or soft tissue tumor, surgical options such as amputation, rotationplasty, and limb-sparing procedures are available.[64–66] Limb-sparing procedures may include the use of a custom endoprosthetic device, allograft reconstruction, or autograft reconstruction, or combine the use of endoprostheses and bone grafts.[24] For children who have not reached skeletal maturity, the lower extremity can be reconstructed by using an expandable endoprosthesis or contralateral epiphysiodesis.[24] Use of the expandable endoprosthesis, also referred to as a re-epiphysis prosthesis, is the common choice.[64] After the expandable prosthesis is implanted, the surgeon can lengthen the child's leg without opening the surgical site. Use of this noninvasive procedure decreases the risk of infection and time required for healing. The short-term limitations of the limb-sparing procedure (Table 15.5) include slow wound healing due to use of chemotherapeutic agents, infection, and poor joint range of motion[67,68] (Fig. 15.5). Long-term side effects include the need for frequent surgical revisions due to loosening of the prosthesis, leg length discrepancy, fractures, infection, poor joint range of motion, extensive problems requiring amputation, and local tumor recurrence.[24,64,67–69] Thus, it is important for physical therapists to plan for these types of complications and provide preventative measures if possible such as exercises to prevent contractures and activity recommendations to decrease the wear and tear on the prosthesis, recommending biking and swimming activities versus running and contact sports.

AMPUTATION This surgical procedure results in removal of a portion of an extremity; the extent of the amount of limb removed depends on the tumor's location, type, and size. Amputation is typically performed when it is not possible to make a wide enough excision to achieve clean margins, or when surgery is so extensive that the extremity is no longer functional.[67] After deciding that a child needs an amputation, the surgeon makes every effort to provide the patient with a residual limb that is conducive to the functional use of a prosthetic device. The short-term complications of an amputation may include psychological distress related to a drastic change in body image, slow healing of the surgical site if the child is receiving chemotherapy, inadequate wound coverage, neuropathic pain, phantom limb sensation, and increased energy expenditure for functional activities.[67] Long-term complications include psychological distress related to a drastic change in body image; skin blisters, redness, or bruising on the residual limb due to growth or weight changes; phantom limb pain

TABLE 15.5

Short- and Long-Term Side Effects of Limb-Sparing Procedures, Amputation, and Rotationplasty

Limb-Sparing Procedures		Amputation		Rotationplasty	
Short term	Long term	Short term	Long term	Short term	Long term
Slow wound healing	Multiple surgical revisions	Slow wound healing	Body image difficulties	Slow wound healing	Poor body image
Infection	Leg length discrepancy	Infection	Skin blisters	Infection	Leg length discrepancy
Poor range of motion	Fractures	Inadequate wound coverage	Redness	Increased energy expenditure	Increased energy expenditure
Increased energy expenditure	Infection	Increased energy expenditure	Phantom limb pain		
	Poor joint range of motion	Neuropathic pain	Muscle pain		
	Increased energy expenditure		Increased energy expenditure		
	Converted to amputation				
	Local recurrence				

and sensation; musculoskeletal pain; and increased energy expenditure for activities of daily living.[67]

ROTATIONPLASTY This surgical procedure is sometimes performed in lieu of an amputation; however, it is still considered a form of amputation.[67] Rotationplasty is not the standard of care at many of the children's hospitals in the United States. Rotationplasty removes a femoral tumor while preserving the neurovascular bundle and the distal portion of the lower leg and foot. The lower leg is turned 180 degrees and attached to the proximal femur in such a way that the foot can serve as the functional knee joint and as a weight-bearing surface for a prosthesis. The resultant residual limb does not require multiple surgical revisions and it is longer than if a below-knee amputation had been performed.[24] This longer limb provides the patient with

the chance for higher functional abilities.[70] Furthermore, patients who have undergone rotationplasty can participate in recreational activities and sports, as can patients who have had an amputation.[71,72] Short term, the wound heals poorly; short term and long term, the extremity appears odd. Researchers have studied quality of life in patients who have undergone a rotationplasty and determined that patients do not show reduction in psychosocial adaptation compared with the healthy population.[73,74]

BONE MARROW TRANSPLANTATION AND PERIPHERAL STEM CELL TRANSPLANTATION

Bone marrow transplantation (BMT) or peripheral blood stem cell transplantation (PSCT) is performed for children with leukemia (relapsed ALL or chronic myelogenous leukemia) or other hematologic diseases (e.g., anemia and sickle cell) that involve the bone marrow. The purpose is to replace the patient's bone marrow with his or her own marrow or donor bone marrow capable of producing healthy cells. Bone marrow is typically harvested by the repeated insertion of a large needle into the donor's bone (e.g., the iliac crest) and withdrawal of the marrow. The stem cells, the most immature cell that further differentiates into mature cells, are obtained by taking blood from the donor via a process called apheresis. There are three common forms of BMT or PSCT:

1. Allogeneic transplants from a histocompatible donor
2. Autologous transplants from the patient's own cells
3. Syngeneic transplants from an identical twin

The protocol being used and the policies of the institution where the transplantation takes place will determine

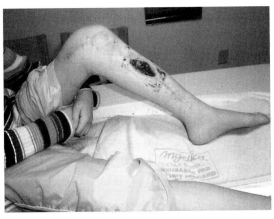

Figure 15.5 ■ *Patient 3 months after a limb-sparing procedure for proximal tibia osteosarcoma, presenting with wound closure problems.*

whether the child receives a BMT or PSCT. The more common procedure currently performed is the PSCT.

Children who receive a BMT or PSCT first receive combination chemotherapy to achieve a state of remission (no identifiable cancer cells in the body). The child is then admitted to the hospital for the conditioning phase. For approximately 1 week, the child receives chemotherapeutic agents (e.g., thiotepa) and total body irradiation, depending on his or her age. The goal of the conditioning phase is to provide complete bone marrow suppression. Because the child's white blood cell, red blood cell, and platelet counts drop, the child requires special care during this period to prevent infection and hemorrhaging. The child then receives an infusion of bone marrow or peripheral stem cells. For approximately 6 weeks, the child stays in an isolated room equipped with a positive-pressure and an air filtration system to help prevent infection. Engraftment, the process by which donor marrow begins to produce healthy cells, typically takes 10 to 17 days.[75] However, until the body produces its own cells, the child will require antibiotics to prevent infection and transfusions of red blood cells and platelets. Children may require red blood cell and platelet transfusions for up to 6 months and may not have adequate white blood cells to fight infection for 6 to 12 months.[75] Thus, physical therapists must be conscientious of the patient's blood count levels to plan for the physical therapy session.

Short term, the bodies of transplant recipients do not produce healthy cells. Therefore, the recipient has an increased risk of infection, bleeding, and severe fatigue. Children who receive allogeneic transplants may develop some form of graft-versus-host disease (GVHD), a process by which the transplanted marrow (graft) starts to attack the patient's (host) organs. There are two types of GVHD: acute and chronic. Acute GVHD can begin as early as the first month after the transplantation, when the engraftment process is taking place. Acute GVHD most commonly affects the skin, the bowel, and the liver; the patient experiences a rash, itchy skin, skin discoloration, dry mouth, mouth ulcers, diarrhea, and weight loss. Chronic GVHD occurs months after the patient receives the transplant and affects the skin and gastrointestinal system. Specific complications may include changes in the skin pigmentation and texture; possible development of joint contractures; dry mouth and ulcer formations; difficulty in swallowing and malabsorption, which may cause the child to lose weight; chronic liver disease; and problems with the eyes such as dryness, pain, and sensitivity to light.[76] The drugs prednisone, cyclosporine, and methotrexate are commonly given to patients to prevent GVHD or to decrease the severity of the reaction.[76] Long-term complications include those that were previously listed under chemotherapy and radiation therapy. Physical therapists will want to evaluate and provide intervention for children with GVHD to assist in the prevention of the development of joint contractures, decreased strength, and functional mobility.

Stem cell rescue is a process by which the child's own stem cells are extracted and stored. The child is then able to receive very high doses of chemotherapeutic agents, after which he or she receives a transfusion of his or her own cells. This procedure allows patients with cancer such as medulloblastoma and neuroblastoma to receive multiple rounds of very high doses of chemotherapy.

Physical Therapy Examination and Evaluation

SYSTEMS REVIEW

Because patients with cancer are often fatigued before the physical therapy examination begins, it is important that the therapist identify areas of concern immediately and focus the examination on those target areas. The systems review is a helpful way to guide the physical therapy examination. As soon as the therapist sees the patient, whether this occurs in the patient's hospital room, the clinic, the child's classroom, or home, he or she can identify key issues. Keeping a list of the essentials in mind helps with speed and thoroughness:

1. Musculoskeletal: obvious joint contractures or foot drop
2. Neuromuscular: signs of pain such as antalgic gait pattern, facial grimacing, guarding an area, increased or decreased muscle tone, facial paralyses, or difficulty hearing when the therapist says "hello;" neurocognitive deficits that will limit the child's ability to follow directions; or impaired balance
3. Cardiovascular and pulmonary: nasal flaring, increased work of breathing or respiratory rate
4. Integumentary: facial skin color that demonstrates possible low hemoglobin or liver function problems, for example, bruising that signals a low platelet count

MEDICAL AND SOCIAL HISTORY

Obtaining a thorough medical and social history is one of the key components of any physical therapy examination. This process helps the physical therapist select the types of questions to ask the patient, directs the specific types of tests and measurements that are chosen, and ultimately guides the plan of care. If the patient's chart is available, it is ideal to obtain the following information before meeting the patient:

1. Diagnoses
2. Disease grade and stage
3. Medical history, including patient's growth and development
4. Current medical treatment, including the types of chemotherapeutic agents the patient is receiving and other medical treatments
5. Current blood values, that is, hemoglobin concentrations, white and red blood cell counts, and platelet counts

However, physical therapists are not always fortunate enough to have the patient's medical chart available before meeting the patient. If the child or caregiver is unable to provide the therapist with the pertinent information, then it is most appropriate to call the physician or nurse.

After obtaining the required medical information, it is important for the therapist to build a rapport with the child and family. This is when the therapist asks about the child's social history. With whom does the child live? Does he or she have any siblings? What grade has he or she completed in school? What sports or other leisure activities does the child enjoy? The therapist will use the answers to these questions as a basis for discussing areas with which the child is having difficulty at home, at school, or in the hospital. Often it isn't until the therapist begins the examination that the child and family realize how much trouble the child is really having with a specific task such as climbing onto a school bus or that he or she is frequently tripping when walking on grass or other uneven surfaces.

TESTS AND MEASUREMENTS

Before the therapist conducts any tests or measurements, it is important that he or she plan the session. To make sure the examination is thorough and comprehensive, the therapist can use a disablement model such as the WHO's International Classification of Functioning, Disability, and Health (body functions/structures, activity, and participation) or the model of the National Center for Medical Rehabilitation Research (pathophysiology, impairment, functional limitation, disability, and societal limitations).[77] In this chapter, the WHO model will be used as a reference. According to the WHO, the term *body function and structure* refers to the physiologic functions of body systems, including the body's psychological functions and anatomic parts, such as organs and limbs and their components. *Activity* refers to the execution of a task or action by an individual and *participation* refers to involvement in a life situation.[77] The WHO model takes into account the interactions between all three components of the model and the child's individual environmental and personal factors. Each child will require an individualized examination based on the specific diagnoses and common side effects of the medical intervention the child received or is receiving. Table 15.6 outlines the key areas of focus in each category. For individual patients, some areas will be more applicable and will require further testing.

BODY FUNCTION AND STRUCTURE (IMPAIRMENTS)

MUSCULOSKELETAL

The musculoskeletal component of the examination is important for children with cancer because they oftentimes have problems with range of motion (ROM), strength, and postural alignment. When performing the ROM examination, the therapist should give particular attention to the joints above and below any area where a surgical procedure has recently been performed. Children will often guard the area around the surgical site because of pain or fear. For example, immediately after a brain tumor resection, a child may have decreased cervical spine ROM or may tilt his or her head laterally to compensate for visual deficits. For a few days after a central line placement, a child may not want to perform full-shoulder flexion or trunk ROM because the chest area is sore. After an aggressive distal femur or proximal tibia limb-sparing procedure, a child's hip, knee, and ankle ROM may be limited. Another important factor to consider when testing a child's range of motion is the type of chemotherapy the child is receiving or has received because agents such as vincristine cause a decrease in active ankle dorsiflexion ROM; over time this decreased ROM can develop into a contracture. Therefore, the therapist will want to focus on the ankle and hand-grip strength in patients receiving vincristine.

When performing the strength component of the examination, the therapist must consider the child's blood count levels. For children with a low platelet count, the typical manual muscle test and dynamometry is not appropriate. However, the therapist can observe the child's functional strength abilities while performing activities such as walking, climbing stairs, and performing transitional movements such as sit to stand.

NEUROMUSCULAR

When examining a child's neuromuscular system (i.e., conducting tests of pain, muscle tone, balance, motor control, vision, sensation, and sensory integration), it is important for the therapist to consider the complex interplay of the neuromuscular system with all the other systems in the body, the environment, and the task. If a child with a brainstem glioma presents with increased or decreased muscle tone or stiffness in the right lower and upper extremity, the therapist must consider how this impairment affects the child's active and passive range of motion, isolated muscle strength, proprioception, functional abilities, and activities of daily living, while also taking into account the child's cognitive abilities, age, family support, and motivation.

It is important that the physical therapist determine whether a child is experiencing pain, and if so, to identify the location, intensity, quality, onset/duration, and aggravating and alleviating factors. Pain is measurable in all individuals regardless of age. Depending on the patient's age and cognitive abilities, a variety of tools are available: (1) the FLACC (Face, Legs, Activity, Cry, Consolability) scale for infants to children 5 years of age; (2) the FACES scale for patients 5 to 13 years of age; and (3) self-reporting numeric scales (0 to 10) or a visual analog scale for children older

TABLE 15.6			
Recommended Tests and Measurements			

Body Function and Structure		Activity	Participation
Musculoskeletal	**Integumentary**	**Ambulation**	**Quality of Life**

Range of motion
    Goniometer
    Functional range
        of motion
	Skin
	    Temperature
	    Color
		Quality of gait pattern
		
		Assistance required
			School
			Work
			Play

Strengthening
    Manual muscle test
    Handheld goniometer
    Functional abilities
	Texture
	
	Wound
	    Healing
	    Drainage
	    Smell
		Forearm crutches
		Axillary crutches
		Walker
		Wheelchair
		Orthoses
		Prosthesis
			Sports
			Marriage
			Travel
			Palliative care
			Talking

Postural alignment	Scar mobility	Manual guidance Locomotion and develop- mental skills Walking Sit to stand Stand to sit	Questionnaires SF-36 PedsQL
Neuromuscular	**Cardiopulmonary**	Pull to stand Creeping Crawling Rolling Stair climbing	

Pain
    FLACC scale
 	
FACES scale
Visual analog scale
	Endurance
	    2-, 6-, 9-minute run/walk
	        tests
	
	Rate of perceived exertion
	    Physiological Cost Index		

Type of pain
    Neuropathic
    Nociceptive
	Heart rate
	Respiratory rate
		Standardized tests
		    Peabody Developmental
		        Motor Scales
		    Pediatric Evaluation of
		        Disability Inventory	

Muscle tone and
    motor control
    Ataxia
    Spasticity
    Hypotonicity
	Cervical and thoracic
	    asymmetry
	Nasal flaring
	Belly breather
	Increased work of
	    breathing
		Balance and coordination
		    Single-limb stance
		    Timed up and down stairs
		    Timed up and go
		    Start/stop on oral cue
		    Tandem walking
		    Walking on uneven
		        surfaces (grass, hills)
		    Dual-task activities	

Clonus Paresis			

Visual exam
    Vision
    Tracking			

Diplopia Eye–hand coordination			

Sensation
    Light touch
    Sharp dull
    Two-point discrimination			

Sensory integration			

than 13 years of age. A child may experience nociceptive pain and/or neuropathic pain. Nociceptive pain, commonly described as aching or throbbing pain, is typically caused by bone, joint, muscle, skin, or connective tissue damage from the disease itself, from medications such as steroids, or from surgery. In contrast, neuropathic pain is typically described as burning, tingling, or piercing, and it is caused by injury to a nerve, either from surgery, chemotherapeutic agents, or radiation therapy.[78–80]

INTEGUMENTARY

Examination of the integumentary system tells the therapist a great deal about a child. The color and texture of the skin alone may offer the therapist some information that will lead to further examination. For example, pallor suggests anemia; jaundice, liver dysfunction; dry and itchy skin, graft-versus-host disease; cold skin, poor circulation; hot skin, infection; drainage with a foul odor, infection; blisters, poorly fitted brace; red/blistered skin, radiation burns; and ulcers, pressure sores. Physical therapists will want to examine the mobility of a scar and note any scar adhesions. Physical therapists play a critical role in the identification and management of the integumentary issues that children with cancer may experience. The physical therapist must take the time to thoroughly examine the integumentary system, document the findings, and communicate and coordinate the plan of care with the physician.

CARDIOPULMONARY

Children with cancer may experience cardiopulmonary complications due to the effects of chemotherapy, radiation, prolonged bedrest, generalized fatigue, or skeletal abnormalities caused by a tumor, surgery, or radiation therapy. Therefore, the physical therapist must perform a comprehensive respiratory, skeletal (rib cage), and endurance examination. A good starting point is observation of the child, which will reveal increased work of breathing, nasal flaring, respiratory rate, and skeletal asymmetries that affect the cardiorespiratory system. More detailed assessments will include the use of a pulse oximeter to obtain a child's resting heart rate before he or she performs an endurance examination, and the therapist calculates his or her target heart rate range.

The child's age and abilities will guide the type of endurance tests the therapist chooses. For infants and toddlers, endurance testing may include observation of skin color, vital signs, and breathing patterns while the child is playing. For testing of the older child and adolescent, more structured methods are available such as a treadmill test at a variety of levels, step tests, and run-walk tests including the 2-, 6-, and 9-minute tests.[81-83] While the child is performing the endurance tests, the therapist can monitor the child's heart and respiratory rates. Tools are available to examine the energy required to perform specific tasks. The physiologic cost index is an objective way to calculate a child's energy expenditure. The rating of perceived exertions scale is a subjective scale of how hard the child reports that he or she is working.[84-88]

ACTIVITY (ACTIVITY LIMITATIONS)

AMBULATION AND LOCOMOTION

Children with cancer may experience difficulties with ambulation and locomotion as a result of the disease and treatment effects. These deficits may occur due to the effects of drugs such as vincristine that cause foot drop, weakness due to nerve root impingement, bone pain from the build-up of

blast cells in the bone marrow, or structural changes from a limb-sparing or amputation procedure. The therapist will first identify the child's primary means of mobility, whether it is walking, crawling, or using a wheelchair. Second, the therapist will identify the amount of assistance or the type of assistive device required for the patient to perform the task. Third, the therapist will examine the quality of the gait pattern or other means of mobility.

BALANCE AND COORDINATION

Balance and coordination deficits are common in children who have had a central nervous system or peripheral nervous system tumor or who have experienced side effects of chemotherapy or radiation therapy, surgical alterations of the skeletal system, or weakness from prolonged inactivity. As previously stated in the neuromuscular section, therapists must consider other systems (e.g., vision, hearing, sensation, muscle tone, and cognition) and environmental factors when examining a child's balance and coordination abilities. A few common tests (Table 15.6) include eyes open or closed, single-limb stance, timed up and down stairs, timed up and go, dual-task activities, and tandem walking.[89,90]

PARTICIPATION (PARTICIPATION RESTRICTIONS)

The most important component of the examination is identification of how the child's body structure/function and activity limitations are affecting the child and the family at home, work, school, or play. This can be achieved by using oral communication, observation, and structured questionnaires. Two commonly used pediatric-specific questionnaires are the PedsQL and the Short Form 36.[91,92] Often a therapist will ask children and parents how things are going at home, and the reply is "just fine;" however, it is the role of the physical therapist to focus the child and family on specific tasks such as getting in and out of bed, eating at the dinner table with the family, bathing, going to the mall with friends, going to school, climbing stairs at school, walking to class at school, and participating in sports. It is also important to discuss with the child and caregiver the child's level of involvement in activities because the child may feel isolated, lonely, and left out when he or she returns to school.[93]

Diagnosis, Prognosis, and Plan of Care

The physical therapy diagnosis and prognosis for pediatric cancer will vary depending on the specific type of cancer, medical intervention, and family dynamics. The following physical therapy diagnoses are common for patients with cancer: pain (neuropathic/nociceptive), fatigue, decreased range of motion, decreased strength, decreased endurance, developmental delays, poor wound closure, decreased functional mobility, and decreased participation in community activities (Table 15.7). For each patient, the plan of care and goals will require individual consideration depending on the child's unique circumstances. The physical therapist's role is to assist children with cancer in the prevention of secondary complications of the cancer and medical interventions; to promote health, wellness, fitness, and normal development; to limit the degree of disability; to promote rehabilitation; and to restore function in patients with chronic and irreversible disease.[94] To fulfill this role, the physical therapist should provide physical therapy intervention for children with cancer with an equal emphasis

---

TABLE 15.7 ▶▶ ▶▶ ▶▶ ▶▶ ▶▶ ▶▶ ▶▶ ▶▶ ▶

Possible Physical Therapy Diagnoses Based on Medical Diagnosis

Medical Diagnosis	Physical Therapy Diagnosis	Possible Causes
Leukemia/lymphoma	Pain	Peripheral neuropathy, bone pain from build-up of blast cells in the bone marrow, joint, and bone mainly due to osteonecrosis
	Decreased sensation	Peripheral neuropathy, nerve root compression
	Decreased strength	Peripheral neuropathy, steroids, inactivity
	Decreased range of motion	Peripheral neuropathy, osteonecrosis necrosis
	Decreased endurance and fatigue	Inactivity, chemotherapy, radiation therapy, stem cell transplant
	Decreased functional mobility	Decreased strength, endurance, pain
	Decreased participation in community activities	Self-confidence, fear, other social concerns such as friendships and previously listed impairments, limited handicapped-accessible accommodations
Central nervous system and peripheral nervous system tumor	Pain	Tumor impingement (spinal cord or peripheral nerve root impingement), peripheral neuropathy or surgical pain
	Decreased sensation	Peripheral neuropathy, central nervous system damage
	Decreased strength	Tumor impingement, surgical pain, fear, immobility, inactivity
	Decreased range of motion	Surgical incision site, decreased motor control, abnormal muscle tone
	Decreased balance and coordination	Poor motor control, ataxia, paralysis/paresis, decreased vision, vestibular dysfunction
	Decreased functional mobility	Visual deficits, decreased strength, endurance
	Decreased participation in community activities	Previously listed impairments and limited handicapped-accessible accommodations
Bone and soft tissue tumors	Pain	Tumor impingement, surgical pain, neuropathic pain, chemotherapy, osteoporosis
	Decreased sensation	Surgical nerve damage, chemotherapy
	Decreased strength	Immobility, nerve damage, central nervous system metastases
	Decreased range of motion	Immobility, nerve damage, scar adhesions
	Open wound	Failure of incision site to close, infection

on body structure/function impairments, activity limitations, and participation restrictions.[95] The time line for physical therapy intervention and the child and caregiver's goals will depend on the individual child and the medical diagnosis and prognosis.

PHYSICAL THERAPY INTERVENTION

The evidence to support the need for physical therapy services for children with cancer is overwhelming. Furthermore, our clinical experience has clearly demonstrated that physical therapy intervention for children with cancer is beneficial on all levels of care from body function/structure limitations to activity limitations to participation limitations. Despite the documented cases of children with cancer who have had complications with range of motion, strength, endurance, decreased balance, and functional activities, the effects of a comprehensive physical therapy program for children with cancer have not been well documented in the literature. The few studies specifically related to physical therapy intervention for children with cancer have been focused primarily on children with leukemia. On the basis of results of these studies, children currently receiving medical intervention for acute lymphoblastic leukemia demonstrate significant improvements in lower extremity strength and ankle dorsiflexion range of motion when they participate in a physical therapy program.[41,49,96] Furthermore, the literature also supports the following benefits of exercise for adults with cancer: improved hemoglobin concentrations, reduced duration of neutropenia and thrombocytopenia, reduced severity of diarrhea and pain, reduced duration of hospitalization, reduced reports of nausea, decreased emotional distress, increased lean body weight, improved physical performance, improved functional capacity, improved quality-of-life index, improved flexibility, decreased fatigue, improved concentration, and increased skeletal mass.[97–108]

COORDINATION, COMMUNICATION, AND DOCUMENTATION

Because of the rapidly changing needs of children with cancer, it is important that the physical therapist take the time to appropriately coordinate, communicate, and document all aspects of the physical therapy care. Physical therapy coordination, communication, and documentation require different approaches, depending on the location of services such as inpatient, outpatient, and school-based services. Regardless of the location of services, it is oftentimes challenging to coordinate appointment times around the child's nap, a procedure that requires sedation, and other medical appointments; to identify the child's blood counts before physical therapy; and to talk with the physician or nurse if changes are observed. It is imperative in order to maximize the physical therapy session that the physical therapist take responsibility in all three of these areas.

PATIENT/CLIENT INSTRUCTION

A primary role of the physical therapist is to provide information, to educate, to motivate and inspire, and to instruct patients, caregivers, and siblings. Fulfillment of this role is essential in optimizing the benefits of physical therapy services. Therefore, a responsibility of the physical therapist is to empower the child and family to take an active role in improving the child's health and well-being. The physical therapist must discuss with the child and family activities that are of interest to them and offer positive encouragement for the activities the child can do.

Physical therapy interventions must be age appropriate, and most importantly, meaningful to the child and caregiver. Physical therapy instruction for a child with cancer may consist of showing a child how to get out of bed for the first time after surgery; helping him or her learn how to properly use an assistive device, orthosis, or prosthesis; or helping him or her perform specific therapeutic exercises. The physical therapist may deliver the instructions orally or by manual guidance, visual demonstration, or written handouts. Through child, family, and therapist collaboration, ideas are generated on how the child and family can participate in activities together, with the goal of enhancing the child's performance, functioning, and, ultimately, quality of life.

PROCEDURAL INTERVENTION

Each intervention session between the therapist and a child with cancer is unique because of the complexity of the disease, the medical intervention, and the individual needs of the child and family. A physical therapy session may require modifications because the child has low blood counts, fever, pain, headache, vomiting, diarrhea, generalized fatigue, or drainage from a wound, or because the child has a specific request. Therefore, the physical therapist should be prepared to modify the intervention session on the basis of the child's needs at that moment, keeping in mind the short- and long-term goals of the therapy. Physical therapy interventions (Table 15.8) may include nonpharmacologic pain management, therapeutic exercise, aerobic exercise, gait training, or a fitting for an assistive device, wheelchair, orthosis, or prosthesis. Most importantly, the pediatric physical therapists must be creative.

TABLE 15.8 》》 》》 》 》 》 》 》 》

Suggested Physical Therapy Interventions

Area of Focus	Intervention	Frequency
Pain	Modalities	As needed
	Ice, heat, massage	
	Positioning	
	Assistive device	
	Neuropathic pain	
	Compression stocking	
	Deep pressure	
	Physician-prescribed medications	
	Gabapentin, Elavil, morphine	
Strengthening	Therapeutic exercises	3–5 days a week
	Functional activities	
	Stair climbing	
	Squats	
Stretching	Continuous passive motion machine	Five times a week to daily
	Splinting, bracing, orthotic	
	Manual stretching, self-stretching	
Aerobic/endurance	Walking	5 days a week
	Treadmill	
	Bike	
	Stair stepper	
	Swimming	
	Dancing	
Manual techniques	Manual guidance	As needed
	Neurodevelopmental treatment	
	Self-directed	
Motor learning principles	Knowledge of performance	As needed
	Knowledge of results	
	Blocked practice	
	Random practice	

CASE STUDIES

CASE STUDY 1

ACUTE LYMPHOBLASTIC LEUKEMIA
History

Three-year-old Emily presented to her pediatrician with excessive bruising, accompanied by reports of wanting her parents to carry her rather than having to walk. She has no significant past medical history and was performing all age-appropriate skills until 3 weeks ago. Her white blood cell count was high. Analysis of bone marrow aspirate and cerebrospinal fluid from a lumbar puncture showed an overproduction of blast cells and CNS involvement. Emily's disease was diagnosed as acute lymphoblastic leukemia, and she was referred to a hospital approximately 60 minutes from her hometown to receive treatment. She was enrolled on a standard risk protocol to receive combination chemotherapy (prednisone, dexamethasone, vincristine, daunorubicin, doxorubicin, L-asparaginase, methotrexate, cyclo phosphamide, and cytarabine). Chemotherapy will last approximately 2.5 years and be administered in four main phases: induction, CNS preven-

tive therapy, consolidation, and reinduction and maintenance therapy. Today Emily's blood counts were mildly low (WBC 4.6 [normal range, 4.9 to 12.9/mm^3]; RBC 3.2 [normal range, 3.90 to 5.30/mm^3]; Hbg 10.0 [normal range, 11.5 to 14.0]; platelet 98,000 [normal range, 190,000 to 490,000]) (St. Jude Children's Research Hospital normal blood value ranges for a 3 year-old child).

Emily lives at home with her mother, father, and two older brothers. She enjoys playing with her dolls, riding her bike, and going to the playground. She attended a preschool 2 hours a day, 3 days a week, before her diagnosis. Emily's mother works out of the home, and her father is an accountant. Emily's parents report that their daughter has not attended preschool in 8 weeks.

Emily was referred to the physical therapy department 3 weeks after her initial diagnosis, with the goal of increased functional mobility. Her parents were very concerned because Emily was not walking.

Physical Therapy Systems Review

Emily is bright and was very comfortable talking with the physical therapist when her father was holding her. She appeared fearful of movement. Her muscle tone appears within normal limits to mildly low. Vision, hearing, and sensation appear intact. She doesn't appear to have any pain while her father is holding her. She is mildly pale with a few healing bruises. Her respiratory rate and breathing pattern appear normal at rest.

Physical Therapy Tests and Measures

Emily presented with full active range of motion (AROM) in her neck, trunk, upper extremities, and lower extremities. Her strength was examined while she was playing with toys and was grossly 4 (0 to 5 scale). Emily tracked right/left/up/down.

She followed directions when spoken to at a normal voice level. Her sensation was within normal limits (WNL) as measured by light touch, and her muscle tone was WNL. Emily had no pain, as measured by the FLACC scale, when she was sitting and playing; however, when she was in a standing position, her FLACC pain score was 5, indicating pain in her lower extremities. Emily's skin color was mildly pale, and she presented with three large bruised areas, which were healing. Emily's skin around her central line was clean and dry. Emily presents with decreased endurance, as indicated by her increased work of breathing and increased heart and respiratory rates while she performed functional tasks such as transitioning from sitting to standing and ambulating.

Emily ambulated independently for 2 feet, slowly with a short step length, and then began to cry. Emily stood independently with her hand on a bench and cruised right and left for 3 feet. Emily transitioned from sitting on a bench to standing with moderate assistance and from standing to sitting on the floor by half-kneeling with her hand on her knees and then on the floor, with minimal assistance for balance. She crawled on her hands and knees for a distance of 4 feet independently. She would not attempt to ascend a step.

Physical Therapy Diagnosis

- Nociceptive pain caused by increased blast cell production in the bone marrow and arthralgia from high dose-methotrexate and intrathecal cytarabine
- Decreased strength from inactivity
- Decreased endurance from inactivity
- Decreased functional mobility due to pain, limited strength, and nausea
- Decreased participation in play and nonattendance at school

Physical Therapy Prognosis

Emily is expected to have a full recovery from her physical therapy diagnoses. After she receives chemotherapy for a few more weeks, she should have no more bone pain from her initial disease. Over the next 3 months, Emily will increase her strength and endurance so she can participate in family activities.

GOALS AS DETERMINED WITH EMILY AND HER FAMILY

- At 1 week, ambulate independently with a rolling walker
- At 4 weeks, ambulate independently without assistance; transition from ring sitting to standing independently; ascend and descend three steps with one hand on a rail

- At 6 weeks, ascend and descend three steps independently; jump up independently with both feet leaving the floor 1 inch
- Ongoing goals including family independently assisting Emily with the exercise program

Plan of Care

Emily will receive physical therapy three times a week for the first 2 weeks. She is scheduled to be an inpatient for a week while she receives chemotherapy. The frequency of her physical therapy will then be decreased to two times a week for 2 weeks, and then one time a week. As soon as Emily is ambulating independently and performing age-appropriate gross motor skills, she will receive physical therapy services on an as-needed basis only. The plan for physical therapy services with Emily will involve educating Emily and her family in the following areas: activities to regain function; normal development; resuming activities that are important to Emily and her family such as going to the park and riding their bikes together as a family; and future concerns such as the development of peripheral neuropathy or osteonecrosis. The physical therapist may find that Emily could benefit from a referral to occupation therapy to assist with fine motor skills or activities of daily living with a focus on age-appropriate developmental skills.

Physical Therapy Patient-Related Instruction

Activity: Ankle dorsiflexion passive range of motion and family instruction on signs and symptoms of peripheral neuropathy due to vincristine (foot drop, tripping, poor grip strength)—Frequency: Five times a week. Intensity: Mild stretch. Duration: Hold for 30 seconds.

Activity: Strengthening exercises—Frequency: Five times a week. Intensity: Fun, functional, strengthening activities such as squatting to pick up a toy off the ground; tossing a ball overhead, from the midchest region, and underhand; painting a picture while standing at the kitchen table, squatting to pick up a different color marker; and doing ankle pumps while listening to music. Duration: Throughout the day because she will not tolerate long periods of exercise at one time; therefore, three sets of 10 repetitions are recommended.

Activity: Ambulation with a walker—Frequency: When she needs to transition from one activity to another. Intensity: Short distances to start and build up. Duration: Throughout the day.

Activity: Aerobic exercise, tricycle riding—Frequency: 7 days a week. Intensity: Slow and controlled. Duration: 5 minutes to start and build up to 10 minutes. She should be wearing a helmet (Fig. 15.6).

Physical Therapy Procedural Intervention

The physical therapist will help Emily perform ankle dorsiflexion stretching and review procedures for ensuring proper alignment with Emily's parents. The therapist will encourage

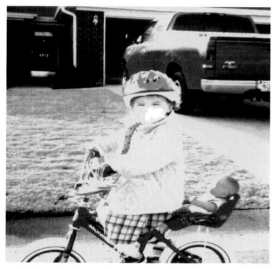

Figure 15.6 ▪ Emily playing outside on her bike.

Emily to play a game such as basketball that requires her to transition from standing to squatting to pick up the ball, walking over to the basket, and tossing the ball into the basket. This activity will assist Emily with her upper and lower extremity strength and ambulation skills. While Emily rides a tricycle, the therapist will monitor her heart rate with a pulse oximeter and visually observe her respiratory rate, skin color, and breathing pattern. During the physical therapy session, the therapist will be able to determine Emily's improvements in range of motion, strength, endurance, and functional mobility, and then make recommended suggestions to Emily and her family on how to modify her home or inpatient exercise program.

Episode of Care

Three months after Emily received the initial diagnosis of ALL, she met all her previously set goals. However, 1 month later, she developed peripheral neuropathy, as indicated by frequent tripping while she was walking and running. The physical therapy examination indicated that Emily had weak intrinsic musculature in her feet and hands and decreased active ankle dorsiflexion strength. Emily's doctors decreased her dose of vincristine to reduce the effects of the peripheral neuropathy, and the physical therapist provided Emily with bilateral solid ankle–foot orthoses to help prevent falls and to protect the alignment of her ankle structure. Emily continued to perform her ankle dorsiflexion stretching and strengthening exercises as previously recommended. Fourteen months after the diagnosis of ALL, she developed severe pain in her right foot. Emily's mother was very concerned because this was the initial symptom of ALL; however, it did not signal a return of leukemia, but was a symptom of avascular necrosis that had developed in her calcaneus. Her physician modified Emily's corticosteroid dose and recommended that she use her walker again for a few weeks. After 1 month, Emily no longer required the use of the walker to ambulate

and was pain free unless she ambulated for long distances. When Emily completed her medical intervention, she no longer needed to use an ankle–foot orthosis. Emily has osteopenia due to the effects of chemotherapy with methotrexate and corticosteroids. She is now in kindergarten, riding her bike, and playing with her friends without difficulty. Emily still runs more slowly and not as smoothly as her friends, but she is hopeful her running will improve.

CASE STUDY 2

OSTEOSARCOMA
History

John, a 14-year-old boy with no significant medical history, presented to his pediatrician with leg pain after a soccer injury. John's physician referred him to the physical therapy department for treatment of a left hamstring strain, three times a week for 6 weeks. After 2 weeks, the physical therapist noticed that John's condition was not improving and called the physician. The physician ordered a CT scan of John's left lower extremity; imaging results indicated a large mass. The physician then ordered a biopsy of the mass; on the basis of the results, he diagnosed John's condition as osteosarcoma of the left distal femur. John had no signs of metastatic disease. John lives in a large metropolitan city with a well-known children's hospital, where he is scheduled to begin 3 to 4 months of neoadjuvant chemotherapy (ifosfamide, carboplatin, and doxorubicin). John went to one session of physical therapy to review training on how to use forearm crutches for a non–weight-bearing left lower extremity. Previous physical therapy had consisted of training on use of axillary crutches and left knee AROM exercises. A central line was surgically placed. After 4 months of chemotherapy, John was re-evaluated by his orthopedic surgeon and oncologist. John, his family, and the doctors agreed that John would receive a limb-sparing procedure, specifically an expandable endoprosthesis because John is still growing. After the surgical procedure, the physician requested that the physical therapist provide John with a continuous passive motion (CPM) machine in the surgical recovery room. The physician also requested that physical therapy services start postoperative day 1 for functional mobility training, left knee ROM therapeutic exercises, and family education.

John's blood test results were within normal limits on postoperative day 1 (WBC 10.2 [normal range, 4.2 to 12.2/mm³]; RBC 4.75 [normal range, 4.50 to 5.30/mm³]; Hbg 14.2 [normal range, 12.5 to 16.5]; platelet 250,000 [normal range, 170,000 to 430,000]) (St. Jude Children's Research Hospital normal blood value ranges for a 16-year-old boy).

Social History

John lives at home with his mother and two younger brothers. He is in the eighth grade in school and enjoys playing soccer and basketball and motorcycle riding. John's mother has a full-time job outside the home, and he sees his father only once every few months.

Physical Therapy Systems Review

When the physical therapist arrived in John's hospital room, he was in bed. A Foley catheter, central venous line, and pain pump had been placed. He was receiving an analgesic through an epidural catheter in his lumbar spinal area to assist with lower extremity pain management. His mom and both brothers were present. John was alert and oriented, but reluctant to begin physical therapy.

Physical Therapy Tests and Measures

John presented with full active range of motion in his neck, upper extremities, and right lower extremity. John's CPM had been set at 0 to 45 degrees of motion after his surgery the previous night, and the settings had not been changed. The therapist removed John's left leg from the CPM and performed gentle passive range-of-motion exercises; the left hip and ankle demonstrated a full range of motion and 50 degrees of left knee flexion. He had decreased trunk mobility due to the placement of his epidural catheter. His strength was 5/5 as measured by manual muscle testing in bilateral upper extremities and right lower extremity. John's strength in the left lower extremity was limited due to pain and fear of movement. With moderate assistance for support of John's left lower extremity, he flexed his left hip to 90 degrees and actively dorsiflexed his left ankle to the neutral position.

He followed directions spoken at a normal voice level. He had lost sensation to light touch in his bilateral lower extremities due to the effects of the epidural. John reported pain in his left lower extremity as a 3 on the 0 to 10 self-report scale. His incision was covered with dressings.

John required minimal assistance to protect the epidural while transferring from a supine to sitting position in his bed. He required maximum assistance for support of his left lower extremity to scoot to the edge of the bed. The physical therapist placed a hinged knee brace, which was locked in extension, on John's left lower extremity before John got out of bed. With the brace locked in full-knee extension, John then transferred from sitting on the edge of bed to standing by using his forearm crutches. He required minimal assistance for balance and maximum assistance for support of his left lower-extremity to maintain non–weight bearing. John ambulated 5 feet to a chair in his room and transferred from standing to sitting with maximum assistance for support of his left lower extremity.

Physical Therapy Diagnosis

- Nociceptive pain from the surgical site
- Neuropathic pain from nerve damage during surgery
- Decreased strength from change in alignment of the muscle pull
- Increased energy expenditure with functional activities such as walking

- Decreased functional mobility due to pain, limited strength and balance, and nausea from the anesthesia
- Decreased participation in school, sports, and socialization with friends

Physical Therapy Prognosis

John's strength and functional mobility are expected to improve. He may continue to lack full-knee extension secondary to the changes in the biomechanical alignment of his knee structure.

GOALS AS DETERMINED WITH JOHN AND HIS FAMILY

John will transfer from a supine position to sitting independently (the same day his epidural catheter is removed). John will transfer from a sitting to a standing position with forearm crutches and non–weight bearing on the left lower extremity, with stand-by assistance (3 days). John and his mother are able to independently use the CPM and don and doff John's lower extremity brace. John will independently ambulate 50 feet with forearm crutches and non–weight bearing on left lower extremity (4 days). John will ascend and descend 12 steps with one hand on the rail and one hand on a forearm crutch, non–weight bearing on left lower extremity with contact guard assistance for safety (6 days).

Plan of Care

John will receive physical therapy daily while in the inpatient unit. After he is transferred home, he will return for outpatient physical therapy five times a week for 1 month, and then be followed once a week to make modifications to his home exercise program.

Physical Therapy Client-Related Instruction

The physical therapist will provide John and his mother with instruction on the use of his equipment, exercises, and safety.

Activity: Instruction on use of the CPM and how to increase the range of motion by 10 degrees each day

Activity: Instruction on donning and doffing the lower extremity brace, which John is to wear when getting out of bed and during ambulation

Activity: Instruction on active left lower extremity range-of-motion exercises

Activity: Transfer training

Activity: Gait training on non–weight-bearing left lower extremity

Physical Therapy Procedural Intervention

The physical therapist will provide John with manual guidance, tactile cues, and oral instruction to achieve his goals.

Episode of Care

John was discharged from the hospital postoperative day 5. He began outpatient physical therapy 2 days after his discharge from the hospital. He reported pain as a 6 on the 0 to 10 numerical scale; therefore, the physical therapist called the pain team working with John, and the team increased his short-acting pain medication. He delayed resumption of chemotherapy until 3 weeks after surgery to allow his surgical incision time to heal. Therefore, the physical therapist had to check the computer during each session to check John's blood counts to determine the appropriate physical therapy intervention for that day. For example, if John's platelet count was less than 50,000, he would not use weights for strength training. Instead, he would perform active range-of-motion exercises for stretching his left knee.

After 6 weeks of outpatient physical therapy that included strengthening and stretching exercises, John achieved 100 degrees of passive left knee flexion and 92 degrees of active left knee flexion. He had a knee extension lag of approximately 20 degrees. John's full active range of motion in his left knee was 20 to 92 degrees of knee flexion.

His left lower extremity strength was hip flexion/extension/abduction/adduction 5/5, hip internal rotation 4−/5, hip external rotation 4/5, knee extension 3+/5, knee flexion 4−/5, and ankle dorsiflexion/plantar flexion/inversion/eversion 5/5. John's orthopedist approved full weight bearing on his left lower extremity. Therefore, gait training and exercises to help John shift onto the left lower extremity were added to the physical therapy sessions, which continued to be focused on range of motion, strength, and weight.

John used the CPM for 6 weeks at night only. When he was not performing his exercises during the day, he wore his knee brace unlocked to continue to work on increasing his knee flexion range of motion. After he completed the use of the CPM, John wore his knee brace at night locked in full extension to assist him in preventing the development of a knee flexion contracture because he still did not have full active knee extension range of motion.

After 1 month of physical therapy five times a week, John's sessions were decreased to one time a week because he was independent in his exercise program and showing signs of progress. He had achieved active knee flexion to 110 degrees and continued to lack 10 degrees of active knee extension to achieve full extension. He ambulated with a mild lateral trunk deviation to the left; however, with oral cues, he could ambulate with his trunk in the midline position. He could ascend and descend 12 stairs, alternating feet to step slowly with his hand on the rail for minimal support. John now wore the lower extremity brace only to sleep in at night, and he wore a small knee brace during the day to provide tactile cues and comfort to his left lower extremity.

Eight months after John's surgery, he completed his chemotherapy. John and the physical therapist noticed he had increased trunk flexion to the left. John had grown over the past 8 months. As a result, his prosthesis needed to be lengthened. After it was lengthened, John's left lower extremity was sore, and he required gentle knee range-of-motion exercises and the use of crutches for 2 days. He then returned to his normal prelengthening functioning.

Twelve months after John's surgery, he came to the physical therapist once every 3 months for check-up visits. He had returned to school and was planning to swim on his high-school swim team.

REFERENCES

1. Centers for Disease Control. Cancer Prevention and Control. Available at: http://www.cdc.gov/cancer. Accessed January, 2005.
2. Ries LAG, Eisner MP, Kosary CL, et al. SEER Cancer Statistics Review, 1975–2001. Available at: http://www.seer.cancer.gov/csr/1975_2001/. Accessed January, 2005.
3. Landier W, Ghatia S, Eshelman DA, et al. Development of risk-based guidelines for pediatric cancer survivors: the children's oncology group long-term follow-up guidelines from the children's oncology group late effects committee and nursing discipline. J Clin Onocol 2004;22:4979–4990.
4. Jemal A, Murray T, Samuels A, et al. Cancer Statistics, 2003. CA Cancer J Clin 2003;53:5–26.
5. American Cancer Society. Available at: www.cancer.org. Accessed 2005.
6. Smith MA, Ries LAG, Gurney JG, et al., eds. Cancer Incidence and Survival Among Children and Adolescents: United States SEER Program 1975–1995. NIH Pub No 99-4649. Bethesda, MD: National Cancer Institute, SEER Program, 1999:17–34.
7. McBride ML. Childhood cancer and environmental contaminants. Can J Public Health 1998;89(Suppl 1):S53–S62, S58–S68.
8. Muts-Homshma S, Muller H, Geracost J. Klinefelter's syndrome and acute non-lymphocytic leukemia. Blut 1981;44:15.
9. Shearer P, Parham D, Kovnar E, et al. Neurofibromatosis type I and malignancy: review of 32 pediatric cases treated at a single institution. Med Pediatr Oncol 1994;22:78–83.
10. Woods W, Roloff J, Lukens J, et al. The occurrence of leukemia in patients with Schwachman syndrome. J Pediatr 1981;99:425.
11. Margolin JF, Steuber CP, Poplack DG. Acute lymphoblastic leukemia. In: Pizzo PA, Poplack DG, eds. Principles and Practices of Pediatric Oncology. 4th Ed. Philadelphia: Lippincott Williams & Wilkins, 2002:489–544.
12. Golub TR, Arceci RJ. Acute myelogenous leukemia. In: Pizzo PA, Poplack DG, eds. Principles and Practices of Pediatric Oncology. 4th Ed. Philadelphia: Lippincott Williams & Wilkins, 2002:545–590.
13. Strother DR, Pollack IF, Fisher PG, et al. Tumors of the central nervous system. In: Pizzo PA, Poplack DG, eds. Principles and Practices of Pediatric Oncology. 4th Ed. Philadelphia: Lippincott Williams & Wilkins, 2002:751–824.
14. Gurney JG, Smith MA, Bunin GR. CNS and miscellaneous intracranial and intraspinal neoplasms. In: Ries LAG, Smith MA, Gurney JG, et al., eds. Cancer Incidence and Survival Among Children and Adolescents: United States SEER Program 1975–1995. NIH Pub No 99-4649. Bethesda, MD: National Cancer Institute, SEER Program, 1999:51–63.
15. St. Jude Children's Research Hospital. Available at: www.stjude.org. Accessed January, 2005.
16. Thapar K, Taylor MD, Laws ER, et al. Brain edema, increased intracranial pressure, and vascular effects of human brain tumors. In: Kaye AH, Laws ER, eds. Brain Tumors: An Encyclopedic Approach. London: Churchill Livingston, 2001:189–215.
17. American Brain Tumor Association. Available at: www.abta.org. Accessed January, 2005.
18. Percy CL, Smith MA, Linet M, et al. Lymphomas and reticuloendothelial neoplasms. In: Ries LAG, Smith MA, Gurney JG, et al., eds. Cancer Incidence and Survival Among Children and Adolescents: United States SEER Program 1975–1995. NIH Pub No 99-4649. Bethesda, MD: National Cancer Institute, SEER Program, 1999:35–49.
19. Hudson MM, Donaldson SS. Hodgkin's disease. In: Pizzo PA, Poplack DG, eds. Principles and Practices of Pediatric Oncology. 4th Ed. Philadelphia: Lippincott Williams & Wilkins, 2002:637–660.

20. Magrath IT. Malignant non-Hodgkin's lymphomas in children. In: Pizzo PA, Poplack DG, eds. Principles and Practices of Pediatric Oncology. 4th Ed. Philadelphia: Lippincott Williams & Wilkins, 2000:661–706.

21. Brodeur BM, Maris JM. Neuroblastoma. In: Pizzo PA, Poplack DG, eds. Principles and Practices of Pediatric Oncology. 4th Ed. Philadelphia: Lippincott Williams & Wilkins, 2002:895–938.

22. Goodman GT, Gurney JG, Smith MA, et al. Sympathetic nervous system tumors. In: Ries LAG, Smith MA, Gurney JG, et al., eds. Cancer Incidence and Survival Among Children and Adolescents: United States SEER Program 1975–1995. NIH Pub No 99-4649. Bethesda, MD: National Cancer Institute, SEER Program, 1999:65–72.

23. Wexler LH, Crist WM, Helman LJ. Rhabdomyosarcoma and the undifferentiated sarcomas. In: Pizzo PA, Poplack DG, eds. Principles and Practices of Pediatric Oncology. 4th ed. Philadelphia: Lippincott Williams & Wilkins, 2002:939–972.

24. Hosalkar HS, Dormans JP. Limb sparing for pediatric musculoskeletal tumors. Pediatr Blood Cancer 2004;42:295–310.

25. Gurney JG, Swensen AR, Bulterys M. Malignant bone tumors. In: Ries LAG, Smith MA, Gurney JG, et al., eds. Cancer Incidence and Survival Among Children and Adolescents: United States SEER Program 1975–1995. NIH Pub No 99-4649. Bethesda, MD: National Cancer Institute, SEER Program, 1999:99–110.

26. Link MP, Gebhardt MC, Meyers PA. Osteosarcoma. In: Pizzo PA, Poplack DG, eds. Principles and Practices of Pediatric Oncology. 4th Ed. Philadelphia: Lippincott Williams & Wilkins, 2002:1051–1090.

27. Ginsberg JP, Woo SY, Johnson ME, et al. Ewings sarcoma family of tumors: Ewings sarcoma of bone and soft tissue and the peripheral primitive neuroectodermal tumors. In: Pizzo PA, Poplack DG, eds. Principles and Practices of Pediatric Oncology. 4th Ed. Philadelphia: Lippincott Williams & Wilkins, 2002:973–1016.

28. Gurney JG, Young JL, Roffers SD, et al. Soft tissue sarcomas. In: Ries LAG, Smith MA, Gurney JG, et al., eds. Cancer Incidence and Survival Among Children and Adolescents: United States SEER Program 1975–1995. NIH Publication No. 99-4649. Bethesda, MD, National Cancer Institute, SEER Program, 1999:111–124.

29. Young JL, Smith MA, Roffers SD, et al. Retinoblastoma. In: Ries LAG, Smith MA, Gurney JG, et al. eds Cancer Incidence and Survival Among Children and Adolescents: United States SEER Program 1975–1995. NIH Publication No. 99-4649. Bethesda, MD, National Cancer Institute, SEER Program, 1999:73–78.

30. Hurwitz RL, Shields CL, Shields JA, et al. Retinoblastoma. In: Pizzo PA, Poplack DG, eds. Principles and Practices of Pediatric Oncology. 4th Ed. Philadelphia: Lippincott Williams & Wilkins, 2002:825–846.

31. Bernstein L, Linet M, Smith MA, et al. Renal tumors. In: Ries LAG, Smith MA, Gurney JG, et al., eds. Cancer Incidence and Survival Among Children and Adolescents: United States SEER Program 1975–1995. NIH Publication No. 99-4649. Bethesda, MD, National Cancer Institute, SEER Program, 1999:79–90.

32. Grundy PE, Green DM, Coppes MJ. Renal tumors. In: Pizzo PA, Poplack DG, eds. Principles and Practices of Pediatric Oncology. 4th Ed. Philadelphia: Lippincott Williams & Wilkins, 2002:865–894.

33. Ghasemi Z, Martin T. Laboratory values in the intensive care unit. Newsletter of the acute care/hospital clinical practice section. American Physical Therapy Association, Alexandria, VA. 1995.

34. Balis FM, Holcenberg JS, Blaney SM. General principles of chemotherapy. In: Pizzo PA, Poplack DG, eds. Principles and Practices of Pediatric Oncology. 4th ed. Philadelphia: Lippincott Williams & Wilkins, 2002:237–308.

35. Vainionpaa L, Kovala T, Tolonen U, et al. Vincristine therapy for children with acute lymphoblastic leukemia impairs conduction in the entire peripheral nerve. Pediatr Neurol 1995;13:314–318.

36. Mattano LA, Sather HN, Trigg ME, et al. Osteonecrosis as a complication of treating acute lymphoblastic leukemia in children: a report from the Children's Cancer Group. J Clin Oncol 2000;18(18):3262–3272.

37. Kaste SC, Jones-Wallace D, Rose SR, et al. Bone mineral decrements in survivors of childhood acute lymphoblastic leukemia: frequency of occurrence and risk factors for their development. Leukemia 2001;15:728–734.

38. Galea V, Wright MJ, Barr RD. Measurement of balance in survivors of acute lymphoblastic leukemia in childhood. Gait Posture 2004;19:1–10.

39. Lehtinen SS, Huuskonen UE, Harla-Saari AH, et al. Motor nervous system impairment persists in long-term survivors of childhood acute lymphoblastic leukemia. Cancer 2002;94:2466–2473.

40. Wright MJ, Halton JM, Martin RF, et al. Long-term gross motor performance following treatment for acute lymphoblastic leukemia. Med Pediatr Oncol 1998;31:86–90.

41. Wright MJ, Hanna SE, Halton JM, et al. Maintenance of ankle range of motion in children treated for acute lymphoblastic leukemia. Pediatr Phys Ther 2003;15:146–152.

42. Lesink PG, Ciesielski KT, Hart TL, et al. Evidence for cerebellar-frontal subsystem changes in children treated with intrathecal chemotherapy for leukemia: enhanced data analysis using an effect size model. Arch Neurol 1998;55:1561–1568.

43. Langer T, Martus P, Ottensmeier H, et al. CNS late-effects after ALL therapy in childhood. Part III: neuropsychological performance in long-term survivors of childhood ALL: impairments of concentration, attention, and memory. Med Pediatr Oncol 2002;38:320–328.

44. Reimers TS, Ehrenfels S, Mortensen EL, et al. Cognitive deficits in long-term survivors of childhood brain tumors: identification of predictive factors. Med Pediatr Oncol 2003;40:26–34.

45. Fletcher BD. Effects of pediatric cancer therapy on the musculoskeletal system. Pediatr Radiol 1997;27:623–636.

46. Vainonpaa L. Clinical neurological findings of children with acute lymphoblastic leukemia at diagnosis and during treatment. Eur Pediatr 1993;152:115–119.

47. Yonemoto T, Tatezaki S, Ishii T, et al. Marriage and fertility in long-term survivors of high grade osteosarcoma. Am J Clin Oncol 2003;26:513–516.

48. Bradley WG, Lassman LP, Pearce GW, et al. The neuromyopathy of vincristine in man clinical, electrophysiological and pathological studies. J Neurol Sci 1970;10:107–131.

49. Wright MJ, Halton JM, Barr RD. Limitation of ankle range of motion in survivors of acute lymphoblastic leukemia in childhood: a cross-sectional study. Med Pediatr Oncol 1999;32:279–282.

50. Tanner KD, Reichling DB, Gear RW, et al. Altered temporal pattern of evoked afferent activity in a rat model of vincristine-induced painful peripheral neuropathy. Neuroscience 2003;118:809–817.

51. Jew R, ed. The Children's Hospital of Philadelphia Formulary 2001–2002. Hudson, OH: Lexi-Comp Inc.

52. Gocha Marchese V, Chiarello LV, Lange BJ. Strength and functional mobility in children with acute lymphoblastic leukemia. Med Pediatr Oncol 2003;40:230–232.

53. Wheeler DL, Vander Griend RA, Wronski TJ, et al. The short- and long-term effects of methotrexate on the skeleton. Bone 1995;16:215–221.

54. Harten G, Stephani U, Henze G, et al. Slight impairment of psychomotor skills in children after treatment of acute lymphoblastic leukemia. Eur J Pediatr 1984;142:189–197.

55. Mattano L. The skeletal remains: porosis and necrosis of bone in the marrow transplantation setting. Pediatr Transplant 2003;7:71–75.

56. Krasin MJ, Rodriguez-Galindo C, Billups CA, et al. Definitive irradiation in multidisciplinary management of localized Ewings sarcoma family of tumors in pediatric patients: outcome and prognostic factors. Int J Radiat Oncol Biol Phys 2004;60: 830–838.

57. Oberlin O, Rey A, Anderson J, et al. Treatment of orbital rhabdomyosarcoma: survival and late effects of treatment-results of an international workshop. J Clin Oncol 2001;19: 197–204.

58. Davis AM, O'Sullivan B, Turcotte BR, et al. Function and health status outcomes in a randomized trial comparing preoperative and postoperative radiotherapy in extremity soft tissue sarcoma. J Clin Oncol 2002;20:4472–4477.

59. Grossi M. Management and long-term complications of pediatric cancer. Pediatr Clin N Am 1998;45:1637–1651.

60. Cooper JS, Fu K, Marks J, et al. Late effects of radiation therapy in the head and neck region. Int J Radiat Oncol Biol Phys 1995;31:1141.

61. Jentzsch K, Ginder H, Cramer H, et al. Leg function after radiotherapy for Ewings sarcoma. Cancer 1981;47:1267–1278.

62. Williams KY, Cox RS, Donaldson SS. Radiation induced height impairment in pediatric Hodgkin's disease. Int J Radiat Oncol Biol Phys 1993;28:85–92.

63. Nysom K, Holm K, Fleischer Michaelsen K, et al. Bone mass after allogeneic BMT for childhood leukaemia or lymphoma. Bone Marrow Transplant 2000;25:191–196.

64. Neel MD, Wilkins RM, Rao BN, et al. Early multicenter experience with a noninvasive expandable prosthesis. Clin Orthop Rel Res 2003;415:72–81.

65. Rougraff BT, Simon MA, Kneisl JS, et al. Limb salvage compared with amputation for osteosarcoma of the distal end of the femur. A long-term oncological, functional, and quality-of-life study. J Bone Joint Surg Am 1994;76:649–656.

66. Tunn PU, Schmidt-Peter P, Pomraenke D, et al. Osteosarcoma in children. Clin Orthop Rel Res 2004;421:212–217.

67. Nagarajan R, Neglia JP, Clohisy DR, et al. Limb salvage and amputation in survivors of pediatric lower-extremity bone tumors: what are the long-term implications? J Clin Oncol 2002;20:4493–4501.

68. Renard AJ, Veth RP, Scchreuder HWB, et al. Function and complications after ablative and limb-salvage therapy in lower extremity sarcoma of bone. J Surg Oncol 2000;73:198–205.

69. Jeys LM, Grimer RJ, Carter SR, et al. Risk of amputation following limb salvage surgery with endoprosthetic replacement, in a consecutive series of 1261 patients. Int Orthop 2003; 27:160–163.

70. McClenaghan BA, Krajbich JI, Prone AM, et al. Comparative assessment of gait after limb-salvage procedure. J Bone Joint Surg Am 1989;71:1178–1182.

71. Fuchs B, Sims FH. Rotationplasty about the knee: surgical technique and anatomical considerations. Clin Anat 2004;17: 345–353.

72. Fuchs B, Kotajarvi BR, Kaufman KR, et al. Functional outcome of patients with rotationplasty about the knee. Clin Orthop Rel Res 2003;415:52–58.

73. Veenstra KM, Sprangers MAG, Van Der Eyken JW, et al. Quality of life in survivors with Van Ness-Borggreve rotationplasty after bone tumour resection. J Surg Oncol 2000;73: 192–197.

74. Hillman A, Hoffman C, Gosheger G, et al. Malignant tumor of the distal part of the femur or the proximal part of the tibia: endoprosthetic replacement or rotationplasty: functional outcome and quality-of-life measurements. J Bone Joint Surg 1999;81:462–468.

75. Horwitz EM. Bone marrow transplantation. In: Steen G, Mirro J, eds. Childhood Cancer: A Handbook from St. Jude Children's Research Hospital. Cambridge, MA: Perseus Publishing, 2000:155–165.

76. Bain LJ. A Parent's Guide to Childhood Cancer. The Children's Hospital of Philadelphia. New York: Dell Publishing, 1995:89–100.

77. World Health Organization. International Classification of Functioning, Disability, and Health. Available at: http://www.who.int/classifications/icf/en/. Accessed January, 2005.

78. Schechter NL, Berde CB, Yaster M. Pain in Infants, Children, and Adolescents. 2nd Ed. Philadelphia: Lippincott Williams & Wilkins, 2003.

79. Jensen MP, Karoly P, Braver S. The measurement of clinical pain intensity: a comparison of six methods. Pain 1986;27;117–126.

80. Wong DL, Hockenberry-Eaton M, Wilson D, et al. Wong's Essentials of Pediatric Nursing. 6th Ed. St. Louis: Mosby, 2001.

81. Jackson AS, Coleman AE. Validation of distance run tests for elementary school children. Res Q 1976;47:86–94.

82. Steele B. Timed walking tests of exercise capacity in chronic cardiopulmonary illness. J Cardiopulm Rehabil 1996;16: 25–33.

83. Health Related Physical Fitness: Test Manual. Reston, VA: American Alliance for Health, Physical Education, Recreation and Dance, 1980.

84. Butler P, Engelbrecht M, Major RE, et al. Physiological cost index of walking for normal children and its use as an indicator of physical handicap. Dev Med Child Neurol 1984;26: 607–612.

85. Nene AV. Physiological cost index of walking in able-bodied adolescents and adults. 1993;7:319–326.

86. Chin T, Sawamura S, Fujita H, et al. The efficacy of physiological cost index (PCI) measurement of a subject walking with an Intelligent Prosthesis. Prosthet Orthot Int 1999;23:45–49.

87. Marchese VG, Ogle S, Womer RB, et al. An examination of outcome measures to assess functional mobility in childhood survivors of osteosarcoma. Pediatr Blood Cancer 2004;42:41–45.

88. Grant S, Aitchison T, Henderson E, et al. A comparison of the reproducibility and the sensitivity to change of visual analogue scales, Borg scales, and Likert scales in normal subjects during submaximal exercise. Chest 1999;116:1208–1217.

89. Habib Z, Westcott S. Assessment of anthropometric factors on balance tests in children. Pediatr Phys Ther 1998;10:101–108.

90. Zaino CA, Gocha Marchese V, Westcott SL. Timed up and down stairs test: preliminary reliability and validity of a new measure of functional mobility. Pediatr Phys Ther 2004; 16:90–98.

91. Varni JW, Seid M, Kurtin PS. Reliability and validity of the pediatric quality of life inventory version 4.0 generic core scales in healthy and patient populations. Med Care 2001;39:800–812.

92. Ware JE, Snow KK, Kosinski M, et al. SF-36 Health Survey Manual and Interpretation Guide. Lincoln, NE: Quality Metric Inc., 2000.

93. Eiser C, Vance YH. Implications of cancer for school attendance and behavior. Med Pediatr Oncol 2002;38:317–319.

94. Guide to physical therapist practice. 2nd ed. Phys Ther 2001; 81:9–744.

95. Marchese VG, Chiarello LA. Relationships between specific measures of body function, activity, and participation in children with acute lymphoblastic leukemia. Rehabil Oncol 2004; 22:5–9.

96. Marchese VG, Chiarello LA, Lange BJ. Effects of physical therapy intervention for children with acute lymphoblastic leukemia. Pediatr Blood Cancer 2004;42:127–133.

97. Dimeo FC, Tilmann, MHM, Bertz H, et al. Aerobic exercise in the rehabilitation of cancer patients after high dose chemotherapy and autologous peripheral stem cell transplantation. Cancer 1997;79:1717–1722.

98. Dimeo FC, Stieglitz RD, Novelli-Fischer U, et al. Effects of physical activity on the fatigue and psychological status of cancer patients during chemotherapy. Cancer 1999;85:2273–2277.

99. Dimeo FC, Fetscher S, Lange W, et al. Effects of aerobic exercise on the physical performance and incidence of treatment-related complication after high-dose chemotherapy. Blood 1997;90:3390–3394.

100. Winningham ML, MacVicar MG, Bondoc M, et al. Effects of aerobic exercise on body weight and composition in patients with breast cancer on adjuvant chemotherapy. Oncol Nurs Forum 1989;16:683–689.

101. MacVigar MG, Winningham ML, Nickel JL. Effects of aerobic interval training on cancer patients' functional capacity. Nurs Res 1989;38:348–351.

102. Young-McCaughan S, Sexton D. A retrospective investigation of the relationship between aerobic exercise and quality of life in women with breast cancer. Oncol Nurs Forum 1991;18:751–757.

103. Courneya KS, Keats MR, Turner AR. Physical exercise and quality of life in cancer patients following high dose chemotherapy and autologous bone marrow transplantation. Psychooncology 2000;9:127–136.

104. Courneya KS, Friedenreich CM, Sela RA, et al. The group psychotherapy and home-based physical exercise (group-hope) trial in cancer survivors: physical fitness and quality of life outcomes. Psychooncology 2003;12:357–374.

105. Hayes S, Davies PSW, Parker T, et al. Quality of life changes following peripheral blood stem cell transplantation and participation in a mixed-type, moderate-intensity, exercise program. Bone Marrow Transplant 2004;33:553–558.

106. Hayes S, Davies PSW, Parker T, et al. Total energy expenditure and body composition changes following peripheral blood stem cell transplantation and participation in an exercise program. Bone Marrow Transplant 2003;31:331–338.

107. Mock V, Burke MB, Sheehan P, et al. A nursing rehabilitation program for women with breast cancer receiving adjuvant chemotherapy. Oncol Nurs Forum 1994;21:899–907.

108. Courneya KS, Friedenreich CM. Relationships between exercise during treatment and current quality of life among survivors of breast cancer. J Psychosoc Oncol 1997;15:35–56.

16

Rehabilitation of the Child with Burns

Suzanne F. Migliore

The purpose of this chapter is to provide a basic description of pediatric burn care and to discuss the therapist's role in providing interventions for a child with a thermal injury—from the acute phase through the rehabilitation phase.

The examinations and interventions for children with thermal injuries are unique. Certainly, the treatment that is appropriate for adults with burn injuries is not necessarily applicable to children with these same injuries and vice versa. Moreover, the treatment for a 9-month-old baby may differ from that for a 3-year-old child, which, in turn, may be different from the approach used for a 10-year-old child. The information presented will be applicable for the pediatric physical therapist across the continuum of care.

The role of the therapist is broadly addressed. The specific role of the therapist is defined, in part, by the individual setting and also may be dependent on the particular facility's medical and surgical techniques and approach.

Epidemiology

According to the National Center for Health Statistics, trauma accounts for 43% of all deaths from ages 1 through 4, 48% of all deaths from ages 5 through 14, and 62% of all deaths from ages 15 through 24. According to the American Burn Association (ABA), over 1.1 million burn injuries occur yearly that require medical attention. Approximately 50,000 of these injuries require hospitalization and 25,000 require burn unit admissions. Each year over 4500 of these people die.[1] According to the National SAFE KIDS Campaign, the fire and burn injury death rate among children ages 14 and under declined 63% from 1987 to 2001.[2]

The Centers for Disease Control and Prevention (CDC) tracks intentional and unintentional injuries for all age ranges and all injury types. In 2002, fire/burn injuries ranked third as a cause of unintentional deaths for the age ranges 1 to 4, 5 to 9, and 10 to 14; fourth as a cause for the age range less than 1 year; and seventh for the age range 15 to 24. Fire/burn injuries rank anywhere from fifth through 10th for violence-related injury deaths (abuse/homicide) for children under the age of 14. The CDC also reported that unintentional fire/burn injuries accounted for over 150,000 injuries in 2002 for children under the age of 18.[3] Table 16.1 gives a summary of fire/burn injuries by age group.

Etiology

There are numerous causes of burns. They include thermal, which are attributed to residential fires; automobile accidents; playing with matches; improper handling of firecrackers; and scalds caused by kitchen or bathroom accidents. Chemical burns occur due to contact, ingestion, inhalation, or injection of acids, alkalis, or vesicants. Electrical burns happen when there is contact with faulty electrical wiring, electrical cords, or high-voltage power lines.[4]

The mechanism of thermal injury may most closely correlate to the child's age. For example, toddlers will often sustain a scald burn due to pulling hot liquids off of surfaces (e.g., boiling water off of a stove, hot tea off of a table); they also sustain unintentional scald burns from bathtub accidents, where the home's water heater temperature is set too high.

A tap water temperature of 140°F will cause a scald burn in under 5 seconds; at 150°F it would take only 1.5 seconds.[5] Examples of household product temperatures include percolated coffee at 180°F and hot grease or hot oil at approximately 400°F. This age group is also at risk for electrical burns due to putting objects into uncovered electrical outlets or by chewing on wires leading to electrical products. Flame burns from playing with matches and contact burns due to touching hot objects (iron/stove/curling irons) happen with the school-age group. As children grow and become more adventurous, the mechanism of burn injury correlates to the risks these children and adolescents

take. The mechanisms of injury correlating to these age groups include improper handling of fireworks and experimenting with gasoline and other chemicals.[6] Overall, a greater number of boys than girls are burned in all age groups.[3]

Young children (especially those younger than 4) have a higher mortality rate than young adults. As one might expect, mortality increases with severity (extent and depth) of injury and concomitant injuries such as inhalation, neurologic, or orthopedic injuries. The reasons for higher mortality rates were suspected to be due to decreased physiologic reserve, thinner skin, difficulties with vascular access, and difficulty with fluid management. Sheriden et al. looked at mortality rates among children who sustained burns from 1974 to 1980 and 1991 to 1997. They found that survival rates have improved significantly for children, even those with large total body surface area (TBSA) burns.[7]

CHILD ABUSE AND NEGLECT

According to the National Clearinghouse on Child Abuse and Neglect, over 896,000 children suffered some form of abuse or neglect in 2002. Physical injuries accounted for greater than 50% of these injuries, inclusive of intentional burns (e.g., immersion, iron) and those sustained due to neglect (e.g., pulling pot off of a stove, unmonitored bathtub). Boys sustained more overall abuse or neglect than girls, although overall the number per 1000 children was down significantly from 1990. Those children of American Indian, Alaskan, or African American decent had higher rates of being abused or neglected. The perpetrators of the abuse were greater than 80% of the time parents, followed by other relatives, unmarried partners, and others.[8]

Up to 8% of infants and children admitted to the hospital for burns are victims of abuse. Suspicion of abuse arises when the injuries are non–splash related, linear demarcations (e.g., glove/stocking distribution), or burns to the buttocks and no other portion of the body (i.e., dipped into hot water). Contact burns with symmetric shapes may also signify intentional burns (e.g., circular lines consistent

TABLE 16.1 ►►►►►►►►►►►►►►►

Fire/Burn Injuries by Age Group

	Age Groups				
Type of Injury	**<1 Year of age**	**1–4 Years of age**	**5–9 Years of age**	**10–14 Years of age**	**15–18 Years of age**
Unintentional fatal (2002)	40	226	153	101	187
Unintentional nonfatal (2003)	11,306	58,931	22,760	17,918	31,571
Intentional fatal (2002)	1	15	11	9	<15
Intentional nonfatal (2003)	287	629	563	305	1637

Source: National Center for Injury Prevention and Control. WISQUARS. 2002 United States Unintentional and Intentional Injuries. Available at: www.cdc.gov. Accessed January 2005.

with a stovetop burner). Children with inflicted burns are more likely to have burns on both hands, feet, and legs, and there may be a higher TBSA involved.[9] In the hospital setting, suspicion of abuse or neglect is investigated by an interdisciplinary team including physicians, nurses, social work, psychology, and physical therapy. Factors in a child's case that may indicate abuse or neglect include:

- Child is brought for treatment by an unrelated adult
- An unexplained delay of 12 or more hours in seeking treatment
- Inappropriate parental affect: Parents appear inattentive to child; lack empathy; may appear to be under the influence of alcohol or drugs
- Attribution of guilt for injury to the patient's sibling or to the patient
- An injury that is inconsistent with the description of the injury
- History of injury that is inconsistent with the developmental capacity of the patient
- History of accidental or nonaccidental injury to the patient or siblings
- History of failure to thrive
- Historical accounts of the injury that differ with each interview
- Injury localized to genitalia, perineum, and buttocks (because of frequency with which injury occurs related to toilet training)
- "Mirror image" injury of extremities (Fig. 16.1)
- Inappropriate affect of child; child appears withdrawn with flattened affect
- Evidence of unrelated injuries, for example, scars, bruises, welts, fractures

All states have laws requiring that certain professionals, including physical therapists and occupational therapists, report suspected cases of child abuse. The physical therapist will aid in the determination of abuse by doing a thorough examination and evaluation of the burn mechanism, size, location, and depth of injury.

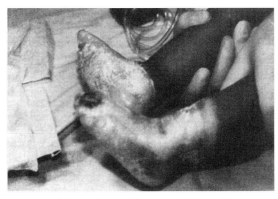

Figure 16.1 ▪ "Mirror image" burns to bilateral feet and lower legs, a pattern consistent with abuse via dunking in hot water.

 Prevention

Because of the high incidence and common pattern of distribution of types of burn injuries among children of various age groups, prevention efforts have been directed toward educating parents, children, and others as to how these injuries occur and how they can be prevented. The National SAFE KIDS Campaign was the first (and only) national organization dedicated to prevention of childhood injuries. It was founded in 1988 and has over 600 SAFE KIDS coalitions and chapters across the United States. Injury prevention efforts in the area of thermal injuries include distribution of smoke alarms and assistance in amending plumbing codes to include "antiscald" technology and a maximum water heater temperature of 120°F.[2]

Injury prevention is commonly called the three E's: education, engineering (including environmental change), and law enforcement.[10] Such prevention initiatives led to changes in the laws for children's sleepwear, smoke detector use, and setting water heaters to less than 120°F.[10]

Several suggestions for preventing pediatric burn injuries include the following:

- Lowering water heater temperature settings to 120°F or lower
- Keeping cords to coffee pots and cups with hot liquids out of reach of young children
- Keeping young children in a safe place during food preparation and serving
- Turning pot handles toward the back of the stove and cooking on rear burners when possible
- Supervising children in the bathtub and testing bath water with a liquid crystal thermometer before placing the child in the tub
- Keeping young children in a safe place when using appliances such as a clothes iron or curling iron, and allowing these items to cool while out of the reach of children
- Discouraging the use of infant walkers
- Placing safety caps on electrical outlets
- Teaching children that matches are tools, not toys
- Teaching older children and adolescents about the dangers of high-voltage wires and about the dangers of and safe use of gasoline and other flammable liquids
- Teaching children about the dangers of fireworks
- Fire department education including "stop, drop, and roll" and identifying a home escape route in the chance of a house fire[5,11]

Additionally, other prevention efforts have focused on federal regulations mandating the use of flame-retardant fabrics and materials in such articles as children's sleepwear and mattresses to help decrease the number and severity of burns resulting from the ignition of these items. In April 1996, the Consumer Product Safety Commission relaxed the standard for children's sleepwear flammability, which became effective January 1, 1997. The change allows the sale of tight-fitting sleepwear and infant sleep wear for those 9 months and younger even if the clothing does not meet the flammability standard previously applicable. As of June 2000, all manufactured or imported sleepwear must be flame resistant or snug fitting and a warning label must be attached to each item.[12]

Structures and Functions of the Skin

The skin, like the heart and lungs, is a vital organ of the body. In fact, it is the largest organ of the body, varying in thickness from 0.5 mm in the eyelids to 4 mm in the palms and soles.[13] The skin is composed of the more superficial and thinner (20 to 400 μ) layer, the epidermis, and of the deeper and thicker (440 to 2500 μ[14]) layer, the dermis. The dermis can be divided into two layers, the more superficial papillary dermis and the deeper reticular dermis. The depth classification of the burn will be determined by the structures involved. In the basal layer of the epidermis are granules of melanin that give skin its color. The dermis is vascular, and the epidermis, although avascular, has its deeper layers nourished by fluid from the dermis (Fig. 16.2). Contained in the skin are sweat glands, hair follicles, sebaceous glands, and, on the fingers and toes, nails. Sensory nerves and sympathetic fibers to vessels, to arrector pili muscles, and to sweat glands abound in the skin.[13] The skin helps regulate body temperature, preserves body fluids, protects against infection (by serving as a barrier and also by having certain bactericidal abilities), protects against radiation, and acts as a barrier to help protect vital organs and other body structures against external objects and fluids. Because of nerve endings that sense touch, pain, and temperature, the skin aids in both protective and discriminatory sensation. The skin also assists in vitamin D production. The skin, along with its appendages, can help reveal an individual's race, age, sex, and health. Ridges in the skin on the fingertips give each person a unique set of fingerprints. The skin on the face, with fluctuations in blood flow (e.g., blushing) and with the action of the underlying muscles, can express an individual's emotions. Whenever the skin is significantly damaged or destroyed, these functions may become impaired. Because the skin is an organ, when the skin is damaged or destroyed, there are not only local but also systemic effects.[13]

Classification of Burns

Burns can be classified by depth of tissue involvement and by size via the percentage of total body surface area and by mechanism of injury. For purposes of triage, they are also classified as minor, moderate, or major.

BURN DEPTH

Burns can be classified according to the depth of skin damaged or destroyed (Fig. 16.3). Superficial burns (formerly referred to as first-degree burns) are most commonly sunburn. They will heal without scar formation or pigment changes. Deeper burns are classified as partial-thickness burns (formerly known as second-degree burns) or as full-thickness burns (previously referred to as third-degree burns). Partial-thickness burns can be either superficial or deep. Superficial partial-thickness burns involve the epidermis and the papillary dermis. Nails, hair, oil and

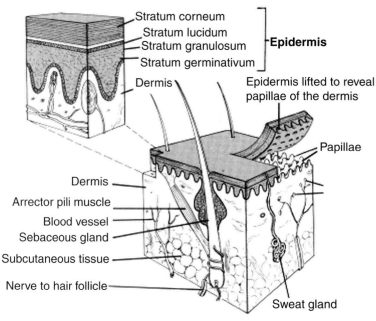

Figure 16.2 ■ Structure of the skin.

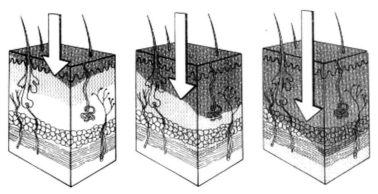

Figure 16.3 ■ Depth of burn injury.

sweat glands, and nerves are spared. They are painful, appear red, and frequently present with blisters. Superficial partial-thickness burns will heal in about 2 weeks or less without scarring.[15]

Deep partial-thickness burns injure structures down into the reticular dermis. Structures affected include nails, hair follicles, and the function of sebaceous glands. They are waxy-white in appearance and are pliable. Such burns may be insensitive to light touch but painful to deep pressure. If they become infected, dry out, or have impaired circulation, deep partial-thickness burns can convert to full-thickness wounds. Deep-partial thickness burns will heal spontaneously by epithelial cells from remaining dermal appendages, but the time required for healing may be 3 to 6 weeks or longer, and such burns heal with scar tissue that can hypertrophy and contract. Although deep partial-thickness burns will heal spontaneously without skin grafting, because of the prolonged healing time and frequently poor functional and cosmetic outcome, as well as other reasons listed later, many surgeons elect to excise and graft these wounds when possible and indicated.

Full-thickness burns, by definition, destroy the full thickness of the skin. Such burns can appear as cherry red, white, or brown and leathery, and thrombosed veins may be visible. Hairs can be easily extracted owing to the death of hair follicles.[15] Because the nerves have been destroyed, full-thickness burns are anesthetic to touch. (This does not mean that there is no pain associated with such burns. Activation of the nerves around the periphery of the burn, exposure of the wound to air by removal of dead tissue, or manipulation of the wound can cause extreme pain.) Full-thickness burns will not heal without skin grafting. Even with skin grafting, such burns may result in scar contraction and hypertrophy. Figure 16.4 demonstrates both deep-partial and full-thickness burns to the shoulder and chest.

The actual depth of injury may not be accurately or easily determined on the first day, even by the most experienced clinician. Burn injuries frequently present with varying depths of involvement and usually are not of uniform depth; such factors as how the injury occurred, the thickness of body skin in the area of the burn, and whether or not the individual was wearing clothes have a bearing on the depth of injury. The skin of infants and young children is thinner than that of adults, so, for example, a hot liquid that would cause a superficial, partial-thickness burn in an adult may cause a deeper injury in an infant or toddler. Knowing the depth of the burn is important in determining triage, resuscitation, wound care and closure, and prognosis.

BURN SIZE

Burns are also classified according to size or TBSA burned. The TBSA is counted as 100%. There are three widely accepted means of determining the extent of body surface area involved. The first is the palmar method, where the palm of an individual's hand is estimated to be about 1% of the TBSA. A second method, more traditionally utilized in the triage of adults, is the "Rule of Nines." According to this rule, in an adult, the head represents 9% of the TBSA, each upper extremity counts as 9%, the trunk represents 36%, each lower extremity represents 18%, and the genitalia is assigned 1%. However, a child's head (especially that of a baby) is larger in proportion to the body than an adult's head is, and a child's lower extremities are smaller in proportion to the body than an adult's lower extremities are.

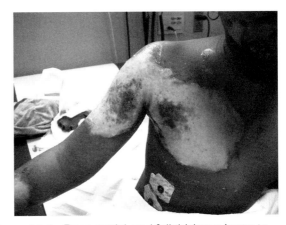

Figure 16.4 ■ Deep partial- and full-thickness burns to right upper extremity and trunk. Darkened areas with no capillary refill and no pain sensation are signs of a full-thickness injury.

For example, the head of a baby who is younger than 1 year of age is counted as 18%, whereas each lower extremity represents 13.5%. Because of such differences, modified versions of the "Rule of Nines" are used to calculate the TBSA burned in children. The most accurate measurement across the age groups and one that has been modified for the pediatric population is the Lund and Browder chart.[15]

The Lund and Browder chart assigns different percentages to body parts, according to the patient's age. Use of a body diagram and the appropriate age-matched percentage will allow for more accurate triage and initial emergency care.[16] The examination form in Figure 16.5 shows the body diagrams and surface area percentages associated with the Lund and Browder chart.

BURN ASSESSMENT

(PATIENT PLATE IMPRINT)

5+ Years   1-5 Years

CAUSE OF BURN: _____

DATE OF BURN: _____ TIME OF BURN: _____

WEIGHT: _____

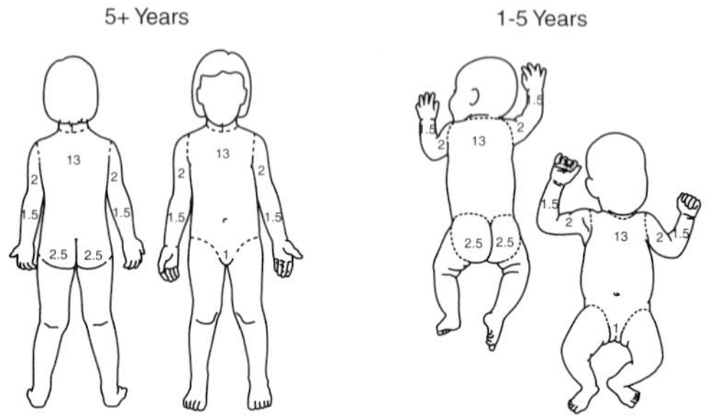

Lund & Browder Chart

Area: *For all body parts except trunk, buttocks, and genitalia, the number in the table represents only the anterior or posterior surface of the body. Need to double number if both anterior and posterior are burned.	Age/Years					% of Body Surface Area Burned: _____		
	0-1	1-4	5-9	10-15	ADULT	PARTIAL THICKNESS	FULL THICKNESS	TOTAL
*Head	9.5%	8.5%	6.5%	5%	3.5%			
*Neck	1%	1%	1%	1%	1%			
Anterior Trunk	13%	13%	13%	13%	13%			
Posterior Trunk	13%	13%	13%	13%	13%			
Right Buttock	2.5%	2.5%	2.5%	2.5%	2.5%			
Left Buttock	2.5%	2.5%	2.5%	2.5%	2.5%			
Genitalia	1%	1%	1%	1%	1%			
*Right Upper Arm	2%	2%	2%	2%	2%			
*Left Upper Arm	2%	2%	2%	2%	2%			
*Right Lower Arm	1.5%	1.5%	1.5%	1.5%	1.5%			
*Left Lower Arm	1.5%	1.5%	1.5%	1.5%	1.5%			
*Right Hand	1.25%	1.25%	1.25%	1.25%	1.25%			
*Left Hand	1.25%	1.25%	1.25%	1.25%	1.25%			
*Right Thigh	2.25%	3.25%	4.25%	4.25%	4.75%			
*Left Thigh	2.25%	3.25%	4.25%	4.25%	4.75%			
*Right Leg	2.5%	2.5%	2.75%	3%	3.5%			
*Left Leg	2.5%	2.5%	2.75%	3%	3.5%			
*Right Foot	1.75%	1.75%	1.75%	1.75%	1.75%			
*Left Foot	1.75%	1.75%	1.75%	1.75%	1.75%			
Signature: _____					TOTAL			
Date: _____								

Figure 16.5 ■ Lund and Browder chart for burn size estimation.

MECHANISM OF INJURY

A third way of classifying burns is according to the mechanism of injury: scald, contact, flash, flame, chemical, radiation, or electrical. Knowing the causative agent or method can be important in giving appropriate treatment. For example, if an individual sustains a chemical burn, knowing which chemical caused the burn is necessary in order to apply the correct antidote and in determining the need for copious water lavage, which would not necessarily be done for an electrical burn or a flame burn. Recognizing the mechanism of injury and correlating the presentation of the burn will aid in ruling out child abuse.

MINOR, MODERATE, AND MAJOR CLASSIFICATIONS

Burns also can be classified as minor, moderate, or major according to guidelines established by the American Burn Association (ABA) for purposes of triage. For example, a minor burn for an adult might be a partial-thickness burn involving less than 15% of the TBSA; such a patient could be treated as an outpatient. A minor burn for a child might be a partial-thickness burn involving less than 10% of the TBSA, but hospitalization might be considered for such a patient. The ABA recommends that an individual with a major burn be admitted or transferred to a burn center.

 Pathophysiology

DIMENSIONS OF INJURY

Regardless of the mechanism of injury, each burn wound consists of three zones that are identified concentrically around the center portion of the injury. The most central area of the burn is the zone of coagulation; this is the area that had the most contact with the heat source. The cells in this zone have been permanently damaged. Extending outwardly is the zone of stasis. The cells in the zone of stasis have decreased blood flow and respond to resuscitation in order to save viable tissue. The outermost zone of burn injury is the zone of hyperemia. These cells have sustained the least damage and should recover within 10 days.[15]

BURN WOUND HEALING

Burn wound healing can be categorized into three phases: inflammation, proliferation, and maturation/remodeling.

INFLAMMATORY PHASE

Once an injury has occurred, the disruption of epidermal and dermal structures signals the healing process to occur. Platelets come in contact with the injured tissue, fibrin is deposited, more platelets are trapped, and a thrombus is formed. There is also a local vasoconstriction that occurs and in combination with the thrombus, it blocks the injured tissue from systemic circulation, thus achieving hemostasis. Once this is achieved, local vasodilation occurs and there is increased capillary permeability.[17] Inflammatory cells including neutrophils arrive at the injured site to control infection. Monocytes arrive at the burn site at about 24 hours after injury and are converted into macrophages that aid in the next stage of wound healing. Macrophages secrete growth factors that are responsible for fibroblast proliferation.[17]

PROLIFERATIVE PHASE

Following the inflammatory phase is the proliferative phase, which is dominated by fibroblast activity. Collagen is deposited at the wound site as early as 48 hours after a burn. Type I collagen is seen by days 4 to 7 after injury. Granulation tissue forms as endothelial cells migrate and will continue until the wound is completely re-epithelialized. Re-epithelialization occurs by cell migration. The cells migrate from the periphery of the wound (e.g., the wound will heal from the outside toward the middle). Re-epithelialization will be more rapid when the stratum granulosum layer of the epidermis is intact, as with superficial partial-thickness burns. The burn wound will remain in this phase until epithelialization is complete or until the wound is surgically addressed (e.g., covered with a skin graft).[17]

MATURATION/REMODELING PHASE

During the remodeling phase of burn wound healing, collagen synthesis and lysis occurs, thus creating scar tissue. During the remodeling phase, the collagen is reorganized into a more compact area. An imbalance in collagen synthesis will result in a hypertrophic or keloid-type scar (discussed later). This is the longest phase of healing and can last up to 2 years.[17]

 Scar Hypertrophy and Contraction

As previously mentioned, there are two common, though often avoidable, sequelae of deep partial-thickness and full-thickness burns: scar hypertrophy and scar contraction. Scar hypertrophy and scar contraction can impede both physical and psychological functioning. Scar hypertrophy is a raised, thick, usually hard, often knotty-appearing area of scar tissue (Fig. 16.6). Scar hypertrophy results from an imbalance of collagen synthesis and collagen lysis. Hypertrophic scars are, at times, also called keloids, although some investigators distinguish between the two. Keloids are hypertrophic scars that grow above and beyond the original perimeters of the injury. Debate persists concerning the distinction between hypertrophic scars and keloids. Linares, in a review of the controversy, concluded that keloids are only extreme variants of hypertrophic scars.[18]

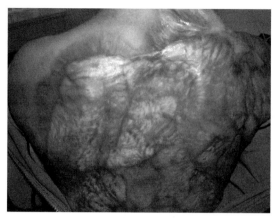

Figure 16.6 ■ Hypertrophic scarring along patient's back following split-thickness skin grafts.

To determine which variables might be predictors for the development of hypertrophic scarring, Deitch et al.[19] considered such factors as the race and age of the patient, the location of the burn, and the length of time before the (ungrafted) burn was healed. The investigation concluded that the length of time required to heal the burn was the most important indicator. One-third of the anatomic sites became hypertrophic if the burns healed between 14 and 21 days. If healing occurred after 21 days, hypertrophic scar incidence increased to 78%.[19] African Americans in the study had a greater incidence of hypertrophic scarring than others if the burn took more than 10 to 14 days to heal. The investigators attributed the increased incidence of hypertrophic scars in certain anatomic sites to wound tension. Hunt[20] concurred that increased tension, which promotes collagen deposition and lessens collagen lysis, may contribute to the formation of hypertrophic scars, evidenced by the appearance of hypertrophic scars in areas of motion, such as the joints (Fig. 16.7). The authors of the first-mentioned study, citing other investigators,[21] also acknowledged that the depth of the wound is related to the incidence of hypertrophic scarring because burns of the reticular dermis are likely to heal with a hypertrophic

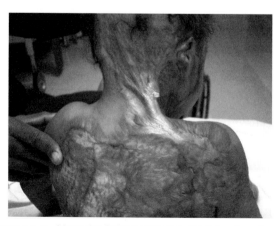

Figure 16.7 ■ Note the keloid scar at right side of neck. Notice the band-like formation.

scar, whereas more superficial burns involving the papillary dermis do not. However, these authors report that it is more accurate to quantify length of healing time rather than to estimate the depth of the wound subjectively. In the study, the age of the patient was not found to correlate with an increased incidence of hypertrophic scarring. However, others[22,23] have suggested that younger patients may have an increased incidence of hypertrophic scars compared with other age groups, probably because of an increased rate of collagen production.

Scar contraction is the pulling or shortening of scar tissue, which can result in the loss of joint motion or skin mobility. Scar contracture is a fixed shortening of the scar tissue that may be amenable only to surgery. Contraction may be attributed to myofibroblasts, cells that have contractile properties, and are found in the healing burn wound.[18] Scar contraction that is not located over a joint can lead to disfigurement, especially if such contraction involves the face. Scar contraction over a joint can lead to loss of joint range of motion (ROM) or posture and gait deviations. Because of the contracting force of scar, which results in loss of skin mobility, a loss of joint ROM also can result from contracting scar tissue that is adjacent to, although not covering, a joint. The scar will contract until it meets an equal or opposing force.[24] What is initially just loss of motion from contracting scar can, if left uncorrected, lead to a gradual shortening of joint capsules, muscles, tendons, and ligaments. A contracting scar in an adult may not cause any loss of motion, whereas that same size scar in a small child may cause a loss of motion.[25]

The processes of scar contraction and hypertrophy begin almost as soon as the burn wound begins healing, although initially they may not be readily visible. Collagen formation begins within 24 hours of the burn injury.[18] There is a high rate of collagen synthesis in the wound,[26] and such activity returns to a normal pace by 6 to 12 months.[27] The scar is initially red because of an increased blood supply, but it usually fades over time. When the scar no longer is actively hypertrophying and contracting, it is said to be mature. The period of scar maturation for most children is approximately 12 to 18 months. For adults, this period may be shorter. While the scar is active, particularly during the first 6 months, the processes of hypertrophy and contraction can be controlled or corrected by nonsurgical approaches, such as pressure, splinting, and ROM exercises, which will be discussed later. As scar maturation progresses, these treatments become less effective in altering scar. After the scar is mature, most nonsurgical treatments are no longer effective, and surgery, if indicated, may afford the only treatment alternative.

◆ Burn Center

In 1999, the ABA published guidelines for the development and operation of burn centers, defined as "a service system based in a hospital that has made the institutional commitment to meet the criteria specified in this guide." The ABA, along with the American College of Surgeons, has set guidelines for centers that provide optimal care for patients with burns. In 1999, there were 38 sites across the United States that qualified for burn center status.[28]

Burn Team

In its guidelines for burn centers, the ABA specifies which personnel should staff the burn center, as well as which specialists and personnel should be on call or available for consultation. (The criteria state that "both physical and occupational therapy should be represented in the burn center staff.") Within the ABA guidelines, each burn center establishes its own burn team. Personnel who comprise the burn team and their specific roles may vary from institution to institution or according to the individual needs of a given patient or the particular phase of healing, although there generally is a core team. The pediatric burn team frequently includes a surgeon, a nurse, an occupational therapist, a physical therapist, a social worker, a respiratory therapist, a dietitian, a child life therapist, a hospital chaplain, a discharge planner, various specialists (pediatrician, pulmonologist, psychiatrist, plastic surgeon, infection control specialist, etc.), and most importantly, the child and family. Because many children do not have a traditional nuclear family, it is often necessary to determine who, in the child's view, comprises the family.[29]

Initial Treatment and Medical Management

The initial treatment and medical management of the pediatric burn patient depend, in part, on the depth, size, and location of the burn; the presence of other concomitant injuries, such as smoke inhalation; the age of the child; and the premorbid health of the child. The injury itself will trigger physiologic responses that, in turn, will affect treatment requirements.

Systems Review

PULMONARY SYSTEM

Establishing and maintaining an adequate airway and breathing are the first concerns when treating a thermally injured patient. If the patient has inhaled steam or noxious gases, intubation may be necessary because bronchospasm and upper airway edema[30] may develop, possibly resulting in airway obstruction within hours.[31] Oxygen is administered if the patient has inhaled high levels of carbon monoxide. The endotracheal tube may be removed once edema has subsided, usually within a few days.[30] Patients

with more extensive airway or lung injuries will require sustained or more involved treatment.

When a patient's respiratory status is evaluated initially, cardiac hemodynamic status is also assessed, and the patient is examined for other injuries such as fractures and lacerations.[32] Prophylactic tetanus toxoid may be administered to help prevent infections. A careful past medical history and a history of the burn incident are recorded. The wounds are evaluated, cleaned, and bandaged.

CARDIOVASCULAR SYSTEM

The circulatory changes that occur following a burn injury have been discussed earlier. These changes are termed *burn shock*. The loss of fluid, increased capillary permeability, and vasodilation that occur all cause decreases in the circulatory volume and reduced cardiac output. Proper fluid resuscitation is key to recovering normal cardiac output. Inadequate fluid replacement can lead to poor tissue perfusion, organ dysfunction, and death.[15]

FLUID RESUSCITATION

Because of the inflammatory process and increased capillary permeability in patients with deep partial-thickness or full-thickness burns, fluid leaves the blood and is dispersed into the interstitial spaces. Patients with burns of less than 10% to 20% of their TBSA, depending on other considerations, may be able to compensate for this fluid shift physiologically through such measures as vasoconstriction and urine retention.[31] Patients with burns involving a greater percentage of TBSA will develop hypovolemic shock and can die if not treated. Replacement of the circulating fluid loss is termed *fluid resuscitation*. Fluids cannot be administered orally to patients with larger area burns because of ileus (obstruction of the bowel), which occurs secondary to shock. Fluids, with electrolytes similar to serum, and colloid are given intravenously. Patients with smaller burns may be able to take fluids orally. However, children, in particular, may be unwilling to drink and therefore may require intravenous fluids. In a few days, with adequate fluid replacement, the fluid in the interstitial spaces returns to the intravascular spaces, and the patient will diurese, signaling successful fluid resuscitation.[31] After fluid resuscitation, the patient may still require the administration of fluids because fluid is also lost through the burn wound and because the patient may be unwilling or unable to take sufficient fluids orally.

A urinary catheter is placed in patients with large burns so as to monitor urine output during resuscitation. Patients with perineal burns may also require catheterization to keep bandages dry or to protect newly placed skin grafts during the skin graft phase.

RENAL SYSTEM

Due to loss of fluid from intravascular spaces, renal vasoconstriction can occur. Renal failure can occur due to decreased renal blood flow and decreased glomerular filtration. With electrical burn injuries, extensive tissue may be damaged, thus releasing myoglobin. The myoglobin may occlude the kidneys, thus leading to renal failure.

CIRCULATORY SYSTEM

Full-thickness burned skin is inelastic. Because of the body's response to injury and fluid resuscitation, the patient will become edematous. This is a systemic response that also occurs in the unburned parts of the body. In the case of circumferential burns of the extremities, the combination of inelastic skin and increasing edema can cause a tourniquet effect, resulting in compromised circulation to the distal extremities. If treatment is not initiated, ischemia and tissue damage or necrosis can occur. Signs of compromise include pallor, decreased skin temperature, delayed capillary refill, numbness/tingling, and decreased chest wall excursion in the case of trunk burns. Compartment pressures of greater than 30 mm Hg also indicate the need for surgical intervention. The trauma surgeon will attempt to relieve the pressure by performing an escharotomy, which is a surgical incision through the burned tissue. These incisions are usually along the lateral and medial sides of the affected extremity. At the chest, longitudinal incisions are made along the anterior axillary lines and a transverse incision at the costal level.[15]

Escharotomy is usually performed within the first 24 to 48 hours of onset of the burn injury. Escharotomies may need to be performed on the chest to allow for adequate chest expansion and breathing in patients with deep circumferential burns of the trunk. Exercise and activities are permitted following escharotomy. When delayed escharotomy results in compartment syndrome, when deep burns involve muscle (as is often the case with electrical burn injuries), and when burns are accompanied by associated skeletal or soft tissue injury, the fascia will need to be released surgically, a procedure termed a *fasciotomy*.[33]

MUSCULOSKELETAL SYSTEM

Due to the association between fire and traumatic injuries, it is not uncommon to have a burn injury and concomitant fracture. Examination of the musculoskeletal injury will often be put on hold while the potential life-threatening injuries are assessed. Patients who are unresponsive or unable to report specific pain may be at risk for having fractures or other musculoskeletal injuries missed upon primary or secondary surveys. The therapist may be the first clinician to discover an undiagnosed musculoskeletal injury. Children likely to have musculoskeletal injuries are those involved in an automobile accident with a resulting fire or those who have jumped from a burning building. Both burns and fractures can cause soft tissue swelling, thus requiring an escharotomy in the case that circulation is compromised (see Circulation). Nonoperative management of fractures includes using a splint or traction. Use of a circumferential cast is discouraged due to swelling and the inability to examine the wounds properly. Internal fixation is also beneficial as it increases the rate of fracture healing. Surgery for internal fixation should occur within 48 hours after injury; otherwise, bacterial colonization is presumed. Surgical fixation of the fracture will allow for reduction in pain at the fracture site and for physical therapy interventions.[34]

Nutrition

In response to the burn injury, the patient is in a hypermetabolic state and caloric and nutritional requirements are greatly increased. The hypermetabolic and inflammatory response caused by a burn is demonstrated by an increase in protein, proinflammatory cytokine, and catabolic hormone levels. These in turn raise energy requirements, which can result in muscle wasting. If this posttraumatic response is prolonged, it can lead to multiple organ dysfunction and death. Raising of room temperatures and nutritional supplementation have been proved efficient in modulating the hypermetabolic responses.[35] Adequate nutrition is necessary to prevent wasting and to promote proper wound healing. The pediatric burn patient, because of the injury and a strange environment, may be unwilling to eat. The severity or location of the burns may make it difficult or impossible to eat. A patient with a larger burn may find it hard to consume the volume of food necessary to obtain sufficient calories. Additionally, the patient will be prohibited from eating on days when a surgical procedure is scheduled in the operating room. Because of such factors, the patient may receive a large portion of nutrition through enteral tube feedings or through peripheral vein infusions. Enteral nutrition is the preferred route of nutritional support since it offers maintenance of the gastrointestinal (GI) mucosal integrity by delivering nutrients into the GI tract. A nutritional assessment should be done upon admission following a thermal injury. This will include looking at medical, nutritional, and medication histories and laboratory data and a patient examination. The clinician will look at plasma protein levels, more specifically albumin and prealbumin. The normal range for serum albumin is 3.5 to 5 g/dL. Low levels of albumin may signify poor potential to heal. Prealbumin is a transport protein for thyroid hormone. Normal serum prealbumin levels range from 16 to 40 mg/dL, with values greater than 16 mg/dL associated with malnutrition. The half-life of prealbumin is 2 to 3 days, thus making it a better predictor of nutritional status.[35a]

Pain Management

Pediatric patients describe their burn injuries as the most painful experience of their life.[36] Sheridan et al.[37] stated that poorly controlled pain and anxiety have adverse psychological and physiologic effects that account for the 30% rate of posttraumatic stress disorder in individuals who suffer severe burns. They also contended that excessive pain and anxiety further fuel the hypermetabolic response by increasing the elaboration of stress hormones.[37] Writing about the psychosocial care of the severely burned child, Knudson and Thomas[38] cited the following research to plead for adequate pain management of burn patients. Studies have shown that medical professionals who treat burn patients underrate the patients' pain when compared with the patients' own estimates of their pain.[39,40] In 2003, Martin-Herz et al.[41] investigated pediatric pain control practices in North American burn centers. Their study was in comparison to one done in 1982, which revealed at that time that 17% of burn units recommended using no opioid analgesics and 8% did not use any analgesics during pediatric wound care.[42] The newer survey revealed significant changes in the use of opioids during pediatric burn dressing changes. Morphine appeared to be the "gold standard" for medicating the child before, during, and after a painful procedure.[41] Twenty-five percent of the responders in the survey utilized psychotropic medications in combination with opioids. Background pain control and breakthrough pain control was also best addressed by IV morphine. Only 8% of centers responding stated that they routinely utilized an anesthesia-based pain service for helping with pain management. Nonpharmacologic adjuvants to pain management were utilized in 77% of centers responding. These techniques included distraction, music/art therapy, and relaxation techniques.[41] The use of child life specialists and music therapists can aid with the nonpharmacologic approach as well as with preparing the child for the procedure. The child's pain and anxiety must be considered and treated appropriately throughout all phases of healing. Age-specific distraction techniques can be seen in Table 16.2.

Medication for pruritus should also be considered as itching can be a source of discomfort, pain, and patient tolerance for interventions. Antihistamines were the most commonly prescribed medications for pruritus. Opioids themselves can cause itching, so careful documentation of the occurrence of itching and whether or not it is related to burn wound healing or medication is important.[41]

Besides specific medications and pain management techniques, the facility and each professional should have a treatment approach that has as a goal caring for the burn patient in a way that causes the least amount of pain. Some suggestions for minimizing patients' pain are made throughout the chapter.

Burn Wound Management

The primary goals of wound management are to provide an optimal environment for wound healing, to provide a healthy tissue bed to receive a skin graft, and to protect healing tissue or a recently placed graft. Such goals are accomplished mainly through removing dead tissue, keeping the wound clean and minimizing bacterial invasion, preventing the wound or new skin graft from drying out, and protecting newly healing tissue or recent skin graft(s) from disruptive mechanical abrasion. There are nonsurgical and surgical interventions that comprise overall burn wound management. Prior to any wound cleansing or dressing changes, the child should be premedicated.

NONSURGICAL INTERVENTIONS

WOUND CLEANSING

HYDROTHERAPY Hydrotherapy is used in some burn centers as a part of wound management. Showering, immersion, or use of a spray table can accomplish it. The purpose of hydrotherapy is to help remove the old topical antimicrobial agent, to clean the wound, to help superficially débride the wound (through the effect of the agitator), to increase circulation in order to promote wound healing, and to provide an environment for exercise. Agitation may be used in the presence of a highly necrotic wound (e.g., road burn). The drawbacks of hydrotherapy are that it can spread infection; it can increase the length of time required for a dressing change; it can increase cost (because of the additional personnel required to perform the procedure and clean the equipment); it can increase edema (especially if a limb is placed in a dependent position); and patients, particularly children, may find it to be traumatic, especially if a bathtub was the mechanism of original injury. Because of the drawbacks of hydrotherapy, some burn centers limit its use to specific wounds or to certain phases of wound healing, or use handheld shower heads to help clean the wound.

Sessions are limited to 30 minutes to decrease the risk of losing excessive sodium through the burn wound. The temperature of the water and room should be elevated so as to not cause hypothermia. Adequate cleansing is achieved

TABLE 16.2	
Non-Pharmacologic Pain Management	
Age Range	**Participation Motivators/ Distraction Techniques**
Under 2 yr	Use parents to help; rattles, bubble blowing, singing, videos
2–7 yr	Singing, looking at a book, videos, magic wand
7–11 yr	Allow them to participate as indicated; headphones for music, videos, sticker chart
11 yr and above	Give precise information regarding the intervention; music, videos, video games, reward chart

by using sterile gauze to remove the old topical agent. Additives should be avoided in the water as wound cleansers have been shown to be cytotoxic.[43]

DRESSING CHANGES

Most burn patients will undergo bandage (also called dressing) changes at least daily. Even very young children can participate in removing their dressings, which may help minimize pain and offer some sense of control and independence in a situation in which they might otherwise feel helpless. Because some of the pain experienced during a dressing change is caused by exposure of the wound to air, such exposure time should be limited. Limiting the exposure time to air will help prevent the tissue from drying out and will also limit exposure to bacteria. To minimize the time required for a dressing change, bandages should be prepared ahead of time so that they may be quickly applied. Health care professionals who wish to observe the patient's wound should be present at the time of the dressing change so that the patient is not waiting with an undressed wound for them to arrive. If the parent desires, and if appropriate, the parent's presence during the dressing change can be beneficial for both the parent and the child. In some cases, however, children may cry more in the presence of a parent because they expect the parent to "rescue" them from the dressing change.

In some burn centers, therapists are responsible for or may assist with daily wound care for both inpatients and outpatients. (It may also be the case that the therapist, before or during performance of outpatient therapy, will need to change the patient's bandage.) During a dressing change, the old bandage is removed and the wound may be superficially débrided (nonviable tissue removed). At the same time the wound is cleaned and examined, ROM is examined without the dressings in place to establish how much ROM the patient should work toward for the remainder of the therapy day.

TOPICAL AGENTS

In a burn injury, the protective barrier of the skin is lost, and the burn wound becomes a host for bacteria. Topical antimicrobial agents play a vital role in helping minimize bacterial colonization of the wound, decrease vapor loss, prevent desiccation, and control pain.[44] Several topical antimicrobial agents may be employed depending on the specific wound and the organisms to be controlled.

Silver sulfadiazine (Silvadene) is the most commonly used topical agent.[4] Silvadene is a white, opaque cream that is painless upon application, has fair eschar penetration, and has a broad antibacterial spectrum.[44] Silvadene can't be used by patients with sulfa allergies.[4] Silvadene has also been shown to cause neutropenia when applied on large surface area burns.[45] Mafenide acetate (Sulfamylon) is another topical agent that can come in liquid or cream form, is painful upon application, has excellent eschar penetration,

and has a broad antibacterial spectrum. Mafenide acetate is utilized on burns of the external ear to reduce suppurative chondritis.[44] Sulfamylon can be used on partial-thickness burns that are resistant to Silvadene and to increase eschar penetration/separation. Sulfamylon is contraindicated for use in a patient with metabolic acidosis.[4] Other topical agents used in burn wound management include silver nitrate, which has broad antibacterial coverage and is applied as a solution on burn wounds or graft sites. Petroleum-based products such as neomycin and bacitracin are used on superficial burns or on areas where the skin is very thin (e.g., eyelids, scrotum).[43]

Another option to topical antimicrobial creams is Acticoat dressing. It has been shown to be more effective than Silvadene and silver nitrate against Gram-negative and Gram-positive organisms. Acticoat is a three-ply gauze that has an absorbent rayon and polyester core. The coating to Acticoat is nonadherent to the wound and is flexible. The child would need to undergo debridement prior to Acticoat placement. A bulky layer of wet gauze is wrapped around the Acticoat and then covered with dry gauze. Daily dressing changes include taking down the gauze dressings, inspecting the Acticoat for slippage from the wound bed, and reapplying wet gauze and dry gauze. Once adhered, the Acticoat is left in place until reepithelialization occurs. This will decrease the risk of infection (from daily wound cleansing) and discomfort associated with dressing changes.[46]

AQUACEL Ag Hydrofiber by Convatec is a moisture-retentive topical dressing that is also being used in the acute management of burns. It consists entirely of carboxymethylcellulose, which forms into a gel upon contact with burn exudate. This gel promotes a moist wound healing environment while still managing moderate amounts of burn exudate.[47] This new hydrofiber with 1.2% ionic silver releases silver within the dressing for up to 2 weeks. It can be applied on an acute burn and left in place until healing occurs, thus decreasing pain and length of hospitalization.[48] Caruso et al. performed a randomized clinical study comparing AQUACEL Ag and silver sulfadiazine for the management of partial-thickness burns. Compared with silver sulfadiazine, AQUACEL Ag was associated with less pain and anxiety during dressing changes. Patients using the traditional silver sulfadiazine dressing had more flexibility and ease of movement during use in comparison with those using AQUACEL Ag. Overall, in this study the AQUACEL Ag group demonstrated greater benefits with requiring fewer dressing changes, less nursing time, and fewer preprocedural opiate medications.[49] These benefits clearly implicate implementation of its use in the pediatric setting where pain reduction and decreased length of hospitalization are overall goals in the patient's plan of care.

FUNCTIONAL DRESSINGS

Dressings should not excessively inhibit motion. The thumb, for example, should not be wrapped into the palm, nor should bandages restrict chest expansion. However, bandages can be used to help position the patient. For example, bulky bandages can be used in place of splints to support the fingers and wrists in infants and toddlers.

Additionally, applying the topical antimicrobial agent to the gauze and then applying the gauze to the wound (instead of applying the topical agent directly to the wound and then applying the gauze) will also help minimize pain during the dressing change. A nonadherent gauze such as Exu-Dry, Adaptic, or Xeroform will decrease the pain associated with dressing removal. A bulky bandage is used to secure the topical agent and nonadherent dressing in place. Tubular netting is then placed over the bulky bandage to secure it in place. The tubular netting can be cut/fabricated into many styles (e.g., sleeve, shirt, stocking) for the specific body part. Figure 16.8 shows a functional dressing for the hand, which allows the child more use of it for play or activities of daily living (ADLs).

Positioning with dressing application should be adhered to. Burns across joints or at the hands or feet require special attention with dressing application. Positioning is utilized to protect the burn wounds, decrease edema, and counteract wound and scar contraction by putting the tissue in an elongated position. For example, burns across the antecubital fossa should be wrapped and splinted into extension. Burns on the plantar/dorsal surface of the foot and calf should be wrapped and splinted into neutral dorsiflexion.[50]

BIOLOGIC DRESSINGS

Advances in burn wound management surround the invention and improvements made in the area of biologic or synthetic dressings. Biobrane is a synthetic dressing that can be used on superficial partial-thickness burns, over autografts, on donor sites, and in the treatment of toxic epidermal necrolysis (TEN). It is a nylon fabric that is combined with a silicone film, where collagen is incorporated. The nylon fabric comes into contact with the burn wound and adheres until re-epithelialization occurs. It is placed on

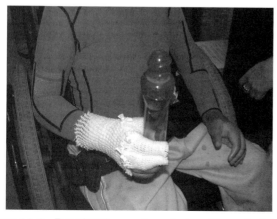

Figure 16.8 ■ Functional wrapping of a hand burn. Individual finger dressings allow for easier movement and performance of activities of daily living.

the burn wounds in the operating room and secured with staples or sutures, and once adhered to the wound, no other dressing is necessary.[43]

SURGICAL MANAGEMENT

Once burn size and depth estimations have been made and the initial burn wound management has commenced, further wound management may include surgery.

Because a superficial partial-thickness burn will heal in approximately 2 weeks with normal skin, the goals of the surgeon in such cases are to keep the wound free of infection, to provide adequate nutrition and fluids, and to manage pain until the wound is healed. Depending on the size and location of the superficial partial-thickness burn, the age of the patient, and the ability of the parent, many of these burns can be treated on an outpatient basis and without surgery.

A deep partial-thickness burn can heal without surgical intervention if adequate medical treatment and wound management are provided. The progression of deep partial-thickness burns will usually take one of two pathways. The first includes the filmy eschar separating from the wound edges, allowing epithelial buds to resurface the wound. The other is following separation of eschar, the wound heals by granulation tissue. The presence of granulation tissue will increase the risk of hypertrophic scarring. This, along with large TBSA of deep partial-thickness burns, makes surgical intervention via grafting more probable.[4] The surgeon may elect to graft the deep partial-thickness burn in a procedure called tangential excision and grafting.[4] Such excision and grafting can be done within the first week of the burn injury and is ideally performed 2 to 5 days after the burn injury (termed *early excision and grafting*). Early excision and grafting may also apply to other wounds, particularly full-thickness wounds, which may be excised to fascia. Tangential excision and grafting of deep partial-thickness wounds during the first week shortens the patient's hospital stay, lessens pain, decreases the incidence of infection, and improves cosmetic and functional outcome (by minimizing the amount of hypertrophic scar tissue development and scar contraction).[51]

There are drawbacks associated with early tangential excision and grafting of deep partial-thickness wounds, however, and not all patients are candidates for this procedure. Early excision and grafting of deep partial-thickness burns usually involves significant intraoperative blood loss that may require substantial transfusion; this may not be recommended for medically unstable patients or those with inhalation injury.[44] When a burn involves a significant percentage of TBSA, and particularly when the burn area consists of both deep partial-thickness and full-thickness burns and there is a limited number of donor sites for skin grafts, excision and grafting of deep partial-thickness burns is generally delayed or such wounds are allowed to heal spontaneously.

SKIN GRAFT AND DONOR SITE

There are several different types of grafts, depending on the source of the skin. An autograft is a piece of skin that is surgically shaved from an unburned part of the patient's body (called the donor site) and placed on the burned area. In the case where infection may be present, or due to a large TBSA, autografting may not be possible. In that case, alternative grafts can be used. These include xenografts and allografts. A xenograft is skin harvested from a pig. They can help protect and facilitate the healing of partial-thickness burns as well as debriding exudative wounds. An allograft is a graft of skin from a cadaver, which has been harvested within 24 hours of death and preserved via cryo-preservation (at a skin bank). These are often used in preparation for autografting to test the "receptivity" of the wound bed for an autograft.[43]

With an autograft, either a full thickness or partial thickness of skin can be harvested. If a full-thickness piece of skin from the unburned donor site were taken and placed on the burned area, the burn would heal, but a wound of similar dimensions to the burn would remain at the donor site. Full-thickness skin grafts (FTSGs) (0.025 to 0.030 inches thick) are used mostly in reconstructive surgery, over pressure points, or anywhere extra skin thickness is needed. More commonly only a partial- or split-thickness (approximately 0.008-inch thick[52]) piece of skin is taken (STSG). Some areas of the body are preferred donor sites because of the thickness, texture, or color of the skin; because they are areas that will heal well; and because they are in a region not usually visible. Common preferred donor sites include the lateral thighs and buttocks. However, when these areas are burned, or in an extensively burned individual, almost any skin on the body can be used. A split-thickness donor site is similar to a superficial partial-thickness burn, with healing occurring within 14 days via re-epithelialization. Removal of the skin that is to be used for grafting is called harvesting. Once the patient has been anesthetized, the skin is shaved from the donor site with an electric knife—known as a dermatome—that has settings to adjust the thickness of skin excised. The procedure is called a sheet graft when the skin is placed "as is" on the excised burned area (also known as the recipient or graft site) (Fig. 16.9). Alternatively, the skin may be placed in a skin mesher before its application to the recipient site. The mesher cuts small slits in the graft, after which the graft is stretched or expanded before placement on the recipient site. Such a graft is known as an expanded mesh graft (Fig. 16.10). The main purpose of meshing is to allow a skin graft to cover a larger area than could otherwise be covered using a sheet graft. The amount of expansion achieved is expressed as a ratio of the expanded to the unexpanded size. For example, an expanded mesh graft that covers one and a half times its original or unmeshed size would be referred to as a 1.5:1 mesh graft. One advantage of a mesh graft is that compared with a sheet graft, there is less likelihood

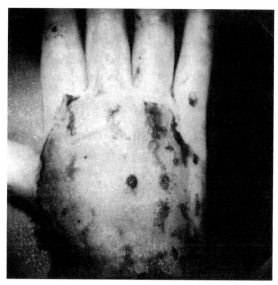

Figure 16.9 ■ *Example of a sheet graft to the dorsum of the hand.*

that hematomas or serous fluid will collect under the graft, causing the graft to be nonadherent. A disadvantage of a mesh graft, particularly a large-ratio mesh graft, is that scarring occurs within the interstices or holes and such scarring can hypertrophy and contract. The permanent meshed pattern of the graft may also be cosmetically unattractive. Because sheet grafts provide a better cosmetic outcome with less contraction and hypertrophy, they are the graft of choice in burns involving less than 30% of TBSA that are not excessively colonized by bacteria and other microbes.[53] Sheet grafts should also be used on the face, neck, and hands, and are often preferred, when possible, for other functional areas of the body, such as the feet and the axillae. The surgeon may secure the graft with surgical staples, stitches, or Steri-strips. The graft usually requires 4 to 7 days to become adherent or to "take." The grafted area is protected during this period by bulky dressings. If the graft site is over a joint, the joint is usually immobilized

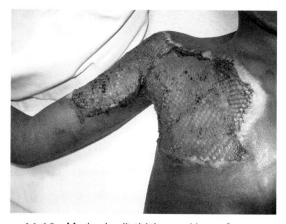

Figure 16.10 ■ *Meshed split-thickness skin graft.*

with a splint during this initial period, and exercise of the joint is discontinued for that same period. Movement or shearing forces can result in graft loss. Other factors that can contribute to graft loss or less than optimal graft take are infection, inadequate nutrition, or a poor graft bed or inadequate debridement.

Donor sites can be "reharvested" once healed, up to three or four times in the case of a large TBSA burn. Harvesting of the skin over irregular surfaces can be achieved by injecting saline to contour such areas.[54]

Before the skin graft can be placed, the burned, necrotic skin, called *eschar,* must be removed. This is usually accomplished surgically, but enzymatic debrider may also be used on partial-thickness wounds. Surgical excision usually extends down to a level of viable tissue. Excision can be effected immediately before placing the skin graft, or, depending on the depth and extent of the wound, it may be accomplished earlier, in a separate operation. If an excised full-thickness wound is not grafted during the same procedure, granulation tissue will develop that will help prepare the site for grafting.

In the case of a burn involving a large percentage of TBSA, even when multiple donor sites are available, the surgeon may elect not to graft the entire burn at once because of the stress of surgery to the patient, particularly if the patient is already medically compromised or unstable. If the grafts do not take, not only is there still a large TBSA burn, but the donor sites are now additional wounds that must be healed, and the donor sites cannot be reused for about 10 days.

CULTURED AUTOGRAFTS AND DERMAL SUBSTITUTES

Several advances in wound healing and surgical techniques during the past decade have improved the outcome and increased survival of burn patients. Among these advances are two that have been shown to increase survival in massively burned individuals who lack sufficient donor sites: cultured autografts and dermal substitutes.

In the 1980s, cultured epithelial autografts (CEAs) or keratinocytes were the newest advancement in wound closure of the severely burned individual. In the case of cultured epithelial autografts, a small piece of unburned skin measuring approximately 1 square inch is taken from the patient and grown in a laboratory. Within several weeks or less, there is enough skin to cover an entire body and this skin can be grafted onto the patient from whom the original sample was taken. However, there are drawbacks and problems with cultured autografted skin. Wound closure must be delayed until the skin is grown, and the rate of graft take, depending on the occurrence of graft site infection, varies from 15% to 80%.[55] CEAs, lacking tensile strength, are fragile and easily cut or bruised.[50] Standard therapy regimens, in particular those involving ROM and mobilization, frequently must be altered or their imple-

mentation delayed. The cost of the CEA can also be high. Although dermal regeneration appears to occur below CEAs over 4 to 5 years,[56] the skin lacks hair follicles and sweat glands. Sensory nerves and pigmentation are also absent.[57] Some of the problems associated with the use of CEAs have been mitigated recently by combining a CEA with cadaver skin that has had the antigenic epidermis removed.

In the mid-1990s, cultured composite autografts (CCAs) were developed. Cultured composite autografts consist of autologous keratinocytes, which form a multilayered epidermal component, and fibroblasts, which form an extracellular dermal matrix. The rate of CCA take is reported to be 80%, and the CCA is durable. Dermal elements, such as hair follicles and sweat glands, are lacking in cultured composite autografted skin. The product is expensive; however, the resulting decreased hospitalization from the use of CCA may offset the high cost.[58]

Several dermal substitutes or dermal analogs are now available for use after decades of research. One such substitute, Integra (Integra LifeSciences Corp., Plainsboro, NJ) is an artificial dermis composed of two layers: a dermal replacement layer of bovine tendon collagen and a substitute epidermal layer of silicone.[50] Integra is placed on the excised wound. The porous dermal replacement layer serves as a matrix for the infiltration of elements from the wound bed that then construct a neodermis. While the patient's own neodermis is being constructed, the bovine collagen dissolves. During the period of neodermis construction, about 2 weeks, the silicone epidermal layer acts to control moisture loss from the wound. Once neodermis construction is complete or later, the surgeon removes the silicone layer and replaces it with very thin autografts from the patient. One major benefit of Integra is that there is no scar formation associated with its use. Other benefits are that it is immediately available for use and it allows for immediate postexcisional wound coverage, early ambulation and rehabilitation, delayed autografting of the neodermis if necessary, more rapid healing and better cosmetic outcome of donor sites because of ultrathin autograft use, and the ability to save certain donor sites for use on cosmetically sensitive areas.[59] Some disadvantages of Integra are that it lacks hair follicles and sweat glands. However, sensory function returns at the same level and time course as it does following normal STSG autografting.[60] Integra is expensive, but such expense may be justifiable if the use of Integra can decrease morbidity and mortality and improve outcome. The high cost of the product may be offset by the lower costs associated with its use if it can hasten wound closure and decrease the rehabilitation needs and future reconstructive needs of the patient.

Another dermal replacement product that is also available for use is allografted skin, AlloDerm (AlloDerm, LifeCell Corp., The Woodlands, TX), which, once the antigenic epidermis and antigenic cells from the dermis are removed, leaves a dermal matrix that will accept an ultrathin

STSG. Less scarring and contraction result with the use of AlloDerm and an ultrathin STSG than with an STSG alone, and the use of ultrathin grafts with the AlloDerm results in quicker healing and less scarring of donor sites.[50] The color of the combined AlloDerm and STSG closely matches that of the surrounding skin. As is the case with Integra, the high cost of AlloDerm may be offset by the lower costs of decreased length of stay and fewer rehabilitation needs or future reconstructive surgeries.

Physical Therapy Examination

The physical therapist plays a crucial role in the rehabilitation of the pediatric burn patient. The therapist's goals for the pediatric burn patient are to assist with burn wound management, maintain or increase active and passive range of motion, manage soft tissue contours, maintain or increase strength and endurance, promote normal development and function, and inhibit loss of motion, deformity, hypertrophic scarring, and contractures. The physical therapist is involved in the entire continuum of care for children with thermal injuries from the acute through the rehabilitative and reconstructive phases. The therapist is a member of the burn team and consults with other team members, including the patient and parents, when providing interventions and assisting with the plan of care.

EXAMINATION/EVALUATION

Depending on the setting the physical therapist is working in, the thermal injury will be in a different phase of healing (e.g., inflammation, proliferation, and maturation). You may be examining a new burn, one that has undergone excision and grafting, one that is healing following a graft, or one that has begun to demonstrate scarring months after the original injury.

HISTORY

Either via reviewing the patient's chart or conducting a detailed patient/parent interview, there are key pieces of information needed. These pieces include the date of injury, the mechanism of injury, what the child was wearing, what was done immediately at the scene prior to emergency services arriving, and what medical or surgical interventions the child has had. The circumstances of the injury, as well as the pattern of the burn, will assist the team in ruling out child abuse. Knowing what the child was wearing may help give a better idea of why a burn appears the way it does. For example, knowing whether a patient had clothing on that wasn't fire retardant or had a diaper on that spared the groin area will assist the therapist in a full evaluation. Since there are still many home remedies for burns, it is important to ask the family members what first

aid was provided at the scene. If there was clothing on, was it removed? Was water poured on the area? Did you put any ointment or other substance on the burn? Many people still put ice, oils, ointments, or even butter on burns as these remedies have been passed down from generation to generation; however, these can affect the healing process and influence the evaluation of the burn. Another part of the history examination is the social history. What type of structure the child lives in, who lives in the home, what grade the child is in, and what mode of transportation the child takes are all questions to ask to assist with early discharge planning. If the child was burned in a house fire, is the home inhabitable, or does the family need assistance to secure safe housing prior to discharge? For the patient in the rehabilitation setting, return to and reintegration into the school setting need early planning to assist teachers and students in what to expect upon their return. Past medical history or developmental history that may influence the patient's recovery or physical therapy interventions is also important to document.

REVIEW OF SYSTEMS

CARDIOPULMONARY The circulatory changes that occur following a thermal injury are called burn shock. Cardiac output is decreased due to fluid losses, vasodilation, and decreased circulating volume. Fluid resuscitation is key to leveling off the normal resting values of cardiac output.[15] Children who demonstrate singed hair of the face or hairline, oral edema and blisters, hoarseness, and carbonaceous sputum have signs and symptoms of inhalation injury and need close monitoring of their respiratory status. They will require 100% oxygen or even intubation to protect their airway and provide adequate respiratory support.[15] The physical therapist in the acute care setting needs to be aware of normal vital signs, oxygen saturation, and the effects of interventions on these parameters. Severe thermal injuries will result in decreased pulmonary function, which can last several years. The initial obstructive phase develops into a restrictive pattern as seen on pulmonary function tests.[61] Other factors that could influence pulmonary function include chest wall burns and the need for a tracheotomy. Suman et al.[61] reported increased pulmonary function in children who underwent exercise tolerance interventions, recommending it be a component of a comprehensive outpatient intervention program for children following thermal injuries.

NEUROMUSCULAR Depending on the depth of the burn, circulatory compromise can result from edema formation. The patient is at risk for compartment syndrome (see Escharotomy), which can affect nerves and muscle viability.[15] The patient is also at risk for peripheral nerve compression due to immobility and improper positioning (e.g., peroneal nerve compression with externally rotated lower extremities).

MUSCULOSKELETAL If the patient was involved in a motor vehicle accident with vehicle fire or needed to jump from a burning home, he or she is at risk for fracture. These fractures may not be initially found if the patient is unresponsive and the initial trauma survey is concentrated on the thermal injury. With a deep hand burn, flexor or extensor tendons may be exposed, which require careful attention as to not cause the tendon to rupture. One complication that often occurs in children following a thermal injury is heterotopic ossification, most often found in the elbow. Other joints affected may be the hip and shoulder, even if not directly affected by the thermal injury, but which may occur due to immobility. In the acute phase, a ramification of heterotopic ossification is pain, while further into the child's recovery, function is limited. Surgical intervention is often required to improve range of motion as well as ADLs such as feeding and self-care.[62]

INTEGUMENTARY As discussed previously, the examination of the integumentary system needs to include burn depth estimation as well as determining the TBSA involved. The physical therapist can utilize a body diagram to make notations on the areas that are burned, as well as graft sites or scars that are present. The Lund and Browder chart should be utilized to determine TBSA. Identifying structures of the skin as well as tissue type, capillary refill, and mechanism of injury will aid in determining burn depth (see Burn Depth Estimation).

For a child following skin grafting, upon removal of the postoperative dressings, examination of the graft adherence can be described in percentage of graft "take." For example, for an STSG that has completely adhered and with no signs of open wound, the graft has 100% take.

Scar-rating tools may be helpful in a more comprehensive examination/evaluation of burn scars. One such tool is the Vancouver Scar Scale (VSS) (Fig. 16.11). This visual examination tool rates the scar according to its pigmentation, vascularity, pliability, and height, assigning a score for each. The scores can then be compared over time.[63] In addition to such tools, the patient's perception of his or her scar should be taken into consideration.[64]

One other component of the integumentary review needs to be an examination of the nonburned skin. The acutely burned child may be immobile, due to medical instability. Careful inspection of nonburned skin needs to be done on at least a daily basis, as the immobile child is at risk for pressure ulcers. Contributing factors, in addition to immobility, are decreased nutrition, altered levels of consciousness, and altered sensory perception in the case of compartment syndrome. Areas at risk for pressure ulcers include the occiput, sacrum, and heels. Splints utilized for joint position and preservation can also be the cause of pressure ulcers due to improper fit or application, or due to volume shifts from edema. Daily inspection of the skin and fit of splints is part of the acute care therapist's examination and subsequent interventions. A skin risk assessment scale that is utilized in the pediatric population is the Braden Q scale. It was adapted from the Braden scale, which was established for determining adults at risk for pressure sores. This scale is often done by the bedside nurse, but can be implemented by any member of the health care team.[65]

Another important component to the integumentary examination is the use of photography. In addition to the body diagrams, a photo may allow for further evaluation, once the burn has been covered by dressings. A photograph will also allow another clinician to view the wound, if he or she missed the dressing change, thus not subjecting the child to another unnecessary dressing change. Advantages of using digital photography (over 35-mm film) include image verification, immediate printing, and ease of collecting a series of photographs to document change. Photography can also be utilized as a communication tool between therapists and nurses in the case of specific dressing or splint application.[66]

TESTS AND MEASURES

PAIN Before your examination, the child's pain management should be a priority. Children following an acute burn suffer from pain not only from the original injury, but also from daily procedures including dressing changes and therapy. These procedures stimulate the nociceptive afferent fibers on a daily basis during their recovery.[67] Before physically examining the child (or during interventions), pain needs to be evaluated. Pain scales are readily available and valid for evaluating pediatric pain. One such self-reporting scale is the Wong-Baker FACES scale, where the child can pick from six different faces (no hurt to hurts as much as you can imagine) with a resultant score of 0 to 10.[68] For children older than age 7, a self-reporting numeric scale of 0 to 10 can be used (ask the child to rate the pain on a scale of 0, no pain, to 10, the worst pain ever). For children who are unresponsive or unable to use one of the self-reporting scales, a behavioral scale should be used. The FLACC pain scale is a behavioral pain scale that has been validated for the evaluation of postoperative pain in children. FLACC is an acronym for five categories: Face, Legs, Activity, Cry, and Consolability. Each category is scored 0 to 2, with a maximum score of 10. Analgesia should be considered for scores above 3, with narcotics utilized for scores above 7.[69] Documentation of the pain score is done daily by the therapist before, during, and after the interventions as well as periodically by nursing in the acute care setting.

SENSATION Sensory testing begins during examination of the acute burn. The patient's ability to detect touch or pain at the burn site indicates the depth of the burn. Areas that are insensate or are not painful despite the burn may indicate a full-thickness injury. As discussed earlier, in the acute phase of a burn, edema formation may be rapid and

VANCOUVER GENERAL HOSPITAL
OCCUPATIONAL THERAPY DEPARTMENT

BURN SCAR ASSESSMENT
PATIENT NAME:

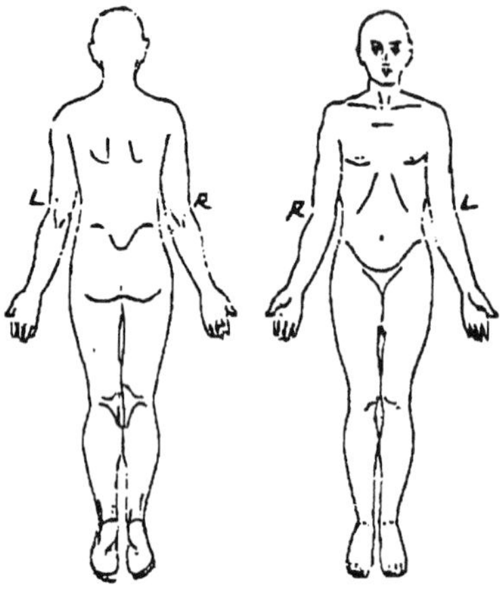

PIGMENTATION (M)

0   normal—color that closely resembles
    the color over the rest of one's body
1   hypopigmentation
2   hyperpigmentation

VASCULARITY (V)

0   normal—color that closely resembles
    the color over the rest of one's body
1   pink
2   red
3   purple

PLIABILITY (P)

0   normal
1   supple—flexible with minimal resistance
2   yielding—giving way to pressure
3   firm-inflexible, not easily moved,
    resistant to manual pressure
4   banding—rope-like tissue that
    blanches with extension of scar
5   contracture—permanent shortening of
    scar producing deformity or distortion

HEIGHT

0   normal—flat
1   < 2 mm
2   < 5 mm
3   > 5 mm

Scale in mm

Date	Scar #	Pigmentation	Vascularity	Pliability	Height	Total	OT init

Figure 16.11 ■ Vancouver Scar Assessment Scale.

extensive. This edema formation can be severe enough to compromise blood flow to the extremities and lead to compartment syndrome. Careful examination of skin color, temperature, and the presence of numbness/tingling are necessary.[15] Children with increased lower extremity edema or groin edema may assume a position of external rotation. This in turn can compress the peroneal nerve, causing numbness, tingling, or footdrop. For children in the later stages of healing, or in the scar maturation phase, careful examination of sensation will aid in planning interventions. Children with foot burns, who lack normal sensation due to the depth of the burn or in the case of a graft on the plantar surface of the foot, need to be instructed in safety

concerns of going barefoot. Children and their parents must be aware of the dangers of walking barefoot and need to do careful skin inspection if they do to look for any cuts or infections.

RANGE OF MOTION On initial examination of the acute burn, careful attention should be given to examining ROM of all affected and unaffected joints. If the patient can participate, active-assistive ROM is beneficial to give the child some form of control while also allowing you to get some idea of what his or her ROM limits are. Passive range of motion (PROM) can be performed but with caution in the acute phase and especially in a child who may be unresponsive. Aggressive PROM is contraindicated over exposed tendons/joints due to the risk of rupture. Care must also be taken at the shoulder so as not to cause joint or brachial plexus injury.

In the remodeling phase of healing, daily examination of ROM with the bandages removed is a necessity. Seeing the ROM without the dressings allows the clinician to view the healing structures and to examine any scar tissue for blanching. Blanching tissue signifies the end of the ROM prior to tearing the skin.[50] Once blanching is noted, the clinician has a clear idea of what ROM to expect from the patient for the rest of the day during all therapies. Pushing the patient past the point of blanching will lead to a painful episode of tearing the skin; this in turn will create a new open wound that needs to be dressed.

For patients well into the scar maturation phase, ROM of joints that have scars needs to be done in multiple planes of movement to fully assess the ROM and scar blanching. For example, a child with a scar on the anterior shoulder may not show limitation in straight plane movements, but may with overhead activities such as throwing a ball. Taking the shoulder and subsequent scars through multiplanar motions will give you a more thorough examination.

MOBILITY/GAIT If the patient is allowed to mobilize, examine his or her level of independence with getting in and out of bed, getting out of a chair, and ambulating. With lower extremity burns, the child may demonstrate an antalgic gait, and may need an assistive device. Following grafts, the child may have pain/limitations at the donor sites, which are frequently on the upper legs, thus impeding mobility and gait. During the scar maturation phase, truncal and leg scars may inhibit normal walking or running patterns.

ACTIVITIES OF DAILY LIVING A thorough examination must also include the child's ability to participate in ADLs. Depending on the age of the child, the level of participation at baseline will be different. For example, the toddler may be able to remove clothes/shoes, but will need assistance with donning the same. The adolescent is expected to be independent with all ADLs. The child's ability to participate in ADLs also may include dressing changes in the acute phase, as well as scar management and donning compression garments during the scar maturation phase.

◆ **Interventions**

PAIN MANAGEMENT

Prior to performing any interventions with the child following a thermal injury, his or her pain must be assessed. As discussed earlier, utilize one of the self-reporting or behavioral pain scales to assess the child's pain level. There will be different types and causes of pain with the patient with burns, including those associated with the injury itself, wound care techniques, debridement, grafting, and therapies. Depending on the type and timing of interventions, pain assessment would determine the need for a pharmacologic approach, nonpharmacologic approach, or one that combines the two.[70] Intervention strategies include premedicating the child prior to procedures that may be painful or anxiety provoking. Drugs that may be used include nonsteroidal anti-inflammatory agents, which reduce pain and modify the systemic inflammatory response. Opiates have been proven to be useful in the alleviation of burn pain. Benzodiazepines are utilized for the role of anxiety control. Ketamine, a dissociative anesthetic, is also widely used to provide comfort and has an amnesic effect so the child does not have memory of the painful procedure.[70]

Nonpharmacologic interventions include cognitive-behavioral therapy; relaxation training; hypnosis and guided imagery; biofeedback; distraction; and art, music, and play therapies.[70] If your institution has child life specialists, they should be included in either preparing the child for the procedure or aiding in distraction during the procedure. If you do not have access to a child life specialist or music therapist, you should be prepared, prior to providing interventions, with age-appropriate distraction activities. These may include bubbles, books, and magic wands for younger patients and portable radio/compact disc players, video games, or DVDs for older patients.

WOUND CARE

ACUTE MANAGEMENT

Depending on the institution you work in, the mode of wound cleansing and dressing application will already be established. The physical therapist may play a primary role in wound care or an adjunctive role if nursing has the lead role in cleaning the wounds and providing dressing application. Daily or twice-daily dressing changes may be ordered in the early stages of burn wound management.

Preparation for wound cleansing and dressing change include premedicating the patient, coordinating all staff that need to examine the patient, and preparing the room and supplies. The room temperature should be at least 86°F to minimize heat loss and lower the metabolic rate of the child.[15] Local wound care can occur in a hydrotherapy (whirlpool) setting or more commonly with saline. Wounds should be gently cleansed to remove old topical agents and devitalized tissue and to decrease pain.[71] Wound beds should not be scrubbed to the point of bleeding, although bleeding may occur in the healing epithelium. Removal of blisters that are intact is controversial. Some believe that the area under the blister is sterile and can remain intact, unless it becomes very tense or erythematous. Others believe that the blisters that remain may interfere with ongoing examination process. Guidance from your trauma or plastic surgeon may dictate your institution's policies.

Once the wound is cleansed, timely application of the topical agent and dry dressings will aid in decreasing the pain felt by the child when the wounds are left open to the air for prolonged periods.

Ideal burn dressings will serve multiple functions. They will be nonadherent to the healing wound; absorb exudates; provide a warm, moist environment for healing; protect the wounds from further damage; and allow for functional use of the affected area.[71] Functional wrapping of the affected areas is often best done by the physical therapist. The physical therapist can suggest positions for extremities or affected joints to be placed in, and then have the bandage applied in order to maximize function. Examples of this include wrapping the elbow into extension with a burn that covers the antecubital fossa, individually wrapping fingers and toes, and positioning the ankle in neutral dorsiflexion to avoid a plantar flexion contracture if wrapped incorrectly, inhibiting movement.

There are several layers to a good burn dressing. The contact layer is just that; it comes in contact with the burn and is low to nonadherent. The topical agent (most commonly Silvadene) should be applied onto the contact layer, and not applied directly to the burn site due to pain concerns. Examples of a contact layer dressing include Exu-Dry, Conformant, Xeroform, and Adaptic. The next layer is the intermediate absorbent layer and is usually dry gauze or absorptive pads (Exu-Dry). The outermost layer serves to hold the other two layers in place and includes rolls of gauze or tubular elastic netting. The netting can be made into garments, thus securing the bandages from slipping and exposing the burns. Tape should be avoided as it makes it more difficult to remove the dressing and can also migrate onto good or burned tissue, thus creating pain and anxiety at dressing removal.[71] Ongoing wound/skin management includes the use of moisturizing cream, sunscreen, and occasionally dressings if there is an open wound that occurs.

SPLINTING AND POSITIONING

The purpose of splinting and positioning during the acute phase is to help control edema, provide support for edematous extremities, and inhibit contraction and loss of motion. It is often not necessary to splint children at this time except in the case of older children and adolescents and those who are extensively burned. Care must also be taken to prevent pressure sores in these children as they are at high risk due to moisture and immobility. Pressure sores in the burn population can occur due to hypovolemia, decreased oxygenation, prolonged bedrest, or poorly fitting splints. Causes of pressure ulcers are attributed to shear, friction, and unrelieved pressure. The most common sites for pressure ulcers are the sacrum/coccyx and heels, with other areas at risk being the ankle, buttocks, and occipital area. The child who requires surgical intervention is also at risk during the operation if appropriate pressure-relieving devices are not used.[65]

For positioning in bed during the first few days of hospitalization, the child who is on bedrest must have appropriate devices in place. Heel and elbow protectors can be used as well as gel pillows for bony prominences. An interdisciplinary approach to proper positioning is key to tackling this problem. Appropriate positioning programs and devices are only effective when implemented correctly. Education and communication between therapists and nurses will aid in this process.

When utilizing splints, the therapist must take into consideration the skin integrity, edema formation, and fit of the device. As reviewed earlier, the zone of stasis is an area that lies immediately beneath the burn and has a compromised state of circulation; this area is sensitive to increased pressure. If splints or elastic bandages are applied too tightly, the zone of stasis could convert to a deeper burn. Care must also be taken when using devices on nonburned areas as they too could cause skin breakdown. Splints made to prevent contractures or protect structures during the early phase of wound healing must be monitored daily to ensure proper fit. They may need to be adjusted daily to accommodate for edema formation or changes in dressings. As edema increases, splints or elastic bandages holding the splints in place can cause increased compression, leading to a pressure sore. Meticulous skin inspection during dressing changes must occur during the edema formation stage and as the burn heals in order to ensure proper fit.[65]

In bed, positioning needs to begin as soon as the child is admitted, either to an intensive care unit or regular unit. For patients who are on bedrest, care must be taken to avoid shear forces. The Agency for Healthcare Research and Quality has made recommendations to minimize shear. These include avoiding placing the head of the bed higher than 30 degrees for any prolonged time. The skin and fascia of the torso tend to remain static while the deep fascia and skeleton slide toward the bottom of the bed when the head is raised. The skin on the scapula and buttocks is then put on traction, thus causing a shearing force. With sufficient traction, blood supply is compromised and a pressure ulcer can develop. Transferring the patient in/out of bed to a stretcher should be performed via a lifting technique rather than sliding him or her across the support surfaces, again to further decrease the risk of shear.

Repositioning the patient in bed should occur at least every 1 to 2 hours, if the patient is medically stable. Keeping to the lower limits of this timeframe will be helpful as different tissues have different tolerances to ischemia from pressure.[65]

There is an axiom that states that the position of comfort—flexion—is the position of contracture for burn patients. Patients are thus splinted or positioned to counteract contracting forces. As mentioned previously, it is often not necessary to splint children during the acute care phase, although the therapist may elect to begin splinting and positioning children with severe burns or older children and adolescents later in this phase. The neck should

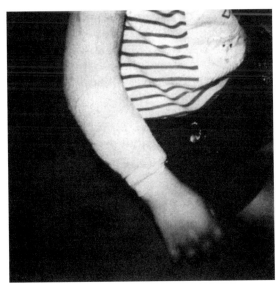

Figure 16.12 ■ Elbow extension splint to prevent or correct elbow flexion contracture.

be positioned in a neutral position or slight extension. Pillows under the head are prohibited because they promote cervical flexion. The shoulders should be positioned in approximately 90 degrees of abduction and in slight protraction. Elbows should be placed in extension and supination (Fig. 16.12). Wrist/hands should be positioned in slight wrist extension, slight metacarpophalangeal (MCP) joint flexion, proximal interphalangeal/distal interphalangeal extension, and thumb abduction (Fig. 16.13). Hips are placed in neutral extension and slight abduction, neutral rotation. Knees are placed in full extension; ankles are in neutral dorsiflexion (no plantar flexion). All of these anti-contracture positions can be attained either with the use

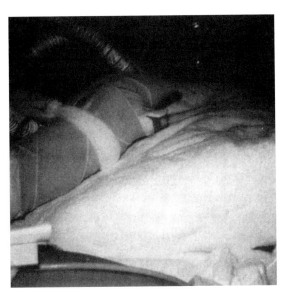

Figure 16.13 ■ Example of a hand splint to prevent contractures.

of towel rolls, splints, or other positioning devices that are commercially available.[50] Splints are fabricated over a uniform layer of dressings in order to ensure proper day-to-day fit and are monitored closely due to the edema issues discussed earlier.

Specialized splints can be fabricated for specific body parts. Airplane splints are made for axillary burns. Microstomias are special devices to assist in mouth/lip stretching. A Multi-Ring Watusi collar is a flexible neck orthosis that allows circumferential pressure to the neck. It assists with gaining ROM and is easier to fabricate than traditional thermoplastic splints.[72]

CASTING

Casting may be used during both the acute and rehabilitation phases to maintain position in pediatric patients when a splint position is difficult to sustain. For example, it may be preferable to immobilize the MCP joints in flexion while allowing active use of the distal joints.[73] Serial casting is effective in correcting contractures in both pediatric and adult burn patients in whom other methods of regaining motion have failed, in noncompliant patients,[74–76] in patients whose splints easily slip or are removed, or in those for whom other methods, such as dynamic splinting, cannot be used.[76] Serial casting can eliminate or delay the need for reconstructive surgery.[76] Once motion is regained through serial casting, it needs to be maintained through continued casting or splinting and ROM exercise. Depending on the particular patient and the phase of healing, casts made of either plaster or synthetic materials may be used. Soft Cast, a synthetic casting material, is particularly useful for children because it sets quickly. In addition, although the child cannot remove it, the therapist can simply unwrap it rather than using a cast saw, which might frighten the child.

RANGE OF MOTION

Active ROM exercises during the emergent phase help control edema and initiate early motion. Muscle contraction serves as a pumping mechanism to aid venous and lymphatic return.[77] As stated previously, ROM exercises should be performed during dressing changes when the bandages do not restrict motion, the therapist can see the limitations in motion resulting from edema, the wound can be viewed, and the patient has received pain medication.

Active ROM exercises should commence upon admission and continue throughout the rehabilitative and scar management phases. Active exercise will aid in decreasing edema as well as preserving muscle, tendon, and joint function. Activities that are fun will assist the child in participating in active exercise. Such activities could include catching/throwing a ball overhead for upper extremity/shoulder burns, playing baseball (for trunk rotation), and riding a bike (for lower extremity burns). Activities of daily living can also be implemented to gain active ROM. Stepping into/out of a tub requires increased hip/knee ROM; reaching up onto a counter or into a cabinet requires good shoulder ROM. Those patients with true weakness due to deconditioning or nerve damage may require assistance with active ROM exercises. Both active and active-assisted exercises provide sensory feedback, increase circulation, maintain muscle function, and allow for preserving fine and gross motor skills.[50]

Hand burns require specific therapeutic interventions. Early use of the injured hand in ADLs increases the child's independence and return to play activities. Active and passive motion exercises will aid in tendon gliding by minimizing adhesions. Blocking and resistive exercises during the scar maturation phase will prevent the maturation of adhesions, which can limit function.[78]

PROM exercises are implemented for children who are unable to move on their own. They maintain elasticity of joint structures, muscle, and tendons and help to minimize the formation of contractures. Stretching exercises can be achieved either via traditional PROM by the therapist or by the patient using a self-stretch premise. Self-stretching can be achieved by using overhead pulleys for shoulder ROM or a towel stretch for ankle dorsiflexion. Stretching, no matter what phase it is done in, needs to be slow, gentle, and sustained. Remember that blanching of tissue/scar is the sign of the appropriate stretch. PROM could be performed in the operating room if the child is undergoing a surgical procedure. For a child that is resistant to all stretching, active ROM, or positioning, the opportunity to examine ROM under anesthesia is invaluable. Caution must be taken, however, to protect joints from subluxation or dislocation during this exam.[50]

MASSAGE

Massage of scar tissue and skin grafts helps maintain motion by freeing restrictive bands and increasing circulation.[79] Massage may also be helpful in decreasing itching. Initially, only gentle massage should be employed, because the newly healed tissue is often too fragile to tolerate much friction. Many children enjoy massage because it decreases itching, but other children find massage painful or will not sit still for such treatment. Although all patients should have scar tissue and skin grafts lubricated by thoroughly rubbing in lotions—preferably two to three times each day—the therapist may select particular areas of concern for massage and may also instruct the parent in massage of these areas. Massage should be done before specific ROM exercises, especially passive ROM exercises.

AMBULATION

Once cleared by the physician, mobility should commence as soon as possible. For patients with donor sites on their legs, premedicating them may allow for less pain during mobility. For those patients with lower extremity burns or grafts, elastic bandage compression is necessary to give vascular support prior to ambulating. Following a lower extremity graft, the child will be on bedrest for 5 to 7 days. Once cleared to get up (usually after the first dressing change), gradual mobility may begin. Ace wrapping or use of an elastic cotton bandage (Tubigrip) should be applied to the lower extremities. To begin, the child is wrapped and then allowed to dangle the extremity for approximately 1 minute. The extremity is returned to an elevated position, the wrap taken off, and the graft inspected for signs of color change, bleeding, or breakdown. The child may progress with a dangling protocol, where he or she sits at the edge of the bed for up to 15 minutes four times a day prior to ambulating. This will decrease the risk of pooling of blood, which could cause graft failure. Once dangling has been successful, ambulation may begin, again with careful monitoring of color, discomfort, tingling, edema, bleeding, or breakdown.[80]

EXERCISE

Sakurai et al. have studied the benefits of exercise in children who have been burned. They found increased physical functioning, muscle mass, strength, and cardiovascular endurance.[81] Exercise that incorporates repetitive movement of extremities and increased core body temperature, thus increasing blood flow, may alter scar elasticity and increase ROM. Celis et al.[82] found that a supervised exercise program produced beneficial outcomes in children with thermal injuries. They found a decreased number of scar releases needed for functional improvement in comparison to their control group.[82]

Children who have sustained an inhalation injury as well as thermal injury are at risk for decreased exercise tolerance due to decreased pulmonary function. Children may have an initial obstructive pattern of disease, which can last up to 2 years after the initial injury. This obstructive pattern then develops into a restrictive pattern for up to 8 years after burn. Suman et al.[61] looked at the effects of an exercise program in severely burned children. The subjects did resistance and aerobic training 3 days per week. They found increases in pulmonary function improvements and subsequent improved exercise tolerance due to the exercise program.[61]

Cucuzzo et al.[83] compared the efficacy and effects of an exercise program versus traditional outpatient therapy in burned children. They did an in-house program with a general conditioning prescription for exercise. This program included moderate-intensity, progressive resistance training with aerobic and general conditioning exercises for 1 hour three times per week. Strength training utilized free weights and aerobic training included motorized treadmill, stationary bike, or independent walking. Their results showed that severely burned children could participate safely in this type of supervised exercise program, as their study group showed gains in strength and functional outcomes.[83]

SCAR MANAGEMENT

Following burn wound healing, or skin grafting, scar formation may occur. Skin and scar care progresses from the initial open wound phase into the scar maturation phase as the wounds heal. Once the wounds or grafts have healed, it is important to keep the skin well moisturized. Application of a moisturizer throughout the day will decrease the risk of skin cracks and decrease itching. Massaging in the lotion with enough pressure to create blanching may assist in releasing the scar tissue and increase ROM.[50] Avoid putting too much pressure too soon on the scars as blisters can form, thus requiring massage to be discontinued. It is thought that massage helps to break up collagen fibers, which in turn will soften the scar.[84]

Compression has also been utilized to combat the formation of hypertrophic scarring. Early compression can begin once the wounds or grafts have healed. Compression can begin in the form of Ace wrapping, elastic cotton tubular stockings, or adhesive wraps (for hands/fingers) (Figs. 16.14 and 16.15). Once edema has stabilized and the grafts or burns are completely healed, the child may be measured for a custom compression garment. Pressure garments have four main functions. They restore function, relieve symptoms, prevent scar recurrence, and promote an aesthetic appearance. Pressure results in the reduction of intercollagen fibers, which helps to flatten the excessive collagen that is deposited during the proliferative phase. Pressure amounts for these garments should be 24 mm Hg or above and applied for a minimum of 12 months. Pressure garments are worn for 23 hours a day, allowing removal for bathing/skin care. Pressures over 24 mm Hg occlude vessels, which leads to hypoxia and fibroblast degeneration and altered collagen synthesis. This process then helps flatten the scar.[84] Early application of pressure is necessary for optimal outcomes. Pressure is applied as soon as re-

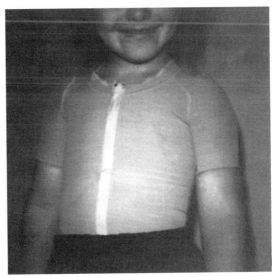

Figure 16.15 ■ Child wearing the temporary compression vest from Figure 16.14.

epithelialization has occurred and continues through the maturation phase. Children are issued two sets of garments due to the constant wear and the need for the garments to be washed. They will need to be refit periodically due to wear from usage, growth, or surgical interventions.[85] Several commercially available options are made for children, with a wider variety of colors and appliqués to try to increase patient use (Fig. 16.16).

To apply uniform pressure over convex or concave areas, foam, rubberized materials, or thermoplastic splinting material may be used as inserts under the garments. Areas often needing more custom pressure include web spaces, the palm of the hand, the interscapular area, and the central face.[50] Silicone linings and inserts have also been used as an adjunct to compression therapy. The mechanism of action by silicone is hydration and occlusion of the scar. Silicone elastomers (putty) were made to solve concavity problems, especially in web spaces. Benefits of using silicone sheets

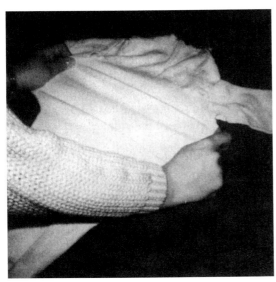

Figure 16.14 ■ Example of a compression vest made out of tubular elastic netting.

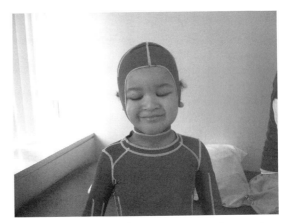

Figure 16.16 ■ Example of custom compression mask and jacket.

include comfort in application and little to no hindrance of movement. Disadvantages include frequent renewing of the sheets, loss of mobility when used over a joint, and excessive sweating.[86] Most manufacturers of compression garments offer some form of silicone lining that can be sewn directly into the garment over specified areas.

Facial burns require special attention due to the importance of cosmetic appearance following a burn. Children with facial burns will have the social stigma of looking different and have long-term psychological impact of disfigurement. Compression therapy for the face can occur in three different ways. Custom compression garments are available for the face, but usually cover the entire face and head, thus "hiding" the deformities. Clear plastic masks allow the clinician to see the pressure applied to the scars directly under the mask; however, the child's face and scars are fully visible. A third option is a silicone mask held in place with a facial pressure garment.[87]

The transparent plastic face mask was introduced in 1979 by Rivers et al. as an alternative to the elastic face mask to control facial scarring (Fig. 16.17).[88] As its name implies, the transparent face mask is a piece of hard, transparent plastic in the form of a custom-fitting face mask secured to the face by means of straps. The mask is constructed by forming heated plastic over a modified positive mold of the patient's face. In the past, the mold would need to be done in the operating room with the child anesthetized due to having to use plaster and not having the patient move. New digital scanning technology has made that procedure obsolete. The Total Contact Scanner, by Total Contact Inc. (www.totalcontact.com), is a digital surface scanner, which allows for noncontact scanning. This system uses a low-power helium-neon laser projected from the moving scanner head to the patient's face. The scan is transmitted to a computer, which captures all the surface data. This data is then sent to the company, which produces a positive mold, over which a negative mold of the plastic/silicone face mask is made. The therapist can then adjust the fit of the mask by making the necessary changes to the positive mold and reheating the mask. The time and resources saved by not having the patient undergo anesthesia are quite beneficial.

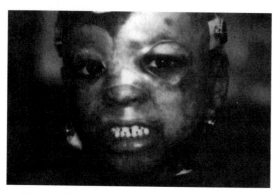

Figure 16.17 ■ Transparent face mask for facial burn compression.

The advantages of the transparent face mask versus the elastic face mask are as follows:

- The mask can be constructed and applied to the patient within 24 hours. (There is no waiting for the elastic garment to return from the manufacturer.)
- The therapist can see exactly where pressure is being adequately applied by observing blanching of the scar. The transparent mask can be adjusted accordingly by the therapist to increase or decrease pressure in specific areas.
- The patient's face is visible to other people and is not covered by a "mask."
- The transparent mask usually does not require the construction and exact placement of inserts.
- The transparent face mask may cause fewer problems with head growth and malocclusion than the elastic mask.

There are also several disadvantages of the transparent face mask, including the following:

- Although both types of mask often have to be replaced as the child grows and the mask wears out, the cost of a new transparent mask is probably greater.
- The plastic used to construct the transparent mask is rigid, permits little movement of the facial muscles, and often limits mandible motion.
- The transparent mask may not cover as many areas on the head as the elastic mask. (However, the transparent mask can be used with a chin strap or alternated with an elastic mask.)
- Perspiration is increased underneath the transparent mask, and plastic may be more uncomfortable than elastic.

There are some documented drawbacks to the use of compression devices. The elastic chin strap may also cause at least a temporary recession of the mandible,[89] and it, in combination with a neck conformer, may cause increased proclination of maxillary and mandibular incisors.[90] The elastic face mask may impede head growth in very young children[91] and may cause abnormal recession of mandibular growth.[92] Both the elastic face mask and the plastic face mask may affect facial growth.[90] Elastic shirts may cause regressed skeletal growth of the thoracic cage,[92] and elastic gloves may cause narrowing of the palmar arch.[92] However, the burn injury and/or the acute or reconstructive therapy, as well as the grafted skin and scar tissue, may also contribute to these problems.[91–93] When the face mask or elastic chin strap is used, the child's head growth, facial growth, and dentition should be monitored.

PATIENT/CLIENT-RELATED INSTRUCTIONS

Throughout the continuum of care for a child following a burn injury, the child and caregivers will need ongoing teaching. Initially the parents may help with burn dressing changes, application of splints, and exercises. As the child returns to home and school, the caregivers must assume all care including skin and graft care, scar management, night splints, day splints, compression garments, massage, and being mom or dad to other siblings in many cases. When possible, practicing interventions in a controlled setting may help parents be more comfortable than carrying out the intervention on their own child. This can occur in a classroom-type setting where parents can practice on mannequins or each other, gain confidence, and then work with their own child. Children who are old enough to follow directions and a schedule are able to learn their self-care and often prefer to have control over parts of their care. A written home program for exercises, splint application, and compression garment wearing schedules will aid in the caregiver's carryover.

 ## Outcomes

Children who suffer a burn injury, especially one of extensive TBSA, have cosmetic and functional impairments that may never be completely corrected. Psychosocial implications for children include acceptance by their family, peers, and schoolmates, with potentially disfiguring and disabling effects of their original injury. A study done by Sheridan et al. in 2000[94] showed that massively burned children do not necessarily suffer from a poor quality of life. Even though they can't be returned to their preburn status, appearance, and function, their acute care team, support after discharge, and family support can produce satisfying long-term outcomes for children with massive burns.[94]

The child who sustains a burn injury undergoes long-term hospitalization, painful procedures and rehabilitation, and lifelong disfigurement. Landolt et al. in 2002[95] also looked at predictors of quality of life in pediatric burn survivors. Their results also demonstrated an almost normal outcome concerning health-related quality of life. One of the main predictors of outcome was the importance of the family environment. The overall quality of life and psychological adjustment were best predicted by greater family cohesion, higher expressiveness, and fewer conflicts within the family. The second most important variable to predicting quality of life was age at injury. Children burned at a younger age had a better quality of life at follow-up. Younger children may more easily deal with their scars and integrate their disfigurement into their developing body image. Older children may have more difficulties with the need of changing their body image. Their study noted that there was a quality-of-life scale pending from the American Burn Association.[95]

The impact of a thermal injury on the family and siblings was reviewed by Mancuso et al. in 2003.[96] Sibling research has shown that their relationships among themselves are among the most significant in preparing a child for adulthood. Their studies revealed that siblings had fewer signs of internalizing problems and were less withdrawn and showed fewer depressive symptoms and fewer somatic problems than the control group. Compared to the control group, those siblings of children with moderate to severe injuries did have more difficulties with social competence. This corresponds with the severity of injury causing an increased duration of care, potentially more absence of parents, and more family attention to the injured sibling. The siblings appeared to do well at school and the social competence piece may have been related to their ability to have friends at their home, in light of the disfigurement of their sibling. Even under stressful events, the well siblings are adjusting socially, emotionally, and behaviorally.[96]

 ## Burn Camp

Just as there are camps for children with various diseases or disabilities (e.g., diabetes camp, spina bifida camp, etc.), there are also about 40 burn camps in North America that offer a variety of programs for children who have sustained burn injuries. Several of these camps are coordinated or staffed by therapists, or therapists are encouraged to attend the camp to help with programs or to assist campers. The purpose of most of the camps is to provide a safe, recreational environment in which children with burns can interact with one another, build self-esteem, learn new skills, and have fun.

SUMMARY

Physical therapists play a vital role on the interdisciplinary burn care team. They function in many different roles from acute burn wound management, to positioning, splinting, ROM, and functional mobility, to scar management and return to home and school. Pediatric physical therapists in any setting across the continuum of care need to be prepared to provide interventions for these children as well as be advocates for their psychosocial needs upon re-entry into the community. Ongoing continuing education and mentorship will provide the best experience to gain clinical competence in the area of care for the child with thermal injuries.

CASE STUDIES
CASE STUDY 1

JADE

Jade is a 6-year-old girl who was admitted to her local hospital following an accident at home. Jade was leaning over a candle in her mom's bedroom when her braids caught on fire and set her shirt on fire. Her mom put out the flames with a blanket and removed her shirt immediately, calling 911 in the process. Jade received emergency care within minutes and was transported to the hospital. She was referred to physical therapy on postburn day 1.

Upon initial examination, she appeared to have superficial partial-thickness burns to her face and deep partial-thickness

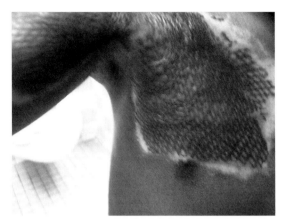

Figure 16.18 ■ Healed meshed split-thickness skin graft (same patient from Figure 16.4)

burns to her arm and chest, with some questionable areas of deeper burns at her right upper chest and arm (Fig. 16.4). She received local wound care and ongoing burn depth estimation as structures evolved. On postburn day 2, the areas at the upper right chest and upper right arm appeared to have a brown coloration and no capillary refill and did not cause her pain upon palpation. It was determined at that time that these areas were full-thickness injuries, and the plastic surgeon decided upon skin grafting. On postburn day 6 she underwent excision of the eschar and split-thickness grafting with her right thigh as the donor site (Fig. 16.10). She was immobilized in the operating room with an airplane splint to protect the graft from shearing as well as to maintain preoperative ROM.

On postoperative day 5, the dressings were taken down with 100% graft take (Fig. 16.18). She was allowed to mobilize on postoperative day 5, with pain limiting her right lower extremity ROM from the donor site. She required assistance with ambulating short distances. She remained in the airplane splint until postoperative day 7 when she began gentle active-assisted ROM exercises. She was discharged on postoperative day 8 to home, with follow-up therapy for ROM and scar management. She was also seen by occupational therapy for ROM, splinting, and ADLs as well as compression garments.

CASE STUDY 2

FRANKIE

Frankie is a 3-year-old boy who was involved in a house fire, sustaining 60% TBSA burns to his face, trunk, upper extremities, and lower extremities. He developed severe compartment syndrome, sepsis, and respiratory complications in addition to his massive burns. He was treated at a local burn center. During his acute hospitalization, he developed decreased circulation to both feet and required bilateral below-knee amputations. He underwent local wound care and multiple grafting

procedures to achieve wound closure. After a prolonged hospitalization, he was transferred to our rehabilitation hospital for further care.

Initially he had multiple open wounds that required daily dressing changes as well as graft care. He had significant loss of ROM at both knees (stuck in extension) as well as limited ROM at his upper extremities. He underwent serial casting of both knees into flexion, which was quite successful in achieving functional ROM. He required occupational therapy and physical therapy to regain the use of his hands, ADLs, bed mobility, and preparation for prosthetic training. He began prosthetic training but had a setback as he developed an open wound at the end of one stump and accentuated growth of his fibula faster than his tibia on the other stump. This precluded gait training for several months.

Once his open wound had healed, new liners and sockets were developed to relieve pressure on both areas and he was cleared to begin standing. He began a standing program both static at the edge of a mat and in a mobile prone standing frame. He had stubbies, which he tolerated well, and began ambulation about 4 days after starting standing (Fig. 16.19). He progressed to platforms on his pylons and quickly to SACH feet. He is ambulating 200 feet with a rolling walker and supervision (Fig. 16.20). His lack of normal knee flexion is limiting his ability to transition as well as ascend and descend stairs. Due to nerve damage to his left hand, he was unable to utilize Lofstrand crutches and worked toward independent ambulation without an assistive device. He continues to work on fine motor skills with occupational therapy (Fig. 16.21).

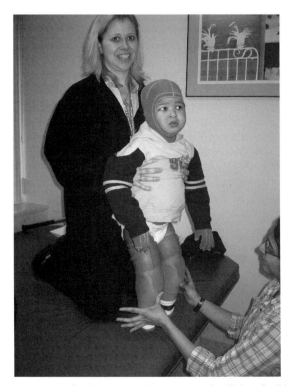

Figure 16.19 ■ Patient attempting to stand utilizing Stubbies as prostheses.

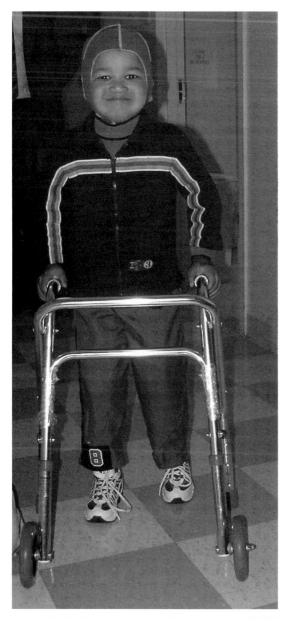

Figure 16.20 ■ Patient progressed to pylons and SACH feet and was able to ambulate with supervision with a rolling walker.

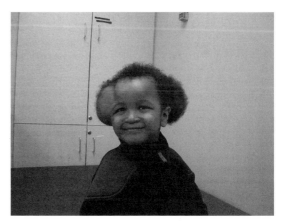

Figure 16.22 ■ Patient with tissue expanders in his scalp.

He has developed several sites of hypertrophic and keloid-type scarring at his face, neck, upper extremities, trunk, and lower extremities (Fig. 16.7). He is utilizing custom compression garments with a mask, jacket, and pants. His new prosthetic liners are actually custom fit and are providing excellent compression for his lower extremities while being worn. While out of the prostheses, he has a custom compression garment that he tolerates well (Fig. 16.16). He has undergone injections of steroids at his keloid scar on his neck and had a z-plasty done to release the neck scar. He participated in our day hospital rehabilitation program for 5 months and then transitioned to outpatient care. He required scar revision surgery for the back and side of his head/neck. For this, he underwent tissue expander placement (Fig. 16.22) at his scalp. This enabled the surgeon to have enough non–burn/scar tissue to cover the previous defect. (Fig. 16.7). Once the tissue expanders were removed, the scarred tissue was excised and the nonscarred tissue moved into its place (Fig. 16.23).

He is now independently ambulating community distances with new prostheses and Impulse feet by Ohio Willow Wood (Fig. 16.24). This energy-storing foot has allowed him to

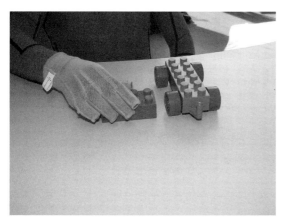

Figure 16.21 ■ Patient using play to increase hand function.

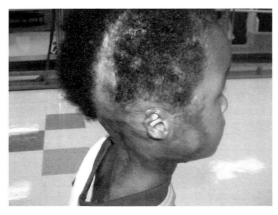

Figure 16.23 ■ Patient status after tissue expander removal and corrective surgery

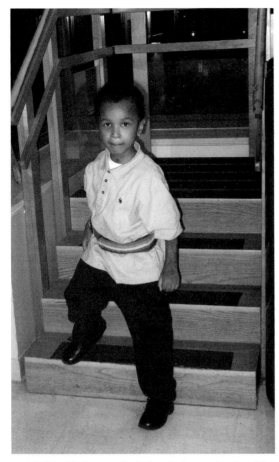

Figure 16.24 ■ Patient ambulating independently with bilateral prostheses.

achieve better heel strike and push-off during the gait cycle. He can now ascend and descend a full flight of stairs and practice bus steps with supervision. Frankie transitioned into a kindergarten class this past fall and is doing well. He will receive school-based physical therapy services as well as continue with outpatient services to address his ongoing scar management and prosthetic needs.

REFERENCES

1. National Institute of General Medical Sciences (NIGMS). Fact Sheets: Trauma, Burn, Shock, and Injury: Facts and Figures. Available at: www.nigms.nih.gov. Accessed January 2005.
2. National Safe Kids Campaign. Injury Facts, Trends in Unintentional Childhood Injury Prevention. Available at: www.safekids.org. Accessed January 2005.
3. National Center for Injury Prevention and Control. WISQUARS: 2002 United States Unintentional and Intentional Injuries. Available at: www.cdc.gov. Accessed January 2005.
4. Johnson RM, Richard R. Partial thickness burns: identification and management. Adv Skin Wound Care 2003;16(4):178–187.
5. Thompson RM, Carrougher GJ. Burn prevention. In: Carrougher GJ, ed. Burn Care and Therapy. St. Louis: Mosby, 1998:497–524.
6. Burn Foundation. NIH Health Interview Survey. Available at: www.burnfoundation.org. Accessed January 2005.
7. Sheriden RL, Remensnyder JP, Schniter JJ, et al. Current expectations for survival in pediatric burns. Arch Pediatr Adolesc Med 2000;154(3):245–249.
8. U.S. Department of Health and Human Services. Child Maltreatment 2002: Summary of Key Findings. Available at: www.nccanch.hhs.gov. Accessed January 2005.
9. Zenel J, Goldstein B. Child abuse in the PICU. Crit Care Med 2002;30(11S):S515–523.
10. Dowd MD, Keenan HT, Bratten SL. Epidemiology and prevention of childhood injuries. Crit Care Med 2002;31(11S): S385–392.
11. Parmet S, Lynm C, Glass R. Burn injuries. JAMA 2003;290 (6):850.
12. Consumer Product Safety Commission. Children's Sleepwear Regulations. Available at: www.cpsc.org. Accessed January 2005.
13. Lockhard RD, Hamilton GF, Fyfe FW. Anatomy of the Human Body. Philadelphia: JB Lippincott, 1969.
14. Moncrief, JA. Grafting. In: Artz CP, Moncrief JA, Pruitt BA, eds. Burns: A Team Approach. Philadelphia: W. B. Saunders, 1979:275.
15. Merz J, Schrand C, Mertens D, et al. Wound care of the pediatric burn patient. AACN Clin Issues Adv Pract Acute Crit Care 2003;14(4):429–441.
16. Lund CC, Browder NC. The estimation of areas of burns. Surg Gynecol Obstet 1944;79:352.
17. Rutan RL. Physiologic response to cutaneous burn injury. In: Carrougher GJ, ed. Burn Care and Therapy. St. Louis: Mosby, 1998:1–33.
18. Linares HA. Pathophysiology of the burn scar. In: Herndon DN, ed. Total Burn Care. London: W. B. Saunders, 1996:383–397.
19. Deitch EA, Wheelahan TM, Rose MP, et al. Hypertrophic burn scars: analysis of variables. J Trauma 1983;23:895–898.
20. Hunt TK. Fundamentals of Wound Management in Surgery— Wound Healing: Disorders of Repair. South Plainfield, NJ: Chirurgecom, 1976.
21. Parks DH, Evans EB, Larson DL. Prevention and correction of deformity after severe burns. Surg Clin North Am 1978;58: 1279–1289.
22. Ketchum LD. Hypertrophic scars and keloids. Clin Plast Surg 1977;4:301–310.
23. Peacock EE, Madden JW, Trier WC. Biological basis for the treatment of keloids and hypertrophic scars. So Med J 1970; 63:7–55.
24. Larsen D, Huang T, Linares H, et al. Preventions and treatment of scar contracture. In: Artz CP, Moncrief JA, Pruitt BA, eds. Burns: A Team Approach. Philadelphia: W. B. Saunders, 1979: 467–468.
25. Hulnick SJ, burn director, St. Christopher's Hospital for Children. Personal communication with LG DeLinde, 1988.
26. Diegelmann RF, Rothkop LC, Cohen LK. Measurement of collagen biosynthesis during wound healing. J Surg Res 1975;19: 239–243.
27. Barnes MK, Morton LF, Bennett RC, et al. Studies on collagen synthesis in the mature dermal scar in the guinea pig. Biochem Soc Symp 1975;3:917–920.
28. American Burn Association Verification Committee. Verified Burn Centers 2004. Available at: www.ameriburn.org. Accessed January 2005.
29. American Burn Association. Hospital and pre-hospital resources for optimal care of patients with burn injury: guidelines for development and operation of burn centers. J Burn Care Rehabil 1990;11:98–104.
30. Phillips AW, Cope O. The revelation of respiratory tract damage as a principal killer of the burned patient. Ann Surg 1962;155:1.
31. Jones CA, Feller I, Richerads KE. Nursing care of the burned child. In: Bailey WC, ed. Pediatric Burns. Chicago: Year Book Medical Publishers, 1988:67–106.

32. Carvajal HF. Resuscitation of the burned child. In: Carvajal JF, Parks DH, eds. Burns in Children. Chicago: Year Book Medical Publishers, 1988:78.

33. Zuker RM. Initial management of the burn wound. In: Carvajal JF, Parks DH, eds. Burns in Children: Pediatric Burn Management. Chicago: Year Book Medical Publishers, 1988:99–105.

34. Blasier RD. Treatment of fractures complicated by burn or head injuries in children. J Bone Joint Surg 1999;81(A7): 1038–1043.

35. Barret JP, Herndon DN. Modulation of inflammatory and catabolic responses in severely burned children by early burn wound excision in the first 24 hours. Arch Surg 2003;138(2):127–132.

35a. Huckleberry Y. Nutritional support and the surgical patient. Am J Health Syst Pharm 2004;61(7):671–684.

36. Spence NA, Miller M, Hendricks L. Perception of burn injury pain in relation to other painful experiences of the pediatric burn patient: a descriptive study. Child Health Care 1992;21: 163–167.

37. Sheridan RL, Hinson M, Nackel A. Development of a pediatric burn pain and anxiety scale. J Burn Care Rehabil 1997;18: 455–459.

38. Knudson CM, Thomas CM. Psychosocial care of the severely burned child. In: Carvajal JF, Parks DH, eds. Burns in Children: Pediatric Burn Management. Chicago: Year Book Medical Publishers, 1988:345–362.

39. Heidrich G, Perry S, Armand R. Nursing staff attitudes about burn pain. J Burn Care Rehabil 1981;2:259–261.

40. Perry S, Heidrich G, Ramos E. Assessment of pain by burn patients. J Burn Care Rehabil 1981;2:322–326.

41. Martin-Herz SP, Patterson DR, Honari S, et al. Pediatric pain control practices of North American burn centers. J Burn Care Rehabil 2003;24(1):26–36.

42. Perry S, Heidrich G. Management of pain during debridement: a survey of burn units. Pain 1982;13:267–280.

43. Carrougher GJ. Burn wound assessment and topical treatment. In: Carrougher GJ, ed. Burn Care and Therapy. St. Louis: Mosby, 1998:133–165.

44. Sheridan FL. Burns. Crit Care Med 2002;30(11S):S500–S514.

45. Helvig EI, Mann R. Care of the patient with toxic epidermal necrolysis. In: Carrougher GJ, ed. Burn Care and Therapy. St. Louis: Mosby, 1998:401–420.

46. Tredget EE, Shankowsky HA, Groeneveld A, et al. A matched-pair, randomized study evaluating the efficacy and safety of acticoat silver-coated dressing for the treatment of burn wounds. J Burn Care Rehabil 1998;19(6):531–537.

47. AQUACEL Ag. The dual-purpose antimicrobial dressing: absorbency with the power of silver. Available at: www.convatec.com. Accessed January 2007.

48. Caruso DM, Foster KN, Hermans MH, et al. AQUACEL Ag in the management of partial-thickness burns: results of a clinical trial. J Burn Care Rehabil 2004;25(1):89–97.

49. Caruso DM, Foster KN, Blome-Eberwein SA, et al. Randomized clinical study of hydrofiber dressing with silver or silver sulfadiazine in the management of partial-thickness burns. J Burn Care Res 2006;27(3):298–309.

50. Ward RS. Physical rehabilitation. In: Carrougher GJ, ed. Burn Care and Therapy. St. Louis: Mosby, 1998:293–327.

51. Xiao-Wu W, Herndon DN, Spies M, et al. Effects of delayed wound excision and grafting in severely burned children. Arch Surg 2002;137(9):1049–1054.

52. Parks DH, Wainwright DJ. The surgical management of burns. In: Carvajal HF, Parks DH, eds. Burns in Children: Pediatric Burn Management. Chicago: Year Book Medical Publishers, 1988:158, 166.

53. Tompkins RG, Burke JF. Alternative wound coverings. In: Herdon DN, ed. Total Burn Care. London: W. B. Saunders, 1996:164–168.

54. Mozingo DW. Surgical management. In: Carrougher GJ, ed. Burn Care and Therapy. St. Louis: Mosby, 1998:233–248.

55. Heimbach DM. Early excision and grafting: clinical implications. Boots Burn Manage Rept 1992;1:8.

56. Compton CC. Current concepts in pediatric burn care: the biology of cultured epithelial autografts: an eight year study in pediatric burn patients. Eur J Pediatr Surg 1992;2:216–222.

57. Egan M. Cultured skin grafts: preserving lives, challenging therapists. OT Week 1992;6:14.

58. Lifeskin, the Next Generation in Burn Care. Culture Technology, Inc., Sherman Oaks, CA: 1994.

59. Medical Economics of Integra Artificial Skin. Plainsboro, NJ: Integra LifeSciences Corp., 1996.

60. Burk JF. Observations on the development and clinical use of artificial skin: an attempt to employ regeneration rather than scar formation in wound healing. Jpn J Surg 1987;17:431–438.

61. Suman O, Mlcak RP, Herndon DN. Effect of exercise training on pulmonary function in children with thermal injury. J Burn Care Rehabil 2002;23(4):288–293.

62. Gaur A, Sinclair M, Caruso E, et al. Heterotopic ossification around the elbow following burns in children: results after excision. J Bone Joint Surg 2003;85-A (8):1538–1543.

63. Baryza MJ, Baryza GA. The Vancouver Scar Scale: an administration tool and its inter-rater reliability. J Burn Care Rehabil 1995;16:535–538.

64. Martin D, Umraw N, Gomez M, et al. Changes in subjective vs. objective burn scar assessment over time: does the patient agree with what we think. J Burn Care Rehabil 2003;24(4):239–244.

65. Gordon M, Gottschlich, MM, Helvig EI, et al. Review of evidence-based practice for the prevention of pressure sores in burn patients. J Burn Care Rehabil 2004;25(5):388–410.

66. Van LB, Sicotte KM, Lassiter RR, et al. Digital photography: enhancing communication between burn therapists and nurses. J Burn Care Rehabil 2004;25(1):54–60.

67. Abdi S, Zhou Y. Management of pain after burn injury. Curr Opin Anaesthesiol 2002;15(5):563–567.

68. Wong D, Baker C. Pain in children: comparison of assessment scales. Pediatr Nurs 1988;14(1):9–17.

69. Merkel S, Voepel-Lewis T, Malviya S. Pain assessment in infants and young children: the FLACC scale: a behavioral tool to measure pain in young children. Am J Nurs 2002;102(10):55–58.

70. Stoddard FJ, Sheridan RL, Saxe GN, et al. Treatment of pain in acutely burned children. J Burn Care Rehabil 2002;23(2): 135–156.

71. Taylor K. The management of minor burns and scalds in children. Nurs Stand 2001;16(11):45–52.

72. Hurlin FK, Doyle B, Paradis P, et al. Use of an improved Watusi collar to manage pediatric neck burn contractures. J Burn Care Rehabil 2002;23(3):221–226.

73. Flesch P. Casting the Young and the Restless. American Burn Association Meeting, Baltimore, 1991.

74. Jordan MH, Lewis MS, Wiegand LT. Dynamic Plaster Casting for Burn Scar Contracture—An Alternative to Surgery (abstract). American Burn Association Meeting, Orlando, 1984.

75. Bennett GB, Helm P, Purdue GF. Serial casting: a method for treating burn contractures. J Burn Care Rehabil 1989;10: 543–545.

76. Ridgway CL, Daugherty MB, Warden GD. Serial casting as a technique to correct burn scar contractures: a case report. J Burn Care Rehabil 1991;12:67–72.

77. Beasley RW. Secondary repair of burned hands. Clin Plast Surg 1981;8:141.

78. Levin LS, Condit DP. Combined injuries-soft tissue management. Clin Orthop Rel Res 1996;327:172–181.

79. Cyriax JH. Clinical application of massage. In: Licht S, ed. Massage, Manipulation, and Traction. New Haven, CT: Elizabeth Licht Publisher, 1960.

80. Schmitt M, Richard RL, Staley MJ. Lower extremity burns and ambulation. In: Richard FL, Staley MJ, eds. Burn Care and Rehabilitation: Principles and Practice. Philadelphia: F. A. Davis Co., 1994:361–379.

81. Sakurai Y, Aarsland A, Herndon DN, et al. Stimulation of muscle protein synthesis by long-term insulin infusion in severely burned patients. Ann Surg 1995;222:283–297.

82. Celis MM, Suman OE, Huang TT, et al. Effect of a supervised exercise and physiotherapy program on surgical interventions in children with thermal injury. J Burn Care Rehabil 2003; 24(1):57–61.

83. Cucuzzo NA, Ferrando A, Herndon DN. The effects of exercise programming vs. traditional outpatient therapy in the rehabilitation of severely burned children. J Burn Care Rehabil 2001;22(3):214–220.

84. Edwards J. Scar management. Nurs Stand 2003;17(52):39–42.

85. Williams F, Knap D, Wallen M. Comparison of the characteristics and features of pressure garments used in the management of burn scars. Burns 1998;24:329–335.

86. Van den Kerckhove E, Stappaerts K, Boeckx W, et al. Silicones in the rehabilitation of burns: a review and overview. Burns 2001;27(3):205–214.

87. Serghiou MA, Holmes CL, McCauley RL. A survey of current rehabilitation trends for burn injuries to the head and neck. J Burn Care Rehabil 2004;25(6):514–518.

88. Rivers EA, Strate RG, Solem LD. The transparent facemask. Am J Occup Ther 1979;33:109–113.

89. Parks DH, Shriner's Burns Institute, Galveston, TX. Personal Communication with L Grigsby de Linde, 1982.

90. Fricke, N, Dutcher K, Omnell L, et al. Effects of Pressure Garment Wear on Facial and Dental Development (abstract). American Burn Association Meeting, Salt Lake City, UT, 1992.

91. Grigsby L. The Use of the Facemask with Children. Fifth Annual Meeting of the Mid-Atlantic Association of Burn Care Facilities, Philadelphia, 1982.

92. Leung KS, Cheng JCY, Ma GFY, et al. Complications of pressure therapy for post-burn hypertrophic scars. Burns 1984; 10:434–438.

93. McCauley RL, Fairleigh JF, Robson MC, et al. Effects of Facial Burns on Facial Growth in Children (abstract). American Burn Association Meeting, Baltimore, 1991.

94. Sheridan RL, Hinson MI, Liang MH, et al. Long-term outcome of children surviving massive burns. JAMA 2000;283(1):69–73.

95. Landolt MA, Grubenmann S, Meuli M. Family impact greatest: predictors of quality of life and psychological adjustment in pediatric burn survivors. J Trauma 2002;53(6):1146–1151.

96. Mancuso MG, Bishop S, Blakeney P, et al. Impact on the family: psychosocial adjustment of siblings of children who survive serious burns. J Burn Care Rehabil 2003;24(2):110–118.

Cardiac Disorders

Heather Brossman

C ongenital heart defects (CHDs) occur in approximately 1% of live births, or 8 of every 1000 births.[1] There are 25,000 babies born each year with a CHD, and more than 1,000,000 individuals have reached adulthood and are living in the United States with a functionally significant CHD.[2] The mortality rates in infants with CHD have declined dramatically as a result of medical and surgical advances for their care. The decrease in mortality rates has now shifted the focus from mortality to the neurodevelopmental status of these individuals and their associated developmental delays. Some studies have even begun to focus on specific gross motor and fine motor proficiencies in children with CHD.[2-9] As physical therapists, we may encounter infants and children with a cardiac disorder in every setting in which we practice. A physical therapist may see a child with a CHD in the acute care setting preoperatively and/or postoperatively, in rehabilitation settings, in schools and home care, and in the outpatient setting. Physical therapists should know what the congenital heart defect is, how it affects the child's cardiovascular system during exercise, and the complications that are prevalent in this population. It is also important to note that CHDs commonly accompany other genetic disorders causing developmental delays, for which they may see a physical therapist.[10] For example, 30% to 50% of children born with Down syndrome will have a CHD.[11]

Congenital abnormalities of the heart can be detected when the heart is no larger than a peanut and is already fully developed.[12] In most infants with CHD it is speculated that genetic factors played a role in the acquisition of the defect, but the patterns of inheritance are unclear.[13] With the exception of single gene mutation syndromes (e.g., DiGeorge 22q11 deletion), most CHDs have multifactorial inheritance. CHDs are therefore the result of genetic inheritance, maternal conditions, and environmental factors, which interact during the critical developmental stage for the heart—during the first 8 to 10 weeks of gestation. There are numerous types of CHDs, each having its own related risk and relative frequency. Table 17.1 lists the more common of the congenital defects of the heart and their relative frequency in the general population.

In order to understand the various CHDs, one needs to have a clear understanding of normal cardiac development, anatomy, and physiology. It is beyond the scope of this text to review in detail cardiopulmonary physiology; there are numerous excellent pediatric cardiopulmonary texts to which you can refer.[14-16]

Children can also carry a diagnosis of heart failure. Heart failure (HF) in pediatrics is often associated with congenital heart disease, but may also be caused by cardiomyopathy. Congestive heart failure (CHF) is a syndrome with many pathophysiologic and compensatory mechanisms in the body's attempt to maintain the normal ventricular

TABLE 17.1	
Relative Frequency of Congenital Heart Lesions	
Ventricular septal defects	25%–30%
Atrial septal defects	6%–8%
Patent ductus arteriosus (excluding preterm neonates)	6%–8%
Aortic valve stenosis	4%–7%
Coarctation of the aorta	5%–7%
Tetralogy of Fallot	5%–7%
Pulmonary valve stenosis	5%–7%
Hypoplastic left heart	1%–2%
Double-outlet right ventricle	1%–2%
Truncus arteriosus	1%–2%
Total anomalous pulmonary venous return	1%–2%
Tricuspid atresia	1%–2%

From Hoffman J, Kaplan S. The incidence of congenital heart disease. J Am Coll Cardiol 2002;39:1890–1900.

TABLE 17.2	
Clinical Presentation of Congestive Heart Failure	
Onset of rapid breathing	Change in behavior: irritability
Edema	Excessive sweating
Fatigue	Vomiting
Poor feeding	Tachycardia
Oliguria	Peripheral vasoconstriction
Pulmonary/systemic vein engorgement	Wheezing
Tachypnea	Nasal flaring
Chest retractions	
Failure to thrive	

ejection of blood from the heart to the vital organs. Right HF presents with hepatomegaly, peripheral edema, and cyanosis. Left HF presents with pulmonary edema and poor perfusion. The clinical presentations of CHF are listed in Table 17.2.

Heart transplantation may be used for children with cardiac defects as well as for heart failure, as an option for end-stage heart failure.[17] Heart transplantation has its own set of circumstances of which the physical therapist must be aware. Physical therapists mainly need to be aware of the denervation of the heart posttransplantation. Children with a heart transplant don't have "vagal tone" to bring down their heart rate to normal resting values. This results in a higher resting heart rate, a lower maximum heart rate, and reliance on circulating catecholamines to increase heart rate. For the physical therapist this means that warm-ups and cool-downs are vital for exercise, which we will talk about in more detail.

Cardiac System Development

The heart begins to form by day 18 as two tubular structures sitting side by side in the midline of the embryo[11] (see Fig. 17.1). These tubes fuse together and produce the early heart tube by day 21. The heart tube is beating by day 22. The heart twists or loops toward the right side, and folds upon itself by the 24th day with the atrium coming to lie near the embryo's head and the ventricle toward the feet.[12] This is all under genetic control, and when things go wrong here you have what is called a looping defect. By the 27th day, the blood is circulating from the heart to the rest of the embryo. The single chamber atria and ventricle will become partitioned by the end of the fourth week of gestation.[12] The single ventricle will lead into a large single vessel called the truncus arteriosus. At this time the ventri-

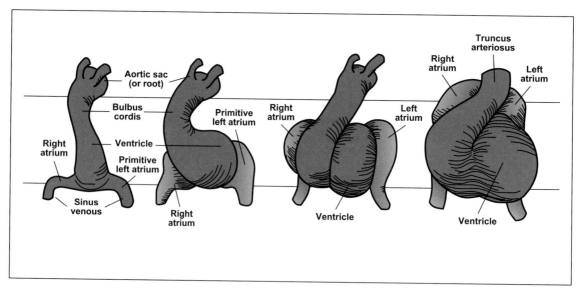

Figure 17.1 ■ Cardiac system development in the fetus.

cles are beginning to separate and the truncus arteriosus develops many changes. A few important events occur: a septum grows vertically, separating the truncus arteriosus into the aorta and the pulmonary artery; the aortic and pulmonary valves develop; and the pulmonary artery comes to lie in front of the aorta and attaches to the right ventricle. Between the 27th and 37th days of development, the atrial wall develops. The foramen ovale remains open to allow blood to pass between the two atria. By 7 weeks, the ventricles are dividing equally. During life in the womb, the right ventricle is the dominant one, with most of the fetal blood bypassing the lungs and reaching the left ventricle through the foramen ovale or the ductus arteriosus, which connects the aorta and pulmonary artery.[10] Development is primarily complete by the 10th week of gestation.[18] This is why the first 10 weeks are called the critical period of cardiac development. Some women may not even know they are pregnant and their embryo has already completed the development of their cardiac structures.[19]

NORMAL FETAL CIRCULATION

The fetal heart has a lack of dependence upon the lungs for respiration. The fetus uses the placenta to obtain oxygen and to get rid of carbon dioxide as a low resistance circulatory pathway (Fig. 17.2). The right and left ventricles exist in a parallel circuit. Blood travels through the umbilical vein through the ductus venosus to the fetal heart via the inferior vena cava to the right atrium, and through the foramen ovale to the left atrium. The superior vena cava leads to the right atrium, to the right ventricle, to the pulmonary artery, to the lungs or ductus arteriosus, bypassing the lungs, into the descending aorta to perfuse the bilateral lower extrem-

ities and body, then travels back to the placenta via the umbilical arteries. The blood traveling through the left ventricle to the aorta perfuses the brain and upper extremities.[19] All of the blood flowing through the various chambers of the heart, as well as the arteries and veins, are rich in oxygen. The vessels of the pulmonary circulation are vasoconstricted in the fetus. Any blood traveling to the lungs, all of which is oxygen rich, will be utilized to develop and nourish lung tissue.

CHANGES ASSOCIATED WITH BIRTH

At birth several things happen to the circulatory system. Figure 17.3 shows normal cardiac anatomy before and after the birth process. As the first breath is taken, the lungs expand with air and lung pressure falls; this allows blood to more easily flow into the lungs.[12] After reaching the lungs, the blood then returns to the left atrium, which causes pressure to be higher on the left of the atrial septum than on the right. This causes the foramen ovale to gradually seal shut anatomically (closed by the third month of life), although it is closed a few hours after birth functionally due to the pressure differential of the two sides of the heart. Once the lungs are filled with air, the oxygen level in the infant's blood rises and causes the muscle wall of the ductus arteriosus to contract, and no blood flows through the ductus.[12] The ductus arteriosus is closed 10 to 15 hours after birth when the partial pressure of oxygen in the blood traveling through the ductus reaches 50 mm Hg.[18] The placenta is then expelled and the fetal heart has separation of oxygenated and deoxygenated blood and relies on the lungs for gaining oxygen and ridding itself of carbon dioxide.

NORMAL CIRCULATION AFTER BIRTH

The heart is two pumps working in unison to propel blood through the blood vessels to the body. The right side of the heart receives deoxygenated blood from the body and pumps it through the pulmonary artery to the lungs. The left side receives oxygenated blood from the lungs and pumps it through the aorta to the body. The tricuspid valve sits between the right atrium and ventricle. The pulmonary valve consists of three semilunar cusps preventing blood from returning to the right ventricle from the lungs. The four pulmonary veins enter the posterior wall of the left atrium with no valves at the openings. The left atrioventricular valve or the mitral valve, which sits between the left atrium and ventricle, allows oxygenated blood from the left atrium to pass into the left ventricle. The left ventricle has three semilunar cusps leading to the aorta. The aortic valve is similar to the pulmonary valve except that its cusps are thicker and placed slightly differently. This valve leads to systemic circulation. The left ventricle has a greater amount of pressure than the right ventricle due to higher systemic pressure of the body versus the lungs. Figure 17.4 demonstrates normal cardiac anatomy.

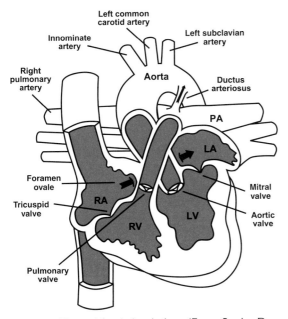

Figure 17.2 ■ Normal fetal circulation. (From Sapire D. Understanding and Diagnosing Pediatric Heart Disease. Norwalk, CT: Appleton & Lange, Prentice Hall, 1991.)

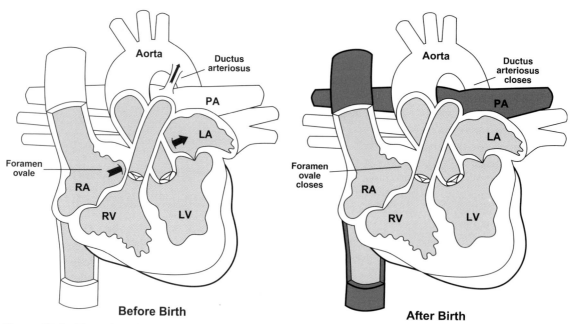

Figure 17.3 ▪ Normal cardiac structures before and after birth. (From Neill C, Clark E, Clark C. From Birth to Adolescence, from Doctor's Office to Playground. The Heart of a Child, What Families Need to Know about Heart Disorders in Children. London and Baltimore: Johns Hopkins University Press, 1992.)

 ## Congenital Heart Defects

At any point in the development of the cardiac system problems can arise leading to a congenital heart defect. It may be a persistent fetal pathway or a problem due to development of the fetal heart itself. CHDs may be cyanotic, meaning they cause oxygen saturations in the blood to be decreased, or acyanotic, meaning they do not alter blood oxygen saturation. Acyanotic lesions can cause issues with blocking the flow of blood to the heart chambers (pressure issue) or with volume of blood traveling through the chambers of the heart back to the lungs (volume issue).

ACYANOTIC CONGENITAL HEART DEFECTS

Acyanotic lesions, which are obstructive, include aortic stenosis, coarctation of the aorta, pulmonary stenosis, and mitral stenosis. Acyanotic lesions, which increase pulmonary blood flow, include patent ductus arteriosus, atrial septal defects, ventricular septal defects, and atrioventricular canal defects. A CHD causing an increase in the volume of blood flowing to the lungs means that there is a communication between the systemic and pulmonary sides of circulation in the heart and results in shunting of fully oxygenated blood back into the lungs. These include atrial septal defects (ASDs), ventricular septal defects (VSDs), atrioventricular septal defects (AVSDs), and patent ductus arteriosus (PDA). Both ASD and VSD are pictured in Figure 17.5. The blood flow is referred to as left-to-right shunt with too much blood to the lungs and no change in arterial blood oxygen saturations. The symptoms for defects that lead to increased blood flow to the lungs include rapid breathing, even when asleep as a consequence of congested lungs; delayed growth, as the extra calories are used by abnormal circulation and rapid breathing (usually growth in weight is more delayed than growth in height); sweating; heart failure; and severe difficulty in feeding.[10]

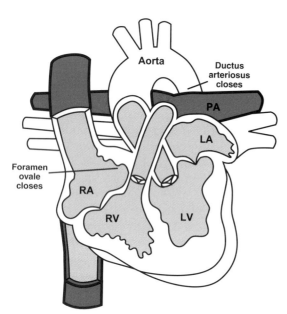

Figure 17.4 ▪ Normal heart anatomy.

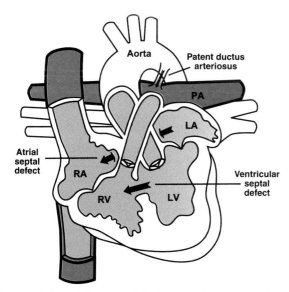

Figure 17.5 ▪ Atrial and ventricular septal defects and patent ductus arteriosus.

ATRIAL SEPTAL DEFECTS

An ASD is a hole in the wall separating the atria. This is most often caused by a patent foramen ovale, which is the oval-shaped hole in the atrial wall that should close soon after birth. The foramen always occurs naturally in the atrial septum in the womb connecting the right and left atria. It is referred to as ostium secundum if the foramen ovale is larger than it should be, or if the flap of tissue that closes it is displaced or deficient. Without closure and over many years, low-pressure shunts at the atrial level result in a gradual enlargement of the right atrium and ventricle. Symptoms include a heart murmur, an overactive right ventricle, and a large pulmonary artery. Surgery is usually performed if the hole is not closed by 2 to 3 years of age, due to risk later in life. Surgery is generally a Dacron patch or a clamshell device implanted via a catheter. It is good to be aware that some surgeons will anticoagulate up to 6 months postoperatively to prevent clotting.

VENTRICULAR SEPTAL DEFECT

The ventricular septum consists of three distinct areas that fuse together to form the singular solid muscle wall of the ventricles. With a VSD some of the oxygen-rich blood in the left ventricle that is supposed to be pumped in the body through the aorta is ejected directly to the right ventricle through a hole in the ventricle wall. With a large defect a lot of blood goes to the lung and causes lung congestion and shortness of breath. A large amount of blood returns back from the lungs to the left heart, which then becomes overburdened and enlarged. Heart failure may even occur causing a backup of fluid in the lungs and other body tissues. For individuals with a large VSD the signs to look for include dyspnea, feeding diffi-

culties, poor growth, profuse perspiration, recurrent pulmonary infections, cardiac failure in early infancy, respiratory distress, and growth failure. One-fifth of all VSDs are small and close spontaneously before the age of 2. If a VSD is not closed by 5 to 7 years of age, it is not likely that it will close without surgery. Surgery is similar to that with the ASD with a Dacron patch to close the hole.

ATRIOVENTRICULAR SEPTAL DEFECT

A complete AVSD involves the portion of the heart where the atrial septum meets the ventricular septum as well as the valves (mitral/tricuspid). The result is a large hole spanning the septum and the presence of one large valve on both sides. Blood flow is excessive in a left-to-right shunt. Symptoms include lung congestion and pulmonary hypertension. The result is a thin child due to the increased work of breathing. It is associated with Down syndrome; approximately 25% of individuals with Down syndrome have an AVSD. This will require surgery in the first few months of life.

PATENT DUCTUS ARTERIOSUS

PDA is associated with maternal rubella and prematurity. It involves a communication between the aorta and the pulmonary artery that remains after birth and allows blood flow between the two vessels. The ductus arteriosus (DA) is a normal pathway in fetal blood circulation that connects the pulmonary artery and the descending aorta. As the amount of oxygen in the blood increases after birth, the body stops producing prostaglandin E_1, which keeps the DA open, and the DA closes hours after birth and is permanently closed in the first few weeks of life. When the shunt does not close it is a PDA, and the pressure differential between the left and right sides of the heart causes too much blood to go to the lungs. The symptoms depend on the size of the opening and the degree of prematurity. A large opening can cause pulmonary congestion, CHF, and edema. No matter how small the hole is, there is a risk of endocarditis. Medically, indomethacin (decreases prostaglandin production) is given to close the PDA in premature infants. In a full-term baby, surgery is usually required if prostaglandins are unable to close the DA[11] (see Fig. 17.5).

A group of acyanotic lesions causes an obstruction to the flow of blood and an increase in pressure. These include coarctation of the aorta, aortic valve stenosis, and pulmonary valve stenosis. These lesions are demonstrated in Figure 17.6 A–C.

COARCTATION OF AORTA

In coarctation of the aorta, the aorta is pinched or narrowed after it leaves the heart. It causes an increase in pressure in the arteries closest to the heart, the head, and the

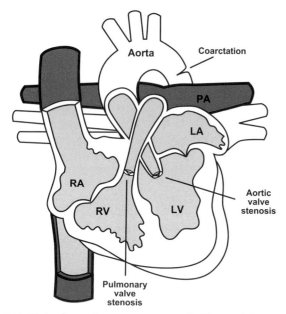

Figure 17.6 ■ *Several common congenital heart defects.*
(A) *Coarctation of the aorta.* **(B)** *Pulmonary valve stenosis.*
(C) *Aortic valve stenosis.*

arms, and low circulation to the lower extremities. This causes upper body hypertension and diminished pulses in the lower extremities. In newborns it is not evident until the ductus arteriosus closes and the resultant obstruction of blood flow from the left ventricle results in heart failure and shock, requiring respiratory support and prostaglandin E_1 to open the ductus. The reason the problem occurs after ductus arteriosus closure is because as the ductus closes, it shortens into a thin cord, and like a noose, pinches off the aorta, making it a narrower tube where the PDA was located. The left ventricle then has to pump blood directly through the constriction, with the result being left ventricular failure. This causes a sudden change from a healthy baby to a baby that is breathing hard, sweating, and wheezing. In an older child, if this is left untreated, symptoms will include headache, leg cramps, a pale appearance, and slow development. Surgery is performed to remove the constriction as shown in Figure 17.6; however in one-third (18%) of individuals undergoing surgery, recoarctation occurs.

CYANOTIC HEART DEFECTS

A cyanotic heart defect is one in which the blood has a decrease in its oxygen saturation. In CHDs that are cyanotic, the lack of oxygen causes the lips, toes, toenail beds, and fingernails to appear blue (*cyanosis* is Greek for blue). Due to the chronic arterial oxygen desaturation, the body stimulates erythropoiesis or increased red blood cell formation, which results in polycythemia. Polycythemia is an overabundance of red blood cells, which increases the viscosity of the blood and increases the risk of cerebrovascular accidents and microvascular problems in these indi-

viduals. The cyanotic heart defects include tetralogy of Fallot (TOF), double-outlet right ventricle, and hypoplastic left heart syndrome as shown in Figure 17.7.

TETRALOGY OF FALLOT

TOF has four basic components and is the most common cyanotic congenital heart defect.[1] The first basic component is a large VSD with blood mixing freely between the two ventricles. The second component is pulmonary stenosis, which causes an obstruction to the lungs or a right ventricular outflow tract obstruction. The third component is an aorta positioned above the VSD (called an overriding aorta). Finally, there is hypertrophy of the right ventricle, caused by the increased pressure from the right ventricular outflow obstruction. Blood flow to the pulmonary artery is obstructed, so oxygen-poor blood finds it easier to enter the aorta than the pulmonary artery. The result is low oxygen levels in the arteries and tissues of the body. This results in cyanosis with symptoms of tiring easily, fainting, and shock.[10] The earlier the surgery can be performed, the better it is for the child's outcome.[19] Figure 17.7 depicts TOF.

DOUBLE-OUTLET RIGHT VENTRICLE

In double-outlet right ventricle (DORV; Fig. 17.8), the aorta and pulmonary artery arise from the right ventricle. The only outlet from the left ventricle is via a VSD into the right ventricle.[13]

HYPOPLASTIC LEFT HEART SYNDROME

Hypoplastic left heart syndrome (HLHS; demonstrated in Fig. 17.9) is the most serious of the congenital malfor-

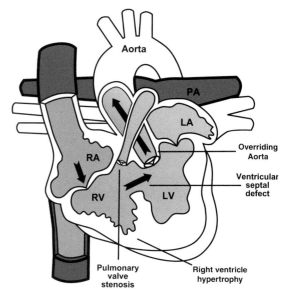

Figure 17.7 ■ Tetralogy of Fallot.

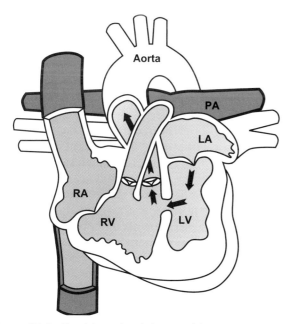

Figure 17.8 ■ Double-outlet right ventricle.

mations with the poorest prognosis. A mild defect means that there is a small left ventricle with some obstruction. A severe defect means a tiny left ventricle and missing (atresia) mitral and aortic valves. The symptoms are usually minimal until the ductus arteriosus closes and the newborn goes into shock and multiorgan failure. Keeping the ductus arteriosus open with prostaglandin E_1 until surgery can be performed keeps the child alive. There are numerous palliative surgeries if the infant survives the initial shock, and cardiac transplantation is often a suggested option.

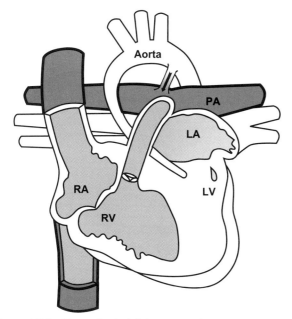

Figure 17.9 ■ Hypoplastic left heart syndrome.

 Heart Transplantation

Heart transplantation is used as an option for end-stage heart failure for children with cardiac defects as well as for cardiomyopathy. Heart failure occurs in some of the children with CHDs postoperatively due to the nature of their artificial circulatory systems. For example, the use of the right ventricle as the main systemic circulation ventricle may cause the right ventricle to fail, as it is not intended to pump against systemic pressures. Some children with high pulmonary pressures from their CHD may need heart and lung transplantation due to the poor condition of their lungs.[20]

Different centers have varied indications for transplantation, but generally transplantation is considered in children with end-stage heart disease that is unresponsive to medical management or when conventional surgical therapy is not considered a realistic or viable option.[13] Transplantation is truly the exchanging of a set of undesirable lethal circumstances for another set of circumstances. Transplantation presents a lifelong risk of graft loss (acute and chronic rejection), graft coronary disease, nonspecific graft failure, and death from infection, oncogenesis, and other organ failure. The most common age for pediatric heart transplantation is within the first year of life.[20,21] For individuals receiving heart transplantation, a CHD is most likely to be the diagnosis.[20] In the first year of life CHDs with a single ventricle, such as HLHS and DORV, have the greatest risk of requiring transplantation.[21] Cardiomyopathy is the diagnosis for 30% of infants who require transplantation.[21] Children from the age of 1 to 10 are most often transplanted due to the cardiomyopathy. Adolescents from age 11 to 17 years have cardiomyopathy as the most frequent reason for transplantation, with only 25% in that age range being transplanted because of CHD.

Survival data suggest that most children who are transplanted will live longer than the cohort from previous years.[20] During the first 30 days after transplantation, graft failure is the leading cause of death. In the first year acute rejection is the leading cause of death, accounting for almost 30% of deaths during this time frame. The graft half-life, (half-life meaning the point in time in which half of all the recipients have died) for infants can't be estimated out to 14 years as greater than 50% of the recipients are still alive.[20] Children from age 1 to 10 have a half-life of 17.5 years, and adolescents have a half-life of 11 years.[20,21] It is thought that there is a survival advantage for infants and children as compared to adolescents.[20]

 Physical Therapy Examination

HISTORY

Your examination begins with the age, date of birth, primary language, and race of the individual you are meeting. It is important to know that families come from all over the world to the centers that perform the delicate operations for these children. As the numbers of centers that perform them are becoming fewer over the years, a family may have traveled a very long distance to come to your center. They may speak a different language, and it is important that the family can understand you; if they cannot, you are responsible for getting an interpreter or you may utilize a phone interpretation service. The family should be an integral part of the care you are providing, and they should be responsible for carrying over the care you are providing. Having the family be a part of the care of their child is one of the most important things you can do as a physical therapist.

The medical and surgical history of the child is also very important and may be very complex. Children born with single ventricle physiologies may have had three stages of palliative surgery prior to meeting you. It is important to get these histories accurate, as they give you a picture of the child's medical course. Medications the child is taking should be documented, including blood thinners (warfarin, Coumadin) and immunosuppression. These medications have side effects such as quick bleeding times, which should be noted for physical therapy treatment. Social history should be documented, as there are numerous family stresses involved with a child who has CHD. There is a very high divorce rate among families with children having CHD.[10] This leads at times to very complicated social situations and custody issues. Family history is also important, as this may be a first child and be a very difficult time of adjustment for the family dynamic, or the parents may have just given birth to a second or third child and are finding that the other two children have milder forms of the same CHD. It is also important to discuss with the family that a child with a CHD is very different from, for example, an uncle who died from atherosclerosis. Developmental history will tell you if the child is receiving early intervention services; other siblings who may be receiving services, giving you an idea of the developmental picture; or, possibly, this child has not received services yet but should have been receiving services. The child's general health status requires you to look at daily schedules, sleep patterns, prior level of function, ability to perform activities of daily living (ADLs), and whether the child is attending school, is home-schooled, or is being tutored. The chief complaints for infants with a CHD or awaiting transplantation are generally poor feeding and failure to thrive. Chief complaints for adolescents are lethargy, fatigue, general malaise, and exercise intolerance. Talk to the family and child about their chief complaint. What do they feel is the main reason for this hospitalization? What has been the clinical course of the current illness and the signs and symptoms as well as precipitating factors?

LABORATORY VALUES

There are numerous lab values that are important to the physical therapist. Cardiac catheterization values tell you the central pressures and oxygen saturations for the child you are working with. These give you a baseline for the degree of mixing between the child's oxygenated and deoxygenated blood, and the degree to which his or her central pressures are altered. As the child's oxygen saturations decrease he or she may have increasing complaints of fatigue, dizziness, lethargy, and general malaise. Figure 17.10 shows normal heart catheterization values for the various chambers of the heart. The values in the circles are the oxygen saturations and the other values are the normal pressures for the various chambers and vessels of the heart.

A cardiac catheterization is an invasive examination where catheters are placed from the vein in the groin to the heart under fluoroscopic guidance into the systemic venous and arterial systems to measure hemodynamic pressures and oxygen saturations. Radiographic material is injected through the catheters to take moving pictures of the heart and its structures. The right ventricle and pulmonary artery are usually about one-fifth that of the left ventricle and aorta. This is due to the high systemic pressure the left side of the heart has to overcome to pump blood out of the aorta. The right side of the heart is the deoxygenated side and generally has oxygen saturations in the 60s; the left side is the oxygenated side with the oxygen saturations in the high 90s (98% to 100%).

AGE-APPROPRIATE ARTERIAL BLOOD GAS VALUES

Arterial blood is the most reliable way to assess O_2 transport (Table 17.3). Hypoventilation causes a shift to the right on the normal curve with an increase in CO_2 and a decrease in pH, causing a respiratory acidosis. Hyper-

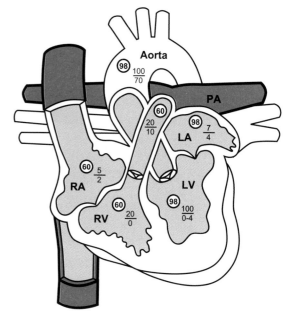

Figure 17.10 ■ Cardiac catheterization values in a normal heart.

TABLE 17.3

Age-Appropriate Arterial Blood Gases

	pH	PCO_2	PO_2
Preterm infant at 1–5 hr	7.29–7.37	39–56	52–67
Term infant at 5 hr	7.31–7.37	32–39	62–86
Preterm and term infant at 5 days	7.34–7.42	32–41	62–92
Children, adolescents, adults	7.35–7.45	35–45	80–100

ventilation causes a shift to the left with a decrease in CO_2 and an increase in pH, causing a respiratory alkalosis. This holds true whether sleeping or running a marathon. A PO_2 of 60 to 80 mm Hg corresponds with a SaO_2 of 90 to 95, which is mild hypoxia. A PO_2 of 40 to 60 mm Hg corresponds with a SaO_2 of 60% to 90%, or moderate hypoxia. A PO_2 of less than 40 mm Hg corresponds with a SaO_2 of less than 60% and is considered severe hypoxia.

GENERAL APPEARANCE

During any physical examination of a child, always discuss with the parents the best way to approach the infant or toddler. For young children, always start with play. Let them explore the equipment you have with you, including stethoscopes or blood pressure cuffs. For adolescents, explain to them what your purpose is for being there and explain to them and their caregiver what you will be doing. Utilize age- and cognitively appropriate descriptions of the activities that you will be performing. This should all come before the actual examination. All vital signs that can be documented before you engage the child should be documented as a baseline resting vital sign prior to engaging the child. Run a resting rhythm strip and document arrhythmia. You should document the child's state of consciousness. Some children with a CHD are very ill and may be on musculoskeletal blockade, due to the inability of their cardiovascular system to tolerate any movement or excitement. A child may also be more lightly sedated. His or her state of consciousness will dictate the level with which the child can cooperate with simple commands appropriate for age, and what you are able to do with the child during your treatment. Document all the equipment in the room including supportive devices such as mechanical ventilation, extracorporeal membrane oxygenation (ECMO), left ventricular assistive devices (LVAD), oxygen masks, nasal cannulas, oxygen hoods, arterial lines, intravenous feeding tubes, nasogastric tubes, chest tubes, pacer wires, central lines, peripheral lines, cardiorespiratory (CR) monitors, and pulse oximetry. We discuss the supportive devices in more detail later in the chapter. Documenting the use of,

as well as the discharge of, these devices gives you a global picture of the child's health and an idea of his or her improving or declining health.

PAIN

Pain should be well documented with age-appropriate pain scales. Pain scales include the Attia,[21] which is utilized for children younger than 1 year of age with a range of 0 to 20, pain being greater than 5. The Children's Hospital of Eastern Ontario Pain Scale (CHEOPS) is utilized for children older than 1 year of age with a range 4 to 13, pain delineated by a score of greater than 8.[22] The Wong-Baker FACES is for children with a cognitive age of 3 to 7 years and uses a visual analog scale (VAS) from no hurt to hurts worst.[23] The FLACC is a behavioral pain assessment scale utilized in children who cannot self-report pain and looks at five categories: Face, Legs, Activity, Cry, and Consolability. Scoring is from 0 to 2 for the category: A 0 is a relaxed and calm behavior, a 1 is an increase in pain behaviors noted, and a 2 is the most pain in each category. Therefore, a total score of 10 means the worst pain; the range of scores is 0 to 10.[24] Finally, there is the visual analog pain scale, with a range of 0 to 10, 0 being no pain and 10 the worst pain ever. The management of pain is very important, as it impacts both movement and respiratory function. You will be better able to treat your patients if they have good pain control. This may mean requesting a directed time for pain medication and scheduling therapy around pain medications. The child's general appearance may include ascites, which is abdominal fluid overload, or peripheral edema due to fluid retained, as the heart is unable to maintain adequate cardiac output. General coloring is important to note: Anemia causes paleness, polycythemia causes plethora, and oxygen desaturation causes a blue color or cyanosis. Document the individual's body type as cachectic, obese, or appropriate for age.

EQUIPMENT AND DEVICES

Supportive devices may include extracorporeal membrane oxygenation (ECMO), mechanical ventilation, or ventricular assistive devices (left ventricular, right ventricular, or biventricular assists). ECMO is similar to a heart–lung machine, supplying an artificial heart and lung outside the body. The machine places oxygen into the blood and removes carbon dioxide, giving the patient's heart and lungs time to rest and heal. ECMO does not cure the disease; it just gives the child some support as he or she heals. Indications for ECMO include acute rejection and respiratory failure. ECMO is generally used for short-term (5 to 15 days) treatment. In Figure 17.11, a child can be seen receiving ECMO. During ECMO a physical therapist will provide a positioning program to maintain midline orientation of the limbs, especially positioning of the feet to prevent foot drop. It is important not to kink the blood flow

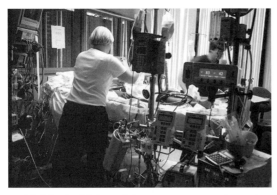

Figure 17.11 ■ A child receiving extracorporeal membrane oxygenation posttransplantation.

circuit; therefore, passive range of motion is often contraindicated. There are many sequelae of ECMO including stroke, necrosis of the extremities (especially distal), and thrombosis. It is important to be aware of these sequelae as a child is coming off of ECMO.

Mechanical ventilation is utilized both pre- and postsurgically for children with CHD. Preoperatively, the ventilator is used to assist with breathing during respiratory distress, and postoperatively, it is used as a bridge to breathing independently. It may be connected to an endotracheal tube or tracheostomy. An endotracheal tube may be placed in the nose or mouth to assist with breathing. Figure 17.12 shows such a situation. Usually these children are unable to vocalize. Suctioning to keep the child clear of secretions is of the utmost value here. Always be sure to clear the tubing of water prior to listening to breath sounds. If physical therapists do not perform suctioning in your venue of work, make sure a person who is able to suction the child is aware of your working with the child in order to keep him or her comfortable during your treatment. You cannot expect gross motor skills to be optimal or to have the child's best performance if you are not prioritizing a clear airway. Providing midline orientation, especially to prevent a head preference, is very important. Some children will try to pull away from the ventilator and will have a head preference to the side away from the ventilator, and some will try to hold still facing the ventilator, afraid to move and pull the tubing, and will have a head preference toward the ventilator. Midline orientation and the full range of motion in the neck are very valuable.

Left ventricular assistive devices (LVADs) are an external device to the body that act to assist the left ventricle to pump blood through systemic circulation. Adults have been using LVADs for many years; only recently have LVADs been used in larger children. More recent technology may allow LVADs to be utilized in small children.

LVADs can be utilized over a long time frame, and are often a bridge to transplantation.[25] There is a wealth of research on LVADs in the adult literature that shows that individuals on an LVAD for longer than 30 days show better recoveries after heart transplantation than individuals on the LVAD for less than 30 days.[1] The LVAD machine gives you a readout on heart rate, stroke volume, and cardiac output. You still need to monitor blood pressure, oxygen saturation, and subjective reports of exertion, pain, and dyspnea. The literature suggests that in best-case scenarios patients should be up and out of bed to a chair 3 days postoperatively, and ambulation should be initiated as muscle strength allows, generally 5 days.[26] A child with an LVAD can be seen ambulating in Figure 17.13. The child who can use the Borg scale of perceived exertion should show a value of between 11 and 13, and exercise should be halted if there is a drop of systolic blood pressure of 20 mm Hg or the patient is symptomatic. We have found that most children with an LVAD feel more comfortable with an abdominal binder in place for upright activities.

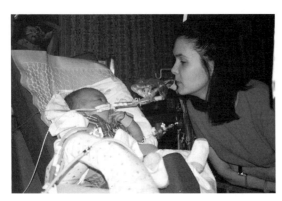

Figure 17.12 ■ A child with mechanical ventilation being provided via nasotracheal intubation as his mother looks on.

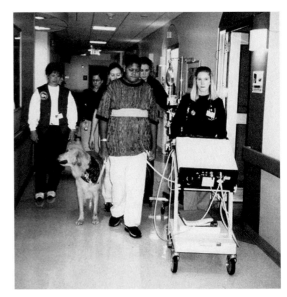

Figure 17.13 ■ A child with a left ventricular assist device ambulating with a physical therapist.

There are numerous lines that a child with CHD may have in place for supportive care. A Broviac catheter is inserted into central circulation and is used to administer medications or fluids, and may be used for drawing blood. A peripherally inserted central catheter is also a central line and is placed more distally to the heart, generally in an arm. Pacer wires are also centrally placed on the heart for emergent needs for electrical intervention for the heart and are usually removed 7 days postoperatively. These lines are to be treated with respect and care. I recommend pinning them to the gown or clothes of the child you are working with during exercise. Nursing units commonly use medical tape around these lines and a pin can be placed through the tape to the gown. Always make sure to remove the pin when you are done treatment.

INTEGUMENT

Examine the state of the integumentary system, beginning with the general appearance of the skin. Does it look glossy, turgid, loose, bruised, or broken down? Anticoagulation can lead to bruising and skin breakdown, and fluid retention can lead to glossy or turgid skin.

Digital clubbing is to be documented and is a sign of hypoxia, where the tip of the distal phalanx becomes bulbus and the nail of the digit exits at an increased angle. It is due to prolonged hypoxemia. Generally it is seen in CHD and is rare in any individual with a cardiomyopathy. An example of clubbing is presented in Figure 17.14.

Document surgical sites and incisions including clamshell, median sternotomy, large thoracotomy, and small thoracotomy incisions for chest tube sites. These sites may be sutured or stapled closed, but occasionally due to edema may be left open with a surgical dressing. How do these scars move? Do they move in all directions, or are they bound to the tissue underneath? Does moving the scars cause discomfort or pain? A typical chest of a child following heart surgery is seen in Figure 17.15.

Examine capillary refill in the extremities. Push down on the nail bed, which should blanch and rebound 1 to 2 seconds after pressure is relieved. Capillary refill ideally should be assessed by compression of the big toe. Children with CHD are at risk for wounds after their surgical procedures due to long operative times with positioning on hard surgical tables at awkward angles in order to access the necessary organs. Children should be examined after each surgical procedure to view their skin over bony prominences. Edema should also be assessed. Peripheral and central edema may be evident with children with CHD. Peripheral edema is due to the inability of the heart to maintain adequate cardiac output. The autonomic nervous system is attempting to increase cardiac output by retaining fluid from the kidneys. This makes the heart work even harder and the fluid accumulates in the periphery in the dependent extremities. Central edema or jugular venous distention results from fluid overload as the fluid is retained centrally because the heart's ability to pump is compromised and fluid backs up into the lungs and venous system.

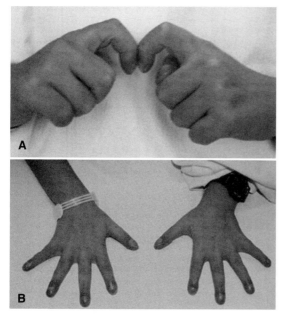

Figure 17.14 ■ A child with digital clubbing and cyanosis in his extremities.

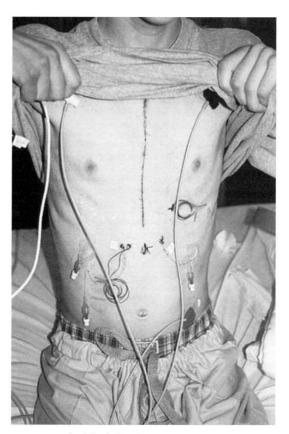

Figure 17.15 ■ A child following transplantation with numerous lines and surgical incisions.

THORAX

Thoracic deformities should be examined, including the pectus excavatum, pectus carinatum, barrel chest, rib flaring, and midtrunk folds. A pectus excavatum may be due to surgical procedures, resulting in the tightening of the upper chest musculature. A pectus carinatum may be due to surgical procedures, resulting in a deformity of the sternum. Barrel chest deformities can be due to the over-inflation of the lung tissue, rib flaring is due to an imbalance of the abdominals with the diaphragm, and a midtrunk fold is due to muscle imbalance of the chest wall to counteract the diaphragm (see Chapter 18). Examination of the rib angles and intercostal spaces for age appropriateness and mobility is important.

To evaluate the thoracic cage of a child with CHD the therapist must have knowledge of what an age-appropriate thoracic cage should look like. Newborns have narrow rib spaces, horizontal ribs, and a triangular shape to their chest wall, with no neck and their chest separate from the abdomen.[27,28] Three- to 6-month-old children will have a normal pectus, more rectangular shape, and horizontal ribs. They will be normal upper chest breathers with only anterior expansion possible.[27,28] Six- to 12-month-old children will have an even more pronounced rectangular shape and lateral expansion will be added to their respiratory repertoire, giving them rib space opening as well as the beginning of gaining a neck. This is a significant stage in the respiratory development of the thorax. There will be a more barrel-shaped appearance of the chest. The rib cage is beginning to be pulled downward due to a more upright posture and the more continuous effects of gravity on the thorax. This change provides the child a better length-tension relationship for the diaphragm and the intercostal muscles. In this stage the diaphragm and all the accessory musculature patterns of breathing are available. This trend in the development of the thorax continues for another year or more as the child shows more midtrunk control, with muscular shortening on one side and lengthening on the other, and wide intercostal spaces.[28] Examining thoracic cage mobility means ascertaining movement of the ribs. Can the child flex laterally? Do the ribs move with respiration? How is abdominal and upper chest movement? Muscular development should be symmetric without hypertrophy of accessory muscles of respiration. An infant with CHD will often have respiratory compromise, which may alter typical muscular function of the chest and, if not addressed, may lead to chest wall deformities. Figure 17.16A–C shows a newborn, 3-month-old, and 8-month-old with normally configured chest walls.

Chest wall movement can be examined by palpation and measurement. By placing your hands over the upper lobe of the lungs with the heel of the hand at the fourth rib, fingertips at the upper trapezii, and thumb at the sternal angle, you may examine symmetry, extent of movement, and general movement. Measure the thoracic circumference with a tape measure at the level of the axilla wrapped around the thorax until it overlaps. Measure the change in circumference during normal inhalation and exhalation. Unpublished data on normal children suggest that the chest wall should move approximately ⅜ inch.[28] Next, move your hands down to the axillary line with palms distal to the nipples. Measure again at the xiphoid process and expect about ⅜ inch of movement. The final level is half the distance between the xiphoid and the umbilicus, and unpublished data suggest ⅛ inch. You will usually observe a larger recruitment pattern from superior to inferior on the thorax.[28]

RESPIRATORY EXAMINATION

Children with CHD will often display respiratory issues as their primary complaint. Sixty percent of individuals with cardiac or thoracic surgeries have pulmonary complications; therefore, this examination in concert with the chest wall examination will give you valuable information for your treatment plan. (See Chapter 18 for more information on respiratory examinations.)

MUSCULOSKELETAL EXAMINATION

An examination of range of motion, postural alignment, and sensation is also necessary. Scoliosis, kyphosis, or a syndromic deviation of the musculoskeletal system may

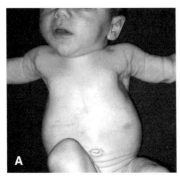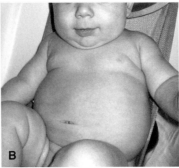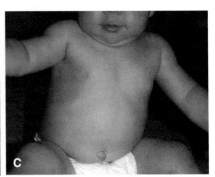

Figure 17.16 ▪ **(A)** A newborn and a normal chest wall shape. **(B)** A normal 3-month-old's chest wall shape. **(C)** An 8-month-old child with a normal chest wall.

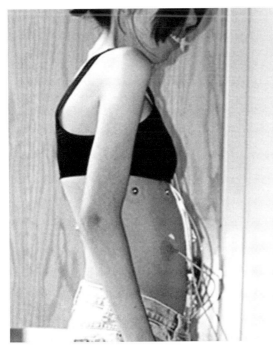

Figure 17.17 ■ A child with Noonan syndrome and its associated postural deviations.

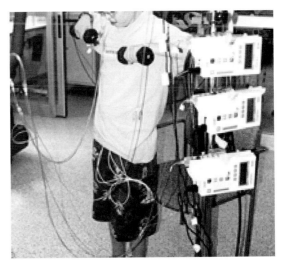

Figure 17.18 ■ A child with a congenital heart defect participating in strength training.

be present and can impact the child's pulmonary system before, during, or after surgery for CHD. Figure 17.17 shows common postural deviations in a child with Noonan syndrome and congenital heart disease including webbing of the neck, pectus excavatum, and facial abnormalities. Children with curvatures of the spine have more difficulty when receiving a lung transplant due to the need for the new lungs to fit in the chest wall cavity; this may lead to atelectasis.

Flexibility can be examined by functional range of motion, a sit-and-reach test, and lateral flexion measurements. Measure from the axilla to the base of the ribs, and then the base of the ribs to the pelvis; it should be a 1:2 ratio.

Peroneal nerve palsies are also important to look for as they can happen during prolonged positioning in the operating room. Children awaiting transplantation with left ventricular failure are at risk for thrombosis and stroke secondary to clot formation in the left ventricle; therefore, after a surgical procedure, it is important to do a full evaluation of the musculoskeletal system.

STRENGTH

Measurement of strength must consider children who are at risk for myopathy, osteopenia, and osteoporosis secondary to steroids preoperatively or following transplantation. Manual muscle testing may not offer an accurate measure of the child's strength. Dynamometry is an excellent objective tool; we have some unpublished data indicating that children with CHD tend to fall in the fifth percentile while

awaiting transplantation (Fig. 17.18). It is important to teach breathing techniques, exhaling on the exertion phase, so the child can perform resistive exercise and learn to avoid Valsalva maneuvers during exertion. An eight-repetition maximum to fatigue is recommended, rather than a one-repetition maximum in an effort to decide on an initial level of resistance. Vital sign monitoring is also an important part of ongoing evaluation during interventions.

VITAL SIGNS

Resting, during treatment, and vital sign monitoring during and after intervention provide invaluable information about the child's cardiovascular response to activity. The trends of the vital signs are very important. A sinus tachycardia is commonly found in response to low cardiac output. After transplantation, patients do not have innervated hearts, which results in a high resting heart rate and a low maximal heart rate. These changes result in a need for warm-up, to increase the heart rate in order to have an effect from the circulating catecholamines in the blood, followed by a cool-down.

FUNCTIONAL MOBILITY

Functional mobility examination includes looking at bed mobility, transfers, balance, gait, and climbing stairs, as well as developmentally appropriate activities. These activities can be evaluated on the first day postoperatively, and again as IV medications are no longer being utilized.

AEROBIC CAPACITY AND ENDURANCE

Aerobic tests in clinical care usually include a 6-, 9-, or 12-minute walk test, with the 6-minute test being the most universally employed. During a 6-minute walk test the child is given specific and age-appropriate directions that once he or she starts walking, the test will run for 6 minutes. You should instruct patients that they are to walk at their own pace, but to try to walk as far as they can to cover the greatest distance possible in the allotted time. Also instruct them that if they need to stop, they may do so, and that if you need to stop them for some reason you will tell them. Patients should let you know if they have chest discomfort, dizziness, severe shortness of breath, unsteadiness, or blurred vision. You should record distance, rates of perceived exertion (RPE), a dyspnea index (DI), and vital signs before, during, and after the testing. According to a paper by Cahalin, performance is thought to depend on motivation, endurance, respiratory function, cardiovascular fitness, and neuromuscular function. Cahalin found that the 6-minute walk test effectively predicted peak oxygen consumption and early survival rates in patients with CHF. Forty percent of his patients who ambulated less than 300 meters died or were admitted to a hospital for inotropic or mechanical support as a bridge to transplantation, and only 12% of those ambulating greater than 300 meters were transplanted.[29] An objective way to assess shortness of breath is by using the ventilatory index scale.[16] This scale asks patients to inhale deeply, then count aloud slowly during the exhalation from 1 to 15 (generally this takes 8 seconds). A level 0 means that they can count aloud to 15 without taking a breath, a level 1 means they take one breath to count to 15, a level 2 means they takes two breaths to count to 15, a level 3 means they take three breaths to count to 15, and a level 4 means they take four breaths to count to 15. You can re-examine patients over time to see if the levels change. Breathlessness can also be examined by counting how many words they are able to speak per normal speaking breath or syllables per breath; normal is eight to 10 words. You can also ask them to hold a vowel sound for a specified time frame while you count; for kids, holding for 10 seconds is considered normal, and for older adolescents, 15 seconds is considered normal (more like adults). A DI (Table 17.4) is a more subjective examination method whereby you ask patients how breathless they feel and they respond with a number from a chart you show them.

The Borg RPE scale (Table 17.5) gives you a picture of overall work. You ask the individual, "How hard do you feel you are working?" This is meant to include overall work, breathing, muscle exertion, and fatigue. You want the patient to integrate information from the peripheral working muscles and joints, the cardiovascular and pulmonary systems, and the central nervous system. A rating of 6 is analogous to no work at all, while a rating of 20 is the hardest work ever done.

Physical Therapy Evaluation, Diagnosis, and Prognosis

You must attempt to integrate all the findings from your examination to determine the individual's physical therapy diagnosis and prognosis. This helps to determine the plan of care and outcomes expected. The goals of your physical therapy plan of care are directly related to your examination findings. The overall objective is to improve the individual's endurance, balance, functional mobility, strength, flexibility, scar and chest wall mobility, and expansion and airway clearance. The physical therapist participates in patient and family education regarding the need for developmentally appropriate activities and encouraging a lifelong commitment to exercise. Long-term objectives include attempting to prevent secondary impairments of muscle atrophy, joint contractures, postural deviations, osteoporosis, respiratory compromise, poor aerobic endurance, obesity, and developmental delay.

Physical Therapy Intervention

Your treatment plan can be generalized to a few categories. Those individuals with functional mobility and strength and endurance compromise will often need three

TABLE 17.5	
Borg Rate of Perceived Exertion Scale	
6	
7	Very, very light
8	
9	Very light
10	
11	Fairly light
12	
13	Somewhat hard
14	
15	Hard
16	
17	Very hard
18	
19	Very, very hard
20	

TABLE 17.4	
Dyspnea Index	
	Score
Breathlessness barely noticeable	1
Breathlessness moderately bothersome	2
Breathlessness severe, very uncomfortable	3
Most severe breathlessness ever experienced	4

or more sessions each week to show improvements in these areas of impairment. Those individuals who need developmental skill building due to developmental delay require twice-a-week physical therapy intervention to improve on these areas.

COORDINATION, COMMUNICATION, AND DOCUMENTATION

INTERDISCIPLINARY TEAMWORK

Physical therapists often recommend consults with other services including genetic counseling, neurology, otolaryngology, orthopedics, feeding team, occupational therapy, or speech therapy. It is important to know your professional limitations and learn to advocate for the child to gain the services he or she deserves. Attending rounds with the medical team in the acute care setting is invaluable, to know where the team stands on a particular child and to offer your unique physical therapy perspective. In the home care and outpatient settings you should contact primary physicians to request laboratory values as necessary and to corroborate medical histories from families.

PATIENT- AND FAMILY-RELATED INSTRUCTION

Family and caregiver education should focus on the family unit as a whole in addition to the specific needs of the child. Maternal perceptions of the child's disease severity have been shown to be a stronger predictor of adjustment of the child to a cardiac disorder than the actual disease severity itself.[30] It is important to emphasize the difference between CHD and adult coronary artery disease. The child should be able to explore and play within boundaries based on his or her specific CHD, not based out of fear of participation. Most children will limit themselves safely and rest when they feel taxed by the motor request.

Enhancement of performance should start with the premise that exercise should be a lifelong habit. Adolescents should be taught to perceive exercise as a responsibility for their own health. Outpatient physical therapy and early intervention programs should be recommended for those who need services regardless of whether their CHD is expected to require surgery or not. The sooner a child is started in services, the better off he or she will be in the long run. Health, wellness, and fitness programs including cardiac rehabilitation programs and YMCA programs are an important component to lifelong health habits.

PROCEDURAL INTERVENTIONS

POSITIONING

Using varied positions will enable the physical therapist to prevent musculoskeletal abnormalities and may help pulmonary parameters as well. Rotation schedules to reduce the possibility of skin pressure and breakdown is important in the early stages of treatment for a child under neuromuscular blockade or sedation. Positioning devices such as Multi-Podus boots help control plantar flexion contractures, address hip rotation, and protect the heel. In addition, molded foot and ankle orthoses, towel rolls, and gel pillows will help prevent secondary integument issues for children with CHD. Providing midline orientation and preventing contractures is a responsibility for the physical therapist before the child is able to move. Scar massage to prevent binding down of scars once healing is occurring and to enhance skin movement as soon as possible will prevent range-of-motion limitations and deformities from surgical scars.

The body has a natural response to changes of position. Body positioning alone can enhance oxygen transport. Infants, even with endotracheal tubes, have an increase in oxygenation in prone versus other positions, especially supine. Small children have better ventilation to the uppermost lung. Larger children have better ventilation to the dependent lung, similar to the adult pattern. A mismatch of ventilation and perfusion is a common cause of arterial hypoxemia. Specific body positioning can more closely match ventilation and perfusion to a specific lobe of the lung. This can be used in two ways: (1) with a lung displaying atelectasis, place the affected lung uppermost to increase ventilation to that lung; and (2) if the lung is overinflated, place that lung down to decrease ventilation to that lung and better match perfusion. In larger children their dependent lung will have better ventilation, similar to the adult situation. Therefore, in cases of atelectasis, place the affected lung dependent to increase ventilation to that lung. If the larger child is having issues with overinflation, place that lung in the superior position to have better ventilation-perfusion matching.[31] Utilize a chart like the one shown in Table 17.6 to place the child in different positions and see where the best ventilation-perfusion matching may be in order to raise SpO_2 and decrease heart rate, blood pressure, and respiratory rate.

THERAPEUTIC EXERCISES

FLEXIBILITY Begin flexibility training with postural awareness and postural training. This may mean using elastic wrap or other tools for tactile cues during upright posture to minimize thoracic kyphosis and rounded shoulders. Flexibility exercises should begin early, including pectoral stretches (Fig. 17.19), Achilles/gastrocnemius/soleus stretches, and stretching over a towel roll for all directions of thoracic cage mobility. Bolsters, balls, and towel rolls for thoracic cage stretching in dynamic or static modes are valuable. Often these stretches need to be held for long periods of time for a sustained stretch, and can be done as "homework" during television time or while playing board games or reading. Active range-of-motion activities for the upper extremities can be initiated during the first post-

TABLE 17.6									
Vital Sign Trends									
Breathing Patterns/Vital Sign Trends		**RR**		**SpO₂%**		**HR**		**BP**	
Position	**Sequence**	1 min	3 min	1 min	3 min	1 min	3 min	1 min	3 min
Supine Side-lying Sitting/upright Prone									

BP, blood pressure; HR, heart rate; RR, respiratory rate.

operative day in the acute care setting. Even children with long-standing inflexibility from numerous surgeries can benefit from the initiation of thoracic cage stretching.

BREATHING EXERCISES Breathing games like bubbles, air hockey, blowing a windmill, sniffing stickers are an excellent

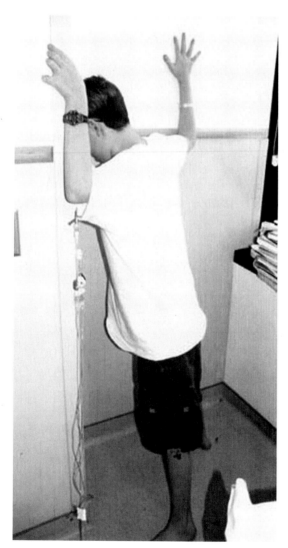

Figure 17.19 ▪ Corner stretches presurgically for a child with a congenital heart defect.

start to improve the child's respiratory status. Belly breathing, inspiratory muscle trainers, incentive spirometers, and deep breathing techniques can be utilized in children as young as 18 months. Finding a strategy that works with the developmental level of the child, and one that the child finds "fun" is the challenge. Some children love bubbles and will attempt to blow a bubble even in the worst of situations. A child as young as 14 months can blow bubbles or a pinwheel with assistance. The major objective is to foster deep breathing to help maintain ventilation. More extensive information about breathing exercises can be found in Chapter 18.

AEROBIC AND ENDURANCE TRAINING Exercise prescription should begin with mode, frequency, duration, and intensity principles. Mode may be a bicycle, a treadmill, or an upper body exerciser (UBE). The frequency should be a minimum of three times a week and up to seven times a week. The duration we find that works the best with the very ill child is multiple short bouts of 3 to 5 minutes, each with rest breaks of 1 to 2 minutes and lower intensity work during this break. Lower intensity may be stretching or weight training or a true rest period if necessary based on RPE and vital signs. The intensity can be determined from the stress test performed prior to training. Generally, an intensity of 60% to 65% of the maximal level of work is a good place to start. Most children who are able to participate will not tolerate more than this amount of work. Their RPE should fall between 11 and 14 on the Borg scale, with a DI between 1 and 2. During their activity they should have their heart rate, blood pressure, RPE, DI, respiratory rate, and SpO₂ monitored. This is also a good time to have patients learn to take their own heart rate, respiratory rate, RPE, and DI. This will help them gain the independence necessary to continue exercise once they leave your facility and move to more autonomous activity.

STRENGTH TRAINING Strength training is an important component of physical therapy for children of an appropriate age. Strengthening will decrease many secondary musculoskeletal effects of corticosteroids. There is a 6- to 8-week postoperative period during which children will have lifting precautions and during which strength training should be deferred. With this caveat, strength training is a valuable tool in the treatment of children with CHD both pre- and postoperatively. The child should always be taught proper breathing techniques with lifting: to breathe out during the exertion portion of lifting and breathe in on the gravity-assisted movement portion. This breathing pattern will prevent a Valsalva maneuver and is very important for keeping blood pressure from rising unnecessarily.

AIRWAY CLEARANCE TECHNIQUES

These topics will be covered in detail in Chapter 18. Positioning to alter the work of breathing and to maximize ventilation and perfusion ratios (noted above) as well as for postural drainage is another first line of defense and should be utilized immediately postoperatively. Positioning programs prevent the prolonged dependency of any one portion of the lung, so that pooling of secretions can be limited/avoided and improved ventilation can be reached. Your evaluation will give you clear information about which position maximizes ventilation–perfusion matching, and this examination should be repeated postoperatively as the child will essentially have a new cardiopulmonary system after surgical repair or transplantation. The therapist must coordinate changes in the infant's position with other nursing procedures to avoid unnecessary stimulation. Infants should never be left in the head-down position alone or placed in the head-down position until over 1 year of age due to the increased likelihood of gastroesophageal reflux. In the side-lying position, place the best lung in the dependent position and the atelectatic lung in the uppermost position to stimulate better ventilation–perfusion matching. Ventilation is increased to the uppermost lung due to chest wall compliance. Mechanical techniques such as percussion, vibration, shaking, and the high-frequency chest wall oscillation are also used but require a short wait postoperatively; other techniques can be utilized more readily.

FUNCTIONAL MOBILITY

Transfer training, gait training, balance training, and stair climbing are functional tasks to be addressed in physical therapy intervention. Transfer training should include ways to move that decrease discomfort and improve independence. This may mean teaching log rolling postoperatively with deep-breathing techniques, or giving a child a "hug pillow" to hold over surgical sites. For small children this may mean teaching family members how to pick up and hold their child in a way to pose as little discomfort as possible. "Timed up and down" stair climbing should start once intravenous or other lines that would interfere are gone. The timed stair climb provides useful test–retest data by which to measure progress and motivate a child having a hard time. Make it a fun game against time, within safe measures of vital signs and balance.

DEVELOPMENTAL ACTIVITY

Play is the means by which young children explore their world. A child with CHD who is awaiting surgery or very ill and hospitalized has little exposure to the world. Age-appropriate play is very important in this population. Although there may be many tubes and wires to deal with in order to change positions or to take the infant out of the crib in the acute care setting, an infant should be exposed to all positions, including prone. Getting the infant accustomed to prone, be it semi-prone over a towel roll or prone on the shoulder of the caregiver, should help the infant developmentally. Prone is the forerunner for many early developmental skills including creeping, crawling, and upper extremity weight bearing. This position is important for children with poor feeding, reflux, and respiratory issues. Families should be encouraged to feel comfortable with prone positioning during awake, alert, calm periods during the day in order to have the infant gain head control and feel comfortable in prone. It is unusual for a child to have difficulty in prone after practice, and prone is seldom a contraindicated position, with the exception of a thoracic wound that is not closed. Figure 17.20 shows

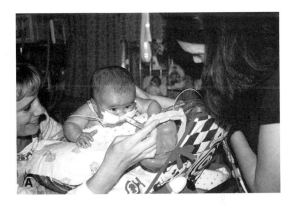

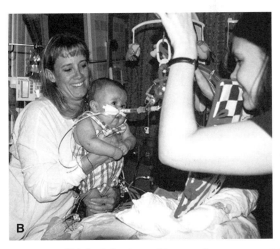

Figure 17.20 ■ **(A)** An infant awaiting cardiac surgery working on prone skills in physical therapy with physical therapist (*left*) and mother very involved. **(B)** Same infant with congenital heart defect working on age-appropriate developmental skills despite receiving mechanical ventilation via nasotracheal intubation.

an infant being placed in prone with the assistance and guidance of the physical therapist and the same infant working on developmental activities.

Crawling should be encouraged in children with CHD as it improves upon all the muscle groups that are impacted by the surgical procedures done to correct or palliate CHD. Children who are ambulatory should be ambulating postoperatively as soon as they are medically stable. Children receiving mechanical ventilation can ambulate with a team effort to maintain their ventilatory support and the safety of their airway. Often this event is a highlight for the child and family, especially if the course of the child's illness has interfered with ambulation for weeks or months. Children with chest tubes can also ambulate with little limitation, and ambulation may help to hasten chest tube removal.

Neurodevelopmental Outcomes of Congenital Heart Disease

The causes of neurodevelopmental problems are multifactorial and involve an interaction of the preoperative, intraoperative, and postoperative events.[5,7] Factors such as the stress of early surgery, long hospitalizations, and overprotective family attitudes may also contribute to developmental lags. There is evidence to suggest that a child with CHD has brain insults prior to any surgical intervention, and that prolonged hypoxemia (oxygen saturations below 90%) before surgery may contribute to developmental delays.[32] As early as 2 months of age, delays in motor and psychological functions were noted in 25% of infants on the Bayley Scales of Infant Development.[7] A study by Majnemer and Limperopoulos assessed infants younger than 2 years of age a mean of 2.8 days before surgery using the Peabody Developmental Motor Scale and found that 40% of these infants had abnormalities preoperatively, which included hypotonia, gross and fine motor delay, behavioral difficulties, and motor asymmetry.[7] Other studies have also found preoperatively abnormal neurobehavioral status in newborns (younger than 1 month), including respiratory difficulties; poorly coordinated suck, swallow, and breathing; tone abnormalities; abnormal posture and activity level; weak cry; and poor auditory and visual orienting responses.[5] Limperopoulos et al. found that over half of the newborns tested with standardized measures had abnormalities including hypotonia, hypertonia, jitteriness, motor asymmetries, and absent suck reflex. Feeding difficulties (34%), poor state regulation (62%), and microcephaly (30%) were also noted.[6]

After surgery, children having CHDs were also likely to display neurologic changes including altered consciousness, seizures, muscle tone abnormalities, dyskinetic movements, and personality changes. Studies have also found mild hypotonia, extensor posturing, cranial nerve abnormalities, and specific motor problems (~50%), whether randomized to predominantly circulatory arrest or to cardiopulmonary bypass intervention.[32] Severe neurologic deficits like cerebral palsy are reported in the range of 5% to 9% of infant cohorts and are considered rare.[4] One year following open heart surgery, 50% of the cohort of Majnemer and Limperopoulos had been one standard deviation below the normative means for gross or fine motor difficulties.[5] Hypotonia and motor delay may contribute to problems with complex perceptual–motor skills at school age.[5] Intelligence quotients (IQs) have also been frequently studied as affected by CHD as compared to the normative mean. Language delays in expressive abilities and vocabulary are also prevalent after surgical correction.[8] Behavior in school-aged children was found to be altered as compared to a group of controls with social and emotional maladjustment. Maternal guilt, anxiety, and overprotectiveness were found to contribute to these difficulties. Goldberg et al. studied a group of infants with CHD and found that these infants were less likely to be securely attached to their mothers and displayed higher avoidant behaviors and greater dependency than a group of healthy peers.[33] They also found that maternal feelings of guilt, anxiety, and maladjustment promoted the behavioral and social problems seen in their children. Individuals with single ventricles (HLHS, DORV) have a higher risk of developmental delays due to the numerous surgeries related to its palliation.[3,7,9] Children undergoing cardiac transplantation after failure to adequately repair or palliate their cardiac condition present with special physical therapy needs as well, and may also present with neurodevelopmental issues.[34]

Family Adjustment

Maternal anxiety and overprotectiveness and social and emotional maladjustment have all been documented in children with CHD. It has been suggested that overprotective parents may contribute to greater dependence in functional skills.[6] In short, the quality of the mother–child relationship is more critical to successful adaptation than the severity of the child's illness. Infancy is a crucial time in the development of healthy psychological function; the presence of CHD may affect the interaction of mothers and their infants. Difficulties with feeding caused mothers to report high levels of frustration and distress and also affect the reaction of mothers and infants at a time when bonding is required. Therapists working on feeding need to be aware of the possibility of distress during these times and must work to support the family members to gain more positive interactions with their infant. Physical therapists should be aware of these interactions and attempt to assist in creating a more positive atmosphere for mothers and their infants. This can be accomplished by something as simple as scheduling therapy services around nap and feeding schedules.

Bergman and Stamm have named the overrestriction and overobservation by parents of a child with a CHD as "cardiac nondisease." The child's reaction and adjustment to his or her illness is directly related to the emotional and behavioral reaction of family members, and family members' reaction is related to the degree of communication with professionals and their comprehension of the child's actual condition.[35]

SUMMARY

There is much a physical therapist can do in the care of a child preoperatively, awaiting transplantation, postoperatively, and posttransplantation to improve functional mobility and developmental skills. Physical therapists are a vital component to the care of all children with cardiac disorders.

CASE STUDY

ADOLESCENT WITH A SIGNIFICANT CARDIAC SURGERY

History of Present Illness
J.T. is a 15-year-old boy who was admitted June 4, 2001, to await heart transplantation secondary to congestive heart failure with poor ventricular function.

General Health Status
Unable to ambulate between classrooms at school, home schooled as of February 2001. Unable to climb stairs at home due to severe dyspnea.

Chief Complaint
Fatigue, shortness of breath, exercise intolerance, inability to keep up with peers.

Medical History
J.T. was delivered at full term; had a 3-week NICU stay with a diagnosis of double-outlet right ventricle, mitral valve atresia, and pulmonary valve stenosis with cyanotic spells.

Surgical History
J.T. underwent atrial septostomy with pulmonary artery bands inserted at 6 months of age. At 13 months of age J.T. had a modified right Blalock-Taussig shunt of 5.0 mm (Fig. 17.21) followed 3 years later with a bidirectional Glenn procedure. Three years later a modified left Blalock-Taussig shunt of 6.0 mm was performed, secondary to persistent cyanosis, in an effort to increase pulmonary blood flow and improve tricuspid valve regurgitation.

Current Medications
Furosemide, dopamine, lidocaine, milrinone, dobutamine, and heparin.

Laboratory Values
Catheterization data: right ventricular pressure 114/8, 78% saturation; aorta pressure 112/77, 81% saturation.

Social History
J.T.'s parents are divorced and have joint custody, although J.T. lives with his father who has remarried. His extended family includes two brothers and their families and a maternal grandmother, all of whom are very involved in J.T.'s care.

Physical Therapy Examination
General appearance: J.T. is a thin teenager who is pale, diaphoretic, and dyspneic. There is both peripheral and central cyanosis. Peripheral edema is absent but there is severe digital clubbing present.
State of consciousness: He is awake, alert, and oriented to person, place, and time.
Pain: Visual analog scale assessment shows no report of pain.

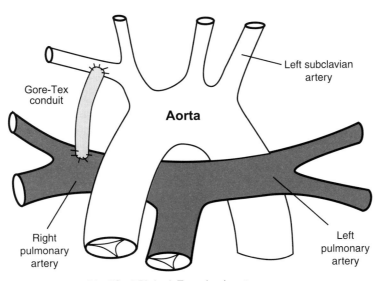

Figure 17.21 ■ Modified Blalock-Taussig shunt.

Supportive devices: Supplemental oxygen by nasal cannula at night.

Vital signs at rest: Heart rate = 116, SpO_2 = 76%, blood pressure in the right upper extremity = 103/57, respiratory rate = 33.

Lines: Peripherally inserted central catheter (PICC) in left upper extremity with IV pole

Abdominal distention: None noted.

Integument: Median sternotomy × 4; left lateral thoracotomy; chest tube sites medial chest wall × 3.

Skin integrity: All wounds well healed. Capillary refill: <5 seconds. Scar mobility: Scars are bound down in numerous areas with poor mobility.

Thoracic Cage Examination

J.T. has a pectus excavatum; superior anterior rib spaces are restricted, but others appropriate for age. There is some superior thorax mobility, but midthorax immobility. There is some asymmetry between the pectoralis majors with no hypertrophy of inspiratory muscles.

Respiratory Assessment

No obvious distress. Respiratory rate is 35 breaths/min. J.T. has a respiratory pattern of primarily diaphragmatic breathing with poor anterior chest wall excursion and no retractions noted. Some inspiratory use of trapezius muscles noted. J.T. can sneeze and cough without splinting required. Auscultation shows decreased breath sounds throughout the lungs but no adventitious sounds and no apneic pauses.

Chest expansion	Third rib	Xiphoid	Umbilicus
Easy breathing	⅛″	⅛″	½″
Maximal breath	½″	1″	1″

Musculoskeletal Examination

Full range of motion (ROM) in the right upper extremity (RUE). PICC line in left upper extremity (LUE) results in decreased end-range for elbow extension and flexion and decreased end-range in horizontal shoulder abduction. Right lower extremity (RLE)/left lower extremity (LLE) show full ROM. Strength ⅘ in both lower extremities; ⅗ in left upper extremity; and ⅘ in right upper extremity. Posture and spinal alignment: forward head posture, rounded shoulders, no scoliosis. Lateral sidebending is symmetric with a 2:1 ratio. Sensation intact throughout to light touch.

Functional mobility: Bed mobility and transfers are independent.

Balance: Higher level balance assessed with no difficulty in tandem walking or single leg stance on each leg.

Gait and stairs: J.T. has slow ambulation cadence with deceased hip flexion, decreased arm swing, and noticeable external rotation of both lower extremities. Stairs were not assessed secondary to IV pole on continuous infusion.

Exercise tolerance testing: Six-minute walk performed with 560 feet with no rest breaks, but J.T. complains of fatigue. Values below before, during, and after 6-minute walk.

Vitals	HRA	SpO_2	BP (RUE)	RR	RPE	DI
Before	116	76%	102/79	23	6	1
During	132	68%	116/69	32	10	2
After	119	74%	100/73	21	6	1

Exercise stress test: Max VO_2=13.4 mL/kg/min; Max heart rate = 136 (65% 205 predicted);8 minutes of activity for a total of 4.6 metabolic equivalents (METS).

Goals

AT 2 WEEKS

- J.T. will ambulate at self-selected pace for 10 minutes without rest break.
- J.T. will increase strength half-grade throughout UE/LE.
- J.T. will increase anterior chest wall expansion ⅛″.
- J.T. will ambulate 720 feet in 6 minutes with vital signs stable.
- J.T. will be independent with pulse monitoring, RPE, and DI.
- J.T. will be sent home with exercise program to include wall squats, corner standing, stretch, gastrocnemius and soleus stretches, hamstring stretches, and ambulation with assistance for IV pole on non–physical therapy days.

Plan of Care

J.T. will be seen 3 days a week to work on the above goals.
Patient and parent education: Given bedside exercise plan, deep breathing, stretching, LE strengthening, endurance activities.

Procedural Interventions

Scar massage: To be performed during bathing routine.

EXERCISE PRESCRIPTION

Aerobic exercise:

- Treadmill warm-up = 0.5 mph @ 0% grade for 3 minutes.
- Treadmill exercise = 1.5 mph @ 0% grade for 10 minutes.

Strength training: 2 lb × 10 repetitions × 2 sets for UE/LE.
Flexibility training: At bedside.

REFERENCES

1. Hoffman J, Kaplan S. The incidence of congenital heart disease. J Am Coll Cardiol 2002;39:1890–1900.
2. Green A. Outcomes of congenital heart disease: a review. Pediatr Nurs 2004;30(4):280–284.
3. Stieh J, Kramer HH, Harding P, Fisher G. Gross and fine motor development is impaired in children with cyanotic congenital heart disease. Neuropediatrics 1999;30:77–82.
4. Limperopolous C, Majnemer A, Shevell M, et al. Functional limitations in young children with congenital heart defects after cardiac surgery. Pediatrics 2001;108(6):1325–1331.
5. Majnemer A, Limperopoulos C. Developmental progress of children with congenital heart defects requiring open heart surgery. Semin Pediatr Neurol 1999;6(1):12–19.
6. Limperopoulos C, Majnemer A, Shevell M, et al. Functional limitations in young children with congenital heart defects after cardiac surgery. Pediatrics 2001;108(6):1325–1331.
7. Limperopoulos C, Majnemer A, Shevell M, et al. Neurodevelopmental status of newborns and infants with congenital

heart defects before and after open heart surgery. J Pediatri 2005;137(5):638–645.

8. Majnemer A, Limperopoulos C, Shevell M, et al. Long-term neuromotor outcome at school entry of infants with congenital heart defects requiring open-heart surgery. J Pediatr 2006; 148:72–77.

9. Majnemer A, Limperopoulos C, Shevell M, et al. Predictors of developmental disabilities after open heart surgery in young children with congenital heart defects. J Pediatr 2002;141:51–58.

10. Neill C, Clark E, Clark C. From Birth to Adolescence, from Doctor's Office to Playground. The Heart of a Child. What Families Need to Know about Heart Disorders in Children. Baltimore: Johns Hopkins University Press, 1992.

11. Walker C. Downs syndrome and congenital heart defects part I: anatomical and functional anomalies, prognosis and treatment. Intens Care Nurs 1991;7:94–104.

12. Larsen WJ. Human Embryology. New York: Churchill Livingstone, 1993 p.157–187;195–229.

13. Nelson W, Behrman R, Kliegman R, et al. Textbook of Pediatrics. 15th Ed. W. B. Philadelphia: Saunders Company, 1996.

14. Frownfelter D, Dean E. Principles and Practice of Cardiopulmonary Physical Therapy. 3rd Ed. St. Louis: Mosby-Year Book, Inc., 1996.

15. Hillegass E, Sadowsky HS. Essentials of Cardiopulmonary Physical Therapy. Philadelphia: W. B. Saunders Company, 2001.

16. Irwin S, Tecklin J. Cardiopulmonary Physical Therapy. 4th Ed. St. Louis: CV Mosby, 2004.

17. Webber S, McCurry K, Zeevi A. Heart and lung transplantation in children. Lancet 2006;368:53–69.

18. Alyn IB, Baker LK. Cardiovascular anatomy and physiology of the fetus, neonate, infant, child, and adolescent. J Cardiovasc Nurs 1992;6(3):1–11.

19. Haziniski MF. Congenital heart disease in the neonate part 1: epidemiology, cardiac development and fetal circulation. Neonatal Netw 1983;1(4):29–35, 42–43.

20. Higgins S, Reid A. Common congenital heart defects: long term follow-up. Nurs Clin North Am 1994;29(2):233–248.

21. Attia J, Amiel-Tison C, Mayer MN, Schider SM. Measurement of postoperative pain and narcotic administration in infants using a new clinical scoring system, Anesthesiology 1987;67 (3A):A532.

22. McGrath PJ, Johnson G, Goodman JT, Schillinger J. CHEOPS: a behavioral scale for rating postoperative pain in children. Adv Pain Res Ther 1985;9:395–402.

23. Wong DL, Baker C. Pain in children: comparison of assessment scales. Pediatr Nurs 1988;14:9–17.

24. Merkel SI, Voepel-Lewis T, Shayevitz JR, et al. The FLACC: a behavioral scale for scoring postoperative pain in young children. Pediatr Nurs 1997;23(3):293–297.

25. Perme C, Southard R, Joyce D, et al. Early mobilization of LVAD recipients who require prolonged mechanical ventilation. Tex Heart Inst J 2006;33:130–133.

26. Humphrey R, Buck L, Cahalin L, et al. Physical therapy assessment and intervention for patients with left ventricular assist devices. Cardiopulm Phys Ther 1998;9(2):3–7.

27. Massery M. Chest development as a component of normal motor development. implications for pediatric physical therapists. Pediatr Phys Ther 1991;3–8.

28. Massery M. If you can't breathe you can't function. Unpublished data.

29. Cahalin L. The 6 minute walk test predicts peak oxygen uptake and survival in patients with Advanced CHF. Chest 1996; 110(2):325–332.

30. Bergman AB, Stamm SJ. The morbidity of cardiac non-disease in schoolchildren. N Engl J Med 1967;276(18):1008–1013.

31. Bhuyan U, Peters AM, Gordon I, et al. Effects of posture on the distribution of pulmonary ventilation and perfusion in children and adults. Thorax 1989;44:480–484.

32. Newburger J, Jonas R, Wernovsky G, Wypij D, Hickey P, Kuban K, et al. A comparison of the perioperative neurologic effects of hypothermic circulatory arrest versus low-flow cardiopulmonary bypass in infant heart surgery. N Engl J Med 1993; 139(15):1057–1064.

33. Goldberg B, Fripp R, Lister G, et al. Effect of physical training on exercise performance of children following surgical repair of congenital heart disease. Pediatrics 1981;68(5):691–699.

34. Suddaby EC, Samango-Sprouse C, Vaught DR, Cluster DA et al. Neurodevelopmental outcome of infant cardiac transplant recipients. J Transplant Coordinat 1996;6(1):9–13.

Evaluation Form for Cardiac Disorders in Pediatrics

PHYSICAL THERAPY CARDIOTHORACIC EXAMINATION

Patient Name: _____

Date: _____ Referring Physician: _____ ❑ IP ❑ OP Location: _____

Diagnosis: _____ Precautions: _____

HPI: _____

_____

_____

_____

PMH: _____

_____

Medications: _____

Social History: _____

Barriers to Learning: ❑ none ❑ language ❑ sensory ❑ physical ❑ cognitive ❑ social ❑ cultural ❑ emotional ❑ motivation

Developmental History/Prior Level of Functioning: _____

TESTS AND MEASURES

General Appearance:

State of Consciousness: ❑ M-S blockade ❑ sedated ❑ awake and alert

Pain: _____ Score: _____ ❑ CHEOPS ❑ Faces ❑ VAS ❑ 0-10

Supportive Devices: ❑ ECMO ❑ mechanical ventilation ❑ LVAD ❑ NC O_2 ❑ NG tube   Chest Tubes: ❑ left ❑ right

Vital Signs at Rest: HR:____ BP:____ SpO_2:____ RR:____ Arrhythmia:_____

Lines: ❑ intracardiac ❑ A-lines ❑ pacer wires ❑ PICC ❑ PIV ❑ broviac ❑ none ❑ other: _____

Cyanosis: ❑ absent   present: ❑ peripheral ❑ central   Diaphoretic: ❑ at rest ❑ with activity ❑ none

Pallor: ❑ none ❑ present   Clubbing: ❑ none ❑ mild ❑ moderate ❑ severe

Peripheral Edema: ❑ none ❑ present   Abdominal Distention: ❑ none ❑ present

Body Type: ❑ obese ❑ cachetic ❑ appropriate for age

Integumentary:

General Appearance: _____

Surgical Sites: ❑ clam shell ❑ median sternotomy   Thoracotomy: ❑ left ❑ right

Skin Integrity: _____

Capillary Refill: _____ Scar Mobility: _____

Thoracic Cage Examination:

Chest Wall Deformities: ❑ none ❑ pectus excavatum ❑ pectus carinatum ❑ barrel chest ❑ rib flaring ❑ midtrunk fold

Rib Spacing: ❑ restricted ❑ increased spacing ❑ appropriate for age ❑ other:_____ Where: _____

Thoracic Cage Mobility: ❑ superior chest ❑ midchest ❑ lateral costal ❑ symmetric ❑ asymmetric Where_____

Degree of Restriction: ❑ mild ❑ moderate ❑ severe Describe: _____

Symmetry of Muscle Development: ❑ symmetric ❑ asymmetric   Hypertrophy: ❑ present ❑ absent

Chest Expansion (inches)

Easy Breathing	Upper	Mid	Lower

Chest Expansion (inches)

Maximal Breath	Upper	Mid	Lower

PHYSICAL THERAPY CARDIOTHORACIC EXAMINATION

Respiratory Assessment:

Respiratory Rate: ___ /minute   Apneic Pauses: ____ sec   Respiratory Pattern: ❏ regular ❏ irregular   ratio I:E _____

Retractions: ❏ suprasternal ❏ substernal ❏ subcostal ❏ intercostal

Work of Breathing: ❏ nasal flaring ❏ head bobbing ❏ stridor ❏ wheezing ❏ grunting

Accessory Muscle Use: ❏ SCM ❏ scalenes ❏ pectorals ❏ serratus anterior ❏ other: _____

Airway Clearance: ❏ sneeze ❏ cough ❏ requires splinting to cough ❏ PDPV ❏ vest

Auscultation: ❏ clear ❏ decreased ❏ adventitious: Where: _____

Breathing Patterns / Vital Sign Trends		RR		SpO$_2$%		HR		BP	
Position	Sequence	1 min	3 min	1 min	3 min	1 min	3 min	1 min	3 min
Supine									
Side-lying									
Sitting/Upright									
Prone									

MUSCULOSKELETAL
Range of Motion/Strength/Sensation

Extremity	Range of Motion	Strength	Sensation	Needs More Assessment
Right Upper				
Left Upper				
Right Lower				
Left Lower				

Posture/Spinal Alignment: ❏ scoliosis_____ ❏ kyphosis_____

Lateral Sidebending: Axilla to base of ribs: _____ inches   Base of ribs to pelvis: _____ inches   Ratio: ___:___

Axilla to base of ribs: _____ inches   Base of ribs to pelvis: _____ inches   Ratio: ___:___

FUNCTIONAL SKILLS: Mobility/Activity Examination

Activity	Comments
Bed Mobility	
Transfers	
Balance	
Gait/Stairs	

PHYSICAL THERAPY CARDIOTHORACIC EXAMINATION

Exercise Tolerance Test: ❏ NA for age

6- or 12-minute walk test: _____feet   Rest: _____   Complaints: _____

Pretest: position _____ SpO_2: _____% HR: _____ BP:_____ Where: _____ RR: _____ RPE: _____ DI: _____	During: position _____ SpO_2: _____% HR: _____ BP:_____ Where: _____ RR: _____ RPE: _____ DI: _____	Posttest: position _____ SpO_2: _____% HR: _____ BP:_____ Where: _____ RR: _____ RPE: _____ DI: _____

Dyspnea Index:
Amount of breathlessness patient perceives

1 - Breathlessness barely noticeable
2 - Breathlessness moderately bothersome
3 - Severe, very uncomfortable
4 - Most severe breathlessness ever experienced

BORG SCALE
(Rate of Perceived Exertion)

6
7   Very, very light
8
9   Very light
10
11   Fairly light
12
13   Somewhat hard
14
15   Hard
16
17   Very hard
18
19   Very, very hard
20

Positioning Recommendation: _____

Other: _____

Patient/Parent Education: _____

EVALUATION/SUMMARY: _____

_____

_____

_____

_____

_____

GOALS: (2 Weeks)

Patient/Parent Goals: _____

1. Patient will tolerate _____ minutes of exercise with vital signs stable.

2. Patient/Parents will be independent with scar massage to surgical site once completely healed.

3. _____

4. _____

PLAN: _____

_____

_____

_____

Signature: _____   Extension: _____   Beeper: _____
        Physical Therapist

18

Pulmonary Disorders in Infants and Children and Their Physical Therapy Management

Jan Stephen Tecklin

U ninformed health professionals may have the misconception that acute respiratory disorders and chronic pulmonary diseases are mainly adult problems. Nonetheless, statistics show that lower respiratory tract disease continues to be a major cause of mortality in children from 1 year of age through 19 years of age.[1] In addition, respiratory viruses and many bacteria continue to cause acute and sometimes fatal respiratory infections in infants and children, although various vaccines against both bacterial and viral agents have decreased the incidence of certain infections. The morbidity statistics are staggering. A recent landmark nationwide survey about asthma indicates that the disorder affects approximately 9.2% of children 18 years and younger, a percentage that represents as many as 7 million children. The disorder is responsible for 21 million days missed from school and 15 million work days missed each year by parents of those children.[2] In the United States, up to 20% or more of children younger than 18 years of age have been reported to have a chronic respiratory problem such as asthma, wheezing, bronchial hyper-

reactivity, cystic fibrosis, and bronchopulmonary dysplasia.[3] Recent data from the Centers for Disease Control and Prevention indicate that in 2004 greater than 12.2% of children had been told that they had asthma at some time and 5.5% had had an asthma attack in the past 12 months.[4] These statistics may seem surprising, but not to the health professional who spends a great deal of time treating children with primary pulmonary diseases or respiratory problems secondary to other conditions.

Initially, this chapter provides background information that will enable readers to understand more completely the fragility of the neonatal and pediatric respiratory system, the process of development of that system, and the need for aggressive treatment of disorders of the system. These introductory topics include growth and development of the respiratory tract and predisposition to acute respiratory failure in children and infants. Physical therapy examination and intervention skills for infants and children with pulmonary disorders follow. Medical information and a discussion of the physical therapy for four major respiratory problems of children—atelectasis, respiratory muscle weakness, asthma, and cystic fibrosis (CF)—are next presented, followed by questions about future research.

Growth and Development of the Lungs

A brief review of the major periods of lung development is useful in discussing the interrelationship between lung and airway growth and specific childhood diseases. A description of lung development also provides insight into some unique aspects of the growth, particularly in number, of pulmonary alveoli.

The earliest sign of lung development occurs during the *embryologic period*, 24 to 26 days after conception. Endodermal tissue of the primitive foregut expands into an anterior lung pouch when the embryo is 4 mm long. During this period in which there is a separation of the trachea and esophagus, aberrations in development may lead to one of several configurations of tracheoesophageal fistulae–abnormal communication between the two structures (Fig. 18.1). Four days later, the future trachea differentiates into right and left bronchial buds, the precursors of each lung. Mesenchymal cellular tissue surrounding the developing bronchial buds will later differentiate to become muscle, connective tissue, and cartilage within the bronchial walls. Also developing from the mesenchyme is vascular tissue that will soon connect the primitive pulmonary artery to the pulmonary veins. Noncellular tissue will provide the elastic and collagen fibers that support the lung structures.[5]

The lung buds continue to grow and subdivide into smaller airways during the fifth to 16th weeks of gestation, termed the *pseudoglandular period* because the lung tissue looks similar to glandular cells. During this period many of the early cells differentiate into specific types of airway cells. Tall bronchial epithelium lines the primitive airways, and there is a burst of growth between the 10th and 14th weeks. Mucus-secreting glands and supportive cartilage appear late in the pseudoglandular period and continue their growth through the canalicular period. Branching and subdivision produces eight to 32 bronchial generations, with the greatest number of divisions occurring in those lung areas that are most distant from the hilum, or root of the lungs.[5] The bronchial tree is complete from the glottis to the terminal bronchioles by the end of the pseudoglandular period and the diaphragm is beginning to form.

The major events that mark the 16th to 26th weeks, the canalicular period, are thinning and flattening of the epithelium that will become the type I pneumocytes or alveolar cells. In addition, a critical occurrence is the appearance of pulmonary capillaries. The capillaries, which protrude into the epithelium, provide close proximity of the blood supply to the airways. Thinning of the epithelium and capillarization provides the apparatus—the air–blood interface—for respiration. Gas exchange can take place by the end of the canalicular period.[5]

At approximately 26 weeks, the energy of the developing lung begins to form outpouchings of the terminal bronchioles called saccules. This *terminal sac* or *saccular* period continues until about 32 weeks, when the alveolar period begins, at which time the saccules branch into many alveolar pockets or ducts. These ducts are in continued proximity to the tiny capillaries formed during the canalicular period. Once sufficient numbers of alveolar/capillary units are present, life may be sustained, provided that the biochemical substance surfactant is present within the alveoli.[5]

Surfactant is a phospholipid material secreted by type II cells that line the pulmonary alveoli. Surfactant reduces surface tension within the alveolus, thus allowing inflation of the alveolus with smaller pressures and less work by the infant than would be needed to inflate a surfactant-deficient alveolus. Surfactant appears at its mature chemical level at approximately 34 weeks of gestation and indicates maturity of the lung by allowing the maintenance of continuous respiration.[6]

The postnatal period is characterized initially by an 18- to 24-month period of rapid growth of both surface area and volume of lung tissue for gas exchange through continued subdivision of the alveolar ducts to form alveolar sacs (i.e., the true alveoli). Of note is that the vasculature grows to an even greater degree than the air spaces in this earlier of the postnatal phases. In the second of postnatal phases there is more parallel growth in the alveoli and capillaries. From the 25 million alveoli present at birth, there is a 12-fold increase by 8 to 10 years, at which time the adult number of approximately 300 million is achieved. Destructive processes within the period of alveolar multiplication may limit the potential for achieving the adult number of pulmonary alveoli.[7]

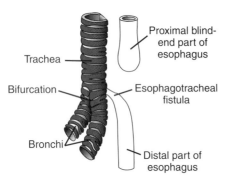

Figure 18.1 ■ Tracheoesophageal fistula. (From Sadler TW. *Langman's Medical Embryology.* 9th Ed. Baltimore: Lippincott Williams & Wilkins, 2002.)

Predisposition to Respiratory Failure

The following information is presented to describe more fully several mechanisms of acute respiratory failure and its rapid development in children and infants. Although acute respiratory failure is not a disease, it is often the final common pathway for many diseases that damage the developing respiratory system.

Several structural and metabolic factors in the pediatric population, although entirely normal, predispose them to acute respiratory failure. Respiratory failure can be defined as a condition in which impairment of gas exchange within the lungs poses an immediate threat to life. Downes and associates were among the first to state that clinical signs and arterial blood gas determinations should be used to monitor infants and children for the development of acute respiratory failure.[8] The arterial blood gas levels compatible with respiratory failure are 75 mm Hg of carbon dioxide and 100 mm Hg of oxygen when the patient is receiving an inspired oxygen concentration of 100%. Respiratory failure exists when either of these arterial levels is reached in the presence of any of the following clinical signs: decreased or absent inspiratory breath sounds, severe inspiratory retractions with accessory muscle use, cyanosis with inspiration of 40% oxygen, depressed consciousness and response to pain, and poor skeletal muscle tone.[8]

The most important general factor predisposing infants and children to acute respiratory failure is their high incidence of respiratory tract infections. During the first several years of life, when immunologic defenses are developing, the child is at risk for infections. This risk increases as the environment of the toddler expands, particularly with early enrollment in daycare, preschool, and other similar exposures to various infectious agents transmitted by classmates, teachers, and other personnel. As the number of children in daycare programs has increased in recent decades, the concurrent increase in the incidence of respiratory infections has been predictable. Indeed, recent research has focused on the economic impact of these infectious episodes and the economic benefits to developing and instituting infection control programs.[9]

Two major structural factors, airway size and poor mechanical advantage for the respiratory muscles, contribute to respiratory failure in a young child. Based upon calculations applied to the work of Effmann et al., the diameter of the tracheal lumen in children younger than 1 year of age is smaller than the diameter of a lead pencil.[10] A large percentage of the young child's peripheral bronchioles are smaller than 1 mm in diameter. A small amount of mucus, bronchospasm, or edema not only can effectively occlude the peripheral airways, but also may obstruct the larger, more proximal bronchi. With sufficient airway blockage, respiratory failure may quickly ensue.

Additional major structural issues that predispose infants and children to respiratory failure involve several items that cumulatively cause poor mechanical advantage to the respiratory bellows of the child's thorax:

- Type I fatigue-resistant muscle fibers are not present in adult proportions in the diaphragm or other ventilatory muscles of the infant until 8 months of age.[11] This lack of fatigue-resistant fibers allows the infant's respiratory muscles to tire quickly, causing alveolar hypoventilation that may lead to respiratory failure.
- There is a greater work of breathing cost that may reach 10% of the basal metabolic rate when the preterm infant must use the diaphragm to distort his or her ribcage in times of stressful breathing. Should the infant have lung disease as well, the increased metabolic demands of the diaphragm may predispose preterm infants to fatigue and may contribute to respiratory failure.[12]
- Poor development of the ability to cough either spontaneously or with direct laryngeal stimulation renders the infant's airways susceptible to obstruction by mucus.[13]
- Horizontal alignment of the infant's ribcage and the round (rather than oval) configuration of the chest provide poor mechanical advantage to the intercostal and accessory muscles of respiration. These muscles lift the ribs and sternum to increase thoracic diameter and lung volume.
- Increased chest wall compliance during infancy can result in sternal retractions associated with increased inspiratory effort during times of illness. The relative lack of stiffness in the infant thorax can simulate a flail chest. Intense inspiratory efforts may paradoxically decrease thoracic volume at a time when just the opposite response is necessary and ventilation is further compromised with the potential for hypoventilation. Developmental changes in the chest wall during the second year of life result in chest wall compliance similar to that of adults.[14]
- The baby's position may affect diaphragmatic excursion. The infant who is in a supine position works harder to ventilate because the abdominal viscera may impede full descent of the diaphragm.

A third important issue for the physical therapist is respiratory metabolism. The high metabolic rate of the child causes increased consumption of oxygen, increased heat loss, and increased water loss secondary to a faster respiratory rate. The range of normal respiratory rates for children is shown in Table 18.1.

In addition to having muscle fibers that are susceptible to early fatigue as noted above, the young child or infant has a relatively poor muscle fuel supply. Glycogen supply in the muscle tissue is small in the infant, and is depleted quickly when muscular activity is increased, which occurs during respiratory distress.[15] The aforementioned general, structural, and metabolic factors, although

TABLE 18.1

Range of Normal Respiratory Rates for Children

Age (Yr)	Mean Respiratory Rate (Range)
1	28 (18–40)
2	25 (19–35)
3	23 (18–32)
4	22 (18–29)
5	21 (17–27)
6	20 (17–25)
8	19 (15–23)
10	18 (15–22)
12	18 (14–21)
14	17 (13–21)
16	17 (12–20)

Adapted from Waring WW. The history and physical examination. In: Kendig EL, Chernick V, eds. *Disorders of the Respiratory Tract in Children*. Philadelphia: W. B. Saunders, 1977:83.

developmentally and chronologically normal and appropriate, may combine to render the young respiratory tract fragile and prone to failure during periods of stress, which are commonly seen in respiratory diseases.

Physical Therapy Examination of Children with Respiratory Disorders

Careful examination of the infant or child with respiratory distress can offer useful information. The younger the patient, the more the therapist may need to rely on careful observation, because the infant or young child cannot participate actively in a chest assessment. An age-appropriate description of the activities that the therapist will be performing should precede the actual physical examination. The following organization of the examination is based upon the Guide to Physical Therapist Practice.[16]

HISTORY

A complete medical chart review should be the first aspect of the physical therapy assessment of a child. The review should provide information regarding the child's medical history; the clinical course of the child's current illness, including signs and symptoms and his or her precipitating factors; any previous treatment for the illness; and a reason for the referral for physical therapy. In addition to the information in the chart, physicians and nurses can often provide invaluable and immediate information regarding the child's current state. The chest roentgenograms are useful in identifying specific areas of the lung or thorax that may be affected by the illness. A complete roentgenographic interpretation is beyond the scope of physical therapy practice.

LIVING ENVIRONMENT

Does the home or other discharge destination provide the space and resources needed for respiratory items such as oxygen, a ventilator, and a suction device?

GENERAL HEALTH STATUS

Has the infant or child displayed a normal developmental history? Have motor milestones been reached at appropriate times? Is there a history of ongoing or recurrent medical problems?

MEDICAL/SURGICAL HISTORY

Have there been recent hospitalizations, illnesses, or surgical interventions of note? Does the patient or parent report comorbidities or past illnesses that may affect the current condition?

CURRENT CONDITION/CHIEF COMPLAINT

What is the recent concern leading to the request for physical therapy? Is this a recurrence of a previous problem? Is the child receiving physical therapy, including airway clearance, at home? What are the patient/family expectations for this episode of care?

FUNCTIONAL STATUS/ACTIVITY LEVEL

Has the child been functioning at an age-appropriate level?

MEDICATIONS

What medications is the child taking, and is there any potential impact on the physical therapy regimen? (Aerosol medications such as bronchodilators and mucolytics may precede airway clearance.)

OTHER CLINICAL TESTS

Review all laboratory values including pulmonary function tests and arterial blood gas values, all imaging information, exercise tests, and any other potentially informative studies.

REVIEW OF SYSTEMS

The systems review is a brief and gross examination—a "quick check"—used to gather additional information and to detect other health problems that should be considered in the diagnosis, prognosis, and plan of care.

CARDIOVASCULAR/PULMONARY SYSTEMS

This brief review of the child should include blood pressure determination, measurement of pulse and respiratory rate, and documentation of any gross indications of edema.

INTEGUMENT

Are the color and integrity of the skin normal? Are any old or new scars apparent? Are current wounds healing properly?

MUSCULOSKELETAL SYSTEM

Measure and record the patient's height and weight. Identify any obvious physical asymmetries. Assess gross muscle strength and range of motion to the degree possible depending upon the age of the child and the ability to cooperate.

NEUROMUSCULAR SYSTEM

Determine whether grossly coordinated and age-appropriate movement or movement patterns are seen.

TESTS AND MEASURES

VENTILATION AND RESPIRATION/ GAS EXCHANGE

Of all the tests and measures administered to the child with pulmonary disease, none is more important than those assessing ventilation and respiration. Many signs and symptoms associated with ventilation and gas exchange have a direct bearing on the interventions that the therapist will choose. A traditional chest examination includes the four classic approaches of inspection, auscultation, palpation, and mediate percussion.

The physical therapist has several objectives related to the chest examination:

- Identify the pulmonary problems and symptoms noted
- Assess coexisting signs of pulmonary disease
- Determine the need for additional tests and measures such as exercise testing when appropriate
- Formulate a prognosis and a plan of care
- Identify treatment goals

INSPECTION   The inspection phase of the chest examination documents clinical characteristics of the presenting symptoms that may indicate what other components of the examination are necessary. Inspection includes:

- Examining the child's general appearance
- Inspecting the head and neck
- Observing the chest
- Considering the child's breath, speech, cough, and sputum

General Appearance   First, the therapist should note the state of consciousness of the child and the level to which the child can cooperate with simple commands. Is the child's body habitus normal, obese, or cachectic? Are there obvious postural issues such as kyphosis, scoliosis, and forward-bent or unusual postures? Children who are dyspneic often assume a forward-bent position.

During the extremity examination, the therapist notes digital clubbing, painful swollen joints, tremor, and edema. Clubbing of the fingers or toes is associated with cystic fibrosis.[17] Painful swollen joints may indicate pseudohypertrophic pulmonary osteoarthropathy[18] rather than the osteoarthritis or rheumatoid arthritis more familiar to physical therapists. Bilateral pedal edema may indicate cor pulmonale or right heart failure in those with long-standing cystic fibrosis and chronic lung disease.[19] The therapist also notes all equipment and monitoring devices used in managing the patient and the impact of those devices on planned interventions (e.g., mechanical ventilator, oxygen hood or mask, intravenous or arterial lines).

Inspection of the Head and Neck   The child's face often shows signs of respiratory distress and oxygen deficit. Of these signs, *flaring of the alae nasi* and *cyanosis* of the mucous membranes are commonly seen in those with acute respiratory distress. *Head bobbing* that coincides with the respiratory cycle may be the result of attempts to use the accessory muscles of inspiration by an infant who has inadequate strength to stabilize the head and neck. *Audible expiratory grunting* is thought to be an effort by the infant and young child to maintain airway patency and prevent airway collapse during expiration. Grunting is most commonly heard during lower respiratory tract disorders.

Examination of the Unmoving Chest   In this portion of the physical examination, the shape and symmetry of the thorax are noted, as are any unusual characteristics of the skin, including rashes, scars, and incisions. The thorax of the infant is more rounded in configuration than the adult thorax and the ribs attach to the vertebrae almost at 90 degrees, which makes further elevation almost impossible.[20] The anteroposterior diameter of the thorax in the infant is likely to be equal to its transverse diameter, whereas in the adult's thorax, there is usually a much greater transverse diameter. Among the more common abnormalities of the thorax are congenital defects including pectus excavatum (or funnel chest) and pectus carinatum (or pigeon breast); barrel chest, usually associated with hyperinflation of the lungs, in which the anterior to posterior measurement of the thorax is greater than the lateral measurement; and the several thoracic deformities associated with scoliosis. Muscle development of the thorax should also be examined for symmetry and for the presence of hypertrophy of the accessory muscles of inspiration, which suggests chronic dyspnea.

Examination of the Moving Chest   Respiratory rate is the first item assessed when examining the moving chest. Counting respirations should be done inconspicuously and is often done when counting the pulse rate. As was previously noted in Table 18.1, the younger the patient, the greater the normal resting respiratory rate. Tachypnea refers to an abnormally high respiratory rate and brady-pnea refers to a low respiratory rate, keeping in mind the normal variation in infant and childhood respiratory rates.

Pattern and regularity of breathing should also be evaluated, particularly in the neonate and in children with neuromuscular disorders. Short periods of apnea are not particularly unusual and may be referred to as periodic breathing in the neonate. True apnea exists when apneic periods exceed 20 seconds. Apnea can be associated with respiratory distress, sepsis, and central nervous system (CNS) hemorrhage. In addition to the rate and regularity, the ratio of inspiration to expiration (I:E) should be determined. This I:E ratio is usually approximately 1:2. Infants and children with obstructive airway disease, such as asthma and bronchiolitis, may have a marked increase in expiratory time; as a result, their I:E ratio may become 1:4 or 1:5. Synchronous motion of the abdomen and thorax should be observed. On inspiration, both thoracic expansion and abdominal bulging should be noted. When this synchrony is lost, a "seesaw" motion of thoracic expansion with abdominal in-drawing occurs on inspiration, with the opposite movements being noted on expiration. The presence of chest wall retractions should be noted. Retractions, or in-drawing, may occur in suprasternal, substernal, subcostal, or intercostal areas. Retractions, seen more frequently in pediatric patients, occur as a result of the compliant thorax of the infant and young child and an increased respiratory effort. During respiratory distress, the muscles of either inspiration or expiration, or both, place sufficient pull on the as yet largely cartilaginous thorax to cause an in-drawing in several areas. When retractions are severe, they may reduce effective inspiration.

Audible sounds during breathing can be heard and may be notable. *Stridor,* a crowing sound during inspiration, suggests upper airway obstruction or possible laryngospasm. Another noise detected during inspiration is *stertor,* a snoring noise created when the tongue falls back into the lower palate. Stertor may be heard in patients with depressed consciousness. During expiration, one may also hear grunting sounds, particularly in infants with respiratory distress. Expiratory *grunting* may represent a physiologic attempt to prevent premature airway collapse. *Gurgling* sounds heard during both ventilatory phases commonly indicate copious secretions in the larger airways.

Evaluation of Coughing and Sneezing   Infants probably use sneezing more than coughing as both a protective and a clearance mechanism for the airway. Older infants and children must be able to cough effectively to clear secretions or other debris from their airway. It is important to determine the ability to cough in a child with neuromuscular disease who may be at risk for retention of secretion and aspiration of feedings and may require some mechanical assistance for secretion removal.

AUSCULTATION   Auscultation (listening to the lungs with a stethoscope) is a useful method of assessment. The stethoscope used for auscultation of the infant and young child is a smaller version of that used for adults (Fig. 18.2). The therapist should warm the stethoscope before using it, and depending on the age of the child, the therapist may show how it is used by demonstrating on a child's doll or on a puppet. Because of the proximity to the thoracic surface of the child's airways, as well as the thin chest wall in the young child and infant, sounds are easily transmitted and anatomic specificity may be reduced. A particular sound, therefore, although heard in one area of the thorax, may not correspond to the lung segment directly below the area in which the sound is heard. As a result, auscultation, particularly in the neonate or premature neonate, may not be as precise as in the older child or adult. Nonetheless, the therapist should attempt to ascertain the presence of normal and abnormal breath sounds throughout the lung fields. The therapist should also try to identify adventitious sounds, such as wheezes, crackles, rubs, and crunches.

Wheezes are musical sounds thought to be produced by airflow through narrowed airways. They may be inspiratory or expiratory and may be monophonic or polyphonic. Expiratory wheezes are probably more common and represent airway obstruction from bronchospasm or secretions.

Crackles are nonmusical sounds that may be heard during inspiration or expiration. They may represent previously deflated airways opening suddenly. Expiratory crackles often denote fluid in the larger airways.

Rubs are coarse, grating leathery sounds that often indicate inflammatory tissues rubbing against one another.

Crunches are crackling sounds often heard over the mediastinum when air has leaked into that area.

The audible sounds of stridor, stertor, and expiratory grunting have been mentioned earlier in this chapter. Because of the ease of transmission of sound through the infant's thorax, the therapist should attempt to correlate

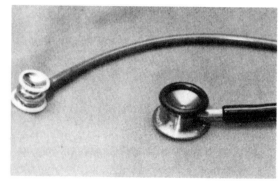

Figure 18.2 ▪ Two sizes of pediatric stethoscopes. (Reproduced by permission from Irwin S, Tecklin JS. *Cardiopulmonary Physical Therapy.* St. Louis: CV Mosby, 1985).

auscultatory findings with roentgenographic changes and other physical findings during the evaluation and treatment planning portion of the patient encounter.[21]

PALPATION Palpation of the thorax in the infant or child can help to identify the following circumstances:

- Position of the mediastinum can be determined via palpation of the trachea.
- Palpation for rhonchal fremitus (the feeling of turbulent airflow around secretions) is also a useful means to localize accumulations of secretion in the larger airways.
- Palpation for local areas of ribcage motion and the symmetry of that motion as the chest expands is also useful in older children.
- The activity of muscles of inspiration can be determined via their direct palpation.

Palpation can also be employed to help identify and localize areas of chest pain in the child.

PERCUSSION This final of the four skills to a traditional respiratory examination enables the therapist to identify areas of abnormal lung density and evaluate the extent of diaphragmatic motion. The technique requires tapping the finger of one hand against the nail of a finger placed firmly in a rib interspace. The actual sound or percussion note can denote air-filled versus non–air-filled lung tissue. The more hollow or resonant the sound, the greater is the likelihood of air-filled lung. The more dull the sound, the more likely it is that the lung is poorly aerated in that specific area.

In addition, percussion can also identify diaphragmatic motion. The percussion note changes from resonant (air-filled) to dull (airless) at the base of the lungs, where the diaphragm is located. The therapist percusses the rib interspaces from lung apex to base. When dullness is encountered, the therapist has the patient exhale fully, causing the diaphragm to ascend. The therapist percusses to mark the highest level of ascent. Next, the patient inspires completely and percussion tracks the descending diaphragm until the limit of descent is identified. Diaphragmatic excursion is the distance traveled between maximum ascent and maximum descent.

AEROBIC CAPACITY AND ENDURANCE

Aerobic capacity and endurance are commonly defined by the term *maximal oxygen uptake*. This measurement is an indication of (1) the ability of the cardiovascular system to provide oxygen to working muscles and (2) the ability of those muscles to extract oxygen for energy generation. Such testing can provide much useful information about the patient, including:

- Identify the baseline ability
- Determine aerobic capacity during functional activities

- Predict the response to physiologic demands during periods of increased or stressful activity
- Recognize limitations in the face of an increased workload

Many modes of testing are used that range from observation of symptomatic responses during a standard exercise challenge to instrumented, technically sophisticated invasive aerobic testing in an exercise laboratory. Exercise testing in a laboratory typically involves progressive and incremental increases in exercise intensity while the patient is walking on a treadmill or riding a bicycle ergometer. Exercise testing sites should have the capacity for continuous electrocardiographic monitoring, periodic heart rate and blood pressure measurement, cutaneous oximetry and arterial blood gas determination, and expired gas analysis; they should also have an oxygen source. In addition, a cardiac defibrillator, other emergency equipment and supplies, and proper personnel for their use must be immediately available in case of cardiopulmonary emergency. Maximal and submaximal testing may be performed. When a formal laboratory is not available or not practical, a 6- or 12-minute timed walking test,[22,23] a shuttle walking test,[24] or a step test[25] are simple alternatives.

ANTHROPOMETRIC CHARACTERISTICS

Assessment of height and weight percentiles, body mass index, and peripheral edema are all important measures of anthropometric characteristics for children with pulmonary disorders. Height and weight along with body mass index values are important in determining physical growth, stature, and nutrition in the child. Nutritional status has a significant impact on lung function and, therefore, exercise capacity in children.[26] Monitoring of cor pulmonale (congestive right heart failure) is an important reason for measuring edema in the child with chronic lung disease. Cor pulmonale often results from long-standing arterial hypoxemia, hypercapnia, and respiratory acidosis, all of which add to right ventricle afterload, leading to right ventricular hypertrophy.[27] Right ventricular failure is associated with peripheral edema, likely manifested as pedal and ankle edema. The physical therapist may use simple girth measurements, volumetric displacement, and figure-of-eight girth measurements to monitor the early development of peripheral edema and its progression.[28] In addition, sudden gross weight gain may indicate the development of cor pulmonale; therefore, periodic weight measurement is useful.

AROUSAL AND COGNITION

The child should be oriented to time and space and should be able to respond both to questions of a cognitive nature and to varied environmental stimuli given the limitations of developmental age. The therapist should determine the general state of consciousness.

ASSISTIVE AND ADAPTIVE DEVICES

Assistive and adaptive devices such as crutches, walkers, wheelchairs, splints, raised toilet seats, environmental control systems, and the like are not inherent needs for most children who have acute or chronic pulmonary problems. Some pulmonary-related devices that children might use include nebulizers, supplemental oxygen by nasal cannulae or mask, mechanical ventilator, tracheotomy tube, and in some cases a port for provision of supplemental nutrition. A major exception to this pattern regards children whose respiratory impairment is secondary to a musculoskeletal or neuromuscular disease for which such devices as walkers, wheelchairs, and others would be appropriate.

CIRCULATION

Two important indicators of potential problems with cardiopulmonary function not previously noted in this chapter include the rating of perceived exertion, commonly quantified with the revised 10-point Borg scale, and quantification of dyspnea. The Borg scale of perceived exertion was originally designed as a scale with a range of scores from 6 to 20. The scale was later revised to a 10-point scale ranging from 0 to 10, with 0 equating to no exertion at all and 10 identifying very strong exertion. The Borg scale correlates well with physiologic measures of maximal oxygen uptake and others. However, recent work has questioned the strength of validity for the Borg scales.[29] There is some indication that the Borg scale has validity in the pediatric and adolescent population, although perhaps not as robust a scale as in adults.[30]

Quantification of dyspnea in children is a new endeavor with very little support in the literature. Prasad et al. described a 15-count dyspnea test in which the child simply inhaled deeply and counted aloud to 15. The authors stated:

> "The 15-count score has been evaluated as an objective measure of breathlessness. It is easy to explain and perform, and can be used by any child capable of counting fluently to 15 in any language. It is best used in conjunction with a subjective score, and either the Borg scale or a visual analog score is appropriate."[31]

A group of visual dyspnea scales for children was published by McGrath et al. in 2005. The descriptive drawings demonstrated and measured throat closing, chest tightness, and effort in a group of 79 children including those with asthma, cystic fibrosis, and no lung disease. The authors stated that the measures appeared to measure the three constructs built into the visual aids.[32]

ENVIRONMENTAL, HOME, AND WORK (JOB/SCHOOL/PLAY) BARRIERS

Major environmental barriers of importance for the child with pulmonary disease involve the physical demands of attending school and playing in various environments. In addition, the therapist should inquire about the presence or absence within the home or school environment of dust, vapors, or other inhalation hazards. These can be evaluated through interviews of the child and parent or caretaker regarding the home, school, and play environments.

INTEGUMENTARY INTEGRITY

The review of systems above will have been useful to the clinician in identifying any existing or potential skin impairments. Major findings are likely to involve pallor or cyanosis in individuals who are hypoxemic. Patients with CF are also likely to exhibit digital clubbing.[33]

MUSCLE PERFORMANCE

Gross muscle performance should be documented in the review of systems. However, because increasing evidence indicates that peripheral muscle dysfunction exists independent of ventilation limitations in persons with CF, the physical therapist must be particularly careful to document and follow strength measures. Studies indicate that chronic lung disease results in muscle weakness, placing voluntary maximal strength measures at about 80% of similar persons without chronic lung disease. Mechanisms leading to this strength deficit have been identified as inactivity that leads to muscle deconditioning, malnutrition, and a myopathic process. Regardless of their cause, it is clear that peripheral muscle strength deficits lead to exercise limitation and intolerance.[34,35]

Muscle performance can be measured in many different ways including manual muscle testing, dynamometry using handheld devices or more sophisticated technology-assisted systems, and functional muscle testing. Functional muscle testing often employs timed walking tests, a shuttle walking test, or a step test.[21-25] Although these several approaches examine more than discrete muscle function, they offer a more practical examination of muscle performance as it occurs during a child's daily activities.

OTHER IMPORTANT TESTS AND MEASURES

Although this chapter deals with disorders of the pulmonary system, the therapist must consider all systems when assessing a child. Neuromotor development and sensory integration testing is often necessary for a child who has experienced periodic or chronic episodes of hypoxemia that often occur with pulmonary disorders. Inadequate oxygenation for a period of time may cause minor or major CNS deficit, resulting in a developmental delay. (Normal development and tests of development are discussed in Chapters 2 and 3 of this text.)

Assessment of pain—both its source and perceived level—is an important part of the examination. Identification of painful areas of the thorax is often accomplished via palpation and questioning the child or parent. If a painful site is identified, it is appropriate for the clinician to use some pain scale or pain diary to determine the patient's level of pain, its attributes, and its effect on daily activity, as well as methods of reducing or modifying the painful stimulus. This issue of an age- and developmentally appropriate rating scale for pain in children has been addressed in the past two decades. The Faces Pain Scale, developed by Bieri, was an early and significant attempt to use a scale that was suitable for children but suffered from having seven faces on the scale and was difficult to correlate with the more commonly employed 5- or 10-point analog pain scales.[36] More recently, Hicks and colleagues revised the scale by Bieri in a manner that it could be more easily compared with either a 5- or 10-point analog pain scale. The revised Faces Pain Scale was not significantly different from either of the analog scales previously noted.[37]

Various postural abnormalities can result from *or* can cause respiratory disorders. Scoliosis with a primary curvature of greater than 60 degrees often results in thoracic restriction and a decrease in lung volumes, as does severe pectus excavatum.[38] Some chronic lung diseases, such as severe asthma and CF, lead to hyperinflated, barreled chest with abducted and protracted scapulae. These possibilities must be considered in the assessment of the child with pulmonary disorders. Common orthopedic disorders, some of which have respiratory complications, are discussed in Chapter 12. Finally, an assessment of the family's knowledge and ability to participate in the child's care is important when planning discharge from the hospital, because many pediatric pulmonary disorders are chronic and will require continuing and effective care at home. The physical therapist is an important family educator and troubleshooter and must participate in formal and informal teaching.

Physical Therapy Evaluation, Diagnosis, and Prognosis of Children with Respiratory Disorders

The physical therapy evaluation and diagnosis should be based on the information acquired during the examination. The evaluation is a clinical judgment based on the findings that provide a diagnosis in the form of a preferred practice pattern. The prognosis refers to the period of time and frequency of visits during the period of physical therapy intervention.

Physical Therapy Interventions for Children with Pulmonary Disease or Respiratory Disorders

Physical therapy for the infant or child with pulmonary disease or respiratory disorder can be categorized into three general areas that often overlap:

1. Airway clearance (AC) for removal of secretions, either by traditional postural drainage with percussion and vibration (PDPV) or more contemporary techniques that will be discussed at some length
2. Breathing exercises and retraining
3. Physical reconditioning including aerobic exercise, strength training, and other types of exercise for the thorax

Of course, the degree to which these three areas are used and the specific interventions employed will depend not only on the disease processes, but also on the age, level of ability, and cooperation of the child. Neonates and infants will be treated almost exclusively with traditional airway clearance procedures including positioning to alter ventilation and perfusion. Simple breathing games and activities can be incorporated into the regimen as needed when the child becomes a toddler. As the child grows older, exercises for breathing retraining, physical reconditioning, and postural exercises become possible. Also, measures for AC that depend on breathing control, such as autogenic drainage, active cycle of breathing, and positive expiratory pressure devices, become more applicable as the older child can coordinate the necessary breathing maneuvers.

AIRWAY CLEARANCE

Removal of secretions from the child's airway is the main goal of AC. Of all types of physical therapy treatment for patients with respiratory problems, AC in its many formats and approaches has been most extensively studied and its efficacy is widely accepted. AC includes traditional methods such as positioning for gravity-assisted drainage of the airways, manual techniques for loosening secretions, and removal of secretions by coughing and suctioning of the airway. AC has also come to include active cycle of breathing techniques, positive expiratory pressure (PEP) devices, oscillating PEP devices (Flutter and Acapella, high-frequency chest wall oscillation [HFWCO]), and intrapulmonary percussive ventilation (IPV). Each of these techniques will be described below.

POSTURAL DRAINAGE WITH PERCUSSION AND VIBRATION

POSITIONING FOR GRAVITY-ASSISTED DRAINAGE Using a working knowledge of bronchopulmonary segment anatomy, the therapist can position the infant or child to drain areas of the lung in which secretions are found during the chest examination. The positions place the segment or lobe of lung to be drained uppermost, with the bronchus supplying that lung area in as close to an inverted position as possible. In adults and older children, specific positioning for segmental drainage often involves the use of treatment tables or tilting beds. In infants and young children, the therapist's lap and shoulder serve as the "treatment table." The infant or toddler can be held and comforted while in each of the 10 drainage positions (Fig. 18.3). When the child reaches 3 or 4 years of age, the transition may be made from lap to treatment table, but many therapists and parents will continue to use the lap for children up to 4 or 5 years of age. Because most families do not have a hospital bed or tilt-table at home, other methods can be used for proper positioning (Fig. 18.4).

One point of caution must be raised regarding tipping infants into traditional head-down positions. In a series of well-designed studies over a period of 8 years, Button et al. clearly demonstrated that infants with CF had significant gastroesophageal reflux and resulting decreased long-term lung function associated with head-down positioning during PDPV.[39,40] With this clear

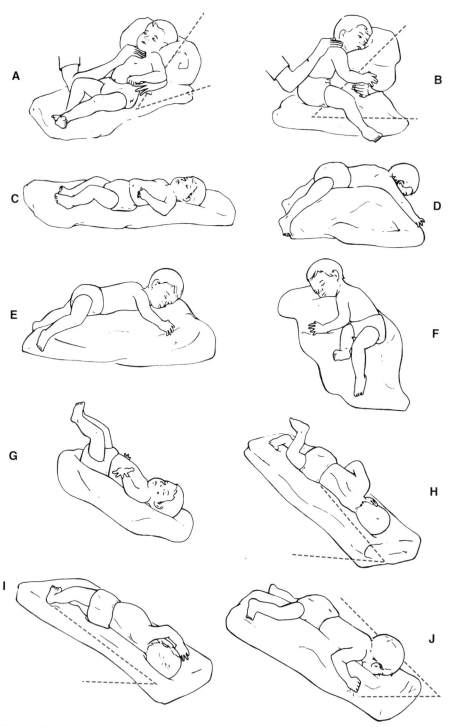

Figure 18.3 ■ Ten positions for postural drainage (*H* and *I* demonstrate lying on the right and left sides). (Reproduced by permission from Irwin S, Tecklin JS. *Cardiopulmonary Physical Therapy*. St. Louis: CV Mosby, 1985.)

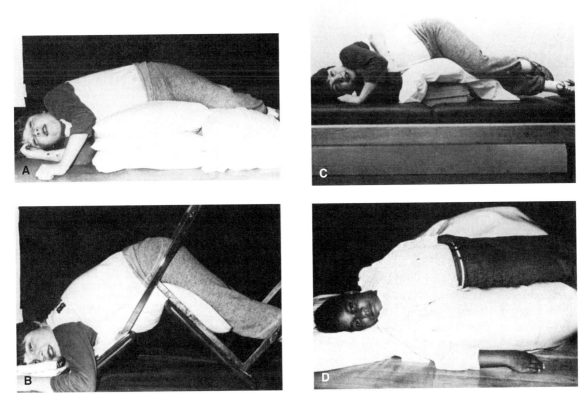

Figure 18.4 ▪ Positioning methods for bronchial drainage at home using bed pillows **(A)**; a desk chair **(B)**; a stack of magazines with a bed pillow **(C)**; and a bean-bag chair **(D)**. (Reproduced by permission from Irwin S, Tecklin JS. *Cardiopulmonary Physical Therapy.* St. Louis: CV Mosby, 1985.)

evidence, the use of head-down positions for PDPV has become unpopular in CF centers around the world.

MANUAL TECHNIQUES OF PERCUSSION AND VIBRA-
TIONS The manual techniques of percussion and vibration are used to loosen or dislodge secretions from the bronchial wall, thus allowing easier removal when the child coughs, sneezes, or undergoes airway aspiration with a suction catheter. Although some obvious differences exist, the techniques used are quite similar to those performed on adults. One of the major differences is the amount of force used for either percussion or vibration. Common sense should dictate that minimal amounts of force should be used on the thorax of a premature infant who weighs 1 to 2 kg or less. Increased amounts of percussion and vibration force can be safely applied as the infant grows and as the bones and muscles of the thorax become stronger.

As with adults, the percussion and vibration should be applied to the area of thorax that corresponds to the lung and airways in which secretions are present. Another difference in the pediatric group is that a therapist's percussing or vibrating hand often covers the entire thorax of an infant or toddler. As a result, other implements have been suggested for percussion and vibration in the infant. Several items used for percussion are shown in Figure 18.5, and different hand configurations for percussion of the infant

are shown in Figures 18.6 to 18.10. Crane has identified the following contraindications for chest percussion in the neonate: a significant drop in transcutaneous (or arterial) oxygen level during percussion, rib fracture or other thoracic trauma, and hemoptysis.[41] Crane also identified various conditions in which percussion should be used carefully in a child, including poor condition of the infant's skin, coagulopathy, osteoporosis or rickets, cardiac arrhythmias, apnea and bradycardia, increased irritability during treatment, subcutaneous emphysema, and subependymal or intraventricular hemorrhage.[41] Vibration, which may be

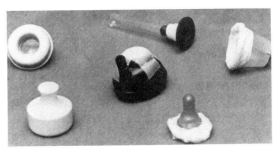

Figure 18.5 ▪ Commercially available and adaptable devices for percussion. (Reproduced by permission from Irwin S, Tecklin JS. *Cardiopulmonary Physical Therapy.* St. Louis: CV Mosby, 1985.)

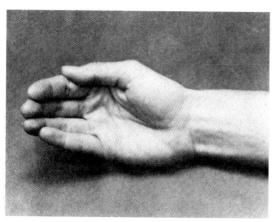

Figure 18.6 ▪ Fully cupped hand for percussion. (Reproduced by permission from Irwin S, Tecklin JS. *Cardiopulmonary Physical Therapy.* St. Louis: CV Mosby, 1985.)

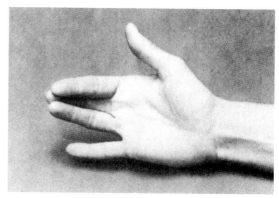

Figure 18.8 ▪ Three fingers cupped for percussion with the middle finger "tented" (anterior view). (Reproduced by permission from Irwin S, Tecklin JS. *Cardiopulmonary Physical Therapy.* St. Louis: CV Mosby, 1985.)

used in addition to or in place of percussion, is a less vigorous technique than percussion. There are few true contraindications to vibration with the exception of hemoptysis and reduced oxygenation during treatment. Because vibration is usually done during the expiratory phase of breathing, and because the infant with respiratory disease often has a rate of 40 or more breaths per minute, it is difficult to coordinate manual vibration with the expiratory phase of breathing. Some persons use various battery-powered vibrators that can be held against the infant's thorax during expiration and then quickly removed during inspiration. The modifications and precautions for both percussion and vibration become fewer as the infant grows, and treatment begins to parallel more closely that used for an adult.

COUGHING AND SUCTIONING Infants and young children will seldom cough on request. Toddlers and school-aged children have the language skills to understand the request for coughing but will often choose not to cough.

Imaginative means, including storytelling, coloring games, and nursery rhymes, have been suggested to entice young children to cooperate.[42] In addition, the author has found that by prompting these young children either to laugh or cry (preferably the former), a useful and productive cough can often be elicited. External stimulation of the trachea ("tracheal tickling") using a circular or vibratory motion of the fingers against the trachea as it courses behind the sternal notch may be another useful technique for removing loosened secretions (Fig. 18.11). However, given the relative small size and fragility of the structures involved with this technique, great care must be employed to avoid injury. Coughing is particularly difficult for the child who has undergone thoracic surgery. Splinting the incision with the hands or with a doll or stuffed animal pressed close to the child's chest promotes the development of an effective cough (Fig. 18.12).

Airway aspiration by suctioning is often needed, particularly in the neonate, to remove secretions. Suctioning must always be done carefully because it has significant

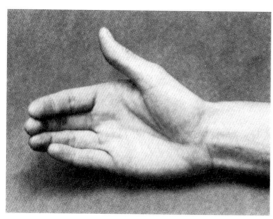

Figure 18.7 ▪ Four fingers cupped for percussion. (Reproduced by permission from Irwin S, Tecklin JS. *Cardiopulmonary Physical Therapy.* St. Louis: CV Mosby, 1985.)

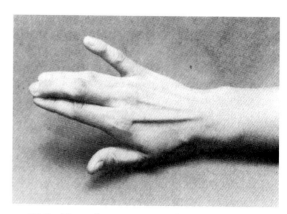

Figure 18.9 ▪ Three fingers cupped for percussion with the middle finger "tented" (posterior view). (Reproduced by permission from Irwin S, Tecklin JS. *Cardiopulmonary Physical Therapy.* St. Louis: CV Mosby, 1985.)

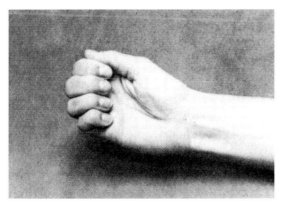

Figure 18.10 ■ Thenar and hypothenar surfaces for percussion. (Reproduced by permission from Irwin S, Tecklin JS. *Cardiopulmonary Physical Therapy*. St. Louis: CV Mosby, 1985.)

risks, even when performed under the best circumstances. Crane has detailed a protocol for endotracheal aspiration.[41] Despite the many protocols available, endotracheal suctioning is always a potential hazard, particularly in the pediatric and neonatal populations.[43]

CONTEMPORARY APPROACHES TO AIRWAY CLEARANCE

During the 1980s and 1990s, several new approaches to AC were developed. Various breathing maneuvers used to

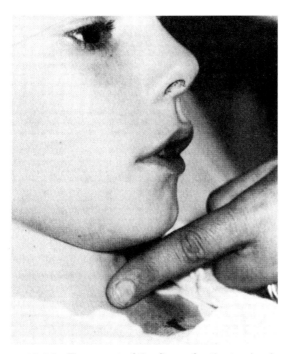

Figure 18.11 ■ Placement of the finger for the tracheal "tickle" maneuver. (Reproduced by permission from Irwin S, Tecklin JS. *Cardiopulmonary Physical Therapy*. St. Louis: CV Mosby, 1985.)

loosen and transport mucus were the common feature of several of these approaches. In addition, these new techniques were all designed in an effort to eliminate the need for an individual other than the patient to perform necessary AC. These approaches were developed primarily for children and young adults with CF, although they are appropriate for all individuals with chronic lung disease that produces copious sputum. The 1990s saw the development of several new AC techniques that employed various modes of oscillation to either the chest wall or the airway lumen. These include oscillatory PEP devices (Flutter and Acapella), intrapulmonary percussive ventilation, and high-frequency chest wall oscillation. Each of these AC techniques will be discussed.

AUTOGENIC DRAINAGE   This approach was introduced by Dab and Alexander, who describe autogenic drainage as follows:

1. The child sits in an upright, or sitting position.
2. The child takes deep breaths at a "normal or relatively slow" rhythm.
3. Secretions move upward as a result of the breathing.
4. When secretions reach the trachea, they are expelled with either a gentle cough or slightly forced expiration.

The authors recommend that slightly forced expiration be used because of their belief that the high transmural pressures that develop during coughing effectively cause airway collapse, thereby rendering the coughing effort ineffective.[44,45]

Current usage of autogenic drainage recommends not deep breathing but tidal breathing at differing lung volumes. That is, the child will breathe at a normal volume but will begin this controlled breathing at a very low lung volume (with most of the resting lung volume previously expelled). After several breaths at low lung volume, the child moves the tidal breathing to a midlung volume and then, following several additional breaths, to a higher lung volume. The movement of air through the smaller to the larger airways is thought to loosen secretions in the smaller more peripheral airways and move them proximally. The child should be taught to suppress active coughing until huff coughing (controlled coughing with an open glottis) can clear the secretions from the respiratory system. Although controlled research is minimal, at least two studies have shown autogenic drainage to be effective and equivalent to other accepted AC techniques.[46,47] The author has worked with many patients in whom this technique has been successful in clearing the airways, particularly with copious thick secretions. A notion has circulated that autogenic drainage is a difficult technique to teach and learn. I believe that this is a highly overstated and essentially incorrect idea. Autogenic drainage is most commonly used for patients who are highly motivated and old enough to control their breathing well.

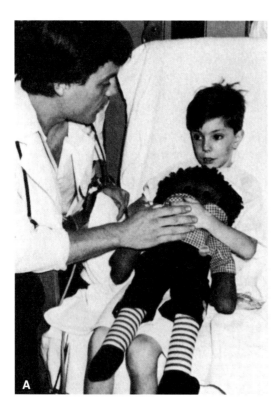
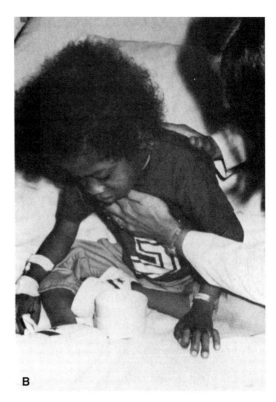

Figure 18.12 ■ **(A)** Incisional splinting during coughing using a favorite stuffed toy. **(B)** Manual compression over the midsternum to facilitate expectoration of sputum. (Reproduced by permission from Irwin S, Tecklin JS. *Cardiopulmonary Physical Therapy*. St. Louis: CV Mosby, 1985.)

FORCED EXPIRATORY TECHNIQUE The forced expiratory technique (FET) was developed in New Zealand, but was popularized in the late 1970s and into the 1980s by Pryor et al., all from Brompton Hospital in London.[48] As with autogenic drainage, the primary benefit derived from FET is that it can be performed without an assistant. Because the Brompton group has expressed great concern about what they believed to be misinterpretations of their original description, their description of FET is provided here in a direct quotation from the original article.

> "The forced expiratory technique (FET) consists of one or two huffs (forced expirations), from mid-lung volume to low lung volume, followed by a period of relaxed, controlled diaphragmatic breathing. Bronchial secretions mobilized to the upper airways are then expectorated and the process is repeated until minimal bronchial clearance is obtained. The patient can reinforce the forced expiration by self compression of the chest wall using a brisk adduction movement of the upper arm."[49]

In a subsequent article that attempts to clarify the various components of FET, the authors place particular emphasis on huffing to low lung volumes in an effort to clear peripheral secretions. In addition, the phrase "from mid-lung volume" has been clarified to mean taking a medium-sized breath before initiating the huffing. The authors

recommend that patients use FET while in gravity-assisted positions, and further suggest that pauses for breathing control and periods of relaxation are part of the overall technique.[49]

Because of continuing differences in interpretation of the FET, it was reconstituted by the Brompton group into series of activities called active cycle of breathing technique (ACBT). The ACBT employs a number of individual skills including controlled breathing, FET, huff coughing, and thoracic expansion exercises. As was the case for the FET, there have been no attempts at controlled research for the ACBT by the individuals who developed the technique, but some data exist to support ACBT.[46,47]

POSITIVE EXPIRATORY PRESSURE BREATHING PEP breathing was developed in Denmark in an attempt to maintain airway patency and employ channels of collateral ventilation to provide airflow distal to accumulated secretions. The airflow in the distal portions of the airway is presumed to dislodge and move secretions proximally toward larger airways. In addition, PEP provides expiratory resistance that appears to stabilize smaller airways, thereby preventing their early collapse during expiration and huff coughing. PEP is thought to be effective in both reducing air trapping and enhancing secretion removal. The original technique relied on breathing through an anesthesia face mask, but more recent devices use mouthpieces.

When using PEP, the therapist attempts to have patients breathe with a level of expiratory pressure of approximately 15 cm H_2O. Devices to provide PEP usually offer varied resistance and have some type of indicator to identify when the 15 cm of pressure has been achieved. The child attempts to maintain that level of pressure throughout the expiratory phase of breathing for 10 to 15 breaths followed by ACBT with huff coughing to clear the secretions. Some recommend using PEP breathing while the child assumes each of the several bronchial drainage positions.[50] Figure 18.13A and B shows commercially available PEP devices (DHD Healthcare, Canastota, NY).

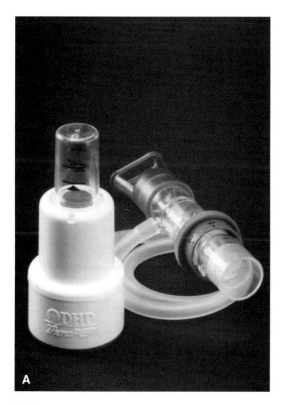

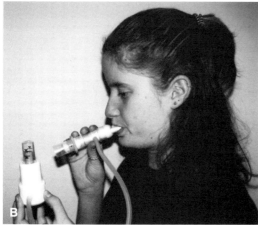

Figure 18.13 ■ **(A)** An example of a positive expiratory pressure device (TheraPEP, DHD Healthcare, Canastota, NY). **(B)** TheraPEP device in use (compliments of A. Tecklin).

FLUTTER The Flutter is a small, handheld pipe-like device that produces an oscillating resistance during expiration. The oscillations are created by a small ball within the device that is moved out of its seat during expiration but then rapidly moves back into its seat through the effects of gravity. The ball is then moved out of the seat again by the continuing force of the expiratory airflow. This repeated movement of the ball rapidly opens and occludes the orifice of the device, which results in the rapid oscillations or vibrations transmitted into the airway. These rapid oscillations are thought to loosen the secretions for ease of removal. As with PEP breathing, airway collapse is reduced by the PEP generated by the device. Use of the Flutter is followed by attempts to clear secretions by ACBT or huff coughing. Figure 18.14 shows the Flutter device (Vario Raw SA, distributed by Scandipharm, Inc., Birmingham, AL). Recent research has shown the Flutter to be an effective AC treatment when compared with PDPV for hospitalized patients with cystic fibrosis.[51]

ACAPELLA This is another small handheld device capable of providing both PEP and oral oscillation. Unlike Flutter, Acapella generates oscillation by using a special valve. A benefit of the Acapella is that it is capable of providing oscillation in any position, thereby being less technique dependent than the Flutter. There are two versions of the device. I recommend the Acapella Choice because it can be disassembled for more complete disinfection and cleaning (Fig. 18.15).

HIGH-FREQUENCY CHEST WALL OSCILLATION HFCWO is a newer means of AC that employs an air pulse generator and a garment (a vest) that has inflatable bladders attached to the compressor by large, flexible tubing. The air pulse generator provides pulses at varying frequencies (5 to 20 Hz) and at varying pressures into the inflatable bladders. The air pulses entering the bladder produce oscillations that are transmitted to the chest wall. Work on dogs by King suggested that the bursts of air produced a shearing force on secretions within the airways and actually increased airflow into and out of the airways.[52] At least one researcher has referred to this air movement as a "staccato cough."[53] These rapidly recurring bursts of air, or staccato coughs, provide a shear force that cleaves the secretions from the walls of the airways. In addition to the shear forces, the air bursts reduce the viscosity of the secretions[54] and move the secretions upward where they can be coughed or suctioned out.[55] All lobes of the lungs are treated at the same time and the patient can sit upright throughout the entire treatment without having to assume the 10 to 12 different positions required for PDPV. Figure 18.16 demonstrates the Med-Pulse Smart Vest (Electromed-USA, New Prague, MN).

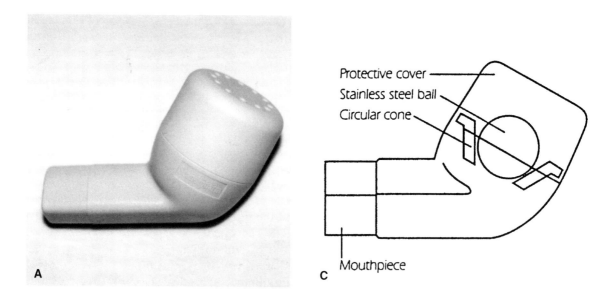

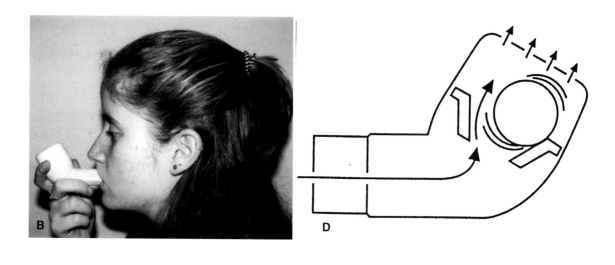

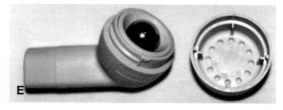

Figure 18.14 ▪ **(A)** Flutter device (VarioRaw SA, distributed by Scandipharm, Inc., Birmingham, AL). **(B)** Flutter device in use (compliments of A. Tecklin). **(C)** Cross section of Flutter device. **(D)** Cross section of Flutter device with representation of oscillating ball. **(E)** Flutter device with oscillating ball.

BREATHING EXERCISES AND RETRAINING

Because many of the commonly used breathing exercises require voluntary participation by the child, the classic methods for teaching improved diaphragmatic descent, increased thoracic expansion, and pursed-lip breathing may not be useful in the infant or young child. Some therapists employ neurophysiologic techniques, such as applying a quick stretch to the thorax to facilitate contraction of the diaphragm and intercostal muscles, to increase inspiration for the baby or young child.

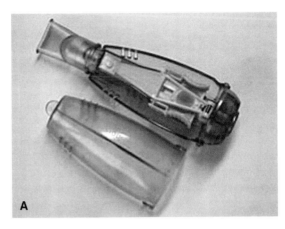

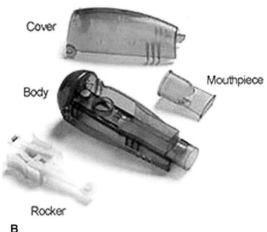

Figure 18.15 ■ **(A)** Acapella Choice airway clearance device. **(B)** Acapella Choice disassembled for cleaning (Smith's Medical, Watford, UK).

The toddler can participate in games that require deep breathing and control of breathing. Asking the child to breathe in time to music or to the beat of a metronome can present the skill of paced breathing. Blowing bubbles from a bubble wand or blowing a pinwheel will help emphasize increased control and prolonged expiration, which may be useful for the child with obstructive disease. Blow bottles may be useful as a means of strengthening the respiratory muscles. The bottles can be set up for inspiration or expiration, and various target levels of water trans-

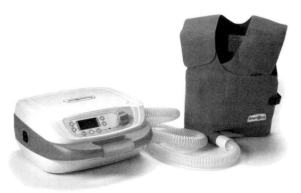

Figure 18.16 ■ The MedPulse SmartVest Airway Clearance System (Electromed, New Prague, MN).

fer can be set for the child. Numerous types of incentive spirometers are also useful for enhancing deep inspiration after either medical or surgical diseases. Incentive spirometry has been studied extensively and is generally considered to be a useful adjunct to postoperative pulmonary care and a means of strengthening respiratory muscles.[56,57] Improving ventilation to the lower lobes by using diaphragmatic breathing and lateral costal expansion also helps reduce postoperative pulmonary complications.[56]

Participation in and cooperation with breathing exercises usually improves as the child grows older. When appropriate, the therapist may use manual contact to teach diaphragmatic breathing, lateral costal expansion, and segmental expansion. Depending on the findings from the assessment of the moving chest, the therapist will choose one or more of these types of breathing exercises. The older child with severe, perennial asthma and the child with CF will often exhibit many of the same characteristics as adults with chronic obstructive pulmonary disease (COPD). Paced diaphragmatic breathing may be very useful for these children and young adults. Reduced energy expenditure of breathing is often considered a benefit of diaphragmatic breathing. Because exercise intolerance becomes a problem for children with asthma and CF, paced diaphragmatic breathing may improve the child's ability to walk, climb stairs, and perform other vigorous physical activities. Pursed-lip breathing may also be useful for breath control in the child with chronic lung disease. Relaxation exercise for the child with asthma is often suggested as a means of reducing breathlessness. Although there is little or no scientific evidence of any change in the pulmonary function of these children with relaxation exercise, there is strong anecdotal evidence of a reduction in the anxiety associated with dyspnea.

PHYSICAL DEVELOPMENT

Activities to improve physical function in the infant or child with a pulmonary disorder may begin in the neonatal nursery. When physiologic conditions permit, physical therapy interventions should be done with the infant removed from the isolette or warming bed. The handling and tactile stimulation provided by the AC session may be helpful adjuncts to the sensorimotor development of the infant, who may spend great amounts of time in a supine position. Of course, this type of movement is not always possible, particularly for the critically ill baby. As the pulmonary condition improves, the infant should begin to receive, in addition to respiratory physical therapy, appropriate intervention to assess and, if necessary, to treat delays in motor development. Chapter 4, devoted to the high-risk infant, describes an approach to this type of child.

PHYSICAL TRAINING

Children with asthma and CF and those with respiratory disease secondary to neuromuscular or musculoskeletal problems represent two distinct groups for whom physical training is important. A case example of each group follows in this chapter. Programs of physical training usually include exercises to improve strength and range of motion (ROM), posture, and cardiovascular endurance.

Strength training is helpful in both groups of children. Children with severe asthma and moderately advanced CF are often limited in strength owing to inactivity and chronic or periodic hypoxemia. In addition, evidence in the past decade has shown that children with CF have weakness in their peripheral muscles associated with diminished maximal workload, even without diminished pulmonary or nutritional status.[58] Darbee and Cerny advocate a strengthening program involving isotonic resistive exercise performed at a high number of repetitions rather than high levels of resistance. They also believe that exercise should stress the shoulder girdle and thoracic musculature as a means of facilitating the respiratory pump.[59] Orenstein et al. demonstrated gains in both upper extremity strengthening exercise and aerobic training, which increased both upper body strength and physical work capacity over a 1-year training program for children with CF.[60] Although data are sparse, one must assume that improving strength in these children will decrease their physical inactivity and disability. Children with diseases such as myopathy, spinal muscle atrophy, and juvenile rheumatoid arthritis will have weakness that prohibits their full participation in normal childhood activities. A carefully planned, judiciously administered strengthening program should help both groups.

Decreased ROM is more commonly a problem for those with neuromuscular/musculoskeletal problems than for those with asthma and CF. Nonetheless, children with asthma and CF have been found to have reduced thoracic motion associated with chronic hyperinflation and may be at risk for both loss of shoulder motion and development of kyphoscoliosis. Exercises for deep breathing, thoracic expansion, segmental expansion, and upper extremity function can help either prevent loss of motion or regain motion that has been lost.

Just as other skeletal muscles respond to training for both endurance and strength, the muscles of inspiration and expiration will respond similarly. Studies of children with chronic lung disease and groups with specific respiratory muscle weakness have shown that significant improvement in respiratory muscle function accompanies breathing activities aimed at either endurance or strength, or both. Inspiratory muscle endurance training and strengthening have resulted in improvement in numerous physiologic indices and have also shown functional and psychosocial benefits.[61,62] Expiratory muscle strengthening may benefit exercise tolerance and surely should enhance the force of expiratory maneuvers, including coughing.[63] These exercises are described later in this chapter.

The child with chronic lung disease will benefit from participation in a program of cardiovascular training or conditioning. Because of the tendency for running to precipitate

exercise-induced bronchospasm in children with asthma, this group of young patients seems to respond much better to swimming programs.[64] Children and young adults with CF participate throughout the United States in organized walking or jogging groups. The popularity of these groups can be traced to Orenstein and colleagues, who first popularized jogging for children with CF and who then studied the benefits for those children.[65] Regardless of the specific exercise or physical reconditioning program, and regardless of the pediatric pulmonary problem, there is a major role for the physical therapist in treating children with lung disease.

The next section of this chapter describes four common disorders of the respiratory tract in children and their physical therapy evaluation and treatment.

Atelectasis

Atelectasis, or incomplete expansion of a lung or a portion thereof, was first described by Laennec in 1819.[66] Primary atelectasis occurs in the neonate as a result of pulmonary immaturity. Secondary atelectasis occurs when gas in a lung segment is reabsorbed without subsequent refilling of that segment. The most common causes of secondary atelectasis in children include external compression of lung tissue, endobronchial obstruction of the bronchial or bronchiolar lumen, and respiratory compromise secondary to musculoskeletal or neuromuscular disorders.[67]

Primary atelectasis in small areas of the newborn lung is a common finding during the first few days of life. The sick neonate with poor respiratory effort and generalized weakness may not fully expand all areas of the lung for several weeks. Major areas of secondary atelectasis may be the result of abnormal thoracic content such as an enlarged heart or great vessels, congenital or acquired lung cysts, diaphragmatic hernia, and congenital lobar emphysema causing external compression of the lung tissue or the airways. The most common type of atelectasis seen by the physical therapist is caused by airway obstruction secondary to secretion of mucus or other debris, including meconium, amniotic content, foreign bodies, and aspirated gastrointestinal contents. In critical care units, a misplaced endotracheal tube may be responsible for a large area of atelectasis. Mobility has been shown to be an important feature in preventing atelectasis, and this is a particularly important issue for those who are acutely ill and unable to move or change position.[68]

MEDICAL INFORMATION

Signs and symptoms of atelectasis depend on the degree of involvement of the lungs. Small areas may be asymptomatic, but common findings in larger areas of atelectasis include decreased chest wall excursion of the affected hemithorax, tachypnea, inspiratory retractions, and cyanosis if the atelectasis is large. The trachea will deviate toward the involved lung because of volume loss, and a dull percussion note, which indicates an airless lung, will be present. By auscultation, breath sounds will be reduced or absent. The roentgenogram will often demonstrate a sharply demarcated area of consolidation, although patchy areas of atelectasis are not uncommon in acute respiratory tract infection.

Medical management of obstructive atelectasis is directed toward removal of the obstructing material. When the atelectasis is associated with an acute infection, therapy to treat the infection will often eradicate the atelectasis. Good hydration will decrease the viscosity of the mucus, thereby aiding in its removal. A bronchodilator may widen the bronchus, thus allowing air past the obstruction to enhance postural drainage with chest percussion, vibration, and coughing. Other airway clearance techniques may also be used including positive expiratory pressure, various forms of oscillation (internal and chest wall), and autogenic drainage. Finally, early patient mobilization while in bed is an important consideration.

When an obstruction is caused by a neoplasm or other structure that occludes the airway or exerts pressure over the lung parenchyma, surgical removal of the item may be indicated. Endobronchial aspiration using a suction catheter may help remove airway debris, and repositioning of a poorly placed endotracheal tube may correct atelectasis. If none of these more conservative measures is successful, particularly in an acute scenario, bronchoscopy, using either a rigid or a flexible bronchoscope with administration of general or local anesthesia, is indicated to remove the intraluminal mucus or debris.

Prognosis is usually good if the underlying disease process is not life threatening and if the duration of the atelectasis has not been prolonged. Permanent damage to the bronchial architecture and lung parenchyma can occur with delayed or incomplete resolution of atelectasis.

PHYSICAL THERAPY EXAMINATION

A thorough review of the patient's chart is necessary to understand fully the pathophysiology of the condition and to identify the type and etiology of atelectasis (primary or secondary). The treatment for each type will include similar efforts to increase respiratory effort, but only secondary atelectasis requires airway clearance.

Review of the roentgenographic findings will identify the location of the atelectasis. The therapist should use the roentgenogram as a clinical tool when treating a patient with atelectasis. Lateral and posteroanterior exposures provide a three-dimensional view of the lung fields to more accurately locate the area of atelectasis. The patient's chest configuration and breathing pattern should be noted. A large atelectasis narrows the rib interspaces and decreases excursion of the involved hemithorax. The muscular pattern of respiration should be noted—diaphragmatic versus

accessory—and the patient's respiratory rate should be determined.

Palpation may indicate a shift of the trachea toward the atelectasis owing to volume loss in the involved lung. The airless lung area has a dull percussion note that helps the therapist locate the atelectasis. Auscultatory findings will vary. The most frequent change is a diminution of breath sounds in the involved area. Complete obstruction of a large or main bronchus associated with the atelectasis may result in complete absence of breath sounds. With patchy or incomplete atelectasis, crackles may be heard for the first of several deep breaths; however, with subsequent deep breaths, the alveoli may open and the crackles may decrease. Other considerations in evaluating the child include the following:

- Mobility—Has the child been on bedrest for an extended time?
- Pain—Can the child take a deep breath and cough effectively?
- Cough—Can the child cough, and does he or she have sufficient strength or neurologic competence?

PHYSICAL THERAPY INTERVENTION

Several studies strongly support physical therapy interventions for the prevention of postoperative atelectasis in adult surgical patients. Therapeutic methods used in these studies included bronchial drainage, percussion, vibration, deep breathing,[69,70] maximal inspiratory efforts,[71] and electrical stimulation of the thorax with direct current.[72] The success of each treatment regimen was unequivocal. (The difference between adults and children in terms of airway cross section and strength of coughing has been previously discussed.)

Finer and associates found a significant decrease in the incidence of postextubation atelectasis in infants who were treated with bronchial drainage, vibration, and oral suctioning when compared with a similar control group treated only with bronchial drainage.[73] Atelectasis after extubation occurs commonly in infants, and is presumably caused by excessive bronchial secretions.

These studies have not evaluated the treatment of atelectasis; however, they have evaluated its prevention, which is the best treatment. Burrington and Cotton have reported the successful use of bronchial drainage, percussion, and coughing, preceded by inhalation of a bronchodilator, in 28 children who had aspirated a foreign body.[74] Of this group, 24 children coughed out the aspirated object after physical therapy. Although atelectasis is not always present with a foreign body in the airway, it is a common radiologic finding. When atelectasis is caused by aspirated material, physical methods can remove the material and relieve the atelectasis.[74]

Controlled studies of physical therapy for the treatment of atelectasis have not been published. The development of a rational approach to treatment should be based on the type and cause of the atelectasis. The methods used in the aforementioned studies are often included in the treatment of a child with atelectasis.

Postoperative atelectasis is often a combination of primary and secondary atelectasis. Secretions are more abundant owing to irritation of the airway by the anesthetic gases and tube manipulations. With incisional pain, and with the generalized weakness that accompanies thoracic or abdominal surgery, the child has a less effective cough and the volume of inspirations is decreased. Deep breathing to achieve maximal inspiration will often be sufficient to resolve small areas of atelectasis. These efforts should be initiated early in the postoperative period—in the recovery room if possible—to prevent atelectasis. Coaching the child to breathe deeply, splinting the incision to reduce pain, and using proprioceptive techniques to facilitate the inspiratory musculature can help the child increase the depth of respiration. Positioning the patient to drain the major lung fields and percussion/vibration followed by attempts to cough will aid in the prevention of pulmonary complications. Incentive spirometers, used as a breathing game, will stimulate deeper inhalations. Percussion and coughing become critical components of the treatment if the patient develops atelectasis despite preventive measures. Aggressive percussion of the chest over the atelectasis and splinted coughing will work to mechanically dislodge and clear the obstructing mucus. Should percussion prove too aggressive and result in increased pain, vibration of the chest is a good alternative intervention. Endotracheal suctioning to remove accumulated mucus and to further stimulate coughing is often employed for postoperative atelectasis. Early ambulation of the patient after surgery and the resultant stress on the respiratory system helps mobilize secretions by causing the patient to breathe deeply.

Children with medical chest conditions develop atelectasis as a result of retained secretions and one of the many types of AC may be employed. These children without incisional pain can often tolerate liberal and more aggressive use of manual techniques. Bronchial drainage with localized percussion will often dislodge the obstructing secretions, and coughing will clear the airway. Other techniques such as ACBT, PEP, intra-airway oscillation, and HFCWO are also likely to be effective in loosening the obstructing debris. Many physicians also suggest nebulized mucolytics and bronchodilators as well as bland aerosols to thin and moisten the secretions and to deliver a bronchodilator. The rationale for these procedures of inhalation is that thinned, moist secretions will drain more easily from a bronchus that is maximally dilated. Data exist to support both of these methods as an adjunct to physical therapy.[75] Primary atelectasis caused by respiratory muscle weakness can be resolved by deep breathing and strengthening of the respiratory muscles and change in position to afford better aeration to the poorly ventilated lung areas.

 Respiratory Muscle Weakness

Respiratory muscle weakness in children, as in adults, may be the result of a disorder affecting any link in the chain of neuromuscular events that produce a contraction of the respiratory muscles. Weakness or paresis of the respiratory muscles may be either mild and transient or severe and irreversible. The underlying pathologic process is the primary determinant of the duration and severity of the weakness. The physical therapist should develop a therapeutic regimen to treat the muscle weakness and to prevent or treat the resultant pulmonary symptoms within the limitations imposed by the disorder.

In the past decade, a growing population of ventilator-dependent children has arisen as a result of improved technology and care for acute and chronic ventilatory failure. These children, too, require physical therapy for problems associated with respiratory pump failure and for the delay in motor skill development caused by reliance on the mechanical ventilator.

MEDICAL INFORMATION

Diffuse pathology of the CNS (e.g., viral encephalitis or barbiturate intoxication) may lead to respiratory failure by paralyzing the voluntary and involuntary portions of the respiratory muscles. Abnormal neural control mechanisms and reflexes may ablate or reduce the physiologic response to chemical and mechanical stimuli. These stimuli may occur within the lungs, brainstem, blood, and cerebrospinal fluid (CSF). Examples of childhood disorders that result in a reduced response to respiratory stimuli are familial dysautonomia, sleep apnea, and obesity-hypoventilation syndrome. Lesions affecting the medullary centers that generate the inspiratory drive may cause marked changes in ventilatory patterns.

Spinal cord lesions above the C-4 level may result in total ventilatory paralysis. Because the phrenic nerve, which innervates the diaphragm, leaves the spinal cord at the C-4 level, a lesion above that level will affect all muscles of respiration. Injury to the high-thoracic or low-cervical cord often results in decreased lung volume and reduced chest wall compliance. Coughing will be inadequate if the abdominal muscles are paralyzed. These factors may cause respiratory insufficiency that may progress to respiratory failure. Acute respiratory care and long-term rehabilitation are essential components of a treatment plan for the child with a spinal cord lesion or injury.

Diseases affecting the efferent portion of the neuromuscular system are not uncommon in children. The progressive loss of anterior horn cells seen in Werdnig-Hoffmann syndrome leads to paralysis and early death secondary to respiratory failure. The result of acute polyneuritis (Guillain-Barré syndrome) is often respiratory paralysis. When this syndrome is fatal, it is usually attributable to respiratory failure. Because recovery from Guillain-Barré syndrome is often complete, the respiratory weakness must be treated aggressively and should include acute and long-term rehabilitation measures.

Degenerative diseases of the muscle (e.g., Duchenne myopathy) are characterized by progressive deterioration of pulmonary function. Adequate arterial oxygen and carbon dioxide values are maintained only through active efforts. Death is usually the direct result of respiratory failure, which often follows the development of pneumonia.

The thoracic cage normally provides for adequate function of the respiratory musculature. Abnormalities of the thorax, such as idiopathic scoliosis, scoliosis secondary to neuromuscular disease, and other specific congenital abnormalities, may result in a loss of mechanical advantage of the respiratory muscles.

The examples just mentioned can cause respiratory muscle weakness or mechanical disadvantage. They may also lead to the requirement for long-term management by mechanical ventilation. Improved technology in recent years, greater use of and acceptance of noninvasive ventilatory support in children, and a change in attitude toward home care have increased the numbers of children receiving long-term mechanical ventilation at home.[76] Mallory and Stillwell identify the physical therapist as a member of the typical team of caregivers for these technology-dependent children.[77] In addition, of the seven rehabilitation goals they have identified for the ventilator-dependent child, six are directly related to physical therapy knowledge, skills, and scope of practice. These seven goals follow:

1. Increase in muscle strength
2. Increase in attention and cognition
3. Decrease in spasticity
4. Increase in chest wall movement
5. Accessory muscle breathing while upright
6. Diaphragmatic breathing
7. Assisted cough

All goals, with the possible exception of the second one, are direct benefits derived from physical therapy.[77]

PHYSICAL THERAPY EXAMINATION

The examination begins with a detailed history of the factors that have led to the respiratory muscle weakness, previous modes of treatment, and other medical information related to the child including appropriate laboratory values, results of imaging studies, and other useful test results. In addition, a socioeconomic history and other pertinent family issues should be considered. A review of systems follows with a "quick check" of integument, cardiovascular/pulmonary system, musculoskeletal, and neurologic reviews.

Tests and measures assessed in a comprehensive physical therapy examination for a child with respiratory muscle weakness include breathing pattern, respiratory muscle strength, chest and shoulder mobility, and airway clearance (see the Case Study). In addition, when appropriate, the therapist should evaluate sensorimotor development of the child, activities of daily living, and ambulatory status.

Determining the breathing pattern is a major part of the examination. Minute ventilation—the product of the respiratory rate and the tidal volume—determines the arterial $Paco_2$. The respiratory rate can be counted for 30 seconds or 1 minute, remembering that the child's normal respiratory rate at rest varies with age (a younger child will have a higher rate).[78] Tidal volume can be easily measured with a spirometer or a Wright respirometer used at the bedside. Similar to respiratory rate, tidal volume varies depending on the child's height. A taller child has a larger predicted tidal volume.[78] The pattern and symmetry of muscular effort must be ascertained. Is the child using primarily the diaphragm, intercostal muscles, accessory muscles, or glossopharyngeal muscles? Is the muscular pattern similar for each hemithorax or is chest wall motion asymmetric? Depending upon the need for and use of various modes of ventilatory support, there may be significant variations in respiratory parameters.

The therapist has several methods by which to evaluate respiratory muscle strength, including measurement of lung volumes, maximal static inspiratory and expiratory pressures, and electromyography. The first two methods are simple and inexpensive, but require the child's full cooperation. With normal lung tissue and without loss of elastic recoil, decreased inspiratory capacity or expiratory reserve volume suggest weakness of the inspiratory or expiratory musculature, respectively.[79] Respiratory failure may be imminent when the vital capacity declines to approximately 30% of predicted values. Maximal inspiratory and expiratory pressures are probably the best and easiest index of respiratory muscle strength. These pressures can be measured with appropriate pressure manometers and digital devices, and can be repeated as often as necessary.[80]

Examination of chest wall mobility includes determining expansion of the chest wall in anteroposterior, transverse, and vertical directions during inspiration. Overall thoracic dimensions can be measured using a tape measure at various bony prominences with comparisons made usually at full inspiration and full expiration. In addition, motion of specific areas of the chest wall can be ascertained grossly in the method identified by Tecklin[21] during inspiration and expiration. ROM in the spine and the shoulder girdle should be examined, including glenohumeral, acromioclavicular, and sternoclavicular joints. Decreased motion at any one of these joints may result in reduced thoracic expansion.

Auscultation of the lungs of a child with respiratory weakness will serve several functions. Breath sounds are the most reliable clinical tool for examining ventilation. Decreased breath sounds will help identify areas that are poorly ventilated. Lung areas with decreased or absent sounds may correlate with decreased chest motion or muscular effort. Breath sounds can help the therapist evaluate the need for airway clearance. If rhonchi and wheezes are heard, airway clearance techniques for removal of secretions are probably necessary. Breath sounds may indicate the resolution or progression of pulmonary complications, such as pneumonia or atelectasis, and the therapist may choose to modify interventions accordingly.

The therapist should evaluate the child's cough. Integral components of a cough are sufficient active inspiration and coordinated closure of the glottis, followed by sudden contraction of the abdominal muscles to markedly increase intrathoracic pressure. With neuromuscular dysfunction, the child may lack any or all cough-related skills. Evaluation of inspiratory effort, glottis closure, and abdominal muscle strength is important in assessing coughing. The child must also be able to coordinate the three components into an effective effort.

Overall strength and mobility, including ambulation and coordination, and the developmental level of the child must be evaluated to plan a realistic rehabilitation program. A child who can actively locomote in some manner is less likely to suffer pulmonary complications and may improve pulmonary function as a byproduct of the rehabilitative effort. An aggressive therapeutic regimen is necessary, both to provide early mobility and to strengthen the respiratory musculature, thus improving ventilatory function.[81]

Evaluation of oral motor function—swallowing and feeding—often requires an interdisciplinary effort by physicians, physical therapists, occupational therapists, speech therapists/pathologists, and nurses. Swallowing must be evaluated for two reasons: Eating is the best way for a child to thrive nutritionally and aspiration of feedings is a major cause of respiratory problems in developmentally delayed and neurologically impaired children.[82] A discussion of aspiration and swallowing function is beyond the scope of this chapter, but a good general overview can be found in Arvedson and Brodsky text.[83]

PHYSICAL THERAPY INTERVENTION

Physical rehabilitation for the child with neurologic impairment should include an exercise program to improve or maintain respiratory function, which is the focus of this section.

Respiratory muscle strengthening should engage both inspiratory and expiratory muscles, including the abdominal muscles that are necessary for effective coughing. A traditional method of "strengthening" the diaphragm by using abdominal weights has not withstood rigorous scientific evaluation.[84] More physiologically appropriate methods of improving inspiratory muscle strength and endurance have been identified by various authors and may include resistive breathing, by breathing through inspiratory resistive loads, and isocapnic hyperpnea.[85]

Respiratory muscle training has become a recognized approach to reduce the progressive decline in respiratory function in children with Duchenne myopathy. A battery of breathing exercises has improved spirometric values in children with Duchenne myopathy, increased respiratory muscle strength and endurance, and shown continuing improvement over a 6-month period of training, with much of the improvement sustained at a point as long as 6 months following the cessation of the formal exercise regimen.[86–88] In addition, active and resistive exercises for the neck will strengthen the accessory muscles of inspiration (i.e., the sternocleidomastoid muscles and scalene muscles). Although accessory muscle use increases the energy cost of breathing, the accessory muscles may provide increased inspiratory volume to prevent respiratory insufficiency in the child with respiratory muscle weakness. Active and resistive exercises for strengthening of the abdomen, which may help develop a strong, effective cough, are well known by physical therapists.

Improving the pattern of breathing of a child with neuromuscular disease may provide two major benefits. First, an improved ratio of alveolar ventilation to dead space ventilation occurs when a slower, deeper pattern of breathing replaces a fast and shallow mode. The therapist may have the child attempt a slower and deeper pattern of breathing using various clinical cues, including counting, a metronome, or a spirogram. Care must be taken to avoid unusually deep breathing, which, owing to increased elastic resistance of the lung parenchyma at high volumes, may increase the work of breathing and negate the expected improvement. Avoiding inefficient or counterproductive muscular effort is the second major benefit of changing the pattern of breathing. A child with respiratory distress may appropriately use the accessory muscles to aid inspiration and may use the abdominal muscles to enhance full expiration. This muscular pattern, however, can become habitual. If the diaphragm provides adequate ventilation, unnecessary muscular effort is exerted if the child continues to use the accessory muscles. Various training methods have been suggested, including relaxation exercises and neurosensory techniques, but little published data support these endeavors, nor do they suggest that short-term changes in muscular patterns during the therapeutic session have a residual effect or replace the inefficient patterns. It must also be noted that upper extremity elevation during tidal breathing results in significant increases in metabolic and ventilatory requirements in those with normal muscular function; therefore, we can assume that those with weakness would have even greater increases in these metabolic and ventilatory requirements.[89] Hence, one must be very observant of respiratory values during upper extremity exercise in those with neuromuscular weakness.

Although the importance of maintaining or improving mobility of the thorax in children has been identified and related treatment plans have been recommended by many authors, few studies of the techniques have been conducted in children with respiratory muscle weakness. Active breathing exercises to improve thoracic mobility have been suggested for localized areas or for the entire chest. Manual stretching of the chest wall has been advocated but has not been tested in this population. Active or passive exercise to improve shoulder girdle mobility in children with paralysis may also improve thoracic excursion. Clinical studies must be undertaken to justify the time-consuming procedures used in the name of respiratory exercises.

Skill at coughing is important because of the smaller airway cross section in children and the predisposition to airway obstruction. Children with muscular weakness often lack an effective cough. Efforts to improve the cough usually involve strengthening of the abdominal muscles. Using sit-ups and straight leg raising has been discouraged because these activities primarily involve the rectus abdominus rather than the strong compressors of the abdominal wall (i.e., the transversalis and oblique muscles).[90] The use of expulsive maneuvers, such as blow-bottles or forced expiratory trials, seems to offer more kinesiologically approximate means of strengthening the cough musculature. Other traditional methods of instruction in coughing rely on a "double cough," "huffing" on expiration, and external stimulation (irritation) of the trachea to elicit a cough.

Because many children with respiratory weakness and resultant inactivity accumulate secretions, airway clearance is an important part of the home treatment program. If the parent suspects an increase in secretions as a result of a respiratory tract infection, the use of aggressive airway clearance may prevent the development of pneumonia or atelectasis. Oral or nasal suctioning may be necessary to maintain a clear airway if a child cannot cough well and if secretions are voluminous. When the child has difficulty raising secretions, some recommend the use of an insufflator–exsufflator device, which alternately provides positive inspiratory pressure followed immediately by negative pressure in an effort to mimic a cough.[91] Parents should be trained in whichever airway clearance and secretion removal techniques are recommended and should have proper equipment at home.

◆ Asthma

There are many definitions of asthma, all with some features in common, but none is agreed on universally. A panel of the National Heart, Lung, and Blood Institute proposed the following definition: "Asthma is a lung disease with the following characteristics: (1) airway obstruction that is reversible (but not completely so in some patients) either spontaneously or with treatment; (2) airway inflammation; and (3) increased airway responsiveness to a variety of stimuli."[92] The chronic inflammatory changes in the airway are responsible for bronchoconstriction, edema within the airways, secretion of mucus, and the chronic nature of the disorder.[93]

MEDICAL INFORMATION

Asthma is among the most prevalent chronic conditions in the United States, affecting approximately 14 million people and 7% of children. Asthma is also an expensive disease whose total cost was estimated in 1990 at more than $6 billion in the United States.[94] Importantly, there has been a notable and troublesome increase in asthma morbidity and mortality since 1977, with the increase seen most significantly in inner cities and among the poor and minority groups, particularly African Americans.[95,96] There is enormous morbidity associated with the condition, as denoted by days lost from school, hospitalizations, and health care costs. Asthma in children is characterized by several factors. Boys seem to predominate over girls by as much as a 2:1 ratio, although this number is not firm. Exercise-induced asthma is very common in children. Children with asthma are often allergic, with the inhaled allergen triggering a type 1 immunoglobin E (IgE)–mediated response. Symptoms may also be provoked by viral infections and emotional problems. Finally, the increasing mortality and continuing high morbidity associated with childhood asthma are attributable, in part, to a growing problem with asthma in the inner city populations.[95–97]

The physiologic changes responsible for the signs and symptoms of asthma are thought to be initiated by the release of one or more chemical mediators from the mast cells and eosinophils within the airways. These inflammatory mediators—histamine, prostaglandin D_2, leukotriene C_4, and others—stimulate a response that increases bronchial smooth muscle contraction, causes mucous secretions from the goblet cells of the bronchial epithelium, and may result in edema of the bronchial wall. The result of all three processes is often an obstruction of the airways. As airway obstruction progresses, expiratory airflow decreases, lung volumes and airway resistance increase, airway conductance decreases, and ventilation/perfusion inequality leads to arterial hypoxemia. The various pathophysiologic aspects of asthma appear to have a major hereditary component. Two phenotypes of childhood asthma have been suggested by Martinez. *Transient wheezing of infancy,* also referred to as *wheezy bronchitis,* often begins in infancy and is associated with viral respiratory infections. The second type, *atopic asthma,* is commonly associated with elevated IgE values and airborne allergens. The former is usually resolved by the early grade-school years, while the latter commonly persists into adolescence.[98,99] A fascinating aspect of asthma in children is the exercise-induced component. With strenuous exercise for a period of time, usually for more than 5 minutes, a child can develop many manifestations of asthma (e.g., dyspnea, wheezing, and airway obstruction) that may reverse spontaneously or with treatment. This exercise component is important to the physical therapist who is developing a conditioning program to increase exercise tolerance in the child with asthma. The exercise-induced response can be modulated by having the child using appropriate oral or inhalation medications before the exercise bout.

MEDICAL MANAGEMENT

Medical management of the child with asthma is commonly divided into treatment of the acute attack and control of chronic asthma. Treatment mainstays for the acute attack include inhaled β_2 agonists such as albuterol and oral or intravenous corticosteroids.[100,101] Supplemental oxygen is used to maintain an SaO_2 of 95%. In severe attacks that appear to be unremitting, subcutaneous epinephrine may be employed.[102] The long-term medical management of asthma has several components: pharmacologic, environmental, and immunologic. The pharmacologic agents used may include sympathomimetic agents delivered orally or by aerosol; oral preparations of theophylline (methylxanthines); anti-inflammatory agents, including inhaled and oral corticosteroids; and cromolyn sodium. Since the third edition of this text was published, a new class of asthma medication has been developed: leukotriene blockers, which inhibit leukotriene production and receptor antagonists that compete with leukotriene for available receptor sites. The medications have been shown to be very effective at asthma control for children aged 2 to 5 years and children aged 6 to 14 years and are generally well tolerated without significant adverse effects.[103] Control of environmental factors plays a major role in asthma therapy. A dust-free environment for the child is imperative, and special air-filtration units may be required for the child's room. Removal of pets from the home, avoidance of tobacco smoke, and careful selection of foods to which the child is not sensitive are also major aspects of environmental control. If the youngster chooses to be active in athletics, care must be taken to avoid levels of activity that may provoke exercise-induced bronchospasm or to use appropriate medication before engaging in asthma-inducing levels of physical exertion.

Another method of long-term therapy for allergic asthma is allergen immunotherapy (AIT). AIT is indicated for patients with demonstrated specific IgE antibodies against clinically relevant allergens. Once identified by skin testing, extracts of these allergens are given in gradually increasing strengths by way of periodic injections. The rationale is that the child's immunologic system will respond to the minute doses of allergen by producing circulating antibodies. Once sufficient levels of antibodies are developed, environmental exposure to the allergen (e.g., pollen or food) will result in limited symptoms because the acquired antibodies will alleviate the allergic response of the child. This type of therapy often needs to be continued for 3 to 5 years.[104]

Nutrition and Asthma in Pediatrics

Colleen Yanni, MS, RD, LDN
Clinical Dietitian
Children's Hospital of Philadelphia

Nutritional risk factors associated with asthma are often related to the pharmacological therapy used (oral steroids and high doses of inhaled steroids) and the severity of the condition. Long-term use of glucocorticoids does have an impact on the bone health and linear growth of children.

Risk Factors	Intervention
Obesity/Excessive Weight Gain	Modify intake to maintain weight Limit intake of high-calorie/fat foods Encourage fruits and vegetables, lean meats, low-fat dairy products Limit juices, avoid sugar-added beverages Increase physical activity
Steroid-Induced Hyperglycemia	Consistent eating pattern/meal schedule Limit juices, avoid sugar-added beverages Plan healthy, balanced meals to avoid excess carbohydrate content
Decreased Bone Density	Ensure adequate calcium, Vitamin D intake; supplementation may be needed Encourage weight-bearing exercise Consider DEXA Scan to assess bone density Minimize glucocorticoid use

(continued)

Nutrition and Asthma in Pediatrics (Continued)

Risk Factors	Intervention
Slowed Linear Growth	Monitor linear growth closely
	Optimize bone density (see above)
	Ensure adequate weight gain and nutrient intake
Fluid and Sodium Retention	Decrease Sodium in Diet
Slowed Weight Gain (Secondary to increased work of breathing)	Increase intake to promote weight gain
	Ensure calorie-dense meals
	Encourage nutrient-dense snacks
	Nutritional supplements may be needed

The effects of antioxidants (vitamin C and E), fatty acids, magnesium, selenium, and sodium have been studied to see the effects they have on the etiology and clinical severity of asthma. Additional studies in this area are still needed before any conclusion and recommendations can be made for any of these nutrients. The main objective when counseling patients with asthma is to reinforce the importance of eating a varied, well-balanced diet and maintaining a healthy body weight based on their age and sex.

SUGGESTED READINGS

Handbook of Pediatric Nutrition; Patricia Queen Samour, Kathy King Kelm & Carol E. Lang; ASPEN Publishers Inc. Co. 1999. Pp 343-353.
Romieu I, Trenga C. Diet and Obstructive Lung Disease. Epidemiol Rev. 2001;23(2):268-287.
Fogarty A, Britton J. Nutritional Issues and asthma. Curr Opin Pulm Med 2000;6:86-9.

PHYSICAL THERAPY EXAMINATION

As with medical care, physical therapy examination and management of children with asthma is largely based on the clinical situation at the time (i.e., whether the child is in an acute, subacute, or chronic stage of the disease). The child with status asthmaticus will generally not tolerate well any maneuvers aimed at AC or physical training. A notable exception is when the patient is intubated and mechanically ventilated, at which time both AC and early stages of physical training should begin.

The physical therapist's examination of a child on a ventilator should include auscultation in an effort to identify secretions and areas of poorly inflated lung. Assessment of the child's position in bed and initial measurement of shoulder ROM are appropriate.

An evaluation of the asthmatic patient in the subacute phases (i.e., when the severe bronchospasm has responded to medication) should include several areas of tests and measures. As noted previously, auscultation of the lungs is very important in determining interventions. Auscultation informs about the need for AC and also reveals the ability to move air through various portions of the lungs. Inspection of the pattern of ventilation and use of accessory muscles should be noted. Measurements of the thorax, including thoracic index, should be made during inspiration and expiration to determine chest mobility. Shoulder-girdle ROM should also be measured. Several

or all of these items are likely to be abnormal as the chest wall has attempted to respond to the physiologic changes to the asthmatic lungs. The therapist must re-examine these items with each session until the ROM, thoracic index, breath sounds, and pattern of breathing are normal.

A long-term rehabilitation plan for the child with asthma must also examine exercise tolerance, strength, and posture. Exercise tolerance may be evaluated by semi-quantitative measures in the physical therapy department or by sophisticated testing in an exercise laboratory. These methods commonly include the 6-minute walk test and its effect upon oxygen saturation, as well as the modified Borg scale.[105] Heart rate during a particular workload and time of recovery to resting heart rate are useful and simple indices of fitness or exercise tolerance. Quantitative strength measurement of major muscle groups can be made with equipment that is readily available in the physical therapy department. Posture can be evaluated using a grid system.[106]

PHYSICAL THERAPY INTERVENTION

There is little, if any, rationale for physical therapy in the child with status asthmaticus or intractable acute asthma. Status asthmaticus usually renders a child too dyspneic, anxious, scared, and physically unable to cooperate with the therapist for AC, breathing retraining, posture and ROM examination, or any rehabilitative endeavors. AC should begin when the status asthmaticus begins to abate and the child can tolerate physical therapy interventions. An exception to this approach is when the child is intubated for mechanical ventilation, in which case the child should receive AC techniques if secretions are problematic.

When the severe bronchospasm begins to wane, accumulated secretions are often encountered in the previously narrowed airways, and aggressive AC is imperative during this subacute stage. Secretions that are not removed quickly predispose the patient to atelectasis and bronchial infection. AC techniques are indicated within the limits of the youngster's tolerance and endurance. Secretion volume, color, consistency, and the child's vital signs before, during, and after treatment should be recorded. When possible, pulmonary function values should also be measured before and after AC.

In the long-term care of asthmatic children, AC instruction for the family is useful, but the techniques are not used routinely as in other conditions, such as CF. Parents must know several AC techniques for use at the first sign of a respiratory infection or increased mucous production. Recent research on AC for children with asthma has focused on pharmacologic approaches to secretion removal rather than traditional physical measures, as are used in many other disorders.[107,108] Nonetheless, it seems reasonable to apply such AC techniques as traditional bronchial drainage with percussion and vibration, autogenic drainage, HFCWO, positive expiratory pressure, and others when children with asthma accumulate large volumes of bronchial secretions.

Breathing training combined with relaxation techniques has been suggested for improvement of respiratory patterns in children with asthma. Several rationales for the use of slow, deep diaphragmatic breathing have been given. The work of breathing can be decreased by slowing the respiratory rate and by decreasing the ratio of dead space ventilation to minute ventilation. Increased diaphragmatic excursion also improves regional ventilation to the lower lobes in persons with architecturally normal lungs.[28] Because many small areas of atelectasis are present in the lower lobes, diaphragmatic breathing to improve lower lobe ventilation may be beneficial in asthma.

As a result of greatly increased residual volume and decreased expiratory reserve volume, the child with severe or perennial asthma often develops a shallow, rapid respiratory pattern that uses the accessory muscle of inspiration. Expiratory obstruction may cause active muscular efforts at expiration, which is of questionable efficacy and exerts unnecessary muscular effort. This abnormal pattern of breathing is energy depleting and inappropriate when an improvement in symptoms occurs and relaxation techniques have been advocated to reduce the anxiety and physical stress associated with asthma. Many anecdotal and verbal reports lend subjective support to the benefits of relaxation techniques along with mental imagery and spiritual healing in patients with asthma. Controlled studies of these alternative approaches have been unable to demonstrate measurable benefits to the individual with asthma.[109-111]

Physical rehabilitation to improve aerobic endurance, work capacity, and strength are major goals in the long-term management of asthmatic children. Children with chronic asthma are often less physically active and fit than their unaffected peers, and both severity of disease and parental beliefs advance this lack of activity and fitness. Exercise-induced bronchospasm may preclude a child with asthma from participating in vigorous exercise and the child may, therefore, be unable to respond to physical demands.[112] Appropriate medication before vigorous exercise may attenuate the bronchospastic response, and the child can derive both the enjoyment and benefits of exercise. A formal physical training program should be preceded by quantitative evaluation of the child's response to strenuous exercise. The initial evaluation determines the level of exercise needed to improve strength and endurance and serves as a baseline against which the results of subsequent studies can be compared to determine progress.[113] Testing can assume the form of clinical testing that often involves the 6-minute walking test, a modified shuttle test, or step test. Testing can also be performed with a complete laboratory evaluation including blood gas and expired gas analysis.

Among the more commonly used methods of training are free running, treadmill running, bicycle ergometry, and swimming. A daily 6-week swimming training program has a beneficial effect on aerobic capacity but not on histamine responsiveness (asthma did not change) in a small group of children with asthma.[114] A larger group of children with asthma performed bicycle ergometry on 3 days each week for a total of 8 weeks. The group who trained for 8 weeks tolerated the training well and completed the course of exercise. There was a trend in the trained group to increased maximal exercise values and an unexpected reduction in corticosteroid use in several of the trained children.[115] Cochrane and Clarke reported the results of a 3-month medically supervised indoor training study of 36 patients with asthma, aged 16 to 40 years. Although the age range largely exceeds childhood, the results are worth noting. Training included an optimal duration and frequency of 30 minutes three times per week, with the target heart rate at 75% predicted maximum. The training sessions were varied to include cycling, jogging, and aerobics. Each session was preceded by a warm-up and followed by a cool-down, including light calisthenics and stretching. Changes in physiologic parameters were compared with those in a nontraining control group of patients with asthma. There were numerous improvements noted in cardiovascular, respiratory, and metabolic function in the training group but not in the control group. Breathlessness was reduced during work levels corresponding to many activities of daily living (ADLs). There was no change in disease severity between the groups. Although exercise-induced asthma cannot be prevented by physical exercise, there can be little doubt of the potential for physical training in individuals with asthma, but strong motivation and good adherence are important factors for the success of an exercise program for children with asthma.[116] In addition to generalized physical training, Weiner et al. reported a double-blind study showing that specific inspiratory muscle training over a 6-month period improved inspiratory muscle strength and decreased asthma symptoms, related hospitalizations, emergency room contacts, absence from school, and medication consumption.[117]

In addition to traditional aerobic, strength, and other exercise training, the use of alternative and complementary medicine (ACM) has become prevalent in recent years. Despite little published research, individuals with asthma and their families have been major consumers of many of these ACM therapies. This phenomenon in the United Kingdom was discussed by Shaw and colleagues with particular attention to patients and parents of children with asthma. They found a wide range of therapies, but the most common were Buteyko breathing (a type of controlled, shallow breathing) and homeopathy. Subjects reported feeling empowered to take greater personal control over their condition rather than depend on medications.[118] As carefully documented in the United States, similar feelings and practices by parents of children with asthma are likely.

Cystic Fibrosis

MEDICAL INFORMATION

CF is the most common life-limiting genetic disorder affecting Caucasians. It is estimated to occur in 1 of every 3500 live births in the United States, and has a carrier rate of approximately 1 in 29 people, with an estimated 900 to 1000 new cases each year.[119] CF is a generalized disorder of the exocrine glands, which, in its fully manifested state, produces high sweat electrolyte concentrations, pancreatic enzyme deficiency, and chronic suppurative pulmonary disease. The clinical presentation of CF varies, but usually includes combinations of productive cough, abnormally frequent and large stools, failure to thrive, recurrent pneumonias, rectal prolapse, nasal polyposis, and clubbing of the digits. Because of its variable presentation, CF is often misdiagnosed as asthma, allergy, celiac disease, and chronic diarrhea. The well-informed health professional should consider CF when any of these symptoms are encountered.

The gene for CF, the cystic fibrosis transmembrane conductance regulator (CFTR), was identified in 1989 on the long arm of chromosome 7.[120,121] Formal identification occurred in 1990 when the secretory defect caused by this gene was corrected in vitro.[122] Although one mutation (ΔF508) is responsible for approximately 75% of all cases of CF, there are more than 1000 mutations of the gene recognized.[123] The major hypothesis of CFTR dysfunction states that the product of the abnormal gene is responsible for a decrease in chloride and water transport across airway epithelial cells, thereby resulting in dehydrated mucus.[124] However, the diversity of organ system involvement in CF suggests that other mechanisms are also associated with the CFTR. Regardless of the specific mechanisms, it is agreed that all exocrine glands are impaired to some degree and the variable dysfunction results in a wide spectrum of symptoms and complications for CF.

When two carriers have a child, there is a 25% chance that the child will have CF, a 50% chance that the child is a carrier of the gene, and a 25% chance that the child will be completely free from the CF gene. Testing for the carrier or heterozygous state is now possible, as is prenatal testing.

The incidence in Caucasians has been mentioned. Although CF is much less common in the Black population, it occurs in 1 in 15,000 births among African Americans.[125] CF is rare in the Asian population. The course of the disease, like its presentation, is variable. Although severe lung and gastrointestinal disease can be fatal for children with CF, survival rates have improved steadily over the last 25 years. In 2005, the Cystic Fibrosis Foundation (CFF) issued a press release indicating that the median age of survival had increased to 36.5 years.[126]

The pulmonary disease associated with CF causes the greatest mortality. Pulmonary involvement in CF begins with the production and retention of thick, viscid secretions within the bronchioles due to the previously noted dehydration of the airway surface fluid. These secretions provide a medium in which bacterial pathogens flourish and begin a cycle of inflammatory changes within the airways. Inflammatory changes and associated infections produce more secretions and additional obstruction, and a vicious cycle is begun. The earliest pathologic changes may be modified with aggressive treatment. With continued reinfection, bronchiolitis and bronchitis progress to bronchiolectasis and bronchiectasis. The latter two processes are largely irreversible and destroy elements within the walls of the airways.

In addition to these destructive processes, hyperplasia of mucus-secreting glands and goblet cells occur within the lungs. Large quantities of thick, purulent mucus are produced, causing the airway obstruction that is common in CF. When the obstruction is partial, a ball-valve process may result in hyperaeration of the lung distal to the obstruction, but complete airway obstruction results in absorption atelectasis distal to the obstruction. Small areas of hyperaeration and atelectasis often exist in adjacent areas and present a "honeycomb" pattern on a chest radiograph. The rapidity of pulmonary progression and success of treatment play major roles in determining the survival of a child with CF. Pulmonary complications often include lobar atelectasis, bronchiectasis, pneumothorax, hemoptysis, pulmonary hypertension, and cor pulmonale. These problems have been known and discussed for decades by others.[127–130]

An important point to note is that the number and percentage of adults with CF have been rising steadily over the past 35 years, resulting in differences in complications and related medical needs from the days when CF was relegated only to the pediatric population.[131] Among the differences in complications and medical needs are decreased bone mineral density, hypertrophic pulmonary osteoarthropathy, problems associated with pregnancy, greater incidence of hepatobiliary disease, and CF-related diabetes mellitus.[132]

MEDICAL MANAGEMENT

Management of CF is directed toward decreasing airway obstruction and pulmonary infection, replacing pancreatic enzymes, aggressively attempting to reverse the nutritional deficiency, maintaining strength and aerobic fitness, and providing appropriate psychosocial and emotional support to the child and family. As the disease progresses, lung transplantation becomes an option and end-of-life care is often necessary. Control of pulmonary infection is the major therapeutic objective. Sputum culture and sensitivity tests to identify pathogens and determine appropriate antimicrobial drugs enable the physician to plan a rational course of medications. The most common bacteria-causing infections in patients with CF are *Staphylococcus aureus* and *Pseudomonas aeruginosa*. The bacterium *Burkholderia cepacia* is largely antibiotic resistant and may be transmitted in epidemic-like fashion. It has been associated in many patients with CF with rapid progression of lung disease, ending in death within several months. It must be noted, however, that not all *B. cepacia* infections react in this manner. The CFF and Centers for Disease Control and Prevention have recommended isolating individuals with this infection in order to prevent epidemic outbreaks. Antimicrobial agents may be given orally, by inhalation, or parenterally for both therapeutic and prophylactic use.[133–135]

Reduction of airway obstruction is the most time-consuming aspect of comprehensive treatment for CF. Reduction of sputum viscosity by aerosolized or oral medications is thought to enhance physical efforts to loosen and drain mucus from the airways. Physical therapy for AC is a major part of the care, as will be described below.

Lung transplantation for those with end-stage disease has been successful for many; however, there is significant morbidity and mortality associated with the procedure. Bronchiolitis obliterans occurs in about one-half of patients about 2 years after transplantation and follows a steady downhill course. The 5-year survival rate for those with CF who have a transplant is approximately 50%.[132]

Replacement of pancreatic enzymes is essential for the 85% of patients with pancreatic dysfunction. Traditionally the recommended diet for patients with CF has included high protein, high calorie, and high salt intake. With effective pancreatic preparations, many children have liberalized their intake of fat. Despite apparent control of pancreatic insufficiency with enzymes, patients with CF may need up to 50% more calories than their age- and weight-matched peers. Continually underweight children, or those who experience weight loss with a progression of disease, may benefit from nocturnal tube feeding and commercial dietary supplements. Supplements must be chosen carefully and added to the diet. A nutritionist's counseling is necessary.

Psychosocial and emotional support for patients with CF and their families is the responsibility of all professionals who work with this population. Issues that must be confronted include chronic life-shortening illness, genetic disease, cost of drugs and care, time-consuming treatments, death of a child, denial, and guilt. Other issues emerge as patients reach adulthood: marriage, occupations, and dependence on others for treatment. A counselor or social worker plays a major role on the CF team, and several publications have addressed the psychosocial aspects of the management of CF. Bluebond-Langner et al. have an outstanding case study–based text on psychological care in CF.[136]

A nationwide network of centers is dedicated to the treatment of CF. These centers are sponsored by the CFF and can reach almost every population center in the United States. The CFF sponsors research projects, fellowships, conferences, fund raising, and other activities in its mandated task of providing the best care for children and adults with CF. Of particular note is the CFF Therapeutic Development Network, which has teamed with several pharmaceutical companies in an effort to develop and market drugs aimed specifically at CF.

Nutrition and the Child with Cystic Fibrosis

Maria D. Hanna, MS, RD, LDN
Clinical Dietitian
The Children's Hospital of Philadelphia

Nutrition-Related Problems	Interventions
GI ISSUES/RISKS	
• Malabsorption	Start/Optimize Pancreatic Enzyme Replacement Therapy (PERT) for patients with Pancreatic Insufficiency (PI)
	High-calorie, high-protein diet (see below)

(continued)

Nutrition for the Child with Cerebral Palsy (Continued)

Nutrition-Related Problems	Interventions
	Consider adjunct therapy (H2 blockers)
	GI referral to rule out other sources (e.g., CF liver disease, bacterial overgrowth, etc.)
• Constipation/DIOS (Distal Intestinal Obstructive Syndrome)	Ensure adequate fluid and electrolytes
	Optimize PERT for patients with PI
	Optimize fiber content of diet
	Increase physical activity
	May require medication
• Gastroesophageal Reflux (GERD)	Small frequent feedings
	May require concentrated infant formula, oral supplements, calorie additives/modulars
	May require medication
	May require supplemental tube feeding
GROWTH FAILURE/MALNUTRITION:	
• Inadequate Calorie Intake	Frequent growth monitoring, dietary and behavioral evaluation and intervention
• Anorexia	
• Behavioral	Structured meals, nutrient-dense snacks
	Avoid grazing, prolonged or skipped meals
	Positive reinforcement for desired behaviors
	Evaluate for comorbidities: GI (see above), CFRD (see below), sinusitis, anemia, pain
	May need Feeding Team referral
• Increased Calorie Requirements	High-calorie, high-protein diet (see below)
• Malabsorption	Calorie-dense foods and oral supplements
• Chronic Infection	Supplemental tube feedings
• Chronic Inflammation	Optimize PERT for patients with PI
• Acute Exacerbations	
• Catch-up Growth	
• Increased Nutrient Requirements	Supplement fat-soluble vitamins (A,D,E,K), monitor levels, correct deficiencies
• Increased losses	High-calorie, high-protein, extra salt diet:
• Increased needs	Encourage varied, balanced diet that includes natural antioxidants (fruits, vegetables, fish, nuts/seeds), adequate sources of
• Decreased intake	calcium, is moderate-to-high in fat and protein; emphasize fluids and salt proactively, especially in warmer weather
	Consider zinc supplementation for patients with growth failure
DRUG/NUTRIENT INTERACTION:	
• Glucocorticoids	Monitor for hyperglycemia, treat CFRD (see below)
• (long term/chronic)	Prevent/treat CF Bone Disease (see below)
CF RELATED DIABETES(CFRD):	Endocrine referral
	High-calorie, high-protein, extra salt diet
	Avoid grazing or skipping meals
	May need to limit sugar-added beverages in-between meals
	Minimize steroid dosing
CF BONE DISEASE:	Optimize nutritional status (BMI>25%ile)
	Optimize absorption/PERT
	Dietary assessment for adequacy of Vitamins D, K, and calcium intake

(continued)

> ## Nutrition for the Child with Cerebral Palsy (Continued)

Nutrition Related Problems	Interventions
	Assess/treat Vitamin D insufficiency or deficiency
	Increase physical activity as tolerated
	DEXA Scan to assess bone density
	Aggressive treatment of pulmonary infection
	Minimize use of glucocorticoids
	Consider Endocrine referral to rule out CFRD, delayed puberty or hypogonadism

SUGGESTED READINGS

Luder E. Cystic Fibrosis and Bronchopulmonary Dysplasia. In Pediatric Nutrition in Chronic Diseases and Developmental Disorders: Prevention, assessment, and treatment. Ekval SW, Ekval V, eds. 2nd ed. New York: Oxford University Press; 2005;363–367.

Wooldridge NH. Pulmonary Diseases. In: Handbook of Pediatric Nutrition. Samour PQ, Helm KK, Lang CE. 2nd ed. ASPEN Publishers, Inc. 1999; 315–332.

PHYSICAL THERAPY EXAMINATION

Physical therapy evaluation for the child with CF is similar to the evaluation for the other disorders discussed in this chapter. Emphasis in CF must be placed on the obstruction by bronchial secretion that causes the numerous pulmonary problems and complications. Auscultation for secretions must be done with the expectation of finding many areas with sonorous wheezes, harsh breath sounds, and crackles (all abnormal breath sounds). The sounds may not change for several days in a patient with advanced disease, and auscultation on an intermittent, rather than daily, basis may be helpful.

A determination of the child's ability to cough and raise secretions is crucial. An acutely ill child with CF who cannot cough effectively risks further deterioration in airway function. The radiograph is useful in identifying specific pockets or patches of developing or advanced lung disease. Many therapists believe that the three-dimensional view of the lungs afforded by posteroanterior and lateral chest films provides specific information to help direct AC treatment. Quantitative evaluation of exercise tolerance provides a basis for planning an aerobic exercise conditioning program at a level appropriate to the child's tolerance. As with other disorders, laboratory testing is the most accurate approach, but clinical testing including the 6-minute walk[137] and the modified shuttle test[138] have been validated and recommended in CF.

An evaluation of the child's muscular pattern of breathing may be accomplished by observation or by palpation. Mobility of the chest wall should be determined for several reasons. A poorly compliant thorax increases the work of breathing. Children with CF often have hyperinflated lungs, and the chest wall may appear barrel shaped and fixed. If chest wall changes occur, the child may have difficulty developing the necessary pressures and flow rates to cough or huff effectively or to increase ventilation during physical stress. Thoracic index, thoracic girth, and rib motion should be determined during full inspiration and full expiration.

Evaluation of the child's posture is essential to identify early changes caused by the hyperaeration and chronic coughing that accompany CF (Fig. 18.17). The thorax assumes a barrel shape, with an increase in the normal thoracic kyphosis. Scapular protraction also becomes evident. With the anatomic changes in the upper thorax that accompany hyperaeration, range of motion of the shoulder girdle must be measured. A comprehensive evaluation should include those postural items that may affect both function and appearance.

PHYSICAL THERAPY INTERVENTION

AIRWAY CLEARANCE

Provision of and instruction in AC techniques is a major role of the physical therapist when treating children with CF. AC can include traditional bronchial drainage, chest percussion, vibration (CPT), and suctioning (if necessary). If specific lung segments have more advanced disease or exhibit increased production of mucus, emphasis for treatment should center on these segments. Early studies of chest physical therapy (CPT) in CF have helped document its efficacy. Lorin and Denning demonstrated that twice the amount of sputum per cough *and* per treatment was obtained when a combined treatment regimen of positioning for gravity drainage, percussion, and vibration was compared with cough alone.[139] Tecklin and Holsclaw documented improvement in forced vital capacity and peak expiratory flow rate after CPT in 26 children with CF.[140]

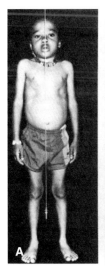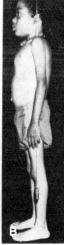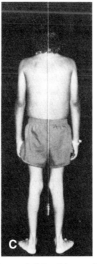

Figure 18.17 ■ Postural abnormalities in a child with cystic fibrosis. **(A)** Anterior view. Notice that the shoulders are held high, especially on the right. This posture appears to offer better mechanical advantage to the accessory muscles for breathing. The lower ribs are flared, and the thorax appears barreled and elongated because of the hyperinflation of the lungs. A full postural evaluation might reveal other, less obvious abnormalities. **(B)** Lateral view. The thoracic kyphosis and barreled chest seen here are common findings in children with obstructive pulmonary disease and hyperinflation of the lungs. **(C)** Posterior view. The shoulders appear high, with a protraction of the scapulae. Notice the enlargement of the thorax in relation to the rest of this patient's body. Pronated feet are also noticeable. (Reproduced by permission from Irwin S, Tecklin JS. *Cardiopulmonary Physical Therapy*. St. Louis: CV Mosby, 1985.)

Feldman and associates found remarkable improvement in flow rates at low lung volumes 45 minutes after treatment in nine patients with CF. In Feldman's study, the isovolume flow rate near 25% of forced vital capacity increased from baseline by 70% 45 minutes after treatment.[141] These changes in small airway flow rates are consistent with the results of Motoyama.[142]

Desmond et al. employed a crossover design to determine whether pulmonary function decreased over a 3-week period during which physical therapy was withheld. There was a statistically significant decrease in flow rates that was reflective of small airway function, forced expiratory flow (FEF, 25% to 75%) and Vmax60 (total lung capacity [TLC]), each of which declined by 20% after 3 weeks of no therapy. These values returned to their prior levels shortly after resumption of physical therapy.[143]

NEWER AIRWAY CLEARANCE TECHNIQUES

As individuals with CF have grown older, to the point where the median age of survival is now more than 36 years, the importance of independent self-treatment has grown. The following AC modalities have become universally applied as either substitutes or adjuncts to CPT. An exhaustive review by Williams of the world's literature on various physical therapy methods demonstrated that the most effective form of treatment has yet to be established.[144] Although there are methodologic flaws in the many studies reported, it appears clear that the alternative techniques offer benefits consistent with CPT and are particularly useful in that several provide total independence in self-care without the need for an assistant to provide the manual techniques of percussion and vibration.

AUTOGENIC DRAINAGE Autogenic drainage has been shown to improve pulmonary function and result in increased secretion removal when compared with PEP breathing and CPT.[145,146] One of the drawbacks with autogenic drainage is that some individuals have difficulty learning and performing the technique, particularly children under 7 years of age. Those who are able to participate report good acceptance and use of the procedure and independence in its use.

FORCED EXPIRATORY TECHNIQUE/ACTIVE CYCLE OF BREATHING The FET was popularized at the Brompton Hospital in London, where, although the studies appear to support the FET, the weak or absent statistical analyses, the small numbers of subjects, and other opportunities for experimental bias raise questions about the objectivity and validity of the work. Verboon et al. found no difference in pulmonary function in eight subjects who received either FET and postural drainage or FET alone. However, if one of eight subjects who produced minimal amounts of sputum is deleted from the analysis, the 24-hour sputum collection in Verboon's study actually favors CPT over FET.[147]

The Brompton group updated the FET by adding breathing control techniques, huffing, and thoracic expansion exercises in various sequences. This newer approach, called active cycle of breathing, was shown to be an effective form of AC.[148]

POSITIVE EXPIRATORY PRESSURE MASK Several studies have found that the efficacy of the PEP mask was equivalent to CPT. McIlwaine et al. compared two groups of subjects with CF who were assigned randomly to a PEP group or a conventional therapy group. At the end of 12 months, the PEP group had small improvements in pulmonary function (forced vital capacity [FVC], forced expiratory volume in 1 second [FEV₁], and FEF$_{25-75}$), whereas the conventional group showed small declines in those values.[149] In a second study, McIlwaine et al. found improved pulmonary functions during a 12-month period in which PEP mask breathing was compared to oscillating PEP in the form of the Flutter (discussed below). PEP was found more effective, despite the fact that PEP with oscillation was the modality of comparison. It seems odd that two similar forms of the same modality of AC would be so different in their results.[150]

FLUTTER The Flutter is another attempt to offer a measure of independence to young adults with CF. The Flutter was compared with voluntary coughing alone and postural drainage during 15-minute treatment sessions in 17 subjects with CF of varied severity. The Flutter appeared far superior in its ability to help subjects raise secretions. However, few would agree that a 15-minute postural drainage session, using up to 10 positions, represents a treatment comparable to those performed and recommended by most physical therapists.[151] Several subsequent studies of the Flutter found no difference between the device and other modalities of airway clearance. It appears that the Flutter is well accepted by some patients and is equivalent to the effects on sputum clearance and pulmonary function of other types of airway clearance.[152]

HIGH-FREQUENCY CHEST WALL OSCILLATION HFCWO has gained great acceptance throughout many CF centers in the United States. Warwick and Hansen examined the efficacy of HFCWO in a long-term study of 16 subjects with CF. All but one of the subjects showed improvement in their respiratory impairment during the trial.[153] Subsequent evaluations of HFCWO demonstrated that the technique was at least as beneficial to subjects with CF as conventional physical therapy and PEP breathing.[154,155] HFCWO has provided an efficacious, independent means for older children and adults with CF to continue treatments without an assistant to provide manual techniques. Despite its cost (more than $10,000), HFCWO has been shown to be cost effective and is now being covered by a very large number of third-party payers in the United States.[156]

In summary, the use of gravity-assisted bronchial drainage with manual techniques as the "gold standard" for children with CF is no longer the rule. There are numerous effective techniques for AC in children with CF. The choice of procedures should fall largely on properly informed patients and family members who are ultimately responsible for this time-consuming daily procedure.

DIRECTED COUGHING At least three studies have examined the efficacy of directed coughing for secretion removal in CF. Each study compared coughing alone with conventional therapy and found that the benefits derived did not differ among the approaches.[157–159] The study by DeBoeck and Zinman, however, found that flows at low lung volume, which are usually indicative of small airway function, were significantly improved with conventional physical therapy.[157]

MODIFICATIONS OF AIRWAY CLEARANCE PROCEDURES

Modifications of usual treatment procedures are often necessary for acutely ill children or for those with certain complications. In a patient with major hemoptysis, more vigorous forms of AC should be discontinued temporarily because the physical maneuvers may dislodge a blood clot

and prolong the bleeding. If the area of hemoptysis can be identified, the child should be positioned to drain the accumulated blood.

Pneumothorax is often a complication of CF and is commonly treated with an intrapleural chest tube with suction. FET, PEP, autogenic drainage, and directed coughing may enable the continued treatment for removal of excessive secretion. AC for the noninvolved thorax should be continued. With advanced destruction of the lung, the child with end-stage disease will not tolerate drainage positions and will often be unable to participate in AC techniques that involve control of breathing due to extreme dyspnea. Vibration during coughing and manual support of the chest may enhance the huffing or coughing effort in the terminal stage of CF. Improvement of diaphragmatic excursion, decreased use of accessory muscles, and relaxation are often advocated for children with CF. The rationale for using these measures in patients with CF is similar to that for those with asthma: decreased work of breathing, decreased dead space ventilation, and reduced anxiety. The efficacy of these treatments has not, however, been tested by appropriate clinical trials.

PHYSICAL EXERCISE

Formal and informal methods of exercise testing and physical conditioning have been recommended for children with CF.[129] Cropp and associates showed that in children with CF, with the exception of those with advanced lung disease, the *cardiovascular* response to exercise was normal during incremental testing on a cycle ergometer.[130] However, the *ventilatory* response to exercise was abnormal because those with CF who had decreased pulmonary function increased their ventilation more than did normal controls at all levels of stress. The authors stated that the relative increase in minute ventilation in subjects with CF was necessary to overcome the airway obstructive element of the disease. Another significant finding is that children with CF engage in less vigorous physical activities than their healthy non-CF peers, despite having good lung function. Physical therapists and others must encourage both patients and parents to understand the benefits of participating in regular vigorous exercise.[160] Children with advanced disease are likely to develop oxygen desaturation and carbon dioxide retention during exercise. These changes in arterial gas levels are indicative of the inability to increase ventilation sufficiently during exercise.[161] These changes can be altered with O_2 supplementation during exercise because this approach minimizes O_2 desaturation and enables patients with CF to exercise more safely despite reduced ventilatory and cardiovascular work.[162] Marcus and colleagues demonstrated that patients with advanced CF who exercised with an FIO_2 of 30% worked longer, had higher maximal oxygen consumption, and experienced less oxygen desaturation than while exercising at room air.[163]

Muscle fatigue as an additional limiting factor in physical exercise was identified by Moorcraft et al. in 78 of

104 subjects with CF who reported that muscular fatigue was a significant limiting factor during peak exercise testing.[164] In an effort to add support to recommending regular exercise for individuals with CF, Moorcraft and associates planned a randomized 1-year unsupervised home exercise program. The active group of subjects were encouraged to exercise by participating in lower or whole body aerobic exercise (walking, jogging, cycling, swimming, playing an appropriate sport) and an upper body exercise that more likely included weight training. They found a training effect, demonstrated by reduced blood lactate levels and heart rate, and improvements in pulmonary function.[165]

The relevance of these findings is that physical training and reconditioning, in a formal or informal program, in a treatment center or at home are safe and beneficial in all patients except those with severe lung disease. Even those with severe disease have been shown to benefit from an exercise program if supplemental oxygen is provided. Treadmill walking or running, cycle ergometer training, free running or walking, and strengthening exercises are useful methods of increasing cardiovascular fitness, endurance, and general muscular strength.

SUMMARY

This chapter has attempted to provide a summary of unique characteristics of lung disease in children, growth and development of the respiratory system, and the reasons why children and infants are predisposed to acute respiratory failure. Assessment of the child with pulmonary disease and treatments aimed at reducing the severity of pulmonary disease in infants and children have been reviewed. Four major respiratory disorders have been described, along with a discussion of appropriate physical therapy assessment and management. Published evidence for the physical therapy methods has been reviewed. Physical therapy for children with lung disease has been shown to be efficacious, depending on the treatment employed and the problems addressed.

CASE STUDY

H.E., a 14-year-old Caucasian boy with a history of Duchenne muscular dystrophy diagnosed at 4 years of age, was referred for pulmonary physical therapy evaluation. This case study will focus on the cardiovascular/pulmonary needs of this patient.

EXAMINATION

History
H.E. was a full-term infant who appeared to be developing normally until approximately 3 years of age, when his par-

ents noted that he had difficulty rising easily from the floor and could not easily ascend stairs. Upon stating their concerns to the pediatrician, H.E. was sent for laboratory testing and a muscle biopsy. The testing indicated abnormally high serum creatinine kinase, and a muscle biopsy was performed. The resulting diagnosis of Duchenne muscular dystrophy was made. He was referred to a large children's hospital for follow-up and continuing care. As the years progressed, H.E.'s weakness became more pronounced and he developed some of the classical physical characteristics including increasingly severe lumbar lordosis, several contractures including plantar flexion, and hip and knee flexion contractures. He was still ambulatory, although he and his mother reported that the distance was steadily decreasing and the speed was getting slower.

Review of Systems
Integument: There were no obvious or stated problems in this area.
Musculoskeletal: Numerous contractures in the lower extremities were obvious along with severe lumbar lordosis. Elbow contractures were also noted, although not as severe as those of the lower extremities. There was obvious weakness, particularly in the shoulders and hip musculature.
Neuromuscular: Ambulation, balance, and transfers were all significantly abnormal and limited. H.E. currently functions from a power wheelchair.
Cardiovascular/pulmonary: Heart rate, respiratory rate, and blood pressure were all within normal limits.

Communication, affect, cognition, language, and learning style appeared unimpaired.

Tests and Measurements
GENERAL SUMMARY OF FUNCTION
At the time of his referral, an examination of overall physical function revealed that H.E. could ambulate 25 feet in 20 seconds, could roll from a prone to a supine position and back to a prone position, and had adequate sitting balance. He was unable to run, ascend or descend stairs, rise from the floor or from a chair, sit up from a supine position, or assume a posture on all fours. A modified manual muscle examination indicated strength that was graded from "poor" to "absent" for all isolated muscle groups, with the exception of wrist extensors, which were graded as "fair" to "good." H.E. could function from an electric wheelchair, and he could ambulate slowly using a walker with supervision.

VENTILATION, RESPIRATION/GAS EXCHANGE
H.E.'s breathing pattern was examined and was found to be a diaphragmatic pattern with appropriate intercostal muscle use while at rest and during exertion; his accessory respiratory muscles became active during inspiration and expiration. His respiratory muscle strength was measured using maximum static inspiratory pressure (MSIP), inspiratory capacity (IC), and slow inspiratory vital capacity (IVC). The MSIP was 60% of predicted values; the IC was 45% of predicted values;

and the IVC was 45% of predicted values. His maximal static expiratory pressure, a measure of expiratory muscle strength, was 35% of predicted values.

Chest wall expansion was determined with a tape measure and found to be approximately 2.5 cm at maximal inspiratory effort. Passive motion was adequate at the glenohumeral joints. Coughing was evaluated as being weak and questionably functional. As previously noted, his limited inspiratory capacity and reduced expiratory pressures were largely responsible for the impaired cough.

EVALUATION, DIAGNOSIS, AND PROGNOSIS

Based on the data gathered specific to his current pulmonary issues, H.E. would receive a classification at cardiovascular/pulmonary pattern 6E ventilatory pump dysfunction or failure. This would be a pattern specific to his respiratory muscle impairment for which he was referred. His prognosis would be 8 to 10 weeks of care with episodes of physical therapy two times per week for the first several weeks, then reduced to weekly.

INTERVENTIONS

Coordination, communication, and documentation would focus upon interaction with the muscular dystrophy center at the children's hospital where H.E. is followed. Patient instruction would focus on instruction of H.E. and his parents and other caregivers regarding a home exercise program to improve his respiratory muscle strength, enhance his coughing, and provide for airway clearance as needed. In addition, they would be trained in proper airway clearance and assisted cough techniques including various devices to support airway clearance.

Procedural Interventions

THERAPEUTIC EXERCISE

Active cycle of breathing to enhance diaphragmatic excursion, maximal inspiration, and forced expiratory technique to aid in improving ventilation to the lower lobes, maintain/improve chest expansion, and aid in secretion removal

Continuing with ongoing strength training and range-of-motion exercise with emphasis on thorax and shoulder girdle to maintain thoracic compliance

Inspiratory muscle and expiratory muscle strengthening using simple handheld devices to maintain/increase respiratory muscle strength

Airway clearance as needed using high-frequency chest wall oscillation with SmartVest or airway oscillation with either Acapella or Flutter device; should secretion removal become problematic, equipment for airway aspiration or insufflation–exsufflation recommended

REFERENCES

1. Kochanek KD, Murphy SL. Deaths: final data for 2002. Natl Vital Stat Rep 2004;53(5):1–115
2. Children and Asthma in the United States. Glaxo Smith Kline.
3. Yeatts K, Davis KJ, Sotir M, et al. Who gets diagnosed with asthma? Frequent wheeze among adolescents with and without a diagnosis of asthma. Pediatrics 2003;111(5 Pt 1): 1046–1054.
4. Bloom B, Dey AN. Summary Health Statistics for U.S. Children: National Health Interview Survey, 2004. National Center for Health Statistics. Vital Health Stat 2006;10(227).
5. Haddad GG, Fontan JJP. Development of the respiratory system. In: Berman RE, Kliegman RM, Jensen HB, eds. Nelson's Textbook of Pediatrics. 17th Ed. Philadelphia: Saunders, 2004:1357–1359.
6. Avery ME. Hyaline membrane disease. Am Rev Respir Dis 1975;111:657–688.
7. Polgar G, Weng TR. The functional development of the respiratory system. Am Rev Respir Dis 1979;120:625–695.
8. Downes JJ, Fulgencio T, Raphaely RC. Acute respiratory failure in infants and children. Pediatr Clin North Am 1972;19: 423–445.
9. Ackerman SJ, Duff SB, Dennehy PH, et al. Economic impact of an infection control education program in a specialized preschool setting. Pediatrics 2001;108(6):E102.
10. Effmann EL, Fram EK, Vock P, et al. Tracheal cross-sectional area in children: CT determination. Radiology 1983;149(1): 137–140.
11. Keens TG, Ianuzzo CO. Development of fatigue-resistant muscle fibers in human ventilatory muscles. Am Rev Respir Dis 1979;119:139–141.
12. Guslits BG, Gaston SE, Bryan MH, et al. Diaphragmatic work of breathing in premature human infants. J Appl Physiol 1987;62(4):1410–1415.
13. Leith DE. The development of cough. Am Rev Respir Dis 1985;131(5):S39–42.
14. Papastamelos C, Panitch HB, England SE, et al. Developmental changes in chest wall compliance in infancy and early childhood. J Appl Physiol 1995;78:179–184.
15. Pagliara AS, Karl IE, Haymond M, et al. Hypoglycemia in infancy and childhood. J Pediatr 1973;82:365–379.
16. Guide to physical therapist practice. Phys Ther 2001;81:S114.
17. Nakamura CT, Ng GY, Paton JY, et al. Correlation between digital clubbing and pulmonary function in cystic fibrosis. Pediatr Pulmonol 2002;33(5):332–338.
18. Nathanson I, Riddlesberger MM Jr. Pulmonary hypertrophic osteoarthropathy in cystic fibrosis. Radiology 1980;135(3): 649–651.
19. Boat TA. Cystic fibrosis. In: Berman RE, Kliegman RM, Jensen HB eds. Nelson's Textbook of Pediatrics. 17th Ed. Philadelphia: Saunders, 2004:1447.
20. Gaultier C. Respiratory muscle function in infants. Eur Respir J 1995;8:150–153.
21. Tecklin JS. The patient with airway clearance dysfunction. In: Irwin S, Tecklin JS, eds. Cardiopulmonary Physical Therapy–A Guide for Practice. St. Louis: Mosby, 2004:290–292.
22. Li AM, Yin J, Yu CC, et al. The six-minute walk test in healthy children: reliability and validity. Eur Respir J 2005;25(6): 1057–1060.
23. Gulmans VA, van Veldhoven NH, de Meer K, et al. The six-minute walking test in children with cystic fibrosis: reliability and validity. Pediatr Pulmonol 1996;22(2):85–89.
24. Tomkinson GR, Leger LA, Olds TS, et al. Secular trends in the performance of children and adolescents (1980–2000): an analysis of 55 studies of the 20m shuttle run test in 11 countries. Sports Med 2003;33(4):285–300.
25. Narang I, Pike S, Rosenthal M, et al. Three-minute step test to assess exercise capacity in children with cystic fibrosis with mild lung disease. Pediatr Pulmonol 2003;35(2):108–113.
26. Steinkamp G, Wiedemann B. Relationship between nutritional status and lung function in cystic fibrosis: cross sectional and longitudinal analyses from the German CF quality assurance (CFQA) project. Thorax 2002;57(7):596–601.

27. Palevsky HI, Fishman AP. Chronic cor pulmonale. Etiology and management. JAMA 1990;263:2347.

28. Mawdsley RH, Hoy DK, Erwin MP. Criterion-related validity of the figure-of-eight method of measuring ankle edema. J Orthop Sports Phys Ther 2000;30:149.

29. Chen MJ, Fan X, Moe ST. Criterion-related validity of the Borg ratings of perceived exertion scale in healthy individuals: a meta-analysis. J Sports Sci 2002;20(11):873–899.

30. Pfeiffer KA, Pivarnik JM, Womack CJ, et al. Reliability and validity of the Borg and OMNI rating of perceived exertion scales in adolescent girls. Med Sci Sports Exerc 2002;34(12): 2057–2061.

31. Prasad SA, Randall SD, Balfour-Lynn IM. Fifteen-count breathlessness score: an objective measure for children. Pediatr Pulmonol 2000;30(1):56–62.

32. McGrath PJ, Pianosi PT, Unruh AM, et al. Dalhousie dyspnea scales: construct and content validity of pictorial scales for measuring dyspnea. BMC Pediatr 2005;5:33.

33. Nakamura CT, Ng GY, Paton JY, et al. Correlation between digital clubbing and pulmonary function in cystic fibrosis. Pediatr Pulmonol 2002;33(5):332–338.

34. de Meer K, Jeneson JAL, Gulmans VAM, et al. Efficiency of oxidative work performance of skeletal muscle in patients with cystic fibrosis. Thorax 1995;50:980–983.

35. de Meer K, Gulmans VA, van Der Laag J. Peripheral muscle weakness and exercise capacity in children with cystic fibrosis. Am J Respir Crit Care Med 1999;159(3):748–754.

36. Bieri D, Reeve R, Champion G, et al. The Faces Pain Scale for the self-assessment of the severity of pain experienced by children: development, initial validation and preliminary investigation for ratio scale properties. Pain 1990;41:139–150.

37. Hicks CL, von Baeyer CL, Spafford PA, et al. The Faces Pain Scale-Revised: toward a common metric in pediatric pain measurement. Pain 2001;93(2):173–183.

38. Koumbourlis AC, Stolar CJ. Lung growth and function in children and adolescents with idiopathic pectus excavatum. Pediatr Pulmonol 2004;38(4):339–343.

39. Button BM, Heine RG, Catto-Smith AG, et al. Postural drainage in cystic fibrosis: is there a link with gastro-esophageal reflux? J Paediatr Child Health 1998;34(4):330–334.

40. Button BM, Heine RG, Catto-Smith AG, et al. Chest physiotherapy in infants with cystic fibrosis: to tip or not? A five-year study. Pediatr Pulmonol 2003;35(3):208–213.

41. Crane L. Physical therapy for the neonate with respiratory disease. In: Irwin S, Tecklin JS, eds. Cardiopulmonary Physical Therapy. 3rd Ed. St. Louis: CV Mosby, 1995.

42. DeCesare J. Physical therapy for the child with respiratory dysfunction. In: Irwin S, Tecklin JS, eds. Cardiopulmonary Physical Therapy. 3rd Ed. St. Louis: CV Mosby, 1995.

43. Morrow BM, Futter MJ, Argent AC. Endotracheal suctioning: from principles to practice. Intensive Care Med 2004;30(6): 1167–1174.

44. Dab I, Alexander F. Evaluation of a particular bronchial drainage procedure called autogenic drainage. In: Baran D, Van Bogaert E, eds. Chest Physical Therapy in Cystic Fibrosis and Chronic Obstructive Pulmonary Disease. Ghent, Belgium: European Press, 1977;185–187.

45. Dab I, Alexander F. The mechanism of autogenic drainage studied with flow volume curves. Monogr Paediatr 1979;10: 50–53.

46. Miller S, Hall DO, Clayton CB, et al. Chest physiotherapy in cystic fibrosis: a comparative study of autogenic drainage and the active cycle of breathing techniques with postural drainage. Thorax 1995;50(2):165–169.

47. Savci S, Ince DI, Arikan H. A comparison of autogenic drainage and the active cycle of breathing techniques in patients with chronic obstructive pulmonary diseases. J Cardiopulm Rehabil 2000;20(1):37–43.

48. Pryor JA, Webber BA, Hodson ME, et al. Evaluation of the forced expiratory technique as an adjunct to postural drainage in treatment of cystic fibrosis. BMJ 1979;2:417–418.

49. Partridge C, Pryor J, Webber B. Characteristics of the forced expiratory technique. Physiotherapy 1989;75:193–194.

50. Hofmyer JL, Webber BA, Hodson ME. Evaluation of positive expiratory pressure as an adjunct to chest physiotherapy in the treatment of cystic fibrosis. Thorax 1986;41:951–954.

51. Gondor M, Nixon PA, Mutich R, et al. Comparison of Flutter device and chest physical therapy in the treatment of cystic fibrosis pulmonary exacerbation. Pediatr Pulmonol 1999;28(4): 255–260.

52. King M, et al. Tracheal mucus clearance in high-frequency oscillation: effect of peak flow bias. Eur Respir J 1990;3:6.

53. Warwick W. High frequency chest compression moves mucus by means of sustained staccato coughs. Pediatr Pulmonol 1991; Suppl 6:283, A219.

54. Tomkiewicz RP, Biviji A, King M. Effects of oscillating air flow on the rheological properties and clearability of mucous gel simulants. Biorheology 1994;31(5):511–520.

55. King M, Phillips DM, Zidulka A, et al. Tracheal mucus clearance in high-frequency oscillation. II: chest wall versus mouth oscillation. Am Rev Respir Dis 1984;130(5):703–706.

56. Shearer MO, Banks JM, Silva G, et al. Lung ventilation during diaphragmatic breathing. Phys Ther 1972;52:139–147.

57. Wetzel J, Lunsford BR, Peterson MJ, et al. Respiratory rehabilitation of the patient with spinal cord injury. In: Irwin S, Tecklin JS, eds. Cardiopulmonary Physical Therapy. 3rd Ed. St. Louis: CV Mosby, 1995:590.

58. de Meer K, Gulmans VA, van Der Laag J. Peripheral muscle weakness and exercise capacity in children with cystic fibrosis. Am J Respir Crit Care Med 1999;159(3):748–754.

59. Darbee J, Cerny F. Exercise testing and exercise conditioning for children with lung dysfunction. In: Irwin S, Tecklin JS, eds. Cardiopulmonary Physical Therapy. 3rd Ed. St. Louis: CV Mosby, 1990:570.

60. Orenstein DM, Hovell MF, Mulvihill M, et al. Strength vs aerobic training in children with cystic fibrosis: a randomized controlled trial. Chest 2004;126(4):1204–1214.

61. Keens TG, Krastins IRB, Wannamaker EM, et al. Ventilatory muscle endurance training in normal subjects and patients with cystic fibrosis. Am Rev Respir Dis 1977;116:853–860.

62. Enright S, Chatham K, Ionescu AA, et al. Inspiratory muscle training improves lung function and exercise capacity in adults with cystic fibrosis. Chest 2004;126(2):405–411.

63. Weiner P, Magadle R, Beckerman M, et al. Comparison of specific expiratory, inspiratory, and combined muscle training programs in COPD. Chest 2003;124(4):1357–1364.

64. Weisgerber MC, Guill M, Weisgerber JM, et al. Benefits of swimming in asthma: effect of a session of swimming lessons on symptoms and PFTs with review of the literature. J Asthma 2003;40(5):453–464.

65. Orenstein D, Franklin BA, Doershuk CF, et al. Exercise conditioning and cardiopulmonary fitness in cystic fibrosis. Chest 1981;80:392.

66. Laennec RTH. Forbes J, trans. Diseases of the Chest. 4th Ed. London: 1819.

67. Rosenfeld R. In: Behrman RE, Kliegman RM, Jensen HB. Nelson Textbook of Pediatrics. 17th Ed. Philadelphia: Saunders, 2004:1459–1461.

68. Gentilello L, Thompson DA, Tonnesen AS, et al. Effect of a rotating bed on the incidence of pulmonary complications in critically ill patients. Crit Care Med 1988;16(8):783–786.

69. Thoren L. Postoperative pulmonary complications: observations on their prevention by means of physiotherapy. Acta Chir Scand 1954;107:193–205.

70. Stein M, Cassara EL. Preoperative pulmonary evaluation and therapy for surgery patients. JAMA 1970;211:787–790.

71. Bartlett RH, Gazzinga AB, Graghty JR. Respiratory maneuvers to prevent postoperative complications. JAMA 1973;224:1017–1021.

72. Hymes AC, Yonehiro EG, Raab DE, et al. Electrical surface stimulation for treatment and prevention of ileus and atelectasis. Surg Forum 1974;25:222–224.

73. Finer MN, Moriartey RR, Boyd J, et al. Postextubation atelectasis. A retrospective review and a prospective controlled study. J Pediatr 1979;94:110–113.

74. Burrington JD, Cotton EK. Removal of foreign bodies from the tracheobronchial tree. J Pediatr Surg 1972;7:119–122.

75. Tecklin JS, Holsclaw DS. Bronchial drainage with aerosol medication in cystic fibrosis. Phys Ther 1976;56:999–1003.

76. Jardine E, O'Toole M, Paton J Y, et al. Current status of long term ventilation of children in the United Kingdom: questionnaire survey. BMJ 1999;318:295–299.

77. Mallory GB, Stillwell PC. The ventilator-dependent child: issues in diagnosis and management. Arch Phys Med Rehabil 1991;72:43–55.

78. Polgar G, Promadhat V. Pulmonary Function Testing in Children. Philadelphia: W. B. Saunders, 1971.

79. Derenne JP, Macklem PT, Roussos CH. The respiratory muscles: mechanics, control, and pathophysiology. Part III. Am Rev Respir Dis 1978;118:581–601.

80. Black LF, Hyatt RE. Maximal respiratory pressures: normal values and relationship to age and sex. Am Rev Respir Dis 1969;99:696–702.

81. Braun NMT, Rochester DF. Muscular weakness and respiratory failure. Am Rev Respir Dis 1979;119:123–125.

82. Williams HE. Inhalation pneumonia. Aust Paediatr J 1973;9:279–285.

83. Arvedson JC, Brodsky L. Pediatric Swallowing and Feeding: Assessment and Management. 2nd Ed. San Diego: Singular Publishers, 2001.

84. Merrick J, Axen K. Inspiratory muscle function following abdominal weight exercises in healthy subject. Phys Ther 1981;61:651–656.

85. McCool FD, Tzelepis GE. Inspiratory muscle training in the patient with neuromuscular disease. Phys Ther 1995;75(11):1006–1014.

86. Siegel IM. Pulmonary problems in Duchenne muscular dystrophy: diagnosis, prophylaxis, and treatment. Phys Ther 1975;55:160.

87. Martin AJ, Stern L, Yeates J, et al. Respiratory muscle training in Duchenne muscular dystrophy. Dev Med Child Neurol 1986;28:314–318.

88. Wanke T, Toifl K, Formanek D, et al. Inspiratory muscle training in patients with Duchenne muscular dystrophy. Chest 1994;105:475–482.

89. Couser JI Jr, Martinez FJ, Celli BR. Respiratory response and ventilatory muscle recruitment during arm elevation in normal subjects. Chest 1992;101(2):336–340.

90. Watts N. Improvement of breathing patterns. Phys Ther 1968;48:563–576.

91. Miske LJ, Hickey EM, Kolb SM, et al. Use of the mechanical in-exsufflator in pediatric patients with neuromuscular disease and impaired cough. Chest 2004;125(4):1406–1412.

92. National Heart, Lung and Blood Institute National Asthma Education Program Expert Panel Report. Guidelines for the Diagnosis and Management of Asthma. Bethesda, MD: NHLBI, 1991.

93. Lemanske RF, Busse WW. Asthma. JAMA 1997;278:1855–1873.

94. Blaiss MS. Outcomes analysis in asthma. JAMA 1997;278:1874–1880.

95. Lang DM, Polansky M. Patterns of asthma mortality in Philadelphia from 1969 to 1991. N Engl J Med 1994;331:1542–1546.

96. Cloutier MM, Wakefield DB, Hall CB, et al. Childhood asthma in an urban community: prevalence, care system, and treatment. Chest 2002;122(5):1571–1579.

97. Weiss KB, Gergen PJ, Crain EF. Inner-city asthma: the epidemiology of an emerging US public health concern. Chest 1992;101(suppl):362S–367S.

98. Martinez FD. The natural history of asthma during childhood. In: Silverman M, ed. Childhood Asthma and Other Wheezing Disorders. London: Arnold, 2002:29–36.

99. Grigg J. Management of paediatric asthma. Postgrad Med J 2004;80(947):535–540.

100. Plotnick L, Ducharme F. Combined inhaled anticholinergics and ß2 agonists for initial treatment of acute asthma in children (Cochrane Review). In: Cochrane Library. Issue 4. Oxford: Update Software, 2002.

101. Rowe B, Spooner C, Ducharme F, et al. Early emergency department treatment of acute asthma with systemic corticosteroids (Cochrane Review). In: Cochrane Library. Issue 4. Oxford: Update Software, 2002.

102. Lemanske RF, Busse WW. Asthma. JAMA 1997;278:1855–1873.

103. Knorr B, Franchi LM, Bisgaard H, et al. Montelukast, a leukotriene receptor antagonist, for the treatment of persistent asthma in children aged 2 to 5 years. Pediatrics 2001;108(3):E48.

104. Theodoropoulos DS, Lockey RF. Allergen immunotherapy: guidelines, update, and recommendations of the World Health Organization. Allergy Asthma Proc 2000;21(3):159–166.

105. Gunen H, Hacievliyagil SS, Kosar F, et al. The role of arterial blood gases, exercise testing, and cardiac examination in asthma. Allergy Asthma Proc 2006;27(1):45–52.

106. Oatis C. Kinesiology: Mechanics and Pathomechanics of Human Motion. Philadelphia: Lippincott Williams & Wilkins, 2003.

107. Disse B. Clinical evaluation of new therapies for treatment of mucus hypersecretion in respiratory diseases. Novartis Found Symp 2002;248:254–272;discussion 272–276, 277–282.

108. Rubin BK. The pharmacologic approach to airway clearance: mucoactive agents. Paediatr Respir Rev 2006;7(Suppl 1):S215–219.

109. Manocha R, Marks GB, Kenchington P, et al. Sahaja yoga in the management of moderate to severe asthma: a randomized controlled trial. Thorax 2002;57(2):110–115.

110. Cleland JA, Price DB, Lee AJ, et al. A pragmatic, three-arm randomised controlled trial of spiritual healing for asthma in primary care. Br J Gen Pract 2006;56(527):444–449.

111. Epstein GN, Halper JP, Barrett EA, et al. A pilot study of mind-body changes in adults with asthma who practice mental imagery. Altern Ther Health Med 2004;10(4):66–71.

112. Lang DM, Butz AM, Duggan AK, et al. Physical activity in urban school-aged children with asthma. Pediatrics 2004;113(4):e341–346.

113. Joyner BL, Fiorino EK, Matta-Arroyo E, et al. Cardiopulmonary exercise testing in children and adolescents with asthma who report symptoms of exercise-induced bronchoconstriction. J Asthma 2006;43(9):675–678.

114. Matsumoto I, Araki H, Tsuda K, et al. Effects of swimming training on aerobic capacity and exercise induced bronchoconstriction in children with bronchial asthma. Thorax 1999;54(3):196–201.

115. Neder JA, Nery LE, Silva AC, et al. Short term effects of aerobic training in the clinical management of moderate to severe asthma in children. Thorax 1999;54:202–206.

116. Cochrane LM, Clarke CJ. Benefits and problems of a physical training programme for asthmatic patients. Thorax 1990;45: 345–351.

117. Weiner P, Azgard Y, Ganam R, et al. Inspiratory muscle training in patients with bronchial asthma. Chest 1992;102:1357–1361.

118. Shaw A, Thompson EA, Sharp D. Complementary therapy use by patients and parents of children with asthma and the implications for NHS care: a qualitative study. BMC Health Serv Res 2006;6:76.

119. Cystic Fibrosis Foundation, Patient Registry 2004 Annual Report, Bethesda, MD, 2005.

120. Rommens JM, Iannuzzi MC, Kerem B, et al. Identification of the cystic fibrosis gene: chromosome walking and jumping. Science 1989;245:1059–1065.

121. Riordan JR, Rommens JM, Kerem B, et al. Identification of the cystic fibrosis gene: cloning and characterization of complementary DNA. Science 1989;245:1066–1073.

122. Kerem B, Rommens JM, Buchanan J, et al. Identification of the cystic fibrosis gene: genetic analysis. Science 1989;245: 1073–1080.

123. Braun AT, Farrell PM, Ferec C, et al. Cystic fibrosis mutations and genotype-pulmonary phenotype analysis. J Cyst Fibros 2006;5(1):33–41.

124. Matsui H, Grubb BR, Tarran R, et al. Evidence for periciliary liquid layer depletion, not abnormal ion composition, in the pathogenesis of cystic fibrosis airways disease. Cell 1998;95(7): 1005–1015.

125. Hamosh A, Fitzsimmons SC, Macek M Jr, et al. Comparison of the clinical manifestations of cystic fibrosis in black and white patients. J Pediatr 1998;132(2):255–259.

126. Cystic Fibrosis Foundation, Bethesda, MD. Press release 2005.

127. Holsclaw DS. Common pulmonary complications of cystic fibrosis. Clin Pediatr 1970;9:346–355.

128. Goldring RM, Fishman AP, Turino GM, et al. Pulmonary hypertension and cor pulmonale in cystic fibrosis of the pancreas. J Pediatr 1964;65:501–524.

129. Holsclaw DS, Grand RJ, Shwachman H. Massive hemoptysis in cystic fibrosis. J Pediatr 1973;76:829–838.

130. Flume PA, Yankaskas JR, Ebeling M, et al. Massive hemoptysis in cystic fibrosis. Chest 2005;128(2):729–738.

131. Widerman E, Millner L, Sexauer W, et al. Health status and sociodemographic characteristics of adults receiving a cystic fibrosis diagnosis after age 18 years. Chest 2000;118(2): 427–433.

132. Yankaskas JR, Marshal B, Sufian B et al. Cystic Fibrosis Adult Care: Consensus Conference. Chest 2004;125:1S–39S.

133. Smyth A. Prophylactic antibiotics in cystic fibrosis: a conviction without evidence? Pediatr Pulmonol 2005;40(6):471–476.

134. Sermet-Gaudelus I, Le Cocguic Y, Ferroni A et al. Nebulized antibiotics in cystic fibrosis. Paediatr Drugs 2002;4(7):455–467.

135. Smyth A, Walters S. Prophylactic antibiotics for cystic fibrosis. Cochrane Database Syst Rev. 2003;(3):CD001912.

136. Bluebond-Langner M, Lask B, Angst DB, eds. Psychological Aspects of Cystic Fibrosis. Oxford University Press, 2001.

137. Gulmans VA, van Veldhoven NH, de Meer K, et al. The six-minute walking test in children with cystic fibrosis: reliability and validity. Pediatr Pulmonol 1996;22(2):85–89.

138. Bradley J, Howard J, Wallace E, et al. Reliability, repeatability, and sensitivity of the modified shuttle test in adult cystic fibrosis. Chest 2000;117(6):1666–1671.

139. Lorin MI, Denning CR. Evaluation of postural drainage by measurement of sputum volume and consistency. Am J Phys Med 1971;50:215–219.

140. Tecklin JS, Holsclaw DS. Evaluation of bronchial drainage in patients with cystic fibrosis. Phys Ther 1975;55:1081–1084.

141. Feldman J, Traver GA, Taussig LM. Maximal expiratory flows after postural drainage. Am Rev Respir Dis 1979;119:239–245.

142. Motoyama EK. Lower airway obstruction. In: Mangos JA, Talamo RD, eds. Fundamental Problems of Cystic Fibrosis and Related Diseases. New York: Intercontinental Medical Book Corp, 1973.

143. Desmond KF, Schwenk F, Thomas E, et al. Immediate and long-term effects of chest physiotherapy in patients with cystic fibrosis. J Pediatr 1983;103:538–542.

144. Williams MT. Chest physiotherapy and cystic fibrosis. Why is the most effective form of treatment still unclear? Chest 1994;106:1872–1882.

145. Pfleger A, Theissl B, Oberwalder B, et al. Self-administered chest physiotherapy in cystic fibrosis: a comparative study of high-pressure PEP and autogenic drainage. Lung 1992;170: 323–330.

146. Giles DR, Wagener JS, Accurso FJ, et al. Short-term effects of postural drainage with clapping vs autogenic drainage on oxygen saturation and sputum recovery in patients with cystic fibrosis. Chest 1995;108(4):952–954.

147. Verboon JML, Bakker W, Sterk PJ. The value of forced expiration technique with and without postural drainage in adults with cystic fibrosis. Eur J Respir Dis 1986;69:169–174.

148. Miller S, Hall DO, Clayton CB, et al. Chest physiotherapy in cystic fibrosis: a comparative study of autogenic drainage and the active cycle of breathing techniques with postural drainage. Thorax 1995;50(2):165–169.

149. McIlwaine PM, Wong LT, Peacock D, et al. Long-term comparative trial of conventional postural drainage and percussion versus positive expiratory pressure physiotherapy in the treatment of cystic fibrosis. J Pediatr 1997;131(4):570–574.

150. McIlwaine PM, Wong LT, Peacock D, et al. Long-term comparative trial of positive expiratory pressure versus oscillating positive expiratory pressure (flutter) physiotherapy in the treatment of cystic fibrosis. J Pediatr 2001;138(6):845–850.

151. Konstan MW, Stern RC, Doershuk CF. Efficacy of the Flutter device for airway mucus clearance in patients with cystic fibrosis. J Pediatr 1994;124:689–693.

152. Gondor M, Nixon PA, Mutich R, et al. Comparison of Flutter device and chest physical therapy in the treatment of cystic fibrosis pulmonary exacerbation. Pediatr Pulmonol 1999;28(4): 255–260.

153. Warwick WJ, Hansen LG. The long-term effect of high frequency chest compression therapy on pulmonary complications of cystic fibrosis. Pediatr Pulmonol 1991;11:265–271.

154. Braggion C, Cappeletti LM, Cornacchia M, et al. Short-term effects of three chest physiotherapy regimens in patients hospitalized for pulmonary exacerbations of cystic fibrosis: a cross-over randomized study. Pediatr Pulmonol 1995;19: 16–22.

155. Tecklin JS, Clayton R, Scanlin T. High frequency chest wall oscillation vs. traditional chest physical therapy in cystic fibrosis - a large one-year, controlled study. Pediatr Pulmonol 2000; 30(S20):304–305.

156. Ohnsorg F. A cost analysis of high-frequency chest-wall oscillation in cystic fibrosis. Am J Respir Crit Care Med 1994; 149(4 pt 2):A669.

157. DeBoeck C, Zinman R. Cough versus chest physiotherapy: a comparison of the acute effects on pulmonary function in patients with cystic fibrosis. Am Rev Respir Dis 1984;129: 182–184.

158. Rossman CM, Waldes R, Sampson D, et al. Effect of chest physiotherapy on the removal of mucus in patients with cystic fibrosis. Am Rev Respir Dis 1982;126:131–135.

159. Bain J, Bishop J, Olinsky A. Evaluation of directed coughing in cystic fibrosis. Br J Dis Chest. 1988;82:138–148.

160. Nixon PA, Orenstein DM, Kelsey SF. Habitual physical activity in children and adolescents with cystic fibrosis. Med Sci Sports Exerc 2001;33(1):30–35.

161. Cerny FJ, Pullano TP, Cropp GJ. Cardiorespiratory adaptations to exercise in cystic fibrosis. Am Rev Respir Dis 1982; 126(2):217–220.

162. Nixon PA, Orenstein DM, Curtis SE, et al. Oxygen supplementation during exercise in cystic fibrosis. Am Rev Respir Dis 1990;142(4):807–811.

163. Marcus CL, Bader D, Stabile MW, et al. Supplemental oxygen and exercise performance in patients with cystic fibrosis with severe pulmonary disease. Chest 1992;101:52–57.

164. Moorcraft AJ, Dodd ME, Howarth C, et al. Muscular fatigue, ventilation, and perception of limitation at peak exercise in adults with cystic fibrosis. Pediatr Pulmonol 1996;Suppl 13: 306(abstr 349).

165. Moorcroft AJ, Dodd ME, Morris J, et al. Individualised unsupervised exercise training in adults with cystic fibrosis: a 1 year randomised controlled trial. Thorax 2004;59(12): 1074–1080.

Physical Therapy in the Educational Environment

Karen Yundt Lunnen and Rita F. Geddes

 ervices for children with disabilities in the educational setting are guided by comprehensive federal legislation, the Individuals with Disabilities Education Improvement Act (IDEIA). In the legislation, physical therapy is considered a related service and may be required to enable a child with a disability to benefit from special education. The educational environment is a rewarding one and challenges physical therapists to use the best of their professional abilities within a unique context.

Background

Physical therapists have been practicing in the educational environment in the United States since the 1930s. During those early years, children with physical disabilities were usually segregated in special orthopedic schools or in separate classrooms within the school building. The primary diagnoses that physical therapists were involved with were poliomyelitis, tuberculosis of bones and joints, birth anomalies, and cerebral palsy.[1] Typically, children with intellectual impairment or more severe disabilities did not have access to public education.

Often, physical therapists were employed as "special teachers, with the same privileges and responsibilities."[1] They met the same educational requirements as teachers and had, in addition, "a course in physical therapy from an approved school."[1] Many also had a background in physical education. Physical therapy departments were generally fully equipped treatment areas with whirlpools, parallel bars, treatment mats, and so on. Pratt described physical therapy in the educational setting at that time as a "rich and happy field" where the physical therapist had the "privilege of seeing the whole child" and where opportunity existed not only to see a child in his or her individual treatment session, but also to "follow the child in his peer groups."[1] Physical therapists experienced "great satisfaction in having an active part in the physical and social adjustments which are accomplished over a long period."[1]

Physical therapists practicing in educational environments were already addressing the benefits of including children with disabilities in activities with "normal" children. DeYoung spoke of an orthopedic school housed under the same roof as the high school allowing a "complete curriculum for little cripples."[2] Hutchinson, in 1937, commented that "it is easier for the crippled child to grow normally when he is in association with regular school children."[3] Yet, for approximately 30 more years, segregation for those with physical handicaps and exclusion for those with mental retardation or severe physical disabilities was the prevailing norm.

In the 1960s and 1970s, parents and other advocates became active in the so-called normalization movement and found support from John F. Kennedy's administration.

Several landmark decisions in the Supreme Court in the early 1970s paved the way for subsequent legislation guaranteeing the rights of those with disabilities. It is essential that physical therapists understand this legislation at both a federal and state level, because it has directed the provision of special education for children and defined the role of the physical therapist in the educational environment.

The first significant civil rights legislation for individuals with disabilities was PL 93-112, the Rehabilitation Act of 1973.[4] Section 504 of the Rehabilitation Act states that "no otherwise qualified disabled individual would be excluded from the participation in, be denied the benefits of, or be subjected to discrimination under any program or activity receiving federal financial assistance."[4] Section 504 paved the way for subsequent legislation impacting the provision of special education for children with disabilities in the public schools.

In 1975, the U.S. Congress passed the Education for All Handicapped Children's Act (PL 94-142),[5] which was the template for dramatic changes in the responsibility of public schools to educate children with disabilities. PL 94-142 provided for a "free appropriate public education" for all children with disabilities from the age of 6 to 21 years (or from 5 years if that was the age in a particular state when children normally began their participation in public school).[5] Special education and related services provided in accordance with an individualized education program (IEP) were emphasized to address each child's unique needs. Related services encompassed a broad range of support services including physical therapy.

Further provisions of PL 94-142 described a number of important new concepts for the public education of children with disabilities that remain part of the current legislation.

1. *Zero reject:* No child is excluded from receiving a free appropriate public education regardless of the type or severity of his or her disability.
2. *Least restrictive environment:* School systems are required to ensure that "to the maximum extent appropriate, children with disabilities are educated with children who are non-disabled; and that special classes, separate schooling or other removal of children with disabilities from regular classes occurs only when the nature or severity of the disability is such that education in the regular classroom with the use of supplementary aids and services cannot be achieved satisfactorily."[5]
3. *Parent participation:* Parents or primary caregivers are essential members of the team approach to evaluation, planning, and intervention and are assured various rights.
4. *Nondiscriminatory evaluation:* Evaluation of a child is free from racial or cultural bias, no one test is used as the sole criterion for placement decisions, and the test is administered in the child's native language.

5. *Individualized Education Program:* Every child receiving special education must receive an individualized education program. This is a comprehensive individualized plan developed by a multidisciplinary team in cooperation with the parents that outlines the special education and related service needs of the child.

The government built into PL 94-142 the requirement that it be periodically reviewed, revised, and reauthorized. Over the past several decades, several amendments have been made to PL 94-142 and other legislation has been introduced that has impacted services for children with disabilities (Table 19.1).

The impact of this legislation on the delivery of services in the educational environment for children with a wide range of disabilities has been dramatic. The reader is urged to explore further the interesting progression of federal mandates over time. However, the remainder of this chapter will focus on IDEIA and the framework it provides for the education of children with special needs. The full text of the legislation is available at http://www.ed.gov/policy/speced/guid/idea/idea2004.html.

IDEIA impacts the education of almost 7 million American children with disabilities and the cost is staggering.[16] The federal government promised to pay the increased cost of educating a child with a disability compared to a general education student, which was 40% of the average per pupil expenditure.[16] The actual federal allocation has always been less than half the amount promised, however, resulting in a significant burden for the states. A large number of professional organizations have formed a funding coalition and developed a proposal for full funding by the federal government that could be phased in over a predetermined time period.[17]

The overall purpose of IDEIA is to "ensure that all children with disabilities have available to them a free appropriate public education that emphasizes special education and related services designed to meet their unique needs and prepare them for further education, employment, and independent living."[14] The purpose has changed little since PL 94-142 but notable is the inclusion of *all* children and the emphasis on planning for a child's lifetime.

IDEIA has four major sections: (1) General Provisions, (2) Assistance for All Children with Disabilities, (3) Infants and Toddlers with Disabilities, and (4) National Activities to Improve Education of Children with Disabilities (including personnel development).[14] In substantiating the reauthorization of IDEIA, Congress noted the overall success of the federal legislation to assure access to a free appropriate public education and to improve educational outcomes for children with disabilities. Cited as impediments to the success of the legislation were low expectations and "insufficient focus on applying replicable research on proven methods of teaching and learning

TABLE 19.1

TABLE 19.1

Legislation Impacting Provision of Services for Children with Disabilities in Educational Environments

Year Enacted	Title of Legislation	Impact
1986	PL 99-457 Education of the Handicapped Act Amendments[6]	Expanded the provisions of PL 94-142 to include infants and toddlers (birth to 3 yr) and preschool children (3–5 yr)
1988	PL 100-360 Medicare Catastrophic Coverage Act[7]	Allowed Medicaid funds to pay for needed services identified in the formal education plan. The intent of this act was to improve access to therapy for children by allowing federal resources other than education to pay for some related services.
1988	PL 100-407 Technology-Related Assistance for Individuals with Disabilities Act (Tech Act)[8]	Mandated that states address policies, practices, and structures to promote access to appropriate assistive technology (AT). Public schools were obligated to provide needed AT services and/or devices.
1990	PL 101-336, The Americans with Disabilities Act (ADA)[9]	Extended comprehensive civil rights protection to individuals with disabilities. The law's major impact on public education was the provision that all public buildings must be accessible.
1991	PL 102-119 Individuals with Disabilities Education Act Amendments (IDEA)[10]	Supported most of the provisions of PL 94-142 and PL 99-457 with amendments that expanded or modified the provisions of the law in other areas
1997	PL 105-17 Individuals with Disabilities Education Act Amendments of 1997[11]	Reauthorization of IDEA Supported most of the provisions of earlier legislation and expanded or modified other provisions
1998	PL 105-394 Assistive Technology Act of 1998[12]	Reauthorization of PL 100-407 (Tech Act)
2002	PL 107-110 No Child Left Behind Act[13]	Addressed quality of education for all children; included annual testing and mandate for adequate progress
2004	PL 108-446 Individuals with Disabilities Education Improvement Act of 2004 (IDEIA)[14]	Reauthorization of PL 102-119 (IDEA) Current legislation in effect until 2010
2004	H.R. 4278 Assistive Technology Act of 2004 (Putting Technology into the Hands of Individuals with Disabilities)[15]	Reauthorization of PL 105-394

for children with disabilities."[14] Overall tenets supported by IDEIA include[14]:

- having high expectations for children and "ensuring their access to the general education curriculum, to the maximum extent possible"[14];
- strengthening the role and responsibility of parents;
- providing appropriate special education and related services;
- supporting the development and use of assistive technology to maximize accessibility;
- supporting high-quality, intensive preservice preparation and professional development for all personnel who work with children with disabilities;

- recognizing the increasing number of racial and ethnic minorities and the need for equitable treatment and for increased participation of minorities in the teaching profession; and
- emphasizing the importance of effective transition services to promote independence and success in employment or further education after leaving public education.

◆ Service Provision for Children Ages 3 to 21 (Part B)

Part B of IDEIA addresses the provision of services for children ages 3 to 21 years and includes a set of operational definitions that are important to understand.[14] A few key definitions are included in Display 19.1.

EDUCATIONAL TEAM

IDEIA stipulates that assessment, planning, and service delivery must be provided by a "multidisciplinary team of qualified professionals and the parent of the child."[14] More specifically, the IEP team must include the parent(s), a regular education teacher, a special education teacher, a representative of the local educational agency (LEA), and "at the discretion of the parent or LEA, other individuals who have knowledge or special expertise regarding the child, including related services personnel as appropriate."[14]

The federal legislation labels teams as "multidisciplinary," although the description of membership, roles, and responsibilities is closer to what most would define as a transdisciplinary or collaborative team model. In the transdisciplinary model, team members jointly assess the child; parents are full and active participants; a primary service provider is assigned to implement the plan with the family; information, knowledge, and skills are continuously shared among team members; and there is a commitment to teach, learn, and work together across disciplinary boundaries to implement a unified service plan.[18] The collaborative model is a combination of a transdisciplinary team functioning in an integrated service delivery model.[19,20]

The role release that is required for meaningful team function is still difficult for physical therapists practicing in the school setting. In a survey of physical therapists practicing in educational environments, Effgen and Keppler[21] found that although they recognized the importance of collaborative team interaction, most physical therapists practicing in educational settings performed evaluations independently of other team members, reported findings separately, conducted evaluations outside the classroom, and provided treatment as a direct service, also outside the classroom. One reason that physical therapists gave for not fully embracing a collaborative team model was concern about legal issues related to standards of professional practice. However, Rainforth[22] examined the physical therapy practice acts in each state and concluded that "documents that define legal and ethical practice of physical therapy allow for, and even encourage, role release in educational settings."

When the Education for All Handicapped Children's Act was passed in 1976, there was suddenly a legal mandate for physical therapy services in the public schools and therapists to provide those services were in high demand and short supply. The Section on Pediatrics was created, at least in part, to define the competencies required to practice in the educational environment and to establish a process for specialty certification in pediatric physical therapy.[23] An American Physical Therapy Association (APTA) task force

---

⟫ DISPLAY 19.1

Key Definitions from Part B of the Individuals with Disabilities Education Improvement Act

Child with a disability	A child ". . . with mental retardation, hearing impairments (including deafness), speech or language impairments, visual impairments (including blindness), serious emotional disturbance, orthopedic impairments, autism, traumatic brain injury, other health impairments, or specific learning disabilities . . . who, by reason thereof, needs special education and related services"[14]
Child with a disability for a child aged 3 through 9 (or any subset of that age range)	". . . may, at the discretion of the State and the local educational agency, include a child experiencing developmental delays, as defined by the State and as measured by appropriate diagnostic instruments and procedures, in 1 or more of the following areas: physical development, cognitive development; communication development; social or emotional development; or adaptive development . . . who, by reason thereof, needs special education and related services"[14]
Related services	". . . transportation, and such developmental, corrective, and other supportive services (including speech-language pathology and audiology services, interpreting services, psychological services, physical and occupational therapy, recreation, including therapeutic recreation, social work services, school nurse services designed to enable a child with a disability to receive a free appropriate public education as described in the individualized education program of the child, counseling services, including rehabilitation counseling, orientation and mobility services, and medical services, except that such medical services shall be for diagnostic and evaluation purposes only) as may be required to assist a child with a disability to benefit from special education, and includes the early identification and assessment of disabling conditions in children"[14]
Special education	". . . specifically designed instruction, at no cost to parents, to meet the unique needs of a child with disability"[14]
Supplementary aids and services	". . . aids, services and other supports that are provided in regular education classes or other education-related settings to enable children with disabilities to be educated with non-disabled children to the maximum extent appropriate . . ."[14]

established competencies for physical therapists in early intervention that were published in 1991.[24] APTA's Section on Pediatrics and the special interest group on school-based physical therapy within the section provide valuable resources on a variety of topics that can be accessed on their webpage (www.pediatricapta.org) (Table 19.2).

The qualifications of personnel working with children who have disabilities received increased emphasis in the 2004 reauthorization of IDEA and is a matter of increasing concern to various agencies and associations. The Association for Persons with Severe Handicaps (TASH), an international association of people with disabilities that advocates broadly for inclusion, developed a Resolution on Preparation of Related Services Personnel for Work in Educational Settings.[25] The resolution addresses both entry-level and advanced competencies in a comprehensive manner.

REFERRAL

Referral for evaluation to determine if a child is a child with a disability (as defined by the law) can be made by a parent, a state agency, or local educational agency. Referral for a related service, including physical therapy, can be initiated by anyone on the child's team, but an IEP must be developed for the student before initiation of a related service. The referral process can be cumbersome, especially for a child who is not already receiving special education services. Physical therapists may screen a child as a preliminary step and help direct the process of subsequent referral in that way. If a student is determined ineligible for special education, a physical therapist may (at the discretion of the local educational agency) offer limited consultation to the classroom teacher, physical education teacher, or parent.

If the state practice act for physical therapy requires physician referral for a client to access physical therapy, it is necessary to obtain that medical referral in addition to the procedural steps outlined by legislative guidelines. In states with direct access, a physician referral is not necessary unless dictated by a third-party payer (e.g., Medicaid). A physician referral is recommended for students with complex medical needs to formalize a process for needed communication with the referring physician. Children with disabilities are frequently served by a variety of professionals and social agencies. Communication with others involved in providing care for the child outside of the educational environment is crucial regardless of the decision about medical referral.

ASSESSMENT/EVALUATION

IDEIA requires a "full and individualized initial evaluation" to determine whether the child has a disability and, if so, whether the disability limits in some way the student's ability to benefit from special education or participate optimally in the educational environment.[14] An evaluation requires parental consent and must be completed within 60 school days after receiving consent. A variety of assessment tools and strategies must be used to gather functional, developmental, and academic information. Progressively more importance has been given in the federal legislation to using technically sound instruments that are nondiscriminatory and administered in the language and form most likely to yield accurate information, by appropriately trained personnel, according to the purpose for which reliability and validity were established and in accordance with instructions specific to the instrument.

A physical therapy evaluation may be part of the initial evaluation to determine eligibility for special education/related services or may be a recommendation of the team after eligibility has been established. A physical therapy evaluation should include traditional elements as suggested by the *Guide to Physical Therapist Practice*[26] or other models. The evaluation should also include an assessment of the student's ability to participate in and benefit from the educational environment. This would include transportation on the school bus; entering and exiting the bathroom and toileting; eating; and negotiating hallways, doors, distances, stairs, and so on. At least one standardized measure, either norm referenced or criterion referenced, is recommended.

TABLE 19.2	
Resources for School-Based Physical Therapists Through the American Physical Therapy Association's (APTA) Section on Pediatrics	
APTA Section on Pediatrics	List of evaluation/assessment tools
	Legislative information about IDEIA
	Brochure, *Providing Services Under IDEA 2004*
	Links to Internet resources
	Manual, *Providing Physical Therapy Services Under Parts B and C of the Individuals with Disabilities Education Act (IDEA)*
APTA Pediatric Listserv	Ongoing e-mail discussion forum for current issues in pediatric physical therapy. Available to all members of Section on Pediatrics
APTA Section on Pediatrics School-Based Special Interest Group	National organization working to provide opportunities for school-based physical therapists to confer, meet, and promote high standards of practice
Pediatric Physical Therapy	Monthly peer-reviewed publication of Section on Pediatrics

Summaries of assessment instruments available to use with children who have developmental delays are available in Chapter 3 and in other published materials. Instruments in common use in the educational environment are:

1. *Bruininks-Oseretsky Test of Motor Proficiency,* Second Edition[27]—a standardized, norm-referenced test for children from 4 to 21 years of age who range from those who are developing normally to those who have moderate motor skill deficits. The complete battery assesses eight areas: (1) fine motor precision, (2) fine motor integration, (3) manual dexterity, (4) bilateral coordination, (5) balance, (6) running speed and agility, (7) upper limb coordination, and (8) strength. Together the items provide a comprehensive index of motor proficiency plus separate measures of both gross and fine motor skills. A test kit contains all items necessary for administration. The test requires approximately 45 to 60 minutes to administer. A Short Form that includes a subset of items from the complete battery can be used as a screening tool. Clinical validity studies have been conducted on children with high-functioning autism, developmental coordination disorder, and mild to moderate retardation.

2. Gross Motor Function Measure[28]—a criterion-based observational measure designed and validated for use by pediatric physical therapists as an evaluative measure for assessing change over time in gross motor function of children with cerebral palsy, head injuries, or Down syndrome. It is appropriate for children whose motor skills are at or below those of a 5-year-old child without motor disability. Motor function is assessed in five dimensions: (1) lying and rolling, (2) sitting, (3) crawling and kneeling, (4) standing, and (5) walking, running, and jumping.

3. School Function Assessment[29]—a criterion-referenced standardized survey instrument that utilizes the responses of one or more individuals familiar with the child's function in the educational environment as the basis for scoring. Items cover a comprehensive array of functional behaviors categorized in five areas: (1) participation, (2) task supports, (3) activity performance, (4) physical tasks, and (5) cognitive/behavioral tasks. The content is specifically relevant for children with physical or sensory impairments and can reveal patterns of strength and weakness. Individual items are worded in behavioral, measurable terms that allow them to be easily converted to IEP goals. Completing the whole assessment can be time consuming (approximately 2 hours), but this is strongly recommended as a baseline. Individual sections can also be administered separately.

4. Mobility Opportunities Via Education (MOVE)[30]—a full curriculum developed specifically for children with severe/profound disabilities over the age of 7 who have not developed the physical skills necessary to sit independently, bear weight on their feet, or take reciprocal steps (although the target population has since expanded). The curriculum is designed as a comprehensive, interdisciplinary approach to teach students basic, functional motor skills needed for adult life in home and community environments. The Top-Down Motor Milestone Test, part of the MOVE curriculum, is an interview-based assessment tool that rates a child's performance in 16 categories of basic motor function.

5. School Outcomes Measure[31]—a new minimum data set, comparable to the Functional Independence Measure for Children (WeeFIM)[32] but specific to the educational environment, that can be used to measure outcomes of students receiving school-based occupational or physical therapy. The authors (McEwen et al.) have published information on the content validity and interrater reliability and are continuing to determine psychometric properties of the measure.[31] The measure should be an important contribution to the need for increasing accountability.

It is especially important in an educational environment that the physical therapist interpret the results of testing for other team members. Depending on their background, team members may have varying levels of understanding about concepts and terms common to a physical therapist. Documentation of the testing must also be written in language that can be understood by nonmedical personnel.

An ecologic assessment is an approach that focuses on the activities necessary for a student to function in various environments and the skills required to perform the specified activities.[33] Brown and colleagues[34] pioneered work on ecologic assessment, developing an inventory to guide the development of functional goals and objectives. Linehan et al.[35] found that teachers had higher expectations for students who had an ecologic assessment report (student's observed competencies in his or her daily environment) as compared with a developmental assessment report (student's mental and developmental ages).

DETERMINING ELIGIBILITY FOR RELATED SERVICES UNDER IDEIA

Determining who is eligible for related services in the educational environment is often a challenging process. It is important to remember that related services support the educational process and not the medical well-being of the child, and that related services are provided to help a child benefit from special education. Under the provisions of IDEIA, if a child does not need special education, he or she is not eligible to receive related services. Decisions about educational relevance are made by the team. Eligibility determination varies from state to state.

Borkowski and Wessman[36] surveyed representatives from each American state. Only four states used eligibility criteria that were more specific than those specified in IDEA. Faced with financial constraints, shortages of physical therapy personnel, and legal accountability, many states struggle to improve the objectivity of the process for determining eligibility without losing the mandate for individualized program plans. Criteria or guidelines are customarily not mandatory but help structure decisions about prioritizing who receives physical therapy, the type of services, and the frequency and duration of services.

In the Waukesha Delivery Model,[37] students are assigned to one of four levels of service based on the rate of change in the student's physical or functional status. Each level defines the purpose of the intervention, the intensity of service, and personnel responsibilities for the delivery of service. Students exhibiting more rapid rates of change receive a greater amount of the therapist's time and direct involvement. "Cognitive referencing," or "performance discrepancy criteria,"[38-40] is a controversial model that presumes a positive correlation between cognitive and motor development and an upper limit for development based on a child's cognitive abilities. Children are eligible for physical therapy services only if motor skills are significantly lower than cognitive abilities. Both models limit intervention for children with severe intellectual impairment and accompanying physical disabilities.

The use of specific criteria or models to determine eligibility can add objectivity and consistency to a difficult process. Giangreco[41] cautions, however, that research does not support the use of these models and unless they are used judiciously, they can negate the individualized approach to evaluation and program planning that the law requires. Each child with a disability has unique needs that must be meshed with the contextual differences in the environments in which he or she functions.

REHABILITATION ACT

The Rehabilitation Act[4] is a federal statute designed to ensure that individuals with disabilities are provided equal opportunities. Provisions of the Rehabilitation Act are generally broader than those in IDEIA and it is often used as justification to expand a student's eligibility for related services within the educational environment and/or the scope of intervention. It ensures that students with disabilities receive an appropriate education even if special education is not required and it is an important source of support and funding for children who do not qualify for services under other legislative acts.

INDIVIDUALIZED EDUCATION PROGRAM

If the team identifies the student as being eligible for special education services, then the process progresses to IEP development. An IEP must be developed within 30 calendar days of the determination of eligibility. In developing the IEP, the law emphasizes the importance of considering the strengths of the child, the concerns of the parents for enhancing the education of their child, the results of the initial (or most recent) evaluation, and the academic, developmental, and functional needs of the child. The written program must include the following:

1. Statement of the child's present levels of academic achievement and functional performance, including how the child's disability affects the child's involvement and progress in the general education curriculum (or for preschool children, the child's participation in appropriate activities)
2. Statement of measurable annual goals, including academic and functional goals designed to enable the child to make progress in the general education curriculum and meet each of the child's other educational needs that result from the child's disability
3. Description of the child's progress toward meeting the annual goals
4. Statement of the special education and related services and supplementary aids and services (based on peer-reviewed research to the extent practical) to be provided
5. Explanation of the extent, if any, to which the child will not participate with nondisabled children in the regular class and in other activities
6. Statement of accommodations that are necessary to measure the academic achievement and functional performance of the child on state- and districtwide assessments
7. Projected date for the beginning of the services and modifications described and the anticipated frequency, location, and duration of those services and modifications
8. Beginning no later than the first IEP to be in effect when the child is 16, and updated annually, appropriate measurable postsecondary goals based on age-appropriate transition assessments related to training, education, employment, and, where appropriate, independent living skills, and the transition services needed to assist the child in reaching those goals

On the U.S. Department of Education website is a sample form that outlines the IEP content required by IDEIA (http://www.ed.gov/policy/speced/guid/idea/model form-iep.doc).[42] An IEP must be reviewed at least annually and revised as appropriate. IDEIA provides the option to develop "a comprehensive multi-year IEP, not to exceed 3 years, that is designed to coincide with the natural transition points for the child."[14] These transitions include the transition from preschool to elementary, elementary to middle school, middle school to secondary, and secondary to postsecondary activities. The use of a multiyear IEP is being piloted in 15 states.

A number of procedural safeguards are stipulated and states must establish mechanisms for due process, mediation, and appeal. States are required to establish quantifiable indicators in specified priority areas and to report data on outcomes. A continuing area of federal focus is evidence that education is occurring in the least restrictive environment and that no discriminatory activity is occurring in relation to minorities.

Service Provision for Infants/ Toddlers (Part C)

Part C of IDEIA describes infants and toddlers with disabilities and the services provided for them. IDEIA recognizes that significant brain development occurs in the first 3 years of life and that early intervention is important to enhance development, reduce educational costs to society, and maximize the ability of individuals with disabilities to live independently.

The basic tenets of IDEIA are the same for this age group as for older children, but there are important differences. Since the providers of early intervention services were much more diverse, the federal government allowed more discretion at the state level in Part C. Every state must use the federal assistance "to develop and implement a statewide, comprehensive, coordinated, multidisciplinary, interagency system . . ." coordinated by an Interagency Coordinating Council.[14] The council must meet at least quarterly and its composition must include parents (no less than 20% of the members), public or private providers of early intervention services (no less than 20% of the members), and at least one representative from the state legislature, the state Medicaid program, and the state welfare agencies responsible for foster care, children's mental health, and homeless children.

IDEIA mandates that states must develop specific policies and procedures for children under 3 years who have experienced substantiated abuse or neglect or who have been affected by the abuse of illegal substances or withdrawal symptoms as a result of prenatal drug exposure. APTA has published an excellent resource for physical therapists, *APTA's Guidelines for Recognizing and Providing Care for Victims of Child Abuse.*[43]

The services identified for early intervention are expansive and include physical therapy; occupational therapy; speech therapy; assistive technology devices and services; psychological services; family training and counseling; diagnostic medical services; special instruction; social work; vision; hearing; and related transportation. As for older children, an important stipulation is that services should be provided in a natural environment, which for infants and toddlers is typically in the home or in daycare centers. Important definitions in Part C are shown in Display 19.2.[14]

EVALUATION UNDER PART C

The same federal mandates and guidelines for evaluation apply under Part C. For this younger population, however, physical therapists may use other assessment instruments, including:

1. *Bayley Scales of Infant and Toddler Development,* Third Edition (Bayley III)[44]—a standardized, norm-referenced test recently revised to measure a child's competency in five major developmental domains that correspond with those stipulated in IDEIA: cognitive, language, motor, social–emotional, and adaptive behavior (the latter two assessed by parental response to a questionnaire).

2. *Peabody Developmental Motor Scales 2*[45]—a standardized, norm-referenced test of motor skills in children from birth to 5 years of age. Six subtests assess motor skills in the following areas: reflexes, stationary, locomotion, object manipulation, grasping, and visual motor integration. A motor activities program with instructional objectives, reasons for teaching the skill, examples of related skills as they occur in the natural environment, and suggested instructional strategies supplements the assessment.

3. *Pediatric Evaluation of Disability Inventory*[46]—a functional assessment instrument for the evaluation of children with disabilities from age 6 months to 7 years. Based on interviews with a primary caregiver, the inventory measures functional status and change in three domains: self-care, mobility, and social function. Scoring is done to indicate functional skill level, the amount of caregiver assistance required, and modifications or adaptive equipment used.

INFANT FAMILY SERVICE PLAN

The Infant Family Service Plan (IFSP) is the equivalent of the IEP for older children. The IFSP must be developed by a multidisciplinary team that includes the parents and must

---

>> **DISPLAY 19.2**

Key Definitions from Part C of the Individuals with Disabilities Education Improvement Act

At-risk infant or toddler	". . . an individual under 3 years of age who would be at risk of experiencing a substantial developmental delay if early intervention services were not provided to the individual"
Infant or toddler with a disability	". . . an individual under 3 years of age who needs early intervention services because the individual is experiencing developmental delays, as measured by appropriate diagnostic instruments and procedures, in 1 or more areas of cognitive development, physical development, communication development, social or emotional development, and adaptive development . . ." or "has a diagnosed physical or mental condition that has a high probability of resulting in developmental delay; and . . . may also include, at State's discretion, at risk infants . . ."
Developmental delay	Defined by each state

include a description of appropriate transition services (e.g., transition from Part C to Part B at 3 years of age). The IFSP must be evaluated once a year but should be reviewed with the family at 6-month intervals or more often when appropriate. Timeliness of assessment, IFSP development, and beginning of services are crucial. The IFSP must include at a minimum the following elements[14]:

1. Statement of the infant's or toddler's present levels of physical development (vision, hearing, motor, and health), cognitive development (thinking, reasoning, learning), communication development (responding, understanding, using language), social or emotional development (feelings, playing, interacting), and adaptive development (bathing, feeding, dressing, etc.) based on objective criteria
2. Statement of family's resources, priorities, and concerns related to enhancing the development of the family's infant or toddler with a disability
3. Statement of the measurable results or outcomes expected to be achieved for the infant or toddler and family, and the criteria, procedures, and timelines used to determine the degree to which progress toward achieving the results or outcomes is being made and whether modifications or revisions of the result or outcomes or services are necessary
4. Statement of specific early intervention services based on peer-reviewed research necessary to meet the unique needs, including frequency, intensity, and method of delivering services
5. Statement of natural environments in which early intervention services will appropriately be provided
6. Projected dates for initiation of services and the anticipated length, duration, and frequency of the services
7. Identification of the service coordinator from the profession most immediately relevant to the needs of the infant or toddler and family
8. Steps to be taken to support the transition of the toddler with a disability to preschool or other appropriate services (which must include a formal plan and team conference 3 to 9 months prior to anticipated transition)
9. Provision for parental consent

 ## Program Development/ Intervention Under Parts B and C

MEANINGFUL COLLABORATION WITH PARENTS

Parents' involvement in the planning process facilitates focus on meaningful functional goals for the child and family and consideration of the child's unique needs within a broader context. Physical therapists share with other professionals the responsibility of ensuring that parents are aware of their rights and encouraged to be active participants in program planning for their children. A meta-analysis of 31 studies indicates that the most effective early

intervention programs are those that focus on parents' involvement in their child's care.[47] Adherence to the principles of family-centered care requires that every effort be made to customize communication to the unique needs of each family member. Parents may feel overwhelmed by the planning process and may need guidance to facilitate their meaningful involvement in planning. Several instruments are available that lend structure and guidance to the process: (1) McGill Action Planning System (MAPS),[48] (2) Choosing Options and Accommodations for Children (COACH),[49] (3) Canadian Occupational Performance Measure,[50] and (4) Planning Alternative Tomorrows with Hope (PATH).[51]

INDIVIDUALIZED EDUCATION PROGRAM/INFANT FAMILY SERVICE PLAN GOALS AND OBJECTIVES

IDEIA requires "measurable annual goals" as part of the IEP and a statement of the "measurable results or outcomes expected to be achieved" for the infant or toddler and family as part of the IFSP.[14] Short-term objectives are not required by current federal legislation, although state regulations may vary. Ideally, IEP/IFSP goals are developed by the team in a collaborative process and not by specific disciplines in isolation. Writing meaningful goals is an important framework for the delivery of services but can be challenging (Table 19.3). Well-developed goals and objectives should be[41,52]:

1. Educationally relevant
2. Functional (i.e., will increase a student's ability to interact with people and objects within the daily environment and would have to be performed by someone else if the student could not)
3. Stated as behaviors the student will demonstrate (i.e., not what will be done with the student)
4. Measurable (including performance criteria, conditions, and time frame)
   Note: A skill is measurable if it can be seen and/or heard, can be directly counted (frequency, duration, or distance measures), and lends itself to determination of performance criteria. The conditions for performance should be clearly stated.
5. Practical (i.e., work on the skill can be integrated into daily routines)
6. Linked to assessment that is valid and reliable when possible
7. Generalizable (i.e., the identified skill represents a general concept as opposed to a particular task, allows for individual adaptations and modifications for a variety of disabling conditions, and can be generalized across settings, materials, and people)

INCLUSIVE EDUCATION

IDEIA requires that states develop policies and procedures to ensure, to the maximum extent appropriate, that children

TABLE 19.3			
Components of an Individualized Education Program Goal and Examples			
Condition	**Student**	**Activity**	**Criteria**
Describe when and where the activity will take place	Name the student	Describe the desired activity and the level of prompting/assistance	Indicate the performance level for achievement
When transitioning between activities in the classroom	Tiffany	Will stand from her classroom chair given verbal prompts	In at least one out of three consecutive trials.
When preparing to leave the classroom	Joey	Will independently get in line with his peers	In at least two out of three consecutive trials.

with disabilities, including children in public or private institutions or other care facilities, are educated with children who are not disabled, and special classes, separate schooling, or other removal of children with disabilities from the regular educational environment occurs only when the nature or severity of the disability of a child is such that education in regular classes with the use of supplementary aids and services cannot be achieved satisfactorily. The terminology used in Part B is "least restrictive environment" and in Part C is "natural environment." The IEP or IFSP must identify the least restrictive or natural environment where services will be provided or justify why services might be provided in a more isolated environment. Noonan and McCormick[54] state that "successful inclusion is enormously complex" and give two essential requirements for meaningful inclusion practices: (1) that participants believe in inclusion and (2) that teachers and other providers have the necessary skills.

Establishing the necessary supports so that every student with a disability is able to participate to the maximum extent possible in the general education environment is beneficial to students with and without disabilities. It presents unique challenges, however, to all service providers. The most appropriate placement might be any of the following: (1) a regular classroom with an aide; (2) a primary placement in a classroom for children with special needs but inclusion for music, mealtimes, and other activities as appropriate; (3) an alternative school with specialized services and processes for children with similar diagnoses (e.g., autism); or (4) home-based services (e.g., a medically fragile child).

MODELS OF SERVICE DELIVERY

Various authors use different terminology to describe models of physical therapy service in the educational setting, but categories commonly referred to are (1) direct, (2) indirect (monitoring), and (3) consultation.[40] Although these are described separately below, they often occur together as complementary components of a comprehensive intervention plan for an individual student.

- *Direct service* involves hands-on intervention directly from a physical therapist or physical therapist assistant. Scheduling is one of the limitations of the direct service model, because if a child is receiving physical therapy, he or she is not participating in the normal academic curriculum.

 Direct service can be offered in an isolated manner (e.g., in a separate physical therapy treatment area) or integrated (provided within the context of normal routines/activities in least restrictive or natural environments). Research, although limited, supports more positive outcomes with integrated intervention, and the mandates in IDEIA for service in inclusive environments make it preferable for direct physical therapy to be integrated. The needs of individual children, however, may be better served in an isolated area. This might be true for a child who is easily distracted or in a classroom where the therapy might be distracting for other children. The need for special equipment or safety concerns may be other factors.
- *Indirect service* (monitoring) involves establishing a management program for a student, instructing others to carry it out, and monitoring the process to ensure positive outcomes. The indirect model requires that physical therapists can effectively teach others and that they can sell their "product" (i.e., the functional importance of the recommended intervention). A study by Otto and Effgen, although limited in scope, suggested that inactive stability behaviors occur naturally at high rates and are easily integrated into a classroom routine, but that movement activities like walking, creeping, or transferring require more direct assistance before they will be integrated and practiced.[56]
- *Consultation* involves a partnership between the physical therapist and the recipient of the information exchange. The expected outcome of consultation is that "the school environment (human and nonhuman) changes in ways that enable a student to succeed at school despite the limitations imposed by a disabling condition."[55] Bundy described consultation as "extraordinarily powerful" and recommended it as the primary form of service delivery for most students.[55]

Decision making about the delivery of physical therapy services is a complex process, guided by numerous considerations. Kaminker et al.[57] conducted a nationwide survey of pediatric physical therapists to explore their recommendations for the models, contexts, frequency, and intensity of service delivery and the factors that influenced their decision making. Therapists were asked to make clinical decisions based on four clinical cases that varied by age, cognitive ability, and condition. Respondents had a strong preference for direct services, especially for the younger children, and for services delivered in a combination of natural (integrated) and isolated settings. Factors that strongly impacted their decision making were the students' functional levels and the students' goals. Factors with minimal impact included administrative influence and budgetary constraints. A follow-up study by some of the same authors investigated the impact of geographic region on decision making and results indicated considerable variability in recommendations across regions.[58]

In a survey of pediatric physical therapists practicing in early intervention, McWilliams and Sekerak[59] found that in typical practice, therapists selected an in-class model more often than an out-of-class model, but that physical therapists are less likely to select an in-class model than occupational therapists, speech and language pathologists, or special educators. A more recent study by Nolan et al.[60] surveyed pediatric occupational and physical therapists and results indicated that 55.3% of children received the majority of services in isolated settings and 24.7% received the majority of services in integrated settings, with the remainder equally blended between the two models. More evidence is needed to guide best-practice recommendations.

ROLE OF THE PHYSICAL THERAPIST ASSISTANT

The Section on Pediatrics addressed the role of the physical therapist assistant in the provision of pediatric physical therapy in a formal position statement that was approved by the APTA Board Review Committee in April 1997.[61] The statement supports the qualifications of physical therapist assistants to assist in the provision of pediatric physical therapy services with the exception of services for children who are physiologically unstable. The physical therapist assistant can play a valuable role in the educational environment.

In 2004, a school-based physical therapist posed a question to the North Carolina Board of Physical Therapy Examiners (NCBPTE) about supervision of the physical therapist assistant in the educational setting.[62] The NCBPTE ruled that "the physical therapist must *see and assess* the patient/client no less frequently than every 30-days and that this reassessment may *not* be defined as

a conversation between a physical therapist and physical therapist assistant in which they review the IEP goals, the effectiveness of the therapeutic interventions being used, and the need, if any, for a direct visit with the student or any changes."[63] This example reflects only one state's determination but highlights the importance of knowing state practice guidelines.

ASSISTIVE TECHNOLOGY

Appropriate assistive technology for individuals with disabilities empowers those individuals to have greater control over their lives and to participate more fully in their home, school, and work environments and in their communities. As defined in IDEIA, an assistive technology device is ". . . any item, piece of equipment, or product system, whether acquired commercially off the shelf, modified, or customized, that is used to increase, maintain, or improve functional capabilities of a child with a disability."[14] Assistive technology devices include such items as communication devices, adaptive equipment (e.g., standers, wheelchairs), environmental control devices, adapted computers, and specialized software.[14]

An assistive technology service is ". . . any service that directly assists a child with a disability in the selection, acquisition, or use of an assistive technology device. Such term includes: evaluation of the child's needs; acquisition of device (e.g., purchase or lease); selection, design, fit, adaptation, application, maintenance/repair; coordinating other services/interventions; training or technical assistance for child/family and service providers or employers."[14]

Physical therapists are often involved with other team members in the selection and use of assistive technology, and it is a crucial role. Thousands of items are available from a variety of vendors and the cost is typically high. It is imperative that decisions about assistive technology consider the individual needs of a child and family; the environment in which the equipment is to be used; sources of funding; training for caregivers; safety; evidence to support its use; and the potential for the technology to be used by other children. Therapists should be aware of assistive technology resources in the state, which might include specialists to assist with evaluation and selection of appropriate devices or centers that will lend equipment on a trial basis.

TRANSITION PLANNING

IDEIA identifies two critical transition periods for children with disabilities and mandates effective results-oriented planning by the IEP or IFSP team. The identified periods are the transition from early intervention services covered under Part C to the preschool programs covered under Part B and the transition from school to community living.

Transition typically results in new personnel working with the child and family, a new environment, and a new lead agency with new policies and processes. It can be very stressful for both children and families.

The goal of transition planning should be to ensure continuity of service, minimize disruption to the student and family, and promote optimum service delivery. For transition from early intervention (Part C) to public school, STEPS (Sequenced Transition to Education in the Public Schools) is a helpful model.[63] Components of the STEPS model include creation of a responsive administrative structure, active involvement of families, preparation of the child, and training for staff so that they can effectively facilitate the process. Physical therapists can and should play an active role in transition planning. A study by Myers and Effgen[64] provided some preliminary data on physical therapists' participation in early childhood transitions. In their survey of pediatric physical therapists, they found varying levels of participation across settings, but the majority of respondents (54.8%) believed they were not participating fully in the transition process. Perceived barriers included a lack of time and lack of administrative support for their involvement. Only 16.6% of the respondents had received training on transition.

RE-EVALUATION

General guidelines for re-evaluation of a child with a disability are not more frequently than once a year and at least every 3 years unless the parent and local educational agency agree to a different schedule. Physical therapists must use their clinical judgment to determine an appropriate schedule for re-evaluation. This will vary depending on the nature of the child's problems, the goals established, and whether a physical therapist assistant is involved in service delivery.

Terminating physical therapy services for children in school settings can be challenging because multiple factors must be considered and the physical therapist must remain focused on the overall purpose of related services under IDEIA, to allow the child to benefit from special education. Effgen[65] found that therapists generally based their decision to terminate physical therapy services on the child's attainment of functional goals without influence from school administrators.

DOCUMENTATION

Although requirements for documentation are not stipulated in IDEIA and practice acts and Medicaid requirements vary from state to state, therapists are encouraged to document every contact, especially if a physical therapist assistant is involved in the provision of care or Medicaid or other third-party payment is involved. Using an electronic format and/or flow charts may streamline the process.

EXTENDED SCHOOL YEAR

The IEP team can consider the necessity of related services outside of the regular school year if it is determined that a child served under Part B will experience substantial regression or loss of functional abilities if services are suspended (typically over the summer months) or if the child failed to make adequate progress toward his or her annual IEP goals.

REIMBURSEMENT FOR SERVICES

The mandate of IDEIA is to provide free and appropriate education to qualified individuals with disabilities, but the cost can be staggering to local education agencies. PL 100-360 was enacted in 1988 to allow states to utilize Medicaid funds to supplement the cost of providing related services for eligible children. Rules and regulations about Medicaid eligibility and allocation of funds vary from state to state but are frequently restricted to direct service, which can limit the ability of providers to select a delivery mode that is most appropriate and is the most efficient use of resources. Private insurance may also be billed if parents give informed consent to do so, but it is important that they are aware of specifics of their policy so that they do not negatively impact long-term coverage (e.g., a policy that has lifetime caps on therapy services).

 Role of the Physical Therapist in Program-Related Areas

The majority of the functions and roles assumed by physical therapists in the public school setting that have been described so far have been student related. Physical therapists can also make significant contributions to program-related needs. Physical therapists may assist others in the educational setting to:

- identify architectural barriers and plan for accessibility modifications;
- establish guidelines and child-specific modifications for the transport of children with disabilities on school-owned vehicles (e.g., buses);
- promote acceptance of students with disabilities by both educational personnel and students;
- plan recreational areas for accessibility;
- contribute to the development of safety procedures for emergency evacuation of students with disabilities;
- collaborate with physical educators to develop "mutually supportive and effective motor programs"[66];
- participate with others in various prevention activities, including screening programs (e.g., musculoskeletal for athletes and patients with scoliosis; developmental); prevention and treatment of sports-related injuries; prevention of neck and back pain secondary to backpack use[67]; development of conditioning programs; and/or educational programs for coaches, parents, and students;

• Promote independence through general environmental modifications.

Frequently, physical therapists are the liaison between the educational and medical communities. They may provide background information about various conditions, interpret medical reports, facilitate communication between educational and medical personnel, and assist with access to resources in the medical community.

Physical therapists may also be expected to provide educational personnel with information about physical therapy and topics related to intervention with children who have physical disabilities. Hardy and Roberts[68] recommend conducting a survey of educators' interests and needs to structure in-service education programs that are meaningful. Topics of interest identified from the authors' survey of special educators included specific student disabilities, classroom adaptations, referral guidelines, physical therapist roles and responsibilities, and the difference between an occupational therapist and a physical therapist. A helpful resource is an article by Dole, Collaborating Successfully with Your School's Physical Therapist, that was published by the Council for Exceptional Children.[69]

Management functions are important in the educational environment to ensure that decisions affecting job descriptions, delivery of care, supervision, and so on are compatible with best-practice models. It is not possible, as it was in the 1930s, for physical therapists to have the same job description and qualifications as teachers. Shortages are common, and therapists must understand and communicate to school administrators recruitment and retention strategies for physical therapists that are often very different from those for educational personnel. In a survey of physical therapists practicing in educational settings, the areas of job dissatisfaction most frequently mentioned were lack of continuing education opportunities, insufficient peer contact, lack of an identified place to work, lack of time allotted for administrative tasks and meetings, and too much travel.[70]

A variety of other management tasks are essential as a framework for best practice, and time should be negotiated to ensure that they can be given adequate attention. Efficient systems should be in place for documentation, record keeping, and billing, and these components should be reviewed on a regular schedule. Job descriptions should be comprehensive, state essential functions, and form the basis for annual performance evaluations of individual physical therapists. A physical therapist should have his or her clinical performance evaluated by another physical therapist, which may require special, formalized arrangements. Both the job descriptions and performance evaluations should be reviewed annually. A plan for program evaluation, quality assurance, and peer review should be in place and reviewed regularly (at least annually). Agreement should be reached on reasonable caseloads and guidelines for determining eligibility for physical therapy as a related

service. Lines of communication and authority should also be clearly established.

Many references are now available to guide the physical therapist in the educational environment.[71-73] Many states have also published guidelines for physical therapy in the schools. Other resources include the APTA's Section on Pediatrics (which has a special interest group for therapists working in the educational environment) and the Council for Exceptional Children.

 Points to Ponder

The educational environment presents ongoing challenges for the team of professionals who serve children with disabilities. Policies and procedures vary from state to state and even within districts. Therapists struggle on a daily basis to make the "right" decisions that most appropriately address the needs of individual students within the context of federal regulations. Below are examples of some of the kinds of questions that therapists must address.

• Do we have evidence to support many of the common recommendations in the school setting—for example, manual stretching to increase range of motion or prevent contractures and supported standing in various types of adaptive equipment?
• Do we have reliable, valid assessment tools and evidence-based intervention options for children with severe/ profound disabilities?
• For many children with severe/profound disabilities, acquiring basic motor skills (e.g., head control) may be a primary focus of an educational plan. Do these children warrant more attention from physical therapists or less?
• Do we have evidence to support our prognosis for potential functional gains that can appropriately guide decisions related to frequency and duration of intervention?
• Can life skills like riding a bicycle be justified within an educational program plan?
• Should a school-based physical therapist increase services for a child on his or her caseload who receives surgical intervention?

SUMMARY

The educational environment is a challenging and rewarding environment for the physical therapist. To be effective in the public school setting in the United States, a physical therapist must have an understanding of the federal legislation that has shaped the delivery of special education for children from infancy to young adulthood. Most significant was PL 94-142, passed in 1975, which mandated physical therapy as a related service and created a variety of conceptually new ways of thinking about the educational needs of children with disabilities. Local, state, and federal rules and regulations must be understood and adhered to.

Physical therapists must be willing and able to participate actively as part of a collaborative team and to consider parents an integral part of that team. They must acknowledge that their intervention is limited to the educational needs of the child. They must utilize models of service delivery that most effectively address the individualized needs of each child. Practice in the educational environment requires the knowledge, skills, and abilities of a specialist in pediatric physical therapy, but with the grounding to always be able and willing to interpret physical therapy intervention so that it is understood and appreciated by nonmedical personnel. The rewards include the benefits of functioning as part of a team, following a child long term, and having the opportunity to observe the child in his or her daily functions within the school environment.

CASE STUDIES

CASE STUDY 1

AMY

A 13-year-old student named Amy has spastic cerebral palsy and multiple disabilities including moderate to severe cognitive impairments and severely limited motor abilities. Her age-equivalent performance of motor skills is less than 12 months. While attending Amy's IEP meeting, her parents asked for physical therapy for 30-minute range-of-motion sessions three times per week to prevent worsening of joint contractures.

What Factors Should the IEP Team Consider When Discussing the Parents' Request?

The primary factor to be determined in consideration of the request is whether or not limitations in Amy's range of motion impact her performance at school or her ability to participate in her educational program. Therefore, the IEP team should examine Amy's goals and performance at school in an effort to examine the educational impact of Amy's range-of-motion deficits. If Amy's limitations are relatively minor, do not affect her ability to access her curriculum, have not progressed significantly, and do not predispose her to significant complications that could potentially impact her education, then the IEP team would likely conclude that addressing range-of-motion issues would not be educationally relevant. If, however, the limitations are more severe and interfere with Amy's school performance (e.g., inability to reach for a switch), then the maintenance of joint range of motion may be deemed educationally relevant. In this case the team would then progress through the IEP process and determine how the maintenance of range of motion can best be met in Amy's school environment.

Is There Evidence in the Literature to Support or Refute This Requested Service?

Prevention of contractures in children can involve flexibility exercises, positioning, serial casting/splinting, pharmacologic management, or surgery. Evidence to support these intervention strategies is not strong, especially stretching exercises and positioning for children with neurologic conditions.[76] Without strong evidence, therapists find it difficult to justify either a regular program of stretching exercises/positioning or no intervention. Research is needed if we are to advocate appropriately for children and make effective recommendations to educational personnel.

Can a Nonskilled Employee Perform Passive Range of Motion?

Issues to consider are the severity of the contracture, evidence of joint involvement, or other risk factors that might include osteopenia or osteoporosis and behavior problems.

Is There a Way to Incorporate Range-of-Motion Activities into Functional Tasks?

It is preferable to incorporate intervention strategies into the child's daily routine as often as possible and to promote consistency across personnel and settings. Proper positioning in a stander during specified activities in the regular school day might be the most appropriate way to maintain range in key joints while also gaining the benefits of weight bearing. Research indicates that weight bearing at least 7.5 hours per week prevents calcium reabsorption in the bones[77] and that prolonged stretching is preferable to maintain muscle lengths and prevent joint contractures.[76]

CASE STUDY 2

RASHEEN

A 10-year-old student named Rasheen has normal cognitive function and spastic quadriplegic cerebral palsy. He is independent with powered mobility in school including the classroom, hallways, playground, cafeteria, bus, and special classes. Rasheen has a stander that he uses on a daily basis at school and he needs only minimal assistance for transfers into/out of the stander. Rasheen participates in physical education class with accommodations, adaptations, and occasional adult assistance. Rasheen has access to assistive technology that allows him to be independent with his classwork and he has peer buddies who help him with classroom set-up. Given his diagnosis and prognosis, Rasheen is not a candidate for independent ambulation.

Would Rasheen Likely Qualify for Physical Therapy Services?

Since Rasheen's disability affects his independence and performance in the educational environment, the IEP team would likely recommend physical therapy as a related service.

What Would Likely Be the Primary Focus of Physical Therapy Intervention for Rasheen in the Educational Environment?

Rasheen's services would focus on maximizing his independence at school including goals to improve his independence with activities of daily living such as feeding, toileting, and transfers.

Would Physical Therapy Likely Be Provided in a Direct, Indirect, or Consultative Model of Service Delivery?

The IEP team's decision about the most appropriate model of service delivery would be based on a complex interplay of factors and would need to be reassessed frequently as circumstances changed. Rasheen is likely to receive direct, indirect, and consultative services. Using independent toileting as an example, the physical therapist might work with Rasheen in a direct model to determine the most efficient way for Rasheen to accomplish independent toileting and work directly with Rasheen to develop the component motor skills required. Then, in an indirect model, the physical therapist might instruct classroom personnel on the toileting strategies for Rasheen to use on a daily basis and monitor his progress and address any questions or concerns weekly or biweekly. Consultation with administrative personnel might occur when determining the most appropriate bathroom modifications.

Do You Expect that Rasheen Would Receive Additional Physical Therapy Services on an Outpatient Basis (i.e., Outside the Educational Environment)? If So, What Would Be the Primary Focus of Rasheen's Outpatient Services?

Outpatient services for Rasheen might be recommended to intensify intervention when working on a particular functional skill or following a medical intervention like implantation of a Baclofen pump to manage spasticity. The outpatient physical therapist might also take a more active role in developing and monitoring a comprehensive home program for prevention of contractures that would involve adaptive equipment for the home environment and night splinting. Regardless of the circumstances, Rasheen's parents, physician, and therapists should all work collaboratively to comprehensively address his needs.

How Might the Focus of Rasheen's Services Change as He Progresses Through Middle School and High School?

As Rasheen approaches middle school and high school, planning for the school to adulthood transition will play a larger role in his educational programming. Exploring Rasheen's vocational interests and linking them to his physical abilities will become increasingly important. Investigating potential living arrangements, identifying community agencies, and examining recreational options will also need to be addressed via transition planning. Increased emphasis on his academic coursework to meet his long-term goals may warrant a decrease in direct physical therapy services and a gradual shift to more indirect and consultative services.

REFERENCES

1. Pratt RE. Physical therapy in schools for crippled children. Phys Ther Rev 1950;30:233.
2. DeYoung R. Child cripples get full course at Morton High. Phys Rev 1932;24.
3. Hutchinson E. The physical therapist looks at the school child. Phys Rev. 1944;24:6–9.
4. Section 504 of the Rehabilitation Act. U.S. Congress. Senate, 1973.
5. Education for All Handicapped Children Act. Public Law 94-142. U.S. Congress. Senate, 94th Congress, 1975.
6. Education of the Handicapped Act Amendments of 1986, Public Law 99-457. U.S. Congress. Senate, 99th Congress, 1986.
7. Medicare Catastrophic Coverage Act, Public Law 100-360, 1988. Individuals with Disabilities Education Act of 1990, Public Law 102-119. U.S. Congress. Senate, 102nd Congress, 1988.
8. Technology-Related Assistance for Individuals with Disabilities Act, Public Law 100–407, 1988.
9. Americans with Disabilities Act, Public Law 101-336, 1990.
10. Individuals with Disabilities Education Act Amendments, Public Law 102-119, 1991.
11. Individuals with Disabilities Education Act Amendments of 1997, Public Law 105-17, 1997.
12. Assistive Technology Act of 1998, Public Law 105-394, 1998.
13. No Child Left Behind Act, Public Law 107-110, 2002.
14. Individuals with Disabilities Education Improvement Act of 2004, Public Law 108-446, 2004.
15. Assistive Technology Act of 2004, H.R. 4278, 2004.
16. Rotherham AJ. The politics of IDEA funding. Education Week 2002;Oct 9.
17. IDEA Funding Coalition, IDEA funding: time for Congress to live up to the commitment–mandatory funding proposal. 2006. Available at: http://www.nea.org/specialed/coalitionfunding 2002.html. Accessed May 6, 2006.
18. Ogletree BT, Bull J, Drew R, et al. Team-based service delivery for students with disabilities: Practice options and guidelines for success. Intervention School Clinic 2001;36(3):138–145.
19. Rainforth B, York J. Collaborative Teams for Students with Severe Disabilities. 2nd Ed. Baltimore: Paul H. Brookes, 1997.
20. Thousand JS, Villa RA. Collaborative teaming: a powerful took in school restructuring. In: Villa RA, Thousand JS, eds. Restructuring for Caring and Effective Education: Piecing the Puzzle. Baltimore: Paul H. Brookes Publishing, 2000:254–292.
21. Effgen SK, Keppler S. Survey of physical therapy practice in educational settings. Pediatr Phys Therapy 1994;6:15–21.
22. Rainforth B. Analysis of physical therapy practice acts: implications for role release in educational environments. Pediatr Phys Ther 1997;9:54–61.
23. DeHaven GE. Is selective hearing an occupational hazard in physical therapy? Phys Ther 1974:54: 1301–1305.
24. Effgen SK, Chair, APTA Task Force. Competencies for physical therapists in early intervention. Pediatr Phys Ther 1991;3:77–80.
25. Association for Persons with Severe Handicaps. TASH Resolution on Inclusive Quality Education, Baltimore: TASH, 2000. Available at: www.tash.org.
26. American Physical Therapy Association. Guide to Physical Therapist Practice. 2nd Ed. Alexandria, VA: American Physical Therapy Association, 2001.
27. Bruininks RH, Bruininks D. Bruininks-Oseretsky Test of Motor Proficiency. 2nd Ed. Minneapolis, MN: American Guidance Service Publishing, Pearson Assessments, Pearson Education, 2005.
28. Russell DJ, Rosenbaum PL, Gowland C, et al. Gross Motor Function Measure. Hamilton, Ontario: Gross Motor Measures Group, 1990.

29. Coster W, Deeney T, Haltiwanger J, et al. School Function Assessment. San Antonio, TX: The Psychological Corporation, Harcourt Brace Assessment, 2000.

30. Blanton KF. M.O.V.E.: Mobility Opportunities Via Education. Bakersfield, CA: MOVE International, 1991.

31. McEwen IR, Arnold SH, Hansen LH, et al. Interrater reliability and content validity of a minimal data set to measure outcomes of students receiving school-based occupational therapy and physical therapy. Phys Occupat Ther Pediatr 2003;23(2):77–95.

32. Granger CV, Hamilton BB, Kayto R. Guide for the Use of the Functional Independence Measure for Children (WeeFIM) of the Uniform Data Set for Medical Rehabilitation. Buffalo, NY: Research Foundation, State University of New York, 1989.

33. Orelove FP, Sobsey D. Designing transdisciplinary services. In: Orelove FP, Sobsey D, eds. Educating Children with Multiple disabilities: A Transdisciplinary Approach. 3rd Ed. Baltimore: Paul H. Brookes, 1996:1–33.

34. Brown L, Branston MB, Hamre-Nietupski S, et al. A strategy for developing chronological age-appropriate and functional curricular content for severely handicapped adolescents and young adults. J Spec Educ 1979;13:81–90.

35. Linehan SA, Brady MP, Hwang C. Ecological versus developmental assessment: influences on instructional expectations. JASH. 1991;16(3):146–153.

36. Borkowski MA, Wessman HC. Determination of eligibility for physical therapy in the public school setting. Pediatr Phys Ther 1994;61–67.

37. Waukesha Delivery Model: Providing OT/PT Services to Special Education Students. Milwaukee: Wisconsin Department of Public Instruction, 1987.

38. Carr SH. Louisiana's criteria of eligibility for occupational therapy services in the public school system. Am J Occup Ther 1989; 43(8):503–506.

39. Baker BJ, Cole KN, Harris S. Cognitive referencing as a method of OT/PT triage for young children. Pediatr Phys Ther 1998;10:2–6.

40. Cole KN, Mills PE, Harris SR. Retrospective analysis of physical and occupational therapy progress in young children: an examination of cognitive referencing. Pediatr Phys Ther 1991;3: 185–189.

41. Giangreco MF. Related service decision-making: a foundational component of effective education for students with disabilities. Phys Occup Ther Pediatr 1995;15(2):47–68.

42. Office of Special Education Programs, Office of Special Education and Rehabilitative Services, U.S. Department of Education. 2006. Model Form: Part B: Individualized Education Program. Available at: http://www.ed.gov/policy/speced/guid/idea/modelform-iep.doc. Accessed 5/1/06.

43. American Physical Therapy Association. APTA's Guidelines for Recognizing and Providing Care for Victims of Child Abuse. Alexandria, VA: APTA, 2005.

44. Bayley N. Bayley Scales of Infant and Toddler Development. 3rd Ed. San Antonio, TX: Harcourt Assessment, 2005.

45. Folio R, Fewell R. Peabody Developmental Motor Scales. 2nd Ed. Austin, TX: Pro-Ed, 2000.

46. Haley SM, Coster WJ, Ludlow LH, et al. Pediatric Evaluation of Disability Inventory. Boston, MA: Center for Rehabilitation Effectiveness, Boston University, 1992.

47. Shonkoff JP, Hauser-Cram P. Early intervention for disabled infants and their families: a quantitative analysis. Pediatrics 1987;80:650–657.

48. Vandercock T, York J, Forest M. The McGill Action Planning System (MAPS): a strategy for building the vision. J Assoc Persons Severe Handicaps 1989;14:205–215.

49. Giangreco MG, Cloninger CJ, Iverson VS. Choosing Outcomes and Accommodations for Children (COACH): A Guide to Educational Planning for Students with Disabilities. 2nd Ed. Baltimore: Paul H. Brookes Publishing, 1998.

50. Law M, Baptiste S, Carswell A, et al. Canadian Occupational Performance Measure. 4th Ed. Ottawa, Ontario, Canada: Canadian Association of Occupational Therapists, 2005.

51. Pearpoint J, O'Brien J, Forest M. PATH: Planning Alternative Tomorrows with Hope. Toronto, Ontario, Canada: Inclusion Press, 1992.

52. Notari-Syverson AR, Shuster SL. Putting real-life skills into IEP/IFSPs for infants and young children. Teaching Exceptional Children (a publication of the Council for Exceptional Children). 1995;27(2):29–32.

53. Dole R, Arvidson K, Byrne E, et al. (2003). Consensus among experts in pediatric occupational and physical therapy on elements of individualized education programs. Pediatr Phys Ther 2003;15:159–166.

54. McCormick L. Assessment and planning: the IFSP and IEP. In: Noonan MJ, McCormick L, eds. Young Children with Disabilities in Natural Environments: Methods and Procedures. Baltimore: Paul H. Brookes, 2006:47–76.

55. Bundy AC. Assessment and intervention in school-based practice: answering questions and minimizing discrepancies. Phys Occup Ther Pediatr 1995;15(2):69–87.

56. Otto DS, Effgen SK. Occurrence of gross motor behaviors in integrated and segregated preschool classrooms. Pediatr Phys Ther 2000;12:164–172.

57. Kaminker MK, Chiarello LA, O'Neill ME, et al. Decision making for physical therapy service delivery in schools: a nationwide survey of pediatric physical therapists. Phys Ther 2004;84: 919–933.

58. Kaminker MK, Chiarello LA, Chiarini Smith JA. Decision making for physical therapy service delivery in schools: a nationwide analysis by geographic region. Pediatr Phys Ther 2006;18: 204–213.

59. McWilliams RA, Sekerak D. Integrated practices in center-based early intervention: perceptions of physical therapists. Pediatr Phys Ther 1995;7:51–58.

60. Nolan KW, Mannato L, Wilding GE. Integrated models of pediatric physical and occupational therapy: regional practice and related outcomes. Pediatr Phys Ther 2004;16:121–128.

61. Section on Pediatrics. Utilization of Physical Therapist Assistants in the Provision of Pediatric Physical Therapy. Approved by the APTA Board Review Committee, April 1997.

62. Public Schools of North Carolina, Memorandum September 7, 2004, from Mary N. Watson, Director, Exceptional Children Division, reporting on decision of NCBPTE on the Supervision of Physical Therapy Assistants.

63. Rous B, Hemmeter ML, Schuster J. Evaluating the impact of the STEPS model on development of community-wide transition systems. J Early Intervent 1999;22:38–50.

64. Myers CT, Effgen SK. Physical therapists' participation in early childhood transitions. Pediatr Phys Ther 2006;18:182–189.

65. Effgen SK. Factors affecting the termination of physical therapy services for children in school settings. Pediatr Phys Ther 2000; 12:121–126.

66. Pediatric Special Interest Group, Pennsylvania Physical Therapy Association. Guidelines for the Practice of Physical Therapy in the Educational Setting, November 1993.

67. Mehta TB, Thorpe DE, Freburger JK. Development of a survey to assess backpack use and neck and back pain in seventh and eighth graders. Pediatr Phys Ther 2002;14:171–184.

68. Hardy DD, Roberts PL. The educational needs assessment on physical therapy for special educators: enhancing in-service programming and physical therapy services in public schools. Pediatr Phys Ther 1989;1:109–114.

69. Dole RL. Collaborating successfully with your school's physical therapist. Teaching Exceptional Children. 2004;36(5):28–35.

70. Effgen SK, Keppler S. Survey of physical therapy practice in educational settings. Pediatr Phys Ther 1994;6:15–21.

71. Martin KD, ed. Physical Therapy Practice in Educational Environments: Policies and Guidelines. American Physical Therapy Association, Alexandria, VA: APTA, 1990.

73. McEwen I. (1999). Providing Physical Therapy Under Parts B and C of the Individuals with Disabilities Education Act (IDEA). Alexandria, VA: American Physical Therapy Association, 1999.

74. David K. IDEIA PL 108-446 Impact on Physical Therapy Related Services. Section on Pediatric, American Physical Therapy Association, 2005. Available at: http://www.pediatricapta.org/members/school.cfm. Accessed 5/1/06.

75. Rapport MJ. Laws that shape therapy services in educational environments. Phys Occup Ther Pediatr. 1995;15(2):5–32.

76. Stuberg W, DeJong S. Contracture management of children with neuromuscular disabilities. Presentation at Combined Sections Meeting, American Physical Therapy Association, San Diego, Feb. 4, 2006. Available at http://www.ed.gov/policy/speced/guid/idea/modelform-iep.doc. Accessed 5/1/06.